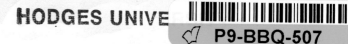
Mosby's ESSENTIAL SCIENCES for THERAPEUTIC MASSAGE

Anatomy, Physiology, Biomechanics, and Pathology

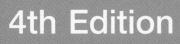

SANDY FRITZ, MS, NCTMB

Founder, Owner, Director, and Head Instructor
Health Enrichment Center
School of Therapeutic Massage and Bodywork
Lapeer, Michigan

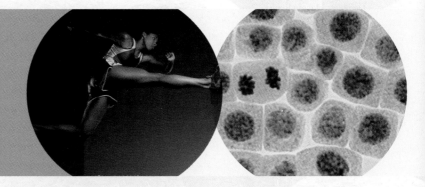

4th Edition

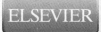

ELSEVIER
MOSBY

3251 Riverport Lane
Maryland Heights, MO 63043

MOSBY'S ESSENTIAL SCIENCES FOR THERAPEUTIC MASSAGE   ISBN: 978-0-323-07743-9

Notice

Neither the Publisher nor the Author assume any responsibility for any loss or injury and/or damage to person or property arising out of or related to any use of the material contained in this book. It is the responsibility of the treating practitioner, relying on independent expertise and knowledge of the patient, to determine the best treatment and method of application for the patient.

The Publisher

ISBN: 978-0-323-07743-9

Vice President and Content Strategy Director: Linda Duncan
Executive Content Strategist: Kellie White
Senior Content Development Specialist: Jennifer Watrous
Content Coordinator: Emily Thomson
Publishing Services Manager: Julie Eddy
Project Manager: Rich Barber
Designer: Maggie Reid

Photo credits
Cover: Dimarion, Patrick Hermans
Title page: Jiri Vratislavsky

Printed in China

Last digit is the print number: 9 8 7 6 5 4 3 2 1

Working together to grow
libraries in developing countries

www.elsevier.com | www.bookaid.org | www.sabre.org

ELSEVIER   BOOK AID International   Sabre Foundation

Contents

SECTION I: FUNDAMENTALS

Chapter 1   The Body as a Whole, 1
Chapter 2   Mechanisms of Health and Disease, 23
Chapter 3   Terminology: Scientific, Medical, Social, and Cultural Communication, 57

SECTION II: SYSTEMS OF CONTROL

Chapter 4   Nervous System Basics and the Central Nervous System, 98
Chapter 5   Peripheral Nervous System, 133
Chapter 6   Endocrine System, 167

SECTION III: KINESIOLOGY AND BIOMECHANICS

Chapter 7   Skeletal System, 192
Chapter 8   Joints, 234
Chapter 9   Muscles, 283
Chapter 10   Biomechanics Basics, 468

SECTION IV: REMAINING BODY SYSTEMS

Chapter 11   Integumentary, Cardiovascular, Lymphatic, and Immune Systems, 550
Chapter 12   Respiratory, Digestive, Urinary, and Reproductive Systems, 603

Appendix A   Muscle Quick Reference Guide, 651
Appendix B   Diseases/Conditions and Indications/Contraindications for Massage Therapy, 663
Appendix C   Clinical Reasoning Activities, 686

Glossary, 689
Works Consulted, 699
Index, 703

Dedication

For more than 10 years I have been blessed with the support and friendship of Jennifer Watrous, Senior Developmental Editor for Elsevier publishing. Jennifer was just a "baby" in her career with Elsevier when she was assigned to me as an Associate Developmental Editor. I am a good author, but I do have my quirks and can present editors with challenges, many of which stem from having dyslexia. Jennifer has lost patience with me only a few times over the years and even then maintained a sense of humor and extraordinary support. Jennifer has contributed in many different ways to the quality of this and other textbooks that I write. As I write this, she recently achieved a richly deserved career advancement and will no longer function as part of my editorial support. This edition of the text will be her last formal work in a long line of projects together. I feel as if one of my kids has graduated from school and is moving forward into her professional future, and I am very proud of Jennifer. I feel it is a small expression of my gratitude to dedicate this edition of *Mosby's Essential Sciences for Therapeutic Massage* to Jennifer Watrous, and I look forward to watching her career expand. Thanks, Jennifer.

Acknowledgments

This text is reviewed, revised, and written by teachers seeking a more efficient and gentle way to help students understand and use this information. Credit and appreciation are given to the authors of the reference texts consulted in the development of this textbook. Without their efforts, this book never could have been written. Thanks also goes to those who reviewed the manuscript. Their dedicated attention adds to the quality of this text.

Special thanks goes to the following people/groups:

To Sandra K. Anderson, for her role as the Lead Reviewer and Consultant of this edition.

To Joseph E. Muscolino, for his thorough review of the bone, joint, and muscle chapters.

And to the staff at Elsevier for all of their wonderful support: Kellie White, Jennifer Watrous, Joe Gramlich, Linda Duncan, Emily Thomson, Abby Hewitt, Julie Burchett, Laura Loveall, Rich Barber, Julie Eddy, and Maggie Reid.

LEAD REVIEWER AND CONSULTANT

Sandra K. Anderson, BA, LMT, NCTMB
Co-Owner, Tucson Touch Therapies
Tucson, Arizona

REVIEWERS

Celia Bucci, MA, LMT
Clinical Massage Therapist
Chicago, Illinois

April Christopher, RN, RVT
Valley Vascular Consultants
Huntsville, Alabama

Teresa Cowan, MP, DA
Department Chair of Health Science, Baker College of
    Auburn Hills
Auburn Hills, Michigan

Laura Weir Danso, MS, LMT
Arizona School of Integrative Studies
Clarkdale, Arizona

Angelica De Geer, BA, BFA, CA, LMT
Dental Hygienist (Sweden)
Instructor, Massage Therapy Midwest Institute
Earth City, Missouri

Gautam J. Desai, DO, FACOFP, CPI
Associate Professor, Department of Family Medicine
Kansas City University of Medicine and Biosciences College
    of Osteopathic Medicine
Kansas City, Missouri

Lisa Erawoc, LMT, Certified Aromatherapist
Author
Instructor, Everest College
McLean, Virginia

Bruce Froelich, JD, NCTMB
Member, American Massage Therapy Association
Program Director for Therapeutic Massage
Baker College
Auburn Hills, Michigan

Julie Goodwin, BA, LMT
Author
Bodywork Instructor, Cortiva Institute—Tucson
Tucson, Arizona

Jarrod Harrall, DO
Board Certified, ABFM
CAQ Sports Medicine, AOASM
Overland Park, Kansas

Christopher V. Jones, LMT, NCTMB
Member, American Massage Therapy Association
Vice-Chair, NCB Exam Committee
Fitchburg, Massachusetts

Joseph C. Muscolino, BA
New York, New York

Joseph E. Muscolino, DC
Instructor, Purchase College, State University of New York
Purchase, New York
Owner, The Art and Science of Kinesiology
Stamford, Connecticut

James R. Nieland, BS, DC
Chiropractic Physician/Adjunct Faculty
Wilkes Community College
Wilkesboro, North Carolina

James O'Hara, MS, MA
Curriculum Developer, National Holistic Institute College of
    Massage Therapy
California Campuses

Roberta L. Pohlman, PhD
Associate Professor, Biological Sciences
Wright State University
Dayton, Ohio

Monica J. Reno, AAS, LMT
Massage Therapist, MVP Sportsclubs
The Villages, Florida

Dawn M. Saunders, BS, LMT, RMTI
Owner and Director, Albuquerque School of Massage
    Therapy & Health Sciences
Albuquerque, New Mexico

Jeffrey A. Simancek, BS, CMT, NCBTMB
Owner/Therapist, Wolf Tracks Massage Therapy
Irvine, California

Michael M. Steeves, BS, RN
Central Maryland School of Massage
Frederick, Maryland

Renee Stenbjorn, CMT (Virginia), LMT (Oregon and Washington, DC), BS, MPA
Massage Therapist, Instructor, and Director of Research Development
Potomac Massage Training Institute
Washington, DC

Deanna L. Sylvester, BS, LMT
Campus President, Cortiva Institute—Tucson
Tucson, Arizona

Melissa C. Wheeler
Faculty Training Coordinator, National Holistic Institute
Emeryville, California

Jeffery B. Wood, LMT, COTA/L, BS
Massage Therapy Program Director, Withlacoochee Technical Institute
Inverness, Florida

Preface

M osby's Essential Sciences for Therapeutic Massage, 4th edition, presents comprehensive science essentials—anatomy, physiology, biomechanics, and pathology—with a focus on clinical application for a specific population: future massage professionals. This population views the body in a holistic manner. Because philosophy and practices from ancient healing wisdom often form the basis for massage modalities, an introduction to the common thread of ancient healing wisdom is carried throughout the text. This wisdom is related directly to body structure and function and does not represent any particular spiritual discipline.

Two themes were woven through this text in its development and revision:

1. Dynamic balance, or homeostasis
2. Analysis and reasoning. This theme honors both the scientific model of cause and effect and the larger picture of intention, intuition, possibilities, and the feelings of the people involved

This textbook presents the objective facts and information about human beings as they currently exist. Information is not static, but dynamic and like life, ever-changing. Teachers and students are encouraged to question and explore the information to make it their own.

Of course, there is no single correct way to use this book. The sections do not need to be presented in any specific order; however, Chapter 1 does set the stage for learning. The activities, exercises, and workbook sections can all be used at your discretion.

This text is designed for a 500- to 1500-hour curriculum (approximately 15 to 30 credits). A more generalized approach will need to be taken with the shorter curriculums, while additional class time will allow for a more in-depth integration process. Since the text is student-friendly and self-directed, much of the work can be assigned in a self-study format. To support the process of self-directed learning, a comprehensive and professionally designed online course is available to accompany this textbook, called *Massage Online for Essential Sciences*. The use of the online course with this textbook creates a hybrid learning process that combines online and classroom learning. Whether the educational program uses the online course as actual class hours or as a homework-type supplement to the textbook, it will provide the student with resources that are not able to be incorporated into a textbook platform. For example, the online course contains many high-quality animations that are supportive of retention for the students. It is strongly encouraged that the online course be used to support and expand science education for massage therapy students.

WHO WILL BENEFIT FROM THIS BOOK?

The format of this text has been designed to address various learning styles and approaches of therapeutic massage students. Throughout the text are activities that assist the student in transferring new information from short-term to long-term memory and in developing clinical reasoning skills. These activities do not have only one correct answer. Instead, they are designed for the student to use what is familiar from past experiences as a vehicle to transport the new or unfamiliar information to a level of understanding through a gentle and effective learning process. This enhances the student's ability to utilize creative problem-solving skills. Because there is seldom only one correct way to do anything, developing a process to determine the most effective decision at the time is important. This may seem uncomfortable for some at first, but an example is often provided to give the student direction within the activities.

Understanding is the learning goal of this text. Memorization is not the goal. Instead, the activities identify fundamental material and ask the student to manipulate it in a personal way to enhance the learning process.

The bulk of this text is designed as reference material. The information was selected to best serve the beginning and intermediate student of therapeutic massage and to reflect current competencies of the profession. Decisions were made as to what to include based on the author's experiences of many years of training entry- and intermediate-level therapeutic massage students, current research, and the guidance of several expert reviewers who analyzed the manuscript content.

A conversational tone has been used whenever possible, and supported by metaphors and practical applications relating specifically to massage therapy. Indications and contraindications for clinical massage practice have also been included. The word *indication* in the context of this book is defined as when treatment is appropriate and beneficial. The word *contraindication* encompasses both avoidance and cautions for the application of treatment. This practical feature allows the student to take the knowledge from the classroom straight into actual therapy. The result is a user-friendly text that relates to daily professional life for the massage therapist.

ORGANIZATION

Mosby's Essential Sciences for Therapeutic Massage is a solid, Western-based scientific text focused specifically on the massage curriculum. The text is heavily illustrated in full color to provide the best visual representation of anatomy and physiology concepts. In addition to anatomy and physiology, the book includes sections on pathologic conditions with suggestions for referral protocols and indications and contraindications for therapeutic massage. The text is clinically relevant, enabling the student to see how material applies to real practice.

The linear flow of this book begins in Section I, with an introduction to the fundamentals and a big-picture look at the body, health, disease, terminology, and a clinical reasoning model.

Section II, "Systems of Control," presents the mechanisms of physiologic function and control by the nervous system and endocrine system. This is a major deviation from traditional presentations and is presented based on more than 20 years of teaching experience indicating that if the systems of control are understood first, then it is much easier to understand the rest of the body's anatomy and physiology.

Section III, "Kinesiology and Biomechanics," represents the core portion of the text from a movement science perspective, and the topics include the musculoskeletal system, kinesiology, and biomechanics. If this information flow seems out of order, the instructor may decide to simply switch the presentation of Sections II and III.

The last section covers the remainder of the body systems, including the integumentary, cardiovascular, lymphatic, and immune systems, as well as the digestive, respiratory, urinary, and reproductive systems. Only the information most applicable to the therapeutic massage student is presented in these chapters.

Three appendices conclude the book with valuable resources for the student. Quick reference charts for muscles and pathology comprise Appendices A and B. The muscle chart is an abbreviated, simplified description of the main muscles and referred pain patterns encountered during massage application. The pathology chart is a quick reference of conditions and the indications and contraindications for massage, including illustrations of common conditions. These give students at-a-glance references for muscle and pathology issues commonly encountered by massage therapists. Appendix C contains two additional clinical reasoning activities to review material from the book.

Anatomy, Physiology, Biomechanics, and Pathology—Comprehensive and Specifically Designed for the Massage Therapy Student

Welcome to the Fourth Edition!

Terminology: Scientific, Medical, Social, and Cultural Communication

CHAPTER 3

http://evolve.elsevier.com/Fritz/essential

CHAPTER OBJECTIVES

After completing this chapter, the student will be able to perform the following:
1. Identify the importance of terminology essential for the practice of therapeutic massage.
2. Use medical terminology to interpret the meanings of anatomic and physiologic terms.
3. Define terms used to describe regions of the body and surface anatomy.
4. Define terms used to describe the positions of the body and the parts of the body in relation to other body parts.
5. Describe kinesiology, body planes, and terms of movement.
6. Describe and use quality-of-life terminology.
7. Explore terminology used in indigenous and cultural-based healing systems.
8. Use a charting method that incorporates a clinical reasoning/problem-solving model.

CHAPTER OUTLINE

LANGUAGE OF SCIENCE AND MEDICINE, 59
   Word Elements Used in Medical Terms, 59
   References, 59
   Abbreviations, 62
GENERAL STRUCTURAL PLAN OF THE BODY, 63
   The Body Map, 63
   Kinesiology, 69
QUALITY-OF-LIFE TERMINOLOGY, 76
ANCIENT HEALING PRACTICES, 76
   Points and Meridians, 85
   Jing Luo, 87
   Yin/Yang Theory, 87
   Organ Relationships, 88
CLINICAL REASONING AND CHARTING, 89
   Charting/Documentation, 90
   Database, 91
   Analyzing the Data, 91
   Treatment Planning, 91
SUMMARY, 92

KEY TERMS

Activities of daily living Normal daily living activity including self-care, such as eating, bathing, dressing, grooming, going to work, housekeeping duties, and leisure activities.
Acupuncture The practice of inserting needles at specific points on meridians, or channels, to stimulate or sedate energy flow to regulate or alter body function. A branch of Chinese medicine, acupuncture is the art and science of manipulating

the flow of Qi, the basic life force; and of xue, the blood, body fluids, and nourishing essences.
Biomechanics The principles and methods of mechanics applied to the structure and function of the human body.
Charting The process of keeping a written record of a client or patient. The most effective charting methods follow clinical reasoning, which emphasizes a problem-solving approach. Many systems of charting are used, but they all have similar components based on the POMR (problem-oriented medical record) and SOAP (subjective, objective, analysis/assessment, and plan).
Combining vowel A vowel added between two roots or a root and a suffix to make pronunciation of the word easier.
Disharmony Distortions in health that result when the functions or systems are neither balanced nor working optimally. In Chinese medicine, disharmony can be created by the imbalance of the Six Pernicious Influences or the Seven Emotions.
Kinematics (kin-i-MAT-ics) A branch of mechanics that involves the aspects of time, space, and mass in a moving system.
Kinesiology (ki-nee-zee-OL-o-je) The study of movement that combines the fields of anatomy, physiology, physics, and geometry and relates them to human movement.
Kinetics (ki-NET-ics) The forces causing...
Mechanics The branch of physics dea... forces and the motion produced by...
Medical terminology Terms used to a... human body, medical treatments a... processes of health care in a science...
Motion A change in position with resp... frame or starting point.
Prefix A word element added to the b... change the meaning of the word.
Qi (chee) Also spelled Chi, Qi refers t...
Quality of life Individuals' perceptions... the context of the culture and value... live and in relation to their goals, e... and concerns.
Root A word element that contains th... word.
Suffix A word element added to the e... the meaning of the word.
Terminology A vocabulary used by pe... specialized activity or field of work. ... meaning of words used in a langua...
Word elements The parts of a word: t...
Yin/yang Yin and yong are terms used... relationships. Yin/yang refers to the... between opposing forces and the c...

ALL CHAPTERS HAVE BEEN REVISED AND UPDATED to reflect changes in curriculum standards and to include new research

CHAPTERS ARE DIVIDED INTO 15- to 30-MINUTE TEACHING AND STUDY SECTIONS with objectives that relate directly to chapter and section objectives

EXTENSIVELY REVISED Chapter 3: Terminology: Scientific, Medical, Social, and Cultural Communication orients students in the language of their profession

LANGUAGE OF SCIENCE AND MEDICINE

SECTION OBJECTIVES

Chapter objectives covered in this section:
1. Use medical terminology to interpret the meanings of anatomic and physiologic terms.

After completing this section, the student will be able to perform the following:
• Identify three word elements used in medical terms.
• Use a medical dictionary.
• Combine word elements into medical terms.
• Identify abbreviations used in health care and their meanings.

Medical terminology uses terms derived from Latin or Greek to accurately describe the human body, medical treatments and conditions, and processes of health care in a science-based manner.

Most scientific and medical terms are derived from fundamental elements from Latin or Greek, the commonly accepted language bases. These elements are combined to form scientific terms, which include medical terms. Once you know the meaning of the fundamental elements, a term can be interpreted easily by separating the word into its elements: prefix, root, and suffix.

Each of the following sections includes a list of some of the more common word elements. These lists are not meant to be all-encompassing, but they provide enough examples for you to gain a general understanding of most of the terms encountered by therapeutic massage professionals.

Word Elements Used in Medical Terms
Prefixes

A **prefix** is an element placed at the beginning of a word to change the meaning of the word. A prefix cannot stand alone; it must be combined with another word element. A vowel,

called a **combining vowel**, often is used to join word elements. The combining vowel most often used is o, but occasionally i or another vowel is used. Table 3-1 presents a list of the more common prefixes and some examples of accompanying combining vowels. These prefixes will help you to recognize and understand scientific and medical terminology.

Roots

The **root** (or stem) word element provides the fundamental meaning of the word. Roots are combined with prefixes and suffixes to form medical and scientific terms. In medicine the root word often refers to a part of the body. As with prefixes, a combining vowel often is added when two roots are combined or when a suffix is added to a root. The combining vowel usually is o, but occasionally it is i. Table 3-2 presents some of the more common root words and their accompanying combining vowels.

Suffixes

A **suffix** is a word element that is added to the end of a root to change the meaning of the word. Suffixes cannot stand alone. The suffix is the starting point when interpreting scientific terms. Roots that end in a consonant require a combining vowel when a suffix is added. If the root ends with a vowel and the suffix begins with a vowel, the vowel at the end of the root is deleted. Table 3-3 presents a list of some of the more common suffixes.

References

A medical dictionary is a necessity. A good dictionary holds an enormous amount of information and is the place to begin research and clarify the meanings of words and topics. When selecting a medical dictionary, you should choose one that is encyclopedic and illustrated. Consider using *Mosby's*

THIS TEXT IS DESIGNED WITH Federation of State Massage Boards Licensing Exam and National Certification Exam specifically in mind, and keeps pace with changes in therapeutic massage education as mandated by the Commission On Massage Therapy Accreditation (COMTA)

KEY TERMS are identified, defined, and have pronunciation guidance when helpful at the beginning of each chapter, providing the terminology reinforcement necessary to fully understand anatomy and physiology, and its relationship to massage practice

Illustrations that Illuminate

MORE THAN 170 BRAND-NEW, HIGH-QUALITY MUSCLE ILLUSTRATIONS added to the comprehensive muscle atlas offer greater detail by clearly showing muscle shapes and the locations of their attachments. Each muscle is then fully explained with a list of its attachments, actions, trigger points, and more

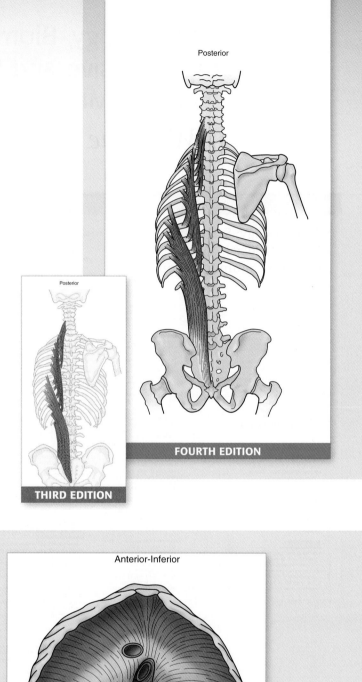

Posterior

FOURTH EDITION

Posterior

THIRD EDITION

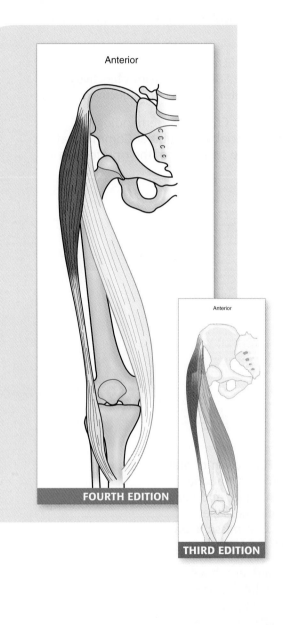

Anterior

FOURTH EDITION

Anterior

THIRD EDITION

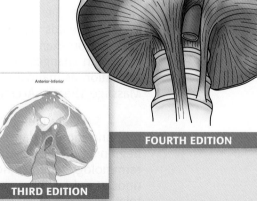

Anterior-Inferior

FOURTH EDITION

Anterior-Inferior

THIRD EDITION

Forearm Supination

Assesses for strength and endurance in the isolation position and tension or shortening in the pronation pattern

Muscles Involved

Supinator

Biceps brachii

Range of Motion

0 to 90 degrees

Position of Client

Seated, arm at side and elbow flexed to 90 degrees, and forearm in neutral or midposition

Examiner stabilizes at elbow with one hand and grasps forearm above wrist with other hand.

Isolation and Assessment

Client supinates the forearm until the palm faces the ceiling while examiner resists the motion.

Forearm Pronation

Assesses for strength and endurance in the isolation position and tension or shortening in the supination pattern

Muscles Involved

Pronator teres

Pronator quadratus

Flexor carpi radialis

Range of Motion

0 to 80 degrees

Position of Client

Seated, with arm at side and elbow flexed to 90 degrees, and forearm in neutral position

Examiner stabilizes at elbow with one hand and grasps forearm at wrist with other hand.

Isolation and Assessment

Client pronates the forearm until the palm faces downward while examiner resists the motion.

FOURTH EDITION

ASSESSMENT PROCEDURES now feature FULL-COLOR PHOTOS of clients being tested for posture, gait, and muscle firing patterns for greater visual clarity

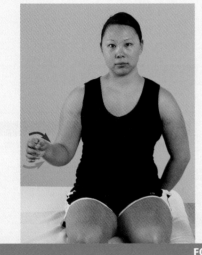

Forearm pronation

THIRD EDITION

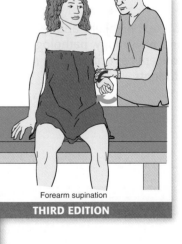

Forearm supination

THIRD EDITION

Features Focused on Knowledge Building

ACTIVITIES THROUGHOUT offer students the opportunity to review and test their skills

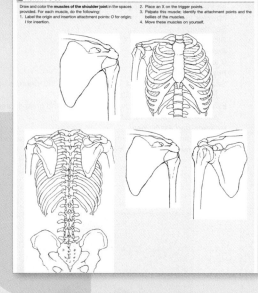

NEW LEARNING HOW TO LEARN chapter introductions prepare students for optimizing their learning experience

LEARNING HOW TO LEARN

At the beginning of each chapter you will find this feature. The information and suggestions will help you learn the skills and become your own best teacher. Lifelong learning is necessary to be successful as a massage therapist, and these skills will support your career success.

Study Tips

Learning is best accomplished in manageable chunks. These pieces of information entail 15 to 30 minutes of reading, doing activities, and reviewing. At the end of each chunk it is important to take a 5- to 10-minute break to give your brain, eyes, and ears a rest. When you study, plan to spend 30 to 90 minutes and divide these sessions into 15- to 30-minute segments, implementing brain breaks as you go along.

Here is an example of a 30-minute study period:
- Reading, doing activities, and reviewing: 15 minutes
- Brain break: 5 minutes
- Reading, doing activities, and reviewing: 10 minutes
- End of study period

A 60-minute study period could be scheduled as follows:
- Reading, doing activities, and reviewing: 30 minutes
- Brain break: 10 minutes
- Reading, doing activities, and reviewing: 20 minutes

...period could be scheduled as follows:
...ivities, and reviewing: 30 minutes

...ivities, and reviewing: 30 minutes

Practical Application

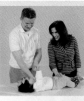

Massage therapy can be supportive during pregnancy, labor, delivery, lactation, and the eventual return of the body to a nonpregnant state. Massage can even support conception by creating relaxation in the body. During the pregnancy the main goal is stress management, sleep support, and management of some of the muscular and skeletal discomforts of pregnancy.

PRACTICAL APPLICATION boxes throughout the text highlight and reinforce anatomy and physiology, pathology, and biomechanic concepts specifically for massage therapy students

Workbook Section

All Workbook activities can be done online as well as here in the book. Answers are located on evolve.

Short Answer

1. List the parts of the neuron.

2. Explain the function of the nerve cell.

8. Describe common pathologic conditions of the CNS.

9. List the drugs that influence the CNS.

10. Explain the influence of therapeutic massage on the CNS.

Fill in the Blank

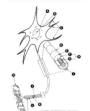

MOTOR (EFFERENT) NEURON

Axon (use twice)
Cell body
Dendrites
Myelin sheath (use twice)
Nerve fiber

WORKBOOK SECTIONS at the end of each chapter encourage critical thinking with short answer and fill-in-the-blank questions, matching and labeling exercises, and more

INDICATIONS/CONTRAINDICATIONS for Therapeutic Massage

Massage and bodywork are contraindicated locally over a trauma area until healing is complete. Very light, subtle methods of touch therapies (e.g., a gentle laying on of hands) may be beneficial in diminishing pain. The process usually is calming and soothing, which encourages healing through stress management. Bodywork methods are beneficial in supporting the rest of the body during the healing process, especially in managing compensation patterns caused by immobilization of an area and in helping the client learn the use of crutches and canes.

INDICATIONS/CONTRAINDICATIONS FOR THERAPEUTIC MASSAGE boxes prepare students for when to continue with a massage or refer a client to another health professional

Take Part in an Evolution of Learning

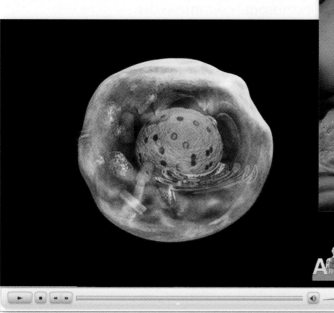

The accompanying Evolve site (http://evolve.elsevier.com/Fritz/essential/) includes more than 100 scientific animations, bringing to life biologic functions and medical procedures for enhanced student learning.

- Find answers and electronic versions of the Workbook sections on Evolve
- Cadaver dissection footage allows students the chance for thorough investigation of the human body
- Additional special features include posture and gait assessment video clips, certification and licensure exam review questions, critical thinking questions following case studies, drag-and-drop labeling exercises, terminology flashcards, categorizing and matching activities, games that review material in a fun and engaging manner, weblinks for further research, and a comprehensive muscle identification activity

- Scientific animations bring body functions to life
- Electronic coloring book gives students the opportunity to study body structure in more detail
- "Brain Breaks" provide ideas for much-needed pauses when studying
- A comprehensive online course is sold separately to accompany this textbook, which greatly enhances the student's learning experience and supports the instructor in presenting the science content to massage therapy students. The first module of the online course is provided complimentary on the Evolve website. Check it out!

Go to www.evolvesetup.com for a quick demonstration on how you can start using Evolve today!

NOTE TO THE STUDENT

It is our greatest hope that the material in this book will come alive with the careful guidance of a skilled teacher and with the patient commitment of a dedicated student. The online course is available for purchase to you even if it is not incorporated in your school curriculum. If, after you check out Module 1 on Evolve, you desire to access the full course, go to http://us.elsevierhealth.com and search for Massage Online for Essential Sciences.

Have fun with the book!

Sandy Fritz

Detailed Contents

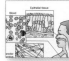

SECTION I
FUNDAMENTALS

Chapter 1: The Body as a Whole, 1
ANATOMY AND PHYSIOLOGY, 4
CHARACTERISTICS OF LIFE, 5
ORGANIZATION OF BODY STRUCTURE, 6

Chapter 2: Mechanisms of Health and Disease, 23
HOMEOSTASIS, 24
FEEDBACK LOOPS, 27
BIOLOGICAL RHYTHMS, 28
MECHANISMS OF DISEASE: PATHOLOGY, 29
PAIN, 37
MECHANISMS OF HEALTH: STRESS, 45
THE LIFE CYCLE, 49

Chapter 3: Terminology: Scientific, Medical, Social, and Cultural Communication, 57
LANGUAGE OF SCIENCE AND MEDICINE, 59
GENERAL STRUCTURAL PLAN OF THE BODY, 63
QUALITY-OF-LIFE TERMINOLOGY, 76
ANCIENT HEALING PRACTICES, 76
CLINICAL REASONING AND CHARTING, 90

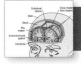

SECTION II
SYSTEMS OF CONTROL

Chapter 4: Nervous System Basics and the Central Nervous System, 98
NERVOUS SYSTEM BASICS: OVERVIEW OF THE NERVOUS SYSTEM, 100
NERVE CELL STRUCTURE, 101
NERVE CELL FUNCTIONS, 103
CENTRAL NERVOUS SYSTEM, 111
PATHOLOGIC CONDITIONS, 123

Chapter 5: Peripheral Nervous System, 133
BASICS OF THE PERIPHERAL NERVOUS SYSTEM, 134
REFLEX MECHANISMS, 139
AUTONOMIC NERVOUS SYSTEM, 147
FIVE BASIC SENSES, 152
PATHOLOGIC CONDITIONS OF THE PERIPHERAL NERVOUS SYSTEM, 158

Chapter 6: Endocrine System, 167
OVERVIEW OF ENDOCRINE GLANDS AND TISSUES, 168
ENDOCRINE GLANDS, TISSUES, AND THEIR HORMONES, 171
PATHOLOGIC CONDITIONS, 181

SECTION III   KINESIOLOGY
AND BIOMECHANICS

Chapter 7: Skeletal System, 192
SKELETAL SYSTEM BASICS, 193

BONES, 194
BONY LANDMARKS, 197
DIVISIONS OF THE SKELETON, 199
INDIVIDUAL BONY FRAMEWORK BY REGION, 202
PATHOLOGIC CONDITIONS, 214

Chapter 8: Joints, 234
JOINT OVERVIEW, 235
JOINT MOTION, 244
IDENTIFICATION AND PALPATION OF SPECIFIC JOINTS, 253
INTEGRATING JOINT MOVEMENT INTO MASSAGE, 270
PATHOLOGIC CONDITIONS OF JOINTS, 273

Chapter 9: Muscles, 283
TERMINOLOGY, 284
MUSCLE STRUCTURE AND FUNCTION, 286
CONNECTIVE TISSUE COMPONENT OF MUSCLE, 298
INDIVIDUAL MUSCLES, 304
PATHOLOGIC CONDITIONS, 458

Chapter 10: Biomechanics Basics, 468
BIOMECHANICS, 469
KINETIC CHAIN, 476
ASSESSMENT BASED ON BIOMECHANICS, 494
PATHOLOGIC CONDITIONS, 537

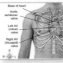

SECTION IV
REMAINING BODY SYSTEMS

Chapter 11: Integumentary, Cardiovascular, Lymphatic, and Immune Systems, 550
INTEGUMENTARY SYSTEM, 552
CARDIOVASCULAR SYSTEM, 562
LYMPHATIC SYSTEM, 583
IMMUNE SYSTEM, 589

Chapter 12: Respiratory, Digestive, Urinary, and Reproductive Systems, 603
RESPIRATORY SYSTEM, 604
DIGESTIVE SYSTEM, 613
URINARY SYSTEM AND FLUID ELECTROLYTE BALANCES, 626
REPRODUCTIVE SYSTEM, 634

Appendix A: Muscle Quick Reference Guide, 651
Appendix B: Diseases/Conditions and Indications/Contraindications for Massage Therapy, 663
Appendix C: Clinical Reasoning Activities, 686

Glossary, 689
Works Consulted, 699
Index, 703

CHAPTER

1

The Body as a Whole

http://evolve.elsevier.com/Fritz/essential

CHAPTER OBJECTIVES

After completing this chapter, the student will be able to perform the following:
1. Define the terms *anatomy* and *physiology*.
2. Define the characteristics of life.
3. List and discuss the levels of organization of the body.
4. Explain the importance of understanding the relationships among the structures and functions of the body as a whole.

CHAPTER OUTLINE

ANATOMY AND PHYSIOLOGY, 4
  Structure and Function, 4
CHARACTERISTICS OF LIFE, 5
ORGANIZATION OF BODY STRUCTURE, 6
  Chemical Level, 6
  Organelle Level, 11
  Cellular Level, 13
  Tissue Level, 13
  Organ Level, 18
  System Level, 18
  Organism Level: The Body as a Whole, 18
SUMMARY, 19

KEY TERMS

Active transport The transport of substances into or out of a cell using energy.

Adenosine triphosphate (ATP) (ah-DEN-o-seen tri-FOS-fate) A compound that stores energy in the muscles. When ATP is broken down during catabolic reactions, it releases energy.

Anabolism (ah-NAB-o-lizm) Chemical processes in the body that join simple compounds to form more complex compounds of carbohydrates, lipids, proteins, and nucleic acids. The processes require energy supplied from adenosine triphosphate.

Anatomy (ah-NAT-o-mee) The study of the structures of the body and the relationships of its parts.

Apical surface (AY-pi-kuhl) The surface of an epithelial cell that is exposed to the external environment.

Atom The smallest particle of an element that retains and exhibits the properties of that element. Atoms are made up of protons, neutrons, and electrons.

Atrophy (AT-ro-fee) A decrease in the size of a body part or organ caused by a decrease in the size of the cells.

Basal surface (BA-sal) The tissue surface that faces the inside of the body.

Basement membrane A permeable membrane that attaches epithelial tissues to the underlying connective tissues.

Carbohydrates (kar-bo-HY-drates) Sugars, starches, and cellulose composed of carbon, hydrogen, and oxygen.

Cardiac muscle fibers (KAR-de-ak) Smaller, striated, involuntary muscle fibers (cells) in the heart that contract to pump blood.

Catabolism (kah-TAB-o-lizm) Chemical processes in the body that release energy as complex compounds are broken down into simpler ones.

Cell The basic structural unit of a living organism. A cell contains a nucleus and cytoplasm and is surrounded by a membrane.

Collagen (KOL-ah-jen) A protein substance composed of small fibrils that combine to create the connective tissue of fasciae, tendons, and ligaments. Collagen constitutes approximately one fourth of the protein in the body.

Collagenous fibers (ko-LAJ-uh-nuhs) Strong fibers with little capacity for stretch. They have a high degree of tensile strength, which allows them to withstand longitudinal stress.

Connective tissue The most abundant type of tissue in the body. It supports and holds together the body and its parts, protects the body from foreign matter, and is organized to transport substances throughout the body.

Compounds Substances made up of different kinds of atoms.

Cytosol (SI-to-sol) The fluid that surrounds the nucleus or organelles inside the cell membrane.

Cytoplasm (SI-to-plasm) Material enclosed by the cell membrane.

Cytoskeleton (SI-to-skel-e-ton) A framework of proteins inside the cell providing flexibility and strength.

Developmental anatomy How anatomy changes over the life cycle.

Diffusion (di-FU-zhun) Movement of ions and molecules from an area of higher concentration to that of a lower concentration.

Deoxyribonucleic acid (DNA) (dee-OK-see-RYE-bo-noo-KLEE-ik) Genetic material of the cell that carries the chemical "blueprint" of the body.

Elastic fibers Connective tissue fibers that are extensible and elastic. They are made of a protein called elastin, which returns to its original length after being stretched.

Element (EL-a-ment) Substance containing only a single kind of atom.

Endocytosis (EN-do-sy-TO-sis) The cellular process of engulfing particles located outside the cell membrane into a cell by forming vesicles.

Endoplasmic reticulum (EN-do-PLAS-mic re-TIC-u-lum) A network of intracellular membranes in the form of tubes that is connected to the nuclear membrane.

Energy The capacity to work. Work is movement or a change in the physical structure of matter.

Epithelial tissues (ep-i-THEE-lee-al) A specialized group of tissues that cover and protect the surface of the body and its parts, line body cavities, and form glands. Epithelial tissue usually is found in areas that move substances into and out of the body during secretion, absorption, and excretion.

Exocytosis (EX-o-sy-TO-sis) The movement of substances out of a cell.

Gross anatomy The study of body structures visible to the naked eye.

High-energy bonds Covalent bonds created in specific organic substrates in the presence of enzymes.

Homeostasis (ho-me-o-STA-sis) The relatively constant state of the internal environment of the body that is maintained by adaptive responses. Specific control and feedback mechanisms are responsible for adjusting body systems to maintain this state.

Hypertrophy (hye-PER-tro-fee) An increase in the size of a cell, which results in an increase in the size of a body part or organ.

Impermeable (im-PER-me-abl) The quality of not permitting entry of a substance.

Inorganic compounds Chemical structures that do not have carbon and hydrogen atoms as the primary structure.

Interphase (IN-ter-faze) The period during which a cell grows and carries on its internal activities but is not yet dividing.

Ion pumps Carriers that transport charged particles into or out of a cell using energy.

Lipids (LIP-idz) Organic compounds that have carbon, hydrogen, and oxygen atoms but in a different proportion than that of carbohydrates.

Lysosome (LY-so-som) Cell organelle that is part of the intracellular digestive system.

Matrix (MAY-triks) The basic substance between the cells of a tissue. Matrix is composed of an amorphous ground substance consisting of molecules that expand when water molecules and electrolytes bind to them. Fibers make up the other component of matrix.

Meiosis (my-O-sis) A type of cell division in which each daughter cell receives half the normal number of chromosomes from the parent cell, forming two reproductive cells.

Membrane A thin, sheetlike layer of tissue that covers a cell, an organ, or some other structure; that lines a tube or a cavity; or that divides or separates one part from another.

Metabolism (me-TAB-o-lizm) Chemical processes in the body that convert food and air into energy to support growth, distribution of nutrients, and elimination of waste.

Metabolites (me-TAB-o-lyts) Molecules synthesized or broken down inside the body by chemical reactions.

Microvilli (MY-kro-VIL-li) Small projections of the cell membrane that increase the surface area of the cell.

Mitochondria (MY-to-KON-dre-a) Rod- or oval-shaped cell organelles that provide energy for cellular activity.

Mitosis (my-TOE-sis) Cell division in which the cell duplicates its DNA and divides into two identical daughter cells.

Molecule (MOL-e-kyool) A combination of two or more atoms. A molecule is the smallest portion of a substance that can exist separately without losing the physical and chemical properties of that substance.

Muscle tissue A specialized form of tissue that contracts and shortens to provide movement, maintain posture, and produce heat.

Nervous tissue A specialized tissue that coordinates and regulates body activity. It can develop more excitability and conductivity than other types of tissue.

Nutrients Essential elements and molecules that are obtained from the diet and that are required by the body for normal body function.

Organelles (or-gan-NELLZ) The basic components of a cell that perform specific functions within the cell.

Organic compounds Substances that have carbon and hydrogen as part of their basic structure.

Osmosis (oz-MO-sis) Diffusion of water from a region of lower concentration of solution to a region of higher concentration of solution across the semipermeable membrane of a cell.

Passive transport Transportation of a substance across the cell membrane without the use of energy.

Phagocytosis (FA-go-sy-TO-sis) The process of endocytosis followed by digestion of the vesicle's contents by enzymes present in the cytoplasm.

Phospholipid bilayer (FOS-fo-LIP-id) Cell membrane made up of lipids, carbohydrates, and proteins.

Physiology (fiz-ee-OL-o-jee) The study of the processes and functions of the body involved in supporting life.

Proteins (PRO-teens) Substances formed from amino acids.

Regional anatomy The study of the structures of a particular area of the body.

Reticular fibers (ri-TIK-u-lar) Delicate, connective tissue fibers that occur in networks and support small structures, such as capillaries, nerve fibers, and the basement membrane. Reticular fibers are made of a specialized type of collagen called reticulin.

Ribonucleic acid (RNA) (RYE-bo-noo-KLEE-ik) A type of nucleic acid. It is transcribed (copied) from DNA by enzymes. RNA carries information from DNA to ribosomes, where it is read and translated so cells can make the proteins necessary for body functions.

Skeletal muscle fibers Large, cross-striated cells that make up muscles connected to the skeleton; under voluntary control of the nervous system.

Smooth muscle fibers Muscle fibers that are neither striated nor voluntary. These muscle cells help regulate blood flow through the cardiovascular system, propel food through the digestive tract, and squeeze secretions from glands.

Surface anatomy The study of internal organs and structures as they can be recognized and related to external features.

Systemic anatomy The study of the structure of a particular body system.

Tissue (TISH-yoo) A group of similar cells that work together to perform a common function.

The study of the human body and its structures and functions is fascinating. For students of massage, the body is the territory of our work. This text provides a map of our territory. A map is a representation of an object, but the map is not the object any more than this textbook is your body. The goal is to give you information you can use to make

At the beginning of each chapter you will find this feature. The information and suggestions will help you learn the skills and become your own best teacher. Lifelong learning is necessary to be successful as a massage therapist, and these skills will support your career success.

Study Tips

Learning is best accomplished in manageable chunks. These pieces of information entail 15 to 30 minutes of reading, doing activities, and reviewing. At the end of each chunk it is important to take a 5- to 10-minute break to give your brain, eyes, and ears a rest. When you study, plan to spend 30 to 90 minutes and divide these sessions into 15- to 30-minute segments, implementing brain breaks as you go along.

Here is an example of a 30-minute study period:
- Reading, doing activities, and reviewing: 15 minutes
- Brain break: 5 minutes
- Reading, doing activities, and reviewing: 10 minutes
- End of study period

A 60-minute study period could be scheduled as follows:
- Reading, doing activities, and reviewing: 30 minutes
- Brain break: 10 minutes
- Reading, doing activities, and reviewing: 20 minutes
- End of study period

A 90-minute study period could be scheduled as follows:
- Reading, doing activities, and reviewing: 30 minutes
- First brain break: 10 minutes
- Reading, doing activities, and reviewing: 30 minutes
- Second brain break: 10 minutes

- Review of content studied: 10 minutes
- End study period

The best way to give the brain a break is by moving the body. Get up and stretch, go outside for a short walk, do some breathing activities such as singing or blowing bubbles. Have a drink of water, brush your teeth, wash your face with cool water, fold some laundry, do the dishes, make your bed. Do something that does not require too much thinking. More brain break suggestions are located on Evolve.

If you are using the online course that accompanies this textbook (and that is a great idea even if you are not required to use it), it makes sense to devote one of the study periods to completing the accompanying segment in the online course. Studying in this way will support your brain by providing repetition of information in novel and different ways. **The first module of the online course that accompanies this chapter is provided on your complimentary Evolve site at http://evolve. elsevier.com/Fritz/essential, so you can experience how helpful it is.**

An effective study schedule for a day would be a 30-minute, 60-minute, and 90-minute period separated by at least an hour or more. Whether you have the 90-minute period in the morning, afternoon, or evening will depend on your family and work schedule and whether you are more alert and focused in the morning or the evening.

Okay, now that you have some guidelines to follow while studying, take a 5- or 10-minute break. Stay on focus, and get back to studying as soon as the break is over.

Box 1-1 **Critical Thinking and Clinical Reasoning**

Massage is mindful, *not* mindless. Excellent massage therapists have two things in common:
1. They use critical thinking.
2. They apply critical thinking to clinical reasoning.

In general, clinical reasoning and critical thinking are similar concepts: Critical thinking is a process of systematic thought that is analyzed and assessed for clarity, accuracy, relevance, and logic. It is the rational examination of ideas, opinions, assumptions, beliefs, conclusions, statements, and actions to identify bias, error, limitations, omissions, and data accuracy that have the potential to create flawed information. Critical thinking is very similar to the scientific method. The scientific method is an objective, consistent, and self-checking process used to identify causes, effects, and relationships between intervention and outcome without opinion, bias, or flawed concepts.

Clinical reasoning is using critical thinking in the therapeutic setting. Clinical reasoning is a thinking process supporting the best judged action in a specific situation.

Clinical reasoning is a method of thinking that follows a sequence (see Appendix C):
1. Investigate the problem.
2. Gather assessment information and factual data.
3. Create a list of possible causes and solutions.
4. Ask questions about (analyze) each of the possible causes and potential solutions.
5. Inquire about the values, beliefs, and feelings of the people involved.
6. Develop a plan.
7. Implement the plan.
8. Evaluate and adjust the plan.

---

decisions as you work with each person you touch. The science aspect of your massage therapy studies is as important as the mechanics of giving a massage. The more familiar we are with the body and its functions, the better able we are to use the methods of therapeutic massage that will most benefit our clients. It is the scientific information that supports your ability to use critical thinking and clinical reasoning during the practice of massage (Box 1-1).

This textbook is written specifically for massage students and provides the information and supports thinking skills you will need to be excellent massage therapists. It covers all the information found in general anatomy and physiology textbooks. However, the scientific information in *Mosby's Essential Sciences for Therapeutic Massage* is based on its relevance to your future practice as a massage therapist. This means that some areas, such as bones, joints, and muscles, are covered in more detail than other areas, such as the urinary system.

There are no shortcuts to becoming a great massage therapist. How well you understand the workings of the human body will determine your ability to serve your future clients.

One of the most important skills you will learn is *where* to find information based on the many *what* and *how* questions you will ask.

You can learn this information in a practical way so that you can formulate and ask intelligent questions related to the practice of massage therapy. You do not have to memorize everything. Instead, question everything and investigate the available resources to find an answer to your question.

This first chapter provides information about the body as a whole because massage professionals deal with the wholeness of each client they serve. The first chapter of the online course that corresponds to this text is available for free at http://evolve.elsevier.com/Fritz/essential in the Chapter 1 folder.

ANATOMY AND PHYSIOLOGY

SECTION OBJECTIVES

Chapter objectives covered in this section:
1. Define the terms *anatomy* and *physiology.*
Using the information presented in this section, the student will be able to perform the following:
- Define *anatomy.*
- Define *physiology.*
- Describe five categories of anatomic study.
- Describe three physiologic fields of study.
- Relate traditional Chinese medicine theory of *yin* and *yang* to Western theory of structure and function.

Anatomy and physiology are two distinct yet interrelated biologic studies that combine to present the operation of the body as a whole organism. **Anatomy** is the scientific study of the structures of the body and the relationship of its parts. **Physiology** is the scientific study of the processes and functions of the body that support life.

The word *anatomy* means to "cut apart." Anatomy is a broad field with many subdivisions, each of which is a comprehensive study in itself. The following categories are examples of these divisions and subdivisions:
- *Developmental Anatomy:* How anatomy changes over the life cycle
- *Gross Anatomy:* The study of body structures large enough to be visible to the naked eye
- *Regional Anatomy:* The study of all the structures of a particular area
- *Systemic Anatomy:* The study of the body divided into the systems that contribute to the same function
- *Surface Anatomy:* The study of the internal organs and structures as they are recognized from and related to the overlying skin surface

The term *physiology* is a combination of two Greek words: *physis*, which means "nature," and *logos*, which means "science." Physiology, the study of the way the body works, can be divided into the following three fields:
- *Organizational Physiology:* The study of the body organization (e.g., cellular physiology)
- *Pathophysiology:* The study of disease and the functional changes in the body during the course of an illness.
- *Systemic Physiology:* The study of body systems (e.g., cardiophysiology)

Structure and Function

Structure (anatomy) and function (physiology) cannot be separated any more than a person can be separated into body, mind, and spirit. Structure and function form a continuum; structure guides function, and function can modify structure.

The concepts of anatomy and physiology are examples of the duality of wholeness. Duality means two opposite states, both of which are parts of unity or wholeness. This concept applies to scientific studies. Opposite aspects of the whole become the foundation for understanding the interplay between structure and function. With regard to structure, for example, you will learn terms for the front and back of the body as well as the top and bottom and inside and outside. *Pathology* can be simply defined as too much or not enough of a body function. Assessment procedures compare normal structure and function with abnormal structure or function. Abnormal is more easily identified if you know what normal is.

The duality of balance is also expressed by the regulatory functions of the body. Maintaining a healthy balance in the body is part of homeostasis. **Homeostasis** is a condition in which the body's internal environment remains relatively constant within physiologic limits. It is maintained by adaptive responses. Specific control and feedback mechanisms are responsible for adjusting body systems to maintain this state.

The duality of wholeness is often how we make sense of our inner and outer worlds. There are many sayings that express this concept. For example, "No rain, no rainbows;" or, "There cannot be light without darkness." Even your brain compares sensation. Cold is understood as relative to the sensation of hot. Muscles work in groups, whereby one group causes a movement such as kicking a ball, and another group of muscles reverses the movement by bringing the leg back. Basic concepts of massage intervention can be as simple as lengthening short tissue and shortening long tissue to ultimately create balance.

The idea of wholeness is presented in many cultures and religions as well as in science. Because the foundation of massage has evolved from various cultural systems, it is prudent to provide information about overlapping cultural theories. Throughout this textbook we will explore ways of thinking about body structure and function based on systems that relate to the practice of massage therapy. We will consider systems from China and India that have a deep and enduring history and wisdom. The first concept to consider is the foundation of traditional Chinese medicine (TCM). The cultural terms in this text, such as *yin* and *yang*, represent physiologic functions; they are not part of any specific religious system.

Yin and Yang

Duality of wholeness is represented in the yin and yang concept expressed in Asian terminology (Figure 1-1). For example, the dual aspects of yin and yang combine to form a dynamic unit; many functions of body physiology are complementary, as described by yin/yang principles. Yin corresponds to the Western concept of structure and yang to

Table 1-1 Yang Qualities Versus Yin Qualities	
Yang Qualities	**Yin Qualities**
Day	Night
Immaterial	Material
Produces energy	Produces form
Hot	Cold
Sun	Moon
Expansion	Contraction
Energy	Matter
Above	Below
Fire	Water
Hollow	Solid
Hard	Soft
Superior	Inferior

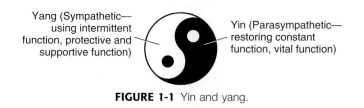

Yang (Sympathetic—using intermittent function, protective and supportive function)

Yin (Parasympathetic—restoring constant function, vital function)

FIGURE 1-1 Yin and yang.

function—opposite but complementary qualities. Yang is said to contain the seed of yin, and yin the seed of yang. These seeds are represented by the small black and white spots in the yin/yang symbol (see Figure 1-1). Nothing can be totally yin or totally yang (Table 1-1). The human body and all its functions can be understood through this concept of the relationship of opposites that creates wholeness. We will use this concept as one of the main themes throughout this text (Activity 1-1).

Practical Application

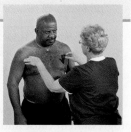

Students of therapeutic massage must be well versed in gross anatomy. The most effective application of massage methods depends on the practitioner's ability to locate, recognize, and understand the structure the hands are manipulating. Knowing the location of a muscle is not enough; we also must know how muscles function and what effects massage and other soft-tissue approaches have on the function of that muscle, as well as the effect of the muscle on the whole body.

Understanding organizational and systemic physiology is important in order to understand how and why methods of bodywork are beneficial. Although we touch the anatomy, the physiology produces the benefits of the massage.

We need to understand how stimulating physiologic changes can influence structure as part of the dynamic process of change that unfolds constantly in our bodies and in our lives as a whole (Activity 1-2).

It is also important to know the historical and cultural roots of massage and understand the basic concepts of the

---

ACTIVITY 1-1

Taking no more than 60 seconds, list as many examples as you can of sets of opposites that together reflect wholeness. Two examples are given to get you started.

Example: black/white, up/down

Your Turn

ACTIVITY 1-2

Consider this statement: As the tree is bent, so it grows.

How does the statement reflect the influence of function on a structure?

Your Turn

Stand up and stretch. Each time you move, notice what parts of your body move toward each other and what parts move away from each other. For example: Bend over and reach for your toes. Notice how your chest moves toward your legs and your head moves away from your low back. Notice how both actions must occur for any movement to happen.

theoretical foundation of these systems. All human beings have a similar anatomy and physiology regardless of their place of birth, cultural influences, and genetic makeup. What is different is the language and the theories. We need to understand that usually the apparent differences among massage and bodywork systems amount to differences in terminology only. These different words used for similar concepts can become confusing unless they are clarified early in massage therapy education. Throughout this text, examples and content about various bodywork system terminology will be compared with the anatomy and physiology terms and concepts used in this book.

CHARACTERISTICS OF LIFE

SECTION OBJECTIVES
Chapter objectives covered in this section:
2. Define the characteristics of life.
Using the information presented in this section, the student will be able to perform the following:
• List and define 13 characteristics of life.

What constitutes life? No single criterion defines it. Instead, characteristics of life consist of the following:

• ***Maintenance of Boundaries:*** Keeping the internal environment distinct from the external environment
• ***Movement:*** The ability to transport the entire being, as well as internal components, throughout the body
• ***Responsiveness:*** The ability to sense, monitor, and respond to changes in the external environment

- *Conductivity:* The movement of energy from one point to another
- *Metabolism:* A chemical reaction that occurs in cells to effect transformation, production, or consumption of energy
- *Growth:* A normal increase in the size and/or number of cells
- *Respiration:* The absorption, transport, and use or exchange of respiratory gases (oxygen and carbon dioxide)
- *Digestion:* The process by which food products are broken down into simple substances to be used by individual cells
- *Absorption:* The transport and use of nutrients
- *Secretion:* The production and delivery of specialized substances for diverse functions
- *Excretion:* The removal of waste products
- *Circulation:* The movement of fluids, nutrients, secretions, and waste products from one area of the body to another
- *Reproduction:* The formation of a new being; also the formation of new cells in the body to permit growth, repair, and replacement

Each characteristic of life is related to the sum of all the physical and chemical reactions that occur in the body. Physiology, or function, characterizes life.

We can study form (structure) without life, such as in cadaver dissection, but we can study physiology only in terms of living dynamics. This text represents the study of life and the dynamic process of living. Therefore anatomy and physiology are presented together (Activity 1-3).

ORGANIZATION OF BODY STRUCTURE

SECTION OBJECTIVES

Chapter objectives covered in this section:
3. List and discuss the levels of organization of the body.
4. Explain the importance of understanding the relationships among the structures and functions of the body as a whole.

Using the information presented in this section, the student will be able to perform the following:
- Describe the sequence of simple-to-complex structures of the body.
- Define each of the following: Chemical Level, Organelle Level, Cellular Level, Tissue Level, Organ Level, System Level.

From the simplest to the most complex, the structures of the body are able to perform their functions in a logical and well-coordinated manner (Figure 1-2). This organization is one of the vital characteristics of body structure and function.

Patterns of dysfunction also present a logical order of progression in a well-coordinated manner. Disease processes usually begin at the most basic level and, if left uninterrupted, progress to complex, multisystem involvement. On careful assessment the logic of the progression can be identified. With this information an intervention process can interrupt the dysfunctional process effectively and move the body toward logical, well-coordinated patterns of health.

✎ ACTIVITY 1-3

Reflect on the characteristics of life as a metaphor for characteristics of your personal life. Then answer the following:
1. Maintenance of boundaries: What are your professional (external) and personal (internal) boundaries?
   _____
2. Movement: How efficient is your movement along the path of life?
   _____
3. Responsiveness: How do you recognize, monitor, and respond to changes in your life?
   _____
4. Conductivity: What is your explanation for how you make something happen? How do you energize?
   _____
5. Metabolism: How do you create your energy and adjust your use of energy in your life?
   _____
6. Growth: How do you measure personal and professional growth?
   _____
7. Respiration: How effectively do you breathe?
   _____
8. Digestion: Describe how you take large, complex concepts and break them into smaller, more understandable pieces.
   _____
9. Absorption: How do you learn? How do you use your learning?
   _____
10. Secretion: How do you teach? How do you reach a diverse population?
   _____
11. Excretion: How do you dispose of those aspects of life that no longer serve you?
   _____
12. Circulation: How do you move physically and mentally in professional relationships?
   _____
13. Reproduction: How do you maintain, restore, and permit new growth in yourself?
   _____

Our bodies work toward balance, which reflects a logical progression of cause and effect. When we understand the patterns of effective function and dysfunction, we can create a map to follow for a return to balance and health.

Both living and nonliving things have certain elements in common that link them and others that differentiate and distinguish them. For this reason a study of anatomy and physiology must begin with an investigation of the basic chemical and physical components. Understanding the basic units of the foundation of life is necessary because massage therapy does influence the client's tissues on a chemical and cellular level.

Chemical Level

Each substance has chemical and physical properties that give it a unique identity. Chemical properties are those that demonstrate the way the substance reacts with other

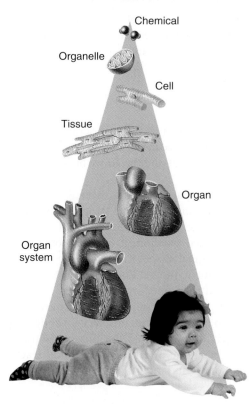

Chemical

Organelle

Cell

Tissue

Organ

Organ system

Organism

FIGURE 1-2 Organizational scheme of the body.

Table 1-2	Elements Found in the Body: Their Symbols and Percentage of Body Weight		
Element (Atomic Number)	Symbol	Weight in Body (%)
Oxygen (8)	O	65.0
Carbon (6)	C	18.6
Hydrogen (1)	H	9.7
Nitrogen (7)	N	3.2
Calcium (20)	Ca	1.8
Phosphorus (15)	P	1.0
Potassium (19)	K	0.4
Sodium (11)	Na	0.2
Chlorine (17)	Cl	0.2
Magnesium (12)	Mg	0.06
Sulfur (16)	S	0.04
Iron (26)	Fe	0.007
Iodine (53)	I	0.0002

substances or the way it responds to a change in the environment.

Physical properties are characteristics such as color, taste, texture, and odor. For example, salt is a chemical. Salt is used to dry food because the chemicals in salt attract water. This is a chemical property. We also can identify salt because of the way it tastes. This is a physical property.

Atoms and Molecules

An **atom** is a small particle of an element. An **element** is a substance composed of a single kind of atom. Atoms are made up of smaller particles called *protons, neutrons,* and *electrons.* Protons, which carry a positive charge, and neutrons, which have a neutral charge, form the nucleus of an atom. They attract electrons, which are negatively charged particles that travel around the nucleus in specific orbital patterns. The atoms most commonly found in living things are hydrogen, carbon, nitrogen, and oxygen.

Electrons are involved in all chemical reactions that bond atoms to make a molecule. A **molecule** is a combination of two or more atoms. It is the smallest part of a substance that can exist independently without losing the physical and chemical properties of that substance. The function of a molecule is related to its structures. The structure of a molecule depends on the patterns of the chemical bonds.

Molecules can form elements or **compounds,** which are substances made up of different types of atoms (Table 1-2). These substances, called *matter,* exist as solids, liquids, or gases, depending on the attraction of the molecules. When the molecules exist close together, the substance is solid; conversely, when the molecules are farthest apart, they form a gas.

Chemical Bonds

The forces that hold atoms together in a molecule are chemical bonds. They occur through chemical reactions. The most important structural feature in a chemical reaction is the stability of the outer shell of the atom, where the electrons are located. Shells, or electron shells, are envelopes or layers of electron orbit patterns. If the outer shell is full and does not react chemically, the atom is inert.

If the outer shell of an atom is not full, the atom is chemically reactive. An atom can achieve a state of maximal stability by forming one of the following three types of bonds to fill the outer electron shell.

Ionic Bond

An atom can gain or lose electrons to fill or empty its outer shell. When this happens, the atom is no longer electrically neutral because the ratio of protons to electrons is no longer equal. The atom becomes an electrically charged ion with a negative charge (anion) or a positive charge (cation). Negatively and positively charged ions attract each other to form a stable union. Soluble negatively charged molecules with ions that conduct electrical currents are called *electrolytes.* This type of bond is important in nerve and brain function.

Covalent Bond

When two or more atoms share electrons, a covalent bond is created—the most stable kind of association that atoms can form with one another. This sharing completes the outer shell. Carbon dioxide (CO_2) is an example.

Polar Covalent Bond

Molecules with polar covalent bonds, called *polar molecules,* are electrically neutral because they have the same number of protons and electrons. However, the electrons can be arranged in the shells so that one side of the molecule is more negative and the other side more positive. Water is an example of a polar molecule. Polar molecules attract each other, with the positive side of one attracting the negative side of a different molecule. A strong attraction exists between water molecules, and this attraction is called *hydrogen bonding*. Hydrogen bonds help create larger molecules such as **proteins** and **deoxyribonucleic acid (DNA)** (Activity 1-4, Box 1-2).

✎ ACTIVITY 1-4

Describe a professional, social, or personal relationship that represents the properties of each of the three types of bonds.

Example
Polar covalent bond: A stray cat lives in my barn. The cat feeds with my other barn cats, but I don't think of the cat as part of my family. The weak bond that we have could be broken easily if the cat were drawn to the neighbor's barn and chose to leave.

Your Turn
1. Ionic bond
2. Covalent bond
3. Polar covalent bond

Chemical reactions take place when chemical bonds are formed and broken and new ones are formed. In a chemical reaction the number of atoms remains the same, but the atoms become linked in a different way, forming a new substance (Figure 1-3).

Metabolism

Metabolism is the word we use to describe all the physiologic processes that take place in our bodies. Metabolism is how we convert the food we eat and the air we breathe into the energy we need to function.

Energy is the capacity to work. *Work* is defined as a movement or a change in the physical structure of matter. Energy exists in two forms: potential and kinetic. If an elastic band is held in a stretched position, it has the potential energy to return to its original shape. Kinetic energy occurs when the elastic band actually moves. Energy is constant; it is not lost but is converted from one form to another.

In the body, during chemical reactions, most of the energy is converted to heat and maintains the core body temperature. For example, if the body is cold, the muscles contract and relax quickly, increasing the metabolism (chemical reactions) and producing more heat.

Box 1-2   What Are DNA and RNA?

DNA, or deoxyribonucleic acid, is the hereditary material in humans and almost all other organisms. The human genome is composed of all the DNA within a cell. Nearly every cell in a person's body has the same DNA. Most DNA is located in the cell nucleus (where it is called *nuclear DNA*), but a small amount of DNA can also be found in the mitochondria (where it is called *mitochondrial DNA, or mtDNA*).

The information in DNA is stored as a code made up of four chemical bases: adenine *(A)*, guanine *(G)*, cytosine *(C)*, and thymine *(T)*. Human DNA consists of about 3 billion bases, and more than 99% of those bases are the same in all people. The order, or sequence, of these bases determines the information available for building and maintaining an organism, similar to the way in which letters of the alphabet appear in a certain order to form words and sentences.

DNA bases pair up with each other, A with T and C with G, to form units called *base pairs*. Each base is also attached to a sugar molecule and a phosphate molecule. Together, a base, sugar, and phosphate are called a *nucleotide*. Nucleotides are arranged in two long strands that form a spiral called a *double helix*. The structure of the double helix is somewhat like a ladder, with the base pairs forming the ladder's rungs and the sugar and phosphate molecules forming the vertical sidepieces of the ladder.

An important property of DNA is that it can replicate, or make copies of itself. Each strand of DNA in the double helix can serve as a pattern for duplicating the sequence of bases. This is critical when cells divide because each new cell needs to have an exact copy of the DNA present in the old cell (see illustration).

Ribonucleic acid (RNA) is a molecule that consists of a long chain of nucleotide units similar to DNA. RNA is transcribed (copied) from DNA by enzymes. RNA carries information from DNA to organelles called *ribosomes* that can read RNAs and translate the information so that the cell can make the proteins necessary for body function.

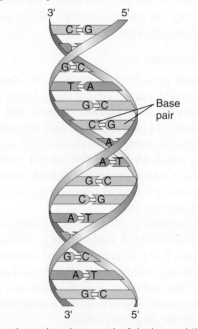

Cytosine and guanine always pair. Adenine and thymine always pair. *C*, Cytosine; *G*, guanine; *A*, adenine; *T*, thymine.

Figure modified from Copstead-Kirkhorn LE, Banasik JL: *Pathophysiology*, ed 4. Philadelphia, 2010, Saunders. Text from The U.S. National Library of Medicine: What is DNA? *Genetics Home Reference, Handbook, Cells and DNA*, available at http://ghr.nlm.nih.gov/handbook/basics/dna. Accessed April 19, 2011.

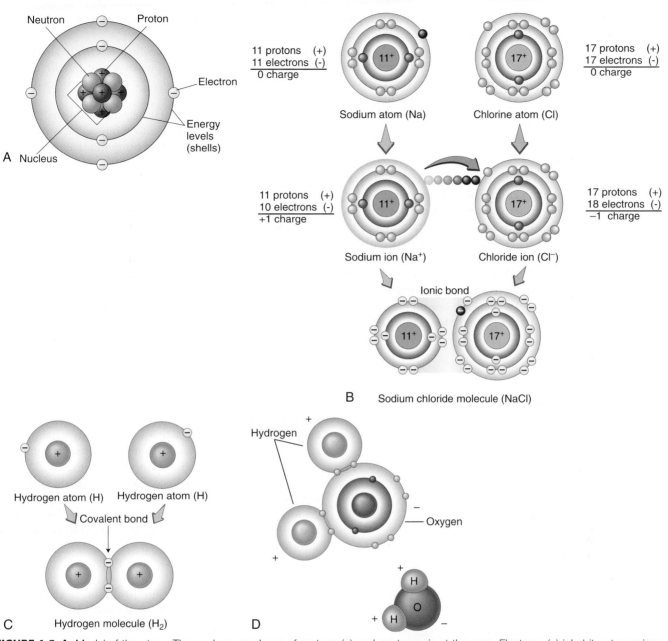

FIGURE 1-3 A, Model of the atom. The nucleus, made up of protons (+) and neutrons, is at the core. Electrons (−) inhabit outer regions called *energy levels*. **B,** Ionic bonding. The sodium atom donates the single electron in its outer energy level to a chlorine atom that has seven electrons in its outer level; now each atom has eight electrons in its outer shell. Because the electron-to-proton ratio changes, the sodium atom becomes a positive sodium ion and the chlorine atom becomes a negative chloride ion. The positive-negative attraction between these oppositely charged ions is called an *ionic bond.* **C,** Covalent bonding. Two hydrogen atoms move together, resulting in overlapping of their energy levels. Neither atom gains nor loses an electron; rather, the two atoms share the electrons, forming a covalent bond. **D,** Water is a polar molecule, as shown in the diagram. The two hydrogen atoms are nearer one end of the molecule, giving that end a partial positive charge. The opposite end of the molecule has a partial negative charge. (**A** to **C,** From Thibodeau GA, Patton KT: *Structure and function of the body,* ed 13, St Louis, 2008, Mosby. **D,** From Thibodeau GA, Patton KT: *Anatomy and physiology,* ed 6, St Louis, 2007, Mosby.)

The body stores potential energy as high-energy compounds. Chemical reactions form these compounds or break them down. **Metabolites** are molecules synthesized or broken down inside the body by chemical reactions.

The two forms of chemical reactions are as follows:

- *Anabolism:* Chemical reactions that use energy as they join simple molecules to form more complex molecules of carbohydrates, lipids, proteins, and nucleic acids

- *Catabolism:* Chemical reactions that release energy as they break down complex compounds. Hydrolysis is a catabolic reaction that uses water to break down larger molecules. Dehydration is an anabolic reaction involving the removal of water while small molecules combine to create larger ones.

The energy used in anabolism and catabolism comes from **adenosine triphosphate (ATP),** the primary carrier of chemical energy in cells. ATP contains many **high-energy bonds** that, when broken, supply energy for the work of the body.

Enzymes are proteins that speed up chemical reactions but are not consumed or altered in the process. Enzyme activity is altered by factors such as temperature, acidity, and alkalinity. Enzyme activity is commonly lower in cold and acidic conditions.

Acidity and Alkalinity

The body has to maintain a balance between acidity and alkalinity to support normal function. The acidity or alkalinity of a solution is measured in terms of pH (Figure 1-4). pH is actually a measure of hydrogen ion concentration in a solution. Deionized, distilled water is considered to have a pH of 7, which is neutral. Tap water could be a little higher or a little lower. If the pH is lower than 7, the fluid has more hydrogen ions and is acidic. If a solution has a pH higher than 7, it has fewer hydrogen ions and is alkaline. Each line on the pH scale is a factor of 10. Therefore a pH of 8 is 10 times more alkaline

than a pH of 7; a pH of 5 is 100 times more acidic than a pH of 7.

The pH of the body is 7.4, which is slightly alkaline. For the enzymes of the body to be active and for the chemical reactions to proceed normally, the pH has to be maintained at this level.

Buffers are compounds that help maintain the hydrogen ion concentration. Proteins, hemoglobin, and a combination of bicarbonate and carbonic acid compounds are examples of buffers present in body fluids.

Inorganic and Organic Compounds

Inorganic compounds are chemical structures that do not have carbon and hydrogen atoms. **Organic compounds** are chemical structures that have carbon and hydrogen atoms. Much of our body consists of organic compounds. The food we eat is made mostly of organic compounds called *nutrients*. When we digest them, we are catabolizing them. A variety of nutrients in the diet are required by the body for normal function. Organic compounds important in the body are carbohydrates, proteins, fats or lipids, nucleic acids, and vitamins. Inorganic nutrients the body needs are water and minerals.

Carbohydrates

Carbohydrates make up 2% to 3% of our body weight. Sugars and starches are examples. Carbohydrates may be simple or complex. They supply most of the energy for cells.

Simple sugars, such as glucose and fructose, dissolve easily in water and are transported easily in blood. Complex sugars are formed by the combination of two or more simple sugars and must be broken down by the digestive tract before being absorbed into the body.

Lipids

Lipids are fats. Lipids make up 10% to 12% of our body weight. Lipids are insoluble in water and have to be transported in the blood by special proteins. Lipids are used to form important structures, such as cell membranes and certain hormones, and are an important source of energy. When lipid supply exceeds demand, lipids are stored as fat reserves for future use or as important body insulators. Fatty acids, glycerides, steroids, and phospholipids are examples of lipids found in the body.

Proteins

Proteins make up about 20% of body weight. Proteins consist of chains of molecules called *amino acids*, and chains of amino acids called *peptides*. In our bodies about 20 amino acids are significant. Each amino acid has a different chemical structure that determines its properties. Proteins form the structural framework of the body.

Enzymes that facilitate chemical reactions are proteins. The blood contains proteins in the plasma, and they are used to transport gases (hemoglobin) and hormones (plasma proteins). The antibodies, part of the body's defense system, are proteins, too. Many hormones are proteins.

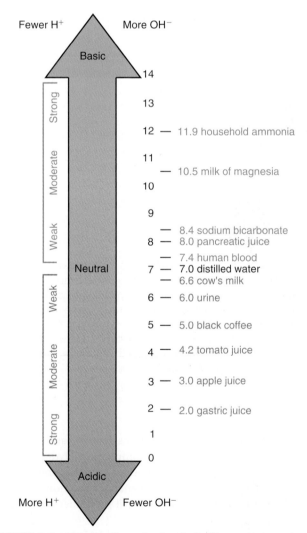

FIGURE 1-4 pH scale. (From Applegate E: *The anatomy and physiology learning system,* ed 4, St Louis, 2011, Saunders.)

Nucleic Acids

Nucleic acid is the major component of ova (eggs) and sperm; it conveys information about the genetic cycle. Two types of nucleic acid exist: deoxyribonucleic acid (DNA) and ribonucleic acid (RNA) (See Box 1-2).

Practical Application

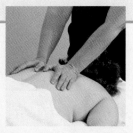

In the study of therapeutic massage, remain mindful of the basic chemical foundations of life and the dynamic processes of change. Change is balanced by stability. We function according to a continual process in which old bonds are being broken and new ones are being formed during every millisecond of our lives, whether in cellular functions or social relationships. Each time we apply massage to a client's body, we become part of the stimuli that activate chemical reactions within that body.

The yin and yang concept of the balance of positives and negatives and of the duality of wholeness that provides stability during change is related to the balance in chemical relationships. A more detailed study of the electrical and chemical levels of life, beyond this basic overview, would be valuable not only for an appreciation of the elegance in the simple physical basis of life but also for an understanding of the metaphor in terms of the way we relate to our clients, our families and friends, and the people of this world.

Organelle Level

Molecules combine in specific ways to form **organelles,** the basic structures found in cells (Figure 1-5). Each type of organelle performs a specific function within the cell. The cell is just a very small version of the human as a whole, and an organelle's function is unique, as are the functions of our body systems. Some of these functions include digestion, respiration, and creating immunities.

More than two dozen organelles have been identified, but the following list includes only the most common ones.

Cell Membrane

Also known as the *plasma membrane,* the cell membrane is the outer boundary of a cell. The membrane is composed of lipids, carbohydrates, and proteins and is called the **phospholipid bilayer.** Its molecules are arranged in such a way that they resemble a sandwich. The function of the cell membrane is to contain the inside of the cell and allow the transport of certain substances into and out of the cell by means of various proteins embedded in the cell membrane. Proteins on the surface of the cell act as markers that identify the cell or work as receptors for chemical signals.

The cell membrane is **impermeable** if it does not allow substances to pass through it; the membrane is selectively permeable if it stops one substance from entering the cell but freely allows another to pass through. Electrical charge, chemical composition, and the size and shape of a substance determine whether the cell membrane will allow it to pass through. Transport of substances across the cell membrane without use of energy is called **passive transport.** Types of passive transport are diffusion, osmosis, filtration, carrier-mediated transport, and vesicular transport.

Diffusion is the movement of ions and molecules from an area of higher concentration to an area of lower concentration.

Osmosis is the diffusion of water from a region of lower solution concentration to a region of higher solution concentration across a semipermeable membrane.

Filtration occurs when hydrostatic pressure forces water across a semipermeable membrane. This occurs in the body when filtration moves fluid out of capillaries and into the renal tubules of the kidney to form urine.

Carrier-mediated transport occurs when integral proteins bind to specific ions or other substances, such as glucose and amino acids, and carry them across the cell membrane into the cell.

Vesicular transport is when small membrane-lined sacs form as the cell membrane folds to form vesicles that surround a substance and move it into or out of the cell. Bringing substances into the cell by forming vesicles is **endocytosis;** transporting substances out of the cell is **exocytosis.**

Active transport of substances across a cell membrane requires energy in the form of ATP. Active transport uses energy to create **ion pumps.** The most common ion pump is the sodium-potassium pump. Under normal circumstances, the extracellular fluid (outside the cell) contains more sodium than the intracellular fluid (inside the cell); but the extracellular fluid contains less potassium than the intracellular fluid. The sodium-potassium pump, by using energy, pumps sodium out and potassium in so as to maintain homeostasis. Cells are negatively charged inside and positively charged outside. This difference in charges, known as the *transmembrane potential,* is maintained by ionic pumps that move substances by means of active transport. The maintenance of transmembrane potential is important because it is necessary for many functions, such as muscle contraction, secretion by glands, and the transmission of nerve impulses.

Cytoplasm

The material enclosed by a cell membrane is called **cytoplasm.** It contains the nucleus and organelles. The fluid portion of the cytoplasm is called *intracellular fluid* or **cytosol.** Cytoplasm, which is not classified as an organelle, is the medium that surrounds all the organelles. The fluid portion, or cytosol, contains many protein enzymes that function as catalysts in the cell processes. The **cytoskeleton** is internal scaffolding that anchors the organelles and allows the cells to move and to maintain or change their shape.

Endoplasmic Reticulum

Endoplasmic reticulum is a network of interconnected tubes, flattened sacs, and channels distributed throughout the cytoplasm. Rough endoplasmic reticulum is found in cells in which large amounts of proteins are made. Smooth

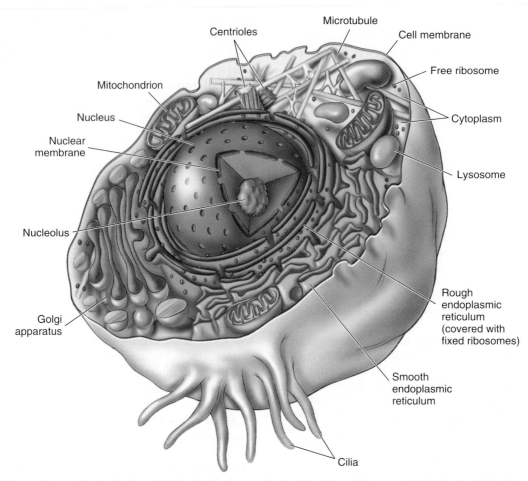

Centrioles

Microtubule

Cell membrane

Mitochondrion

Free ribosome

Nucleus

Cytoplasm

Nuclear
membrane

Lysosome

Nucleolus

Rough
endoplasmic
reticulum
(covered with
fixed ribosomes)

Golgi
apparatus

Smooth
endoplasmic
reticulum

Cilia

FIGURE 1-5 Generalized cell. (From Herlihy B: *The human body in health and illness,* ed 4, St Louis, 2011, Saunders.)

endoplasmic reticulum is involved in the metabolism of lipids (fats); it also assists in eliminating toxicity caused by drugs and in deactivating steroids. Smooth endoplasmic reticulum of muscle cells (sarcoplasmic reticulum) uses large amounts of calcium to trigger muscle contractions.

Golgi Apparatus (or Complex)

The Golgi apparatus processes and packages protein and some carbohydrates for distribution to other parts of the cell or for secretion from the cell.

Lysosomes

Lysosomes contain enzymes that function as the digestive system of the cell. These enzymes are enclosed in membranes to keep them from breaking down the cell itself.

Microvilli

Microvilli are small fingerlike projections of the cell membrane that serve to increase the surface area. They are found in cells that are involved in absorbing substances from the extracellular fluid.

Mitochondria

The **mitochondria** may be the largest and one of the most numerous of the organelles. They produce ATP, which provides energy for cell activity.

Peroxisomes

Peroxisomes are similar to lysosomes, except that they help to detoxify the cell of substances such as alcohol and hydrogen peroxide.

Ribosomes

Often the most numerous of the organelles, ribosomes are the sites where amino acids are combined to create various proteins.

Nucleus

The nucleus controls the daily activities of the cell and all cellular reproduction. Usually the largest of the organelles, the nucleus contains the chromosomes (threads of DNA). DNA is a double-helix strand held together by hydrogen bonds. The nitrogenous bases adenine, thymine, cytosine, and guanine are arranged in different ways to form the genetic code of DNA. The lineup of these bases that provide the code for a specific protein is known as a gene. A gene exists for every type of protein manufactured in the body. Inside the nucleus is the nucleolus, which contains RNA structures that form ribosomes. The nucleus has the information needed for the manufacture of more than 100,000 proteins, and it controls which proteins are synthesized and in what amounts during a given time (Activity 1-5).

✍ ACTIVITY 1-5

Develop a metaphor for each organelle (think of its function).

Example
The nucleus is the mom of the cell; or, the nucleus holds the building plans for a house.

Your Turn
1. Nucleus
2. Ribosomes
3. Endoplasmic reticulum
4. Mitochondria
5. Lysosomes
6. Golgi apparatus
7. Cytoplasm
8. Cytosol
9. Cytoskeleton

Cellular Level

A **cell** is the basic structural unit of an organism. It is also the primary functional unit, and it has properties maintained by the organelles that reflect the characteristics of life:
- Maintenance of boundaries
- Movement and responsiveness
- Conductivity
- Growth
- Respiration
- Digestion
- Absorption
- Secretion
- Excretion
- Circulation
- Reproduction
- Metabolism

Cells are self-regulating, which allows them to adjust to constant changes and to interact with their surroundings. Cells are surrounded by a dilute saltwater solution called *interstitial fluid*. Interstitial fluid is a type of extracellular (outside the cell) fluid. Fluid found inside cells is called *intracellular fluid*. Disease is most likely to appear when cellular homeostasis has been lost.

Chemically, a cell is composed of carbon, hydrogen, nitrogen, oxygen, and trace amounts of several other elements. Cells are made of approximately 15% protein, 3% lipids, 1% carbohydrates, 1% nucleic acids, and 80% water. Although cells are diverse in size and shape, almost all of them have the same parts and general form. Cells are surrounded by cell membranes. All cells contain cytoplasm and organelles.

Cell metabolism involving catabolism and anabolism can be identified and measured in terms of our recurring theme, the duality of wholeness.

The life cycle of a cell involves a series of changes from the time it is formed until it reproduces. The cycle can be divided into two major periods:
1. Growth, or **interphase**, during which the cell carries on most of its activities
2. Reproduction (**mitosis**), or cell division, in which the cell reproduces itself by dividing in half. **Meiosis** is a form of mitosis that halves the number of chromosomes in reproductive cells (ova or sperm) before they combine and multiply.

Cell division is regulated by growth factors found in the extracellular fluid that bind to receptors in the cell membrane and trigger cell division. Growth factors are hormone-like regulatory chemicals. The main growth factors are growth hormone; nerve growth factor; epidermal growth factor; and erythropoietin, which stimulates the production of red blood cells.

Cell division is suppressed by repressor genes. If the rate of cellular growth exceeds that of repression, tissues enlarge. If cell growth is uncontrolled, a tumor or neoplasm results.

Cells change size in response to hormones, nutrient availability, and changes in their functions. **Atrophy** is a decrease in the size of a cell. **Hypertrophy** is an increase in the size of a cell.

Muscle cells in particular can adapt their sizes to their functions. Hypertrophy most often occurs when a person is continually using muscle cells, such as in weight training; atrophy occurs in underused muscle cells, such as when a muscle is immobilized while a broken bone is healing.

Cell Differentiation

No matter what a cell does or where it is located in the body, its basic maintenance functions are the same: nutrition, metabolism, respiration, excretion, organization, and responsiveness. When a cell must adapt to perform specialized duties, the structure of the cell and in turn some of the specialized functions are modified. This form of specialization is referred to as *cell differentiation*. For example, fat cells are modified to store energy, but they have lost the functions of contraction and secretion. Muscle cells have well-developed functions of contractility but diminished functions of secretion and reproduction.

Tissue Level

A **tissue** is a group of similar cells that are specialized to perform a specific function. The cells of a tissue are embedded in or surrounded by material called the **matrix**. The amount and configuration of matrices differ with the type of tissue and the amount of containment or support needed for the tissue.

In most cases, cells connect directly with one another, which allows for better, more stable intercellular communication. Desmosomes are small contact points; they are filaments that extend between cells and act as welds. Gap junctions are formed when channels of the cell membranes adhere to one another. Tight junctions are the type of configuration implied by the name: whole membranes fused together around the cells to create nonpermeable structures. The exception is blood plasma, which is a liquid matrix. Plasma maintains tissue structure but does not hold it in a solid mass.

The four principal types of tissue—epithelial, connective, muscle, and nervous—can be identified by their structures and functions.

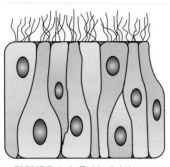

FIGURE 1-6 Epithelial tissue.

Epithelial Tissues

Epithelial tissues cover and protect the surface of the body as well as cover and line certain internal structures (Figure 1-6). They line cavities; form glands; and specialize in moving substances into and out of the blood during secretion, absorption, and excretion. Because they endure a considerable amount of wear and tear, epithelial cells reproduce constantly. If a person is suffering from stress overload or any homeostatic imbalance, the condition often is seen first in the epithelial tissues because of the fast turnover of cells. For example, a skin wound should heal quickly because skin is made of epithelial tissue. However, if someone is stressed, wound healing may be much slower.

Typically, little matrix material is found in epithelial tissues. The matrix present tends to form continuous sheets of cells, with the cells held closely together. The surface of most epithelial tissue is not in contact with other tissues but is exposed to the external or internal environment. This surface is the **apical surface.** The other surface faces the inside of the body and is known as the **basal surface.**

A permeable, thin **basement membrane** attaches epithelial tissues to the underlying connective tissues. Because epithelial tissues contain no blood vessels, they must obtain oxygen and other nutrients by means of diffusion from capillaries in the connective tissues.

The epithelial tissues make up three types of membranes; each membrane has epithelial tissue on the surface and a specialized connective tissue layer underneath. A **membrane** is a thin, sheetlike layer of tissue that covers a cell, an organ, or a structure; lines tubes or cavities; or divides and separates one part from another. There are three types of membranes:

1. *Cutaneous Membranes:* Cutaneous membranes cover the surface of the body, which is exposed to the external environment. The largest cutaneous membrane, more commonly known as our skin, accounts for about 16% of our body weight.
2. *Serous Membranes:* Serous membranes line body cavities not open to the external environment and cover many of the organs. These membranes secrete a thin, watery fluid that lubricates organs so as to reduce friction as they rub against one another and against the walls of the cavities. Serous membranes line the peritoneal, pleural, and pericardial cavities. The peritoneal cavity is around the intestines, the pleural cavity is around the lungs, and the pericardial cavity is around the heart.

3. *Mucous Membranes:* Mucous membranes are found on the surfaces of tubes that open directly to the exterior, such as those lining the respiratory, digestive, urinary, and reproductive tracts. The film of mucus secreted by these membranes coats and protects the underlying cells.

Practical Application

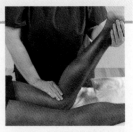

Therapeutic massage focuses on the skin as the primary point of touch. Of particular importance is the sensory function of the touch receptors in the skin. Touch is discussed more extensively in Chapter 11. Passive and active methods of joint movement support the normal function of the synovial membranes, which are connective tissue membranes. The synovial membranes secrete synovial fluid; they line all synovial joints.

Connective Tissue

Connective tissue is the most abundant tissue in the body and is the most widely distributed of the four primary types of tissue. Connective tissue is specialized to support and hold together the body and its parts, to transport substances through the body, and to protect the body from foreign substances. All forms of connective tissue are made of matrix, fibers, and cells.

The properties of the connective tissue cells and the composition and arrangement of the matrix elements account for the amazing diversity of connective tissues. Very exciting research is being conducted to learn more about the structure and function of connective tissue. This research may eventually explain some of the ways massage provides benefits (Box 1-3).

Connective tissue cells commonly are spaced far apart, and the space between cells is filled with large amounts of matrix. It consists of protein fibers embedded in an amorphous mixture of huge protein-polysaccharide ("proteoglycan") molecules. Within the matrix of connective tissue is a shapeless ground substance containing molecules that expand when combined with electrolytes and water molecules. The matrix of connective tissue may be 90% ground substance. The remainder is made up mainly of one or more of the following fibers:

• *Collagenous Fibers:* Collagenous fibers are tough and strong and have minimal stretch capability. They have a high degree of tensile strength, meaning they can withstand longitudinal stress. These fibers occur in bundles. Because of their color, they are referred to as *white fibers.* **Collagen** makes up more than one quarter of the protein in the body. As we age, the molecular structure of collagen changes, and this accounts for the appearance of changes in our tissues.
• *Reticular Fibers:* Reticular fibers are delicate fibers found in networks that support small structures, such as capillaries, nerve fibers, and the basement membrane. These fibers are made of a form of collagen called *reticulin.*

Box 1-3 **Connective Tissue Research, Acupuncture, and Massage**

Acupuncture appears to affect connective tissues. In 2001 researcher Dr. Helene Langevin of the University of Vermont found that when acupuncture needles were inserted and twisted in acupuncture points, connective tissue wrapped around the needles, offering an explanation for the phenomenon called "needle grasp." Needle grasp results in mechanical signals at the cellular level by pulling on the cell wall and then into the cytoskeleton, stimulating cellular function (Langevin, 2001).

There is an unusually high overlap between the sites of acupuncture points and connective tissue planes. Loose connective tissue forms a network extending throughout the body, including subcutaneous and interstitial connective tissues that seem to be involved in the integrative functions of the body.

The many mechanisms by which cells convert mechanical stimulus into chemical activity are referred to as *mechano-transduction*. Mechanical stimuli can lead to a wide variety of cellular and extracellular events. Loose connective tissues may function to transmit mechanical signals to and from the fibroblasts and immune, vascular, and neural cells present within these tissues. It has also been shown that cellular responses to mechanical stimuli can include cell contraction, signaling pathway activation, and gene expression.

These results have potential relevance to the mechanisms of treatments applying brief mechanical stretch to tissues, such as myofascial release. Massage application creates a similar type of mechanical stretch. As mechanical loading (tension) within the matrix increases, the mechanisms that the cells use to remodel the matrix change. Fibroblasts in matrices under tension or relaxed respond differently to growth factor stimulation. Cell division is also influenced by switching between mechanically loaded and unloaded conditions (Grinnell, 2000).

Bottom line: Pull on connective tissue to change the shape of the tissues, which mechanically stimulates cells.

References: Grinnell F: Fibroblast–collagen-matrix contraction: growth-factor signalling and mechanical loading, *Trends Cell Biol* 10(9):362-365, 2000.
Langevin HM, Churchill DL, Cipolla MJ: Mechanical signaling through connective tissue: a mechanism for the therapeutic effect of acupuncture. *FASEB J* 15:2275-2282, 2001.

- *Elastic Fibers:* Elastic fibers are extensible and elastic. Found in the stretchy tissues, they are made from a protein called *elastin*, which has the ability to return to its original length, much like an elastic band does after being stretched. Because of their color, these fibers are called *yellow fibers*.

Each major type of connective tissue has a fundamental cell type that secretes the matrix and fibers (Table 1-3).

A watery ground substance creates a fluid connective tissue such as blood. By changing the proportion of collagen and elastic and reticular fibers, the tissue can be made as tough as a tendon or as flexible as the tissue that covers muscles. Calcium salts added to the ground substance make the tissue become rigid, like bone.

Connective tissue can be manipulated by the application of heat, cold, stretching, and activity. Connective tissue is thixotropic, which means that the substance in question solidifies

Table 1-3 — Connective Tissue Cell Types

Cell Type	Matrix and Fibers
Fibroblast	Connective tissue
Chondroblast	Cartilage
Osteoblast	Bone
Hemocytoblast (hematopoietic stem cell)	Blood

when cold or undisturbed but becomes more fluid when warmed or stirred (gelatin is an example). If not stretched and warmed by muscular activity, connective tissue tends to stiffen and become less flexible.

Therapeutic massage stretches and moves tissue and generates heat to make connective tissue more fluid, allowing greater mobility and encouraging blood flow.

The collagen fibers of connective tissue tend to bind together by means of hydrogen bonding when they are in a state of disuse or chronic pressure. Inflammation is a factor in the bonding process known as *adhesion* in which tissues are abnormally joined together. The result is also called an *adhesion*. Nerves and blood vessels may get caught in adhesions; the result is reduced range of motion and pain. Manipulation by massage helps slow the formation of adhesions and also helps the alignment of the collagen fibers, reducing friction and allowing more optimal movement.

Although connective tissue is found in all areas of the body, some areas contain more than others. The brain has little connective tissue, whereas ligaments, tendons, and skin have high concentrations of it. The number of blood vessels in connective tissue varies. Cartilage has none, but other types of connective tissue have a large number of blood vessels.

Connective tissue contains cells that help with repair, healing, and storage as well as other cells that help with defense. Fibroblasts, which make fibers, and mesenchymal cells, which make ground substance, repair injured tissue. Connective tissue disease is discussed in greater detail in Chapter 8.

Three other types of cells are also commonly found in connective tissue:

1. *Macrophages* are large, irregularly shaped cells. They develop in the bone marrow and move throughout the connective tissue, searching for microorganisms, damaged cells, and foreign particles. When these targets are found, the macrophages dispose of them by ingesting and digesting them, a process known as **phagocytosis.**
2. *Mast cells* also develop in bone marrow. Their functions focus on releasing chemicals such as heparin and histamine, as part of the inflammatory response, the allergic response, and pain.
3. *Adipose cells* are large cells stored in white or brown fat in the dermis, which is the deep layer of the skin. Adipose cells are also found in other parts of the body. When clustered together, they are known as *adipose tissue*.

Types of Connective Tissue

Descriptions of the structure and function of four types of connective tissue follow.

Dense Regular Connective Tissue

Structure: The matrix consists mainly of collagen fibers produced by fibroblasts, with fibers oriented in parallel. The ligaments and tendons formed by this type of tissue have a small number of cells, and blood flow to the area is limited.

Function: Dense regular connective tissue provides strength and resistance while allowing some degree of stretch.

Dense Irregular Connective Tissue

Structure: Collagen and elastin fibers are interwoven and oriented in an irregular pattern to create the matrix. The tissue has little blood flow and is concentrated in the dermis, in the joint capsules and surrounding muscles, and in some organs.

Function: Dense irregular connective tissue can withstand intense pulling forces and resist impact.

Loose (Areolar) Tissue

Structure: A loose, irregular configuration of fibroblastic cells, macrophages, and lymphocytes is contained within a fine network of mostly collagen and elastin. Fluid-filled spaces separate the cells and fibers from one another.

Function: Areolar tissue is distributed throughout the body and is the substance on which most epithelium rests. Areolar tissue is the packing material between glands, muscles, and nerves; it attaches the skin to the underlying tissues and supplies nourishment because of its high level of vascularity.

Adipose Tissue

Structure: Adipose tissue is composed of fat cells with little matrix between the cells. Support is provided by reticular and collagenous fibers. Most adipose tissue is found in the buttocks, anterior abdominal wall, breasts, arms, and thighs.

Function: The storage and release of fat are regulated by stimulation by hormones and the nervous system. Adipose tissue is a source of fuel; it helps insulate and pad organs and tissues, and it stores fat-soluble vitamins.

Types of Cartilage

Cartilage is composed of chondrocytes surrounded by an extensive matrix. Collagen gives cartilage its flexibility, and the strength and water-binding capacity of the ground substance make cartilage rigid, yet able to spring back when compressed. Because cartilage has little blood flow, it heals slowly. The three types of cartilage are hyaline cartilage, fibrocartilage, and elastic cartilage.

Hyaline Cartilage

Structure: Hyaline cartilage is semitransparent and has a milky bluish color and a strong and solid matrix, and is flexible and insensitive.

Function: Hyaline cartilage is found at the ends of bones in most synovial joints, where it provides additional weight-bearing support or attaches to other bones, as occurs with costal cartilage. Hyaline cartilage provides the support and flexibility found in the trachea, lungs, and nose.

Fibrocartilage

Structure: Fibrocartilage is composed of large amounts of dense fibrous tissue and small amounts of matrix, an arrangement that creates a more rigid structure than does hyaline cartilage. Fibrocartilage is found mainly in the symphysis pubis, the joint between the left and right pubic bones, intervertebral disks, between adjacent vertebrae of the spinal column, and tendon attachments.

Function: Fibrocartilage can withstand compression and impact forces, diffusing the force so that it is not focused on specific areas of the bone.

Elastic Cartilage

Structure: As its name implies, elastic cartilage is a flexible form of hyaline cartilage with a large concentration of elastic fibers.

Function: Elastic cartilage provides flexibility and support to the external ear and the larynx (voice box).

Other Forms of Connective Tissue

Bone

Structure: Bone is the most rigid of the connective tissues because of its hard, mineralized matrix.

Function: Bone provides the framework for supporting the body, protects the internal organs, serves as storage for minerals, and produces blood cells.

Blood

Structure: Blood cells float within an extremely loose matrix, a fluid known as plasma, which contains no fibers.

Function: Blood helps maintain homeostasis by transporting substances, resisting infection, and maintaining heat.

Connective Tissue Membranes

Connective tissue membranes are composed of various types of connective tissue. They are classified as synovial membranes.

Synovial membranes line the joint spaces in the mobile joints. This type of membrane also is found in bursae, which are protective sacs found near joints; between layers of muscle and connective tissue; and wherever the body needs extra protection. Synovial fluid is a thick lubricant secreted by these membranes to keep themselves slippery.

Figure 1-7 shows all of the types of tissue, cartilage, and fiber discussed so far in this chapter.

Muscle Tissue

The main characteristic of **muscle tissue** is its ability to provide movement by shortening through contraction. Contraction assists in maintaining posture and produces heat. Contraction results from the action of contractile proteins found inside muscle cells. Muscle cells are longer than they are wide, creating a distinctive pattern that resembles fibers; for this reason the cells often are referred to as *muscle fibers*.

Muscle tissues may be categorized by their appearance, function, and location as follows:

Skeletal muscle fibers are large, cross-striated cells that make up muscles connected to the skeleton. They are controlled by the nervous system, and their actions are voluntary.

Cardiac muscle fibers, which are found in the heart, are smaller, striated fibers. Their structure is not as organized as that of skeletal muscles.

Smooth muscle fibers are neither striated nor voluntary. Found in the organs and viscera, they help regulate blood flow

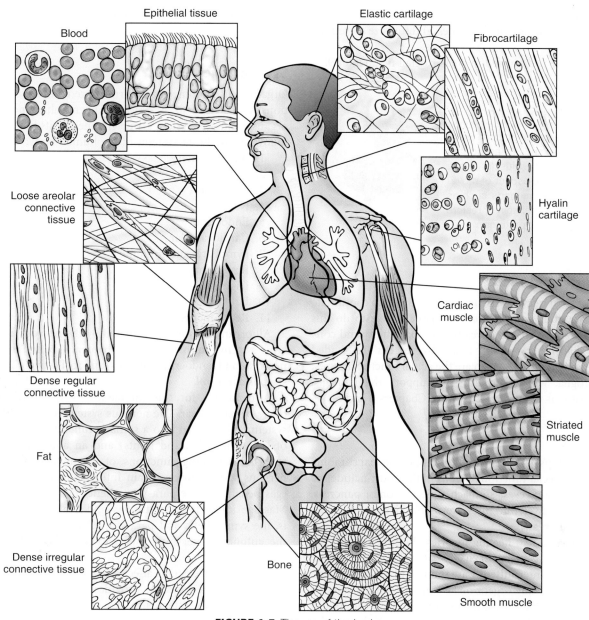

FIGURE 1-7 Tissues of the body.

Practical Application

Many of the benefits of massage and bodywork therapies derive from the effects of these treatments on the connective tissue. Most methods affect the consistency of the ground substance and the directional pattern of the fiber configuration and networks. The gel of the ground substance is considered thixotropic, which means that it liquifies when agitated and returns to a gel state as it stands. Connective tissue is responsive to mechanical forces. Manipulating connective tissue seems to soften the ground substance and increase the water-binding capacity, which makes the tissue more pliable (i.e., induces a more liquid state).

Piezoelectricity is the electrical charge that accumulates in certain solid materials in response to applied mechanical strain. When an electrical current is passed through collagen, a slight

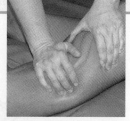

deforming of the structure results because of the piezoelectric property of the collagen. When collagen itself is compressed, stretched, or twisted, it produces minute electrical currents. Researchers recognize that some forms of electrical stimulation enhance bone growth, but the exact reason that bodywork methods could cause this effect on collagen is under investigation. The innate ability of the body to generate electrical current may provide some insight into the inherent energy flow through the body described by ancient healing practices. That energy can be called *Qi* or *Prana,* among other names, and may be considered the life force or the enlivening energy.

through the cardiovascular system, move substances such as food and waste through the intestines, and squeeze secretions from glands.

Muscle tissue is discussed in greater detail in Chapter 9.

Practical Application

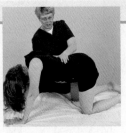

The major elements of soft tissue are the muscle and its associated connective tissue. Muscle tissue provides the active aspect of movement. Soft-tissue methods such as massage seek to maintain or restore effective movement patterns.

Nervous (Neural) Tissue

The functions of **nervous tissue** (Figure 1-8) are to coordinate and regulate body activity. Nervous tissue is able to do this because it is specialized to develop more excitability and conductivity than other types of tissue. Nerve cells are divided into two types: neurons, which are the actual functional units, and neuroglia, which connect and support the neurons. Nervous tissue is discussed in depth in Chapters 4 and 5.

Organ Level

Organs are groups of two or more kinds of tissue that combine to perform a special function. Organs in the body include the heart, lungs, brain, eyes, stomach, spleen, bones, pancreas, thyroid, kidneys, liver, intestines, uterus, bladder, and skin (the largest human organ).

According to Asian healing theories, the functions of the organs can be associated with energy patterns. Organs that are hollow and work intermittently are thought of as yang organs. Extensions of the yang organs make contact with the exterior of the body. Examples include the stomach, with the mouth opening to the exterior, and the bladder, which empties through the urethra. Organs that are solid and must work all the time to maintain homeostasis are yin organs. Instead of filling and emptying, they store the various essences of life extracted from the food and air. Examples include the heart and lungs. The relationships of the organs are presented in the

five-element (phases) meridian theory, which is explained in Chapter 3.

System Level

Organs that combine to perform more complex body functions are referred to as *systems*. The number and types of organs found in a system are determined by its functions. The following are the 11 systems of the human body:

1. Integumentary
2. Skeletal
3. Muscular
4. Nervous
5. Endocrine
6. Cardiovascular
7. Lymphatic and immune
8. Respiratory
9. Digestive
10. Urinary
11. Reproductive

All organ systems are regulated by the nervous and endocrine systems. In this textbook Chapters 4, 5, and 6 cover the nervous and endocrine systems and collectively are called *systems of control.*

A metaphor for this interaction is the gas pedal and brake pedal in a car. The nervous system is the main control system. It is divided into a somatic function (the movement of bones, muscles, and joints) and an autonomic function (the life-sustaining functions of organs). The autonomic nervous system divides again into the sympathetic division (gas pedal) and the parasympathetic division (brake pedal). Massage interacts with the gas and brake functions—that is, the sympathetic and parasympathetic systems balance in the autonomic nervous system to help the body maintain homeostasis.

All the organ systems affect one another:

- The digestive system provides fuel for energy that all other organ systems use.
- The cardiovascular system keeps all other organ systems functioning by supplying blood, nutrients, and oxygen to body cells.
- The respiratory system brings in the oxygen that the cardiovascular system delivers to body cells.
- The skeletal system provides physical protection and structural support for other organ systems.
- The urinary system is essential to maintaining fluid and pH balance within all organ systems. This allows them to function optimally.
- The integumentary (skin) and immune systems prevent infections that could affect all other organ systems.

Organism Level: The Body as a Whole

We are more than the sum of our parts. Each part of the body works with the other parts to support the whole. The mutually dependent nature of cells and the organization of complex systems allow us the endless possibilities of diversity that we experience. The cooperation, interdependence, and respect

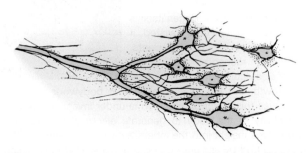

FIGURE 1-8 Nervous tissue. (From LaFleur Brooks M: *Exploring medical language: a student-directed approach,* ed 5, St Louis, 2002, Mosby.)

the body displays for itself could be a wise metaphor for the larger organism of the world in which we are the cells—fundamental units of life. After the overview information has been developed in Chapters 1, 2, and 3, this text discusses each of the systems individually.

SUMMARY

This chapter has laid the foundation for the study of anatomy and physiology. The relationship among structure, function, and homeostasis, in terms of Western and Asian thought, has been presented. The biologic organization of life, from the parts of the atom to the systems of the body, has been laid out sequentially, and each level reveals the components that build the next level of body organization. If a massage therapist is going to plan and organize competently an effective massage session that meets the outcome goals of the client, the therapist must have knowledge of the structure and function of the human body. On this foundation we will continue to build levels of knowledge as our study of the human body progresses.

⊖volve

http://evolve.elsevier.com/Fritz/essential

1-1 Complete a crossword puzzle with definitions of anatomy and physiology terms and clues.

1-2 Review the structures of the cell in a drag n' drop labeling exercise

1-3 Further test your knowledge of cell parts in a fill-in-the-blank exercise

1-4 Match names of tissues to their images

1-5 Test your comprehension of the organizational scheme of the body by completing a sequencing problem

Additional Resources:

Weblinks

Audio Glossary

Remember to study for your certification and licensure exams! Review questions for this chapter are located on Evolve.

Access Module 1 of *Massage Online for Essential Sciences for Therapeutic Massage,* offered complimentary on Evolve in Chapter 1 resources.

Workbook Section

All Workbook activities can be done online as well as here in the book. Answers are located on ⊖volve.

Short Answer

1. Why is the understanding of the relationship between anatomy and physiology important to the massage therapist?

_____
_____
_____
_____
_____

2. Explain the relationship of yin and yang to anatomy and physiology.

_____
_____
_____
_____
_____

3. List and define the 13 characteristics of life.

1. _____
2. _____
3. _____
4. _____
5. _____
6. _____
7. _____
8. _____
9. _____
10. _____
11. _____
12. _____
13. _____

4. List and explain the seven levels of organization of the body.

1. _____
2. _____
3. _____
4. _____
5. _____
6. _____
7. _____

Fill in the Blank

(1) _____ is the scientific study of the (2) _____ of the body and the relationship of its parts. (3) _____ is the scientific study of the processes and (4) _____ of the body that support life.

(5) _____ is the study of body structures large enough to be visible to the naked eye. (6) _____ is the study of all of the structures of a particular area. (7) _____ is the study of the body divided into its systems.

(8) _____ is the study of internal body structures as they can be recognized and related to the overlying skin surface.

An (9) _____ is the smallest particle of an element that retains the properties of that element. (10) _____ are the smallest parts of a substance that can exist independently without losing the physical and chemical properties of that substance.

(11) _____ refers to the chemical reactions in the body. A chemical reaction that releases energy as it breaks down complex compounds into simpler ones is (12) _____.

(13) _____ is a chemical reaction that uses energy as it joins simple molecules together to form more complex molecules. The energy molecule of the body is adenosine triphosphate, or (14) _____.

(15) _____ are proteins that speed up chemical reactions but are not consumed or altered in the process. The (16) _____ / _____ of a solution is measured in terms of pH. (17) _____ are the basic structures of the cells, and they perform specific functions within the cell.

(18) _____ is the movement of ions and molecules from an area of higher concentration to that of a lower concentration. Bringing substances into the cell by forming vesicles is (19) _____, and transporting substances out of the cell is (20) _____.

A (21) _____ is the basic structural and functional unit of a living organism. (22) _____ is the period when the cell grows and carries on most of its activities. (23) _____ occurs when the cell divides, the process by which the cell (24) _____ itself.

(25) _____ is a special form of mitosis that halves the number of chromosomes in (26) _____ cells. (27) _____ is an increase in the size of a cell; (28) _____ is a decrease in cell size.

A (29) _____ is a group of similar cells that usually have a similar embryologic origin and that are specialized for a particular function. The tissue surface that faces the inside of the body is known as the (30) _____ surface.

(31) _____ tissue covers and protects the surfaces of the body; lines body cavities; specializes in moving substances into and out of the blood during secretion, excretion, and absorption; and forms many glands. A (32) _____ is a thin, sheetlike layer of tissue that covers a cell, an organ, or a structure; that lines tubes or cavities; or that divides and separates one part from another.

(33) _____ tissue is specialized to support and hold together the body and its parts, to transport substances through the body, and to protect it from foreign substances. Within the (34) _____ of connective tissue is a shapeless or amorphous ground substance containing molecules that expand when bound with electrolytes and water molecules. Of all the hundreds of different protein compounds in the body, (35) _____ is the most abundant, accounting for more than one fourth of the protein in the body.

(36) _____ fibers are strong fibers with minimal stretch capacity. They have a high degree of tensile strength, which allows them to withstand longitudinal stress.

(37) _____ fibers are delicate connective tissue fibers that occur in networks, which support small structures such as capillaries, nerve fibers, and the basement membrane.

(38) _____ fibers are extensible and elastic. They are made from a protein called *elastin,* which returns to its original length after being stretched.

(39) _____ tissue provides movement, maintains posture, and produces heat.

(40) _____ muscle fibers are made up of large, cross-striated cells connected to the skeleton and under voluntary control of the nervous system.

(41) _____ muscle fibers are small, striated, involuntary fibers that enable the heart to pump blood.

(42) _____ muscle fibers are neither striated nor voluntary. They help to regulate blood flow through the cardiovascular system, propel food through the gut, and squeeze secretions from glands.

Problem Solving

Read the problem presented. There is no correct answer; rather, this exercise assists the student in developing the analytical and decision-making skills necessary in professional practice. After reading the problem thoroughly, follow the six steps below:

1. Identify the facts presented in the information.
2. Identify the possibilities presented ("what-if" statements), or develop your own possibilities that relate to the facts.
3. Evaluate each possibility in terms of the logical cause and effect and pros and cons.
4. Consider the effects on the persons involved.
5. Write each answer in the space provided.
6. Develop your solution by answering the final question posed.

Problem

The study of anatomy, physiology, and the mechanisms of health and disease can be fascinating as well as overwhelming and frustrating. The student must absorb and understand a tremendous amount of information and remember many details. Textbooks do not always agree, and new research results change the information constantly. Frequently, the information does not seem relevant to the career choice or the broader topic the student is studying, but this textbook is specially designed to focus on content that is important for massage therapy practice. As a result, the wonder, fascination, and importance of the information about the body can continue throughout your studies.

Question

What can you do to avoid becoming overwhelmed and to remain excited as you learn about the body?

The first response is provided as a guide to get you started. Fill in at least two more statements.

Facts

1. The student must learn a tremendous amount of information.
2. _____
3. _____

Possibilities

1. The student may not know what should be committed to memory.
2. _____
3. _____

Logical Cause and Effect

1. The student studies only to pass the test.
2. _____
3. _____

Effect

1. The student feels overwhelmed.
2. _____
3. _____

What can you do to avoid becoming overwhelmed and to remain excited as you learn about the body?

_____

_____

Assess Your Competencies

Review the following Chapter 1 Objectives:

1. Define the terms *anatomy* and *physiology.*
   - Define anatomy.
   - Define physiology.
   - Describe five categories of anatomical study.
   - Describe three physiologic fields of study.
   - Relate traditional Chinese medicine theory of yin and yang to Western theory of structure and function.
2. Define the characteristics of life.
   - List and define 13 characteristic of life.
3. List and discuss the levels of organization of the body.
4. Explain the importance of understanding the relationships among the structures and functions of the body as a whole.
   - Describe the sequence of simple-to-complex structure of the body.
   - Define each of the following:
     Chemical Level
     Organelle Level

Cellular Level
Tissue Level
Organ Level
System Level

Next, on a separate piece of paper or using an audio or video recorder, prepare a short narrative that reflects how you would explain this content to a client and how the information relates to how you would provide massage. When read or listened to, the narrative should not take more than 5 to 10 minutes to complete. Simpler is better. Use examples, tell stories, and use metaphors. It is important to understand that there is no precisely correct way to complete this exercise. The intent is to help you identify how effectively you understand the content and how relevant the application is to massage therapy. An excellent learning activity is to work together with other students and share your narratives. Also share these narratives with a friend or family member who is not familiar with the content. If that person can understand what you have written or recorded, that indicates that you understand it.

This chapter's activity is completed for you as an example. You are on your own for the rest of the chapters.

Example

Massage is done on the body, which is the anatomy. The effects of massage occur because of the ways the physiology and functions of the body respond to the massage. The anatomy is like the hardware of a computer; for example, the computer has a keyboard, a mouse, and a screen. The physiology is how it works. For example, I touch a key on the keyboard (similar to performing a massage method), which activates an electrical signal that tells the computer to do something (the result of massage). On a computer the anatomy can break, as when a key is stuck, or there can be some sort of problem in the programming, as when a virus is attached to an e-mail. This is the physiology. There are lots of words that can describe the same thing. A chair remains a chair, regardless of what language you use—English, Chinese, Spanish, or sign language. *Yin* and *yang* are other names that describe the concepts of anatomy and physiology. The anatomy refers to the parts, but the physiology is what makes things alive. You can have anatomy without physiology. This happens all the time, or else we would not be able to do cadaver dissections to learn about the body parts. But all of the activities of life—breathing, digesting, eliminating, reproducing, and the rest—can happen only when we are alive. When the characteristics of life stop, we are physically dead. The body begins with cells, and these cells eventually decide on their purpose in life. Then all the cells that have the same purpose gather together and cooperate like a village. Once the village is in place (tissues, for example), the specialized departments are organized—police, social services, parks and recreation. These departments are similar to the body's systems, and the ways in which they are organized are like the people in each department. Each one has a special job. For example, the respiratory system is the air-quality department. In this way the little village becomes a town with everything the residents need.

This is only an example. There are many different ways to complete this learning activity. Yes, it can be confusing to do this, but that is all right. Out of confusion comes clarity. By the time you've done this 12 times, once for each chapter, you will be much more competent.

Further Study

Using additional resource material, locate the information presented in this chapter, and then elaborate on it by writing a paragraph of additional information on each of the following based on those additional resources:

Atoms

_____
_____
_____
_____

Molecules

_____
_____
_____
_____

Chemical bonds

_____
_____
_____
_____

Metabolism

_____
_____
_____
_____

Adenosine triphosphate (ATP)

_____
_____
_____
_____

Organelles

_____
_____
_____
_____

Cells

_____
_____
_____
_____

Tissue types

_____
_____
_____
_____

Membrane types

_____
_____
_____
_____

Mechanisms of Health and Disease

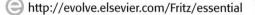

CHAPTER OBJECTIVES

After completing this chapter, the student will be able to perform the following:

1. Define *homeostasis* and *adaptive capacity*.
2. Relate the concept of homeostasis to traditional Chinese medicine and Ayurveda.
3. Define and relate feedback loops to homeostatic self-regulation mechanisms.
4. List and define biologic rhythms and their influence on health.
5. Define disease terminology.
6. Identify major risk factors for disease development.
7. List sources of disturbances in homeostasis.
8. Describe the body's response to homeostatic disturbances.
9. Define pain, and list the types of pain.
10. Describe methods used for pain management.
11. Define stress and the factors contributing to the stress response.
12. Describe ways to manage stress.
13. List the stages in the cycle of life.

CHAPTER OUTLINE

HOMEOSTASIS, 24
    Homeostasis, Traditional Chinese Medicine, and
        Ayurveda, 25
FEEDBACK LOOPS, 27
BIOLOGICAL RHYTHMS, 28
MECHANISMS OF DISEASE: PATHOLOGY, 29
    Causes of Disease, 30
PAIN, 37
    Pain Sensations, 37
    Somatic and Visceral Pain, 40
    Referred Pain, 40
    Phantom Pain, 42
    Pain Threshold and Tolerance, 43
    Pain Management, 43
MECHANISMS OF HEALTH: STRESS, 45
    Stress and Stress Management, 45
THE LIFE CYCLE, 49
    The Aging Process, 50
    Longevity, 50
SUMMARY, 51

KEY TERMS

Acute pain Pain that is usually temporary, of sudden onset, and easily localized. Acute pain can be a symptom of a disease process or a temporary aspect of medical treatment.

Afferent (AF-er-ent) Toward a center or point of reference.

Anaplasia (an-ah-PLAY-zee-a) Meaning "without shape," the term describes abnormal or undifferentiated cells that fail to mature into specialized cell types. Anaplasia is a characteristic of malignant cells.

Benign (be-NINE) Usually describing a noncancerous tumor that is contained and does not spread. More broadly, it can also be defined by a term such as "nonthreatening" to cover instances when the word is not associated with cancer.

Biologic rhythms The internal, periodic timing component of an organism, also known as a *biorhythm*.

Cancer Malignant, nonencapsulated cells that invade surrounding tissue. They often break away, or metastasize, from the primary tumor and form secondary cancer masses.

Chakra (CHUHK-ra) A wheel-like energy center believed to receive, assimilate, and express life force energy.

Chronic pain Pain that continues or recurs over a prolonged time, usually for more than 6 months. The onset may be obscure, and the character and quality of the pain may change over time.

Circadian rhythms (sur-KAY-dee-uhn) Biologic rhythms that work in a 24-hour period to coordinate internal functions such as sleep.

Dosha (DOH-sha) Physiologic function; described in Ayurveda.

Efferent (EF-er-ent) Away from a center or point of reference.

Entrainment (en-TRAIN-ment) A coordination or synchronization with an internal or external rhythm, especially when a person responds to certain patterns by moving in a manner that is coordinated with those patterns.

Etiology (e-tee-OL-o-jee) The study of the factors involved in the development of disease, including the nature of the disease and the susceptibility of the person.

Fistula (FIS-tu-la) A tract that is open at both ends, through which abnormal connections occur between two surfaces.

Health A condition of homeostasis resulting in a state of physical, emotional, social, and spiritual well-being; the opposite of disease.

Hyperplasia (hye-per-PLAY-zee-a) An uncontrolled increase in the number of cells of a body part.

Inflammation (in-flah-MAY-shun) A protective response of the tissues to irritation or injury that may be chronic or acute. The four primary signs are redness, heat, swelling, and pain.

Kapha dosha Physiologic function that blends the water and earth elements.

Neoplasm (NEE-o-plazm) The abnormal growth of new tissue. Also called a tumor, a neoplasm may be benign or malignant.

Opportunistic pathogens (PATH-uh-jen) Organisms that cause disease only when immunity is low in a host.

Pain An unpleasant sensation. Pain is a complex, personal, subjective experience with physiologic, psychological, and social aspects. Because pain is subjective, it is often difficult to explain or describe.

Pathogens (PATH-uh-jens) Disease-causing organisms; are a type of infectious agent.

Pathogenicity (PATH-o-jen-ISS-i-tee) The ability of an infectious agent to cause disease.

Pathology (pah-THOL-o-jee) The study of disease as observed in the structure and function of the body.

Phantom pain A form of pain or other sensation experienced in a missing extremity after a limb amputation.

Pitta dosha Physiologic function that combines fire and water.

Sinus A tract leading from a cavity to the surface.

Somatic pain (so-MAT-ik) Pain that arises from the body wall. Superficial somatic pain comes from the stimulation of receptors in the skin, whereas deep somatic pain arises from stimulation of receptors in skeletal muscles, joints, tendons, and fasciae.

Stress Any external or internal stimulus that requires a change or response so as to prevent an imbalance in the internal environment of the body, mind, or emotions. Stress may be any activity that makes demands on mental and emotional resources.

Ultradian rhythms Biologic rhythms that repeat themselves at a rate that ranges from 90 minutes to every few hours.

Vata dosha Physiologic function formed from ether and air.

Virulent (VIR-u-lent) A quality of organisms that readily cause disease.

Visceral pain (VIS-er-al) Pain that results from the stimulation of receptors or an abnormal condition in the viscera (internal organs).

LEARNING HOW TO LEARN

Learning new information usually requires that you understand the meaning of unfamiliar terms. When content in the textbook seems complicated and overwhelming because of all the new terms, your brain needs more frequent breaks. For example, you might want to study for 10 minutes and break for 10 minutes. Sweep the floor, put on some music and dance—move your body to rest your brain. More brain breaks are provided on Evolve.

When you are learning the meaning of new terms, it is helpful to review the list just before bed, sleep on all the information, and then review the material again first thing in the morning.

The goals of Chapter 2 are to provide a context for understanding why it is important to understand the anatomy, physiology, kinesiology, biomechanics, and pathology of the human body. Most students ask the question, "Why do I have to know this stuff?" This chapter will begin to provide the answers to that question. The start of the answer is, "Because you want to be able to intelligently explain the benefits of massage."

Massage therapy clients most often request that massage provide the following types of outcomes:
- Stress management
- Support for health and healing
- Increased mobility
- Relief from pain

It is common for a client to want all four of these outcomes to be achieved, along with the unspoken outcomes of pleasurable, safe, nurturing, compassionate, nonjudgmental touch. All of these outcomes are necessary for health and well-being. All of these fundamental massage-based outcomes are also directly or indirectly related to an understanding of the mechanisms of health and disease.

Massage therapy application typically follows the following sequences:

General →specific→general

Surface→deep→ surface

This textbook is organized in the same way. The first three chapters present a general and surface overview of body organization, health and disease, and the language of science (medical terminology). Chapters 4 through 10 explore the human body in specific and deep detail as it relates to massage therapy. Finally, Chapters 11 and 12 are more general and cover content in a broader manner, highlighting information about the body that is important for understanding the influences of therapeutic massage and general health maintenance.

Chapter 1 set the stage as an overview and introduction to the study of the body in structure and function. This chapter provides a wider view of how anatomy and physiology affect each of us in daily life.

It may be necessary to use a medical dictionary to look up unfamiliar terminology. The brief overview of anatomy and physiology in Chapter 1 should provide enough of a basis for understanding this chapter; however, it is a great learning experience to explore terminology by looking up definitions.

Once you have understood the importance of anatomy and physiology in relation to how we function, the relevance of the more detailed study in future chapters becomes clear. If you are using the online course that accompanies this textbook, it will support your learning process by providing an interactive, enjoyable, and expanded learning experience.

HOMEOSTASIS

SECTION OBJECTIVES

Chapter objectives covered in this section:
1. Define *homeostasis* and *adaptive capacity.*
2. Relate the concept of homeostasis to traditional Chinese medicine and Ayurveda.

After completing this section, the student will be able to perform the following:
- Define homeostasis in relation to adaptive capacity.
- Compare Asian yin/yang theory to homeostasis.
- Explain how the Asian five-element theory describes homeostasis.
- Explain how the Ayurvedic theories describe homeostasis.

Our body cells survive and thrive in a healthy condition only when the temperature, pressure, and chemical composition of their fluid environment remain relatively constant. The overall structures of our bodies do not change noticeably from moment to moment. We go to bed at night, and unless major trauma has occurred, our bodies function pretty much the same when we wake up. This consistency is due to the constant balancing activities of our physiology.

Recall from Chapter 1 that homeostasis is the relatively constant internal body state maintained by the physiology of the body. Regulatory mechanisms constantly adjust and adapt to keep our body's temperature and chemical composition in balance within our internal fluid environment. When this balance is interrupted, homeostasis is altered, and the body is more susceptible to a disease process.

One definition of *stress* is any stimulus, internal or external, that creates an imbalance in the internal environment. If we are exposed to stress, certain mechanisms attempt to counteract the responses to that stress and bring the conditions back into balance. Thus the body of a person exposed to stress could respond before any awareness of the stress occurs and bring itself back into a balanced state or homeostasis. This ability is called *adaptation*. If this does not occur, homeostasis is lost and dysfunction begins.

Health can be described as the effectiveness of the body's ability to maintain homeostasis. This ability can be referred to as *adaptive capacity*. Dysfunction and disease can happen when there is reduced adaptive capacity.

Reduced adaptive capacity results from the following:

- Too much demand to adapt, such as being in a car accident and the injury of a loved one
- Not enough ability to adapt because of poor nutrition, sleep disturbances, and so forth
- Dysfunction in the body's organ systems, such as an inability to make the hormone insulin.

Intervention to support return to health involves the following:

- Reduce the demands.
- Support healthy lifestyle changes.
- Use medical treatment such as medication or surgery to replace lacking substances or correct dysfunction.

Homeostasis, Traditional Chinese Medicine, and Ayurveda

Homeostasis is the delicate maintenance of the balance of yin and yang (discussed in Chapter 1). No matter how complicated, the signs and symptoms of disease can be explained in terms of yin and yang relationships, the foundation of traditional Chinese medicine (TCM) (Box 2-1).

Box 2-1	Characteristics of Yin and Yang
Fire is yang.	Hard is yang.
Water is yin.	Soft is yin.
Hot is yang.	Excitement is yang.
Cold is yin.	Inhibition is yin.
Restlessness is yang.	Rapidity is yang.
Excessive fatigue or sleepiness is yin.	Slowness is yin.
Dry is yang.	Transformation/change is yang.
Wet is yin.	Conservation/storage is yin.

Modified from Maciocia G: *The foundations of Chinese medicine,* ed 2. Edinburgh, 2005, Churchill Livingstone.

Asian Five-Element Theory

Most healing arts describe the balanced state of homeostasis in their own terminology. Besides the organ relationship of yin and yang, the Asian five-element theory is a metaphor for the life elements of fire, earth, metal, water, and wood. These elements are found in nature, and their characteristics are reflected in our bodies in a similar way as the characteristic of life was described in Chapter 1.

Each element can support or control another to support balance. Fire is hot and consumes, but it needs fuel, which is wood. This metaphor describes how our food is used as fuel to provide energy for body function or metabolism. The fire breaks down the wood to release the energy. Think of how your body uses the process of catabolism to break apart large molecules into smaller units that are used by the body.

After the fire burns the wood, ash is left over and feeds the earth. We do the same thing as our body eliminates the leftovers from digestion and metabolism. These organic and inorganic substances return to the earth and there will form organic and inorganic or metal materials. Metal can also be thought of as minerals. Our bodies need certain minerals to function properly. For example, zinc and iron are minerals necessary for health. Metal in the law of five elements must be taken from the earth and concentrated.

Fire and water are used to separate the metal from the earth. Think of how water is used to separate gold from the earth and fire is used to melt iron ore. As the fire concentrates the metal, water is separated and becomes the next element of the five elements. Water in some form is necessary for life as we understand it. You can live quite a long time without food but not very long without water. Water is necessary for our food/fuel (wood) to grow in the earth. Metals become tools strong enough to harvest the wood to maintain the fire.

Although these examples of relationships found in nature are not exactly the same as the physiology of the body, they are helpful to describe the way the body functions, using concepts that are already familiar to us.

We can find examples of five-element imbalances in our world today. An excess of mining, for example, is disturbing the stability of the earth. Without tree roots to hold the earth in place, water washes away the soil, which is the food for the plants. We are burning (fire) energy (fuel) faster than the earth can renew it, and the waste that results far exceeds what the earth can purify and return to the soil. The waste enters the water, making it unfit to drink. It is not difficult to understand that our planet is becoming unable to maintain homeostasis. Just as we get sick when homeostasis is lost, the world in which we live will get sick if it is unable to maintain balance (Figure 2-1).

Ayurvedic Theories

Ayurveda is the ancient and indigenous healing system native to India. Ayurveda is thought to have appeared in India nearly 5000 years ago. It emerged from an ancient body of knowledge called the *Vedas,* which is a Sanskrit word meaning "knowledge."

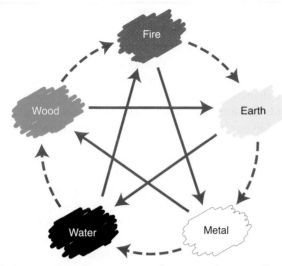

FIGURE 2-1 Five-element wheel--→Supports→Controls. (From Anderson SK: *The practice of shiatsu,* St Louis, 2008, Mosby.)

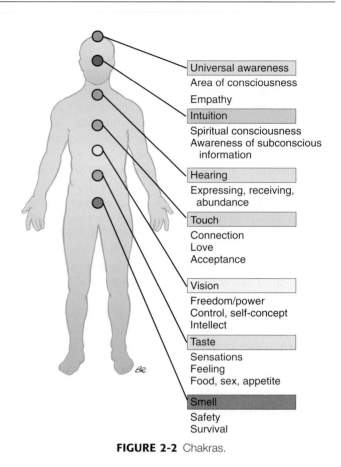

FIGURE 2-2 Chakras.

The word *Ayruveda* means knowledge or science of life. Many of the beliefs and practices of Ayurveda are similar to those of ancient Chinese medicine. One premise of Ayurveda is that the body is a projection of consciousness. Similar underlying principles are fundamental to other ancient healing practices, and more current methods include behavioral medicine and mind/body approaches.

Ayurveda is based on the premise that an individual is made up of five primary elements. The elements differ from the Asian model, but the whole picture of balance is similar. The Ayurvedic elements are ether (space), air, fire, water, and earth.

In this ancient healing system, elements can combine to create various physiologic functions called **doshas.** The **Vata dosha** is formed from ether and air. Vata governs the principles of movement and is seen in nerve impulses, circulation, respiration, and elimination.

The **Pitta dosha** is a combination of fire and water and represents the process of transformation. Metabolic transformation begins at a cellular level and moves up through all body functions. One example of Pitta is the transformation of food into usable nutrients.

The **Kapha dosha** blends the water and earth elements. These elements hold our cells together and build our muscles, fat, and bones. They also form some of the protective lining and fluids, such as the mucosal stomach lining and cerebrospinal fluid.

We are created with our own unique proportions of Vata, Pitta, and Kapha, which allow for the great diversity of human beings.

Healing systems indigenous to India are also based on the chakra system. A **chakra** is a wheel-like energy center believed to receive, assimilate, and express life force energy. The location of these spinning wheels of bioenergetic activity (life force) is thought to emerge from the major nerve ganglia of the spinal column, beginning on the posterior (back) side of the body and radiating through the body to the front. There are seven major chakras, beginning with the first chakra at the

top of the head. The seven major chakras correlate with the endocrine system on a physical level, with basic states of consciousness on a mind level and a process of life fulfillment on a spiritual level (Figure 2-2).

The three doshas of Ayurveda or the five elements of TCM must be balanced for us to maintain healthy bodies. A person's character is an expression of the harmonious and smooth interaction among these doshas or elements.

The same concept of balance found in Eastern healing systems is the foundation of the body/mind relationship in

Practical Application

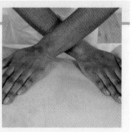

Some of you learning from this textbook may wonder about the benefits of knowing information about TCM, Ayurveda, chakras, or other ancient culture–based healing systems. You may be asking yourself, "What does this information have to do with anatomy, physiology, and pathology?" On a practical level, the current practice of massage therapy is built on the foundation of these ancient healing traditions. The way that anatomic and physiologic functions are named and explained can add insight to the study of what can be called *Western science.* Scientists are actively researching the Western-scientific basis of the ancient healing traditions. Health care systems are now commonly encompassing integrated health care practice that blends many health care traditions, including the wisdom of the ancient systems.

health and disease that has developed in Western science in recent years. It is important to realize that regardless of the healing system, the physiology and the processes are the same; only the terminology is different.

FEEDBACK LOOPS

SECTION OBJECTIVES

Chapter objectives covered in this section:

3. Define and relate feedback loops to homeostatic self-regulation mechanisms.

After completing this section, the student will be able to perform the following:

• Explain how stress causes adaptation.
• List the three components of a feedback loop.
• Define the terms *afferent* and *efferent*.
• Describe negative and positive feedback loops

Self-regulation requires interaction and communication by way of a well-developed control system. This control system is called a *feedback loop*. Every system in the body contributes to maintaining homeostasis, but the nervous and endocrine systems are the most important. Nerve impulses or chemical messengers transmit the information needed to maintain homeostasis through these feedback loops.

Each feedback loop is made up of the following:

1. A sensor mechanism that responds to the change in homeostasis. This change is referred to as a *stimulus*. The sensor usually creates an electrical or chemical signal.
2. An integration or control center that analyzes and integrates all signals received and, if necessary, initiates a response
3. An effector mechanism that responds to information from the control center and creates a change to bring back homeostasis

The terms *afferent* and *efferent* are directional terms. They are used to describe the movement of a signal from a sensor to an integrating or control center or, in reverse, the movement of a signal from the control center to some type of effector mechanism. **Afferent** means that a signal is traveling toward a particular center or point of reference. **Efferent** means that a signal is traveling away from a particular center or point of reference. Effectors are the various organs of the body that can reestablish homeostasis by changing hormone balance, blood flow, breathing rate, and so forth.

The term *negative feedback* refers to the feedback that reverses the original stimulus, stabilizes physiologic function, and helps us maintain our constant internal environment. Most feedback loops are of this type. For example, increasing and maintaining the tension in a muscle help us to relax the muscle later. During massage sometimes we will tell the client to contract a shortened muscle, actually making it shorter. This increase in stimulus is processed in the central nervous system (the brain and spinal cord) as *too much* shortening. The signal sent from the central nervous system back out to the effector, the muscle, is for it to stop contracting so much. Then the shortened muscle can be lengthened back to its normal position, and balance is restored.

Positive feedback enhances the original stimulus and thus maintains or accelerates a disturbed state of homeostasis. Therefore the purpose of positive feedback is not to maintain a stable internal environment. Instead, it continues the disturbed state of homeostasis until something outside the loop stops it.

One example of a positive feedback loop is the contractions during labor and delivery of a baby. Owing to the release of certain hormones, the contractions become stronger and stronger until the baby is born. The birth of the baby is what eventually stops the feedback loop.

Another example of a positive feedback loop is the way in which the body responds to invading pathogens. **Pathogens** are disease-causing organisms. The body's immune system has specialized cells called *lymphocytes* that respond to these pathogens. Because of certain hormones and chemicals released by body tissues, lymphocytes know to attack the pathogens. Additionally, these lymphocytes stimulate even more lymphocytes to respond and attack the pathogens. This buildup of lymphocytes is a positive feedback loop that continues until the infection is contained. It is the containment of the pathogens that eventually stops the feedback loop.

One type of continuing positive feedback loop may become harmful if it does not cease when the cycle no longer serves a purpose. An example of this is a muscle spasm that causes pain, which results in increased spasm. This is referred to as the *pain-spasm-pain cycle*. Pain creates protective spasm, which in turn increases pain (Figure 2-3). The cycle

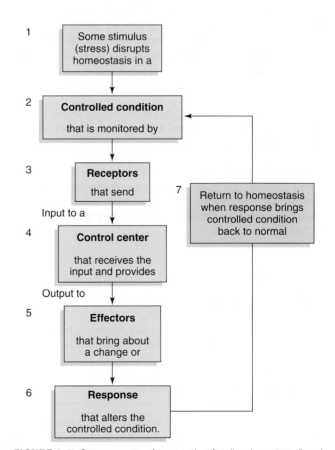

FIGURE 2-3 Components of a negative feedback system (loop).

✎ ACTIVITY 2-1

Many mechanical systems in our homes, automobiles, and work environments have feedback mechanisms. Identify one and, on a separate piece of paper, diagram the flow pattern, labeling the sensor mechanism, control center, and effector mechanism. Show afferent and efferent message pathways.

continues until some sort of intervention, such as massage therapy, stops it.

The systems of control become the physiologic foundation for self-regulation. Self-correcting systems use feedback loops to influence their expression. The body can use this information to coordinate activities (negative feedback), which allows us to remain in a relatively constant state while being immersed in the waves of change (Activity 2-1).

Practical Application

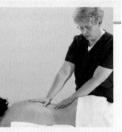

When the body is not able to maintain homeostasis, there are two main problems: *too much* of something and *not enough* of something. We can begin to think about how massage can support homeostasis by using these two principles.

Therapeutic massage can support or stimulate homeostatic processes. The stimuli resulting from the methods are received by the receptors of the nervous or endocrine system, which send signals through afferent pathways for interpretation in the control centers of the central nervous system. Messages are returned by way of efferent pathways to the effector targets, where the response is to reestablish balanced function, such as relaxing or tightening a muscle, softening or firming connective tissue, or reducing or increasing the arousal responses of the autonomic nervous system—whichever restores homeostasis.

More simply, if some function is excessive, or too much, we want to decrease it. When a function is deficient, or not enough, we want to increase it.

Massage approaches are often nonspecific; the stimuli used usually disrupt the general existing pattern of too much or not enough. This disruption requires a response through the feedback mechanism. The objective is to reestablish homeostasis in the same way that we push a reset button on a machine.

BIOLOGICAL RHYTHMS

SECTION OBJECTIVES

Chapter objectives covered in this section:
4. List and define biologic rhythms and their influence on health.
After completing this section, the student will be able to perform the following:
• Define three major biologic rhythms.
• Relate biologic rhythms to health and disease.

Biological rhythms are the internal, periodic timing components of an organism generated within the body. **Circadian rhythms** work in a 24-hour period to coordinate internal

✎ ACTIVITY 2-2

Map your own body rhythms for a 24-hour period. Write in any other rhythms you recognize.

Rhythm	Time
Waking	_____
Elimination (bladder and bowel)	_____
Food	_____
Alert phase (mental and physical peak)	_____
Fatigue phase (mental and physical low)	_____
Elimination	_____
Food	_____
Alert phase	_____
Fatigue phase	_____
Elimination	_____
Food	_____
Alert phase	_____
Fatigue phase	_____
Elimination	_____
Food	_____
Alert phase	_____
Fatigue phase	_____
Elimination	_____
Sleep	_____

functions such as sleep. **Ultradian rhythms** repeat themselves every 90 minutes to every few hours, whereas seasonal rhythms are annual functions, such as feeling more alert in the spring and wanting more sleep in winter. Some forms of depressive disorders—as well as many sleep, neurologic, cardiovascular, and endocrine disorders—recently have been associated with biologic rhythm dysfunction. Many of the conveniences we use have put us out of sync with the natural rhythms of light and dark, the seasons, and the cycles of the moon (Activity 2-2, Figure 2-4).

The biologic rhythms of the body are interconnected and kept balanced by negative feedback loops. Synchronization of the rhythms of the heart, respiration, and digestion promotes this balance, or homeostasis, to support a healthy body. For example, balance between portions of the nervous system influences the heart and vascular systems, which in turn modulate heart rate and blood pressure. Nasal reflexes, stimulated by the movement of air through the nose, rhythmically interact with the heart, lung, and diaphragm (Timmons, 1994).

The various mental and emotional stressors we encounter daily stimulate the sympathetic nervous system, the part of the nervous system that responds by means of fight-or-flight reactions. The central nervous system integrates the information; slows down our brain waves; and decreases the release of cortisol, a hormone released during the fight-or-flight response. This stimulates the parasympathetic nervous system, the part of the nervous system involved in relaxation and restoration of the body.

Biologic rhythms can be affected by the rhythms of music, by repetitive sounds such as a bubbling brook and a breeze in the trees, or by visual patterns. Chaotic or abrupt noise can be a disruptive factor, whereas surf and similar nature sounds usually have a calming effect.

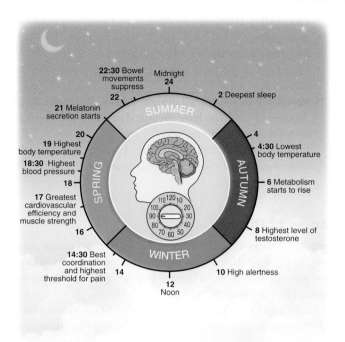

FIGURE 2-4 Biological rhythms. Circadian rhythms work in a 24-hour period and involve body functions such as sleep. Ultradian rhythms repeat themselves every few hours and influence functions such as appetite. Seasonal rhythms are annual functions such as feeling more alert in the spring and wanting more sleep in winter.

Practical Application

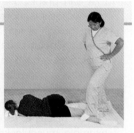

When a person experiences positive emotional states, the tendency is for the biologic rhythms to begin to oscillate together; this is called *entrainment*. **Entrainment** is the physical phenomenon of resonance tendency, in which oscillating bodies move in a synchronized, harmonic manner. Research on entrainment dates to 1665, when Dutch scientist Christian Huygens noticed that when several clocks are placed near each other, their pendulums became synchronized.

We can enhance entrainment processes by using techniques that shift the conscious mind to focus on our breathing patterns and heart rates. Many disciplines quiet the mind and body during meditation. Examples include yoga, which focuses attention on the breath, and Qigong, which focuses on the point below the navel. These systems center attention on body areas that have known biologic oscillators. The Ayurvedic chakra system correlates with biologic oscillators.

Studies have shown that the rhythmic physiologic patterns of a dog's or cat's breathing or heart rate can benefit elderly persons. The rhythmic patterns of drumming, clapping, singing, chanting, and movement in our religious and social rituals interact with biologic patterns, resulting in a calming or exciting organization or disruption of body rhythms.

The rhythmic and ordered approach used in massage and bodywork methods seems to have effects similar to those just mentioned, especially when provided by a calm and focused practitioner. The length of application seems to be important

ACTIVITY 2-3

The following exercise demonstrates the entrainment process as part of your understanding of your own body rhythm.

First, take your pulse to measure heart rate.

Next, measure your respiration rate by counting the number of breaths taken in a 60-second period.

Now play some music and listen to it for about 5 minutes. Retake your pulse and recount your respiration rate.

Notice whether any changes have occurred.

Repeat the exercise two more times with different types and tempos of music.

Preassessment
Pulse rate _____
Respiration rate _____

Music
Type _____
Beats per minute _____

Postassessment
Pulse rate _____
Respiration rate _____
Describe the change _____
_____
_____
_____

Music
Type _____
Beats per minute _____

Post assessment
Pulse rate _____
Respiration rate _____
Describe the change _____
_____
_____
_____

Post assessment
Pulse rate _____
Respiration rate _____
Describe the change _____
_____
_____
_____

Music
Type _____
Beats per minute _____

as well. A session that lasts between 45 and 90 minutes falls within the ultradian rhythm pattern, thus working within the natural balance of the body.

Researchers are currently examining the possibility that disease processes result from disruptions in body rhythms as well as from the effects of work environments that directly disturb or alter natural body rhythms (Activity 2-3).

MECHANISMS OF DISEASE: PATHOLOGY

SECTION OBJECTIVES

Chapter objectives covered in this section:
5. Define disease terminology.
6. Identify major risk factors for disease development.
7. List sources of disturbances in homeostasis.
8. Describe the body's response to homeostatic disturbances.

After completing this section, the student will be able to perform the following:
- Define terms that relate to disease.
- Discuss risk factors in disease development.
- List the nine causes most likely to disturb homeostasis.
- List the five types of pathogenic organisms and infectious agents.
- Define two types of tumors.
- Explain the factors known to play a role in cancer development.
- Define the inflammatory response.
- List the four primary signs of the inflammatory response.

Massage, other forms of soft-tissue bodywork, exercise, and movement therapies focus on maintaining health—a balanced state of physical, emotional, social, and spiritual well-being, or homeostasis. As discussed previously, health results from the effective adaptation of the organism to change. When a disease process disturbs homeostasis, a variety of feedback mechanisms usually attempt to return the body to health. Disease occurs when the demand to adapt exceeds the ability of the body, and imbalance results. In acute conditions the body recovers its homeostatic balance within the normal healing cycle. In chronic diseases the normal state of balance may never be restored.

The following terms are used to describe disease:

- *Pathology* is the study of disease.
- *Disease* can be described as an abnormality in the function of the body, especially when the abnormality threatens well-being.
- *Epidemiology* is the field of science that studies the frequency, transmission, occurrence, and distribution of disease in human beings.
- *Etiology* is the study of all the factors involved in causing a disease.
- *Idiopathic* is a term that refers to diseases with undetermined causes.
- *Pathogenesis* describes the development of a disease. For example, flu begins with a latent or nonactive stage, during which the virus becomes established. When a disease is infectious, this stage is called the *incubation stage*. After the disease develops and has run its course, body functions return to normal during the convalescence stage.
- *Diagnosis* occurs when a licensed medical professional categorizes a disease by identifying its signs and symptoms.
- *Signs* are objective changes that can be seen or measured by someone other than the client.
- *Symptoms* are the subjective changes noticed or felt only by the client.
- *Acute Diseases* have a specific beginning and signs and symptoms that develop quickly, last a short time, and then disappear.
- *Chronic Diseases* have a vague onset, develop slowly, and last for a long time, sometimes for life. Some chronic disorders are initiated by an acute injury/disease.
- *Subacute* refers to diseases that have characteristics that fall between those described as acute or chronic.
- *Syndromes* are groups of signs and symptoms that identify a pathologic condition, especially when they have a common cause.
- *Communicable Diseases* can be transmitted from one person to another. Communicable diseases are infectious diseases that spread through contact with infected individuals; also called a *contagious disease*. Contact with the bodily secretions of such individuals, or with objects that they have contaminated, can also spread this kind of disease. Infectious diseases are airborne and can be caught at any time. Diseases can also be transmitted by bites from insects and other creatures.

- *Congenital Diseases* are present at birth, not acquired during life.
- *Inherited Diseases* are due to genetics.
- *Prognosis* is the expected outcome in a client who has a disease.
- *Remission* is the reversal of signs and symptoms that may occur in clients who have chronic diseases. Remission can be temporary or permanent.
- *Pharmacology* deals with the preparation and the actions of medications and their uses in treating or preventing a disease.

Causes of Disease

Certain predisposing conditions may make a disease more likely to develop. Usually called risk factors, these conditions may put one at risk for a disease but do not actually cause a disease (Box 2-2 and Activity 2-4).

According to Thibodeau and Patton (2007), disturbances in homeostasis may come from many different sources:

Box 2-2 | **Major Risk Factors for Disease Development**

1. Genetic factors: Several types of genetic risk factors exist. Body type (somatic type) is an example of a genetic trait that can predispose a person to disease. For example, osteoporosis is more prevalent in Caucasian women with slight builds. A family history of disease processes and causes of death usually can reveal possible familial genetic traits. Steps, such as changes in diet and lifestyle, can be taken to support the body against the genetic tendency toward a disease process.
2. Age: Biologic and behavioral factors increase the risk for certain diseases to develop at certain times in life. For example, musculoskeletal problems are common between ages 30 and 50.
3. Lifestyle: The way we live and work can put us at risk for some diseases. Many researchers believe that the high-fat, low-fiber diet common among people in developed nations increases their risk for certain types of cancer. Smoking, excessive use of alcohol, lack of exercise, and poor sleep habits are examples of unhealthy lifestyles.
4. Stress: Stress may be defined as any substantial change in a person's routine or any activity that causes the body to adapt. Stress makes demands on mental and emotional resources. Research has shown that as stresses accumulate, an individual becomes increasingly susceptible to physical, mental, and emotional problems and accidental injuries.
5. Environment: Some environmental situations put us at greater risk for getting certain diseases. For example, living in a place that has high concentrations of air pollution may increase the risk for respiratory problems.
6. Preexisting conditions: A primary (preexisting) condition can put a person at risk for a secondary condition. For example, a viral infection can compromise the immune system and make the person more susceptible to a bacterial infection.

Evolve Activity 2-3

✎ ACTIVITY 2-4

Using the various factors, including risk factors that disrupt homeostasis, do a personal health assessment.

Example

Genetic mechanisms: My family has a history of strokes, heart attacks, and joint problems.

Physical and chemical agents: I grew up in an environment with heavy secondary cigarette smoke.

Nutrition: I do not eat enough fresh vegetables, and I eat on the run all the time.

Degeneration: I have degenerative disk problems.

Immune hypersensitivity: I have some allergies to pollens.

Immune deficiency: I get upper respiratory problems when my immune system is depressed.

Viruses: I am susceptible to flu, colds, and herpes simplex when stressed and tired.

Fungi: I used to get yeast infections in my teens and 20s.

Protozoa: N/A.

Pathogenic animals: N/A.

Tumors and cancer: N/A.

Inflammatory response: I have chronic inflammation in my back.

Environment: I work in a clean environment with natural light. I live in an area I like, but my sleep is sometimes interrupted by highway noise.

Age: I am in my 40s and am experiencing age-related hormonal changes and weight gain.

Lifestyle: My lifestyle is extremely busy with demands from many persons. I work 60 to 70 hours per week, but I am able to maintain a regular sleep schedule. I exercise moderately, eat too much fat, have never smoked, and do not drink alcohol or use drugs.

Stress: I am a single parent of three. I have many persons in my life with many different needs. I have many agencies to answer to and feel stressed by the bureaucratic expectations.

Preexisting conditions: I have disk dysfunction, an endocrine problem, inner ear balance syndrome, breathing-pattern disorder, and dyslexia.

Considering this information, how would you rate your personal health history on a scale of 1 to 10, with 10 being excellent health? To what types of disease processes do you feel you are most susceptible? What could you do to support your personal homeostasis?

Example

In general my health is good, an 8 on the scale. The inner ear problem creates physiologic confusion and nausea that add to my stress levels. The back and endocrine problems have stabilized but have to be managed. The breathing pattern disorder is under control. I take fairly good care of myself and use some nutritional supplements to balance my diet. If I get enough sleep and exercise, I do better. I feel that I am most susceptible to cardiovascular disease, joint problems, and osteoporosis. Continued attention to diet and exercise, coupled with therapeutic massage to manage my back and my stress level, seems to be working.

Your Turn

Genetic mechanisms:

Physical and chemical agents:

Nutrition:

Degeneration:

Immune hypersensitivity:

Immune deficiency:

Viruses:

Fungi:

Protozoa:

Pathogenic animals:

Tumors and cancer:

Inflammatory response:

Environment:

Age:

Lifestyle:

Stress:

Preexisting conditions:

Considering this information, how would you rate your personal health history on a scale of 1 to 10, with 10 being excellent health? To what types of disease processes do you feel you are most susceptible? What could you do to support your personal homeostasis?

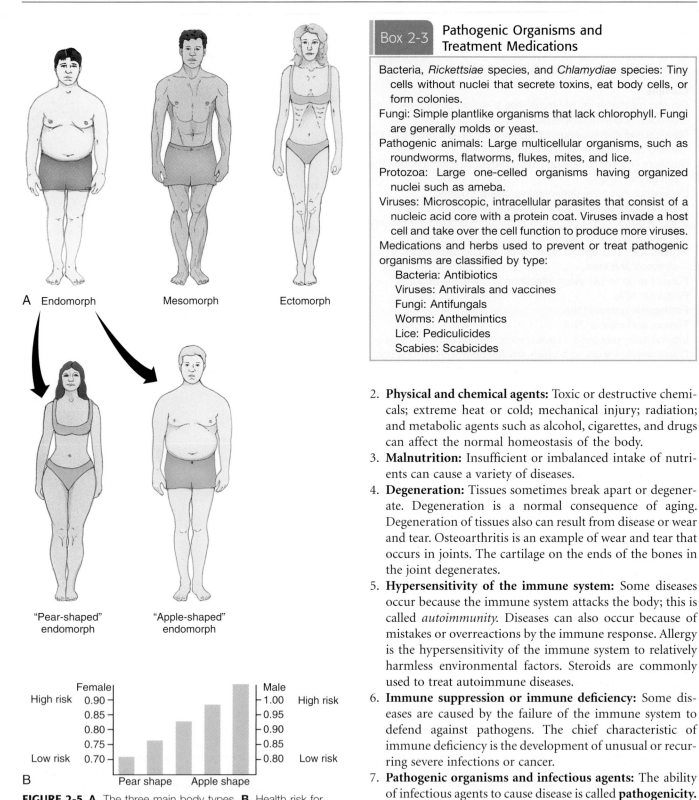

A   Endomorph   Mesomorph   Ectomorph

"Pear-shaped"   "Apple-shaped"
endomorph   endomorph

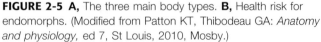

B   Pear shape   Apple shape

FIGURE 2-5 A, The three main body types. **B,** Health risk for endomorphs. (Modified from Patton KT, Thibodeau GA: *Anatomy and physiology,* ed 7, St Louis, 2010, Mosby.)

1. **Genetic mechanisms:** Altered or mutated genes can cause abnormalities. Predisposition is the genetically determined tendency toward disease development. Genetic disease is caused directly by genetic abnormality. Body type is also determined by genetics (Figure 2-5).

2. **Physical and chemical agents:** Toxic or destructive chemicals; extreme heat or cold; mechanical injury; radiation; and metabolic agents such as alcohol, cigarettes, and drugs can affect the normal homeostasis of the body.

3. **Malnutrition:** Insufficient or imbalanced intake of nutrients can cause a variety of diseases.

4. **Degeneration:** Tissues sometimes break apart or degenerate. Degeneration is a normal consequence of aging. Degeneration of tissues also can result from disease or wear and tear. Osteoarthritis is an example of wear and tear that occurs in joints. The cartilage on the ends of the bones in the joint degenerates.

5. **Hypersensitivity of the immune system:** Some diseases occur because the immune system attacks the body; this is called *autoimmunity.* Diseases can also occur because of mistakes or overreactions by the immune response. Allergy is the hypersensitivity of the immune system to relatively harmless environmental factors. Steroids are commonly used to treat autoimmune diseases.

6. **Immune suppression or immune deficiency:** Some diseases are caused by the failure of the immune system to defend against pathogens. The chief characteristic of immune deficiency is the development of unusual or recurring severe infections or cancer.

7. **Pathogenic organisms and infectious agents:** The ability of infectious agents to cause disease is called **pathogenicity.** An organism that lives in or on another organism to obtain nutrients from it is called a *parasite.* Organisms that easily cause disease are **virulent,** and organisms that cause disease only when the immunity is low are **opportunistic pathogens.** The presence of microscopic or larger parasites may interfere with the normal body functions of the host and cause disease (Box 2-3).

8. **Tumors and cancer:** Abnormal tissue growths resulting from uncontrolled cell division called **hyperplasia** results

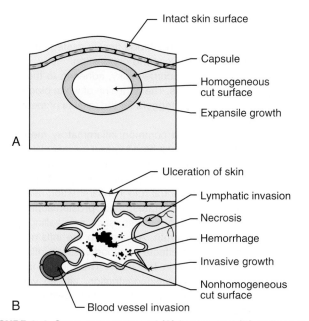

A

- Intact skin surface
- Capsule
- Homogeneous cut surface
- Expansile growth

B

- Ulceration of skin
- Lymphatic invasion
- Necrosis
- Hemorrhage
- Invasive growth
- Nonhomogeneous cut surface
- Blood vessel invasion

FIGURE 2-6 Gross appearance of **(A)** benign and **(B)** malignant tumors.

in a **neoplasm,** or tumor. Tumors can cause a variety of physiologic disruptions. A tumor is named according to its tissue type; a lipoma, for example, is a benign tumor of adipose (fat) tissue.

A **benign** tumor is contained and encapsulated. Benign tumors are relatively harmless, remain localized within the tissue from which they arose, and usually grow slowly. Benign tumors can become serious if the location and size interferes with body functions by blocking of functional tissue or can cause pain by pressing on pain-sensitive structures.

A malignant tumor (**cancer**) is a nonencapsulated mass that invades surrounding tissue. In addition, malignant cells have the ability to break away from the primary tumor and form secondary cancer masses. This ability of cells to break away is called *metastasis*. The cells most commonly migrate by way of the lymphatic system or blood vessels. Cancer cells that do not metastasize can spread another way by growing rapidly and extending the tumor into nearby tissues. Malignant tumors can replace part of a vital organ with abnormal tissues, a life-threatening situation (Figure 2-6). For example, osteosarcoma is cancer of the bone.

Generally speaking, cells that divide many times display increased mutation (change) rates. Cells in the lymphatic system, epidermis, bone marrow, and gastrointestinal tract are more prone to develop cancer than cells of organs that do not divide rapidly, such as nerve and muscle tissue. The mechanism of all cancers is a mistake or problem in cell division called *anaplasia*.

Anaplasia is the reproduction of abnormal and undifferentiated cells that fail to mature into specialized cell types. The result is tissue not related to the needs of the body and not contributing to the body.

Mature specialized cell types display boundary recognition, so they do not invade surrounding tissue. Abnormal

From Thibodeau GA, Patton KT: *The human body in health and disease*, ed 5, St Louis, 2010, Mosby.

undifferentiated cancer cells lack the ability to recognize boundaries and therefore invade and destroy surrounding tissue.

Certainly, a life metaphor is reflected in mature versus undifferentiated (immature) cell behavior. Even at the cellular level, it is important to grow up and follow a life purpose, living in a way that respects the boundaries of others. When we do not know who we are, we have no purpose in life and act in an immature manner that invades others' boundaries; we function as a cancer in their lives (Box 2-4).

Cancer specialists, or oncologists, have summarized some major signs of early stages of cancer. Early detection of cancer is important because it is during the development of primary tumors, before metastasis and the development of secondary tumors have begun, that cancer is most easily treatable. Several warning signs of cancer are listed in Box 2-5.

Surgery, radiation, and medication usually are used in a cancer treatment program. Chemotherapy medications used to treat cancer are called *antineoplastics*. Most of the drugs in this category prevent the growth of rapidly

Box 2-6 Inflammatory Process

Inflammation is a complex process that involves (1) changes in blood circulation, (2) changes in vessel wall permeability, (3) a white blood cell response, and (4) the release of inflammatory mediators.

Changes in blood flow involve the relaxation of smooth muscle cells in arterial walls so that blood moves into capillaries, creating redness, swelling, and warmth of the tissue. The first response of arterioles (small arteries) to an injury is *vasoconstriction*. Vasconstriction is the narrowing of the hollow center of a blood vessel. Vasoconstriction lasts only a few seconds and is followed by *vasodilation*. Vasodilation is the enlarging of the hollow center of a blood vessel. This results in the flooding of the capillary network with arterial blood. The influx of blood dilates the capillaries, which cannot actively regulate blood flow. From the capillaries the pressure is transmitted to venules (small veins). Increased pressure in the capillaries and venules forces plasma through the vessel wall into the surrounding tissue, leading to edema.

The permeability of the capillaries and venules changes in response to inflammation because of (1) increased pressure inside the congested blood vessels; (2) slowing of the circulation, which reduces the supply of oxygen and nutrients to cells; (3) adhesion of white blood cells and platelets (cells involved in blood clotting) to vessel walls; and (4) the release

of inflammatory mediators. The blood flow in dilated capillaries and venules is slow, which leads to congestion.

The white blood cells become sticky, adhering to the lining of the capillaries and venules. The adhesion of white blood cells is one of the most common triggers for the release of mediators of inflammation.

The most important and common inflammatory mediators are histamines (which increase blood vessel permeability); bradykinin (which, among other functions, elicits pain); and arachidonic acid and its derivatives, such as prostaglandins. Arachidonic acid plays a central role in inflammation related to injury and many diseased states, and prostaglandins are responsible for inflammation features, such as swelling, pain, stiffness, redness, and warmth. As a group the inflammatory mediators have numerous effects on blood vessels, inflammatory cells, and other cells in the body. The most important effects are vasodilation or vasoconstriction, altered vascular permeability, activation of inflammatory cells to destroy pathogens, pain, and fever.

The process of prostaglandin synthesis can be blocked by aspirin. The antiinflammatory effects of corticosteroid hormones are caused primarily by the inhibition of arachidonic acid formation.

---

dividing cells. One of the side effects is that they affect epithelial cells, which also rapidly divide, and as a result, antineoplastic drugs interfere with the function of the epithelial tissues and tissue repair.

9. **Inflammatory response:** The body commonly responds to homeostatic disturbances by initiating the inflammatory response, which may occur as a response to any tissue injury. The inflammatory response is a normal mechanism that usually speeds recovery from an infection or injury. Disease symptoms can occur when the inflammatory response activates at inappropriate times or is abnormally prolonged or severe, resulting in damage to normal tissues (Box 2-6).

Inflammation also may accompany specific immune system reactions. It occurs only in living tissue; necrotic or dead tissue cannot generate an inflammatory response. For example, a gangrenous foot cannot become inflamed. Because the body cannot combat infection in necrotic tissue, a foot that is affected by gangrene must be amputated.

The inflammatory response has four primary signs (Figure 2-7):

- *Heat and Redness:* As tissue cells are damaged, they release inflammation chemicals (mediators), such as histamine, prostaglandins, and compounds called *kinins*. Some inflammation mediators (histamine and bradykinin) cause blood vessels to dilate, increasing blood volume in the tissue. Increased blood volume produces the heat and redness of inflammation. This response is important because it allows white blood cells (immune system cells) to travel quickly and easily to the site of injury. These cells attach themselves to the pathogens to

Box 2-7 Types of Inflammatory Exudates

Exudates vary in the composition of proteins, fluid, and cell contents and in the types of cells. Inflammatory exudates contain important proteins such as fibrin and immunoglobulins (antibodies). If the skin is slightly burned, a blister forms that is filled with clear exudate, indicating a low protein content. These are known as *serous exudates*.

Sometimes, inflammation results in fibrous exudates that are thick and sticky because of a meshwork of proteins present in the exudates. This type of inflammation can increase adhesion and scar tissue in the area.

Yellow-white fluid in an infected inflamed area is called *pus* or *purulent exudate*. Purulent exudates may collect in different ways, such as in a capsule surrounding the injury, to form an abscess. If the body's immunity level is low, the purulent exudates may spread over a large surface of tissue.

If the fluid that collects is blood-tinged, the blood vessels are injured or the tissue is crushed, resulting in hemorrhagic exudates.

---

be destroyed, especially if they are tagged with antibodies, which are proteins that mark pathogens.

- *Swelling and Pain:* Some inflammation mediators increase the permeability of blood vessel walls, allowing water to move through them. As water leaks out of the vessel, tissue swelling, or edema, results. The pressure caused by edema triggers pain receptors. The fluid that accumulates in inflamed tissue is called *inflammatory exudate* and has the beneficial effect of diluting the irritant that is causing the inflammation. Inflammatory exudates are removed slowly by lymphatic vessels (Box 2-7).

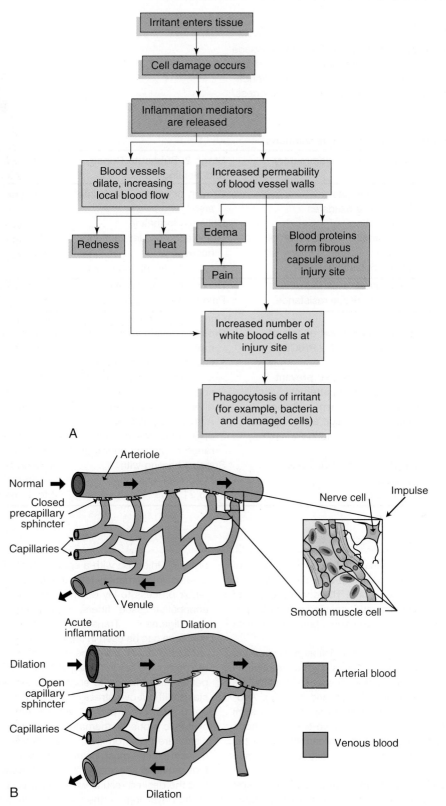

FIGURE 2-7 A, Inflammatory response. **B,** Circulatory changes in inflammation. Relaxation of the precapillary sphincter in the arterioles results in the flooding of the capillary network and dilation of capillaries and postcapillary venules. (**B,** Modified from Damjanov I: *Pathology for the health professions,* ed 3, Philadelphia, 2006, Saunders.)

Practical Application

By understanding the process of tissue healing, the massage therapist is able to support the normal progress of the inflammatory response. The following chart provides recommendations for massage intervention during the tissue healing process.

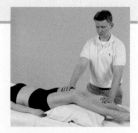

Stages of Tissue Healing and Massage Interventions

	Stage 1: Acute Inflammatory Reaction	Stage 2: Subacute Repair and Healing	Stage 3: Maturation and Remodeling
Characteristics	Vascular changes Inflammatory exudates Clot formation Phagocytosis, neutralization of irritants Early fibroblastic activity	Growth of capillary beds into area Collagen formation Granulation tissue; caution necessary Fragile, easily injured tissue	Maturation and remodeling of scar Contracture of scar tissue Collagen aligns along lines of stress forces
Clinical signs	Inflammation Pain before tissue resistance	Decreasing inflammation Pain during tissue resistance	Absence of inflammation Pain after tissue resistance
Massage intervention	Protection Control and support effects of inflammation: Use PRICE methods Promote healing and prevent compensation patterns: • Passive movement midrange • General massage and lymphatic drainage with caution Support rest with full-body massage 3 to 7 days	Controlled motion Promote development of mobile scar: • Cautious and controlled soft-tissue mobilization of scar tissue along fiber direction toward injury • Active and passive, open- and closed-chain range of motion, midrange Support healing with full-body massage 14 to 21 days	Return to function Increase strength and alignment of scar tissue: • Cross-fiber friction of scar tissue coupled with directional stroking along the lines of tension away from injury • Progressive stretching and active and resisted range of motion; full range Support rehabilitation activities with full-body massage 3 to 12 months

Practical Application

Sometimes creating controlled inflammation over an area of chronic soft-tissue inflammation can jump-start the body into a resolution process and support healing. The controlled use of inflammation can stimulate healing and, coupled with appropriate rehabilitation, is an effective approach when dealing with these situations.

Some soft-tissue methods can be used deliberately to create mild and controlled inflammation. Methods such as transverse friction create a localized inflammatory response to stimulate tissue reorganization in areas of adhesion and scarring. Acupuncture and moxibustion (a type of heat application to skin) cause mild inflammation. Certain connective-tissue methods and stretching methods can pull apart microadhesions in the soft tissue, resulting in inflammation that signals the tissue repair process.

Controlled therapeutic inflammation is also used to stabilize ligaments that are lax because of overstretching, degeneration,

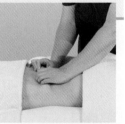

or injury. Injection with a solution that creates inflammation tells the tissue repair process to lay down additional connective-tissue fibers, reinforcing the ligament. Transverse friction massage can be used in areas that are accessed easily from the surface of the body. The key in these methods is to use just enough therapeutic inflammation to encourage the body to restore homeostasis without overstressing the system. These methods should not be used in a person with systemic inflammation, such as systemic lupus erythematosus, or when tissue repair mechanisms are compromised, as in fibromyalgia. Proper training in these methods must include a clear understanding of anatomy that provides specificity, the exact application of technique so that the desired results will be obtained, and an understanding of the physiology of the inflammation and healing processes.

Bacteria and damaged cells are held in the lymph nodes and destroyed by white blood cells. This causes the lymph nodes to enlarge when they process a large amount of infectious material.

The normal inflammatory response is the process that heals the body. The goal is to promote regeneration, which is replacement of dead cells with living functional cells, and keep replacement of functional tissue with scar tissue to a minimum (Boxes 2-8, 2-9, and Figures 2-8 and 2-9).

However, if the inflammation lasts too long or becomes too widespread, the result is an inflammatory disease. More information on the inflammatory response is presented in Chapter 11.

Box 2-8 Tissue Repair

The processes of inflammation eventually eliminate the irritant causing the problem. Tissue repair can then begin. Tissue repair is the replacement of dead cells with living cells.

Tissues have two cell types: Parenchymal cells perform the tissue functions, and stromal cells provide the tissue structure. In a type of tissue repair called *regeneration,* just the parenchymal cells are involved. The new cells are similar to those that they replace. Another type of tissue repair is replacement, and it involves stromal cells. The new cells are formed from connective tissue. These stromal cells are different from those they replace, and the result is a scar. Collagen is the chief constituent of scar tissue. The factors that promote collagen formation are vitamin C and adequate nutrition, in particular protein intake. Often, fibrous connective tissue replaces the damaged tissue, resulting in a condition called *fibrosis.* Most tissue repairs are a combination of regeneration and replacement.

Cells regenerate to different degrees and at different rates. *Labile cells* regenerate easily and quickly; these include the cells of the lymphatic system, epidermis, bone marrow, and gastrointestinal tract. *Stable cells,* the most common cell type, regenerate at slower rates; these include the cells of the parenchymal, or epithelial, portion of an organ or gland and the connective tissue, or stroma. For example, intestinal cells regenerate in 1 to 2 days, liver cells in 3 to 5 days, and kidney cells in 7 to 14 days.

Total tissue repair can take 4 weeks or longer. Permanent cells, such as nerve and muscle cells, do not regenerate well, if at all, and when they do regenerate, the process is slow, taking months. Bone regenerates extremely well. Massage practitioners should wait at least 30 to 45 days before working aggressively on an area of tissue repair so as not to disturb the repair formation. Moderate mobilization of the healing tissue supports tissue repair.

Box 2-9 Inflammatory Disease

Local inflammation occurs in a small area. If the irritant spreads throughout the body or causes changes in other areas, the inflammation is said to be *systemic.* When inflammation becomes chronic and stays active for a longer period than benefits the body or is more intense than seems necessary, it may be called an *inflammatory disease.* Systemic inflammations that may become diseases include arthritis, asthma, eczema, and bronchitis.

Chronic Inflammation

Chronic inflammation persists from 6 weeks to years. Medically, inflammation is considered chronic if the area is infiltrated by white blood cells, if growth of new capillaries occurs, and if fibroblasts are in the area. Chronic inflammation is implicated in many disease processes, from arthritis to autoimmune disease. Chronic inflammation may cause development of fibrosis. The fibroblasts produce collagen and fibrous tissue, causing fibrosis and resulting in scar tissue and adhesion

formation. Chronic inflammation may also cause a *sinus* or a *fistula.* A **sinus** is a tract leading from a cavity to the surface. A **fistula** is a tract that is open at both ends and allows an abnormal connection between two surfaces. For example, fistulae may form between the bladder and the vagina.

Chronic inflammation may lead to ulcer formation when the surface covering of an organ or tissue is lost because of cell death and is replaced by inflammatory tissue. The most common locations of ulcers are the stomach, intestines, and skin.

Treatments

Antiinflammatory and steroid medications are used to treat inflammation. Antihistamines and aspirin can be used to suppress inflammatory responses. Ice and other forms of cold hydrotherapy may also be beneficial if the inflammation is localized, such as with a shoulder bursitis or ankle sprain.

PAIN

SECTION OBJECTIVES

Chapter objectives covered in this section:
  9. Define pain, and list the types of pain
  10. Describe methods used for pain management.
After completing this section, the student will be able to perform the following:
• Describe pain sensations.
• Describe the difference between hurt and harm.
• Define acute and chronic pain.
• Describe five common pain sensations.
• Discuss the pain-spasm-pain cycle.
• Define somatic and visceral pain.
• Identify viscerally referred pain patterns.
• Define referred pain.
• Define phantom pain.
• List factors that influence pain threshold and tolerance.
• Recommend or teach various pain management strategies.

Pain is a complex, private, abstract experience that is difficult to explain or describe. Pain is the number-one symptom or complaint that causes people to seek health care. Its effective management is a major challenge. Defining pain in descriptive and measurable terms is not easy because pain has physiologic, psychological, and social aspects.

Pain Sensations

We need the sensations we get from pain to keep us safe. These sensations give us enough information about potential tissue damage to help us protect ourselves from greater damage. Pain often initiates a person's search for medical assistance. The subjective description and indication of the location of the pain help pinpoint the underlying cause of disease.

The receptors for pain, called *nociceptors,* are simply the branching ends of the dendrites of certain sensory neurons. Neurons are nerve cells, and dendrites are branches from the

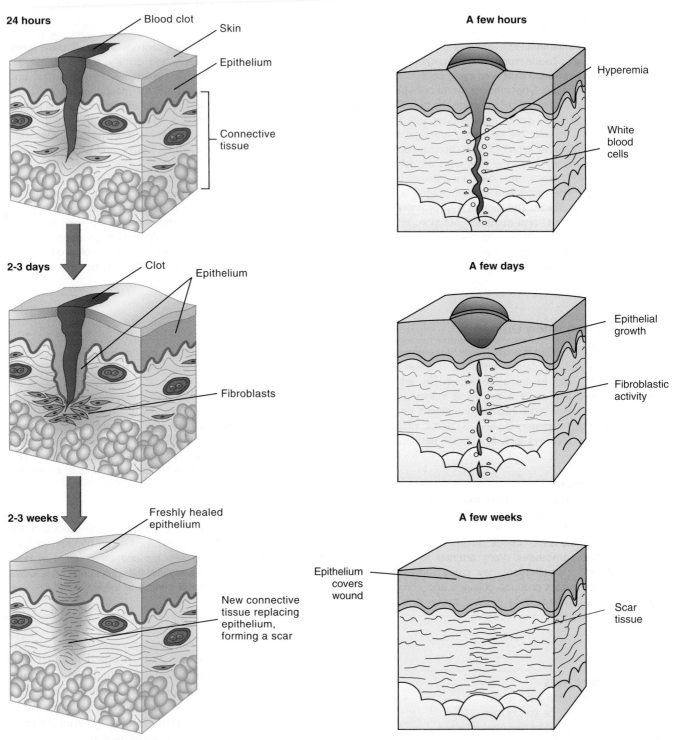

FIGURE 2-8 Skin wound healing. Healing of skin wounds reflects mechanisms of healing in general. This figure illustrates healing of superficial wounds by primary intention and deeper wounds by second intention. Wound healing is accelerated by bringing the edges of the wound together through the use of bandaging and sutures. If this were a muscle injury (strain), muscle spasming around the site of the injury would bring the ends closer together to encourage healing. (Modified from Thibodeau GA, Patton KT: *Anatomy and physiology,* ed 6, St Louis, 2007, Mosby.)

neuron cell body. Pain receptors are found in practically every tissue of the body, and they may respond to any type of stimulus. When stimuli for other sensations, such as touch, pressure, heat, and cold, reach a certain intensity, they too may cause the sensation of pain. Stimulation of pain receptors also occurs during distention or dilation of a structure, prolonged muscular contractions, muscle spasms, inadequate

blood flow to an organ, and the presence of certain chemical substances.

Injured tissue releases bradykinin, which causes the release of inflammation-producing chemicals such as histamine and prostaglandins. Inflammatory mediators make nociceptors more sensitive to the normal pain response. This increased sensitivity to pain is called *hyperalgesia.*

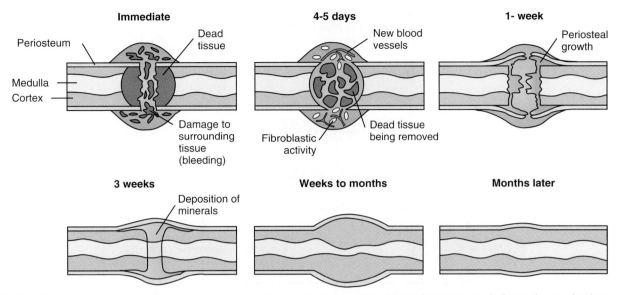

FIGURE 2-9 Bone fracture healing. The basic mechanisms involved in the healing of bone fractures are similar to the mechanisms involved in the healing of skin or other tissue. Adequate blood supply, nutrition, and rest are necessary for appropriate healing. A deficiency in protein, essential fatty acids, vitamin C, or zinc delay healing. The acute inflammatory process also supports healing; therefore the use of antiinflammatory medicine in the first week after the injury can slow down the healing process.

| Box 2-10 | Hurt and Harm: What Does the Pain Mean? |

To understand the meaning of pain, we need to understand the two meanings of pain. Pain hurts. Pain should occur when the body is harmed. Harm means that there is danger and potential damage.

Most acute pain indicates harm. This can be a bad thing or a good thing. Breaking a bone is usually a bad thing, and the pain indicates harm. The pain that occurs from the surgery to fix the broken bone does occur because of tissue damage, but the result is ultimately a good thing.

Chronic pain hurts but is not productive. Chronic pain accomplishes nothing that is beneficial. It does not warn us of danger or tissue damage. Chronic pain is not fatal, but the sensation of pain is confusing, making individuals think something is very wrong. Chronic nonproductive pain can make an affected person miserable.

Pain receptors, because of their sensitivity to all stimuli, perform a protective function by identifying changes that may endanger the body. Pain receptors adapt only slightly or not at all. Adaptation is the decrease or disappearance of the perception of a sensation, even though the stimulus is still present. An example is getting used to our clothes soon after dressing. If adaptation to pain occurs, the stimuli cease to be sensed and irreparable damage can result.

Sensory impulses travel along nerves to the spinal cord and brain. Recognition of the kind and intensity of most pain occurs in the cerebral cortex (the decision-making part of the brain). Some awareness of pain also occurs at subcortical levels (under the cortex, the instinctual part of the brain). The experience of pain is both conscious and subconscious, allowing us to decide what the pain means (Box 2-10).

The subconscious part of the brain experiences pain and interprets it as harm whether or not actual damage is occurring. The problem is that pain is often more about hurt than actual harm. The conscious part of the brain can identify what is causing the pain and coordinate the changes necessary to alleviate the harm or understand the hurt. Sometimes we hurt (i.e., after surgery or because of an old injury), but we are not in any danger (harm). If we experience chronic pain, such as back pain (hurt), we must come to grips with the realization that the pain is not productive and does not harm us, even if it does hurt. Conscious understanding of the pain experience allows us to get on with living in spite of the pain.

Acute Pain

Acute pain is a symptom of a disease condition or a temporary aspect of medical treatment. Acute pain acts as a warning signal because it can activate the sympathetic (fight-or-flight response) nervous system. Acute pain is usually temporary, of sudden onset, and easily localized. We can describe the pain, which often subsides with or without treatment.

Chronic Pain

Chronic pain is not only a symptom of a disease condition; it is identified as a major health problem. Approximately 25% of the population is affected. **Chronic pain** is a symptom that persists or recurs for indefinite periods, usually for longer than 6 months. Chronic pain frequently has an obscure onset, and the character and quality of the pain change over time. The pain usually is diffuse and poorly localized and often requires the efforts of a multidisciplinary health care team for its effective management.

The term *intractable pain* means that chronic pain persists even when treatment is provided or when chronic pain exists without active disease. This is the greatest challenge for all health care providers. Temporary symptomatic relief from this type of pain may be provided by soft-tissue approaches.

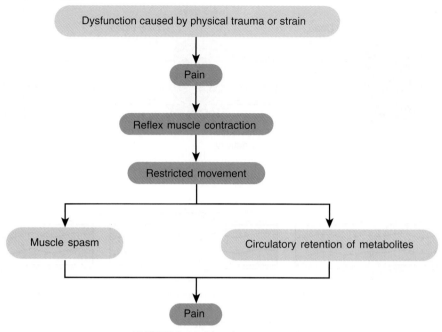

FIGURE 2-10 Muscle spasm cycle.

Specific Types of Pain

- *Pricking or Bright Pain:* This type of pain exists when the skin is cut or jabbed with a sharp object. The pain is short-lived but intense and easily localized and is sometimes termed *superficial somatic pain.*
- *Burning Pain:* This type of pain is slower to develop, lasts longer, and is localized less accurately (e.g., when the skin is burned). This type of pain often stimulates cardiac and respiratory activity.
- *Aching Pain:* Aching pain occurs when the visceral organs are stimulated. The pain is constant, is not well localized, and commonly is referred to areas of the body distant from where the damage may be occurring. Aching pain is important because it may be a sign of a life-threatening disorder in a vital organ.
- *Deep Pain:* The main difference between superficial and deep pain is the nature of the pain evoked by noxious stimuli. Unlike superficial pain, deep pain is poorly localized, is nauseating, and is commonly associated with sweating and changes in blood pressure. Deep pain initiates the reflex contraction of nearby skeletal muscles. This reflex contraction is similar to the muscle spasm associated with injuries to bones, tendons, and joints. The steadily contracting muscles become ischemic (lacking in oxygen), and ischemia stimulates the pain receptors in the muscles. The pain, in turn, initiates more spasms, setting up a vicious circle. Recall the pain-spasm-pain cycle in the discussion about positive feedback loops (Figure 2-10).
- *Muscle Pain:* If a muscle contracts rhythmically in the presence of an adequate blood supply, pain usually does not result. However, if the blood supply to a muscle is occluded (closed off), the same rhythmic contraction soon causes pain. The pain persists even after the contraction until blood flow is reestablished. If a muscle with a normal blood supply is made to contract continuously without periods of relaxation, it begins to ache because the maintained contraction compresses the blood vessels supplying the muscle, reducing the blood supply.

Somatic and Visceral Pain

There are two other ways to look at pain: somatic and visceral. **Somatic pain** arises from the stimulation of receptors in the skin (superficial somatic pain) or from stimulation of receptors in skeletal muscles, joints, tendons, and fasciae (deep somatic pain). **Visceral pain** results from the stimulation of receptors in the viscera, which are internal organs.

Superficial somatic pain is transmitted along finely myelinated (a fatty insulation) A delta nerve fibers at a fast rate (metaphor: a highway or expressway). Deep somatic pain and most visceral pain are transmitted slowly by unmyelinated (no insulation) C nerve fibers (metaphor: a dirt road).

This difference in the transmission of pain signals explains why superficial somatic stimulation transmitted on A delta fibers can block or mask deep somatic or visceral pain. Stimulation of more A fibers than C fibers blocks the C fiber transmission from entering the spinal cord. If the signal does not enter the spinal cord, it cannot be felt as pain.

Methods of touch and pressure and most methods of movement are transmitted on A fibers; any stimulus of this type increases A-fiber transmission, blocking pain signals. Treating pain in this way is called *counterirritation* (Figure 2-11).

Referred Pain

The ability of the cerebral cortex of the brain (the thinking part of the brain) to locate the origin of pain is related to past experience. In most instances of somatic pain and in some instances of visceral pain, the brain accurately projects the pain back to the stimulated area.

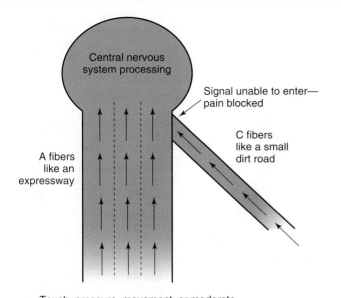

FIGURE 2-11 Gate-control theory of pain (based on Melzack and Wall's gate-control theory of pain).

The visceral pain also may be felt in a surface area far from the stimulated organ. This phenomenon is called *referred pain*. In general, the area to which the pain is referred and the visceral organ that is stimulated receive their nerves from the same section of the spinal cord. Because of this association, the brain may misinterpret the source. For example, the pain of a heart attack is typically felt in the skin over the heart and along the left arm. The same factor is at work in the referred pain in the shoulder caused by gallstones. Figure 2-12 illustrates cutaneous (skin) regions to which visceral pain may be referred. If the client has a recurring pain pattern that resembles the patterns on the chart, the client should be referred to a physician for an accurate diagnosis.

Irritation of the viscera frequently produces pain that is felt not in the viscera but in some somatic structure that may be a considerable distance from the viscera. Such pain is said to be referred to the somatic structure. Deep somatic pain also may be referred, but superficial pain is not. When visceral pain is local and referred, it sometimes seems to radiate from the local to the distant site.

Visceral pain, like deep somatic pain, initiates reflex contraction of nearby skeletal muscle. Because somatic pain is

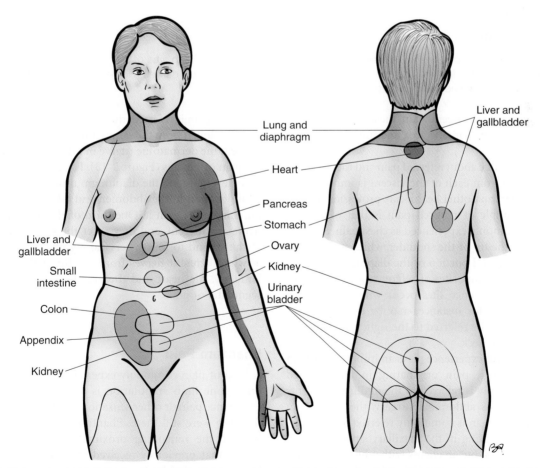

FIGURE 2-12 Referred pain. The diagram indicates cutaneous areas to which visceral pain may be referred. The professional encountering pain in these areas should refer the client for diagnosis to rule out visceral dysfunction. (From Fritz S: *Mosby's fundamentals of therapeutic massage,* ed 5, St Louis, 2013, Mosby.)

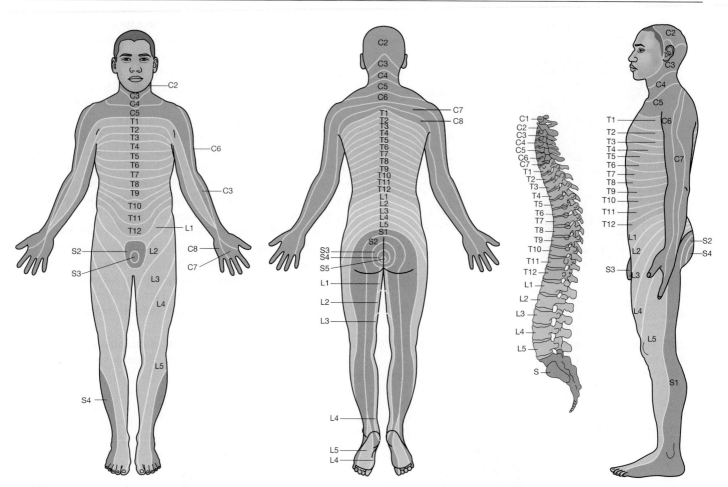

FIGURE 2-13 Dermatomal map: posterior, anterior, and lateral views. A dermatome is an area of skin in which sensory nerves derive from a single spinal nerve root. In the figure, the boundaries of dermatomes are sharply defined. However, for each individual there is an overlap of innervation between adjacent dermatomes.

much more common than visceral pain, the brain has learned to project the pain to the somatic area and initiate the reflex contraction there.

Obviously, knowledge about referred pain and the common sites of pain referral from each of the viscera is important to massage practitioners and other health care professionals. The most common example of referred pain is that of a heart attack, which is commonly experienced as chest pain. Another example is pain in the tip of the shoulder, which may be due to irritation in the central portion of the diaphragm.

However, remember that sites of reference are not stereotyped, and unusual reference sites occur with considerable frequency. Heart pain, for instance, may be experienced as purely abdominal, may be referred to the right arm, and may even be referred to the neck.

As previously noted, experience plays an important role in referred pain. Although pain originating in an inflamed abdominal organ usually is referred to the midline, in clients who have had previous abdominal surgery, the pain of an inflamed abdominal organ is commonly referred to their surgical scars. Pain originating in the maxillary sinus usually is referred to nearby teeth, but in clients with a history of traumatic dental work, such pain is regularly referred to the previously traumatized teeth. This is true even if the teeth are distant from the sinus.

When pain is referred, the reference is usually to a structure that developed from the same embryonic segment or is located in the same dermatome (nerve map) as the structure in which the pain originates (Figure 2-13). For example, during embryonic development, the diaphragm moves from the neck to its adult location in the abdomen and takes its nerve supply, the phrenic nerve, with it. One third of the fibers in the phrenic nerve are afferent, and they enter the spinal cord at the level of the second to fourth cervical segments, the same location at which afferent nerves from the tip of the shoulder enter. Similarly, the heart and the arm have the same embryonic segmental origin.

Phantom Pain

A kind of pain commonly experienced by persons who have undergone limb amputation is called **phantom pain.** They experience pain or other sensations in the extremity as though the limb were still there. Phantom pain is believed to occur because the remaining proximal portions of the sensory nerves that previously received impulses from the limb are being stimulated by the trauma of the amputation. Stimuli from these nerves are interpreted by the brain as coming from the nonexistent (phantom) limb. New research about phantom pain indicates connection to established patterns in the brain as a cause.

Pain Threshold and Tolerance

Pain may be brought on by mechanical, electrical, thermal, or chemical stimuli. We do not appear to adapt to pain or accommodate it. We all have about the same threshold for pain.

A pain threshold occurs when stimulation becomes intense enough to initiate the firing of pain receptors.

Pain tolerance is the response to pain. It varies considerably and is influenced greatly by cultural and psychological factors. Pain tolerance is modified by age and emotional and mental states.

Subjective measurements of pain intensity are more reliable than observable measurements. Only the person in pain can determine the severity being experienced. Pain is rarely the same at all times. Pain is perceived differently over time, and it differs with various precipitating and aggravating factors.

The cause, the severity, and the type of pain must be identified if it is to be treated optimally. Assessing the severity and degree of pain is difficult because pain cannot be measured objectively; a thorough history has to be obtained and a systematic physical assessment carried out. The following questions might be asked:

- Is the pain acute or chronic?
- What is the location of the pain?
- What is the quality of pain (e.g., sharp, burning, pricking)?
- How intense is the pain?
- When does the pain occur (i.e., what is the timing?)?
- What factors affect the intensity of the pain? (Activity 2-5).

✍ ACTIVITY 2-5

List three personal factors that could change your pain tolerance.

Examples

Things that could increase pain tolerance:
1. Reading a good book
2. Going for a walk
3. Practicing relaxation techniques

Things that could decrease pain tolerance:
1. Being tired and upset with the kids
2. Driving in heavy traffic
3. Loud music

Your Turn

Things that could increase my pain tolerance:
1.
2.
3.

Things that could decrease my pain tolerance:
1.
2.
3.

Pain Management

Acute pain usually is caused by tissue injury. Inflammation is commonly present. In many instances the PRICE type of treatment is used, especially if the injury is minor. PRICE stands for *p*rotection, *r*est, *i*ce, *c*ompression, and *e*levation. Short-term use of an analgesic medication, which changes pain perception, is effective (Box 2-11).

Management of chronic pain is more difficult. Some options work for certain individuals and not for others. The following pain management strategies can be used alone or in combination for both acute and chronic pain.

Transcutaneous Electric Nerve Stimulation

Electrodes attached to a small portable unit are used to stimulate the skin surface over the area of pain. Transcutaneous electric nerve stimulation stimulates large A delta fibers in the skin and, according to the gate-control theory, the fibers inhibit pain-conducting fibers in the spinal cord. Research has shown that low-voltage doses of electricity increase the levels of endogenous (made in the body) opioids, such as endorphins, enkephalins, and dynorphins, in the body.

Acupuncture

Acupuncture is performed by inserting thin needles into the skin along acupuncture meridians. One of the ways acupuncture works is that it releases endogenous opioids.

Acupressure

Acupressure stimulates acupuncture points without using needles. Pressure is applied to the points with the thumb, a finger, or a blunt instrument. The physiologic explanations are the same as for acupuncture.

Placebo Response

The placebo response involves the use of any treatment process that produces a positive response. Because of a person's belief that the treatment will be effective, rather than because of the pain-killing properties of the method, 20% to 40% of persons in whom pain has been induced by stimuli have reported pain relief with the use of placebos.

Distraction and Imagery

Distraction is focusing the attention on stimuli other than pain. Imagery consists of using the imagination to create or remember a mental picture that is relaxing and relieves pain.

Box 2-11   PRICE

Protection prevents further injury
Rest speeds up healing
Ice numbs pain receptors, constricts blood vessels, and reduces swelling (edema)
Compression reduces bleeding, if any, and edema
Elevation allows gravity to help with lymphatic drainage and reduces edema

Biofeedback

Biofeedback is a technique in which a person is made aware of body functions by means of external measuring equipment, such as a computer-generated image of blood pressure. It allows control of the function at the conscious level. Likewise, nerve fibers in the cerebral cortex that can inhibit the impulses ascending in the pain pathways can be controlled to produce pain relief. This kind of treatment is especially useful in treating migraines, tension headaches, and other forms of pain in which muscle tension is involved.

Aromatherapy

Essential oils are lipid extracts from various parts of plants. They can penetrate the skin quickly or be inhaled to stimulate the olfactory nerve. *Olfaction* refers to sense of smell. The olfactory nerve links parts of the brain that involve emotions and endocrine function. Therefore aromas can have profound effects on the mind and emotions. Essential oils can be used as compresses, for inhalation, in baths, and with massage oils.

Music Therapy

Music has been used to reduce pain. The pain relief may result from a reduction in anxiety, the inhibition of pain pathways, distraction, or an increase in endorphins that is produced by the music. However, music therapy can also aggravate pain, so preferences in music must be considered before using music during massage.

Hypnosis

Hypnotic techniques alter the focus of attention and enhance imagery by using suggestions. Individuals vary widely in their abilities to be hypnotized.

Heat

Heat can be used to reduce pain. Heat dilates local blood vessels and increases the blood flow. The increase in blood flow can reduce pain by washing away pain-producing chemicals. Temperature receptors are stimulated by heat, and the impulses are carried by large myelinated nerve fibers that may inhibit the pain fibers. Heat softens collagen fibers, making them more pliable, which allows joints, tendons, and ligaments to be stretched farther before the pain receptors are stimulated.

Cold

Cold relieves pain by decreasing swelling through vasoconstriction, by decreasing stimulation of pain nerve endings, and by stimulating the release of endogenous opioids.

Massage

Massage can have an analgesic effect. Various methods help speed up the drainage of pain-producing substances from the area. Release of histamine and direct stimulation cause local blood vessels to dilate and wash away toxins, remove edema, and bring oxygen to the area. Massage can reduce muscle spasm, improve blood flow, and remove pressure on pain receptors. The touch and pressure sensations carried by large myelinated fibers can inhibit pain fibers. Massage also is used as distraction. The relaxing music that is often used also helps. Special techniques that help reduce adhesions can free nerves that may be producing the pain.

Other Forms of Therapy

Art, prayer, meditation, and laughter are other forms of therapy that are being used effectively for pain management.

Medical Treatment

Pain-killing medications are called *analgesics*. Oral analgesics such as aspirin reduce inflammation and inhibit transmission of pain impulses. They are nonaddictive. Narcotic analgesics such as morphine are addictive, and tolerance may develop. Narcotics (opioids) are used in individuals in whom relief cannot be obtained by other means, especially those suffering from cancer pain and those whose life expectancy is limited.

Surgical techniques are used to remove the cause or block the transmission of pain. Because damage to nerve cell bodies produces irreversible changes, surgery is used as a last resort.

To have sufficient information for dealing with clients in pain, it is helpful to have a pathology text and a reference text of pharmaceuticals. Texts written for nurses are likely to provide the most useful information on these subjects. Suggestions are included in the Works Consulted list at the back of this book.

Practical Application

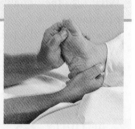

Pain is a complex problem with physical, psychological, social, and financial components. The vast differences in the experience of pain by human beings suggest that natural neural mechanisms must exist to modulate pain transmission and perception. Beta-endorphins, enkephalins, and endorphins are natural opiates. They are released when the body is in pain, and they reduce the perception of pain. Stimulus-induced forms of analgesia, such as acupuncture, massage, other forms of bodywork, hydrotherapy, and exercise, are believed to tap into these natural opiate pathways. The counterirritations produced by touch and movement therapies are effective in pain management because they trigger the release of endorphins and enkephalins. The massage professional, as part of a health care team, can contribute valuable manual therapy for various painful conditions by means of direct tissue manipulation and reflex stimulation of the nervous system and the circulation. Touch and movement, when used as therapeutic interventions, may help reduce the need for pain medication, thus minimizing its side effects. When a client is in intense pain, the massage therapy must be monitored by a physician or other appropriate health care professional.

Most persons experience less extreme pain occasionally throughout their lives. Massage approaches may provide temporary symptomatic relief of moderate pain brought on by daily stress, thus reducing or eliminating the use of over-the-counter pain medications. However, if any pain persists, the client should be referred to a physician.

MECHANISMS OF HEALTH: STRESS

SECTION OBJECTIVES

Chapter objectives covered in this section:

11. Define stress and the factors contributing to the stress response.
12. Describe ways to manage stress.

After completing this section, the student will be able to perform the following:

- Define health.
- Define stress.
- Identify factors contributing to the stress response.
- Describe effects of excessive stress.
- Explain how humans adapt to stress.
- Manage stress.

A state of good health is supported by a balanced lifestyle. On the continuum of imbalance, disease reflects a state of "too much" or "not enough." Health is that state of "just right," or homeostasis.

Health is influenced by many factors, including inherited and constitutional conditions. Lifestyle, activity level, rest, loving relationships, exercise, diet, empowering beliefs and attitudes, self-esteem, authentic personality, and freedom from self-hindering patterns all support health. Individuals need to understand their own bodies, minds, and spiritual selves as they seek balance. It is this that allows the body to maintain a dynamic state of homeostasis (Activity 2-6).

Stress and Stress Management

Maintaining and supporting good health requires effective management of stress and stressors. A stressor is not always a negative event. A wedding and a funeral may be equally stressful.

Both exposure to intense or extreme stressors (too much) and deprivation of necessary stimuli (too little) can cause imbalance and thus many problems. Too much heat, cold,

✎ ACTIVITY 2-6

This activity affords you an extensive look at your health profile. Complete the following statements by providing three different responses to each statement.

Example

My lifestyle supports health in the following ways:
1. I am involved in work that I love.
2. I am surrounded by information.
3. I am financially stable.

My lifestyle does not support health in the following ways:
1. I work too many hours.
2. I am overwhelmed by too much to know and understand.
3. I have a lot of debt.

Your Turn

My lifestyle supports health in the following ways:
1. _____
2. _____
3. _____

My lifestyle does not support health in the following ways:
1. _____
2. _____
3. _____

My activity level supports health in the following ways:
1. _____
2. _____
3. _____

My activity level does not support health in the following ways:
1. _____
2. _____
3. _____

My rest pattern supports health in the following ways:
1. _____
2. _____
3. _____

My rest pattern does not support health in the following ways:
1. _____
2. _____
3. _____

My relationships support health in the following ways:
1. _____
2. _____
3. _____

My relationships do not support health in the following ways:
1. _____
2. _____
3. _____

My aerobic exercise supports health in the following ways:
1. _____
2. _____
3. _____

My aerobic exercise does not support health in the following ways:
1. _____
2. _____
3. _____

My diet supports health in the following ways:
1. _____
2. _____
3. _____

My diet does not support health in the following ways:
1. _____
2. _____
3. _____

My beliefs and attitudes support health in the following ways:
1. _____
2. _____
3. _____

My beliefs and attitudes do not support health in the following ways:
1. _____
2. _____
3. _____

Continued

✎ ACTIVITY 2-6—cont'd

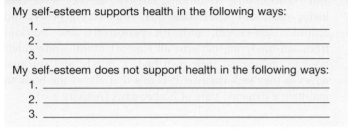

My self-esteem supports health in the following ways:

1. _____
2. _____
3. _____

My self-esteem does not support health in the following ways:

1. _____
2. _____
3. _____

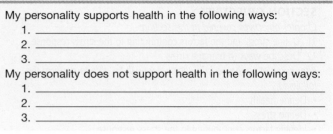

My personality supports health in the following ways:

1. _____
2. _____
3. _____

My personality does not support health in the following ways:

1. _____
2. _____
3. _____

✎ ACTIVITY 2-7

In Figure 2-14, *A*, fill in the boxes with those stressors that you can manage. In *B*, again fill in the stressors from *A*, and add some additional stressors. In *C*, fill in the stressors you listed in *B* and add two more that would make the load too heavy. In *D*, identify the stressors that you can manage yourself. Write those in the boxes carried by the figure representing you. Identify two stressors that can be eliminated by putting them in the trash basket. Then identify two stressors that you can have someone help you with, and write them in the boxes carried by the figure representing social support.

noise, activity, exercise, food, or social demands or not enough food, touch, social interaction, or sleep can be detrimental to health. Detrimental effects of stress occur because of our continuing need to respond or change our bodies to maintain homeostasis (Figure 2-14 and Activity 2-7).

What Is Stress?

Hans Selye called the response of the body to stress "the general adaptation syndrome." General adaptation is a uniform and consistent general response to perceived stimuli. Selye suggested that it be divided into three stages (Selye, 1978) (Box 2-12 and Figure 2-15).

- The first stage is the alarm reaction, also called the *fight-or-flight response,* which is the initial reaction of the body to the perceived stressor.
- The second stage is known as the *resistance reaction;* the secretion of regulating hormones (cortisol) allows the body to continue fighting a stressor long after the effects of the alarm reaction have dissipated.
- The third stage is the *exhaustion reaction;* it takes place if the stress response continues without relief.

The autonomic nervous system (see Chapter 5) is responsible for monitoring, regulating, and coordinating almost all systems of the body—temperature, pH, oxygen levels, volume of blood, blood pressure, intake of food, digestion and absorption of food and water, and excretion of waste products. The response of the autonomic nervous system to a stressor is, in short, the fight-or-flight response. It is triggered by an increase in the activity of the sympathetic nervous system. Some of the manifestations of arousal of the sympathetic nervous system are dilation of the pupils, increased heart rate and blood pressure, increased respiratory rate, dry mouth, and sweating

hands. Gastrointestinal tract activity is diminished. One of the manifestations of stress is the tensing of muscles, particularly in the neck, shoulders, and torso. Prolonged tension causes responses such as stiffness of the neck, backache, headache, and clenching of the teeth. Also, stress inhibits the production of thyroid, reproductive, and growth hormones so as to conserve energy. Therapeutic massage is particularly helpful in managing this aspect of stress.

Perception of Stress

An individual's perception of stress is significant. Anything that is perceived as a threat, whether real or imagined, arouses fear or anxiety. How a person responds is influenced by other conditions, some of which are under conscious control and some of which are not. Physical and mental health; hereditary predisposition and genetics; past experiences; current coping habits, learned and inborn; diet; environment; and social support all determine which stimuli are interpreted as stressors. Most stress management methods support the functions of the parasympathetic autonomic nervous system (rest and restore).

Persons who experience excessive or ongoing stress often say they feel overwhelmed by tension, anger, fear, and frustration and the resulting anxiety. This causes adrenaline levels to rise, blood pressure and heart rate to increase, and breathing to change. Stressed individuals often experience one or more of the following:

- Overbreathing often results in overoxygenation of the blood, which reduces carbon dioxide levels and leads to breathing-pattern disorders. This is discussed in more detail in Chapter 12. This response can mark the beginning of panic attacks.
- Sleep disorders and depression commonly accompany long-term stress. A decrease in memory and the ability to concentrate and solve problems are also common, as are complaints of stomach pain, heart palpitation, fatigue, and muscle aches. Blood levels of glucose and fatty acids rise, and the combination eventually causes plaque to be laid down in the arteries, which causes the development of coronary artery disease. Immune function becomes less effective, and the body is less capable of dealing with pathogens and cancer cells. Susceptibility to infection increases. Water retention caused by certain hormones increases blood volume, which can cause high blood pressure.
- Mood and behavior are affected by stress as well. There is an ongoing interplay between physiologic and psychological stress that is best described by the chicken-and-egg question,

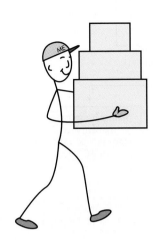
Homeostasis—ability to adapt—but at limit

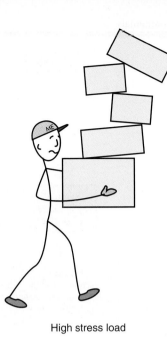
High stress load

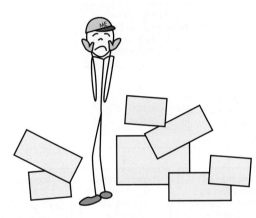
Falling apart—too much to carry and manage

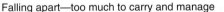
Stress coping. Reduce the load—eliminate
some stressors and add social support

FIGURE 2-14 Stress load. It is not always the type of stress that causes problems, although some types of stress are more demanding than others. It is more the amount of the stress load and the need to balance many different things that cause breakdown. Many stressors cannot be easily altered, but the stress load can be managed through physical mechanisms such as exercise, diet, and relaxation methods that allow the body to better cope with those things that cannot be changed. The stress load can be lightened by eliminating those stressors that are possible to eliminate and asking for help from social support such as family, friends, and co-workers.

Box 2-12 Hans Selye and Stress Research

Hans Selye's groundbreaking research on stress began in 1935 and was formalized in his book *The Stress of Life,* published in 1956. Selye's research laid the foundation for current concepts about stress (Selye, 1978).

Many hormones regulated by the hypothalamus come into play during stress. The hypothalamus has connections with the cortex and limbic system and controls the pituitary gland. The pituitary gland regulates the secretion of hormones by the thyroid gland, adrenal cortex, ovaries, and testes. Thus stress easily becomes an event that affects the whole body.

One of the hormones secreted by the adrenal cortex is cortisol. Cortisol maintains blood glucose levels, facilitates fat metabolism, and affects protein and collagen synthesis. Increased cortisol secretion in stressful situations reduces the immune reaction, and the antiinflammatory effect of cortisol can slow healing as well. In generalized stress conditions, the hypothalamus acts on the anterior pituitary gland to cause the release of adrenocorticotropic hormone, which in turn stimulates the adrenal cortex to secrete glucocorticoid.

Glucocorticoids are a class of adrenal cortical hormones that protect the body against stress and aid in protein and carbohydrate metabolism. Cortisol is an example. Glucocorticoids also provide an antiinflammatory effect, assist in the release of amino acids from muscle, mobilize fatty acids from fat stores, increase the ability of skeletal muscles to maintain contraction and thus avoid fatigue, and increase adenosine triphosphate production.

In addition to causing glucocorticoid release, the adrenal medulla stimulates the release of epinephrine (adrenaline) and norepinephrine to help the body in its response to stress.

However, during periods of prolonged stress, continued release of these hormones may have harmful side effects, such as decreased immune response, lowered blood glucose levels, and altered protein and fat metabolism. These effects, in turn, decrease the resistance to stress. Therefore the continued release of epinephrine and norepinephrine increases the possibility of high blood pressure, decreased digestion, reduced tissue repair, and more

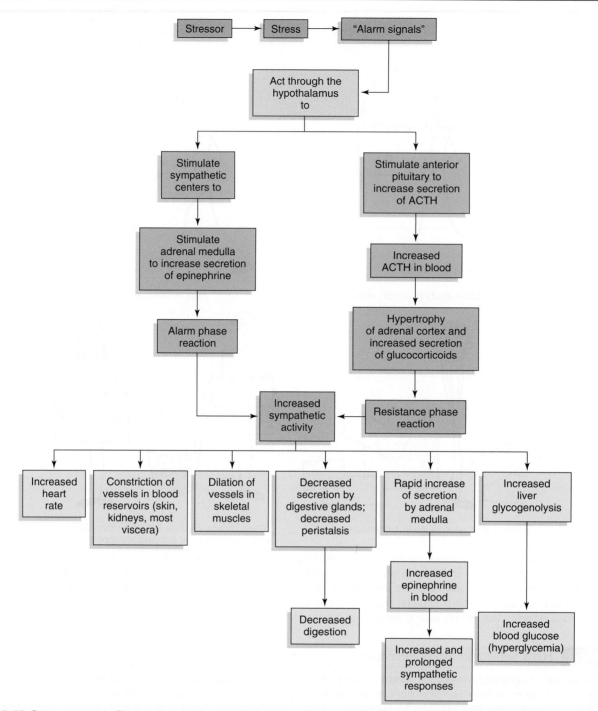

FIGURE 2-15 Stress response. The word *stress* is currently used to refer to any stimulus that directly or indirectly stimulates neurons of the hypothalamus to release corticotropin-releasing hormone. Many hormones regulated by the hypothalamus come into play during stress. The main stress response of the autonomic nervous system can be summed up as the fight-or-flight response and is brought about by an increase in the activity of the sympathetic nervous system. Some of the manifestations of sympathetic arousal are dilation of the pupils, increased heart rate and blood pressure, increased respiratory rate, dry mouth, and sweating hands. One of the manifestations of stress is the tensing of muscles, particularly in the neck, shoulders, and torso. Prolonged tension causes effects such as stiffness of the neck, backache, headache, and clenching of the teeth.

"Which came first?" Certainly, psychological stress can result in physiologic response, and the physiologic stress response alters perception, mood, thought processes, and behavior, thus creating psychological stress. Another consequence of chronic stress is stress-induced disease, although the exact cause-and-effect relationship is often unclear (Box 2-13).

Stress Management

Adaptation

One of the remarkable effects of change, internal and external, is the body's ability to adapt. The body is better able to adapt if changes occur gradually. Sudden changes, along with a

Box 2-13 ## Stress-Induced Disease

Digestive tract: Diseases that may be caused or aggravated by stress include gastritis, stomach and duodenal ulcers, ulcerative colitis, and irritable colon.

Reproductive organs: Stress-related problems include infertility or difficult conception, menstrual disorders or absence of menstrual periods in women, and impotence and premature ejaculation in men.

Bladder: A common stress response is sensitivity or irritability in the bladder, causing bladder urgency, bed-wetting, or incontinence.

Brain: Many mental and emotional problems—including anxiety, psychosis, and depression—may be triggered by stress.

Hair: Some forms of hair loss and baldness have been linked to high levels of stress.

Mouth: Sores, ulcers, and oral lichen planus (thrush) often seem to develop under stress.

Lungs: Asthma symptoms often worsen under high levels of mental or emotional stress.

Heart: Heart rate disturbances and angina attacks often occur during or after periods of stress.

Muscles: Muscle tension and its associated pain are often the result of stress, as are muscle twitches and nervous tics. The muscular tremor of Parkinson's disease is also more marked at such times.

diminished physiologic reserve, can have dramatically negative effects on the body.

Genetic makeup contributes to the effects of stress on the body. It is responsible for how well the organs adapt and respond to stressful situations. With age the ability to adapt diminishes. Individuals who are fit mentally and physically are able to adapt to stress more easily than others. Those who are strongly motivated to live are well known to be capable of surviving the worst onslaughts made on their minds and bodies. Restorative and optimal amounts of sleep are important for restoring energy, regenerating tissue, and coping with stress. Irregular cycles of sleep and wakefulness can reduce immunity and physical and psychological functioning. Proper nutrition protects us from detrimental effects of stress. Poor nutrition is itself a stress-causing agent.

Medical Assistance

More and more individuals are seeking medical assistance to help sort out and identify stress-related symptoms. Because each person responds to stress differently, accurate diagnoses become difficult. This lack of specificity has led to frustration in clients and health care providers, but as more research is done in the area of coping and adaptive capacities, the situation is continuing to improve. In contemporary health care, excessive and long-term stress is now recognized as an important and widespread cause of disease.

Psychophysiology is the study of the interplay between psychological and physiologic stressors and neuroimmunology; it is sometimes referred to as *psychoneuroimmunology,* or the study of the mind-immunity link within the larger field of the mind/body connection.

Additional Stress Management Techniques

Increased openness to, respect for, and understanding of approaches such as massage and other forms of bodywork, along with acupuncture, meditation, and relaxation methods using breathing, biofeedback, music therapy, hypnosis, exercise, and other forms of movement therapy, allow for additional ways of managing stress as well as pain.

The ancient wisdom of indigenous peoples is now being understood through investigation by Western scientific methods. For example, therapeutic massage has been shown to reduce levels of hormones associated with stress and decrease the arousal level of the sympathetic nervous system, resulting in reestablishment of homeostatic balance.

The primary reason for the stress may require a multidisciplinary approach for resolution or effective long-term management, and massage modalities can play a part.

A person's perception of stressful events combined with the amount of stress, not the type of stress, determines the response. Anything that can change the perception of threat to a perception of safety or that can reduce the intensity of the physical stress response will promote mechanisms of good health. These supportive changes include allowing for effective sleep, reducing pain, and establishing a sense of affiliation that supports effective social contact and enhancement of the restorative and self-regulating processes of the body.

The stress response and stress syndrome are discussed throughout the text as they relate to each system studied (Activity 2-8).

Practical Application

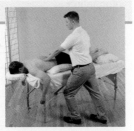

Massage therapy seems to introduce a different sort of stimulus. The body can respond to this stimulus through physiologic coping mechanisms. Because unresolved stress increases the intensity of the stress syndrome, the signals introduced by massage help reset the system. Massage methods are usually pleasurable and comforting, and they can provide a soothing rhythmic pattern with which the recipient's body can entrain.

Massage is based on the premise of providing safe touch that delivers balanced sensory stimulation, thus supporting good health for its recipients. Therefore massage can be an effective stress management tool.

THE LIFE CYCLE

SECTION OBJECTIVES

Chapter objectives covered in this section:

13. List the stages in the cycle of life.

After completing this section, the student will be able to perform the following:

- Define life.
- Define life cycle.
- List six basic phases of the life cycle.
- Define death.
- Identify periods during the life cycle when humans are most vulnerable.
- Explain the aging process.
- Identify behaviors that support longevity.

✎ ACTIVITY 2-8

List three major stressors in your life:

Example: Losing car keys

Your Turn

1. _____
2. _____
3. _____

Now complete the following for each of the listed stressors:

When (the stressor) happens, I feel (What are the physical and emotional sensations you experience?). The result is (What do you do about the feelings?). What I could do to alleviate the stress response is (Identify an activity that would restore homeostasis.).

Example

When I lose my car keys, I feel anxious and frustrated. My neck tenses up, and I start to breathe fast, which makes me feel light-headed, confused, and panicky. The result is that I begin to look frantically for my keys and start to holler at anyone around. What I could do to alleviate the stress response is use a breathing method to reestablish the oxygen/carbon dioxide balance and reverse the overbreathing.

Your Turn

Choose three different stressful situations and fill in the information.

When _____
happens, I feel _____.
The result is _____.
What I could do to alleviate the stress response is
_____.

When _____
happens, I feel _____.
The result is _____.
What I could do to alleviate the stress response is
_____.

When _____
happens, I feel _____.
The result is _____.
What I could do to alleviate the stress response is
_____.

The term *life* can be defined as the expression of the functions (see Chapter 1, "The Body as a Whole") that distinguish living organisms from inorganic matter. The term *cycle* can be defined as a complete set of regularly recurring events in the same sequence within a specified period of time.

The life cycle can be understood as the expression of functions of life that begin and end in an expected and organized pattern.

• A human being is conceived by the joining of two cells, a process that reinforces the yin/yang concept of two opposites blending to make a whole.
• Cells multiply, divide, and differentiate, forming the human being.
• Birth brings forth an independent human, which remains in a dependent functioning state while accelerated growth and development occur.
• The human matures, connects, creates, and contributes.
• The human ages, and function declines.
• The human body dies.

Death can be thought of as the separation of structure (yin) from function (yang). In its purest form, yang is totally immaterial and corresponds to pure energy. Yin in its coarsest and most dense form is totally material and corresponds to matter. Yin and yang are essentially an expression of duality in time.

Dying and gestation, death and birth are similar processes. Metaphorically speaking, birth is anabolic and death is catabolic.

During the beginning and ending of the life cycle—infancy and old age—the body is presented with its greatest challenges to homeostasis The homeostatic mechanisms in infants and children are less regular than those in adults because the young are in the process of creating their bodies. From adolescence through middle adulthood, humans have the most efficient bodily functions (Box 2-14).

The Aging Process

Normal aging affects the repair and replacement of the structural components of the body. Advancing age creates changes in cell numbers and their ability to function effectively. Changes occur in the production of hormones and in the receptors in target tissues that bind those hormones. Some hormonal levels increase, whereas others remain unchanged or decrease.

Many theories on aging exist, but the actual mechanics remain elusive to research. Three areas of research look to the physiologic mechanics of aging, which seem to be associated with the following:

• Cellular changes produced by genetic and environmental factors
• Changes in cellular regularity and central process
• Degenerative extracellular and vascular changes

Examples of decreased functional ability include muscle atrophy; loss of elasticity of the skin; and changes in the cardiovascular, respiratory, and skeletal systems. The term *atrophy* describes the wasting effects of advancing age. In addition to structural atrophy, the functioning of many physiologic control mechanisms also decreases and becomes less precise with advancing age. The aging process is cumulative, progressive, and natural.

Longevity

Any behavior that supports cellular function enhances longevity. Many who live to advanced ages have lived simple lives

Box 2-14 Different Types of Life Cycles

As in any cycle (e.g., night and day, the seasons of the year), there is a repeating pattern of events. All living things move from one life stage to the next, a pattern that is repeated, generation after generation

Biologic
The human biologic life cycle consists of six stages:
- Conception
- Birth
- Growth
- Adult
- Elderly
- Death

Conception: Combining of elements of male (sperm) and female (ovum) to create an embryo. A human begins as a single cell, the tiniest building block of life. The human cells duplicate and specialize and become the baby.

Birth: The baby moves out of the womb. The infant, weighing on average 5 to 10 pounds, takes about 40 weeks from the time that that first cell starts growing.

Infancy: Infancy takes place from birth through the first year of life. The infant is totally dependent on caregivers to remain alive.

Childhood: From 1 year to about 12 years, a human is a child. For the first 2 years after infancy, the child is called a *toddler.*

Adolescence: Humans become adolescents roughly from age 12 to 18 years. In this stage, starting with puberty, boys become men and girls become women. The adolescent is preparing for adulthood, growing to his or her maximum size, and is physically able to reproduce.

Adulthood: The end of adolescence is at 18 to 20 years, at which point adulthood begins. The life cycle usually starts over again during this stage, when, through reproduction, adults give birth to their own children.

Elderly: The time of the life cycle when the body begins to break down. By the time they reach 75 to 80 years of age, human are typically considered elderly.

Death: Death is the final stage of the life cycle. Humans die when their bodies are no longer able to carry on life functions.

Psychological Life Cycle
Psychology provides another way to look at the human life cycle. Not only do we grow through stages physically; we also grow emotionally. We can use Maslow's hierarchy of needs as a model for a psychological life cycle (see illustration).

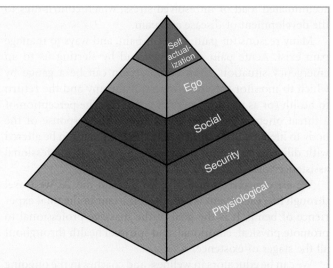

Maslow's hierarchy of needs. (Modified from Finkbeiner BL, Finkbeiner CA: *Practice management for the dental team,* ed 7, St Louis, 2011, Mosby.)

Physiologic: At this stage we are most concerned with survival.

Security: The stage of security is where we stabilize resources to ensure survival.

Social: When we are secure enough to believe we can survive, we are able to develop family and friends.

Ego: The ego stage begins as we seek status within the social structure.

Self-actualization: The stage where we are confident enough in our status, social support, security, and survival that we can begin the process of achieving our life purpose.

Chakra System
A third way to view the cycle of life is by considering the symbolic stages of life referred to in the chakra system:

Root chakra 1: Conception, survival, preservation
Water chakra 2: Gestation, specialization
Solar plexus chakra 3: Birth, willpower
Heart chakra 4: Living, compassion
Throat chakra 5: Dying, communication
Brow chakra 6: Death, transformation, self-realization
Crown chakra 7: Expansion, purpose

---

with a sense of purpose, physical work, and social support. Currently, the usual life span of human beings in Western society is between 80 and 100 years, but in societies that offer proper sanitation, nutrition, and health care, living beyond 100 years is becoming more common.

Life expectancy, or the average life span, has increased; women between the ages of 80 and 100 are the fastest growing segment of many populations. In general, women live longer than men because of the influences of genetics, hormones, immunity, and social roles.

Many scientific advances are increasing the potential for a long and physical life. It remains the responsibility of each of

us to support the potential for a fulfilling, productive, and meaningful life.

SUMMARY

In this chapter, we looked at homeostasis and factors influencing health and disease. Homeostasis consists of balancing mechanisms that are in constant communication with each other in a feedback loop system. Many factors can disrupt homeostasis, yet in most situations the body is able to respond effectively and restore efficient functioning. We are equipped with the ability to deal with many different types of stressors.

However, stress-coping mechanisms can be overloaded by an accumulated load of unresolved stress, which contributes to the development of disease and pain.

Many reasons for pain, types of pain, and ways to manage pain exist. Acute pain can be a friend by alerting us to an emergency situation. Even chronic pain can be a gauge by which to monitor the effectiveness of therapy and the return to health (or as near to health as possible). The perception of a threat often makes a big difference in the response of the body to life events. Perception is something that can be altered with diligent work and awareness coupled with professional assistance when necessary.

We are conceived and born; we live and die. As we travel through life, each event is equally important in the total experience of being. It is the goal of the massage professional to promote physical, emotional, and spiritual health throughout all the stages of existence.

We can be educators in wellness and coaches in the ongoing dynamic of homeostasis by being competent and able to recognize and support health mechanisms in ourselves and the clients we serve. We must assess for and identify disease, be able to refer clients effectively as necessary, and develop appropriate treatment plans for clients with disease processes. We must also proficiently integrate our skills with those of others in the health care community when being supervised by medical professionals. Massage can be a valuable tool in the treatment and management of many health concerns, especially those related to stress. The information in this chapter is essential for the massage professional if she or he is to be able to plan and organize an effective therapeutic massage session.

⊖volve

http://evolve.elsevier.com/Fritz/essential
2-1 Categorize the characteristics of yin and yang
2-2 Answer true/false questions about biologic rhythms and massage
2-3 Play a hangman game that texts your knowledge of pathology terms and definitions
Additional Resources:
  Scientific Animations
  Research Weblinks
Remember to study for your certification and licensure exams! Review questions for this chapter are located on Evolve.

REFERENCES

1. Selye H: *The stress of life*, ed 2, New York, 1978, McGraw-Hill.
2. Thibodeau GA, Patton KT: *Anatomy and physiology*, ed 6, St. Louis, 2007, Mosby.
3. Timmons BH: *Behavioral and physiological approaches to breathing disorders*, New York, 1994, Plenum Press.

Workbook Section

All Workbook activities can be done online as well as here in the book. Answers are located on evolve.

Short Answer

1. Define homeostasis, self-regulatory mechanisms, and body rhythms in relationship to Asian and Ayurvedic theories of health.

2. What are the differences in lifestyles that support health or predispose to disease? Discuss and contrast the mechanisms of disease and health.

Vocabulary

1. Disease

2. Pathology

3. Etiology

4. Health

5. Pharmacology

6. Signs

7. Symptoms

8. Syndrome

9. Acute

10. Chronic

11. Subacute

12. Communicable diseases

13. Pathogenesis

14. Incubation

15. Convalescence

16. Remission

17. Carcinogens

18. Oncologist

19. Tissue repair

20. Regeneration _____
_____
_____

21. Replacement _____
_____
_____

Short Answer

1. List forces that may disturb homeostasis.
_____
_____
_____

2. List the major risk factors in disease development.
_____
_____
_____

3. List the four primary signs of the inflammatory response.
_____
_____
_____

4. Define pain and list the general and specific types of pain.
_____
_____
_____

5. Identify viscerally referred pain patterns.
_____
_____
_____

6. Explain phantom pain.
_____
_____
_____

7. List the factors influencing health.
_____
_____
_____

8. Identify factors contributing to the stress response and the response of the body to stress.
_____
_____
_____

9. List the stages in the cycle of life.
_____
_____
_____

Fill in the Blank

(1) _____ is the relatively constant state maintained by the physiology of the body. (2) _____ signals move toward a particular center or point of reference, whereas (3) _____ signals move away from a particular center or point of reference.

(4) _____ are the internal, periodic timings of an organism that are generated within the body. (5) _____ is the synchronization of rhythms.

(6) _____ is the study of disease. (7) _____ disease is something present at birth, not something acquired during life, whereas (8) _____ disease is acquired naturally, not as a result of circumstance. (9) _____ is the study of all the factors involved in causing a disease. (10)_____ is a term that refers to diseases with undetermined causes.

Uncontrolled cell division is (11) _____ and can result in a (12) _____ or abnormal growth of new tissue called a tumor. A (13) _____ tumor is a contained and encapsulated neoplasm. (14) _____ is the reproduction of abnormal and undifferentiated cells that fail to mature into specialized cell types. (15) _____ is a nonencapsulated malignant cell mass that invades surrounding tissue. The cells have the devastating ability to break away from the primary tumor and form secondary cancer masses called (16) _____.

(17) _____ is a protective response of the tissues to irritation or injury. The inflammatory response has four primary signs: heat, redness, swelling, and pain.

Chronic inflammation may produce a sinus or (18) _____. A (19) _____ is a tract leading from a cavity to the surface. (20) _____ is an unpleasant complex, private, abstract experience. (21) _____ pain can be a symptom of a disease condition or a temporary aspect of medical treatment. The pain acts as a warning signal, activating the sympathetic nervous system, and is usually temporary, of sudden onset, and easily localized. (22) _____ pain persists or recurs for indefinite periods, usually for more than 6 months. The pain frequently has an obscure onset, and the character and quality of the pain change over time. The pain is usually diffuse and poorly localized.

(23) _____ pain arises from stimulation of receptors in the skin, in which case it is called (24) _____ somatic pain, or from stimulation of receptors in skeletal muscles, joints, tendons, and fasciae, in which case it is (25) _____ somatic pain. (26) _____ pain results from stimulation of receptors in the (27) _____ or internal organs. (28) _____ pain frequently is experienced by

persons who have had a limb amputated and experience pain or other sensations in the extremity as though the limb were still there. Pain may be brought on by mechanical, electrical, thermal, or chemical stimuli.

Problem Solving

Read the problem presented. There is no correct answer; rather, the exercise assists the student in developing the analytical and decision-making skills necessary in professional practice. After reading the problem thoroughly, follow the six steps below:

1. Identify the facts presented in the information.
2. Identify the possibilities presented ("what if" statements), or develop your own possibilities that relate to the facts.
3. Evaluate each possibility in terms of the logical cause and effect and pros and cons.
4. Consider the feelings of those involved.
5. Write each answer in the space provided.
6. Develop your solution by answering the question posed.

Problem

Supporting good health is a lifetime commitment. Many factors encountered in day-to-day life threaten the homeostatic mechanisms of the body. Not only do inherent genetic strengths and weaknesses predispose us to disease, but also our learned behaviors influence our perception of events and can determine whether we respond with survival fight-or-flight actions. Behavior often is determined by attempts to manage stress. Sometimes the behavior is resourceful and resolves the situation or brings the understanding that no answer to the problem exists and allows for the development of effective coping strategies. When this happens, the person feels effective, empowered, and resourceful. However, if stress is managed with unresourceful behavior, such as temper tantrums or the use of alcohol, the person feels out of control, and the people with whom the person interacts may feel uncomfortable, helpless, or afraid. In general, people seem to respond to stress management better if they understand the physical, mental, and spiritual components that contribute to good health and a disruption in health. If more education were provided on these topics, maybe we could learn to cope better with what seems to be the increasing stress load in our societies. If the body were better understood, maybe we would take better care of it. Regardless, the inability to cope effectively with stress is becoming a major health concern, the result of which is renewed interest in drugless approaches to dealing with stress and pain management. Such interest will likely create an environment in which bodywork methods are seen as important components in stress management programs.

Question

What information would you need to become an effective educator about stress management methods?
The first response is provided as a guide to get you started. Fill in at least two more statements.

Facts

1. Supporting health is a lifelong commitment.
2. _____
3. _____

Possibilities

1. We could compromise our health by responding in ways that activate the fight-or-flight response.
2. _____
3. _____

Logical Cause and Effect

1. The person may develop behaviors such as alcohol abuse.
2. _____
3. _____

Effect

1. The person may feel out of control.
2. _____
3. _____

Assess Your Competencies

Review the following Chapter 2 objectives:

1. Define *homeostasis* and *adaptive capacity*.
2. Relate the concept of homeostasis to traditional Chinese medicine and Ayurveda.
   - Define homeostasis in relation to adaptive capacity.
   - Compare Asian yin/yang theory to homeostasis.
   - Explain how the Asian five-element theory describes homeostasis.
   - Explain how the Ayurvedic theories describe homeostasis.
3. Define and relate feedback loops to homeostatic self-regulation mechanisms.
   - Explain how stress causes adaptation.
   - List the three components of a feedback loop.
   - Define the terms *afferent* and *efferent*.
   - Describe negative and positive feedback loops.
4. List and define biologic rhythms and their influence on health.
   - Define three major biologic rhythms.
   - Relate biologic rhythms to health and disease.
5. Define disease terminology.
6. Identify major risk factors for disease development.
7. List sources of disturbances in homeostasis.
8. Describe the body's response to homeostatic disturbances.
   - Define terms that relate to disease.
   - Discuss risk factors in disease development.
   - List the nine causes most likely to disturb homeostasis.
   - List the five types of pathogenic organisms and infectious agents.
   - Define two types of tumors.
   - Explain the factors known to play a role in cancer development.
   - Define the inflammatory response.

- List the four primary signs of the inflammatory response.

9. Define pain, and list the types of pain.
10. Describe methods used for pain management.
    - Describe pain sensations.
    - Describe the difference between hurt and harm.
    - Define acute and chronic pain.
    - Describe five common pain sensations.
    - Discuss the pain-spasm-pain cycle.
    - Define somatic and visceral pain.
    - Identify viscerally referred pain patterns.
    - Define referred pain.
    - Define phantom pain.
    - List factors that influence pain threshold and tolerance.
    - Recommend or teach various pain management strategies.
11. Define stress and the factors contributing to the stress response.
12. Describe ways to manage stress.
    - Define health.
    - Define stress.
    - Identify factors contributing to the stress response.
    - Describe effects of excessive stress.
    - Explain how humans adapt to stress.
    - Manage stress.
13. List the stages in the cycle of life.
    - Define life.
    - Define life cycle.
    - List six basic phases of the life cycle.
    - Define death.
    - Identify periods during the life cycle when humans are most vulnerable.
    - Explain the aging process.
    - Identify behaviors that support longevity.

Next, on a separate piece of paper or using an audio or video recorder, prepare a short narrative that reflects how you would explain this content to a client and how the information relates to how you would provide massage. See the example in Chapter 1 on p. 22. When read or listened to, the narrative should not take more than 5 to 10 minutes to complete. Simpler is better. Use examples, tell stories, and use metaphors. It is important to understand that there is no precisely correct way to complete this exercise. The intent is to help you identify how effectively you understand the content and how relevant your application is to massage therapy. An excellent learning activity is to work with other students and share your narratives. Also share these narratives with a friend or family member who is not familiar with the content. If that person can understand what has been written or recorded by you, you obviously understand it. There are many different ways to complete this learning activity. Yes, it may be confusing to do this, but that's all right. Out of confusion comes clarity. By the time you do this 12 times, once for each chapter in this book, you will be much more competent.

Further Study

Using additional resource material (see the Works Consulted list at the back of this book), locate the information presented in this text and elaborate by writing a paragraph of additional information on each of the following:

Feedback mechanism

_____

_____

_____

Tumor development and types

_____

_____

_____

Inflammatory response

_____

_____

_____

Gate-control theory of pain and Melzack and Wall

_____

_____

_____

Pain-spasm-pain cycle

_____

_____

_____

General adaptation syndrome and Hans Selye

_____

_____

_____

Breathing pattern disorder

_____

_____

_____

Life cycle

_____

_____

_____

Terminology: Scientific, Medical, Social, and Cultural Communication

CHAPTER OBJECTIVES

After completing this chapter, the student will be able to perform the following:

1. Identify the importance of terminology essential for the practice of therapeutic massage.
2. Use medical terminology to interpret the meanings of anatomic and physiologic terms.
3. Define terms used to describe regions of the body and surface anatomy.
4. Define terms used to describe the positions of the body and the parts of the body in relation to other body parts.
5. Define kinesiology, body planes, and terms of movement.
6. Describe and use quality-of-life terminology.
7. Explore terminology used in indigenous and cultural-based healing systems.
8. Use a charting method that incorporates a clinical reasoning/problem-solving model.

CHAPTER OUTLINE

LANGUAGE OF SCIENCE AND MEDICINE, 59
  Word Elements Used in Medical Terms, 59
  References, 59
  Abbreviations, 62
GENERAL STRUCTURAL PLAN OF THE BODY, 63
  The Body Map, 63
  Kinesiology, 69
QUALITY-OF-LIFE TERMINOLOGY, 76
ANCIENT HEALING PRACTICES, 76
  Points and Meridians, 85
  Jing Luo, 87
  Yin/Yang Theory, 87
  Organ Relationships, 88
CLINICAL REASONING AND CHARTING, 90
  Charting/Documentation, 91
  Database, 91
  Analyzing the Data, 91
  Treatment Planning, 91
SUMMARY, 92

KEY TERMS

Activities of daily living Normal daily living activity including self-care, such as eating, bathing, dressing, grooming, going to work, housekeeping duties, and leisure activities.

Acupuncture The practice of inserting needles at specific points on meridians, or channels, to stimulate or sedate energy flow to regulate or alter body function. A branch of Chinese medicine, acupuncture is the art and science of manipulating the flow of Qi, the basic life force; and of xue, the blood, body fluids, and nourishing essences.

Biomechanics The principles and methods of mechanics applied to the structure and function of the human body.

Charting The process of keeping a written record of a client or patient. The most effective charting methods follow clinical reasoning, which emphasizes a problem-solving approach. Many systems of charting are used, but they all have similar components based on the POMR (problem-oriented medical record) and SOAP (subjective, objective, analysis/assessment, and plan).

Combining vowel A vowel added between two roots or a root and a suffix to make pronunciation of the word easier.

Disharmony Distortions in health that result when the functions or systems are neither balanced nor working optimally. In Chinese medicine, disharmony can be created by the imbalance of the Six Pernicious Influences or the Seven Emotions.

Kinematics (kin-i-MAT-ics) A branch of mechanics that involves the aspects of time, space, and mass in a moving system.

Kinesiology (ki-nee-zee-OL-o-je) The study of movement that combines the fields of anatomy, physiology, physics, and geometry and relates them to human movement.

Kinetics (ki-NET-ics) The forces causing movement in a system.

Mechanics The branch of physics dealing with the study of forces and the motion produced by their actions.

Medical terminology Terms used to accurately describe the human body, medical treatments and conditions and processes of health care in a science-based manner.

Motion A change in position with respect to some reference frame or starting point.

Prefix A word element added to the beginning of a root to change the meaning of the word.

Qi (chee) Also spelled Chi, Qi refers to the life force.

Quality of life Individuals' perceptions of their position in life in the context of the culture and value systems in which they live and in relation to their goals, expectations, standards, and concerns.

Root A word element that contains the basic meaning of the word.

Suffix A word element added to the end of a root to change the meaning of the word.

Terminology A vocabulary used by people involved in a specialized activity or field of work. Also, the study of the meaning of words used in a language.

Word elements The parts of a word: the prefix, root, and suffix.

Yin/yang *Yin* and *yang* are terms used to describe polar relationships. *Yin/yang* refers to the dynamic balance between opposing forces and the continual process of creation and destruction. Yin/yang reflects the natural order and duality of the whole universe and everything in it, including the individual.

LEARNING HOW TO LEARN

This chapter is about learning a language. As you encounter each new word, translate it into an example you understand. For example, the definition of terminology is as follows: A vocabulary used by people involved in a specialized activity or field of work; also, the study of the meaning of words used in a language. How would you explain this definition to yourself? Maybe you would describe terminology as the words used to describe a unique language people use to understand one another at work or when talking to one another about a task. The learning happens as you try to figure out how to say the same thing differently.

Especially when learning the definition of words, you must review the material over and over again. You need to see the material at least four times—ideally at least six times. Each time you review the same information, you need to do it in a different way. Examples include flash cards, singing the terms and definitions, listening to someone else read them to you, writing the terms and definitions, listening to music while reviewing, and reading the terms and definitions out loud. There are activities in the book and on the Evolve site to help you with novel review methods.

You also need to review the material over several days, and then once every week or so to keep from forgetting. The adage "use it or lose it" is true when it comes to terminology. Remember the brain breaks. Study for about 30 minutes, and then take a short break. Mindless tasks are productive during brain breaks. Water the plants, take out the trash, or do some dishes.

We need to be able to communicate using terms that are meaningful and understandable. For example, the title of this textbook is *Mosby's Essential Sciences for Therapeutic Massage*. The words in this title have a meaning relevant to your massage therapy studies.

The word *essential* means "relevant and necessary." Something is relevant if it is pertinent, connected, and applicable to a given purpose. Our purpose is the study of therapeutic massage. *Science* refers to a system of acquiring knowledge through observation and experimentation to describe and explain natural phenomena. The word *science* comes from the Latin *scientia*, meaning knowledge. Science can be any systematic field of study or the knowledge gained from it. Knowledge is an understanding gained through experience or study through learning facts and information, resulting in the ability to do something. Because the word in the title is *sciences*, it means more than one science (Box 3-1). *Therapeutic* refers to the capability to restore and maintain health. As defined by the Massage Therapy Body of Knowledge (www.mtbok.org), massage therapy is a health care and wellness profession involving manipulation of soft tissue. The practice of massage therapy includes assessment; treatment planning; and treatment through the manipulation of soft tissue, circulatory fluids, and energy fields; this affects and benefits all the body systems for therapeutic purposes including, but not limited to, enhancing health and well-being; providing emotional and

Box 3-1   Branches of Science

Physics is the science that deals with matter and energy and their interactions. Matter makes up physical objects. It deals with the fundamental particles of which the universe is made and the interactions between those particles, the objects composed of them (e.g., nuclei, atoms, molecules), and energy.

Chemistry is the science that deals with the composition, structure, and properties of substances and with the transformations that they undergo. We learned a little bit about chemistry in Chapter 1.

Biology is the science of living organisms and vital processes. It describes the characteristics, classification, and behaviors of organisms; how species come into existence; and the interactions of species with one another and with the environment. We started learning about biology in Chapter 1, and Chapter 2 was all about biology. Much of the information in this textbook is based on biology.

Earth science or geoscience is the study of the planet Earth. Eventually we will even cover a little bit of earth sciences in this book.

physical relaxation; reducing stress; improving posture; facilitating circulation of blood, lymph, and interstitial fluids; balancing energy; remediating; relieving pain; repairing and preventing injury; and rehabilitating. Massage therapy treatment includes a hands-on component and provides information, education, and nonstrenuous activities for the purposes of self-care and health maintenance. The hands-on component of massage therapy is accomplished by use of digits, hands, forearms, elbows, knees, and feet with or without the use of emollients, liniments, heat and cold, handheld tools, or other external apparatus. It is performed in a variety of employment and practice settings.

The purpose of this textbook is to provide you with the applicable knowledge necessary to develop the capability to restore and maintain health through the manual manipulation of soft tissue, circulatory fluids, and energy fields.

Why is the importance of terminology and the study of the sciences essential for the practice of therapeutic massage? Consider the following definitions:

- A word is a speech sound or series of speech sounds that symbolizes and communicates a meaning.
- A term is a word or expression that has a precise meaning peculiar to a science, art, profession, or subject.
- Vocabulary is defined as words used by, or understood by, a particular person or group and technical terms used in a particular field, subject, science, or art.
- Communication is exchange of information.
- Terminology is a vocabulary used by people involved in a specialized activity or field of work and the study of the meaning of words used in a language.
- Terminology is also a language system of communication, with its system of words used to name things in a particular discipline.

Massage professionals work with their clients' anatomy and physiology; this is an aspect of the science of biology. We need to be able to communicate intelligently with clients, colleagues, and other health care professionals. Therefore standard terminology is a must. Without a common language, health care practitioners cannot communicate.

Massage therapists have an ethical responsibility to learn the following:

- To communicate with their clients in a common language
- To understand and communicate across disciplines with other health care professionals
- To communicate cross-culturally so as to appreciate different perspectives on health and healing

This chapter introduces you to the basic concepts necessary to do the following:

- To enable communication in standardized scientific and medical terms
- To consider a model of cross-cultural terminology
- To use a clinical reasoning approach in client care

Terminology relevant to massage is an ongoing study. Terminology is an area of study that requires memorization, which occurs only with repetition and periodic review. It is like learning a new language. To become proficient, you need to speak and use it often.

LANGUAGE OF SCIENCE AND MEDICINE

SECTION OBJECTIVES

Chapter objectives covered in this section:

1. Identify the importance of terminology essential for the practice of therapeutic massage.
2. Use medical terminology to interpret the meanings of anatomic and physiologic terms.

After completing this section, the student will be able to perform the following:

- Identify three word elements used in medical terms.
- Use a medical dictionary.
- Combine word elements into medical terms.
- Identify abbreviations used in health care and their meanings.

Medical terminology uses terms derived from Latin or Greek to accurately describe the human body, medical treatments and conditions, and processes of health care in a science-based manner.

Most scientific and medical terms are derived from fundamental elements from Latin or Greek, the commonly accepted language bases. These elements are combined to form scientific terms, which include medical terms. Once you know the meaning of the fundamental elements, a term can be interpreted easily by separating the word into its elements: prefix, root, and suffix.

Each of the following sections includes a list of some of the more common word elements. These lists are not meant to be all-encompassing, but they provide enough examples for you to gain a general understanding of most of the terms encountered by therapeutic massage professionals.

Word Elements Used in Medical Terms

Prefixes

A **prefix** is an element placed at the beginning of a word to change the meaning of the word. A prefix cannot stand alone;

Practical Application

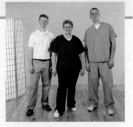

Most students are required to take tests to measure their competency in therapeutic massage. Sometimes the tests are given in school in the form of quizzes and exams. There are mandated licensing tests and voluntary certification tests indicating that you have skills that exceed the entry-level requirements of licensing. All these tests require that you be able to read and understand the questions.

Sometimes test takers become confused because they do not know the meanings of the words in the questions. This is where ongoing study of and practice using medical terminology can really help. If you know the meanings of the word elements that make up the terms, you can figure out what the word means. Even if you are not sure of the definition of the word, you may still be able to make a well-educated guess about the meaning of the question. If you spend time becoming confident with scientific terminology and the meaning of common word elements, it will help you be a more confident test taker.

it must be combined with another word element. A vowel, called a **combining vowel,** often is used to join word elements. The combining vowel most often used is *o,* but occasionally *i* or another vowel is used. Table 3-1 presents a list of the more common prefixes and some examples of accompanying combining vowels. These prefixes will help you to recognize and understand scientific and medical terminology.

Roots

The **root** (or stem) word element provides the fundamental meaning of the word. Roots are combined with prefixes and suffixes to form medical and scientific terms. In medicine the root word often refers to a part of the body. As with prefixes, a combining vowel often is added when two roots are combined or when a suffix is added to a root. The combining vowel usually is *o,* but occasionally it is *i.* Table 3-2 presents some of the more common root words and their accompanying combining vowels.

Suffixes

A **suffix** is a word element that is added to the end of a root to change the meaning of the word. Suffixes cannot stand alone. The suffix is the starting point when interpreting scientific terms. Roots that end in a consonant require a combining vowel when a suffix is added. If the root ends with a vowel and the suffix begins with a vowel, the vowel at the end of the root is deleted. Table 3-3 presents a list of some of the more common suffixes.

References

A medical dictionary is a necessity. A good dictionary holds an enormous amount of information and is the place to begin research and clarify the meanings of words and topics. When selecting a medical dictionary, you should choose one that is encyclopedic and illustrated. Consider using *Mosby's*

Table 3-1 Common Prefixes and Their Meanings

Prefix	Meaning	Prefix	Meaning	Prefix	Meaning
A-, an-	Without or not	Febr(i, o)-	Fever, boil	Onc(o)-	Tumor, mass
Ab-	Away from	Fract-	Break, broken	Ortho(o)-	Straight, erect, correct
Acr(o)-	Extremity, tip	Fund-	Base, bottom	Osm(io, o)-	Smell, odor
Ad-	Toward	Gen-	Beginning, origin, produce	Oxy-	Sharp, acute, acid
Alba-	White	Gluc-	Sweet, sugar, glucose	Palp-	Touch, feel
Ambi-	Both, on sides	Gyn(a, e, eco, o)-	Female	Pan-	All
Ana-	Upward, backward, excessive, through	Hemi-	Half	Para-	Abnormal, near
Andr(o)-	Male	Heter-	Other, different	Path(o)-	Disease, suffering
Ankyl(o)-	Crooked, fused, stiff	Hol-	Whole, all	Pept(o)-	Digestion
Ante-	Before, forward	Hom(eo, o)-	Unchanged, alike, same	Per-	By, through
Anti-	Against, opposed	Hyg(ei, ie)-	Health	Peri-	Around
Audi-	Hear	Hyper-	Excessive, too much, high	Phag(o)-	Eat, consume
Auto-	Self	Hypo-	Under, decreased, less than normal	Pharmaco-	Drugs, poison, medication
Bi-	Double, two	Iatr(o)-	Physician	Physio-	Natural, physical agents
Bio-	Life, living matter	Idio-	Distinct, peculiar to the individual	Poly-	Many, much
Brach-	Short	Immuno-	Protection	Post-	After, behind
Brady(o)-	Slow, short, dull	In-	In, into, within, not	Pre-	Before, in front of, prior to
Carcin(o)-	Cancer, malignant	Infra-	Beneath	Pro-	Before, in front of
Cata-	Down, negative, under, against, lower	Inter-	Between	Pseudo-	False
Caud-	Tail, inferior	Intra-	Within	Quadr(a, i)-	Four
Cent(i)-	Hundred	Intro-	Into, within	Re-	Again
Chron(i, o, us)-	Time, long time	Iso-	Equal, like, identical	Retro-	Backward
Circum-	Around	Juxta-	Adjoining, near to	Schist(o)-	Split, divided
Contra-	Against, opposite	Kyph(o)-	Bend, hump	Scler(o)-	Hard
Counter-	Against, opposite	Lact(o)-	Milk	Semi-	Half
Cry(mo, o)	Cold	Later(al, o)-	Side	Sepsi-	Putrid, rotten
De-	Down, from, away from, not	Leuk-	White	Son(o)-	Sound
Dext-	Right	Levo-	Left	Steno-	Contracted, narrow
Di-	Two, double, twice	Macro-	Large	Strat(i)-	Layer
Dia-	Across, through, apart	Mal-	Bad, illness, disease	Sub-	Under
Dis-	Separation, away from	Mega-	Large	Super-	Above, over, excess
Dys-	Bad, difficult, abnormal	Micro-	Small	Supra-	Above, over
Ecto-	Outer, outside	Mono-	One, single	Therm-	Warm
Endo-	Inner, inside	Multi-	Many	Tract-	Pull down
Epi-	Over, on, upon	Necr(o)-	Death, destruction, corpse	Trans-	Across
Eryth-	Red	Neo-	New	Ultr(a, o)-	Excessive, extreme, beyond
Esthesi-	Sensation	Noct(i, o)-	Night	Uni-	One
Etio-	Cause	Non-	Not	Zyg(o, us)-	Yoke, join, together
Ex-	Out, out of, from, away from	Olig-	Small, scanty		

Table 3-2 Common Root Words and Their Meanings

Root (Combining Vowel)	Meaning	Root (Combining Vowel)	Meaning	Root (Combining Vowel)	Meaning
Abdomin(o)-	Abdomen	Hemat(o)-	Blood	Psych(o)-	Mind
Aden(o)-	Gland	Hepat(o)-	Liver	Pulm(o)-	Lung
Adren(o)-	Adrenal gland	Hydr(o)-	Water	Py(o)-	Pus
Angi(o)-	Vessel	Hyster(o)-	Uterus	Rect(o)-	Rectum
Arteri(o)-	Artery	Ile(o)-, ili(o)-	Ileum	Rhin(o)-	Nose
Arthr(o)-	Joint	Laryng(o)-	Larynx	Salping(o)-	Eustachian tube, uterine tube
Bronch(o)-	Bronchus, bronchi	Mamm(o)-	Breast, mammary gland	Splen(o)-	Spleen

Table 3-2 Common Root Words and Their Meanings—cont'd

Root (Combining Vowel)	Meaning	Root (Combining Vowel)	Meaning	Root (Combining Vowel)	Meaning
Card-, cardi(o)-	Heart	Mast(o)-	Mammary gland, breast	Sten(o)-	Narrow, constriction
Cephal(o)-	Head	Men(o)-	Menstruation	Stern(o)-	Sternum
Chondr(o)-	Cartilage	My(o)-	Muscle	Stomat(o)-	Mouth
Col(o)-	Colon	Myel(o)-	Spinal cord, bone marrow	Therm(o)-	Heat
Cost(o)-	Rib	Nephr(o)-	Kidney	Thorac(o)-	Chest
Crani(o)-	Skull	Neur(o)-	Nerve	Thromb(o)-	Clot, thrombus
Cyan(o)-	Blue	Ocul(o)-	Eye	Thyr(o)-	Thyroid
Cyst(o)-	Bladder, cyst	Ophthalm(o)-	Eye	Tox(o)-	Poison
Cyt(o)-	Cell	Orth(o)-	Straight, normal, correct	Toxic(o)-	Poison, poisonous
Derma-	Skin	Oste(o)-	Bone	Trache(o)-	Trachea
Duoden(o)-	Duodenum	Ot(o)-	Ear	Ur(o)-	Urine, urinary tract, urination
Encephal(o)-	Brain	Ped(o)-	Child, foot	Urethr(o)-	Urethra
Enter(o)-	Intestines	Pharyng(o)-	Pharynx	Urin(o)-	Urine
Fibr(o)-	Fiber, fibrous	Phleb(o)-	Vein	Uter(o)-	Uterus
Gastr(o)-	Stomach	Pnea-	Breathing, respiration	Vas(o)-	Blood vessel, vas deferens
Gloss(o)-	Tongue	Pneum(o)-	Lung, air, gas	Ven(o)-	Vein
Gyn-, gyne-, gynec(o)-	Woman	Proct(o)-	Rectum	Vertebr(o)-	Spine, vertebrae
Hem-, hema-, hem(o)-	Blood				

Table 3-3 Common Suffixes and Their Meanings

Suffix	Meaning	Suffix	Meaning	Suffix	Meaning
-able	Capable of, suitable for	-graph	Diagram, recording instrument	-phylaxis	Protection
-ago	Disease	-graphy	Making a recording	-plasty	Surgical repair or reshaping
-algesia	Pain	-hood	State, quality of, condition	-plegia	Paralysis
-algia	Pain	-iasis	Condition of	-pnea	To breathe
-ase	Enzyme	-ician	One skilled in, one who practices	-porosis	Passage
-asis	State or condition of, usually abnormal	-ism	Condition	-ptosis	Falling, sagging
-cele	Hernia, herniation, pouching	-itis	Inflammation	-rrhage, -rrhagia	Excessive flow
-cide	Kill, causing death	-ity	Quality of, state of	-rrhea	Profuse flow, discharge
-cule	Very small	-ive	Having power to, that which performs	-sclerosis	Dryness, hardness
-cyte	Cell	-ize	To treat by a special method	-scoliosis	Curvature, crooked
-dom	State of being	-kinesis	Motion	-scope	Examination instrument
-duct	Tube, channel	-lemma	Sheath, covering	-scopy	Examination
-eal	Pertaining to	-logy	The study of	-sepsis	Putrefaction
-ease	Condition	-lysis	Destruction of, decomposition	-some	Body
-ectasis	Dilation, stretching	-malacia	Softening	-stasis	Maintenance, maintaining a constant level
-ectomy	Excision, removal of	-megaly	Enlargement	-stenosis	Narrow, tighten, short, constrict
-ema	Swelling, distention	-oid	Form, like, resemble	-stomy, -ostomy	Creation of an opening
-emesis*	Vomiting	-oma	Tumor	-thymia	Thymus gland, mind, soul, emotions

*One of the few suffixes that can stand alone.

Continued

Table 3-3 Common Suffixes and Their Meanings—cont'd

Suffix	Meaning	Suffix	Meaning	Suffix	Meaning
-emia	Blood condition	-opsy	View of	-tomy, -otomy	Incision, cutting into
-ferent	Bear, carry	-osis	Condition	-tonia	Stretching, putting under tension
-feron	To strike	-otomy	Cutting into	-trophic	Related to growth, development, or nutrition
-form	Shape, structure	-paresis	Paralysis	-ule	Little, small
-genesis	Development, production, creation	-pathy	Disease	-uria	Condition of the urine
-globin	Protein	-penia	Lack, deficiency	-version	To turn
-gram	Record	-phobia	An exaggerated fear	-vert	Turn

Table 3-4 Common Abbreviations and Their Meanings

Abbreviation	Meaning	Abbreviation	Meaning	Abbreviation	Meaning
ABD	Abdomen	Dx	Diagnosis	OTC	Over the counter
ADL	Activities of daily living	ext	Extract	P	Pulse
ad lib	As desired	ft	Foot (or feet)	PA	Postural analysis
alt dieb	Every other day	fx	Fracture	PM, p.m.	Afternoon
alt hor	Alternate hours	GI	Gastrointestinal	PT	Physical therapy
alt noct	Alternate nights	GU	Genitourinary	Px	Prognosis
AM, a.m.	Morning	h, hr	Hour	R	Respiration; right
a.m.a.	Against medical advice	H₂O	Water	R/O	Rule out
ANS	Autonomic nervous system	Hx	History	ROM	Range of motion
approx	Approximately	IBW	Ideal body weight	Rx	Prescription
as tol	As tolerated	ICT	Inflammation of connective tissue	SOB	Shortness of breath
BM	Bowel movement	id	The same	SP, spir	Spirit
BP	Blood pressure	L	Left, length, lumbar	Sym	Symmetric
Ca	Cancer	lig	Ligament	T	Temperature
CC	Chief complaint	M	Muscle, meter, myopia	TLC	Tender loving care
c/o	Complains of	ML	Midline	Tx	Treatment
CPR	Cardiopulmonary resuscitation	meds	Medications	URI	Upper respiratory infection
CSF	Cerebrospinal fluid	n	Normal	WD	Well developed
CVA	Cerebrovascular accident, stroke	NA	Nonapplicable	WN	Well nourished
DJD	Degenerative joint disease	OB	Obstetrics		
DM	Diabetes mellitus				

Dictionary of Medicine, Nursing, and Health Professions. The table of contents indicates how expansive the dictionary is and whether it contains a special section on medical terminology. Even with all the electronic technology available, you will still need a good old-fashioned paper medical dictionary for the convenience of access to the reference material.

Electronic reference resources are also helpful. There are excellent sites that provide electronic medical dictionaries, encyclopedias, and other reference materials. Activity 3-1 gives you a chance to create some medical terms of your own.

Abbreviations

Abbreviations are shortened forms of words or phrases. They are used primarily in written communications to save time and space. Table 3-4 lists some of these abbreviations. Most medical dictionaries have a more extensive list of accepted abbreviations. If you are unsure whether an abbreviation is

✐ ACTIVITY 3-1

The beauty of medical terminology is that it allows new words to be created as needed. From the lists of prefixes, root words, and suffixes, make up five silly words and define them.

Example
Oligorhinoscoliosis: *oligo,* small; *rhino,* nose; *scoliosis,* curve

Your Turn

1.

2.

3.

4.

5.

✎ ACTIVITY 3-2

Using the abbreviations in Table 3-4, decipher the message below. (The answers can be found on p. 97.)

Your Turn

In the AM _____ evaluate Hx _____
and ADL _____. Use this information ad lib
_____ to CC _____
of GI _____ and ABD _____
meds _____. Use ROM _____
as tol _____ on the h _____
as PT _____ on the ft _____
to assist R _____. Monitor T _____
and P _____ in the pm _____
and provide H₂O _____ and TLC _____
as requested for OB _____ clients.

acceptable when **charting** and keeping records, write out the full term to ensure accuracy.

Activity 3-2 gives you a chance to put your knowledge of medical abbreviations into practice. Using too many abbreviations creates confusion. Massage therapists need to use the standard abbreviations that are accepted in the profession, not make up abbreviations or use texting abbreviations. These can become outdated quickly, and not everyone understands their meaning.

If you use abbreviations when charting, you should provide an abbreviation key with the clinical notes. Abbreviations are not understood universally, and a key ensures accurate interpretation of your notes by the client or a fellow health care professional (Activity 3-3).

GENERAL STRUCTURAL PLAN OF THE BODY

SECTION OBJECTIVES

Chapter objectives covered in this section:
3. Describe terms used to describe regions of the body and surface anatomy.
4. Define terms used to describe the positions of the body and the parts of the body in relation to other body parts.
5. Define kinesiology, body planes, and terms of movements.

After completing this section, the student will be able to perform the following:
• Explain the structural plan of the human body.
• Identify regions of the body and surface anatomy.
• Locate abdominal quadrants and regions.
• Use proper terms to indicate the positions of the body.
• Use directional terms to describe the relationship of one body area to another.
• Define kinesiology.
• Define the body planes, and demonstrate the movements that occur in each plane.
• Name and demonstrate movement terms.

The Body Map

The layout of a map is fairly universal. North usually is placed at the top, a legend identifies the number of miles per inch, and symbols indicate types of roads and landmarks. The

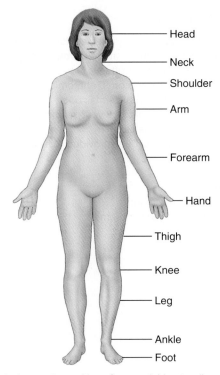

FIGURE 3-1 Anatomic position. Our model is standing upright, facing forward, feet slightly separated, arms hanging at her side with palms facing forward. Structures are named and their positions are described using this standard position. (Modified from Muscolino JE: *Kinesiology: the skeletal system and muscle function,* ed 2, St Louis, 2011, Mosby.)

Evolve Activity 3-2

locations of body areas are also universal. The map of the body begins with the body in the anatomic position (Figure 3-1).

The following information provides the basic knowledge needed to read the body map and provide accurate descriptions to guide others around the body.

Regions of the Body and Surface Anatomy

Regional terms are used to designate specific areas of the body (Activity 3-4). Study Figure 3-2 carefully.

Structural Plan

The structural organization of the body follows a clear plan. Each human being has a vertebral column that supports the trunk and determines the central axis of the body. The spine also supports two body cavities: the dorsal cavity, which holds the brain inside the skull and the spinal cord in the vertebral column; and the ventral cavities, which are the combined thoracic, abdominal, and pelvic cavities (sometimes referred to as the *abdominopelvic* cavity). Human beings are bilaterally symmetric beings, with left and right mirror images. Also, the body is segmented; this is most obvious in the vertebral column, ribs, and spinal cord. The body is designed as a tube within a tube. The digestive system is a tube that lies within the greater tube of the trunk (Figures 3-3 and 3-4).

Terms Related to the Structural Plan

The following terms are used to describe the structural plan of the body:

✎ ACTIVITY 3-3

Using the list in Table 3-4, as well as lists from a medical dictionary and your own imagination, develop a key for abbreviations you plan to use most often.

Think in terms of symptoms, anatomic locations, methods and techniques, directional terms, body movement patterns, assessment, and referrals. As your learning progresses, you may want to expand this list.

Some examples have been provided to help you get started.

Example
Symptoms
- ACP: Acupuncture point
- CFS: Chronic fatigue syndrome
- HA: Headache
- TP: Trigger point

Your Turn

Example
Anatomic Locations
- L-5: Fifth lumbar
- LB: Low back
- SI: Sacroiliac

Your Turn

Example
Methods and Techniques
- CTM: Connective tissue massage
- DP: Direct pressure
- EB: Energy balance
- MET: Muscle energy technique
- MLD: Manual lymph drainage
- SH: Self-help
- STM: Soft-tissue manipulation
- XFF: Cross-fiber friction

Your Turn

Example
Directional Terms
- ant: Anterior
- L: Left
- R: Right
- sup: Superior

Your Turn

Example
Body Movement Patterns
- flex: Flexion
- ROM: Range of motion
- SB: Side bending

Your Turn

Example
Assessment
- inter: Intermittent
- PB: Pain behavior
- WNL: Within normal limits

Your Turn

Example
Referrals
- AP: Acupuncturist
- DC: Doctor of chiropractic
- MD: Medical doctor
- DO: Doctor of osteopathic medicine

Your Turn

- *Soma, Somato:* Root words that mean "the body," as distinguished from the mind. Somatic organs and tissues are associated with the skin and skeleton (e.g., bone and skeletal muscles, extremities, the body wall) and commonly can be controlled voluntarily.

- *Axial:* Areas and organs along the central axis of the body, including the head, neck, trunk, brain, spinal cord, and abdominal organs.

- *Appendicular:* The limbs, joined to the body as lateral appendages.

✎ ACTIVITY 3-4

Stand in front of a mirror, and identify each landmark and point of surface anatomy and body region in Figure 3-2. Say the words out loud.

Write one sentence describing what it feels like to be your own anatomy model.

Example
I felt silly pointing at my body.

Your Turn

Repeat the exercise with a partner. Wearing a swimsuit or exercise wear that exposes more of the surface of the body is helpful.

Write one sentence about what it feels like to be an anatomy model.

Example
The same body parts can look somewhat different on two persons.

Your Turn

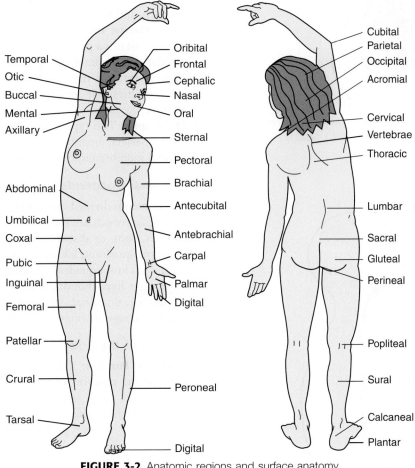

FIGURE 3-2 Anatomic regions and surface anatomy.

• *Torso, Trunk:* Structures related to the main part of the body, including the chest, abdomen, and vertebral cavity. The head and limbs are attached to the trunk.

Posterior Region of the Trunk

The two dorsal cavities are located toward the back of the body. They are as follows:

• *Cranial Cavity:* Found in the skull, containing the brain and related structures.
• *Vertebral Cavity:* Extending from the base of the cranial cavity and containing the spinal cord.

The back, or posterior surface, of the trunk is divided into regions named for the corresponding vertebrae in the spinal column.

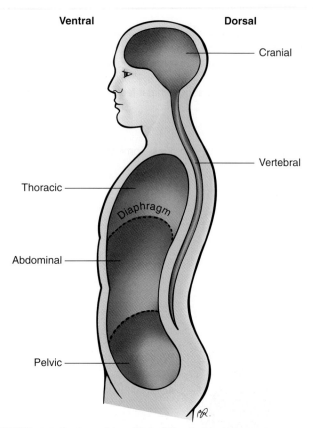

Ventral   **Dorsal**

— Cranial

— Vertebral

Thoracic —

Diaphragm

Abdominal —

Pelvic —

FIGURE 3-3 Body cavities. (From Fritz S: *Mosby's fundamentals of therapeutic massage,* ed 5, St Louis, 2013, Mosby.)

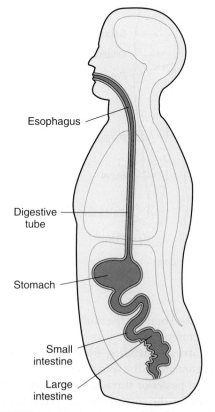

Esophagus —

Digestive tube —

Stomach —

Small intestine —

Large intestine —

FIGURE 3-4 The body as a tube within a tube.

- **Cervical Region:** The neck (7 cervical vertebrae).
- **Thoracic Region:** The chest (12 thoracic vertebrae).
- **Lumbar Region:** The low back (5 lumbar vertebrae).
- **Sacral Region:** The sacrum (5 sacral vertebrae fused into one bone).
- **Coccyx:** The tailbone (4 coccygeal vertebrae fused into one bone).

Anterior Region of the Trunk

Ventral cavities are located in the trunk. They include the following:

- **Thoracic Cavity:** Also known as the *chest;* found between the neck and the diaphragm and surrounded by the ribs. The mediastinum is a part of the thoracic cavity in the middle of the thorax, between the pleural sacs containing the two lungs.
- **Abdominal Cavity:** Also known as the *belly;* located below the diaphragm, enclosed within the abdominal muscles. This cavity contains the liver, kidneys, spleen, pancreas, stomach, and intestines.
- **Pelvic Cavity:** Inferior to the abdomen, inside the pelvic bones; contains a portion of the large intestine as well as the bladder and the internal reproductive organs.
- **Viscera:** Internal organs of the thoracic, abdominal, and pelvic cavities that are considered to be under involuntary control.
- **Membranes:** Two types, associated with the regions of the trunk: parietal membranes, lining the body cavities, and visceral membranes, covering the visceral organs.

Abdominal Quadrants and Regions

The abdomen is divided into four quadrants and nine regions, the names of which are used to describe the location of body structures, pain, or discomfort. The four quadrants are the right upper quadrant, left upper quadrant, right lower quadrant, and left lower quadrant (Figure 3-5, *A).* The nine regions are the right hypochondriac, epigastric, left hypochondriac, right lumbar, umbilical, left lumbar, right iliac, hypogastric, and left iliac regions (Figure 3-5, *B).*

Positions of the Body

- **Anatomic Position:** A term used in Western medicine to describe the position of the body and the location of its regions and parts. The central axis of the body passes through the head and trunk.

Terms related to the position of the body include the following:

- **Anatomic Position:** The body standing upright with the feet slightly apart, arms hanging at the sides, palms facing forward, thumbs outward (see Figure 3-1).
- **Functional Position:** The body standing upright with the feet slightly apart, arms hanging at the sides, palms facing sides of body, thumbs forward.
- **Erect Position:** The body standing.
- **Supine Position:** The body lying horizontally with the face up (Figure 3-6, *A).*
- **Prone Position:** The body lying horizontally with the face down (Figure 3-6, *B).*

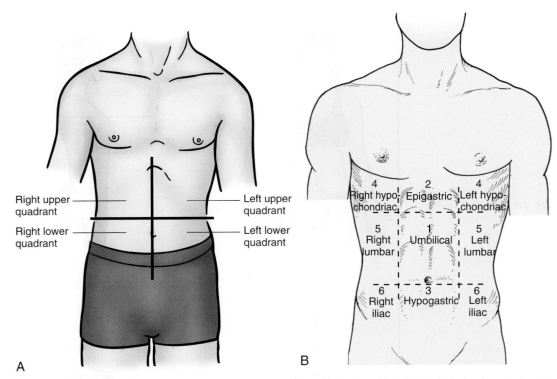

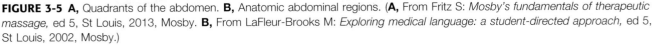

FIGURE 3-5 A, Quadrants of the abdomen. **B,** Anatomic abdominal regions. (**A,** From Fritz S: *Mosby's fundamentals of therapeutic massage,* ed 5, St Louis, 2013, Mosby. **B,** From LaFleur-Brooks M: *Exploring medical language: a student-directed approach,* ed 5, St Louis, 2002, Mosby.)

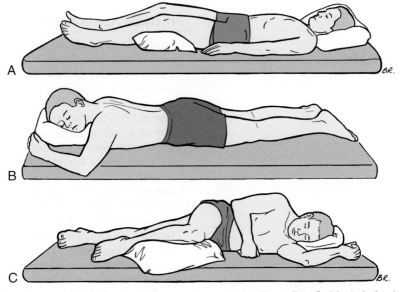

FIGURE 3-6 Positions of the body. **A,** Supine. **B,** Prone. **C,** Lateral recumbent. (From Fritz S: *Mosby's fundamentals of therapeutic massage,* ed 3, St Louis, 2004, Mosby.)

- *Lateral Recumbent Position:* The body lying horizontally on the right or left side (Figure 3-6, *C).*

Directional Terms
Certain terms are used to describe the relationship of one body position to another (Figure 3-7).

The following directional terms, which are organized in pairs of opposites, are derived from some of the prefixes listed in this chapter:

- *Anterior (Ventral):* In front of or in or toward the front.
- *Posterior (Dorsal):* Behind, in back of, or in or toward the rear.

- *Proximal:* Closer to the trunk or the point of origin (usually used on the appendicular body only).
- *Distal:* Situated away from the trunk, or midline, of the body; situated away from the origin (usually used on the appendicular body only).

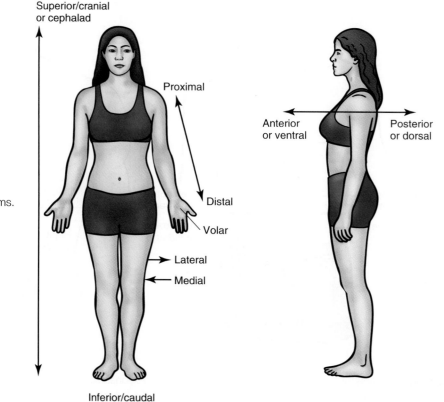

FIGURE 3-7 Directional terms.

- *Lateral:* On or to the side, outside, away from the midline.
- *Medial:* Relating to the middle, center, or midline.

- *Ipsilateral:* The same side.
- *Contralateral:* The opposite side.

- *Superior:* Higher than or above (usually used on the axial body only).
- *Inferior:* Lower than or below (usually used on the axial body only).

- *Volar (Palmar):* The palm side of the hand.
- *Plantar:* The sole side of the foot.

- *Varus:* Ends bent inward; angulation of a part of the body inward toward the midline.
- *Valgus:* Ends bent outward; angulation of a part of the body outward from the midline (e.g., example, bent toward the wall).

- *Internal:* An inside surface or the inside part of the body.
- *External:* The outside surface of the body.

- *Deep:* Inside or away from the surface.
- *Superficial:* Toward or on the surface.

- *Dextral (Dextro):* Right.
- *Sinistral (Sinistro):* Left; *levo* also is used to mean "left."

Practical Application

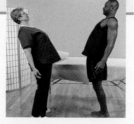

Etymology is the study of the history of words and how their form and meaning have changed over time.

Sometimes terminology is confusing. For example:
- **Varus:** Ends bent inward; angulation of a part of the body inward toward the midline. Derived from the Latin word *varus*, meaning knock-kneed; bent outwards; bandy; bowlegged.
- **Valgus:** Ends bent outward; angulation of a part of the body outward from the midline; for example, bent toward the wall. Derived from the Latin word *valgus*, which means "bowlegged"; knock-kneed, having legs converging at the knee and diverging below.

Varus means bent in. *Valgus* means bent out. Knock-knees look like they are bent in, but it is a valgus deformity, so what is really bent out? The tibia is turned outward in relation to the femur (angulation of the distal part of a limb at a joint), resulting in a knock-kneed appearance, and that is why.

According to the Latin definitions, *varus* and *valgus* both mean bow-legged and knock-kneed. With bowlegs, the knees appear to "bow" out from the body. Knock-knees, on the other hand, occur when the knees appear to bend toward each other.

- **Volar (Palmar):** The palm side of the hand.
- **Plantar:** The sole side of the foot.

The term *volar* is derived from the Latin word *vola*, meaning the hollow of the hand or foot. Now it really gets confusing. The dorsum (back) of the hand corresponds to the dorsum (top) of the foot.

Kinesiology

By definition, **kinesiology** is the study of movement. Kinesiology brings together the study of anatomy, physiology, physics, and geometry as a means to understand human movement. Kinesiology uses principles of **mechanics**, musculoskeletal anatomy, and neuromuscular physiology. Mechanical principles that relate directly to the human body are used in the study of **biomechanics**. This may involve looking at the static (nonmoving) or dynamic (moving) systems associated with various activities. Dynamic systems can be divided into **kinetics** and **kinematics**. Kinetics are the forces causing movement; kinematics are the aspects of time, space, and mass in a moving system.

Motion is a change in position with respect to some reference frame or starting point. If we are going to observe and describe any type of motion, we have to have an agreed-upon starting point (i.e., reference or baseline position) for the following reasons:
- To reduce confusion
- To define positional and motion terms
- To identify the position of the segment in space
- To identify whether motion has occurred

There are two reference points for movement:
- **Anatomic Position:** The body standing upright with the feet slightly apart, arms hanging at the sides, palms facing forward, thumbs outward.
- **Functional Position:** The body standing upright with the feet slightly apart, arms hanging at the sides, palms facing sides of body, thumbs forward.

Body Planes and Movements

The body can be divided into sections by imaginary lines and various planes to identify the particular areas (Figure 3-8).

Movements are described as beginning in or returning to the anatomic position (Figure 3-9). Movement terms define the action as the body part passes through the various planes.
- The sagittal plane is a vertical plane that divides the body into left and right. A midsagittal plane divides the body into equal left and right parts; a parasagittal plane divides it into unequal left and right parts.
- The frontal (coronal) plane also runs vertically but divides the body into anterior and posterior (front and back) parts.
- A transverse plane divides the body horizontally into two sections, described as *superior* (meaning "above") and *inferior* (meaning "below"). The transverse plane runs perpendicular to the frontal and sagittal planes.

A movement that takes a part of the body forward from the anatomic position within a sagittal plane is called *flexion;* movement backward is called *extension.*

Movements in a frontal plane that take a part of the body toward the midline are called *adduction;* movements away are called *abduction.* Lateral flexion, or side bending, of the head, neck, or trunk also takes place in the frontal plane. A movement in a transverse plane that takes a part of the body away from the midline is called *lateral rotation;* movement inward is called *medial rotation.*

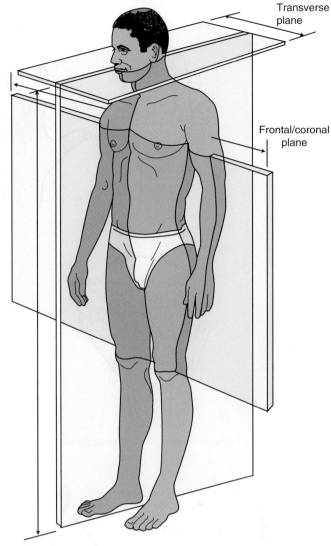

Transverse plane

Frontal/coronal plane

Median/sagittal plane

FIGURE 3-8 Anatomic planes.

Movement Terms

The following terms are commonly used to describe movement in the health care profession:
- *Flexion:* A decrease in the angle between two bones as the body part moves out of the anatomic position. Most flexion movements are forward movements. The major exception is knee flexion. Flexion is a sagittal plane movement. Place the fingers of your left hand on your left shoulder. You have just flexed your elbow joint. Make a fist with your right hand. You have just flexed the joints of your fingers.
- *Extension:* An increase in the angle between two bones, usually moving the body part back toward the anatomic position; most extension movements are backward movements. The exception is knee extension. Extension is a sagittal plane movement.
  - Begin with the fingers of your left hand on your shoulder. Now touch the lateral side of your left leg. You have just extended your elbow.
  - Begin with your right hand in a fist. Now open your hand so your fingers are straight. You have just extended your finger joints.

Text continued on page 74.

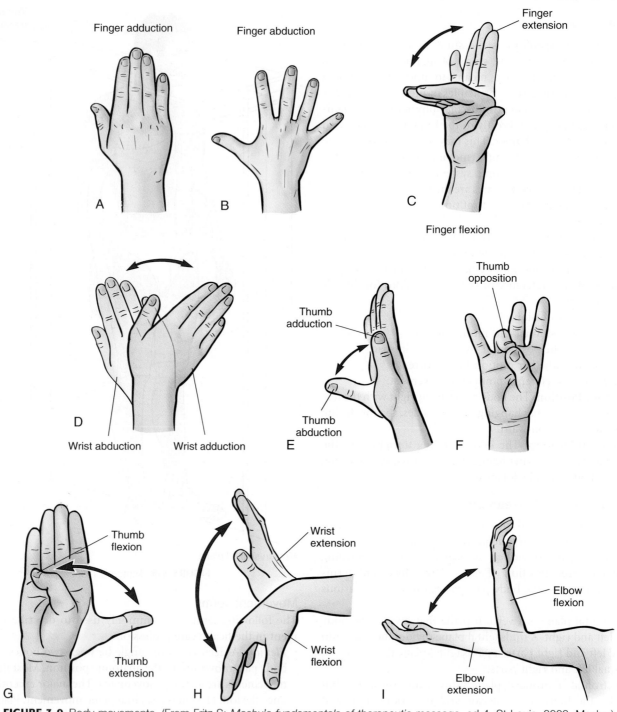

FIGURE 3-9 Body movements. (From Fritz S: *Mosby's fundamentals of therapeutic massage,* ed 4, St Louis, 2009, Mosby.)

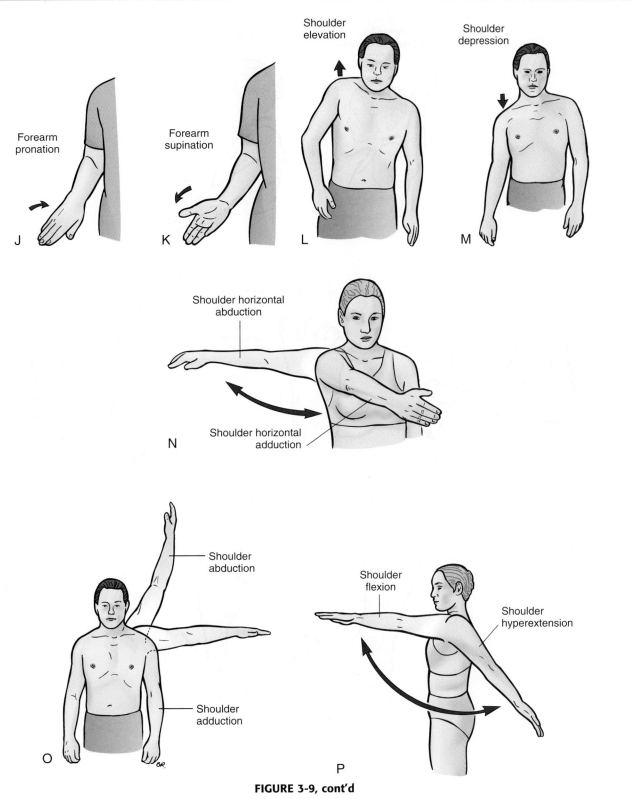

Forearm pronation

Forearm supination

Shoulder elevation

Shoulder depression

J

K

L

M

Shoulder horizontal abduction

Shoulder horizontal adduction

N

Shoulder abduction

Shoulder adduction

Shoulder flexion

Shoulder hyperextension

O

P

FIGURE 3-9, cont'd

Continued

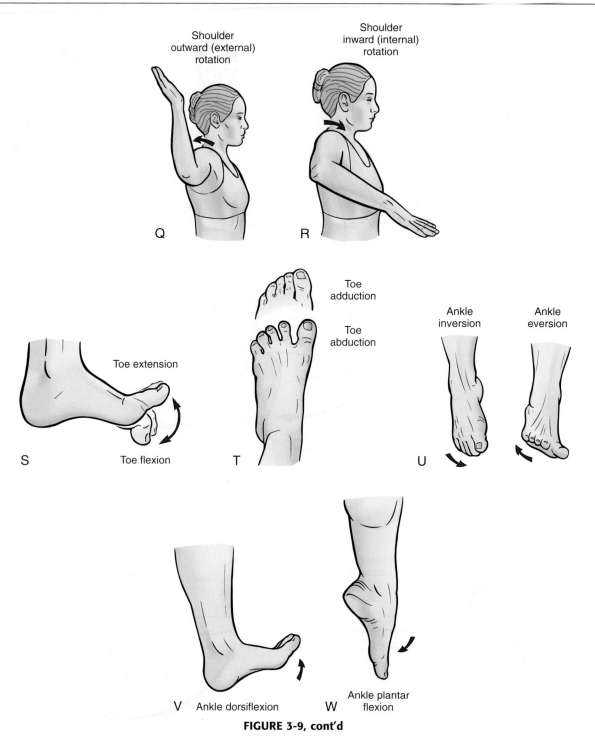

Shoulder outward (external) rotation

Q

Shoulder inward (internal) rotation

R

Toe extension

Toe flexion

S

Toe adduction

Toe abduction

T

Ankle inversion

Ankle eversion

U

V Ankle dorsiflexion

W Ankle plantar flexion

FIGURE 3-9, cont'd

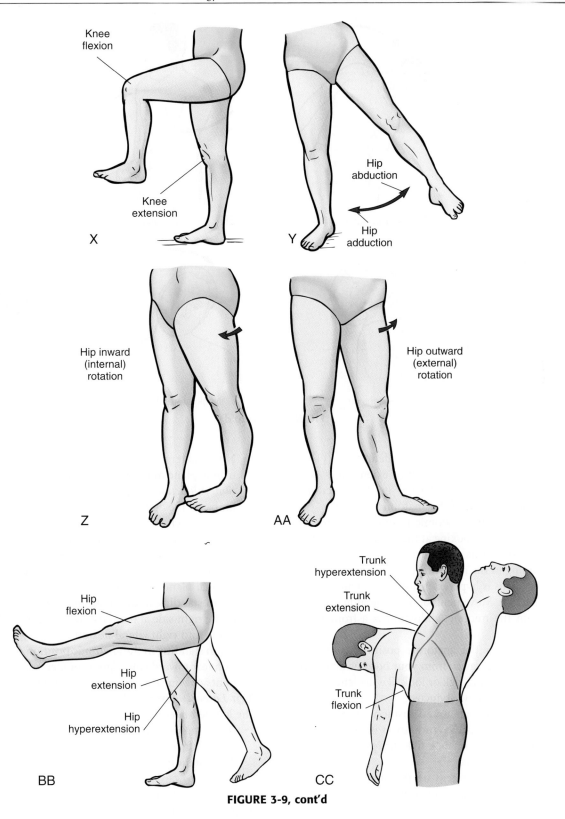

FIGURE 3-9, cont'd

Continued

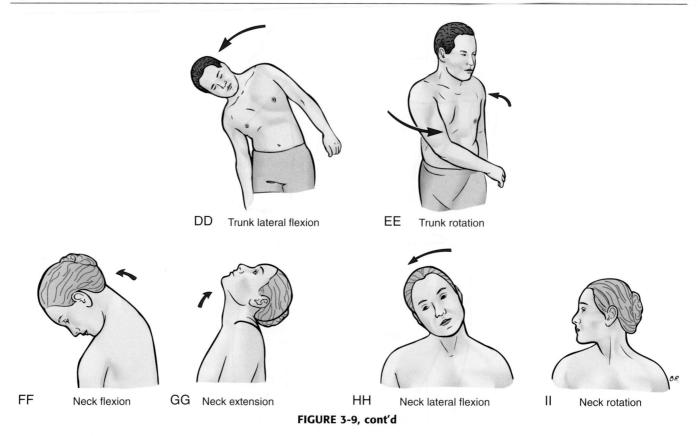

DD   Trunk lateral flexion   EE   Trunk rotation

FF   Neck flexion   GG   Neck extension   HH   Neck lateral flexion   II   Neck rotation

FIGURE 3-9, cont'd

- **Hyperextension:** A term that has two definitions: (1) any extension beyond normal or healthy extension; (2) any extension that takes the part farther in the direction of the extension, farther out of the anatomic position.
  - Begin standing in the anatomic position. Now tip your head back so you are looking at the ceiling. This is hyperextension of the joints of the neck.
  - Begin standing in the anatomic position. Now lean back at the waist. This is hyperextension of the trunk.
- **Abduction (ABD):** Movement of the appendicular body part away from the midline; abduction is a frontal plane movement.
  - Begin standing in the anatomic position. Move your arms out to the side away from your body as if you were going to do a jumping jack or look like the letter Y. Your shoulder joints are now abducted.
  - Begin standing in the anatomic position. Move your legs out to the side away from your body as if you were going to do a jumping jack or look like the letter A. Your hip joints are now abducted.
- **Adduction (ADD):** Movement of the appendicular body part toward the midline; adduction is a frontal plane movement.
  - Begin standing and positioned looking like a Y. Now lower your arms flat to your sides so you look like an I. You have just adducted your shoulder joints.
  - Begin standing and looking like an A. Now bring your legs together so you look like an I. You have just adducted your hip joints.
- **Right Lateral Flexion:** Movement of the axial body part to the right; right lateral flexion is a frontal plane movement.

- NOTE: Lateral flexion terminology is confusing because frontal plane movements are called *abduction* and *adduction*. *Adduction* and *abduction* refer to movement of the limbs, or the appendicular body, not the head, neck, and trunk, which are part of the axial body. Other terms used for lateral flexion are *tilt* and *sidebending*. Lateral flexion of the trunk involves moving the shoulders left or right toward the hips; therefore it is exercised in the frontal or coronal plane of motion.
  - Begin standing in the anatomic position. Now lean (tilt) to the right side at the waist. You have moved your spinal joints into right lateral flexion.
  - Begin standing in the anatomic position. Now move your right ear toward your right shoulder. You have moved the joints of your neck into right lateral flexion.
- **Left Lateral Flexion:** Movement of the axial body part to the left; left lateral flexion is a frontal plane movement.
  - Begin standing in the anatomic position. Now lean (tilt) to the left side at the waist.
  - Begin standing in the anatomic position. Now move your left ear toward your left shoulder. You have moved the joints of your neck into left lateral flexion.
- **Right Rotation:** Partially turning or pivoting the axial body part in an arc around a central axis to the right; right rotation is a transverse plane movement.
  - Begin standing in the anatomic position. Twist your head as if you were attempting to look at your right shoulder. Your cervical (neck) joints have just rotated right.
  - Begin standing in the anatomic position. Twist at the waist as if you were attempting to look behind you and

over your right shoulder. Your spinal (back) joints have just rotated right.

- *Left Rotation:* Partially turning or pivoting the axial body part in an arc around a central axis to the left; left rotation is a transverse plane movement.
  - Begin standing in the anatomic position. Twist your head as if you were attempting to look at your left shoulder. Your cervical (neck) joints have just rotated left.
  - Begin standing in the anatomic position. Twist at the waist as if you were attempting to look behind you and over your left shoulder. Your spinal joints have just rotated left.
- *Medial Rotation:* Partially turning or pivoting a body part located in the appendicular body in an arc around a central axis toward the midline of the body; also called *internal rotation.* Medial rotation is a transverse plane movement.
  - Begin standing in the anatomic position. Now place the palm of your right hand on your low back. You have just medially rotated your right shoulder.
  - Begin in the seated position. Bring your knees together, and move your feet apart. You have just medially rotated your hip joints.
- *Lateral Rotation:* Partially turning or pivoting a body part located in the appendicular body in an arc around a central axis away from the midline of the body; also called *external rotation.* Lateral rotation is a transverse plane movement.
  - Begin standing in the anatomic position. Now place the palm of your right hand on the back of your head. You have just laterally rotated your right shoulder.
  - Begin seated. Place the outside of your left ankle on your right knee. You have just laterally rotated your left hip joint.
- *Circumduction:* Not a movement, but a sequence of movements that turn or pivot the part through an entire arc, making a complete circle. (Note: Circumduction involves no rotation and is a multiplanar movement.)
  - Begin standing in the anatomic position. Raise your arms out to the side (shoulder abduction). Now move your arms in a big circle. You have just circumducted your shoulder joints.
  - Begin standing in the anatomic position. Now stand on your left foot, and make a big circle with the heel of your right foot. You have just circumducted your right hip.
- *Protraction:* Pushing of a part forward in a horizontal plane.
  - Begin standing in the anatomic position. Flex both shoulder joints, bringing your arms out in front of you. Keep elbows straight. Now reach forward with both arms. You should feel your scapula bones move apart in the back. You have just protracted your scapula (shoulder blades).
- *Retraction:* Pulling of a part back in a horizontal plane.
  - Begin standing in the anatomic position. Now move the inside edges (medial border) of your scapula together. You have just retracted your shoulder blades.
- *Elevation:* Moving a part upward (superiorly).
  - Shrug your shoulders by bringing the tips of your shoulders up toward your ears. You have just elevated your scapula.

- *Depression:* Moving a part downward (inferiorly).
  - Begin in the anatomic position. Slide your arms down the side of your legs toward your knees. You have just depressed your scapula.
- *Supination:* Movement of the forearm (at the radioulnar joint, not the elbow joint) that turns the palm anteriorly (upward), as in cupping a bowl of soup.
  - Begin in the seated position. Flex your elbows, and position your hands as if you were going to type on the computer or play the piano. Now turn your hands so the palm of your hand is facing up and you can look at it. You have just supinated your radioulnar joint.
- *Pronation:* Movement of the forearm (at the radioulnar joint, not the elbow joint) that turns the palm posteriorly (downward).
  - Begin in the seated position. Bring your hands together, palms up as if you are making a bowl to hold water. Now turn your hand as if you were going to type or play the piano. You have just pronated your radioulnar joint.
- *Inversion:* Movement of the sole of the foot inward, toward the midline.
  - Note: The subtalar joint (talocalcaneal joint) is a joint of the foot and not the true ankle joint. It is located in the rear foot. The subtalar joint is the area between the calcaneus and talus bones. The true ankle joint (talocrural joint) is made up of three bones. Two bones—the tibia and fibula—are from the lower leg, and the third bone, the talus, is from the foot.
  - Begin in the seated position. Now move your feet so that the bottoms (soles) of your feet touch each other. You have just inverted your feet. It occurs at the subtalar joint.
- *Eversion:* Movement of the sole of the foot outward, away from the midline.
  - Begin in the seated position. Now lift your left leg a little off the floor, and attempt to move your little toe toward the outside of your knee. You have just everted your subtalar joint.
- *Plantar Flexion:* Movement of the foot downward (may also be called *flexion*).
  - Begin standing in the anatomic position. Now raise your body up so you are standing on your toes (think ballet dancer). You have just plantar flexed your true ankle joint (talocrural) joint.
- *Dorsiflexion:* Movement of the foot upward (may also be called *extension*).
  - Begin in the seated position. Lift your feet a little off the floor. Now bring the top of your foot up toward your shin. If you were walking, you would be walking on your heels. You have just doriflexed your true ankle joint.

Movement is necessary for various **activities of daily living (ADLs).** ADLs are things we normally do in daily living, including self-care such as eating, bathing, dressing, grooming, going to work, performing housekeeping duties, and engaging in leisure activities (Activity 3-5). Physical activity involves movement. A common outcome goal for massage is supporting the ability to move without pain and stiffness.

✎ ACTIVITY 3-5

For each of the movements, give an example of a common activity.

Flexion:
Extension:
Hyperextension:
Abduction:
Adduction:
Right Lateral Flexion:
Left Lateral Flexion:
Right Rotation:
Left Rotation:
Medial Rotation:
Lateral Rotation:
Circumduction:
Protraction:
Retraction:
Elevation:
Depression:
Supination:
Pronation:
Inversion:
Eversion:
Plantar Flexion:
Dorsiflexion:

Practical Application

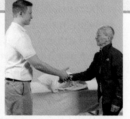

An important aspect of massage is describing clearly the information obtained during the data-collection process. The structural plan of the body and the terms used to describe location, position, and movement provide the language we use during the documentation process. We can clearly communicate with peers and other health care professionals using this common language. When we use these terms in our charting, others should be able to interpret accurately the content recorded in the charts. We can also understand other medical record information if it is written using standardized language. By understanding medical terminology, we can explain information to our clients without using terms that they may not understand. Standardized language supports effective communication.

QUALITY-OF-LIFE TERMINOLOGY

SECTION OBJECTIVES

Chapter objectives covered in this section:
6. Describe and use quality-of-life terminology.
After completing this section, the student will be able to perform the following:
• Define quality of life.
• Use quality-of-life terminology in massage practice.

In Chapter 2 we discussed mechanisms of health and disease. Implied in a state of health is that a person is experiencing a satisfactory quality of life (QOL).

The World Health Organization (WHO) is the directing and coordinating authority for health within the United Nations system. WHO undertook the task of identifying, defining, and assessing the spectrum of life quality The definition of **quality of life** presented by WHO is "... individuals' perceptions of their position in life in the context of the culture and value systems in which they live and in relation to their goals, expectations, standards and concerns."

The categories of QOL have been described and presented in a language that can be used to clearly communicate with clients, peers, and others. Interestingly, the common outcome goals for massage therapy intervention are directly related to quality-of-life categories. These categories are called *domains* by WHO (Box 3-2).

The WHO QOL criteria are divided into six domains:
1. Physical
2. Psychological
3. Level of Independence
4. Social Relationships
5. Environment
6. Spirituality/Religion/Personal Beliefs

There are 24 areas spread among the six domains.

The language provided by WHO and other documents concerning QOL provide a structure for critical thinking, clinical reasoning, communication, and documentation, which is described later in the chapter (Activity 3-6).

ANCIENT HEALING PRACTICES

SECTION OBJECTIVES

Chapter objectives covered in this section:
7. Explore terminology used in indigenous and cultural-based healing systems.
After completing this section, the student will be able to perform the following:
• Explain indigenous health care systems.
• Explain the role of intuition in traditional health care systems.
• Identify terminology from an ancient Chinese healing model.
• Compare terminology used in various healing traditions.

✎ ACTIVITY 3-6

Using the language presented in Box 3-2, develop a list of questions relevant to massage on one of the six domains. Even better, find five other classmates and divide up the six domains, and each of you develop relevant massage questions. Combine the work from all six of you to develop a massage-related quality-of-life assessment form.

Box 3-2   World Health Organization Quality-of-Life Domains

The following information is summarized from the World Health Organization (WHO) Quality of Life (QOL) user's manual. WHO reports are available at http://www.who.int/whr/en/index.html.

Domain I: Physical Domain
Pain and Discomfort
Pain is judged to be present if a person reports it to be so, even if there is no medical reason to account for it. The assumption is made that the easier the relief from pain, the less the fear of pain and its resulting effect on quality of life.

Examples:
- Unpleasant physical sensations such as stiffness, aches, long-term or short-term pain, and itches
- Constant threat of pain
- Extent to which these sensations are distressing and interfere with life

Energy and Fatigue
Energy is the enthusiasm and endurance that a person has in order to perform the necessary tasks of daily living, as well as other chosen activities, such as recreation. Lack of energy becomes fatigue.

Examples:
- Feeling really alive
- Adequate levels of energy
- Fatigued but functioning with effort
- Disabling tiredness due to illness, problems such as depression, and overexertion.

Sleep and Rest
Restorative sleep is necessary for quality of life. Problems with sleep and rest affect the person's quality of life. If sleep is disturbed, reasons can be due either to the person's life and circumstances or to factors in the environment, such as noise or interruption.

Examples:
- Difficulty going to sleep
- Waking up during the night
- Waking up early in the morning
- Being unable to go back to sleep
- Lack of refreshment from sleep

Domain II: Psychological
Positive Feelings
A person's view of and feelings about the future are seen as an important part of life. Does the individual experience enjoyment of the good things in life?

Examples:
- Contentment
- Balance
- Peace
- Happiness
- Hopefulness
- Joy

Thinking, Learning, Memory and Concentration
A person's view of his or her ability to think with clarity of thought and ability to gather and absorb new information and make informed decisions that affect quality of life.

Examples:
- Thinking
- Learning

- Memory
- Concentration
- Confidence
- Confusion
- Forgetfulness

Self-Esteem
Self-esteem is how people feel about themselves and their perception of self-worth. This might range from feeling positive about themselves to feeling extremely negative about themselves.

Examples:
- Feeling of self-efficacy
- Satisfaction with oneself
- Self-control
- Ability to get along with other people
- Educational experience and success
- Ability to respond to change
- Sense of dignity
- Self-acceptance

Body Image and Appearance
The focus is on the person's satisfaction with the way he or she looks and the effect it has on his or her self-concept, including the extent to which "perceived" or actual physical impairments, if present, can be corrected (e.g., by makeup, clothing, artificial limbs). How others respond to a person's appearance is likely to affect the person's body image considerably.

Examples:
- The person's view of his or her body
- Is the appearance of the body seen in a positive or negative way?

Negative Feelings
Although negative feelings are normal, how often, how much, and to what extent a person experiences negative feelings reflect quality of life and affect the person's day-to-day functioning.

Examples:
- Despondency
- Guilt
- Sadness
- Tearfulness
- Despair
- Nervousness
- Anxiety
- Lack of pleasure in life

Domain III: Level of Independence
Mobility
The focus is on the person's general ability to go wherever he or she wants to go without the help of others, regardless of the means used to do so.

Examples:
- Ability to perform mobility tasks (e.g., walking, running, reaching, pushing)
- Ability to get from one place to another
- Ability to move around the home
- Ability to move around the workplace
- Access to transportation services.

Activities of Daily Living
The focus is on a person's ability to carry out activities, which he or she likely needs to perform on a day-to-day basis.

Continued

Box 3-2   World Health Organization Quality-of-Life Domains—cont'd

Examples:
- Ability to perform usual daily living activities
- Self-care
- Wellness level exercise
- Family care
- Work activities
- Caring appropriately for property
- Participation in hobbies and other recreational activities

Dependence on Medication or Treatments

When an individual feels dependent on medication or some sort of treatment, quality of life is affected. A person's real or perceived dependence on medication or integrative and complementary medicines and treatments such as acupuncture, massage, and herbal remedies for supporting his or her physical and psychological well-being can either enhance or hinder quality of life.
Examples:
- Medications or treatment side effects
- Medication or treatment benefits
- Time expended in obtaining treatments
- Convenience of obtaining medication or treatments
- Medication or treatment costs and ability to pay
- Perception of medication or treatment cost/benefit ratio

Working Capacity

Work is defined as any major activity in which the person is engaged. Quality of life can depend on a person's use of his or her energy for work, satisfaction with the work, and ability to work.
Examples:
- Work for pay
- Desire to work but not employed
- Unpaid work
- Voluntary community work
- Full-time study
- Care of children
- Household duties

Domain IV: Social Relationships
Personal Relationships

The extent to which people feel they can share moments of both happiness and distress with loved ones and a sense of loving and being loved affect quality of life.

Experience Companionship, Love, and Support

- Ability to hug and touch and display other forms of physical affection
- Ability to be hugged and touched and to receive physical affection
- Desire for intimate relationship, both emotionally and physically
- Commitment to caring for and providing for other people
- The ability and opportunity to love, to be loved, and to be intimate

Social Support

Social support occurs when family and friends share in responsibility and work together to solve personal and family problems.
Examples:
- Support of family and friends
- Ability to depend on support in a crisis
- Availability of practical assistance from family and friends
- Approval and encouragement from family and friends

Sexual Activity

For many people sexual activity and intimacy are intertwined. How a person is able to express and enjoy his or her sexuality appropriately and without guilt or value judgment is an aspect of quality of life.
Examples:
- Healthy sexual expression is practiced.
- The individual is physically able to participate in sexual behavior.
- Supportive sexual partners are available.
- Sexual activity is expressed in intimate relationships.
- The individual is able to choose to participate in sexual relationships.
- The individual is free to express the creative forces of sexually in a nonphysical way.

Domain V: Environment
Physical Safety and Security

A threat to safety or security might arise from multiple sources, such as other people, political oppression, and natural disasters, and affects quality of life.
Examples:
- Sense of freedom
- Feeling of safety and security
- Lack of safety and security
- Protection from physical harm

Home Environment

Home is the principal place where a person lives; keeps most of his or her possessions; and, at a minimum, sleeps. The quality of the home is assessed on the basis of being comfortable, as well as affording the person a safe place to reside.
Examples:
- Crowdedness
- Amount of space available
- Cleanliness
- Opportunities for privacy
- Availability of facilities such as electricity, toilet, running water
- The quality of the construction of the building
- The quality of the immediate neighborhood

Financial Resources

A person's perspective on financial resources is an influence on quality of life.
Examples:
- Resources that meet the need for a healthy and comfortable lifestyle
- What the person can afford or cannot afford
- A sense of satisfaction/dissatisfaction with income
- Income that allows independence
- Financial resources that are inadequate to support independence
- The feeling of having enough

Health and Social Care: Availability and Quality

A person's view of the health and social care in the near vicinity, access to that care, and the quality of the care are aspects of quality-of-life experience.
Examples:
- Time it takes to get help
- The availability of health and social services
- The quality and completeness of care

Box 3-2 World Health Organization Quality-of-Life Domains—cont'd

- Access to volunteer and community support organizations
- Access to governmental support organizations
- Access to police, fire, and rescue services

Opportunities for Acquiring New Information and Skills

The ability of a person to fulfill a need for information and knowledge, whether this refers to knowledge in an educational sense or to local, national, or international news, is relevant to a person's quality of life.

Examples:
- Opportunity to learn new skills, acquire new knowledge
- Access to libraries, schools, and organizations involved in learning
- Access to media (television, radio, Internet) to be in touch with what is going on

Participation in and Opportunities for Recreation and Leisure

Quality of life is found in a person's ability, opportunities, and inclination to participate in leisure, pastimes, and relaxation.

Examples:
- Access to parks and recreational faculties
- Ability to see friends and spend time with family
- Time to read, watch television, be entertained, or do nothing

Physical Environment (Pollution/Noise/Traffic/Climate)

A person's view of his or her environment can improve or adversely affect quality of life.

Examples:
- Noise
- Pollution
- Climate
- General aesthetic of the environment

Transport

The availability of transport allows the person to perform the necessary tasks of daily life as well as the freedom to perform chosen activities.

Examples:
- Available and easy to find
- Reliable
- Affordable
- Easy to use
- Multiple modes of transport available (e.g., bicycle, car, bus)

Domain VI: Spirituality/Religion/Personal Beliefs

Spirituality/Religion/Personal Beliefs

A person's personal beliefs affect quality of life. Beliefs can enhance or degrade quality of life.

Examples:
- Ability to cope with difficulties in life
- Give structure to experience
- Ascribe meaning to spiritual and personal questions
- Provide a sense of well-being
- Ability to be hopeful
- Lack of spiritual, religious, and personal beliefs sometimes leading to despondency
- Rigid, imposed spiritual, religious, and personal beliefs sometimes disempowering

Data from WHOQOL User Manual, Geneva, Switzerland, 1998:61-71.

Practical Application

Quality-of-life terminology can become a useful tool for performing and documenting client history and assessment as the initial database for the client is developed. The terminology is also helpful for framing questions used during the history-taking process and developing outcome-based goals for massage. For example, the energy and fatigue content from Domain 1 can be used as part of the subjective aspect of gathering data from the client (see Box 3-2).

Energy and Fatigue

Energy is the enthusiasm and endurance that a person needs to perform the necessary tasks of daily living, as well as other chosen activities, such as recreation. Lack of energy becomes fatigue.

Levels:
- Feeling really alive
- Adequate levels of energy
- Fatigued but functioning with effort
- Disabling tiredness caused by illness, problems such as depression, or overexertion

Questions to ask:
- How would you explain your endurance for performing daily tasks?
- Could you describe your energy level today?

Possible answers:
- Really alive and full of energy
- Adequate
- Fatigued but functioning
- Unable to function because of fatigue.

Follow-up questions:
- What would you be able to do differently if your fatigue decreased and your energy increased?

- What do you believe is causing you to be fatigued?
- How might massage help you have more energy?
- Would an appropriate outcome goal for massage be to reduce stiffness and improve sleep?

The language in each of the domains in Box 3-2 can be used to form useful questions as you communicate with your clients.

The language can also be used to educate clients. For example:

DOMAIN IV—SOCIAL RELATIONSHIPS

Social support: When family and friends share in responsibility and work together to solve personal and family problems, this provides social support.

Examples include the following:
- Support of family and friends
- Ability to depend on support in a crisis
- Availability of practical assistance from family and friends
- Approval and encouragement from family and friends

If a client has been diagnosed with a chronic pain condition, coping mechanisms can be described as follows:

Massage therapy can be helpful in managing chronic pain. In addition, support of family members and friends and their ability to help, especially in a crisis, can be an important aspect of coping. I would be happy to teach some basic massage methods to some of your family members or friends so that they can help you between massage sessions.

Terminology is the major source of confusion between Eastern and Western science. Ancient and indigenous health care systems each have unique terminology. *Traditional medicine* (TM) refers to the knowledge, skills, and practices based on the theories, beliefs, and experiences indigenous to different cultures. Traditional medicine covers a wide variety of therapies and practices and has been used for thousands of years.

The confusion occurs because each system describes the same anatomy or physiology using different words. Western science is a relatively new healing method, one that requires the practitioner to observe, measure, accumulate data, and analyze findings in a clinical manner. It has a particular language. Ancient approaches to healing also have a specific language and require observation, measurement, and accumulation and analysis of data; however, they also validate intuition.

Intuition is defined as knowing something without going through a conscious, problem-solving, rational process of thinking. According to researcher and scientist Hans Selye, nothing can be investigated or validated scientifically unless the researcher first has an idea—that is, uses intuition. Without validation, practical application is limited.

Ancient, or indigenous, healing practices do not separate the body, mind, and spirit as Western science does. Spiritual knowledge is based on intuition—that is, on knowledge that exists but has not been materially or concretely proved—and Western science, until recently, has discounted anything that has not fit within the narrow boundaries of scientific validation. Today technology and advances in research design are revealing the validity of the more subtle aspects of ancient healing wisdom. The gap between ancient and new knowledge is narrowing, and with this development comes the need to understand the terminologies involved in various ways of describing the same thing. These other systems do not separate the body from the emotions or the mind, and now Western mind/body medicine is developing along similar lines.

Watching these older healing theories being discovered, explored, and understood by Western science is exciting. As these systems move closer together in understanding, we all will benefit from the sharing and blending of all types of human knowledge.

As previously mentioned, the general structural plan of the body can be mapped out using standard descriptions and Western terminology. Other healing systems also map the body, but they use their own standards and terms.

Understanding the Chinese system more fully is helpful for the therapeutic massage student because historical and current Chinese medicine has an important influence on massage practice.

The traditional Chinese health system is among the most ancient. It is based on the continual accumulation of knowledge through centuries of experiential observation. The system is similar to those of other cultural healing systems, which also endeavor to promote health by working toward homeostasis rather than by eliminating symptoms (a Western approach).

Practical Application

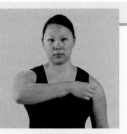

You may be asking yourself why you need to know about these various types of traditional medicine, especially in light of the fact that you are reading a science book. There are many answers to that question, but one of the most important reasons is to appreciate that there are many terms used to describe human anatomy and physiologic processes. As the concept of integrated heath care expands, massage therapists will need to be able to decipher the language of various cultural systems. The process is akin to being bilingual or multilingual. The ability to understand and speak more than one language expands communication possibilities. This textbook provides only a very basic introduction to other health care traditions. The intent is to create an awareness of the similarities and differences in theory and process for some of the various healing traditions.

The Asian systems are used here as examples of terminology components, specifically Chinese medicine. The Asian perspective is based on the meridian system. **Acupuncture** points and the five-element relationship system are used to identify and explain anatomic and physiologic functions.

The yin/yang concept, which was discussed in the previous chapter, is an excellent example of the Asian perspective. In this chapter the specific terminology used in the meridian system and five-element theory is presented in greater detail (Activity 3-7).

In the past treatments used to help in the survival of and recovery from trauma were mostly a matter of luck. Some believe that before the advent of pain-relieving drugs and treatments, a healer would press, rub, or hit the affected part of the body to alleviate the pain. Sometimes the person who had been burned, bruised, or cut would find that the preexisting pain would dissipate and healing would occur.

The earliest concept of acupuncture involved stimulating a painful point by pressing on it, puncturing it, or burning it. The point was referred to as an *Ah shi point*, which can be loosely translated into, "Ah, yes, that's where it hurts." In Western science this method of treatment can be explained by the gate-control theory, in which one set of sensory signals travels faster to the central nervous system and blocks the

| Box 3-3 | Acupuncture for Common Conditions |

World Health Organization (WHO) identified symptoms, diseases, and conditions that have been shown through controlled trials to be treated effectively by acupuncture. The findings of this report found acupuncture beneficial for these common conditions:

Low back pain	Postoperative pain
Neck pain	Stroke
Sciatica	Essential hypertension
Tennis elbow	Primary hypotension
Knee pain	Adverse reactions to radiation or chemotherapy
Sprains	
Facial pain	Allergic rhinitis, including hay fever
Headache	
Dental pain	Depression (including depressive neurosis and depression following stroke)
Temporomandibular joint (TMJ) dysfunction	
Rheumatoid arthritis	Primary dysmenorrhea
Induction of labor	Peptic ulcer
Morning sickness	Acute and chronic gastritis
Nausea and vomiting	

Data from Acupuncture: Review and Analysis of Reports on Controlled Clinical Trials, World Health Organization, 2003, accessed May 5, 2011, at http://apps.who.int/medicinedocs/en/d/Js4926e/5.html

transmission of a different set of sensory stimuli that may be distressing.

With the increasing use of acupuncture, the need for a common language to facilitate communication in teaching, research, clinical practice, and exchange of information became apparent. In 1989 WHO used a group of experts to develop the Standard International Acupuncture Nomenclature, which is now widely used.

Healers identified specific points before they recognized any patterns. The mapping of points eventually developed into various healing systems (Box 3-3).

In Western science acupuncture points have been identified with various anatomic or physiologic locations or functions in the body. Many acupuncture points have been associated with the motor points of the nervous system. (A motor point is the location where a nerve enters a muscle.) Acupuncture points also correspond to Golgi tendon organs and muscle stretch receptors. These same acupuncture points have been shown to have close correlations with trigger points and corresponding pain patterns. (A trigger point is a localized area of deep tenderness and increased tissue resistance.) Pressure exerted on a trigger point causes referred pain in a predictable area (Figure 3-10).

Ancient practitioners may have observed the referred pain pattern as they pressed on and used needles on certain points. Pressure on acupuncture points also affects the levels of dynorphins, enkephalins, and endorphins (pain- and mood-modulating, opiate-like chemicals in the body), which block the transmission of pain signals along nerve fibers.

Ayurveda, a healing tradition from India, also uses points, called *marmas*. They are clustered around joints and also have a high correlation with meridians, acupuncture points, and trigger points.

ACTIVITY 3-8

Palpate one of your forearms and hands with moderate pressure, making sure you cover every inch. Whenever you find an Ah shi point, mark it with a washable marker. Compare the points you have identified on your arm and hand with the point charts in this chapter.

On a separate piece of paper, draw a picture of your arm and the points located on it. Describe what you found.

Point phenomena in the ancient and Western scientific systems have many commonalities; for example, they all share the following characteristics:

1. They are located in a palpable depression.
2. They are associated with a neurovascular formation consisting of free nerve endings, Golgi tendon receptors, spindle cells, Pacinian corpuscles, and lymph or blood vessels that pass through the fasciae.
3. They are located on the surface of alpha and delta fiber afferent, fast-transmitting receptors that are sensitive to sharply pointed stimuli and heat. These points may correlate with the acupuncture points.
4. They are deep to the alpha and delta fibers in the same area; they have intramuscularly placed, C afferent, slow-transmitting fibers, which are more sensitive to chemicals and may correlate with the trigger points.

The mapping of 100 acupuncture points showed them to be located over large nerve trunks and cutaneous neurovascular bundles.

In less technical terms, the points stimulated to create a body change are located in the same areas on top of nerves (Activity 3-8). The more superficial nerves may be the acupuncture points, and the deeper nerves may be the trigger points (Chaitow, 1990) (Figure 3-11).

Western research has produced no great breakthroughs in the understanding of acupuncture until recently. Helene M. Langevin (2006) and her associates have identified that the imperfections in the acupuncture needle actually grab microscopic fascia fibers during insertion and twisting, creating a mechanical force into the tissues that in turn stimulates the mechanoreceptors embedded in the fascia. Sufficient evidence has been acquired to explain many of the effects as being related to chemical functions of the body, especially neurotransmitters and hormones.

Particular effects may be demonstrated after acupuncture treatment. Some of these effects involve alterations in the functions of organs or systems. An analgesic effect and also an anesthetic effect occur. The reflexes involved may not yet be explained fully.

In China acupuncture was used in combination with herbal medicine, dietetic regimens, and psychological guidance. The use of finger pressure on an acupuncture point has been demonstrated to induce the desired feeling of soreness and fullness that is a forerunner of the anesthetic effect. Electrophysiologic studies have showed that deep pressure applied to muscles and tendons has a definite inhibitory effect on the nervous system. Because the body strives toward health, it uses all helpful

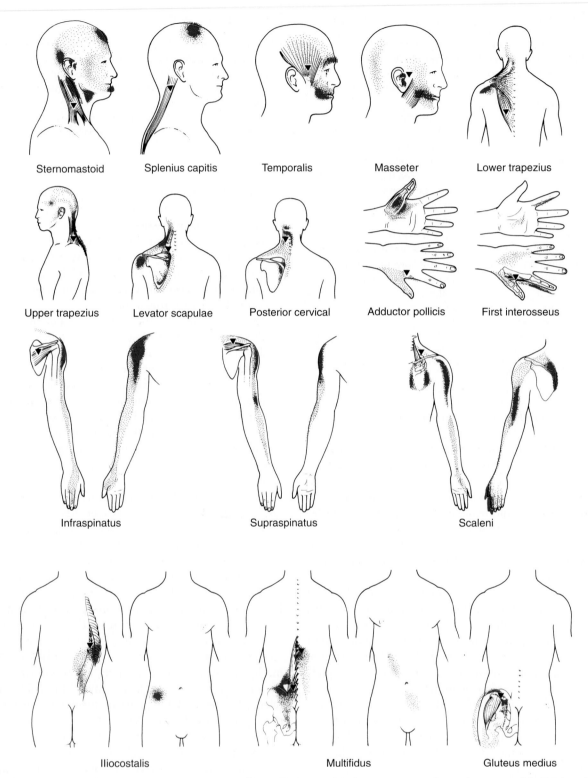

FIGURE 3-10 Common trigger point locations in muscles. (From Chaitow L: *Modern neuromuscular techniques,* ed 2, Edinburgh, 2003, Churchill Livingstone.)

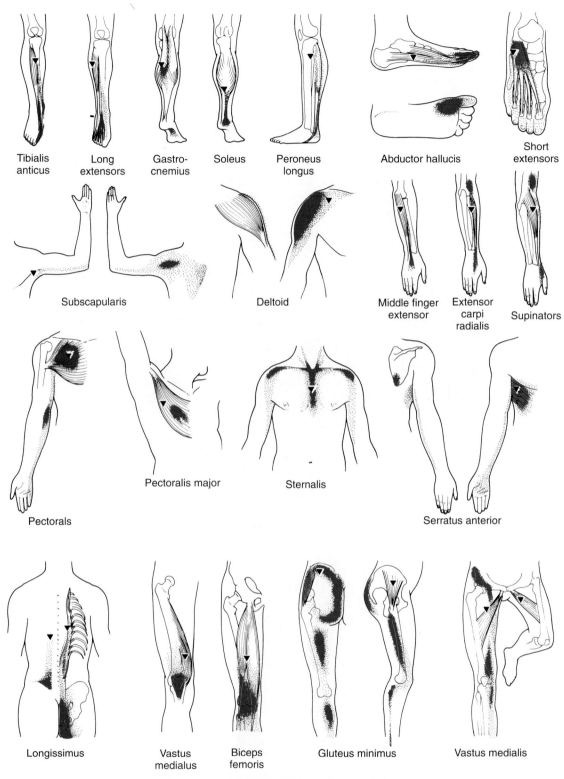

Tibialis anticus · Long extensors · Gastrocnemius · Soleus · Peroneus longus · Abductor hallucis · Short extensors

Subscapularis · Deltoid · Middle finger extensor · Extensor carpi radialis · Supinators

Pectorals · Pectoralis major · Sternalis · Serratus anterior

Longissimus · Vastus medialus · Biceps femoris · Gluteus minimus · Vastus medialis

FIGURE 3-10, cont'd

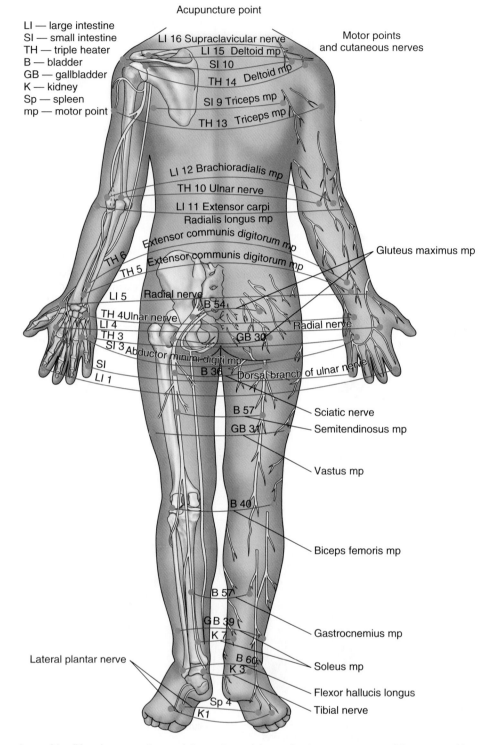

Acupuncture point

LI — large intestine
SI — small intestine
TH — triple heater
B — bladder
GB — gallbladder
K — kidney
Sp — spleen
mp — motor point

Motor points
and cutaneous nerves

LI 16 Supraclavicular nerve
LI 15 Deltoid mp
SI 10
TH 14 Deltoid mp
SI 9 Triceps mp
TH 13 Triceps mp

LI 12 Brachioradialis mp
TH 10 Ulnar nerve
LI 11 Extensor carpi
Radialis longus mp
Extensor communis digitorum mp
TH 6
TH 5 Extensor communis digitorum mp
LI 5 Radial nerve
B 54
TH 4 Ulnar nerve
LI 4
TH 3
SI 3 Abductor minimi digiti mp
SI
B 36
LI 1

Gluteus maximus mp
Radial nerve
GB 30
Dorsal branch of ulnar nerve
Sciatic nerve
B 57
Semitendinosus mp
GB 31
Vastus mp
B 40
Biceps femoris mp
B 57
GB 39
K 7
Gastrocnemius mp
B 60
Soleus mp
K 3
Lateral plantar nerve
Flexor hallucis longus
Sp 4
Tibial nerve
K1

FIGURE 3-11 Comparison of traditional acupuncture points, motor points, and cutaneous nerves of the arm and leg. (From Fritz S: *Mosby's fundamentals of therapeutic massage,* ed 5, St Louis, 2013, Mosby.)

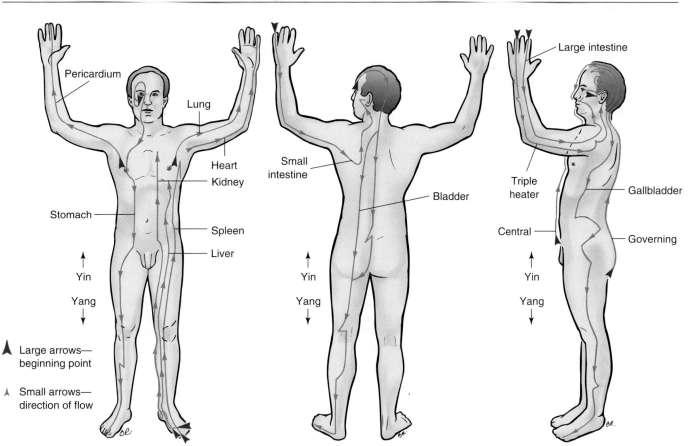

FIGURE 3-12 Typical location of meridians. Meridians tend to follow nerves. Yin and yang meridians are paired as follows:

Pericardium	Triple heater
Liver	Gallbladder
Kidney	Bladder
Heart	Small intestine
Spleen	Stomach
Lung	Large intestine

stimuli to achieve that goal. If, through acupuncture or manual pressure (acupressure), this function can be assisted, health is supported. In addition, an obstruction, or stagnant Qi, may cause problems, and acupuncture is used to help restore the energy.

Points and Meridians

Acupuncture, acupressure, and cupping are based largely on the theory of the channels and network vessels. In traditional Chinese medicine, this system of points and meridians is known as *jing luo,* which usually is translated into English as either "meridians" or "channels and network vessels." This system of acupuncture points, organized as meridians, is the fundamental infrastructure of Chinese anatomy and physiology. Disturbances in the meridians are reflected in abnormalities along their course.

The patterns of acupuncture points on the surface of the body have been charted by practitioners for centuries. They have been grouped together in lines (called *channels* or *meridians*). The actual tracts of each meridian were determined by plotting the various sensations that radiated above or below a point when it was pressed (Figure 3-12). In the past the points most used were located below the elbow and the knee.

Twelve main meridians have been identified. They are bilateral, symmetrically distributed lines of acupuncture points with affinity for or effects on the functions or organs for which they are named (Box 3-4, see also Figure 3-12). In addition to the 12 pairs of bilateral meridians, two meridians lie on the anterior and posterior midline of the trunk and head. Various extra meridians also exist, and they appear to relate to the organs and functions of the body. Other points on the ear surfaces, the hands, and the face have specific reflex effects.

Box 3-4 Meridians

12 Main Meridians

1. The lung meridian (L; yin) begins on the lateral aspect of the chest, in the first intercostal space, and then passes down the anterolateral aspect of the arm to the root of the thumbnail.

   11 points

   Pathologic symptoms: fullness in the chest, cough, asthma, sore throat, colds, chills, and aching of the shoulders and back.

2. The large intestine (LI; yang) meridian starts at the root of the fingernail of the first finger and passes up the posterolateral aspect of the arm over the shoulder to the face, ending at the side of the nostril.

   20 points

   Pathologic symptoms: abdominal pain, diarrhea, constipation, nasal discharge, and pain along the course of the meridian.

3. The stomach (ST; yang) meridian starts below the orbital cavity and runs over the face and up to the forehead, from where it passes down the throat, the thorax, and the abdomen and continues down the anterior thigh and leg to end at the root of the second toenail (lateral side).

   45 points

   Pathologic symptoms: bloat, edema, vomiting, sore throat, and pain along the course of the meridian.

4. The spleen (SP; yin) meridian originates at the medial aspect of the great toe and then travels up the internal aspect of the leg and thigh to the abdomen and thorax, where it finishes on the axillary line in the sixth intercostal space.

   21 points

   Pathologic symptoms: gastric discomfort, bloat, vomiting, weakness, heaviness of the body, and pain along the course of the meridian.

5. The heart (H; yin) meridian begins in the axilla and runs down the anteromedial aspect of the arm to end at the root of the little fingernail (medial aspect).

   9 points

   Pathologic symptoms: dry throat, thirst, cardiac-area pain, pain along the course of the meridian.

6. The small intestine (SI; yang) meridian starts at the root of the small fingernail (lateral aspect) and then travels up the posteromedial aspect of the arm and over the shoulder to the face, where it terminates in front of the ear.

   19 points

   Pathologic symptoms: pain in lower abdomen, deafness, swelling in the face, sore throat, and pain along the course of the meridian.

7. The bladder (B; yang) meridian starts at the inner canthus and ascends, passing over the head and down the back and the leg to terminate at the root of the nail of the little toe (lateral aspect).

   67 points

   Pathologic symptoms: urinary problems, mania, headaches, eye problems, and pain along the course of the meridian.

8. The kidney (K; yin) meridian starts on the sole of the foot, ascends the medial aspect of the leg, and runs up the front of the abdomen to finish on the thorax, just below the clavicle.

   27 points

   Pathologic symptoms: dyspnea, dry tongue, sore throat, edema, constipation, diarrhea, motor impairment and atrophy of the lower extremities, and pain along the course of the meridian.

9. The circulation (C; yin) meridian (also known as *heart constrictor* or *pericardium*) begins on the thorax lateral to the nipple, runs down the anterior surface of the arm, and terminates at the root of the nail of the middle finger.

   9 points

   Pathologic symptoms: angina, chest pressure, heart palpitations, irritability, restlessness, pain along the course of the meridian.

10. The triple-heater (TH; yang) meridian begins at the nail root of the ring finger (ulnar side) and runs up the posteromedial aspect of the arm, over the back of the shoulder, and around the ear to finish at the outer aspect of the eyebrow.

    23 points

    Pathologic symptoms: abdominal distention, edema, deafness, tinnitus, sweating, sore throat, and pain along the course of the meridian.

11. The gallbladder (GB; yang) meridian starts at the outer canthus and runs backward and forward over the head, passing over the back of the shoulder and down the lateral aspect of the thorax and abdomen. The meridian passes to the hip area and then down the lateral aspect of the leg to terminate on the fourth toe.

    44 points

    Pathologic symptoms: bitter taste in mouth, dizziness, headache, ear problems, and pain along the course of the meridian.

12. The liver (LIV; yin) meridian begins on the great toe and runs up the medial aspect of the leg and up the abdomen to terminate on the costal margin (vertically below the nipple).

    14 points

    Pathologic symptoms: Lumbago, digestive problems, retention of urine, pain in lower abdomen, and pain along the course of the meridian.

Midline Meridians

The body has two midline meridians. The conception or central vessel (CV; yin) meridian starts in the center of the perineum and runs up the midline of the anterior aspect of the body to terminate just below the lower lip; it is responsible for all yin meridians (24 points). The governing vessel (GV; yang) meridian starts at the coccyx and runs up the center of the spine and over the midline of the head, to terminate on the front of the upper gum; it is responsible for all yang meridians (28 points).

Jing Luo

The channels and network vessels, or meridian system, form an essential feature of the human body. The jing luo joins the tissues and organs of the body into an organic whole. The word *jing* means "warp; channels; longitude; manage; constant, regular; scripture, classic; pass through." The word *luo* means "something that resembles a net; the subsidiary channels; to hold something in place with a net; to wind or twine."

The jing luo is the network of routes for the circulation of Qi and blood. Through this network the entire body is interconnected: The viscera, bowels, extremities, upper and lower parts, and interior and exterior are brought into communication with one another.

The system is a comprehensive matrix that serves as an energy grid and generates, propagates, stores, and releases information and forces related to the body and its various components. Every place in the body is permeated by and connected with every other place in the body by means of the jing luo system. It is interesting to note that the recently proposed concept of an interconnected fascial web is similar to the Chinese description of jing luo.

The Chinese word concept that we translate into English as *acupuncture point* is composed of elements conveying the sense of body transport or communication hole or portal.

Functionally, acupuncture points seem to have two basic actions: They open, and they close. The names of the many points include words that mean "gate," "pass," and "door." In opening they release information and energy. In closing they store it.

In clinical use the meridian point system is the thoroughfare that allows Chinese medicine to influence the body when the balance of fundamental processes needs to be restored.

Yin/Yang Theory

The yin/yang theory is one of the oldest doctrines in Chinese culture. The words *yin* and *yang* were originally representations of the shady and sunny sides, respectively, of a mountain or a hill. They came to represent two primordial forces that were the fundamental constituents of the universe and everything in it.

When yin and yang were separated from the singularity at the beginning of existence, the resulting potential gave rise to Qi. For the Chinese **Qi** is a vital component of everything; all things are manifestations of Qi.

Often yin and yang are described as being opposites or complementary opposites. In terms of Western science, the notion of opposing forces is a powerful one, echoing throughout religious, moral, and ethical concepts of right and wrong, good and evil. However, in Chinese theory yin and yang are conceived as being in opposition but not in conflict.

Yin and yang nourish each other and foster each other's growth; they restrain each other; they support one another; they penetrate each other; they coexist. Box 3-5 contains other terms that you may encounter.

This brief introduction to the concepts and terminology of Chinese medicine demonstrates how many different words can be used to describe the same thing.

Box 3-5 **Traditional Chinese Medicine Terminology**

The following words describe additional aspects of Chinese medicine:

Cun (also xun) (SOON): A method of measurement that uses a relative standard, usually the length of the second phalange of the second finger of the patient, not the practitioner. Cun is most commonly applied in Asian bodywork and used to identify the location of acupoints on the body

Cupping: A method that uses suction to increase blood flow to an area. As the skin is pulled by the suction, the fascia is influenced.

Disharmony: Distortions in health that result when the functions or systems are neither balanced nor working optimally.

Essential Substances: The fluids, essences, and energies that maintain balance in the body, mind, and spirit. They include the **Qi**, or life force; shen, or spirit; jing, or essence; xue, or blood fluids; and jin ye, or fluids.

Han Re (HAHN RAY): A term meaning "cold" and "heat," respectively. It refers to two of the eight principal syndromes in differential diagnosis. The primary manifestations of yin and yang are symptoms that indicate the predominance of cold or heat. These two signs of disease are considered of primary importance when prescribing herbal ingredients to treat illness.

Jin Ye (SHJINYAY): A general term that refers to all the liquid components of the body other than the blood, although jin

ye is one of the basic substances that becomes blood. Jin ye is found in organs and tissues, where it serves a nutritive function. It is composed of two categorically different substances that form a single entity and can transform into one another.

Jing (SHJING): The yin essence of life that nurtures growth, reproduction, and development.

Liu Fu (LOO FOO): The six bowels; the six hollow organs; a term that is given collectively to the gallbladder, stomach, large intestine, small intestine, and urinary bladder and to the hard-to-define triple-heater (san jiao). In contrast to the five zang (wu zang) organs, the six fu organs are considered to be hollow and to be involved in the transportation of substances (rather than in the storing of essential substances) and in the decomposition of food and elimination of waste. *Liu* means "six;" *fu* means "bowel."

Liu Qi (LOO CHEE): A term that describes the environmental conditions ancient theorists identified as pathogenic factors. This concept also is called the Six Pernicious Influences. *Liu Qi* refers to wind, cold, heat, dampness, dryness, and fire—the six kinds of weather. When changes in weather exceed an individual's tolerance, disease may result. Identifying which of the six Qi are involved in the pathogenesis of a particular disease is an important step in diagnosing body substances (essence, Qi, liquid, humor, blood and vessels, or pulse). Wind diseases are most common in spring, heat

Continued

| Box 3-5 | Traditional Chinese Medicine Terminology—cont'd |

diseases in summer, damp diseases in summer, dryness diseases in autumn, and cold diseases in winter.

Moxibustion: A form of heat therapy in which burning herbs are used to stimulate specific acupuncture points.

Qigong (CHEEGONG): An ancient Chinese art of exercise and meditation that encourages the flow of Qi and supports homeostasis.

Qi Heng Zhi Fu (CHEE HANG SHZEE FOO): Literally, "extraordinary organs," a designation given to a group of organs that resemble the fu organs in structure and the zang organs in function: the bones, blood vessels, gallbladder, and uterus. They are different from the bowels because they do not decompose food or convey waste, and they are different from the viscera because they do not produce and store excess. The gallbladder is an exception because it is classed as a bowel and as an extraordinary organ. It is considered a bowel because it plays a role in the processing and conveyance of food and stands in interior/exterior relationship with its paired viscus, the liver. However, the bile that the gallbladder produces is regarded as a clear fluid rather than as waste; hence it also is classed among the extraordinary organs. The brain, marrow, bone, blood vessels, gallbladder, and uterus are born of the Qi of the earth. They represent the nature of earth and belong to yin. Thus they can store essence and not release it.

Qi Qing (CHEE CHING): The seven effects, which include emotional and mental activities in general. The term considers their potential as pathogenic factors in disease. Ancient theorists recognized that intense or prolonged emotional disturbances can be pathogenic, and they identified seven such states: anger, melancholy, anxiety, sorrow, terror, fright, and excessive joy. Each can disturb the normal function of the Qi, blood, and viscera and thus cause disease.

Qi (CHEE): The life force; also spelled *Chi.*

Shen (SHEN): The eternal dimension of life, the magical or heavenly aspects of being alive; God, deity, divinity or divine nature; supernatural; magical expression, look, appearance; smart, clever.

Si Shi (SEE SHEE): The four seasons; a general term for spring, summer, autumn, and winter in which the third month of summer (the sixth month of the Chinese lunar year) is termed "long summer." The four seasons are correlated with the five phases: spring, wood; summer, fire; long summer, earth; autumn, metal; winter, water.

Wu Xing (WOO ZING): The five phases (elements)—metal, water, wood, fire, and earth. This theoretic structure supports much of traditional Chinese thought. Wu xing is an extension of yin/yang theory; here it is applied to the nature of material substances and to the interrelationships that exist among the various phases of matter. These five phases function metaphorically, providing images that ancient theorists used to organize their thinking about the physical world. The five phases describe a cycle that represents the inherent existence of change and reflects yin and yang movements in nature. The five phases, like yin and yang, are representatives of qualities and relationships (Table 3-5). When combined with the principles of Chinese medicine, they are used to determine the diagnosis and treatment of a dysfunction (Figure 3-13).

Wu Zang (WOO ZANG): Meaning viscera, internal organ, wu zang refers to the solid organs: the heart, liver, spleen, lungs, and kidneys. These organs constitute a category that is distinguished from the six fu organs in structure and function. The zang organs are thought of as solid, essence-containing organs.

Xu Shi (ZOO SHEE): A word that is translated as deficiency and excess, insubstantial and substantial (particularly in the martial arts), replete and deplete, full and empty. *Xu shi* refers to two principles used in estimating the condition of a patient's resistance and the pathogenic factors present.

Xue (ZOO-ay): A word that means the blood itself in the same sense as it is understood in modern physiology. Xue also is used to mean something specific to Chinese medicine: the substantial fraction of the circulatory system that is in a unique relationship with the circulation of Qi.

Ying (YING): Construction (Qi), construction nutriment; one of the substances essential to sustaining vital activities. Ying is derived from digested food and is absorbed by the internal organs. It circulates through the channels as a part of the blood to nourish all parts of the body. It is the essential ingredient of the blood and is responsible for the production of blood and the nourishment of body tissues. The blood (xue) and the ying are inseparable. Thus they often are referred to as *ying xue.*

Zheng Xie (SHZENG ZEE-ay): Righteous and evil, normal and pathogenic; this term refers to a distinction between the normal functions of an organism and the pathogenic changes that accompany and characterize disease.

Organ Relationships

Unlike the Western concept of individual organs, Eastern philosophy considers organ systems. Each system includes an organ, essences, and fluids as they interact with the meridians. Ayurveda, a healing tradition of India, describes body functions in terms of doshas: Vata, Pitta, and Kapha (see Chapter 2). Randolph Stone integrated the two systems and added other energetic methods to develop the polarity system. Ancient healing methods always have treated internal functions by means of external stimulation of the body, using methods such as acupuncture and massage. For centuries practitioners have been using these techniques to reestablish homeostasis within the body, so it is reasonable to think that such practices must have some sort of consistent benefit.

Current research has validated the cutaneous-visceral connections that are an aspect of the practices.

As discussed in Chapter 2, the nerve reflexes of internal organs manifest on the surface of the body, showing up as referred pain. The following are examples of other manifestations of nerve patterns that connect the internal organs with the surface:

- Pain sensations felt on the skin may be referred by internal organs (viscerosomatic reflex).
- Muscular splinting may be noted over an area of internal disturbance.
- The autonomic nervous system influences surface areas of the body.

Table 3-5 Qualities of the Five Elements

| | ELEMENT | | | | |
Phase	Metal	Earth	Fire	Water	Wood
Yin	Lung	Spleen	Heart circulation/ Pericardium	Kidney	Liver
Yang	Large intestine	Stomach	Small intestine Triple-heater	Bladder	Gallbladder
Sense	Smell	Taste	Speech	Hearing	Sight
Organ	Nose	Mouth, lips	Tongue	Ears	Eyes
Liquid	Mucus	Saliva	Sweat	Urine	Tears
Color	White	Yellow	Red	Blue/black	Green
Expression	Weeping	Singing	Laughing	Groaning	Shouting
Extreme emotion	Grief, anxiety	Worry, reminiscence	Shock, overjoy	Fear	Anger
Balanced emotion	Openness, receptivity	Sympathy, empathy	Joy, compassion	Resolution, trust	Assertion, motivation
Taste	Pungent, spicy	Sweet	Bitter, burned	Salty	Sour
Season	Fall	Indian summer	Summer	Winter	Spring
Related activity	Releasing	Thinking	Inspiration	Willpower and intimacy	Planning and decision making
Times	Lung, 3-5 AM	Stomach, 7-9 AM	Heart, 11 AM-1 PM	Bladder, 3-5 PM	Gallbladder, 11 PM-1 AM
	Large intestine, 5-7 AM	Spleen, 9-11 AM	Small intestine, 1-3 PM	Kidney, 5-7 PM	Liver, 1-3 AM
			Triple-heater, 9-11 PM		
			Pericardium, 7-9 PM		

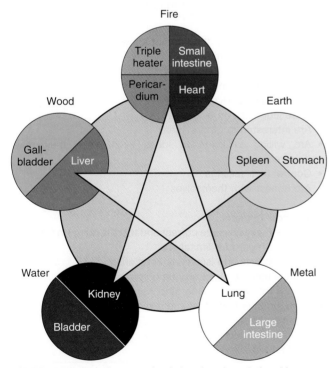

FIGURE 3-13 Five-element wheel showing the relationships among elements and organs. A circle relationship is a creation cycle. A star relationship is a control cycle.

Practical Application

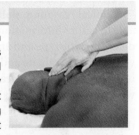

Because trigger points are located in shortened muscle fibers, these fibers must be lengthened to the normal resting length of the muscle, and any shortening of connective tissue must be addressed by using stretching methods. Often the type of point being addressed is not clear; therefore, unless contraindicated, the shortened muscles should be restored to appropriate resting length by means of lengthening and stretching methods. Regardless of the classification or name of the tender point, methods of treatment include some sort of stimulation of the point, often in the form of pressure, to bring about combined neurologic and chemical adjustments in the tissues of the area as well as in the system as a whole. This method restores and adjusts the homeostatic mechanisms. Focusing massage applications over the meridians in the direction of their energy flow can be an effective approach to supporting the body's self-healing abilities. An awareness of Asian theory and practice helps massage practitioners understand the complementary practices involved in Asian disciplines.

• Stimulus causes shifts in endogenous chemicals (those manufactured inside the body), which can affect organ function (somatovisceral reflex).

Theoretic discussions about using surface stimulation to affect the function of internal organs could explain the relationship of meridians and acupuncture points to specific internal physiologic features.

If the multitude of points described in the various health practices were mapped on the body, little space would be left. The case can be made that the entire body is a series of points. All this information can be used to reinforce the idea that events on the inside of the body affect the outside, and vice versa.

CLINICAL REASONING AND CHARTING

SECTION OBJECTIVES

Chapter objectives covered in this section:

8. Use a charting method that incorporates a clinical reasoning/ problem-solving model.

After completing this section, the student will be able to perform the following:

- Describe critical thinking.
- Explain how critical thinking is used in clinical reasoning.
- List the qualities of a critical thinker.
- Describe a problem-oriented medical record.
- Use a SOAP note system to support critical thinking and clinical reasoning.

Effective assessment, analysis, and decision making are essential to meeting the needs of each client. In attempting to individualize treatment, the practitioner often finds that routines or recipe-type applications of massage and bodywork treatments are of limited value or even ineffective because clients' circumstances vary so widely. Therefore the mark of an experienced professional is skill in effective reasoning.

As the volume of knowledge grows and as massage and bodywork treatments become part of the health care system, the massage therapist will find it increasingly important to be able to think through an intervention process and justify the effectiveness of particular massage methods.

Clinical reasoning skills enable massage practitioners to be able to gather information effectively, analyze the information, determine the type and appropriateness of a therapeutic intervention, and evaluate and justify the benefits derived from the intervention. This is a learned skill. Clinical reasoning begins with the broader process of critical thinking.

Critical thinking is a learned skill for logical and objective thinking. Thinking processes are sometimes ineffective. How many times have you thought about a problem; made a decision; implemented the decision; and then, when the results were different than expected, said, "I never thought of that!"

Thinking can be biased, distorted, partial, uninformed, and emotional and leave out very important information and ideas. Flawed thinking is costly—in time, resources (including money), and quality of life. Therefore productive critical thinking, which is systematically learned, is essential for the massage professional's career success.

Because it is natural to have flawed thinking, educators, scientists, and other experts have developed processes such as the scientific method for effective thinking. An example is the documentation process that you learn in massage school. It provides a form, such as a SOAP note, that will act as a map of the critical thinking process. Many activities in this text are designed to teach and reinforce critical thinking.

Clinical reasoning occurs when we use critical thinking skills to make decisions about how we are going to structure a massage to achieve the goals of the client. Clinical reasoning requires a commonly accepted clinical vocabulary. Scientific and medical terminology provides that vocabulary. Because even computers have to speak to each other in a common language, the National Library of Medicine created the Unified

---

Box 3-6 What Is Critical Thinking?

John Dewey was an American psychologist, philosopher, educator, and social activist. In his book *How We Think*, Dewey (1910) defined critical thinking as "reflective thought": to suspend judgment, maintain a healthy skepticism, and exercise an open mind. Critical thinking in education involves students doing things such as asking questions; answering questions; examining a problem; and finding a solution while thinking about the things they are doing by reflecting, contemplating feedback, and evaluating.

When you are thinking critically, you examine a problem, find a solution, think about why you were or were not successful, and learn from your successes and failures.

John Dewey said,

"One thing more, and that is—you who are students really have as great an opportunity as any students of any subject ever had at any time, but it will take a lot of patience, a lot of courage, and, if I may say so, considerable guts!"
—Boydston J, editor: The collected works of John Dewey, 1882-1953, Carbondale and Edwardsville, 1991, Southern Illinois University Press. LW 17:466.)

Box 3-7 Characteristics of Critical and Noncritical Thinkers

Critical Thinkers

- Acknowledge what they do not know
- Recognize their limitations
- Are conscious of their errors
- Think before acting
- Keep curiosity alive
- Base judgment on evidence
- Are interested in others' ideas
- Are willing to listen to ideas even when they may disagree
- Control their feelings
- Are honest with themselves

Noncritical Thinkers

- Believe their views are correct and there is no room for error
- Have no regard for limitations
- See problems and issues as irritations
- Believe their opinions are the only correct ones
- Do not try to understand other views
- Base judgments on first impressions
- Act impulsively
- Are preoccupied with themselves
- Are know-it-alls

Modified from Elsevier: Master Teacher Development Process Online, 2005, Elsevier.

Medical Language System (UMLS) to facilitate the development of computer systems that work as if they "understand" the meaning of the language of biomedicine and health.

It all begins with the critical thinking that is used for clinical reasoning in massage practice, and the recording or documentation of the process uses a common vocabulary (Boxes 3-6 and 3-7).

Charting/Documentation

Charting/documentation is the process of keeping a written record of the clinical reasoning process during professional interactions. Effective charting is more than writing down what happened. It is a clinical reasoning methodology that emphasizes a problem-solving approach to client care. Clinical problems are varied and are not necessarily related to dysfunction; rather, the problem involves ways to achieve therapeutic outcomes for the client.

To reason clinically and document effectively, a practitioner must have a comprehensive knowledge of medical terms and abbreviations and deep familiarity with the anatomy and physiology in clients who are in both balanced and altered states of functioning. Assessment procedures identify deviations from effective and normal functioning, and that information is the basis for formulating the care plan, identifying any contraindications to massage therapy, developing appropriate adaptation to the massage, and evaluating the need for referral.

A commonly used method of charting is the problem-oriented medical record (POMR). A type of problem-oriented medical record that is commonly used by massage therapists is called SOAP notes. The process of critical thinking applied to clinical reasoning is supported by using the SOAP note form.

In the SOAP note charting method, the following pattern is used:

S: Subjective information from the client

O: Objective data based on inspection, palpation, and testing and a record of interventions performed

A: Analysis and assessment of the subjective and objective data; of the effectiveness of the intervention; of the methods used; and of the actions taken during the session

P: Plan, including the methodology to be used in future interventions and the progress of the sessions

The *S* and *O* are the data-collecting (fact-gathering) parts of the SOAP method. The *A* is the most complex of the four parts. Because the method is based on an analytical process, after you have learned it, the method can be adapted easily to any other documentation method. The key is to consider a massage session rationally and comprehensively. A charting method can provide a structure for and a record of the process.

Database

Any problem-solving charting method must begin with a database, which is collected before the process of identifying the client's problems and goals actually has begun. The database consists of all the available information that contributes to client care. It has two parts: (1) information obtained from a history-taking interview with the client and from other pertinent persons, prior records, and health care treatment orders (subjective) and (2) the physical assessment (objective).

The first part of the database, the history-taking interview, provides information about the client's health and the reason for the visit, a descriptive profile of the client, a history of the client's current condition, a history of illness and health, and a history of family illness. The history also contains an account of the client's current health practices and perception of quality of life.

The physical assessment makes up the second part of the database. The extent and depth of this assessment vary from setting to setting, from practitioner to practitioner, and according to the client's situation. Practitioners of therapeutic massage generally use some sort of visual assessment to look for bilateral symmetry and deviations. Functional assessment reveals restricted, exaggerated, painful, or otherwise altered movement patterns. Palpation is used to identify changes in tissue texture and temperature, locate energy changes, and identify areas of tenderness. Various manual tests may be used to distinguish soft-tissue problems from other conditions, such as joint dysfunction.

Analyzing the Data

After collecting the information, the massage practitioner analyzes it, identifying problems to be addressed and goals to be achieved, on the basis of the examination, investigation, and analysis of the data collected. The practitioner then decides on a treatment plan, recording at each session the actions taken and their effectiveness.

Not all therapeutic goals relate to dysfunction. Clients commonly use therapeutic massage to maintain health, manage stress, and fulfill needs for human comfort and pleasure. The same analytical process is used to determine the methods that best meet these client goals.

Detailed steps in that analytic process are presented in Box 3-8.

Treatment Planning

The *P*, or *plan*, section of the SOAP method involves the development and implementation of a treatment plan. After the analysis has been completed, a decision must be made about what will be involved in the treatment plan. The plan is not an exact protocol set in stone but rather a guideline. After implementing the plan, the practitioner reevaluates and adjusts it as necessary.

SOAP may be summarized as follows:

S and *O* are the facts obtained during data collection and what was done during the session.

A is the analysis of the data in *S* and *O* and the research into possibilities, logical causes and effects, consequences, and effects on the persons involved.

P is the decision-making and implementation structure.

The practitioner must be able to collect all data from client history, assessment, and any necessary research. Once all the information is collected, it is analyzed to make decisions about what the data mean and what patterns are represented in the whole person. Because of the amount of information involved and because most human difficulties are multidimensional, involving body, mind, and spirit, all areas must be addressed. In many cases it is necessary to make a referral.

Box 3-8 The Analysis Process

Step 1

What facts have been gathered from the data provided by the client and from research about the situation presented?

What is considered normal or balanced function?

What has happened? (Spell out the events.)

What caused the imbalance? (Can the cause be identified?)

What was done or is being done?

What has worked or not worked?

Step 2

What are the possibilities? (What could all the information mean?)

What does my intuition suggest?

What are the possible patterns of dysfunction?

What are the possible contributing factors?

What are possible interventions?

What might work?

What are other ways to look at the situation?

What do the data suggest?

Step 3

What are the logical progression of the symptom pattern, the contributing factors, and the current behaviors?

What are the logical causes and effects of each intervention identified?

What are the pros and cons of each intervention suggested?

What are the consequences of not acting?

What are the consequences of acting?

Step 4

For each intervention under consideration, what would be the effect on the persons involved—the client, the practitioner, and other professionals working with the client?

How does each person involved feel about the possible interventions?

Is the practitioner within the scope of practice to work with such a situation?

Is the practitioner qualified to work with such a situation?

Does the practitioner feel confident about working with such a situation?

Does a feeling of cooperation and agreement exist among all parties involved?

Effective practice and ethical behavior require a massage therapist to stay within the competencies of a professionally defined scope of practice and a personal level of training, expertise, and experience. Therefore assessment and analysis may indicate a need to refer the client elsewhere or to use a team approach, working in a multidisciplinary cooperative effort to provide the best possible care for each client (Activity 3-9).

The ability to apply what has been learned from the study of anatomy and physiology comes from the reasoning and problem-solving processes. With this skill, the information acquired becomes alive and practical. Effective work with clients is a continual learning process of assessing, deciding on interventions, and analyzing effectiveness through evaluation of progress from session to session. Even in the most basic

Practical Application

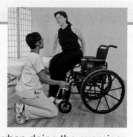

This textbook has been developed on the model of critical thinking and clinical reasoning to ensure that the massage treatment plan developed and implemented has the best chance of success. A model is a pattern to imitate. See if you can identify the clinical reasoning model when doing the exercises and activities that encourage analysis and reasoning. Imitating a model is a good way to begin a learning process. After understanding the model and using it effectively, the student can vary it as necessary to provide the best response to each set of circumstances. A model is a tool, not an absolute.

sessions, when the client's goals are pleasure and relaxation, the practitioner must decide on the best ways to encourage the body to respond to meet those goals.

SUMMARY

A competent massage therapist is able to understand the language of the scientific community as well as the language and underlying philosophy of other healing practices, such as those of Asia. Even though the main focus of this text is Western science, a tremendous amount of overlap exists between Western and Eastern methods, and therapeutic massage is influenced richly by ancient healing practices.

The ancient and indigenous healing traditions share similar philosophies but use different terminology. Two additional examples are the chakra system (described in Chapter 6) and the dosha system (described in Chapter 2). Common to these healing traditions is the use of soft-tissue methods; movement; meditation and inner reflection; exercise; dietary influences, including the use of naturally occurring substances for medicinal purposes; emotional influences; and spiritual connections that make human beings one with their environment and the universe. These ancient systems are often based on metaphors that describe naturally occurring, observable phenomena that are correlated with physical and psychologic function.

Western scientific study is no less colorful, and it weaves a tapestry of its own. It is a young discipline and will eventually reach the harmony of approaches evident in ancient practices. Western methods and ancient healing traditions are not in opposition; rather, they complement one another. Together, they blend ancient wisdom and current understanding as we strive for homeostasis. Because it is impossible to be knowledgeable about every aspect of every healing tradition in the world, it is always better to ask your clients what they think if you are not sure.

Access to texts that describe Eastern and native perspectives on health is beneficial. Those used in the development of this text are listed in the Works Consulted section at the end of this book; that is a good place to begin.

Professional practices, such as charting and writing reports, mandate proficiency in language usage, which is the basis of effective written and verbal communication.

✍ ACTIVITY 3-9

Synthesize the section that you just completed on charting and clinical reasoning by answering the following questions here or on a separate piece of paper. A shortened version of the analysis process is provided for this activity. There is no correct answer; rather, the exercise is intended to assist the student in developing the analytical and decision-making skills necessary in a professional practice. Each section has an example to help you get started.

Step 1

1. What are the facts?
2. What has worked or not worked?

Example

1. Charting is written communication (fact).
2. To chart effectively, a practitioner needs a knowledge base of medical terms and abbreviations and of anatomy and physiology (fact).

Your Turn

Give three more facts about charting and clinical reasoning.

1. _____
2. _____
3. _____

Step 2

1. What are the possibilities?
2. What does my intuition suggest?
3. What are other ways to look at the situation?
4. What do the data suggest?

Example

1. I may need to take a medical terminology class.
2. My instincts suggest that learning about assessment procedures is important.
3. I may need to be careful not to become too analytical.
4. The information suggests that further investigation of problem solving could be helpful.

Your Turn

Give three more possibilities.

1. _____
2. _____
3. _____

Step 3

1. What are the pros and cons?
2. What are the consequences of acting or not acting?

Example

1. The pros of charting include having a continuous log of progress.
2. A consequence of not charting would be a lack of information for reference and for reference by other professionals.

Your Turn

Provide three more consequences.

1. _____
2. _____
3. _____

Step 4

1. What would be the effect on the persons involved: client, practitioner, and other professionals working with the client? Does a feeling of cooperation and agreement exist among all parties?

Example

1. I would feel burdened with the paperwork and frustrated because of my spelling, but the client would feel a sense of caring.

Your Turn

Provide three more effects on the persons involved.

1. _____
2. _____
3. _____

Plan

Now that you have analyzed this information, write down your decisions about charting and problem solving, and then develop an implementation plan based on that decision.

Example

I have come to the conclusion that charting is important and that I need to learn more about it. I want to explore methods other than SOAP. I will need to research charting procedures, and a logical place to begin would be nursing or psychological charting systems. I will go to the library and check information on the computer about charting methods.

Your Turn

⊖volve

http://evolve.elsevier.com/Fritz/essential

3-1 Review the terminology in this chapter with electronic flashcards
3-2 Listen and spell: more terminology review
3-3 Take a memory quiz on the posterior region of the trunk
3-4 Take a memory quiz on the anterior region of the trunk
Additional Resources:
    Scientific Animations
    Weblinks
    Study Tips
    Electronic Coloring Book
Remember to study for your certification and licensure exams! Review questions for this chapter are located on Evolve.

REFERENCES

Chaitow L: *The acupuncture treatment of pain*, Rochester, VT, 1990, Healing Arts Press.

Dewey J: *How we think*, Lexington, Mass, 1982, Health (originally published in 1910).

Langevin HM, Bouffard NA, Badger GJ, et al: Subcutaneous tissue fibroblast cytoskeletal remodeling induced by acupuncture: evidence for a mechanotransduction-based mechanism, *J Cellular Physiol* 207(3):767, 2006.

Workbook Section

Short Answer

1. List and define the three word elements used in medical terms.

_____

_____

_____

_____

_____

2. Break the following words into their word elements, and give the meaning of each element. Then define the word.

Antiseptic _____

_____

_____

_____

Contralateral _____

_____

_____

Subaxillary _____

_____

_____

Neurogenic _____

_____

_____

Bradycardia _____

_____

_____

Neuralgia _____

_____

_____

Contraindication _____

_____

_____

_____

Periosteum _____

_____

_____

_____

Intracephalic _____

_____

_____

Arthroplasty _____

_____

_____

_____

3. Give the meanings of the following abbreviations:

ADL _____

ad lib _____

a.m.a. _____

ANS _____

as tol _____

BP _____

CC _____

c/o _____

Dx _____

h (hr) _____

H₂O _____

Hx _____

IBW _____

ICT _____

id _____

L _____

lig _____

M _____

ML _____

meds _____

n _____

NA _____

OTC _____

P _____

PA _____

PT _____

Px _____

R _____

R/O _____

ROM _____

Rx _____

SOB _____

SP, spir _____

Sym _____

T _____

TLC _____

Tx _____

WD _____

4. Define charting/documentation, and explain the problem-solving model of charting.

_____

_____

_____

_____

_____

5. In what ways do the Asian view and terminology act as a model of indigenous ancient healing practices? Compare the Asian discipline with Western theory and terminology.

_____

_____

_____
_____
_____
_____
_____
_____
_____

6. Write the terms used to describe the position of the body in relation to other body parts.

a. _____ In front of or toward the front of the body or body part

b. _____ Behind, in back of, or in the rear of the body or body part

c. _____ Situated away from the trunk or midline of the body; away from the origin

d. _____ On or to the side, outside, away from the midline

e. _____ Relating to the middle, center, or midline of the body

f. _____ Closer to the trunk or to the point of origin

g. _____ The same side

h. _____ The opposite side

i. _____ Toward the head

j. _____ Toward the tail

k. _____ Higher than or above

l. _____ Lower than or below

m. _____ The circumference or an area away from the center

n. _____ The palm side of the hand; also called palmar

o. _____ The sole side of the foot

p. _____ Bent inward; angulation of a part of the body inward toward the midline

q. _____ Bent outward; bent toward the wall

r. _____ Right

s. _____ Left

t. _____ The inside surface or the inside part of the body

u. _____ The outside surface of the body

v. _____ Far beneath the surface

w. _____ Toward or on the surface

x. _____ The wall of a part of the body

Fill in the Blank

A (1) _____ is part of a word. A (2) _____ is placed at the beginning of a word to alter the meaning of the word. A vowel added between two roots or a root and a suffix to make pronunciation easier is a (3) _____. The (4) _____ word element contains the basic meaning of the word, and the (5) _____ is placed at the end of a root to change the meaning of the word. A shortened form of a word or phrase is an (6)

_____. A (7) _____ is a written record of professional interactions representing a clinical reasoning methodology emphasizing a (8) _____ approach. The (9) _____ is a problem-oriented medical record, and (10) _____ is the acronym (subjective, objective, assessment/analysis, and plan) for the four parts of the written account of the health assessment.

(11) _____ normal daily living activity including self-care such as eating, bathing, dressing, grooming, going to work, housekeeping duties, and leisure activities. By definition, (12) _____ is the study of movement. Mechanical principles that relate directly to the human body are used in the study of (13) _____. (14) _____ is the dynamic balance between opposing forces and the continual process of creation and destruction within the natural order of the universe and of each person's inner being.

(15) _____ is the art and science of manipulating the flow of (16) _____, the basic life force. The patterns that acupuncture points make on the surface of the body have been charted by practitioners of acupuncture for centuries and are grouped together in lines called (17) _____ or (18) _____. In traditional Chinese medicine this system of points and meridians is known as (19) _____. (20) _____ are the fluids, essences, and energies that keep the mind, body, and spirit in balance. (21) _____ is the spirit. Moxibustion uses (22) _____ herbs placed on or near the body to stimulate specific acupuncture points. Unlike the Western concept of organs, Chinese medicine thinks in terms of an (23) _____, which comprises an organ, essences, and fluids as they interact with the meridians.

(24) _____ is an ancient Chinese art of exercise and meditation that supports homeostasis. The Seven Emotions are (25) _____, _____, _____, _____, _____, and _____.

Heat, cold, wind, dampness, dryness, and summer heat are known as the (26) _____. The Seven Emotions and the Six Pernicious Influences are internal triggers of disharmony in (27) _____.

The (28) _____ are five basic processes or phases of a cycle that represent inherent capabilities of change. The Five Elements are (29) _____, _____, _____, _____, and _____.

A (30) _____ is a method of measurement using a relative standard of size and spacing on an individual, regardless of size or shape.

Problem Solving

Analyze the following situation using the problem-solving model, and complete the exercise at the end.

Agreement on terminology is an abiding issue in the sharing of information. Many times, professionals are speaking of the same process, methodology, or diagnosis but approaching it from a different cultural and language base. In one study Mexican Americans refused medical treatment because their explanation of the disease process was discounted. If cultural differences were better understood, such problems might not arise. As researchers and health professionals take a serious look at ancient forms of healing, and as more validity is given to noninvasive methods such as massage, some sort of common language base must be found or we will be unable to speak to one another. Consumers, meanwhile, will remain confused and unable to make informed decisions about the services they want to use. In all these approaches, the body remains the same. Anatomy and physiology do not change.

In the following exercise, the first statement is provided as a guide. Fill in at least two more statements.

Facts
1. Terminology is an abiding issue in the sharing of information.
2. _____
3. _____

Possibilities
1. Schools could teach more cross-cultural terminology.
2. _____
3. _____

Logical Cause and Effect
1. If schools expanded their curricula, more teachers and textbooks would be needed, and the cost of education would rise.
2. _____
3. _____

Effect
1. Persons may find their spiritual belief systems challenged in the study of healing disciplines in which a spiritual practice has an intrinsic part, and they may feel uncomfortable with these philosophies.
2. _____
3. _____

What can you do as a professional to bridge the communication gap?
_____
_____
_____
_____
_____
_____
_____
_____
_____

Quality-of-Life–Based, Massage-Related Outcome Goals

Develop at least three massage-related outcome goals that are related to a client's perception of quality of life.

Example
Reduce use of over-the-counter nonsteroidal antiinflammatory drugs for tension headache by 50%. _____
_____
_____
_____
_____
_____

Assess Your Competencies

Review the following objectives for this chapter:
1. Identify the importance of terminology essential for the practice of therapeutic massage.
2. Use medical terminology to interpret the meanings of anatomic and physiologic terms.
   • Identify three word elements used in medical terms.
   • Use a medical dictionary.
   • Combine word elements into medical terms.
   • Identify abbreviations used in health care and their meanings.
3. Define terms used to describe regions of the body and surface anatomy.
4. Define terms used to describe the positions of the body and the parts of the body in relation to other body parts.
5. Define kinesiology, body planes, and terms of movements.
   • Explain the structural plan of the human body.
   • Identify regions of the body and surface anatomy.
   • Locate abdominal quadrants and regions.
   • Use proper terms to indicate the positions of the body.
   • Use directional terms to describe the relationship of one body area to another.
   • Define kinesiology.
   • Define the body planes, and demonstrate the movements that occur in each plane.
   • Name and demonstrate movement terms.
6. Describe and use quality-of-life terminology.
   • Define quality of life.
   • Use quality-of-life terminology in massage practice.
7. Explore terminology used in indigenous and cultural-based healing systems.
   • Explain indigenous health care systems.
   • Explain the role of intuition in traditional health care systems.
   • Identify terminology from an ancient Chinese healing model.
   • Compare terminology used in various healing traditions.
8. Use a charting method that incorporates a clinical reasoning/problem-solving model.

- Describe critical thinking.
- Explain how critical thinking is used in clinical reasoning.
- List the qualities of a critical thinker.
- Describe a problem-oriented medical record.
- Use a SOAP note system to support critical thinking and clinical reasoning.

Next, on a separate piece of paper or using an audio or video recorder, prepare a short narrative that reflects how you would explain this content to a client and how the information relates to how you would provide massage. See the example in Chapter 1 on p. 22. When read or listened to, the narrative should not take more than 5 to 10 minutes to complete. Simpler is better. Use examples, tell stories, and use metaphors. It is important to understand that there is no precisely correct way to complete this exercise. The intent is to help you identify how effectively you understand the content and how relevant your application is to massage therapy. An excellent learning activity is to work with other students and share your narratives. Also share these narratives with a friend or family member who is not familiar with the content. If that person can understand what you have written or recorded, that indicates that you understand it. There are many different ways to complete this learning activity. Yes, it may be confusing to do this, but that's all right. Out of confusion comes clarity. By the time you do this 12 times, once for each chapter in this book, you will be much more competent.

Further Study

Using additional resource material, do some research on one other ancient healing practice. Identify the major components of the discipline, and correlate it with the Western model presented in this text. Pay particular attention to the following elements:

Healing practice

_____
_____
_____

Soft-tissue methods

_____
_____
_____

Movement and exercise

_____
_____
_____

Meditation and inner reflection

_____
_____
_____

Dietary influences

_____
_____
_____

Use of naturally occurring herbs for medicinal purposes

_____
_____
_____

Emotional influences

_____
_____
_____

Spiritual connections

_____
_____
_____

Metaphor based on naturally occurring phenomenon

_____
_____
_____

Correlation with Western scientific theories

_____
_____
_____
_____

Answers to Activity 3-2

am: morning
Hx: history
ADL: activities of daily living
ad lib: as desired
CC: chief complaint
GI: gastrointestinal
ABD: abdominal
meds: medications
ROM: range of motion
as tol: as tolerated
h: hour
PT: physical therapy
ft: foot (or feet)
R: respiration
T: temperature
P: pulse
pm: Afternoon
H_2O: water
TLC: tender loving care
OB: obstetrics

CHAPTER

4

Nervous System Basics and the Central Nervous System

e http://evolve.elsevier.com/Fritz/essential

CHAPTER OBJECTIVES

After completing this chapter, the student will be able to perform the following:

1. Describe the basic organization of the nervous system.
2. Describe the anatomy of the neuron and neuroglia.
3. Describe the physiology of the neuron and neuroglia.
4. Explain the relationship between neurochemicals and behavior, including pain behavior.
5. Identify the structures and functions of the brain.
6. Identify the structures and functions of the spinal cord.
7. List drugs that affect the central nervous system.
8. Describe common pathologic conditions of the central nervous system and the related indications/contraindications for massage.

CHAPTER OUTLINE

NERVOUS SYSTEM BASICS: OVERVIEW OF THE NERVOUS
SYSTEM, 100
Nervous System Functions, 100
Nervous System Divisions, 100
Nervous System Structure, 100
NERVE CELL STRUCTURE, 101
Neurons, 101
Neuroglia, 102
NERVE CELL FUNCTIONS, 103
Membrane Potential, 103
Nerve Impulse, 104
Synapses and Neurotransmitters, 105
Role of Neurotransmitters, 106
Body Chemistry of Behavior and Pain Behavior, 106
Pain Behavior, 109
CENTRAL NERVOUS SYSTEM, 111
Brain, 111
Spinal Cord, 121
PATHOLOGIC CONDITIONS, 123
Drugs Affecting Central Nervous System Function, 123
Pathologic Conditions, 124
SUMMARY, 128

KEY TERMS

Amyotrophic lateral sclerosis (a-MI-o-TROF-ik) Also called *Lou Gehrig disease.* A progressive disease that begins in the central nervous system and involves the degeneration of motor neurons and the subsequent atrophy of voluntary muscle.

Ascending tracts Tracts in the spinal cord that carry sensory information to the brain.

Axon (AK-son) A single elongated projection from a nerve cell body that transmits impulses away from the cell body.

Brain The largest and most complex unit of the nervous system; the brain is responsible for perception, sensation, emotion, intellect, and action.

Brainstem The inferior, primitive portion of the brain that contains centers for vital functions and reflex actions, such as vomiting, coughing, sneezing, posture, and basic movement patterns.

Catecholamine (cat·e-CHOL·amine) Any of several compounds occurring naturally in the body that serve as hormones or as neurotransmitters in the sympathetic nervous system.

Central nervous system The brain and spinal cord and their coverings.

Cerebellum (sair-e-BELL-um) The second largest part of the brain; the cerebellum is involved with balance, posture, coordination, and movement.

Cerebrospinal fluid (sair-e-bro-SPY-nal) A clear, colorless fluid that flows throughout the brain and around the spinal cord, cushioning and protecting these structures and maintaining proper pH balance.

Cerebrum (se-REE-brum) The largest of the brain divisions; the cerebrum consists of two hemispheres that occupy the uppermost region of the cranium. The cerebrum receives, interprets, and associates incoming information with past memories and then transmits the appropriate motor response.

Dendrites (DEN-drites) Branching projections from the nerve cell body that carry signals to the cell body.

Descending tracts Tracts in the spinal cord hat carry motor information from the brain to the spinal cord.

Dorsal root Also called the *posterior root.* Posterior attachment of a spinal nerve to the spinal cord. Transmits sensory information into the spinal cord.

Enteric nervous system (en-TER–rik) (ENS) A subdivision of the peripheral nervous system (PNS) that controls the digestive system.

Essential tremor A chronic tremor that does not proceed from any other pathologic condition.

Gray matter Unmyelinated nervous tissue in the central nervous system.

Monoplegia (mon-o-PLE-je-a) Paralysis of a single limb or a single group of muscles.

Myelin (MY-e-lin) A white, fatty, insulating substance formed by the Schwann cells that surrounds some axons. Also produced in the central nervous system by oligodendrocytes.

Evolve Activity 4-1

Neurolemma (noo-ri-LEM-mah) Also called *Schwann's membrane, sheath of Schwann,* and *endoneural membrane.* The outer cell membrane of a Schwann cell that encloses the myelin sheath found on certain peripheral nerves. Essential in the regeneration of injured axons.

Neuroglia (noo-ROG-lee-ah) Specialized connective tissue cells that support, protect, and hold neurons together.

Neurons (NOO-ronz) Nerve cells that conduct impulses.

Neurotransmitters (noo-ro-TRANS-mit-erz) Chemical compounds that generate action potentials when released into the synapses from presynaptic cells.

Paraplegia (par-a-PLEE-je-a) Paralysis of the lower portion of the body and of both legs.

Quadriplegia (quad-ra-PLEE-je-a) Paralysis or loss of movement of all four limbs.

Schwann cell (shwon) A specialized cell that forms myelin.

Spinal cord The portion of the central nervous system that exits the skull and extends into the vertebral column. The two major functions of the spinal cord are to conduct nerve impulses and to be a center for spinal reflexes.

Status epilepticus (ep-i-LEP-TIK-us) A medical emergency characterized by a continuous seizure lasting longer than 30 minutes.

Synapse (SIN-aps) A space between neurons or between a neuron and an effector organ.

Ventral root Also called the *anterior root.* Anterior attachment of a spinal nerve to the spinal cord. Transmits motor information away from the spinal cord. One of two roots that attach a spinal nerve to the spinal cord.

White matter Myelinated nerve tissue in the central nervous system.

LEARNING HOW TO LEARN

In this chapter we begin to use the terms and concepts described in the first three chapters. This will help you review what you have learned so far. We will also begin to study a body system, including all of the parts (anatomy), how it works (physiology), and what can go wrong (pathology). There are new terms as well. Learning involves more than memorizing the definitions of the words and being able to identify the parts. Each body system has a specific job in the body. You can begin to use metaphors, examples, and stories to help you learn.

A metaphor is when we relate a quality or characteristic to a person or thing by using a name, image, adjective, or other word normally used for something else to which it is similar. For example: The central nervous system is your body's computer.

"This is like that" is an example of a simile. For instance, the nerves are like the electrical wires in a house.

Stories let you connect the information together. For example: Once upon a time there was a meeting of the nervous system and the endocrine system because of confusion about who did what. The person that used these body systems was not able to sleep. The nervous system was blaming the endrocrine system for too many hormones, and the endrocrine system was blaming the nervous system for being on alert all the time....

It does not matter if the stories are silly.

This is the first chapter in the Systems of Control unit, which consists of Chapters 4, 5, and 6. Chapter 4 provides an introduction to the nervous system in general and then concentrates on the central nervous system. Chapter 5 covers the peripheral nervous system, and Chapter 6 the endocrine system. This content is placed right after the first unit, Fundamentals (Chapters 1, 2, and 3) because the nervous system and the endocrine system act as the main regulators of the body. These systems monitor processes and coordinate body functions. The nervous and endocrine systems receive information, decide what to do, and then tell the rest of the body what to do with it. Systems of control coordinate the smooth function of the rest of the body's systems to maintain homeostasis. Combined, Chapters 1, 2, and 3 have provided enough of a foundation so you can understand how the nervous and endocrine systems perform their important monitoring and regulating functions.

The nervous and endocrine systems transmit information from one part of the body to another, but they do it in different ways. The nervous system transmits information rapidly with a short duration of action by nerve impulses conducted from one body area to another. The endocrine system is a network of ductless glands and other structures that secrete chemicals called *hormones* directly into the bloodstream, affecting the function of specific target organs. The action of hormones is slower and longer lasting than that of nerve impulses. Often, the nervous system initiates a response and the endocrine system sustains it.

However, both systems use chemicals. The nervous system uses **neurotransmitters,** which are chemicals that cross a synapse. A **synapse** is a gap between a neuron and another neuron, muscle cell, or gland. Neurotransmitters carry nerve impulses across synapses. As previously discussed, the endocrine system uses hormones. Many times hormones are the same chemicals. If the chemical is found in the synapses it is called a *neurotransmitter.* If the same chemical is found in the blood, it is called a hormone.

The influence of the nervous system regulates the endocrine system, and the endocrine system influences the nervous system, forming a feedback loop that increases or decreases activity for healthy function. The feedback system and autoregulation, or maintenance of internal homeostasis, are interlinked in all body functions.

As you learn this content, remember that you are learning a new language. Learning all the words, what they mean, and how they are applicable to massage therapy takes effort (Box 4-1). Keep in mind that you may have to review the content

---

Box 4-1 Effort

Effort: derived from French words *esforz* and *esforcier,* meaning "to force out and exert oneself."

"All growth depends upon an activity. There is no development physically or intellectually without effort, and effort means work." —Calvin Coolidge

"Continuous effort—not strength or intelligence—is the key to unlocking our potential." —Winston Churchill

"Education comes from within; you get it by struggle and effort and thought." —Napoleon Hill

"It is astonishing what an effort it seems to be for many people to put their brains definitely and systematically to work." —Thomas A. Edison

"The one thing that matters is the effort." —Antoine de Saint-Exupery

"A little more persistence, a little more effort, and what seemed hopeless failure may turn to glorious success." —Elbert Hubbard

"If I am a cup maker, I'm interested in making the best cup I possibly can. My effort goes into that cup, not what people think about it." —Denzel Washington

"I was determined that if I failed it wouldn't be due to lack of effort." —Heston Blumenthal

"Effort is only effort when it begins to hurt." —Jose Ortega y Gasset

more than once. The Evolve site has review activities and links to other websites that you can use to help integrate this information into the way you think as a massage therapist. This will help you develop critical thinking and clinical reasoning skills.

NERVOUS SYSTEM BASICS: OVERVIEW OF THE NERVOUS SYSTEM

SECTION OBJECTIVES

Chapter objectives covered in this section:
1. Describe the basic organization of the nervous system.
After completing this section, the student will be able to perform the following:
- List the two main divisions of the nervous system.
- List the two main subdivisions of the peripheral nervous system.
- Describe the basic functions of the autonomic nervous system.
- List and define three types of nerve cells.

Nervous System Functions

The nervous system is the most complex of the body systems. There are three main functions of the nervous system:
- Sensing: Collecting data from the environment
- Interpreting: Processing data and formulating a response
- Acting: Telling the body to perform the response

Nervous System Divisions

The nervous system is divided into the following:
- **Central nervous system** (CNS), which is composed of the brain, spinal cord, and coverings
- Peripheral nervous system (PNS), which includes the cranial nerves, spinal nerves, and ganglia
  The PNS has two main subdivisions. These subdivisions combine and communicate to innervate the somatic and visceral parts of the body:
- Somatic: The somatic subdivision monitors and controls bones, muscles, soft tissues, and skin. The word *somatic* is derived from the Greek *somatikos,* meaning "of the body."

- Autonomic: The visceral or autonomic subdivision is associated with the internal glands, organs, blood vessels, and mucous membranes. The word *viscera,* from Latin, is plural of *viscus,* meaning "internal organ." *Autonomic* is from the Greek word *autonomia,* meaning "independence." When you combine the meanings, you get independence of internal organs. The autonomic nervous system was so named because it was originally believed to act independently. However, although it does operate without conscious control, it is actually regulated by parts of the brain.

The autonomic nervous system (ANS) is divided further into the following:
- The sympathetic aspect of the ANS activates arousal responses and expends body resources in response to emergencies, excitement, or exercise. The sympathetic ANS is considered the "flight, fight, fear" system, but any highly emotional state of joy, excitement, or elation is also sympathetic in nature.
- The parasympathetic aspect of the ANS reverses the response of the sympathetic ANS by returning the body to a non-alarm state and restoring body resources. The parasympathetic ANS is considered the "rest and digest" system.

Enteric Nervous System: A Division of the Autonomic Nervous System

Some experts have defined a third aspect of the ANS called the *enteric nervous system. Enteric* means "pertaining to the intestines" and is derived from the Greek word *enterikos,* meaning "intestinal." The **enteric nervous system (ENS)** is a subdivision of the ANS that directly controls the digestive system.

The ENS has been called the "little brain in the gut." It is a network of nerves that is mainly located in the wall of the intestines. It is believed that the ENS contains as many neurons as the entire spinal cord. It also contains multiple plexi, which are groups of intertwined nerves that function together. A large nerve, the vagus nerve, is a cranial nerve that comes directly from the brain. It supplies most of the abdominal viscera, among other structures and organs. The vagus nerve plays an important role in ENS functions (Figure 4-1, Activity 4-1).

Much of the interaction between body and mind takes place through ANS activity. Most indigenous health traditions do not separate the body/mind connection. The concepts of yin and yang are reflected in the ANS, with parasympathetic functions relating to yin and sympathetic functions relating to yang.

Nervous System Structure

The basic structure of the nervous system is the neuron, or nerve cell. The nervous system is composed of more than 100 billion nerve cells. The nerve cell is an impulse-transmitting fiber connecting the CNS with all parts of the body through the PNS. The three basic types of neurons are as follows:
1. Afferent or sensory neurons that carry impulses to the CNS
2. Connecting or associative interneurons that transmit nerve impulses between neurons
3. Efferent or motor neurons that transmit impulses away from the CNS to muscles, organs, and glands

✎ ACTIVITY **4-1**

Study the figure and flow chart. Then, on a separate piece of paper, draw the figure and chart to see how much you recall.

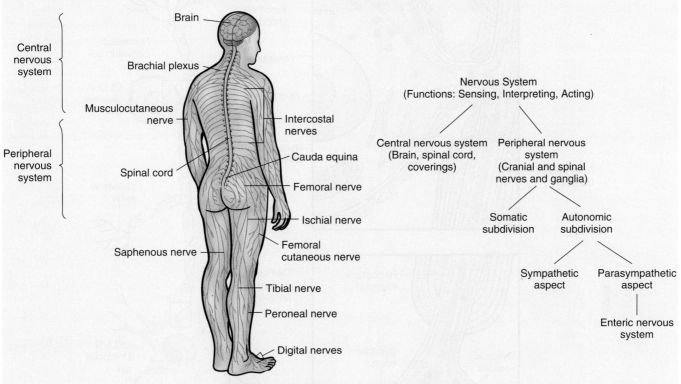

FIGURE 4-1 The divisions of the nervous system.

Practical Application

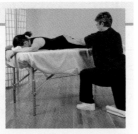

When we give a massage, we are communicating with the sensory neurons. They are receptors. No matter how quickly, slowly, or deeply massage is applied, it activates sensory nerves that send information to the spinal cord and brain. Here the information is interpreted and a decision is made about how to respond to the information. That decision is then sent back to the rest of the body, where commands are issued, such as, "release some chemicals here," "increase circulation there," or "stop contracting and relax." What the body does with the sensory information produced by massage ends up being either a benefit of massage or some sort of adverse outcome.

NERVE CELL STRUCTURE

SECTION OBJECTIVES

Chapter objectives covered in this section:
2. Describe the anatomy of the neuron and neuroglia.
After completing this section, the student will be able to perform the following:
- Describe the two cells in the nervous system.
- Define neurons.
- List the parts of the neuron.
- Define neuroglia.

Two types of cells are found in the nervous system: neuron and neuroglia.

Neurons

Neurons are nerve cells. The function of the neurons is to receive and transmit electrical signals from and to other neurons, muscles, or glands (Figure 4-2). Nerve cells consist of a cell body and its nerve fibers, the axons and dendrites. The cell body contains a nucleus and its organelles. The **dendrites,** which look like small hairs, are extensions of the cytoplasm of the cell. Their job is to receive signals and carry them to the cell body. The **axon** is an elongated projection that carries signals away from the cell body. An axon may have branches (known as *collaterals*) that allow communication among several neurons.

Neurons are identified by structure or functions (Box 4-2; see also Figure 4-2). The simplest way to classify neurons is on the basis of function. A sensory neuron detects stimuli from the internal environment, such as a decrease in water levels of the blood, and from the external environment, such as the warmth of the sun on the skin. These neurons send this information into the CNS. Interneurons, or connecting or association neurons, integrate the sensory information. They analyze it, store some of it, and make a decision for appropriate responses. Motor neurons carry nerve impulses from the CNS out to effectors (muscles and glands) in response to decisions made by the CNS.

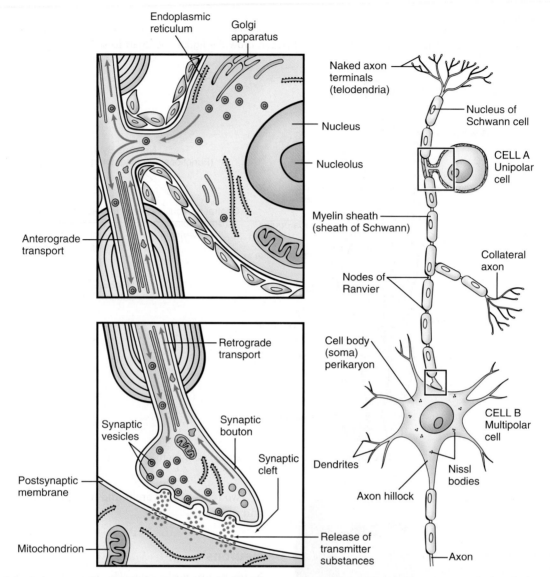

FIGURE 4-2 A typical neuron. An electrical impulse travels along the axon of the first neuron to the synapse. A chemical transmitter is secreted into the synaptic cleft to depolarize the membrane (dendrite or cell body) of the next neuron in the pathway.

Stimulation of the effectors causes muscles to contract and glands to secrete.

Unipolar and bipolar neurons are usually sensory neurons. Multipolar neurons are usually motor neurons or interneurons.

Neuroglia

Neuroglia are specialized connective-tissue cells. The word **neuroglia** means "nerve glue." They provide physical support, protection, insulation, and nutrient exchange pathways between blood and the neurons of the brain and spinal cord. The four types of neuroglia found in the CNS are as follows:

1. Ependymal cells line the walls of the ventricles and form the epithelium, which secretes the **cerebrospinal fluid (CSF).**
2. Astrocytes provide physical and nutritional support for neurons, digest parts of dead neurons, and regulate content of extracellular space.
3. Oligodendrocytes provide the insulation (**myelin**) to neurons in the CNS.
4. Microglia digest parts of dead neurons.

In the PNS Schwann cells form **myelin,** a fatty, insulating protective sheath around the axons of certain neurons. The outer layer of the **Schwann cell** encloses the myelin sheath and is called the **neurolemma.** The neurolemma plays a role in regenerating an injured axon.

Satellite cells surround cell bodies of PNS neurons, enclosing them in structures called *ganglia.* Therefore ganglia are small bundles of nerve cells found in the body (Figure 4-3).

Nerve Repair or Regeneration

If a neuron cell body is damaged, the neuron dies. However, in the PNS if damage occurs only to the axon of a neuron and the neurolemma is not destroyed, the nerve can repair itself. At the point of injury, the myelin sheath and the distal portion of the axon degenerate. A tunnel is formed by the neurolemma from the point of injury to the original destination of the

Box 4-2   **Neurons: Classification by Structure or by Function**

Three structural classifications of neurons:

1. Neurons that only have one projection to form the cell body that includes both the dendrite and axon are called unipolar.

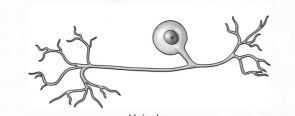

Unipolar

2. Neurons that have only one dendrite and the axon are called *bipolar neurons.*

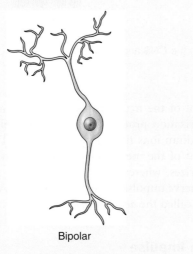

Bipolar

3. Neurons that have multiple dendrites and one axon exiting from the cell body are called *multipolar neurons.*

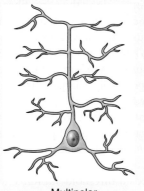

Multipolar

The three functional classifications of neurons are as follows:

1. Sensory or afferent neurons conduct sensory signals to the central nervous system.
2. Interneurons, or connecting or association neurons, act as bridges in the central nervous system to conduct signals from one neuron to another.
3. Motor or efferent neurons conduct motor signals away from the central nervous system to effectors.

axon—another axon, a muscle, or a gland. This tunnel provides a path for the axon to follow as it regenerates. Nerve regeneration can take a long time; just how long is determined by the length of the axon, the location of the injury, the inflammatory response, and the amount of scarring.

In the CNS oligodendrocytes do not create myelin the same way as occurs in the PNS. There is no neurolemma, so no tunnel forms that can guide regrowth of the axon from the injury site. Therefore regeneration in the CNS is limited (Figure 4-4). However, extensive and exciting research is occurring in the area of CNS regeneration and nerve growth factors. In the near future, scientists may identify nerve growth factors that can be used to assist those with spinal cord and brain injuries.

NERVE CELL FUNCTIONS

SECTION OBJECTIVES

Chapter objectives covered in this section:

3. Describe the physiology of the neuron and neuralgia.
4. Explain the relationship between neurochemicals and behavior, including pain behavior.

After completing this section, the student will be able to perform the following:

- Define membrane potential.
- Describe nerve impulse.
- Explain nerve impulse conduction.
- Describe a synapse.
- Describe neurotransmitter functions.
- List common neurotransmitters and other neurochemicals.
- Describe the function of neurochemicals.
- Explain the relationship between neurochemicals and behavior.
- Relate brain chemistry to behavior.

Membrane Potential

Neurons send messages electrochemically. This means that chemicals cause an electrical signal. Chemicals in the body that are electrically charged are called *ions.* Ions can have a positive (+) or negative (−) charge.

A membrane potential, meaning that a nerve impulse could potentially be generated, is created by the different concentration of ions in the fluids inside the neuron and around the outside of the neuron. Sodium ions (Na+) tend to concentrate in the extracellular fluid (outside the cell), and the cell membrane does not allow them to flow into the cell. Potassium ions (K+) predominate inside the cell membrane. When a neuron is at rest, the outside of its cell membrane is positively charged, whereas the inside of the cell is negatively charged. This difference is called the *membrane potential,* and the cell is said to be polarized, meaning that the ions with the negative pole are outside the cell and the ions with the positive pole are inside the cell.

A neuron that is not stimulated but is polarized has a resting potential. This means the neuron is not doing anything; it is resting. However, if it receives a sufficiently strong stimulus, it will generate an impulse.

A stimulus, such as a pressure, light, temperature, or chemical change, results in a brief change in the charge of one

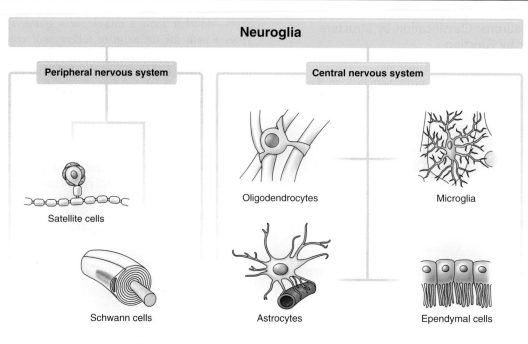

FIGURE 4-3 Types of neuroglia found in the CNS and PNS.

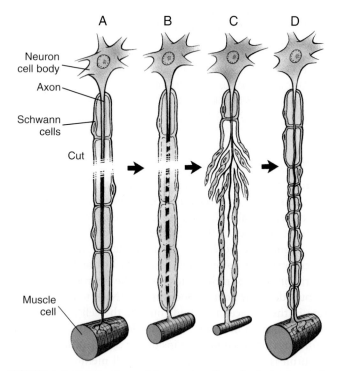

FIGURE 4-4 Repair of a peripheral nerve fiber. **A,** An injury results in a cut nerve. **B,** Immediately after the injury occurs, the distal portion of the axon degenerates, as does its myelin sheath. **C,** The remaining neurolemma tunnels from the point of injury to the effector. New Schwann cells grow within this tunnel, maintaining a path for regrowth of the axon. Meanwhile, several growing axon sprouts appear. When one of these growing fibers reaches the tunnel, it increases its growth rate, growing as much as 3 to 5 mm per day. (The other sprouts eventually disappear.) **D,** The connection of the neuron with the effector is reestablished. (From Patton KT, Thibodeau GA: *Anatomy and physiology,* ed 7, St Louis, 2010, Mosby.)

segment of the neuron; this is called *depolarization.* During depolarization protein channels in the cell membrane open and sodium ions flood into the neuron. The outside of that segment of the membrane becomes negatively charged as it depolarizes, whereas the inside becomes positively charged and a nerve impulse is created. This flip in charges as the ions flow is called the *action potential,* or *nerve impulse.*

Nerve Impulse

An action potential, or nerve impulse, is a progressive wave of electric and chemical activity along a nerve fiber. As the electrical signal continues along the nerve fiber, the nerve impulse depolarizes the next section, causing it to reverse its charges while the previous segment returns to its original polarity or is repolarized. When the nerve segment repolarizes, sodium channels close and potassium channels open, the outside again becomes positively charged, and the inside becomes negatively charged.

The term *excited* is used to describe the segment as the positive and negative charges flip with the action potential, and the term *inhibited* describes the reversal of that action (Figure 4-5).

A neuron needs a threshold stimulus, the minimum level of stimulus needed, to trigger the opening of the first sodium channel. Once that occurs, an "all-or-none" principle applies, meaning that once an impulse starts, it continues down the entire length of the axon; it does not stop partially along the way.

After transmitting an impulse, the neuron cannot immediately fire again; it needs time for the sodium and potassium to return to the original location and repolarize the membrane. This time is called the *refractory period.* The refractory period is the brief period after inhibition when the neuron

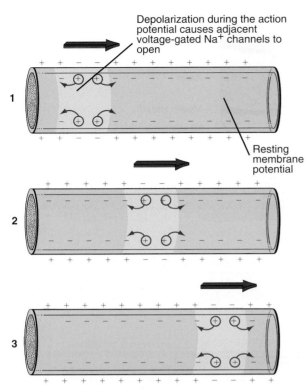

Depolarization during the action potential causes adjacent voltage-gated Na+ channels to open

Resting membrane potential

FIGURE 4-5 Conduction of the action potential. The reverse polarity characteristic of the peak of the action potential causes local current flow to adjacent regions of the membrane *(small arrows)*. This stimulates the voltage-gated Na+ channels to open and thus creates a new action potential. This cycle continues, producing wavelike conduction of the action potential from point to point along a nerve fiber. Adjacent regions of membrane behind the action potential do not polarize again because they are still in their refractory period. (From Thibodeau GA, Patton KT: *Anatomy and physiology,* ed 6, St Louis, 2007, Mosby.)

recovers. The absolute refractory period is the time during which a neuron will not respond to any stimuli. This is followed by the relative refractory period, when the neuron will respond only to a strong stimulus.

Nerve Impulse Conduction

The path of the nerve impulse is different in myelinated (insulated) and unmyelinated nerve fibers. Myelinated nerve fiber conduction is faster than in unmyelinated fibers. In the PNS myelin has gaps in the insulation where the actual nerve is exposed. These gaps, called *nodes of Ranvier,* occur at regular intervals along the length of the nerve fiber. The electrical impulse jumps from gap to gap, greatly decreasing the length of time it takes to travel down the axon. This is called *saltatory conduction.* The term *saltare* means "to dance" and is used to describe the signal jumping from one gap to the next (Figure 4-6).

Synapses and Neurotransmitters

Recall that nerves transmit both electrical and chemical signals. Also recall that the space or junction between two neurons or a neuron and an effector organ is called a *synapse.*

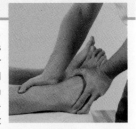

Practical Application

Therapeutic massage methods, such as muscle energy techniques and proprioceptive neuromuscular facilitation, use the refractory period to their advantage. Muscles often resist lengthening by initiating a protective spasm. If the muscle is first contracted and then lengthened, it is less likely to spasm during the refractory period, and the muscle can be restored more easily to a more normal resting length. Because these periods are short, gentle applications of lengthening procedures must be used. Methods that generate any sort of strong stimuli, especially pain, must be avoided. If too strong a stimulus is introduced, instead of relaxing, the muscle will generate nerve impulses and contract, thus resisting any sort of lengthening or stretching methods.

An effector organ produces an effect in response to nerve stimulation.

In a synapse, various chemicals called *neurotransmitters* are used to transfer the impulse across the gap to the next cell. To cross the gap, an electrical signal is transformed to a chemical signal. The neuron sending the signal is referred to as *presynaptic* because it is before the synapse, whereas the neuron or effector organ receiving the signal is postsynaptic, or after the synapse. The actual space in the synapse is called the *synaptic cleft* (Figure 4-7).

At the end of the axon of the presynaptic neuron, small sacs, or vesicles, are present. The vesicles contain neurotransmitters. The vesicles release neurotransmitters in response to the nerve impulse. Once released, these chemicals cross the synaptic cleft and bind with specific receptor sites on the postsynaptic neuron or effector organ. This will either generate another action potential and the nerve impulse continues, or it will prevent another action potential and the nerve impulse stops. This is how, for example, muscle contraction is controlled. Some muscles are stimulated to contract and others are inhibited from contracting, ensuring smooth, sequential movements. Another way to think of this is that the two actions, stimulation and inhibition, work the same way as the gas pedal and brakes in a car.

Neurotransmitters that cause the action potential to be transmitted across the synaptic cleft are considered stimulatory neurotransmitters. Those that slow or prevent the transmission of the action potential are inhibitory neurotransmitters.

Vesicles can store thousands of neurotransmitter molecules. After the neurotransmitters bind and their action is completed, they are broken down immediately by enzymes. They diffuse out of the synaptic cleft or are reabsorbed by the axons. This ensures that only one action potential is transmitted by the release of one portion of neurotransmitters.

In certain instances, medication may be used to interrupt the cycle by stopping the metabolism of the neurotransmitter. It does this by preventing binding to the postsynaptic membrane or by slowing the reabsorption of the neurotransmitter into the presynaptic vesicles.

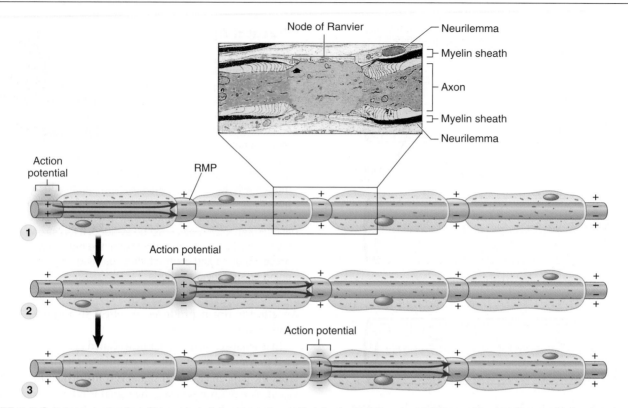

FIGURE 4-6 Saltatory conduction. This series of diagrams shows that the insulating nature of the myelin sheath prevents ion movement everywhere but at the nodes of Ranvier. The action potential at one node triggers current flow *(arrows)* across the myelin sheath to the next node, producing an action potential there. The action potential thus seems to leap rapidly from node to node. The *inset* is a transmission electron micrograph showing a node of Ranvier in a myelinated fiber. *RMP,* Resting membrane potential. (From Patton KT, Thibodeau GA: *Anatomy and physiology,* ed 7, St Louis, 2010, Mosby.)

Role of Neurotransmitters

Neurotransmitters regulate many of the body's activities and senses. At present, more than 50 neurotransmitters have been identified, and many more are suspected to exist. When released into the bloodstream, many of these same chemicals are called *hormones.* Some of the known hormones are thought to work as neurotransmitters, implying a close link between the nervous system and endocrine activity.

Neurotransmitters have three basic chemical categories: amino acids, amines, and peptides. Even a gas such as nitrous oxide can be a neurotransmitter. There are small differences in the actions of these chemicals. For example, peptide chemicals are more complex and can cause a longer effect in the nervous system than a more simple amino acid can.

To be classified as a neurotransmitter, a chemical must have certain characteristics. These characteristics include being found in presynaptic vesicles, being able to be removed from the synaptic cleft, and being capable of stimulating a nerve impulse. Also, it is important to appreciate that it is the receptor that dictates the neurotransmitter's effect.

There are neuromodulator chemicals as well. A neuromodulator chemical is a relatively new concept. A neuromodulator is like a neurotransmitter, but it is not reabsorbed by the presynaptic neuron or broken down in the synapse. Instead, neuromodulators spend a significant amount of time in influencing, or modulating, a nervous system activity. This can have long-lasting effects on the postsynaptic neuron's metabolic activity and on its response to subsequent input. Although many neurotransmitters act as neuromodulators, not all neuromodulators are neurotransmitters (Box 4-3).

Body Chemistry of Behavior and Pain Behavior

Behavior is affected by the type and amount of neurotransmitters released at the synaptic junction. Daily behaviors, such as those involved with pleasure, pain, and survival, are determined by the body's chemistry. Too little or too much of any one neurotransmitter or neuromodulator results in a behavior that takes extra effort to manage.

Behavior seems to be the outward manifestation of attempts at homeostasis, and we seek sensations that stimulate our brains. The issue is one of balance. Neurotransmitters and neuromodulators balance one another. Those that excite are usually paired with those that inhibit. An ongoing dynamic balance exists in this chemical soup, allowing for behavior that is resourceful for each situation encountered. When behavior is effective in achieving some sort of balance, it will be reinforced.

By observing behavior, we can make educated guesses about which neurochemicals are involved. If the behavior is

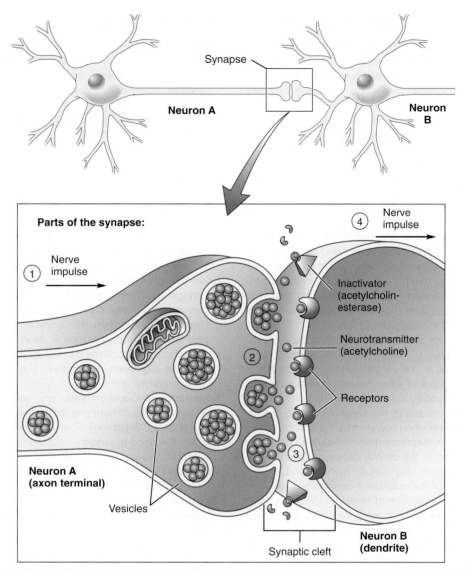

FIGURE 4-7 A synapse is the junction between two nerve cells or a nerve and an effector organ such as an endocrine gland or a muscle. The space in the synapse is called the *synaptic cleft*. (From Herlihy B: *The human body in health and illness,* ed 4, St Louis, 2011, Saunders.)

Practical Application

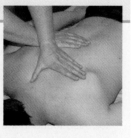

Many words have similar meanings, which can be confusing. Consider this list of terms: neurotransmitters, neuromodulators, neuroactive peptides, peptide transmitters, small-molecule transmitters, chemical messenger, neurochemical.

Neuropeptides are actually neuromodulators that bind to receptors and activate enzymes but are usually listed as neurotransmitters. Endorphin and the other endogenous (made in the body) opioids are considered neuromodulators in the CNS but are often found in neurotransmitter lists. Making this all even more complicated, many hormones that are endocrine chemicals are also considered neurotransmitters and neuromodulators.

Neurochemical refers to a chemical having a neural function. *Chemical messenger* is descriptive as well. This overlapping terminology is confusing when it comes to massage-related research. Some massage therapy research indicates that massage influences neurochemicals, and other research says massage does not affect neurochemicals. However, to interpret the research findings, it is necessary to know what neurochemicals are involved. Are they describing true neurotransmitters such as dopamine or GABA or neuromodulators such as endorphins? When you read research, it is important to know the terminology, even though it can be confusing.

Box 4-3   Important Neurochemicals, Their Primary Actions, and Their Locations

Acetylcholine: Acetylcholine stimulates the skeletal muscles and acts primarily on the parasympathetic nervous system. Acetylcholine can stimulate or inhibit various organs, depending on the receptors to which it is bound. Plentiful in the brain, the chemical is involved in memory. A lack of acetylcholine has been found in many patients diagnosed with Alzheimer's disease, although a cause-and-effect relationship has not yet been established. Myasthenia gravis, which is a disease that causes weakening of skeletal muscles, results from a low level of acetylcholine receptors.

Catecholamine: Several compounds occurring naturally in the body that act as or as neurotransmitters or hormones in the sympathetic nervous system. The catecholamines include epinephrine, norepinephrine, and dopamine. These neurochemicals play an important role in the body's physiologic response to stress and increase the rate and force of muscular contraction of the heart, increasing cardiac output; constrict peripheral blood vessels, increasing blood pressure; elevate blood glucose; and promote an increase in blood lipids by increasing the catabolism of fats.

Epinephrine: Epinephrine can be a stimulant or an inhibitor, depending on the type of receptor bound. Epinephrine is found in several areas of the central nervous system and in the sympathetic divisions of the autonomic nervous system. Epinephrine is also involved in fight-or-flight responses, such as dilation of blood vessels to the skeletal muscles, and is classified as a hormone when secreted by the adrenal gland.

Norepinephrine: Like epinephrine, norepinephrine can excite or inhibit and is found in the central nervous system (especially the hypothalamus and limbic system) and in the sympathetic division of the autonomic nervous system. Norepinephrine causes constriction of skeletal blood vessels, is considered a feel-good neurotransmitter, and is involved in emotional responses. The release of norepinephrine is enhanced by amphetamines. Cocaine stops the removal of norepinephrine from the synapses, such that stimulation of the synapses continues.

Dopamine: Generally excitatory, dopamine is found in the brain and the autonomic nervous system. A feel-good neurotransmitter, dopamine is involved in emotions and moods and in the regulation of motor control and the executive functioning of the brain. Release is enhanced by L-dopa and amphetamines. Deficiencies occur in people with Parkinson's disease and possibly also in those with schizophrenia. Dopamine is part of the endogenous reward/pleasure, craving/seeking behavior system in the brain. Many addictive drugs stimulate dopamine activity, including cocaine, narcotics, and alcohol.

Histamine: Considered a stimulant, histamine is released by the mast cells as part of the inflammatory process. Histamine causes itching at a cellular level and also works as a vasodilator. Also found in the hypothalamus, the chemical regulates body temperature and water balance and plays a role in emotions. Histamine also stimulates pain receptors to sensitize against further stimulation, as in the case of sunburn.

Serotonin: Serotonin usually works as an inhibitor in the central nervous system. It is synthesized into melatonin and affects biologic cycles, sleep, and moods. Insufficient levels can result in anxiety or depression. Serotonin is described as one of the feel-good neurotransmitters.

Gamma-Aminobutyric Acid (GABA): Generally inhibitory and found in the brain, this acid is the most common inhibitory neurotransmitter in the brain.

Glutamate (Glutamic Acid): Generally excitatory and found in the central nervous system, glutamate is thought to be responsible for as much as 75% of the excitatory signals in the brain.

Cholecystokinin: Found in the brain, retina, and gastrointestinal tract, the function of cholecystokinin in the nervous system is unclear and may be related to feeding behavior. Cholecystokinin is a gut-brain peptide.

Endorphins, Enkephalins, Endomorphins, Dynorphins: These endogenous morphines block the brain from feeling pain. Generally inhibitory, they are found in several regions of the central nervous system, retina, and intestinal tract. They inhibit pain by inhibiting substance P. Morphine and heroin mimic their effects. Endorphins and enkephalins seem to play a part in mood regulation, pain/pleasure cycles, and the internal reward system of the body.

Somatostatin: Generally inhibitory, somatostatin inhibits the release of growth hormone and is a gut-brain peptide.

Substance P: Substance P is excitatory and is found in the brain, spinal cord, sensory pain pathways, and gastrointestinal tract. Substance P transmits pain information.

Vasoactive Intestinal Peptide: Found in the brain, some autonomic nervous system and sensory fibers, retina, and the gastrointestinal tract; the function of this peptide in the nervous system is unclear. It plays an important role in the regulation of coronary blood flow, cardiac contraction and relaxation, and heart rate.

Oxytocin: Involved in complex emotional and social behaviors, including attachment, social recognition, aggression, and approach and avoidance behavior toward others. It reduces anxiety, increases feelings of trust, helps establish maternal behavior, and is associated with well-being in relationships. Touch causes the body to produce oxytocin, which produces the desire to touch and be touched. It is also involved with uterine contractions and lactation but as a hormone.

Phenylethylamine (PEA): Helps regulate mood, focus, and stress. Exercise seems to increase PEA levels, causes feelings of happiness, and relieves depression. It aids in the transmission of dopamine and norepinephrine and can enhance aggression.

Nitric oxide: A gas that supports transport of oxygen to the tissues and transmission of nerve impulses. It can function as a neurotransmitter involved in functions of blood flow to heart and erectile tissue (e.g., the penis), the sphincters in the gut, and formation of memory.

destructive, possibly we can introduce other forms of behavior that are less detrimental but result in similar neurotransmitter activity. It is important to recognize that repeated behavior is accomplishing some form of homeostasis—even destructive behavior such as drug addiction, excessive exercise, eating disorders, rage, thrill seeking, crisis orientation, and the deliberate creation of pain.

An attempt to eliminate one form of behavior without replacing it with another way of achieving effective homeostasis almost always results in failure and reversion to old behaviors. Consider the following examples:

Substituting binge eating with movement and aerobic exercise may work because the two operate from a similar neurochemical base. Eliminating binge eating without providing a substitute behavior leaves the individual without a way of achieving chemical balance in the brain and body.

Eating chocolate affects levels of serotonin and phenylethylamine (PEA) (as does the consumption of potato chips, ice cream, and cookies), which are feel-good neurotransmitters. Massage and exercise also stimulate feel good neurotransmitters. However, eating chocolate is faster and easier. Although chocolate may help a person feel good, if that is the only way that the person can feel good, other problems can arise, such as obesity and heart disease.

Changing a behavior from one that is quick and reliable to one that requires more effort is difficult for some people.

The statements "moderation in all things" and "variety is the spice of life" are important and wise advice as far as brain chemistry is concerned. Sprinkled into this mix of expressions are the highs and lows of ecstasy and despair; these feelings are important as well. This wisdom is found in most ancient healing practices. Having many different ways of feeling good is best.

Understanding what is causing us to feel bad is also important. When we can respond deliberately with our behavior to generate appropriate feelings in response to the situation being faced, instead of reacting and relying on only one type of behavior to meet our needs and cope, our neurochemicals work for us instead of against us.

When medication is used to manage various neurochemicals, mood and behavior are affected. The natural functions of the body allow for a wide range of behavior through continual adjustment of the balance among neurotransmitters, neuromodulators, and hormones. When neurochemical levels are held in a more static ratio by medication, it means that feelings, moods, and resultant behaviors are held within the expected parameters.

However, medication alters the ability to have the highs and lows of emotional expression appropriate to daily circumstances. Therefore compliance with taking psychotropic or mood-altering medication often is affected because many people enjoy emotional extremes. These people sometimes miss the range of emotional experiences and stop taking their medications as prescribed, often with devastating results. Careful monitoring by the physician can minimize this situation, but recognizing that it exists is also important (Box 4-4, Activity 4-2).

Box 4-4 Body Chemistry–Related Behaviors

We behave in certain ways to increase or decrease levels of neurotransmitters or hormones (e.g., eating or not eating because we are depressed; exercising or not exercising because we are anxious). On the flip side, if there is some sort of imbalance in the various neurochemicals, we may find ourselves behaving in ways we do not understand.

Extreme and novel behaviors have the biggest influence.

Soap operas are good examples. Little program content tells about day-to-day life in the midrange of emotional or behavioral expression. Television viewers seldom get caught up in stories about making the bed, changing the oil in the car, or going to the market.

Depression may follow when the release of catecholamines is blocked. Anxiety is aggravated by an increase in catecholamines. Have you ever been depressed or become all worked up about something that was really not that important? The depression lifts, and life goes on.

Researchers are currently investigating the effect of serotonin on migraine headaches.

Too much dopamine in the brain may result in hallucinations and can cause mildly erratic behavior, such as that displayed when a person first falls in love or when an extreme of schizophrenic behavior is occurring.

Dopamine levels are thought to be involved in attention deficit hyperactivity disorders.

The presence of cholecystokinin and vasoactive intestinal peptide in the eye and the stomach indicates that there is a connection between what we see and what we eat. These same neurochemicals are in the brain. Could this suggest a connection between food, behavior, and emotions? Anyone who has emotional issues around food certainly would not deny that the food we eat changes the way we feel and influences the behavior connected with those emotions.

The following questions are relevant:

Is the behavior the result of a neurochemical imbalance?

Is the behavior causing a neurochemical imbalance?

Is the behavior attempting to regulate a neurochemical imbalance?

Is the behavior normal but occurring at the wrong time?

Is the behavior normal for the situation?

Pain Behavior

Pain is a protective device for the body and is therefore important to survival. *Pain behavior* refers to the way we act when under the influence of pain and can either result from pain or perpetuate pain. Such behavior is caused by brain chemistry; pain is a complicated neurochemical event. Pain is perceived in the brain. A stimulus that is painful one day may not be painful the next.

Drugs interfere with the production of neurochemicals or block the receptor sites for the various chemicals involved in pain sensations. For example, aspirin interferes with the production of prostaglandin such that it cannot sensitize nerve endings to pain. Anesthetics, including alcohol and barbiturates, depress pain processing so that although the brain senses pain, the person "doesn't care" because his pain perception is altered.

ACTIVITY 4-2

Understanding the neurochemical influences on behavior is important for self-awareness and clinical reasoning when assessing and analyzing a client.

The following is an analysis of an event that resulted in a pattern of behavior.

1. Describe the event in factual terms.

Example

The hood on the car would not close, and I was late for an appointment.

2. Describe your emotions and feelings concerning the event.

Example

I became very frustrated and anxious because I could not drive the car with the hood unlatched.

3. Describe the behavior displayed.

Example

I tried to slam down the hood three or four times and then started to yell at the car.

4. Identify the possible neurotransmitters involved in these feelings and behaviors.

Example

The catecholamines epinephrine and norepinephrine.

5. Indicate mode of action for the neurotransmitters.

Example

Epinephrine and norepinephrine: mostly excitatory, activating sympathetic arousal.

6. Correlate neurotransmitters with the feelings and behaviors.

Example

I was anxious because I was late. Stress levels that increase sympathetic activity were high before I noticed the problem with the car. The increase in the catecholamines would produce or perpetuate the fight-or-flight behavior, resulting in my hitting the car and yelling.

7. Propose a balancing behavior to reset homeostasis, and identify possible neurochemical interaction.

Example

I could have tightened all my muscles for a few seconds and then relaxed them and repeated this three or four times. This would simulate the activity of fighting or fleeing and use up some of the epinephrine. The goal would be to calm down.

Choose an event from your life in which you were unable to alter an inappropriate behavior pattern.

1. Describe the event in factual terms.
2. Describe the emotions and feelings concerning the event.
3. Describe the behavior displayed.
4. Identify the possible neurotransmitters involved in the feelings and behavior.
5. Indicate mode of action for the neurotransmitters.
6. Correlate the neurotransmitters with the feelings and behaviors.
7. Propose a balancing behavior to reset homeostasis, and identify possible neurochemical interaction.

Practical Application

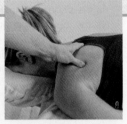

The actions of neurotransmitters are important for many physiologic effects. Many drugs of abuse either mimic neurotransmitters or otherwise alter the function of the nervous system. Barbiturates act as depressants, with effects similar to those of anesthetics. They seem to act mainly by enhancing the activity of the neurotransmitter GABA, an inhibitory neurotransmitter. In other words, when barbiturates bind to a GABA receptor, the inhibitory effect of GABA is greater than before. Opiates such as heroin bind to a particular type of opiate receptor in the brain, resulting in effects similar to those of naturally occurring endorphins. Amphetamines can displace catecholamines from synaptic vesicles and block reuptake of catecholamines in the synapse, prolonging the action of catecholamine neurotransmitters.

A pain-inhibiting system exists within the body. Receptors for opiates (e.g., morphine) are present on the nerves transmitting pain signals. Internal, or endogenous, opiates (e.g., endorphins, enkephalins) produced by the body block pain impulses in various portions of the pathway, probably as a protective device.

The neurotransmitter known as substance P is secreted by pain fibers in the spinal cord but is blocked by enkephalins. Serotonin modulates pain perception. During pregnancy a woman's serotonin level gradually increases until it reaches its highest point at the time of delivery, in preparation for birth pain. Some of the food cravings experienced during pregnancy may be caused by the body's need to increase serotonin levels.

Practical Application

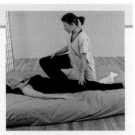

Behavior that causes pain sufficient to increase endorphin and enkephalin activity can result in a pleasant change in mood.

Many forms of touch and movement modalities can cause a "good hurt," and the deliberate use of controlled pain actually can be therapeutic. However, an imbalance is occurring if a person continually creates or seeks pain so as to receive the secondary gain, pleasure. Professional counseling and support are usually required to shift this complex behavior pattern into a more appropriate coping style.

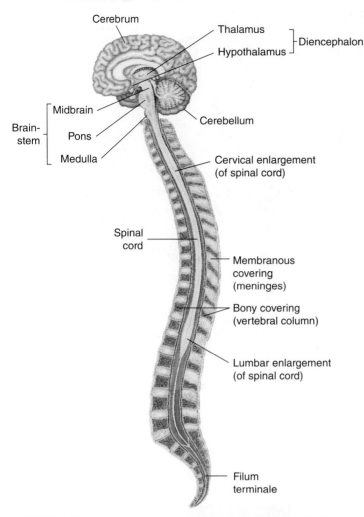

FIGURE 4-8 The central nervous system. (Modified from Patton KT, Thibodeau GA: *Anatomy and physiology,* ed 7, St Louis, 2010, Mosby.)

CENTRAL NERVOUS SYSTEM

SECTION OBJECTIVES

Chapter objectives covered in this section:
5. Identify the structures and functions of the brain.
6. Identify the structures and functions of the spinal cord.
After completing this chapter, the student will be able to perform the following:
• Describe the parts and functions of the central nervous system.
• Describe consciousness and altered states of consciousness.
• Explain the process of memory and learning.

The CNS has two main areas: the brain and the spinal cord (Figure 4-8).

Brain

The **brain** is the largest and most complex unit of the nervous system and is composed of approximately 100 billion neurons, which are packed together inside the skull. Besides intellect, emotions, and actions, the brain interprets, regulates, and coordinates physiologic activities.

Although the brain weighs an average of only 3 pounds, it makes up more than 97% of the nervous system. The neuroglia account for more than half its weight. Composed of more than 85% water, the brain contains a higher percentage of fluid than blood.

The brain is divided into four main areas (Figure 4-9):
1. Cerebrum
2. Diencephalon, the main structures of which are the thalamus and hypothalamus
3. Cerebellum
4. Brainstem, composed of the medulla oblongata, pons, and midbrain

Cerebrum

The **cerebrum**, also called the *forebrain*, is the largest portion of the brain. It is divided into right and left hemispheres, which are connected by the corpus callosum.

The left and right hemispheres oversee motor control. Each receives sensory input from the opposite side of the body: The left hemisphere controls the right side of the body, and the right hemisphere controls the left side.

The term **brain dominance** refers to which hemisphere specializes in language functions and linear thought processing. Most right-handed persons have a dominant left hemisphere. More than 70% of left-handed persons also have a dominant left hemisphere. The right hemisphere concerns itself more with creative and intuitive abilities and imagination. The left side of the brain is working as you are reading this text, whereas the right side jumps in when you daydream or wonder what all the information means (Figure 4-10).

Most of the cerebrum is composed of **white matter.** Because the corpus callosum is composed of myelinated axons, it is white (Figure 4-11). The surface of the cerebrum is covered by the cerebral cortex, a thin layer of matter that is gray because of the presence of dendrites and cell bodies. The basal ganglia are small collections of gray matter in the cerebrum that assist in coordination.

The major functions of the cerebrum are as follows:
• To receive sensory information
• To interpret it
• To associate it with memories, emotions, and past experiences
• To transmit the most appropriate motor impulse in response to the input

Each side of the cerebrum is divided into five lobes, four of which are named for the skull bones lying over them.

Frontal Lobe

The anterior portion of the cerebrum, the frontal lobe is positioned behind the frontal bone and contains the prefrontal cortex (governing personality, intellect, and cognition), the premotor cortex (directing learned motor skills), and the precentral gyrus (managing motor control of muscles). This lobe is responsible primarily for control of the voluntary skeletal muscles and is active during problem-solving moods and activities that involve concentration and planning. An area

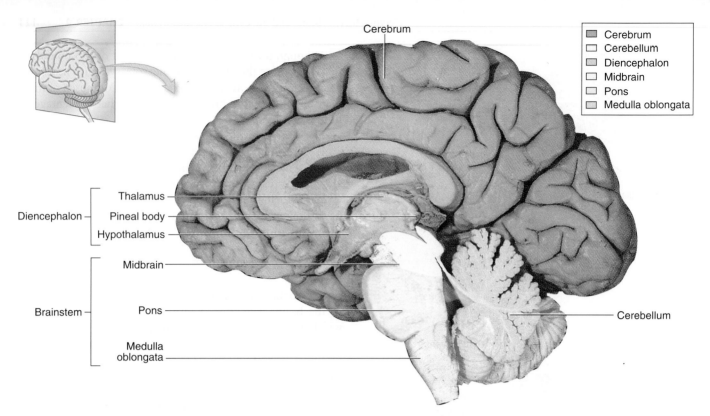

FIGURE 4-9 Divisions of the brain. A midsagittal section of the brain reveals features of its major divisions. (Courtesy of Vidic B, Suarez FR, from *Photographic atlas of the human body,* 1984.)

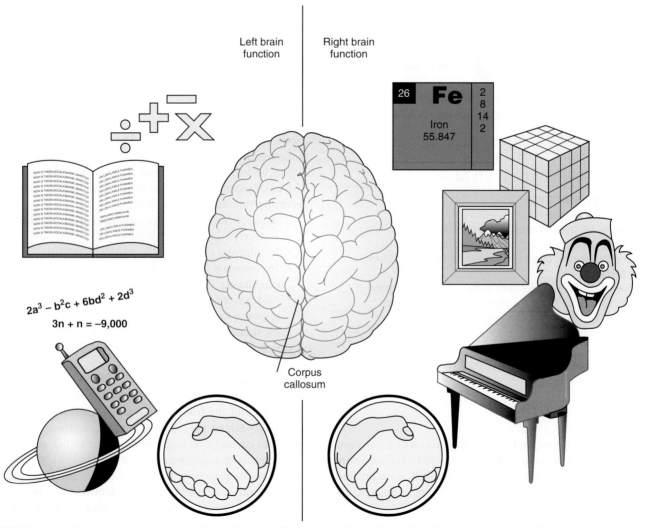

FIGURE 4-10 Left-brain functions and right-brain functions. The handshakes indicate the integrated functions of the left and right brain.

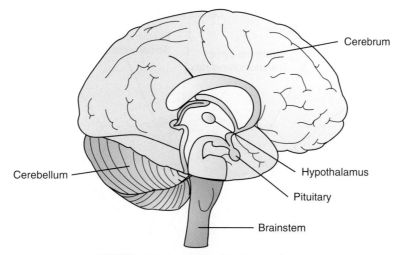

FIGURE 4-11 Location of brain structures.

known as Broca's area is found in the dominant hemisphere and controls the muscle movements involved in speech.

Parietal Lobe

Located next to the parietal bones, the parietal lobe contains the postcentral gyrus, which is the primary sensory area of the brain. This lobe receives and evaluates the sensory information of temperature, pressure, touch, taste, and pain. Its areas of association include speech, thought, and emotions.

Temporal Lobe

Found below the lateral fissure, the temporal lobe is next to the temporal bones. The temporal lobe is responsible for the reception and evaluation involved in hearing and smell. Wernicke's area, which is located in the superior portion of the gyrus of the dominant hemisphere, is involved in understanding language, and it transmits information to the Broca's area in the frontal lobe. Broca's area processes language information comprehended by Wernicke's area and relays it to the precentral gyrus. The areas of association combine complex sensory data (e.g., from music and visual scenes) into comprehensive patterns that form memories.

Occipital Lobe

Located just anterior to the occipital bone of the skull, the occipital lobe is responsible for the mechanical control of eyesight and the integration of visual input with other sensory experiences.

Insula, or Island of Reil

The fifth lobe, the insula (also called the *island of Reil*) is located under the lateral fissure and is the part of the limbic system that gives us a feeling or impression of what is real, true, and important.

The cerebral cortex contains folds called *convolutions,* or *gyri* (singular, *gyrus),* which increase the area available to the cortex. These folds are separated by creases called *sulci.* The deepest sulci are known as *fissures.* These fissures can be used as landmarks when identifying certain areas of the brain.

- The longitudinal fissure divides the cerebrum into right and left hemispheres.

- The central sulcus, or the fissure of Rolando, separates the frontal and parietal lobes.
- The lateral fissure, or the fissure of Sylvius, lies above the temporal lobe and below the frontal and parietal lobes.
- A fifth lobe, the insula, lies deep in the lateral fissure.
- The occipital and parietal lobes are separated by the parietooccipital fissure.

The limbic system is located in the interior of the cerebrum and is important in emotional responses, including fear, rage, and pleasure. Therefore a built-in reward and avoidance process exists in the brain. The limbic system is connected to the hypothalamus by the fornix, a band of fibers consisting of axons (Figure 4-12; Table 4-1).

Integrative or Associative Brain Functions

Integrative or associative functions include all the activities that occur in the cerebrum after sensory signals are received and before motor responses are sent to where those signals originated. These responses include consciousness, language, emotions, memory, and learning mechanisms (Figure 4-13, Box 4-5).

Consciousness

The term *consciousness* can be defined as the capacity for sensation, thinking, memory, and emotion, thereby creating an awareness of self and the environment. There is a continuum of consciousness from a high state of consciousness during which we are alert and hyperaware to a depressed state of consciousness such as a coma. Daily life is usually somewhere between those extremes. The level of consciousness is a measurement of a person's responsiveness to stimuli from the environment. The Glasgow Coma Scale is a neurologic assessment that provides an objective way to record the conscious state of a person that has experienced trauma or illness (Activity 4-3).

Language

Language involves the perception of written and spoken words and the physical ability to speak and write. For 90% of the population, this takes place in the left hemisphere of the cerebrum in the frontal, parietal, and temporal lobes. The ability

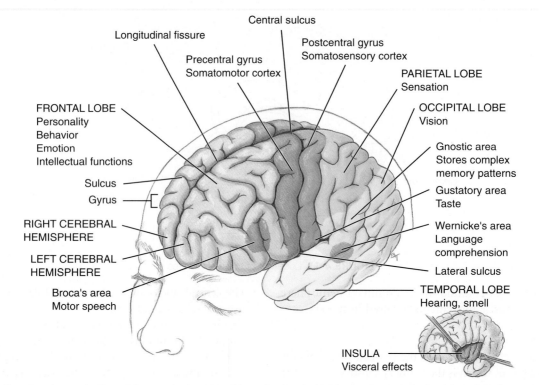

FIGURE 4-12 Functional organization of the cerebral cortex. (From Applegate E: *The anatomy and physiology learning system,* ed 4, St Louis, 2011, Saunders.)

Table 4-1   Functions of the Cerebral Cortex

Functional Area	Anatomic Area	Functional and Performance Components
Frontal Lobes		
Primary motor area	Precentral gyrus	Execution of movement
Secondary association area	Premotor cortex	Planning and programming of movement
		Sequencing, timing, and organization of movement
		Frontal eye field
		Voluntary eye movements
		Broca's area in the left inferior frontal gyrus
		Programming of motor speech
		Supplementary motor area
		Intention of movement
Tertiary association area	Orbitofrontal and dorsolateral prefrontal cortex	Ideation
		Concept formation
		Abstract thought
		Intellectual functions
		Sequencing, timing, and organization of action and behavior
		Initiation and planning of action
		Judgment
		Insight
		Intention
		Attention
		Alertness
		Personality
		Working memory
		Emotion
Parietal Lobes		
Primary somesthetic sensory area	Postcentral gyrus	Fine touch sensation
		Proprioception
		Kinesthesia

Continued

Table 4-1 Functions of the Cerebral Cortex—cont'd

Functional Area	Anatomic Area	Functional and Performance Components
Secondary somesthetic sensory association area	Superior parietal lobule	Coordination, integration, and refinement of sensory input Tactile localization and discrimination Stereognosis
Tertiary association area	Inferior parietal lobule	Gnosis: recognition of received tactile, visual, and auditory input Praxis: storage of programs or visuokinesthetic motor engrams necessary for motor sequences Body scheme: postural model of body, body parts, and their relation to the environment Spatial relations: processing related to depth, distance, spatial concepts, position in space, and differentiation of foreground from background
Occipital Lobes		
Primary visual sensory area	Calcarine fissure	Visual reception (from the opposite visual field)
Visual association area	Brodmann's areas 18 and 19	Synthesis and integration of visual information Perception of visuospatial relationships Formation of visual memory traces Prepositional construction of language comprehension and speech
Temporal Lobes		
Primary auditory sensory area	Superior temporal gyrus	Auditory reception
Secondary association area	Superior and middle temporal gyri (Wernicke's area)	Language comprehension Sound modulation Perception of music Auditory memory
Tertiary association area	Temporal pole, parahippocampus	Long-term memory Learning of higher-order visual tasks and auditory patterns Emotion Motivation Personality
Limbic Lobes		
Tertiary association area	Orbitofrontal cortex in frontal lobe, temporal pole, and parahippocampus in the temporal lobe	Attention
	Cingulate gyrus in frontal and parietal lobes	Motivation Emotions Long-term memory

Modified from Árnadóttir G: *The brain and behavior: assessing cortical dysfunction through activities of daily living,* St Louis, 1990, Mosby.

✎ ACTIVITY 4-3

How could you alter your state of consciousness in a health-enhancing way? Write down two methods.

Example
Listen to gentle music for 15 minutes while rocking in a rocking chair.

Your Turn

Practical Application

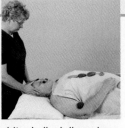

Massage therapy interacts with the cerebral cortex and reticular activating system, the same mechanisms involved in consciousness. Consequently, massage methods often generate the sensations experienced during altered states of consciousness. Most of the major spiritual disciplines have a movement or positional aspect in their practices that contributes to the meditative states experienced by their participants. Some even incorporate touch, which enhances the experience.

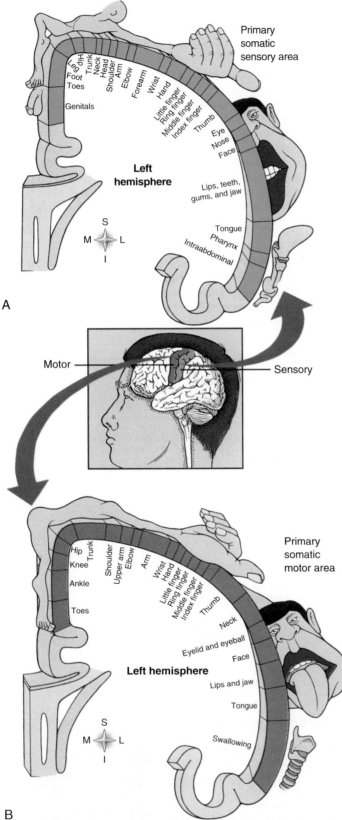

A

B

FIGURE 4-13 Sensory and motor areas of the brain. The surface area is largest for sensory interpretation of the face, lips, and fingers. The motor surface area is largest for the hands and face. (From Thibodeau GA, Patton KT: *Anatomy and physiology,* ed 6, St Louis, 2007, Mosby.)

to apply labels to processes and subjects inside and outside of the body also is tied to sensory systems.

Emotions

We experience and express our feelings and emotions through the limbic system of the brain. Located inside the cerebrum, the limbic system works with other parts of the cerebral cortex. For most of us, the normal expressions of anger, pleasure, fear, and sorrow are under our control. An individual whose limbic system does not interact effectively with the cortex may have episodes of uncontrollable rage or other emotions. Motivation is driven by emotions, especially the pleasure sensations. They cause people to move toward anticipated feelings of pleasure and to move away from negative feelings to avoid situations remembered from past experiences of distress.

Memory

Memory involves the storage of information in the brain, and it is one of our major mental activities. Two types of memory are short-term (recent) memory and long-term memory. Short-term memory is fragile, unstable, and disappears unless it is reinforced and transferred to long-term memory. The activities in this text are designed to assist in the transference of new data from short-term to long-term memory, which can be retrieved days or even years after the initial event.

The temporal lobes are involved with long-term memory, which consists of structural traces in the cerebral cortex called *engrams;* these involve protein synthesis and physical brain changes, resulting in permanent change in the synapses in a specific circuit of neurons. Repeated impulse conduction over a given neuronal circuit seems to produce the synaptic change. Many research findings indicate that the limbic system—the "emotional brain"—plays a key role in memory also. Highly emotional events seem to become stored immediately in long-term memory, indicating neurotransmitter involvement in memory structures (Box 4-6).

Practical Application

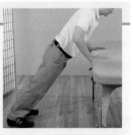

The key to long-term memory is repeated impulses. This text provides opportunities to review information repeatedly. The same information is presented in various and novel forms so that it is more likely to be stored in long-term memory. Learning strategies commonly are focused on circular learning, in which information continues to reappear, reinforcing storage by the neural circuit. Learning that takes place with excitement and enthusiasm, or even with tears and sorrow, is remembered better. Events that create tears of joy are some of the best remembered.

Learning

Learning can be thought of as the best and simplest way to solve a problem. Anatomically and physiologically, learning is the use of multiple synaptic pathways to process information. Advanced learning takes place in the association areas of the

Box 4-5   Consciousness and Altered States of Consciousness

Consciousness is awareness of the environment and our relationship to everyone and everything in that environment. Throughout the day changes take place in our level of consciousness, ranging from asleep to wide awake.

Consciousness depends on excitation of cortical neurons by impulses conducted from the reticular activating system. The reticular activating system consists of centers in the brainstem that receive impulses from the spinal cord and relay them to the thalamus. The thalamus transmits the data to all parts of the cerebral cortex. Substances that stimulate the cerebrum, enhancing alertness, probably act by stimulating the reticular activating system.

We are not always consciously aware of all the functions of our internal body and the external stimuli around us. Subconscious activity occurs beyond the level of consciousness. The ability to not be conscious of all internal and external stimuli and sensations is important. Otherwise, we would be overwhelmed.

Some people have an intensified awareness of ordinary body functions, such as heartbeat, breathing, and stomach noises. This can be very distressing if the person does not know that the sensations are normal. What is abnormal is that the person is aware of these functions. Hypochondriasis is a mental disorder characterized by excessive fear of or preoccupation with a serious illness, despite medical testing and reassurance that no illness exists. Many doctors believe that these individuals may have some sort of abnormal hypersensitivity or inability to filter sensation. Some behaviors associated with autism-type conditions are related to sensation hypersensitivity: smell, touch, sound, and sight.

Altered States of Consciousness

Consciousness may be altered in many ways, including the use of medications, herbs, or foods that change chemical processes; repetitive activities or sounds; and trance. For centuries many cultures and religions have explored altered states of consciousness and have used them readily in defensive actions, healing, and pain control. Meditation, tai chi, and yoga are examples of ancient methods to achieve altered consciousness. States of higher consciousness refers to the primary activity that actually increases alertness and induces relaxation. Research has confirmed this state to be health enhancing.

We can achieve the same result by gardening, drawing, knitting, or playing a musical instrument. Any rhythmic activity that uses a repetitive motion (e.g., drumming) or nature sounds (e.g., a bubbling brook) can quiet or excite, depending on the speed of the rhythm, the nervous system through entrainment and thereby alter the physiologic processes of the body.

The pleasure derived from the sense of well-being experienced during altered states of consciousness can be addictive. Various plants containing chemicals that alter consciousness have been used over the centuries in awareness rituals. Within the confines of cultural and religious ritual, the limited and judicial use of these plants was controlled. Today most, if not all, of the old discipline and structure are nonexistent, and the risk of drug abuse has made the exploration of altered states of consciousness problematic.

During a massage session a beneficial altered state of consciousness can be achieved by both the therapist and the client. When the altered state has been achieved, it should be maintained for at least 15 minutes for optimal therapeutic benefit. The typical time required for the body to respond to the physiologic change is 15 minutes.

Box 4-6   State-Dependent Memory

Sometimes the memory takes the form of state-dependent memory. In state-dependent memory, the engram cannot be accessed unless the state of consciousness is similar to that in effect when the event occurred and was encoded. State-dependent memory can take many forms. Sometimes trauma beyond what the conscious centers can integrate is hidden in state-dependent memory. Any form of therapy that can engage the various states of consciousness, such as hypnosis, biofeedback, and various forms of bodywork, may recreate the state of consciousness that holds the key to the memory structure, allowing it to surface. Depending on the person's coping skills, resources, support systems, and professional services available, this awareness of past experience can be a time of conscious understanding and integration of a part of the person's life. However, without the proper resources this resurfacing of state-dependent memory can be devastating and extremely harmful.

Pleasure states also are encoded in state-dependent memory. Warm feelings such as being held or feelings of exhilaration such as running in the wind on a beautiful spring day can be remembered and in a sense recreated through various forms of bodywork. These are health-enhancing states that support homeostasis.

cerebral cortex, whereas more primitive learning takes place in the brainstem. The ability to read is considered advanced learning, whereas the recognition that something is hot is a more primitive form of learning. Learning involves memory because it is the development of neural structures that remember the way to solve a problem. This process supports survival.

Learning can be thought of as conditioning. Ivan Pavlov's research identified some of the mechanisms of conditioning. In his work an external stimulus was connected to a natural occurrence in the body. Dogs were conditioned by bells being rung at the same time food was being presented. Soon the dogs learned that the bell and food equaled the same thing, whereupon the sound of the bell alone stimulated digestion and eating behaviors. This is behavioral conditioning, which also can be considered learned habit.

The process of learning is conscious, but after a response has been integrated, it commonly becomes unconscious, a habit. Some habits are beneficial, and others no longer serve their original purpose. Breaking a habit is difficult. Learning a new way to do something involves making the thought process take a different path to reach the same result. The body and learned memory tend to resist change, especially because learned behavior is a strong component of primitive survival behavior. In addition, changing learned behavior takes tremendous energy, and the natural tendency of the body is to conserve energy. Unless the habit is causing us to expend resources in a detrimental way for a sufficiently long time to affect survival, rallying the resources of the body necessary to change the behavior is difficult.

Diencephalon

The diencephalon is found between the cerebrum and the midbrain and contains the thalamus, hypothalamus, pineal body, and other small structures.

Thalamus

The thalamus is created from the gray matter of nerve cell bodies deep in the white matter of the cortex. It is a relay station to the cerebrum for all sensory input except smell. Signals from the reticular activating system, discussed in the section on the brainstem, also are sent through the thalamus to the cerebral cortex. The thalamus is also associated with pain, temperature, crude touch, and reflex muscle coordination. Additionally, it associates pleasant and unpleasant feelings with sensory input and then relays information to the limbic system. The thalamus may act as a bio-oscillator involved with internal biorhythm entrainment and supporting internal balance.

Hypothalamus

The hypothalamus lies below the thalamus and above the pituitary gland. It regulates and coordinates functions such as heart rate, blood pressure, aspects of digestion, appetite and satiety, pleasure, temperature, and general coordination of ANS functions. It also produces releasing hormones that affect pituitary gland hormones, which in turn influence important activities such as hunger, appetite, sleep cycles, wakefulness, sexual arousal, and water balance in the body. The hypothalamus is closely associated with the limbic system and is an important link between the nervous and endocrine systems; this allows the mind to affect the body, so it is part of the mind/body connection.

Pineal Body

The pineal body, or gland, is found on the dorsal side of the diencephalon. Approximately 30% of the pineal cells are responsive to external magnetic patterns. The gland functions as an internal biologic clock that regulates daily activities (circadian rhythms) as well as yearly rhythms (circannual rhythms). Exposure to natural sunlight assists these functions. The pineal body needs darkness to convert serotonin into

---

Box 4-7 Sleep

Sleep can be divided into two types: slow-wave sleep and rapid eye movement (REM) sleep.

Four stages of sleep have been defined, stage 4 being the deepest sleep.

Slow-wave sleep produces slow-frequency, high-voltage brain waves and is associated with stages 2 and 3. Such sleep is almost entirely a dreamless part of the sleep pattern. At the deeper levels, the activity of the reticular activating system is depressed in the pons and medulla.

REM sleep is associated with dreaming. At intervals of 90 minutes or so, the closed eyes begin to move rapidly. Repeatedly waking a person at the beginning of REM sleep produces anxiety and irritability. If the person is then allowed to sleep, longer than usual periods of REM sleep and dreaming occur for a few nights to allow for catching up. This process is called *REM rebound*.

Many medications, particularly sleeping pills and tranquilizers, suppress REM and stage 4 sleep. Stopping the drug may result in REM rebound, which is sometimes associated with nightmares. Therefore it is important to use medicines with minimal REM rebound when medication is necessary.

---

melatonin, which seems to be involved with sexual activity. Melatonin also triggers the pituitary gland to release luteinizing hormone, which affects sexual maturity and may be involved in puberty and menopause, and it is involved in sleep patterns (Box 4-7).

Practical Application

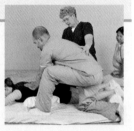

The pleasure center deep inside the hypothalamus involves feel-good neurotransmitters and predisposes a person to addictive behavior to feel good, alter mood, and so forth. Romantic love is a brain bath of norepinephrine and dopamine— feel-good chemicals. Therapeutic massage stimulation also influences the feel-good neurotransmitters. Abuse of substances—including nicotine, alcohol, and caffeine—and extreme indulgence in eating, sex, gambling, exercise, thrill seeking, pain, violence, and crisis creating are feel-good-chemical substitutes. They have the potential to produce addictive behavior because they interact with feel-good neurotransmitters as well. Many psychotropic or mood-regulating medications act on the feel-good neurotransmitters. The use of chemicals or extreme behaviors to produce pleasure often depletes or inhibits the natural production of the chemicals, resulting in a big downslide after a big high. The extremes of pleasure and discomfort create craving and seeking behaviors that support addictive behavior.

Because therapeutic massage stimulates the release of the feel-good neurotransmitters and hormones, inclusion of these therapies has been shown to support the treatment of addictive behavior by replacing a destructive manner of mood alteration with a constructive, more moderate way to feel good. It is essential that the treatment of complex factors such as those found in addiction be monitored and dealt with by means of a multidisciplinary team approach.

Practical Application

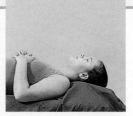

To maintain homeostasis, we need sufficient sleep. During this time of rest, most of the growth and repair of the body take place. Many chronic diseases are associated with disrupted sleep patterns. If sleep possibly can be restored to an effective pattern without the use of medications, often the body can better cope with or even begin to heal a chronic problem over time. Massage is relaxing and conducive to supporting effective sleep patterns, providing benefit to the client and thus decreasing the effects of the chronic problem.

Brainstem

The **brainstem** is considered the primitive portion of the brain and is divided into three main parts: the midbrain, pons, and the medulla oblongata. A fourth area is the reticular formation and its associated reticular activating system. These areas are control centers for vital survival functions and reflex actions, such as sneezing, coughing, vomiting, and balanced movements. Research shows that the brainstem probably processes much of the sensory data generated by massage modalities.

Midbrain

The midbrain, or mesencephalon, is located in the middle of the brain, below the cerebrum and between the thalamus and the pons. The midbrain contains reflex centers for visual and auditory stimuli and correlates information about muscle tone and posture. The midbrain contains an important part of the reticular activating system.

Pons

The pons (pons varolii) is in the middle of the brainstem, between the midbrain and the medulla. The pons assists in the coordinated patterns of breathing, eye movement, and facial expressions and is involved in rapid eye movement (REM) sleep.

Medulla Oblongata

The medulla, or medulla oblongata, connects the pons with the spinal cord and is composed of white matter and the reticular formation, a network of white and gray matter. The fibers handle impulses to lower motor neurons. The fibers on one side of the medulla handle signals to the contralateral side. The medulla regulates the heartbeat, blood pressure, and breathing as well as such reflex actions as coughing and sneezing. Because the medulla controls vital life functions, injury or disease in the medulla is often fatal.

Reticular Activating System

The reticular activating system is a structural and functional part of the reticular formation in the brainstem. It maintains arousal levels in the cerebral cortex and alerts it to changes in homeostasis, thus keeping us awake and alert. The reticular

The vestibular apparatus is a paired organ that is part of the inner ear. Sensations produced in this organ are conveyed to the brain, along with that of hearing, by way of the vestibulocochlear nerve and are related directly to equilibrium, balance, and functions of the cerebellum.

The vestibular apparatus on each side consists of three circular canals that are interconnected and filled with fluid. The canal expands to form fluid-filled structures called *utricles* and *saccules*. The canals, utricles, and saccules have receptors that respond to movement, especially when the head is rotated and when the head moves forward or backward.

Every time the head is moved, the fluid in the semicircular canals is set in motion, generating nerve impulses. The impulses travel to the brainstem and to the cerebellum to provide information about body and head movement, and neurons also provide information to the cranial nerves supplying the eye so that they can adjust eye position according to movement and direction. The motor cortex is stimulated, and the body is able to increase and decrease tone and maintain balance and equilibrium.

The vestibular apparatuses are important for spatial orientation, our sense of position in gravity, which is aided by vision, proprioceptors, and input from touch and pressure receptors.

activating system also helps regulate respiration, blood pressure, heart rate, endocrine secretion, and conditioned reflexes. Epinephrine and amphetamines stimulate reticular activating system conduction, whereas anesthesia and barbiturates depress conduction. Trauma or damage to the reticular activating system can cause a person to become comatose.

Cerebellum

The cerebellum is located in the posterior cranial fossa beneath the posterior portion of the cerebrum. The **cerebellum** is the second-largest part of the brain and consists of a cortex composed of gray matter and an inner portion composed of white matter. Like the cerebrum, the cerebellum has sulci and gyri, and it contains two lateral hemispheres that are connected by the vermis. The cerebellum maintains balance and posture and, with proprioceptive input, coordinates everything from normal movements to the complex activities involved in dancing, performing gymnastics, and giving massage. The cerebellum, limbic system, and other relay centers of the brain have been shown to work on the same circuit (Hooper, 1986) (Box 4-8).

Other Brain Structures

There are many structures in the brain that support the function of the CNS. Three important areas are the ventricles, meninges, and blood vessels.

Meninges

The meninges are three layers of connective tissue membranes that cover and protect the brain and spinal cord (Figure 4-14).

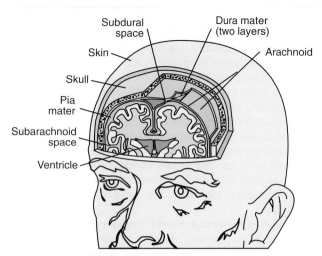

FIGURE 4-14 Meninges of the brain.

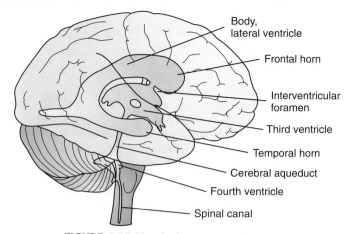

FIGURE 4-15 Ventricular system, lateral view.

Practical Application

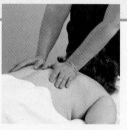

Massage techniques that stimulate the cerebellum, such as rhythmic rocking, have widespread influence. Methods that alter the body's positional sense and initiate specific movement patterns change sensory input from muscles, tendons, joints, and the skin. The output from the cerebellum goes to the motor cortex and brainstem. Stimulation of the cerebellum by alteration of muscle tone, position, and vestibular balance also stimulates the hypothalamus to adjust ANS functions and thus restore homeostasis. Rocking produces movement at the neck and head that influences our sense of equilibrium by stimulating the balance mechanisms of the inner ear. Such mechanisms include the vestibular complex and the labyrinthine righting reflexes, which work to keep our heads level. A close relationship exists between the vestibular nerves and the cerebellum.

Rocking also stimulates muscle-contraction patterns that pass throughout the body. Pressure on the side of the body may stimulate the righting reflexes.

The dura mater is the outermost layer and is made up of a white, tough, fibrous connective-tissue membrane. The dura mater lines the cranial bones and covers the outside of the brain and spinal cord. Portions of the dura mater line the fissures between the left and right hemispheres of the cerebrum and cerebellum and cover the spinal nerve roots. Nerves and blood vessels run through the epidural space next to the dura mater.

The middle layer is the arachnoid mater, a cobweblike membrane containing many blood vessels.

The third layer, the pia mater, is thin and adheres directly to the brain and spinal cord.

The meninges form three spaces that add additional cushioning and protection to the CNS:

- **Epidural space:** Found between the skull and dura mater, this space contains connective tissue, including fat.

- **Subdural Space:** Found between the dura mater and arachnoid membrane, this space is filled with a cushioning serous fluid.
- **Subarachnoid Space:** Found between the arachnoid and pia mater, this space contains the cerebrospinal fluid (CSF).

Classified as one of the circulating fluids of the body, CSF is a colorless, watery substance that flows throughout the brain and around the spinal cord, providing cushioning and protection. CSF maintains homeostasis of the brain environment, including pH balance (Figure 4-15). CSF is replenished continuously from the fluid filtering out of the choroid plexus, a network of brain capillaries. CSF circulates through the brain and around the spinal cord and is returned to the venous system at the dural sinuses.

Ventricles

The ventricles are four fluid-filled chambers found within the brain. There is one in each of the cerebral hemispheres, one positioned just below and between them, and one at the attachment of the cerebrum and the brainstem. CSF fills these ventricles and then passes through several small openings to the subarachnoid space.

Practical Application

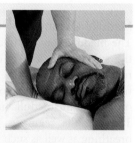

Some methods of bodywork, such as cranial-sacral therapy, are thought to interact with the movement of the meninges, especially the dura mater, and to affect the flow of CSF. In the CNS a rhythm known as the *cranial-sacral impulse* can be observed and palpated.

The effect of bodywork on this rhythm is still under investigation, although entrainment methods that synchronize the motions and rhythms of the body are credited with providing the most benefits. The application is to be done in a quiet, rhythmic manner by a quiet and focused practitioner who adds an additional external influence that allows the body rhythms to synchronize. When synchronization is achieved, homeostatic mechanisms seem to operate more efficiently.

Vessels of the Brain

Blood is supplied to the brain through the middle cerebral arteries, which are a continuation of the internal carotid arteries and the basilar artery. These are created from the two vertebrobasilar arteries. These three brain arteries are connected at the midbrain in the circle of Willis, which is a check-and-balance system that provides blood flow to the brain in case of blockage or damage to any of the three arteries (Figure 4-16). Blood is transported out of the brain by several veins and the dural sinuses, which drain into the internal jugular veins.

Spinal Cord

The two main functions of the spinal cord are as follows:
1. To conduct nerve impulses
2. To integrate spinal reflexes.

The **spinal cord** is made of white and gray matter and is about 17 to 18 inches long in the average person. The spinal cord is oval and, like the brain, has fissures. The anterior median fissure is deeper and wider than the posterior median sulcus (Figure 4-17).

The spinal cord begins at the base of the brainstem, exiting through an opening in the skull called the *foramen magnum.* The spinal cord continues through the vertebral column to the first and second lumbar vertebrae. At this point the pia mater continues on as the filum terminale and connects to the dura mater at the second sacral vertebra; they both end at the coccyx.

There are 31 pairs of spinal nerves that connect with the spinal cord. When they exit the spinal cord, they are considered part of the PNS.

The section of the spinal cord that corresponds to a single pair of spinal nerves is known as a *segment.* The spinal cord has 31 segments:
- 8 cervical
- 12 thoracic
- 5 lumbar
- 5 sacral
- 1 coccygeal

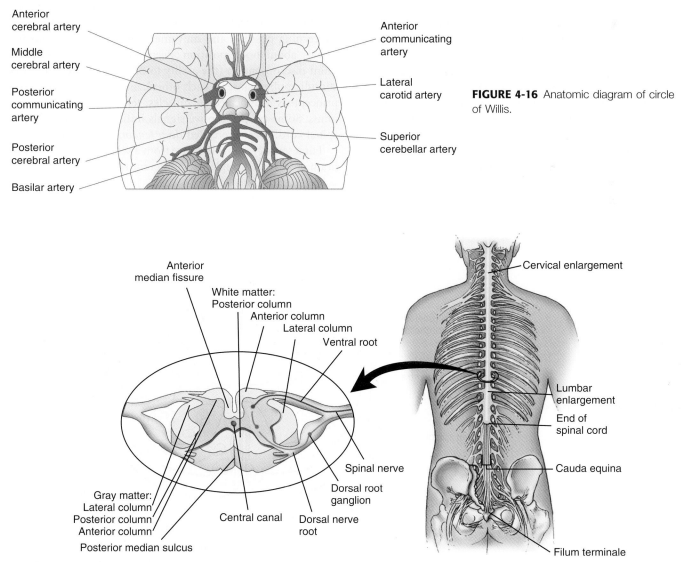

FIGURE 4-16 Anatomic diagram of circle of Willis.

FIGURE 4-17 Spinal cord. The *inset* illustrates a transverse section of the spinal cord shown in the broader view. (From Thibodeau GA, Patton KT: *Anatomy and physiology,* ed 6, St Louis, 2007, Mosby.)

The spinal nerves are indicated easily in relation to the vertebrae. For example, the nerve between the first and second thoracic vertebrae is T1. Spinal nerves exit the spinal cord through intervertebral foramina. Because the spinal cord is shorter than the vertebral column (ending at the second lumbar vertebra), the spinal nerves from the lower lumbar and sacral regions extend to and exit through sacral foramina. The spinal and lower lumbar nerves, which are referred to as *cauda equina,* make the lower end of the spinal cord look like the tail of a horse.

Each spinal nerve is attached to the spinal cord by two roots:

1. The dorsal or posterior root, which carries sensory information
2. The ventral or anterior root, which carries motor information

The **dorsal root** enlarges to form the dorsal root ganglion. Distal to the dorsal root ganglion, the dorsal root joins with the **ventral root** so that the sensory and motor roots are bound together to form a spinal nerve. Spinal nerves are called *mixed nerves* because they contain both sensory and motor nerve fibers.

Gray matter is located inside the spinal cord and extends the entire length. A cross-section shows that the gray matter forms an H pattern.

The dorsal portion of the H forms the dorsal horns and is composed of the cell bodies of association, or interneurons. The anterior portion of the H forms the ventral horns, consisting of the cell bodies of motor nerves. In the center of the gray matter is the central canal containing CSF.

Surrounding the gray matter are pathways of white matter called *tracts,* created from the myelinated nerve fibers. The axons in each tract are limited to one action, such as transmitting specific touch and pain sensations. The tracts ascend to and descend from the brain. The **ascending tracts** conduct sensory impulses such as pain, touch, and temperature up from the spinal nerves through the spinal cord to the brain. The **descending tracts** conduct motor impulses from the brain down the cord to the spinal nerves (Figure 4-18). Figure 4-17 shows the sectional anatomy of the spinal cord in the inset.

Sensory Ascending Tracts

Sensory receptors are found in the skin, the muscles, and all organs. When stimulated by touch, pain, and muscle action, they respond by generating nerve impulses. These signals travel along the nerve fibers from these receptors to the spinal cord, where they cross to the other side and ascend one of the sensory pathways, or tracts, to the thalamus, medulla, or cerebellum. In the brain the sensations are integrated into perceptions or filtered as being unimportant. This sensory information is needed to maintain homeostasis.

Some of the most important sensory information supplied to the client's body during massage comes from sensory receptors, specifically from proprioceptors that sense data concerning position and movement. Sensory fibers transmit signals about body position, deep touch or pressure, two-point discrimination (the ability to differentiate between two stimuli applied close to each other), and vibration. The proprioceptors are located in muscles, tendons, ligaments, and joints. Some proprioceptive signals initiate a response in the spinal cord; these are called *deep tendon reflex arcs.*

For a sensory signal to move from a sensory receptor to the brain, it passes through three different neurons.

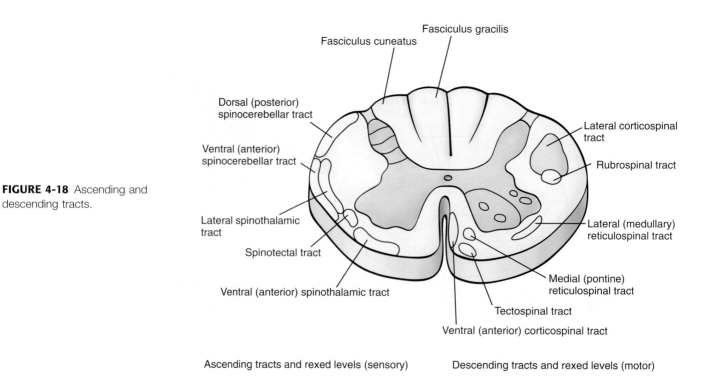

FIGURE 4-18 Ascending and descending tracts.

Fasciculus gracilis

Fasciculus cuneatus

Dorsal (posterior) spinocerebellar tract

Ventral (anterior) spinocerebellar tract

Lateral spinothalamic tract

Spinotectal tract

Ventral (anterior) spinothalamic tract

Lateral corticospinal tract

Rubrospinal tract

Lateral (medullary) reticulospinal tract

Medial (pontine) reticulospinal tract

Tectospinal tract

Ventral (anterior) corticospinal tract

Ascending tracts and rexed levels (sensory)   Descending tracts and rexed levels (motor)

ACTIVITY 4-4

Summarize the ascending and descending functions of the spinal cord.

Ascending
Example:

Descending
Example:

Sends information to
CNS regarding pain

Delivers information
to muscles

The first one, referred to as the *primary,* is a relay from the receptor to the brainstem or the spinal cord. This is part of the PNS and is discussed in detail in the next chapter.

The second neuron extends from the brainstem or spinal cord to the thalamus. The secondary neuron synapses with the tertiary (or third) neuron in the thalamus. The actual crossing of sensory signals from the left to the right side (and vice versa) takes place mostly in the secondary neurons before they enter the thalamus.

The third neuron ends in the postcentral gyrus of the parietal lobe of the cortex. The axons of these third neurons make up the white matter of the cerebrum, referred to as the *internal capsule,* whereas the dendrites and cell bodies make up the gray matter of the cerebral cortex.

Motor Descending Tracts

Motor tracts transmit information regarding adaptive responses and sensory experiences concerned with gross movements, posture, and fine motor skills. One of the main motor tracts is the pyramidal, or corticospinal, tract, which ties in to the voluntary motor system. The pyramidal fibers handle voluntary and reflex signals to the muscles.

The fibers begin in the cortex at the precentral gyrus and descend to the medulla, where they cross to the opposite side of the spinal cord. From that point they descend through the lateral corticospinal tract to the motor neurons of the skeletal muscles. Signals traveling from the CNS to the muscles use the somatic motor pathways.

One important rule to remember is the final common path principle. Each motor unit within a muscle receives impulses that are conducted along a single motor neuron that begins in the anterior gray horn of the spinal cord. This principle is important to health care providers who are exploring muscle dysfunction and its relationship to spinal cord injuries. By identifying a muscle dysfunction, common relationship to the spinal nerve also can be determined (Activity 4-4, Box 4-9).

Upper and Lower Motor Neuron Injury

Injuries to the upper and lower motor neurons result in differing responses in the skeletal muscles. When upper motor neurons are damaged or destroyed by trauma or disease, the result is usually an increase in rigidity and an exaggerated response to reflexes. This is referred to as *spastic paralysis.*

Injuries to the lower motor neurons result in a lack of signal to the muscles, causing absence of movement. This is known as *flaccid paralysis.*

Box 4-9 | The Spinal Cord

The spinal cord has five main motor tracts:
1. Lateral corticospinal tracts: These tracts handle voluntary movements, especially the contraction of small groups of muscles such as those in the hands and feet. They affect muscles on the side of the body opposite from the cerebral cortex.
2. Anterior or ventral corticospinal tracts: These tracts handle the same lateral tracts, but the muscles are on the same side of the body as the cortex. The term *pyramidal tracts* refers to the lateral and anterior corticospinal tracts. The neurons from the cerebral cortex cross through the pyramid areas of the medulla.
3. Lateral reticulospinal tracts: These tracts transmit facilitatory impulses from the medulla through the anterior horn motor neurons to skeletal muscles that handle muscle tone and extensor reflexes.
4. Medial reticulospinal tracts: These tracts carry mainly inhibitory impulses from the pons through the anterior horn motor neurons to skeletal muscles that deal with muscle tone and extensor reflexes.
5. Rubrospinal tracts: These tracts transmit impulses that coordinate body movements and maintain posture. The extrapyramidal tracts are composed of the lateral and medial reticulospinal and rubrospinal tracts. They relay motor signals through the cerebrum, thalamus, brainstem, and cerebellum to the gray matter of the spinal cord. At this point most synapse with interneurons, which then synapse with the lower motor neurons. It should be noted that facilitating and inhibiting signals are sent through these motor neurons.

PATHOLOGIC CONDITIONS

SECTION OBJECTIVES

Chapter objectives covered in this section:
7. List drugs that affect the central nervous system.
8. Describe common pathologic conditions of the central nervous system and the related indications/contraindications for massage.
After completing this section, the student will be able to perform the following:
- Explain the influence of massage methods on CNS pathology.
- Explain how certain drugs affect the central nervous system.

Pathologies related to the CNS can have profound implications for both physical and mental health. While the CNS regulates physiologic functions, it also influences personality and behavior reflecting, in essence, the concept of self. Damage to the brain and spinal cord can be caused by disease or trauma. Various drugs can be used to treat CNS disorders. However, if used inappropriately, these same chemicals can lead to CNS dysfunction.

Drugs Affecting Central Nervous System Function

There are many medications that are used to treat dysfunction in the CNS. The main categories are as follows:
- Analgesic
- Antianxiety (including tricyclics)

Practical Application

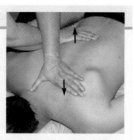

The disability or dysfunction caused by brain and spinal cord injuries is determined by the region and function of the area affected. The prognosis for trauma to the motor neurons is commonly difficult to identify. The use of soft-tissue work and other forms of movement thera-

pies seems to be most beneficial as part of the whole health care picture. Specific recommendations regarding massage are difficult to make solely on the basis of the location of damage because the body compensates by rerouting the interrupted signals. This is why clinical reasoning methods are so important. The ability to process a situation and determine the best intervention methods is essential for the successful therapeutic massage professional.

For example, spastic paralysis results from upper motor neuron injuries. A client with such injuries will have spastic paralysis of the muscles in the affected region. Voluntary control over movement is lost, and limbs may have to be restrained to prevent involuntary movement at inappropriate times. Usually, less muscle atrophy is present, and lymph and blood flow continues because of the working of the muscles. The preferred modalities, when applied to each individual, can moderate some of the random spasms and keep the soft tissues more supple and the joints more mobile, resulting in less rigidity in the muscles.

With lower motor neuron difficulties, the muscles atrophy and actions and reflexes are slow, limited, or nonexistent. Massage and joint movement may be able to replace the mechanical pumping action of normal muscle contraction and assist in moving the blood and lymph. In addition, keeping the soft tissue pliable may lessen any contractures.

- Anticonvulsant
- Antidepressant
- Antiemetic (nausea, vomiting)
- Antihistamine
- Anti-Parkinson
- Sedative/hypnotic
- Antitussive (relieve coughing)
- Antipyschotic
- Opioid

Most drugs of abuse affect CNS functions. Physical dependency (addiction) means that when a drug is withdrawn, severe autonomic excitability occurs. The person thus requires the drug to feel normal. Time, and sometimes medical intervention, is required before the body reestablishes the ability to self-regulate without the drug.

Tolerance, which occurs with stimulants and depressants, means that larger doses of the drug are required for the same effect because the body has adjusted to the current dose. Amphetamines are dangerous because there is no physical dependency; thus the body gives no physical warnings of abuse. Therefore, because of tolerance a person can approach a lethal dose without being aware of it.

Stimulants that affect the neurotransmitters and receptor sites of the cells in the CNS include caffeine, nicotine, amphetamines, and cocaine. Caffeine is a CNS stimulant that enhances the sense of alertness and diminishes the sense of fatigue and boredom. Nicotine first stimulates and then depresses the nervous system by affecting the release of norepinephrine and mimicking the action of acetylcholine. Amphetamines and cocaine stimulate the release of **catecholamines,** primarily norepinephrine and dopamine, from sympathetic neurons. Their effect on the CNS ranges from a feeling of well-being to euphoria to psychosis.

Depressants (e.g., alcohol, narcotics, minor tranquilizers, and barbiturates) act on the cerebral cortex by blocking norepinephrine and dopamine. The paradoxical effect of alcohol as a stimulant results from its ability to inhibit learned behavior and release primitive biologic impulses from inhibitory control. Depressants are also anesthetics. The cortex is depressed first, and then the more primitive centers (brainstem) are depressed as the dosage is increased. Brainstem depression can result in death because respiration and cardiac function are slowed; if the depression continues, they eventually stop.

The hallucinogens include lysergic acid diethylamide (LSD), phencyclidine (PCP), peyote (mescaline), and marijuana (tetrahydrocannabinol). LSD blocks the neurotransmitter serotonin, and PCP blocks acetylcholine. These drugs seem to alter brain function by randomly stimulating and blocking neurotransmitters. A typical action is that smell may be "seen," color may be "heard," and so forth. PCP is considered the most dangerous of the hallucinogens. It uncouples sensory pathways in the brain to produce a sensory deprivation syndrome, creating an increase in body strength accompanied by an acute schizophrenic reaction. Because of high fat solubility and the production of long-acting metabolites, PCP may remain in body tissues for months or even years, causing recurring episodes of violence and psychosis.

Pathologic Conditions

Cerebrovascular Accidents (Strokes)

The most common brain disorder is a cerebrovascular accident (CVA), or stroke. Common causes of CVAs are hemorrhage from a blood vessel in the brain, emboli (blood clots), and atherosclerosis of the cerebral arteries. Atherosclerosis is the formation of cholesterol-containing plaques that block blood flow. Plaque or a portion of a blood clot may break away from a different part of the body and form an embolus that travels to the brain. These conditions deprive the brain of oxygen. Because brain cells consume large quantities of oxygen, any deficit can cause damage quickly.

When a stroke occurs, blood flow to stop part of the brain is interrupted. The location at which the blood flow has been cut off and the length of time the cutoff has lasted determine the damage caused by the stroke.

The following deficits may occur:
- **Hemiparesis:** Partial motor deficit on one side of the body.
- **Quadriplegia:** Total motor deficit in both arms and legs. **Quadriplegia** usually occurs from trauma to the spinal cord but can occur from a stroke.
- **Sensory Losses:** Inability to feel pain, temperature, vibration, and so forth.

The limbs are initially flaccid or relaxed. Later they become spastic or contracted. The forearm in flexion and the leg in extension are common sights because of the unequal innervation of extensors and flexors. The cause of the spasticity is thought to be loss of control of lower motor neurons.

Behavioral changes caused by damage in the association areas of the cortex often are present. If the left hemisphere is involved, language difficulties such as aphasia (difficulty speaking) occur. A stroke in the right hemisphere produces inattention and lack of concern. Confusion may be present if either hemisphere is affected.

A transient ischemic attack (TIA) is a prestroke condition that mimics a stroke. *Transient* means temporary. TIA resolves in less than 24 hours. In some cases, when the deficit lasts longer than 24 hours and then clears completely, the condition is called a *reversible neurologic deficit* or a *residual ischemic neurologic deficit.*

The signs of a TIA are transient blindness in one eye, aphasia, numbness or weakness of the hand or foot, slurred speech, dizziness, ataxia, syncope, and numbness around the lips. The signs may last only a few minutes and then disappear. They are commonly ignored. Because a TIA is often a warning of a major stroke, it is important to know the basic signs of TIA.

Cerebrovascular Disease

Cerebrovascular disease is a gradual buildup of arteriosclerotic lesions (thickened, hardened areas of reduced elasticity) in arteries of the neck and brain. Hypertension is a strong predisposing factor. Arteries commonly affected are the common carotid, internal carotid, and middle cerebral arteries. Complications of cerebrovascular disease are blood clots and hemorrhage, leading to a stroke.

Aneurysm

An aneurysm is a weakening and bulging of any artery, including those in the brain. If the weakened area bursts, bleeding and complications can be fatal. In the brain it can lead to a stroke. Sometimes the rupture of a brain artery is preceded by a series of small leaks that produce transient headaches and neck stiffness. These symptoms are common in many other conditions and in normal stress, so it is important to have a qualified medical professional rule out more serious conditions before assuming that symptoms are minor or only stress related.

INDICATIONS / CONTRAINDICATIONS for Therapeutic Massage

Therapeutic massage in a supervised setting can be supportive during rehabilitation. Its methods are effective in managing the discomfort caused when the functioning portions of the body must work extra hard to compensate for nonfunctioning areas. Stress management is an important part of the long-term management of these conditions. Because anticoagulants are commonly used to prevent further CVAs or TIAs, care must be taken when using soft-tissue methods so that bruising does not occur during therapy. Careful attention should be paid to any symptom of thrombosis, and the type of massage application used should not place heavy pressure over vulnerable vessels so as to avoid the possible mobilization of an embolism.

Central Nervous System Trauma

A sudden blow to the head or intense shaking of the head may or may not involve a fracture. The fracture itself is usually not important; more significant is the possibility of intracranial bleeding or brain swelling (edema). When the bleeding occurs between the dura and arachnoid, it is called a *subdural hematoma;* when the bleeding is located between the skull and dura, it is referred to as an *epidural hematoma.*

Concussion

A concussion is brain trauma that may be mild, moderate, or severe. Symptoms of mild concussions include brief loss of consciousness or a state of confusion. A headache and vomiting may follow the episode. In most cases complete recovery occurs in a matter of a few days to a week, although in rare cases recovery may take longer.

In cases of moderate to severe concussions, a brain contusion, or bruise, may cause swelling of the brain tissues. This is common in traumas known as *closed head injuries.* Prolonged unconsciousness and problems with vasomotor and respiratory functions may be present. After waking, the person may exhibit behavioral and personality changes, amnesia, and motor and sensory disturbances. The prognosis can range from complete recovery to continued deterioration. Because the amount of internal injury may not be immediately recognizable, any person with head injury should be immediately referred to a medical professional.

Cerebral Palsy

Cerebral palsy is a general term for brain damage that takes place before, during, or shortly after birth. Damage may involve the whole brain but usually is limited to the pyramidal tracts, which results in motor function disturbance. The most common symptoms include muscle spasticity especially in the feet, legs, and hands; impaired speech, vision, hearing, and tactile sensations; and seizures. Impaired intellectual function may or may not result.

INDICATIONS / CONTRAINDICATIONS for Therapeutic Massage

Therapeutic massage is an effective part of a supervised comprehensive care program. Massage and other forms of bodywork can help manage secondary muscle tension resulting from the alteration of posture and the use of equipment such as wheelchairs, braces, and crutches.

Spinal Cord Injury

Injuries to the spinal cord can result in a number of neurologic problems. Studies of blood flow and metabolism indicate that spinal cord injury involves not only direct neuronal trauma but also direct and delayed vascular trauma. The most commonly injured sites are at the most mobile segments of the spine, such as the cervicothoracic (C7 to T1) and thoracolumbar (T12 to L1-L4) junctions. About 40% of spinal cord injuries result in complete interruption of function. The rest of the injuries result in the impairment or destruction of certain sensory and motor functions.

Injury to or cutting of the spinal cord is followed by a 2- to 3-week period of spinal shock when all spinal reflex responses are depressed. The spinal reflexes below the cut become exaggerated and hyperactive. The neurons become hypersensitive to the excitatory neurotransmitters, and the spinal neurons may sprout collaterals that synapse with excitatory input. The stretch reflexes are exaggerated, and the tone of the muscle increases.

If spinal cord injury occurs above the third cervical spinal nerve, loss of voluntary movement of all the limbs occurs, and respiratory movements are affected if the phrenic nerve is damaged. The phrenic nerve arises from the third, fourth, or fifth cervical nerve and supplies the diaphragm. If the lesion is lower, only the lower limbs are affected and **paraplegia** results. Should the nerves to only one limb be affected, **monoplegia** results.

One of the complications common among persons with spinal cord injuries is decubitus ulcer. Because voluntary shifting of weight does not occur, the weight of the body compresses the circulation to the skin over bony prominences and produces ulcers.

The function of the autonomic system below the level of the lesion also is affected. Voluntary control of the bladder and rectum is lost if the lesion is above the sacral segments; reflex contractions of the bladder and rectum occur as soon as they become full, resulting in incontinence; and inconsistency of blood pressure can occur. However, paralysis of the muscles of the urinary bladder could also occur, resulting in stagnation of urine and urinary tract infections.

The mass reflex occurs when a slight stimulus to the skin triggers many other reflexes, such as emptying of the bladder and rectum, sweating, and blood pressure changes. Persons with chronic spinal injuries can be trained to initiate these reflexes by stroking or pinching the thigh, triggering the mass reflex and intentionally giving them some control over urination and defecation.

Because of disuse, calcium from bones is reabsorbed and excreted in the urine, increasing the incidence of calcium stones in the urinary tract.

INDICATIONS/CONTRAINDICATIONS for Therapeutic Massage

Massage is an effective part of a comprehensive, supervised rehabilitation and long-term care program. Massage and other forms of bodywork can help manage secondary muscle tension resulting from the alteration of posture and the use of wheelchairs, braces, and crutches. Specifically focused massage can help manage bowel paralysis. The circulation enhancement produced by massage can assist in the management of a decubitus ulcer.

Tumors

A brain tumor rarely develops in a neuron because neurons do not divide. Most tumors are formed from the neuroglia, the tissues of the membranes, and the blood vessels found in and around the brain. Most tumors that develop in the brain are benign. But because no space is available for them to expand, they compress the brain and its supporting tissues, sometimes with fatal results. Malignant brain tumors usually grow from cells of malignant tumors that exist elsewhere in

the body, often from lung and breast cancer. For this reason surgical removal is indicated whenever possible.

Signs and symptoms of tumor-caused compression are as follows:

- The loss of sensory or motor function, mainly on one side of the body
- Personality changes, behavioral changes, or both
- Headaches
- Awkward movement or gait (ataxia)

INDICATIONS/CONTRAINDICATIONS for Therapeutic Massage

Massage therapists should be able to recognize the signs and symptoms of a possible brain compression and refer the client to a medical professional for diagnosis and care. During rehabilitation from surgery, massage can be used as supportive care and to improve any compensation patterns that have resulted from brain damage caused by surgery.

Degenerative Disorders

A variety of degenerative diseases referred to as *dementia* are organic mental disorders caused by chemical imbalance, endocrine dysfunction, or trauma to the brain, and they can result in the destruction of brain neurons. As the degeneration progresses, symptoms such as memory loss, decreased attention span, diminished intellectual capacity, and loss of control of personality or behavior commonly are observed.

Alzheimer's Disease

Alzheimer's disease is a type of dementia in which the brain degenerates, resulting in judgment errors, memory difficulties, and a tendency to become confused. Neuronal tangles and plaque found in brain tissue contain amyloid, a pathologic, insoluble starchlike protein. Neurons essential for memory are particularly vulnerable to this degenerative process. The current theory is that Alzheimer's disease is determined genetically by amyloid B, which is regulated by a gene located in chromosome 21. Deficiencies in neurotransmitters also are implicated in dementia.

INDICATIONS/CONTRAINDICATIONS for Therapeutic Massage

The degeneration seen in Alzheimer's disease may be slowed by therapeutic intervention and medication. Studies indicate that sensory stimulation modalities such as rhythmic massage and movement may provide calming and orienting influences.

Amyotrophic Lateral Sclerosis

Also known as Lou Gehrig's disease, **amyotrophic lateral sclerosis** is a progressive disease that begins in the CNS, involves the degeneration of motor neurons, and eventually results in the atrophy of voluntary muscle. Symptoms of amyotrophic lateral sclerosis include weakness, fatigue, and muscle spasms. The disease is most common in men between 40 and 70 years of age.

Seizures

Seizures, or convulsions, are defined as sudden involuntary muscle contractions. The most common group of seizure

INDICATIONS/CONTRAINDICATIONS for Therapeutic Massage

> Massage is indicated for amyotrophic lateral sclerosis, with caution and under a doctor's supervision. The degrees of pressure and intensity must be adjusted as the disease progresses.

disorders is referred to as *epilepsy,* which occurs when the nerve cells of the cerebral cortex send out uncontrolled signals. In many cases the cause of the neuron stimulation is unknown, but known precipitating factors include hereditary factors, trauma to the head, stroke, brain tumor, and infections.

Minor (absence seizures, formerly known as *petit mal)* seizures may not include actual spasms of the skeletal muscles. Usually seen in children, these seizures are typified by a moment of blankness. Major (tonic-clonic seizures, formerly known as *grand mal)* seizures begin with an aura or sensation, such as a taste, smell, or feeling. The person usually experiences involuntary spasms or continuous tension in the skeletal muscles and loss of consciousness. A sense of confusion and a desire to sleep are common after effects.

Most forms of epilepsy can be controlled by antiseizure medication, commonly phenobarbital or phenytoin (Dilantin). The side effects of the medications can include headache, muscle tension, nervousness, joint pain, and sleeping difficulties. A continuous seizure lasting more than 30 minutes is called **status epilepticus** and is a medical emergency.

INDICATIONS/CONTRAINDICATIONS for Therapeutic Massage

> The side effects of medications may be decreased by the application of massage techniques. Massage therapists must remember that clients who exhibit any exaggerated or increased symptoms should be referred to their prescribing physicians.

Tremors

Tremors are involuntary muscle twitches. They may be minor and occur in a tired muscle, or they may be exaggerated in conditions such as St. Vitus' dance, Huntington's chorea, or Parkinson's disease. They are not a form of epilepsy, although they originate in the CNS.

Essential tremor is a chronic tremor that does not result from any pathologic condition. The tremor is slowly progressive but usually not debilitating. Onset can occur as early as adolescence but usually occurs in midlife. Essential tremor may be an inherited disorder.

Parkinson's Disease

In Parkinson's disease, the neurons that release the neurotransmitter dopamine in the brain degenerate, thus slowing or stopping its release. Parkinson's disease occurs mainly in the elderly; the symptoms include rigidity of the muscles of the limbs, tremors while the person is at rest, a shuffling gait, and a masklike face.

Pharmacologic intervention includes the use of L-dopa (levodopa), the precursor of dopamine; amantadine (Symmetrel), which releases dopamine at the synapse; and benztropine (Cogentin) and trihexyphenidyl (Artane), both of which are anticholinergic drugs.

Chorea

Chorea results from the degeneration of neurons in the basal ganglia. The affected person's normal voluntary movements are replaced by involuntary dancelike motions. The most common forms are St. Vitus' dance and Huntington's chorea, a hereditary disease that also includes a form of dementia.

INDICATIONS/CONTRAINDICATIONS for Therapeutic Massage

> Because massage has been shown to increase dopamine activity, its use is indicated in managing Parkinson's disease and tremor. In addition, secondary muscle tension can be managed effectively by methods such as massage therapy and other forms of soft-tissue manipulation.

Headache

Headaches can be caused by trauma, stress, muscle tension, chemical imbalance, circulatory and sinus disorders, or tumors.

Migraine headache pain is believed to be caused by dilation of the cranial vessels. The pain is knifelike, throbbing, and unilateral. Any visual distortion (e.g., flashing lights) is thought to be caused by vasoconstriction preceding the vasodilation and pain.

Cluster headaches occur on one side of the head, with remissions and recurrences lasting for long periods. They usually occur at night and are associated with other symptoms, such as red eyes and sinus drainage.

Medications used to treat headaches are usually nonsteroidal analgesics such as aspirin, but migraines may not respond to medication after the headache begins. Migraines sometimes may be prevented by the medication ergotamine (a vasoconstrictor) or other vasoconstricting medications. The judicious use of caffeine may reduce migraine symptoms.

INDICATIONS/CONTRAINDICATIONS for Therapeutic Massage

> Massage and other forms of soft-tissue therapy are effective in treating muscle tension headache but are much less effective for migraine and cluster headaches. Soft-tissue therapy can relieve secondary muscle tension headache caused by the pain of the primary headache. Headache is often stress-induced, so stress management in all forms usually is indicated for chronic headache.

Depression

Depression is associated with a decrease in the neurotransmitters norepinephrine, serotonin, and dopamine. Affected persons can be helped by medications such as amphetamines that inhibit the reuptake of norepinephrine and by monoamine oxidase inhibitors that reduce the breakdown of norepinephrine. A class of medications known as *selective serotonin reuptake inhibitors* is also helpful in managing depression.

Anxiety

Anxiety is a normal reaction to stress. When anxiety becomes an excessive, irrational dread of everyday situations, it has become a disabling disorder. Anxiety disorders range from feelings of uneasiness to immobilizing bouts of terror. Symptoms include chronic, exaggerated worry, tension, and irritability that appear to have no cause or are more intense than the situation warrants. Physical signs, such as restlessness, trouble falling or staying asleep, headaches, trembling, twitching, muscle tension, and sweating, often accompany these psychological symptoms. Types of anxiety include the following:

- Panic disorder
- Obsessive-compulsive disorder
- Post-traumatic stress disorder
- Phobias
- Generalized anxiety disorder

Treatment can involve medicines, therapy, or both. Effective treatments include cognitive behavioral therapy, relaxation techniques, and biofeedback to control muscle tension. Medications used to treat anxiety are called *antianxiety drugs*.

INDICATIONS/CONTRAINDICATIONS for Therapeutic Massage

Therapeutic massage is supportive in a multidisciplinary treatment for depression or anxiety because serotonin, among other neurotransmitters, is influenced by massage. Research has also indicated that the perception of anxiety and tendency to be anxious are reduced by the use of massage therapy.

Schizophrenia

Schizophrenia is the most common mental disorder and includes a large group of psychotic disorders characterized by gross distortions of reality; disturbances in language and communication; withdrawal from social interaction; and disorganization and fragmentation of thought, perception, and emotional reaction. No single cause has been identified, but increased dopamine activity in parts of the brain is strongly indicated. A diagnosis of schizophrenia requires the exclusion of other disorders. Management of chronic schizophrenia requires expert multidisciplinary support along with psychopharmacologic and long-term psychosocial intervention.

Because schizophrenia is associated with increased dopamine levels in the brain, the symptoms are moderated by medications that block or reduce the release of dopamine at the synapses. Large amounts of cocaine and certain amphetamines are associated with increased production of dopamine and may mimic schizophrenic behaviors in otherwise normal persons.

Infectious Disease

Most CNS infections are bacterial or viral. An infection of the brain is called *encephalitis*. Infection of the meninges is called *meningitis*. The two diseases may appear separately or together. Both have symptoms of fever, nausea, and vomiting. Encephalitis may affect motor function, cause seizures, and produce behavioral and mood changes. Meningitis, which occurs mainly in the subarachnoid fluid, adds stiffness of the neck to the symptom list. As with other infections, the primary treatment of viral infection is support for general immune function, with antibiotics given for a bacterial infection.

Myelitis is an infection of the spinal cord or brainstem. In the past the poliomyelitis virus was the most common of its type of infection. It affects motor and sensory functions. Because most forms of myelitis result from viruses, treatment supports the body while the immune functions resolve the infection.

INDICATIONS/CONTRAINDICATIONS for Therapeutic Massage

Infectious processes are contraindicated for massage intervention unless closely supervised by appropriate medical personnel. A person with an unusual or unexplained stiff neck should be referred for diagnosis.

SUMMARY

Many of the physiologic effects of therapeutic massage are caused by interactions with the functions of the CNS. Research has shown that applying massage effectively has beneficial influences on the CNS and the associated neurotransmitters and neuromodulators.

Competence in interpreting symptoms and behaviors related to the CNS is necessary to determine the factors causing distressing symptoms. Clinical reasoning skills and problem-solving techniques allow the therapist to select the methods that will encourage the system's return to effective functioning or create a sense of relaxation and well-being. Knowledge of the CNS is important also because it allows the massage professional to practice safely and refer clients who have conditions contraindicated for massage.

This chapter's focus is the components and functions of the CNS. Behavior and the nervous system are linked in the feedback loop pattern. Consciousness is a function of the CNS. Soft-tissue and movement modalities are supportive, maintaining the health of the CNS. Pathologic conditions of the CNS disrupt many types of body functions, and massage methods can provide support in coping with many of these dysfunctions.

evolve

http://evolve.elsevier.com/Fritz/essential

4-1 Sound it Out: Practice nervous system terminology pronunciations.

4-2 Fill-in-the-Blank: Review nerve structure and function material.

4-3 Play a tic-tac-toe game about the CNS.

4-4 Label structures of the brain.

4-5 Read a case study about the nervous system and then answer follow-up questions.

Additional resources

  Scientific animations

  Weblinks

  Study tips

  Electronic coloring book

Remember to study for your certification and licensure exams! Review questions for this chapter are located on Evolve.

REFERENCE

Hooper J, Teresi D: *The three pound universe*, New York, 1986, Dell.

Workbook Section

Short Answer

1. List the parts of the neuron.

_____
_____
_____
_____

2. Explain the function of the nerve cell.

_____
_____
_____
_____
_____

3. Describe neurotransmitter functions, and list the major neurotransmitters.

_____
_____
_____
_____
_____

4. Relate brain chemistry to behavior.

_____
_____
_____
_____
_____

5. Define the major parts and functions of the CNS.

_____
_____
_____
_____
_____

6. Describe consciousness and altered states of consciousness.

_____
_____
_____
_____
_____

7. Explain the process of memory and learning.

_____
_____
_____
_____
_____

8. Describe common pathologic conditions of the CNS.

_____
_____
_____
_____
_____

9. List the drugs that influence the CNS.

_____
_____
_____
_____
_____

10. Explain the influence of therapeutic massage on the CNS.

_____
_____
_____
_____

Fill in the Blank

The central nervous system consists of the brain and (1) _____. (2) _____ are nerve cells that conduct impulses. Neuroglia are specialized (3) _____ cells that support, protect, and hold neurons together. (4) _____ are branching projections from the nerve cell body. Axons are (5) _____ elongated projections from the nerve cell body. An axon may have branches known as (6) _____, allowing communication among neurons. (7) _____ is the outer cell membrane of a Schwann cell that plays an essential part in the (8) _____ of injured axons.

White matter is (9) _____ nerve fibers. Gray matter is formed by nerve cell bodies in the CNS that are (10) _____. (11) _____ is a disease that causes weakening of skeletal muscles and results from a reduction of acetylcholine receptors.

Neurotransmitters are chemical transmitters released in the (12) _____ from presynaptic cells. A synapse is a (13) _____ between neurons. (14) _____ modulates pain perception, and insufficient levels can result in anxiety or depression.

The (15) _____ is the largest and most complex unit of the nervous system and is responsible for perception, sensation, emotion, and intellect. The

(16) _____ is the largest of the brain divisions and occupies the uppermost region of the cranium. It consists of two (17) _____. The cerebrum is covered by a thin layer of gray matter called the (18) _____ that is formed into folds called convolutions or (19) _____. These folds are separated by creases called (20) _____. Underneath the gray matter is the (21) _____, which is made up of complicated pathways of myelinated axons called white matter that connect the gray matter of the left and right hemispheres.

The (22) _____ of the cerebral cortex is the anterior area positioned behind the frontal bone. Its major function is to control the voluntary skeletal muscles in an area called the (23) _____ and is active in functions of problem solving that involve concentration and planning. The (24) _____ is located next to the parietal bones of the skull and contains the (25) _____, which is the sensory area of the brain and which functions with the sensory data reporting of temperature, pressure, touch, and pain. The (26) _____ is positioned next to the temporal bones. The temporal lobe is responsible for the sensory functions of (27) _____ and (28) _____. The occipital lobe is located just anterior to the occipital bone of the skull and is responsible for the control of (29) _____.

The (30) _____ is a group of structures located on the interior of the cerebrum that plays an important role in arousal and emotional responses, endocrine and autonomic responses, and sexual behavior. Every time the head is moved, the fluid in the semicircular canals is set in motion, generating (31) _____ impulses. The impulses travel to the (32) _____ and to the (33) _____ to give information. The cerebellum is the second largest part of the (34) _____ and is involved with (35) _____. The brainstem contains centers for (36) _____ function connected with (37) _____, as well as vomiting, coughing, and sneezing; posture; and basic movement patterns. Located in the (38) _____ are the thalamus, hypothalamus, and pineal gland. The (39) _____ is associated with pain, temperature, touch sensations, crude sensation, and muscular coordination. The (40) _____ is stimulated, and the body is able to increase and decrease tone and maintain balance and equilibrium.

The (41) _____ controls the pituitary gland by producing releasing hormones and is the temperature center, the sexual center, the thirst and hunger center, and the rage and fear center. The pineal gland appears to act as a (42) _____, regulating circadian rhythms. The midbrain or (43) _____ is located between the thalamus and the pons and contains centers for visual and auditory reflexes and for correlating information about muscle tone and posture, as well as visual reflexes. Nerve fibers entering on one side of the (44) _____ cross and exit the other side; therefore one side of the brain controls the opposite side of the body. The (45) _____ regulates heartbeat, blood pressure, breathing, coughing, sneezing, swallowing, and vomiting.

The CNS is surrounded by three membranes called the (46) _____. (47) _____ is a clear, colorless fluid that flows throughout the brain and around the (48) _____, cushioning and protecting these structures.

The spinal cord is the portion of the CNS that exits the skull into the (49) _____. The two major functions of the spinal cord are to conduct nerve impulses and to be a center for (50) _____. (51) _____ are collections of nerve fibers in the CNS having a common function.

Exercise

For the illustration of a neuron pictured, fill in the blanks for each part indicated by a letter, and then color each part.

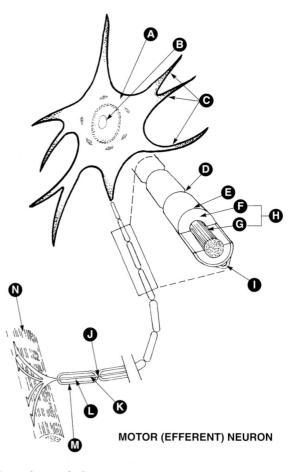

MOTOR (EFFERENT) NEURON

Axon (use twice)
Cell body
Dendrites
Myelin sheath (use twice)
Nerve fiber

Neurolemma (use twice)
Neuromuscular junction
Node of Ranvier (use twice)
Nucleus
Nucleus of Schwann cell

A. _____
B. _____
C. _____
D. _____
E. _____
F. _____
G. _____
H. _____
I. _____
J. _____
K. _____
L. _____
M. _____
N. _____

Problem Solving

Read the problem presented. There is no correct answer; rather, the exercise is intended to assist the student in developing analytical and decision-making skills necessary in a professional practice. After reading the problem thoroughly, follow the six steps below:

1. Identify the facts presented in the information.
2. Identify the possibilities ("what if" statements) presented, or develop your own possibilities that relate to the facts.
3. Evaluate each possibility in terms of the logical cause and effect and pros and cons.
4. Consider the feelings of those involved.
5. Write each answer in the space provided.
6. Develop your solution by answering the question posed.

Problem

Obviously, behavior influences the CNS. It seems to be important for a person to engage in a pleasure-seeking activity that stimulates the feel-good neurotransmitters. Connected with this process is the drive to achieve altered states of consciousness. Today's world places many demands on individuals. Most of these demands are performance based. Time becomes a rare commodity. When this is the case for an individual, the structure for satisfying pleasure needs decreases. Could this situation support the search for quick methods of affecting neurotransmitters? Ancient meditative processes and touch and movement therapies, including exercise, are time consuming. Maybe individuals do not do what they know is beneficial because these methods are cumbersome to integrate into a busy lifestyle. How does one balance the needs for pleasure, excitement, calmness, joy, sadness, love, companionship, and so forth with the time necessary to procure such experiences? One wonders whether this current situation is responsible, at least in part, for extreme behavior and the use of chemicals to create the internal chemical responses that satisfy these needs in a fast and reliable way, regardless of how destructive the long-term consequences may be.

Question

What do therapeutic massage and movement therapies have to offer to satisfy pleasure needs, and how does one efficiently integrate these methods into a busy schedule or begin to justify the time necessary to use the important approaches to CNS health?

Facts

1. Behavior influences the CNS.
2. _____
3. _____

Possibilities

1. Individuals may not take the time to fulfill pleasure needs.
2. _____
3. _____

Logical Cause and Effect

1. Not taking time to fulfill pleasure needs would seem to produce extreme behavior resulting in addictive actions.
2. _____
3. _____

Effect

1. Persons may feel helpless because they do not understand why they do something that initially feels good but ultimately hurts them.
2. _____
3. _____

What do therapeutic massage and movement therapies have to offer to satisfy pleasure needs, and how does one efficiently integrate these methods into a busy schedule or begin to justify the time necessary to use the important approaches to CNS health?

_____
_____
_____

Professional Application

What additional knowledge base would one need to work in CVA rehabilitation and long-term care using therapeutic massage and movement therapies? Where might a practitioner find this information and get additional training?

_____
_____
_____
_____
_____

Assess Your Competencies

Review the following objectives of this chapter:

1. Describe the basic organization of the nervous system.
   - List the two main divisions of the nervous system.
   - List the two main subdivisions of the PNS.
   - Describe the basic functions of the ANS.
   - List and define three types of nerve cells.
2. Describe the anatomy of the neuron and neuroglia.
   - Describe the two cells in the nervous system.
   - Define neurons.
   - List the parts of the neuron.
   - Define neuroglia.
3. Describe the physiology of the neuron and neuroglia.
4. Explain the relationship between neurochemicals and behavior, including pain behavior.
   - Define membrane potential.
   - Describe nerve impulse.
   - Explain nerve impulse conduction.
   - Describe a synapse.
   - List common neurotransmitters and other neurochemicals.
   - Describe the function of neurochemicals.
   - Relate brain chemistry to behavior.
5. Identify the structures and functions of the brain.
6. Identify the structures and functions of the spinal cord.
   - Describe the parts and functions of the central nervous system.
   - Describe consciousness and altered states of consciousness.
   - Explain the process of memory and learning.
7. List drugs that affect the CNS.
8. Describe common pathologic conditions of the CNS and the related indications/contraindications for massage.
   - Explain the influence of massage methods on CNS pathology.
   - Explain how certain drugs affect the CNS.

Next, on a separate piece of paper or using an audio or video recorder, prepare a short narrative that reflects how you would explain this content to a client and how the information relates to the way you would provide massage. See the example in Chapter 1 on p. 22. When read or listened to, the narrative should not take more than 5 to 10 minutes to complete. Simpler is better. Use examples, tell stories, and use metaphors. It is important to understand that there is no precisely correct way to complete this exercise. The intent is to help you identify how effectively you understand the content and how relevant your application is to massage therapy. An excellent learning activity is to work with other students and share your narratives. Also share these narratives with a friend or family member who is not familiar with the content. If that person can understand what you have written or recorded, that indicates that you understand it. There are many different ways to complete this learning activity. Yes, it may be confusing to do this, but that's all right. Out of confusion comes clarity. By the time you do this 12 times, once for each chapter in this book, you will be much more competent.

Further Study

Using additional resource material (see the Works Consulted list at the back of this book) locate the information presented in this chapter, and then elaborate by writing a paragraph of additional information on each of the following:

Nerve cell regeneration

_____

_____

Neuromodulators

_____

_____

Neurotransmitters

_____

_____

Memory

_____

_____

Differences in dominant and nondominant cerebral hemisphere functions

_____

_____

Brainstem function in relationship to survival behavior

_____

_____

Reticular activating system

_____

_____

Spinal cord tracts

_____

_____

Peripheral Nervous System

http://evolve.elsevier.com/Fritz/essential

CHAPTER OBJECTIVES

After completing this chapter, the student will be able to perform the following:
1. Describe the peripheral nervous system.
2. Relate the reflex mechanisms of the peripheral nervous system to massage application.
3. Explain the structure and function of the autonomic nervous system
4. Describe the structure and function of the five basic senses: touch, hearing, vision, taste, and smell.
5. Describe pathologic conditions of the peripheral nervous system and the related indications/contraindications for massage.

CHAPTER OUTLINE

BASICS OF THE PERIPHERAL NERVOUS SYSTEM, 134
  Nerves, 134
REFLEX MECHANISMS, 139
  Types of Reflexes, 140
  Reflex Patterns, 141
  Sensory Receptors of the Somatic Nervous System, 141
  Reflex Arc, 143
  Proprioception: Gamma Motor Neurons and Muscle
    Tone, 146
AUTONOMIC NERVOUS SYSTEM, 147
  Divisions of the Autonomic Nervous System, 147
  Eastern/Western Connection, 150
FIVE BASIC SENSES, 152
  Touch, 153
  Hearing, 153
  Vision, 155
  Taste, 156
  Smell, 157
**PATHOLOGIC CONDITIONS OF THE PERIPHERAL NERVOUS
  SYSTEM,** 158
  Medications That Affect the Autonomic Nervous System, 158
  Pathologic Conditions, 158
SUMMARY, 162

KEY TERMS

Afferent nerves (AF-fer-ent) Sensory nerves that link sensory receptors with the central nervous system and transmit sensory information.

Autonomic nervous system (aw-toe-NOM-ik) A division of the peripheral nervous system composed of nerves that connect the central nervous system to the glands, heart, and smooth muscles to maintain the internal body environment.

Cranial nerves Twelve pairs of nerves that originate from the olfactory bulbs, thalamus, visual cortex, and brainstem. They transmit information to and from the sensory organs of the face and the muscles of the face, neck, and upper shoulders, as well as organs of the thorax and abdomen.

Dermatome (DER-mah-tohm) A cutaneous (skin) section supplied by a single spinal nerve.

Efferent nerves (EF-fer-ent) Motor nerves that transmit motor impulses; they link the central nervous system to the effectors outside it.

Enteric nervous system (ENS) A subdivision of the peripheral nervous system (PNS), which directly controls the gastrointestinal system.

Free nerve endings Sensory receptors that detect itch and tickle sensations.

Kinesthesia (kin-uhs-THEE-zhuh) Sense of movement of body parts.

Mechanical receptors Sensory receptors that detect changes in pressure, movement, temperature, or other mechanical forces.

Mixed nerves Nerves that contain sensory and motor axons.

Myasthenia gravis (my-uhs-THEE-nee-uh) A disease that usually affects muscles in the face, lips, tongue, neck, and throat but can affect any muscle group.

Myotome (MY-o-tohm) A skeletal muscle or group of skeletal muscles that receives motor axons from a particular spinal nerve.

Neurovascular bundle A spinal nerve, artery, deep vein, and deep lymphatic vessel bound together by connective tissue, traveling the same pathway in the body.

Nerve A bundle of axons, dendrites, or both.

Nociceptors (no-se-SEP-tors) Sensory receptors that detect painful or intense stimuli.

Parasympathetic nervous system The energy conservation and restorative system associated with what commonly is called the *relaxation response.*

Peripheral nervous system (pe-RIF-er-al) The system of somatic and autonomic neurons outside the central nervous system. The peripheral nervous system comprises the afferent (sensory) division and the efferent (motor) division.

Plexus (PLEK-sus) A network of intertwining nerves that innervates a particular region of the body.

Polio A viral infection, first of the intestines and then (for about 1% of exposed persons) of the anterior horn cells of the spinal cord.

Proprioceptors (pro-pree-o-SEP-tors) Sensory receptors that provide the body with information about position, movement, muscle tension, joint activity, and equilibrium.

Reflex An automatic, involuntary reaction to a stimulus.

Somatic nervous system (so-MA-tik) A system of nerves that keeps the body in balance with its external environment by transmitting impulses among the central nervous system, skeletal muscles, and skin.

Spinal nerves Thirty-one pairs of mixed nerves, originating in the spinal cord and emerging from the vertebral column; they are part of the peripheral nervous system.

Sympathetic nervous system The part of the autonomic nervous system that provides for most of the active function of the body; when the body is under stress, the sympathetic nervous system predominates with fight-or-flight responses.

Thermal receptors Sensory receptors that detect changes in temperature.

LEARNING HOW TO LEARN

You learn best when you are in a good mood and well rested. We can get into a bad mood when stressed, hungry, tired, sad, worried, or even bored. When we are in a good mood, we are calm, have energy, are alert, can focus, and have a sense of well-being. Things that we can do to support a good mood are eating a nutritious diet, getting natural light and moderate exercise each day, and sleeping well at night. Research suggests that sleep plays an important role in memory, both before and after learning new information. Lack of adequate sleep affects mood, motivation, judgment, and our perception of events. So in order to learn, sleeping throughout the whole night (8 hours) is important. Briefly reviewing before going to sleep is also helpful. The brain takes that information and turns it into a memory.

Remember to study in chunks and give your brain a break. Move your body to rest the brain. Productive mindless activity is beneficial during these brain breaks. Fold laundry, water plants, go outside, or pick up trash while taking a short walk.

This chapter focuses on the anatomy and physiology of the perpherial nervous system. In Chapter 4 we discussed the basic structural plan of the nervous system before specifically describing the neuron and the central nervous system. Remember that the nervous system is divided into the central nervous system (CNS)—composed of the brain, spinal cord, and coverings—and the peripheral nervous system, which includes the cranial nerves, spinal nerves, and ganglia.

The **peripheral nervous system** (PNS) has two main subdivisions. The *somatic subdivision* monitors and controls bones, muscles, soft tissues, and skin. The *visceral* or *autonomic subdivision* is associated with the internal glands, organs, blood vessels, and mucous membranes.

Also remember that the **autonomic nervous system** (ANS) is divided further into two (or three) divisions:

- The **sympathetic aspect** of the ANS activates arousal responses and expends body resources in such a way to respond to emergency situations or any physical activity. The sympathetic ANS is considered the "flight, fight, fear"

system, but any highly emotional state of joy, excitement, and elation is also sympathetic in nature.

- The **parasympathetic aspect** of the autonomic nervous system reverses the response of the sympathetic ANS by returning the body to a non-alarm state and restoring body resources. You can think of the functions as "rest and digest." The parasympathetic nervous system is associated with the "relaxation response."

- The **enteric nervous system** (ENS) is the subdivision of the ANS that directly controls the gastrointestinal system.

This chapter explores the PNS in more depth and further explains the importance of the effects of massage on systems of control.

BASICS OF THE PERIPHERAL NERVOUS SYSTEM

SECTION OBJECTIVES

Chapter objectives covered in this section:

1. Describe the peripheral nervous system.

After completing this chapter, the student will be able to perform the following:

- Describe components of the peripheral nervous system.
- List the cranial nerves, and describe the general function of each.
- Explain the function of spinal nerves.
- Identify the four nerve plexuses.
- Compare and contrast dermatomes and myotomes.

The PNS is responsible for transmitting messages from the sense organs (e.g., nose, ears, eyes) and sensory receptors in the soft tissue and bones to the CNS and then relaying messages from the CNS back to the organs, glands, skeletal muscles, and joints to maintain homeostasis and perform functions to maintain life.

The PNS is composed of the motor nerves, sensory nerves, and ganglia outside the brain and spinal cord. The system consists of 12 pairs of **cranial nerves** and 31 pairs of **spinal nerves,** as well as their various branches in the body. Fibers that innervate the body wall are called *somatic fibers*. Those that supply the internal organs are called *visceral fibers*. The ANS consists of the peripheral nerves involved in regulating cardiovascular, respiratory, endocrine, and other unconscious body functions.

Nerves

A **nerve** is a bundle of axons, dendrites, or both. Recall from Chapter 4 that sensory, or **afferent,** peripheral nerves transmit information to the CNS; motor, or **efferent,** peripheral nerves carry impulses from the brain back to the body. A group of nerve fibers in a nerve is called a *fasciculus*. Nerves may be of the motor, sensory, or mixed type.

- Sensory nerves transmit input from sensory receptors
- Motor nerves innervate or provide action
- Mixed nerves contain sensory and motor fibers

Connective tissues of the nerve (Figure 5-1) include:

- *Epineurium*: Surrounds the entire nerve
- *Perineurium*: Surrounds each fasciculus
- *Endoneurium*: Surrounds and holds each nerve fiber

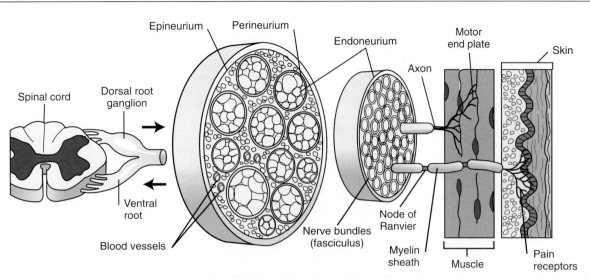

FIGURE 5-1 Peripheral nerve trunk and coverings. (Modified from Thompson JM et al: *Mosby's clinical nursing,* ed 5, St Louis, 2002, Mosby.)

Practical Application

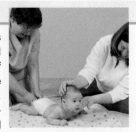

Stimulation of the peripheral nervous system and the responses elicited by this stimulation constitute one of the main physiologic ways massage and bodywork benefit the client. Therefore it is important to thoroughly understand the anatomy and physiology of the peripheral nervous system and the way soft tissue and movement methods interact with the peripheral nervous system.

Cranial Nerves

Twelve pairs of **cranial nerves** enter (sensory) or leave (motor) the olfactory bulbs, thalamus, visual cortex, and brainstem. These nerves are identified by roman numerals (according to their order from the anterior to the posterior brain) and by names (which refer to their function or distribution) (Figure 5-2; Table 5-1).

Disorders of the cranial nerves can result from a stroke, a tumor, or trauma. A lack of function may indicate damage to a particular nerve. The resulting change in action may help locate the lesion (area of damage). For example, the accessory nerves (XI) affect the trapezius and sternocleidomastoid muscles. Dysfunction in either of these muscles may indicate involvement of this nerve.

Practical Application

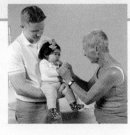

The distribution of the vagus nerve affects many visceral functions. Massage has been shown to support vagus nerve function, especially in premature babies, resulting in better development (particularly in weight gain) and fewer developmental problems.

Spinal Nerves

Recall from Chapter 4 that 31 pairs of **spinal nerves** originate in the spinal cord and emerge from the vertebral column. All contain sensory and motor fibers in the same nerve (forming a mixed nerve), making sensation and movement possible. Each nerve attaches to the spinal cord by way of two short roots on each side, one in front and one in back. The anterior, or ventral, root is motor; the fibers originate in the ventral horn cells and innervate skeletal muscles. The posterior, or dorsal, root is sensory; the fibers originate in the sensory receptors and travel to the dorsal roots of the spinal cord. The dorsal root of each spinal nerve is recognized by a swelling, known as the *dorsal root ganglion,* that contains the cell bodies of the sensory neurons.

Spinal nerves are identified by a letter and a number, which refer to their segment of attachment to the spinal cord (Figure 5-3; Table 5-2). After spinal nerves exit the spinal cord, their nerve pathways generally follow the same pathway as the arteries and deep veins. Deep lymphatic vessels also follow this pathway. Often they are bound by connective tissue into what is called a **neurovascular bundle.**

Nerve Plexuses

Most of the spinal nerves, except those that emerge from the second to twelfth thoracic vertebral spaces, converge in small groups to form an intersecting network known as a *nerve plexus.* Each **plexus** contains fibers that innervate a specific region of the body. Overlap of nerve function prevents total loss of function if just one nerve in the group is damaged. The four major plexuses are the cervical, brachial, lumbar, and sacral plexuses. Thoracic nerves are the motor nerves to the intercostal muscles and sensory nerves from the skin of the thorax.

Cervical Plexus

The cervical plexus, formed from nerves C1 to C4 and part of C5, consists of sensory distribution from the head, front of the neck, and upper part of the shoulders, of motor impulses to many neck and shoulder muscles and the diaphragm (Figure 5-4).

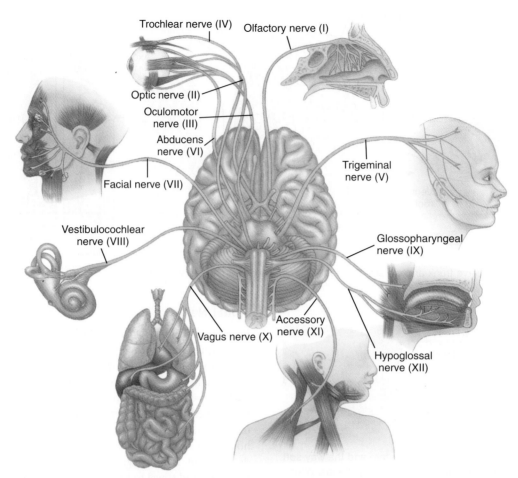

FIGURE 5-2 Cranial nerves. The ventral surface of the brain shows the attachments of the cranial nerves. (From Patton KT, Thibodeau GA: *Anatomy and physiology,* ed 7, St Louis, 2010, Mosby.)

Table 5-1   Cranial Nerves

Nerve	Description
I	The olfactory nerves are sensory and transmit information about taste and smell from the nasal cavity to the cerebrum (into the olfactory bulb of the forebrain).
II	The optic nerves are sensory and transmit information about clarity and field of vision from the retina to the midbrain of the cerebrum by way of the thalamus.
III	The oculomotor nerves are sensory and motor. The sensory portion transmits information about eye movement. The motor portion originates in the midbrain and controls all external eye muscles (except the superior oblique and lateral rectus muscles) and pupil contraction and relaxation.
IV	The trochlear nerves are composed mainly of motor nerves, which begin in the midbrain. They innervate the superior oblique eye muscles. The few sensory neurons provide proprioceptive information about eye movement.
V	The trigeminal nerves arise in the pons. The motor neurons innervate the muscles involved in chewing. The sensory neurons carry information about sensations and proprioception for the head, face, skin of the face, mucosal linings, eyelids, and tongue. The trigeminal nerves are the largest of the cranial nerves.
VI	The abducens nerves arise in the pons. The motor neurons innervate the lateral rectus eye muscle (an eye abductor). The sensory neurons provide proprioceptive information about eye movement.
VII	The facial nerves have motor fibers that arise in the pons and innervate the muscles that produce facial expression and the glands that release tears and saliva. The sensory fibers carry information about taste to the cerebral cortex. Some of the fibers also relay proprioceptive information about the face and scalp.
VIII	The vestibulocochlear nerves are sensory and are divided into two branches. The vestibular branch begins in the semicircular canals of the ear and carries signals for equilibrium to the pons, medulla, and cerebellum. The cochlear branch arises in the organ of Corti and carries impulses for hearing to the pons and medulla.

Table 5-1 Cranial Nerves—cont'd

Nerve	Description
IX	The glossopharyngeal nerves contain sensory and motor neurons. The sensory fibers extend to the medulla from the pharynx and the tongue; they are concerned primarily with taste. Another sensory fiber extends from the carotid sinus in the internal carotid artery and aids in the control of respiration and blood pressure. The motor neurons arise in the medulla and affect saliva production, swallowing, and the gag reflex.
X	The vagus nerves contain sensory and motor neurons. The motor fibers originate in the medulla and carry signals that control the muscles involved in swallowing and speaking. Other motor fibers terminate in the muscles of the digestive and respiratory tracts and in the heart. The sensory fibers arise from the same structures that the motor fibers innervate and carry information about sensations and proprioception of these organs.
XI	The accessory nerves arise in the medulla and are primarily motor neurons for speaking, turning the head, and moving the shoulders. The few sensory neurons relay proprioceptive information from these muscles.
XII	The hypoglossal nerves originate in the medulla and contain mostly motor neurons, which innervate the tongue and throat. A few sensory neurons carry proprioceptive information from the tongue.

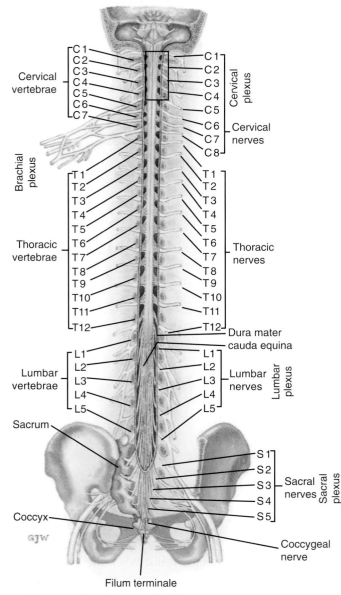

FIGURE 5-3 Spinal nerves. (Each of 31 pairs of spinal nerves exits the spinal cavity from the intervertebral foramina. Notice that after leaving the spinal cavity, many of the spinal nerves interconnect to form networks, called *plexuses.*) (From Vidic B, Suarez FR: *Photographic atlas of the human body,* St Louis, 1984, Mosby.)

Table 5-2 Spinal Nerves

Nerve	Location
Cervical (neck)	Eight pairs: C1 to C8
Thoracic (chest)	Twelve pairs: T1 to T12
Lumbar	Five pairs: L1 to L5
Sacral	Five pairs: S1 to S5 (These exit through the sacral foramina.)
Coccygeal	One pair: Long thoracic nerve

C, Cervical; T, thoracic; L, lumbar; S, sacral.

Brachial Plexus

The brachial plexus, formed from nerves C5 to T1, is organized into three divisions: the superior, middle, and inferior trunks. These divisions supply the skin and muscles of the upper limbs (Figure 5-5).

Thoracic nerves that are not part of the brachial plexus are the motor nerves to the intercostals muscles and sensory nerves from the skin of the thorax.

Lumbar Plexus

The lumbar plexus is composed of nerves L1 to L4.

The lumbar and sacral nerves combine to form the lumbosacral plexus (Figure 5-6). This text presents them separately.

Sacral Plexus

The sacral plexus is created from nerves L5 to S3.

Spinal Nerve Injury

Injury to a nerve can stop the transmission of signals to and from the brain, preventing muscles from working and causing loss of feeling in the area supplied by that nerve. Nerves are fragile and can be damaged by pressure, stretching, or cutting. Pressure or stretching injuries can cause the fibers carrying the information to break and interfere with the nerve function, without disrupting the insulating cover. When a nerve is cut, both the nerve and the myelin sheath are damaged.

When nerve fibers are separated during injury, the distal end of the fiber (farthest from the brain) dies. The proximal end that is closest to the brain and contains the cell body of the fiber does not die, and after some time it may begin to heal. If the myelin sheath was not cut, the nerve fibers may grow down the empty tubes until reaching a muscle or sensory receptor.

Cervical plexus

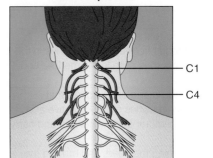

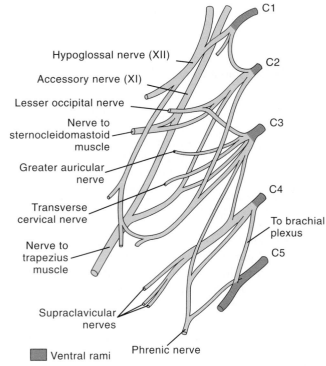

Nerve	Innervation
Ansa cervicalis	Hyoid muscles
Lesser occipital	Skin behind and above the ear
Greater auricular	Skin in front of, below, and over the ear and parotid glands
Transverse cervical	Skin on the anterior portion of the neck
Phrenic	Diaphragm
Supraclavicular	Skin on the shoulders and upper portion of the chest
Segmental branches	Deep neck muscles, midscalenes, and levator scapula muscle

FIGURE 5-4 Cervical plexus. Ventral rami of the first four cervical spinal nerves (C1 to C4) exchange fibers in this plexus found deep within the neck. Some fibers from C5 also enter this plexus to form a portion of the phrenic nerve. (Figure from Patton KT, Thibodeau GA: *Anatomy and physiology,* ed 7, St Louis, 2010, Mosby.)

If both the nerve and sheath have been cut, the growing nerve fibers may grow into a ball at the end of the cut, forming a nerve scar called a *neuroma,* which is painful and can cause an electrical feeling when touched.

Injury to the sensory portion of any spinal nerve causes loss of sensation or altered sensation in the innervated area:
- Hyperesthesia (excessive sensation)
- Hypoesthesia (decreased sensation)
- Paresthesia (numbness, tingling, burning sensation)
- Anesthesia (loss of sensation)

Injury to the motor nerves impairs movement or function and results in the following:
- Impaired movement
- Various forms of paralysis of the muscles served by the damaged nerve
- Gradual weakening
- Wasting away
- Uncontrollable twitching (called *fasciculations*)

When upper motor neurons are damaged, the results include spasticity or stiffness of limb muscles, overactivity of

ACTIVITY 5-1

What could happen if each of the following nerves was damaged?
  Phrenic nerve
  Thoracodorsal nerve
  Radial nerve
  Lateral femoral cutaneous nerve
  Posterior femoral cutaneous nerve

tendon reflexes (e.g., knee and ankle jerks), and loss of the ability to perform fine movements. When the lower motor neurons are damaged, the result is muscle weakness, twitching, loss of muscle tone, flaccid paralysis, diminished or absent reflexes, and progressive atrophy of the muscle (Activity 5-1).

Dermatomes
Dermatomes indicate the relationship between the spinal nerve and skin.

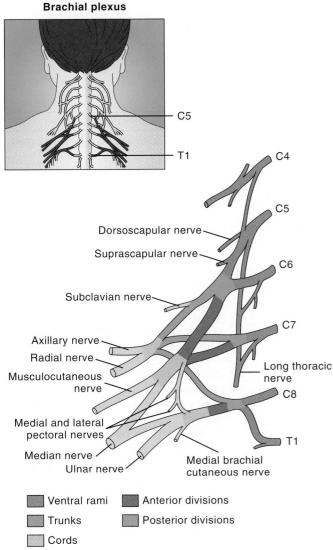

Brachial plexus

Dorsoscapular nerve
Suprascapular nerve
Subclavian nerve
Axillary nerve
Radial nerve
Musculocutaneous nerve
Medial and lateral pectoral nerves
Median nerve
Ulnar nerve
Medial brachial cutaneous nerve

C4
C5
C6
C7
C8
T1

Long thoracic nerve

Ventral rami   Anterior divisions
Trunks   Posterior divisions
Cords

Nerve	Innervation
Dorsoscapular	Superficial muscles of the scapula
Long thoracic	Serratus anterior muscle
Subclavian	Subclavius muscle
Suprascapular	Infraspinatus and supraspinatus muscles
Musculocutaneous	Biceps, brachialis, and coracobrachialis muscles; skin
Subscapular	Subscapularis and teres major muscles
Median	Forearm flexors and palmar surface of the skin of the thumb, index, and middle fingers
Thoracodorsal	Latissimus dorsi muscle
Pectorals	Pectoralis major and minor muscles
Axillary	Deltoid and teres minor muscles and skin
Radial	Triceps and forearm extensors, skin of the forearm and hand, and dorsal surface of the thumb, index, and middle fingers
Medial cutaneous	Skin of the arm
Ulnar	Muscles of the hand and skin of the ring and pinkie fingers

FIGURE 5-5 Brachial plexus. From the five rami, C5 to T1, the plexus forms three trunks. Each trunk subdivides into an anterior and a posterior division. The divisional branches reorganize into three cords, and the cords give rise to the individual nerves that exit this plexus. (Figure from Patton KT, Thibodeau GA: *Anatomy and physiology,* ed 7, St Louis, 2010, Mosby.)

A **dermatome** is a section of skin supplied by a single spinal nerve. Dermatomes are identified by the number of the nerve. Although Figure 5-7 shows a clear boundary for each cutaneous segment, the nerve supplies in adjoining dermatomal segments overlap. Knowledge of the dermatome pattern enables a clinician to locate injuries in the spinal cord and spinal nerves. A correlation can be seen between dermatome patterns and the pathway of traditional Chinese medicine meridians, also known as *channels.*

Myotomes

Myotomes indicate the relationship between the spinal nerve and the muscles innervated by it. A skeletal muscle or group of muscles that receives motor axons from a single spinal nerve is known as a **myotome.** As with dermatomes, the boundaries of myotomes are not always exact; some muscle groups may be innervated by motor axons from more than one spinal nerve.

REFLEX MECHANISMS

SECTION OBJECTIVES

Chapter objectives covered in this section:
2. Relate the reflex mechanisms of the peripheral nervous system to massage application.
After completing this section, the student will be able to perform the following:
• Define a nerve reflex.
• List the sensory receptors involved in reflex action.
• Define a reflex arc.
• Explain motor tone.

A **reflex** is a biological control system that occurs as a response to a stimulus returning the body to homeostasis. A reflex arc is the mechanism of linking stimulus to response. A nerve reflex is usually an involuntary action where the message caused by the stimulus is sent, the brain and spinal cord sense the sensory stimulus, and send a signal (action

Evolve Activity 5-1

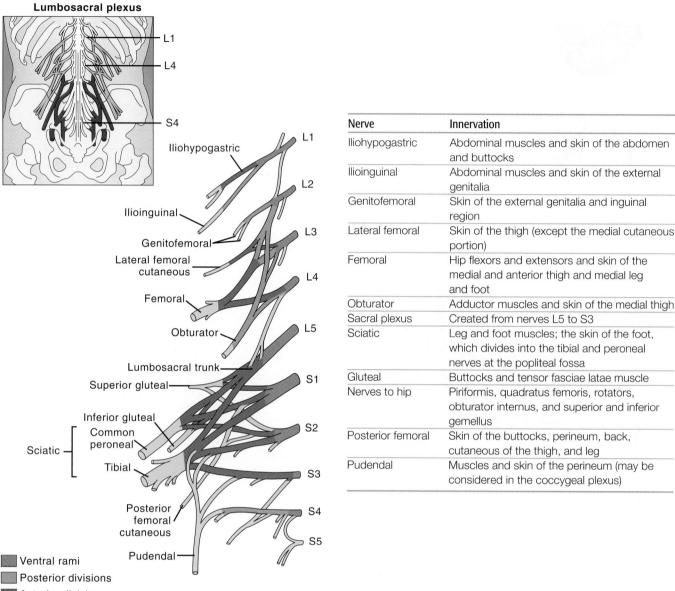

Lumbosacral plexus

Nerve	Innervation
Iliohypogastric	Abdominal muscles and skin of the abdomen and buttocks
Ilioinguinal	Abdominal muscles and skin of the external genitalia
Genitofemoral	Skin of the external genitalia and inguinal region
Lateral femoral	Skin of the thigh (except the medial cutaneous portion)
Femoral	Hip flexors and extensors and skin of the medial and anterior thigh and medial leg and foot
Obturator	Adductor muscles and skin of the medial thigh
Sacral plexus	Created from nerves L5 to S3
Sciatic	Leg and foot muscles; the skin of the foot, which divides into the tibial and peroneal nerves at the popliteal fossa
Gluteal	Buttocks and tensor fasciae latae muscle
Nerves to hip	Piriformis, quadratus femoris, rotators, obturator internus, and superior and inferior gemellus
Posterior femoral	Skin of the buttocks, perineum, back, cutaneous of the thigh, and leg
Pudendal	Muscles and skin of the perineum (may be considered in the coccygeal plexus)

FIGURE 5-6 Lumbosacral plexus. The lumbosacral plexus is formed by the combination of the lumbar and the sacral plexuses, as shown in the *inset*. The ventral rami split into anterior and posterior divisions before reorganizing into the individual nerves that exit this plexus. (Figure from Patton KT, Thibodeau GA: *Anatomy and physiology*, ed 7, St Louis, 2010, Mosby.)

potential) to an effector organ, (muscle) to create an immediate action to counter the stimulus. Involuntary reflexes involve receptors, neurons, interneurons, and the spinal cord. Conditioned learned reflexes also involve the brain. Almost every reflex is polysynaptic, meaning that internal reflex signals cross many synapses. Breaking down these complex patterns is necessary for understanding the automatic and sometimes perpetuating functional and dysfunctional reflex patterns that interact in the continual attempt of the body to maintain homeostasis.

Types of Reflexes

Reflexes are of two types:
• Simple or unconditioned or natural reflex
• Complex or conditioned reflex

Simple or Unconditioned or Natural Reflex

In this type of reflex, the brain is not involved. The receptor is stimulated which is conducted to the spinal cord by the effector. The effector neuron from the spinal cord conducts a response to the muscle or the gland. This causes an immediate reaction. It does not involve any thinking or reasoning. It is a natural response and will occur even in newborn babies. For example, blinking of eyes when strong light falls on the eyes.

Complex or Conditioned Reflex

This type of reflex involves the brain but it is also as fast as the simple reflex. Salivation on smelling one's favorite food is an example of conditional reflex. The individual recognizes the smell and based on a previous experience, the response

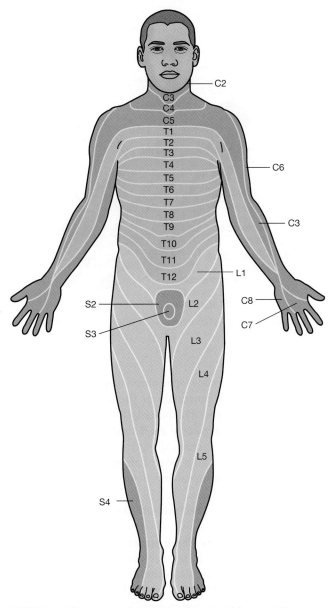

FIGURE 5-7 Dermatomal map *(anterior view)* (also see Figure 2-13).

Some conduct signals to and from the spinal cord to prompt withdrawal of the arm; others carry signals to and from the brain, letting us know when to yell "Ow!"

Almost every reflex is polysynaptic, meaning that internal reflex signals cross many synapses. Breaking down these complex patterns is often difficult but can be a clinical necessity if we are to understand the automatic and sometimes perpetuating responses of functional and dysfunctional reflex patterns that interact in the continual attempt of the body to maintain homeostasis.

Reflex Patterns

Somatosomatic reflexes involve stimulus of sensory receptors in the skin, subcutaneous tissue, fascia, striated muscle, tendon, ligament, or joints, producing a reflex response in segmentally related somatic structures (e.g., from one such site on the body to another segmentally related site on the body, such as the knee jerk that follows tapping the patellar tendon). Massage therapy and hydrotherapy commonly evoke such reflexes.

Somatovisceral reflexes occur where a localized somatic stimulation (from cutaneous, subcutaneous, or musculoskeletal sites) produces a reflex response in a segmentally related visceral structure (internal organ or gland). Vasoconstriction that results from cooling the skin is an example. Massage and hydrotherapy commonly affect these reflexes.

Viscerosomatic reflexes occur when a localized visceral (internal organ or gland) stimulus produces a reflex response in a segmentally related somatic structure (cutaneous, subcutaneous, or musculoskeletal). Viscerosomatic reflexes occur when organ dysfunction produces superficial effects involving the skin (including pain and tenderness). Examples include right shoulder pain in gallbladder disease and cardiac ischemia producing the typical angina distribution of right arm and thoracic pain.

Viscerovisceral reflexes occur when a stimulus in an internal organ or gland produces a reflex response in another segmentally related internal organ or gland, such as the changes in heart rate and blood pressure that relate to baroreceptor stimulation.

Sensory Receptors of the Somatic Nervous System

The **somatic nervous system**, a division of the PNS, primarily affects the skin, muscles, joints, and bones. Our bodies contain many types of receptors located in various areas. Receptors that detect information from outside the body are called *exteroceptors* and are stimulated by actions or changes in our external environment. Two examples are our eyes and ears. Changes in our internal environment stimulate the visceroceptors, or interoceptors. These receptors receive signals monitoring factors such as blood pressure and hunger. Specific to the somatic aspect of the PNS are specialized receptors. In and around the muscles and joints of our body are the proprioceptors, which are affected by changes in position, movement, and tension (Figure 5-8).

(salivation) occurs. The recognition of the previous experience involves the association centers of the brain.

A series of experiments were conducted by Ivan Pavlov, a Russian biologist, which demonstrated *conditioned reflex*. He found that when a bell was rung every time a dog was given food, the dog showed salivation only at the sound of the bell. The ringing of the bell is called the conditioned stimulus. The dog had, thus, 'learnt' to associate the sound of the bell to food and this made it salivate at the sound of the bell.

Reflexes have a fast response time and allow the body to prevent injury by withdrawing or changing position to compensate for the additional stress. Some of these reflexes persist even when injury or disease affects the spinal cord.

Because of the "wiring" of the body, a simple activity that stimulates a few receptors can involve many neurons going to and from muscles and glands. A brief action such as bumping the funny bone (the ulnar nerve) requires many neurons.

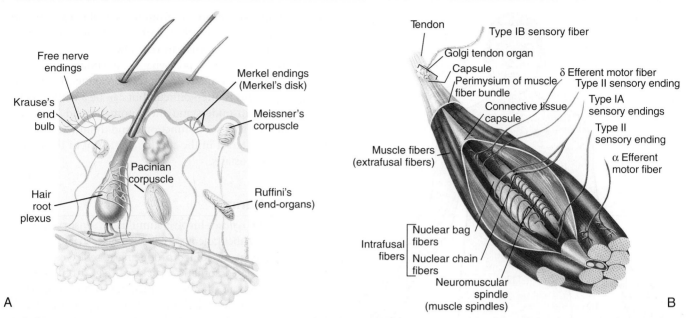

A

B

FIGURE 5-8 Somatic sensory receptors. **A,** Exteroceptors. **B,** Proprioceptors. (Modified from Thibodeau GA, Patton KT: *Anatomy and physiology,* ed 6, St Louis, 2007, Mosby.)

Receptor Adaptation

Most of the time, we are not aware of the subtle changes that stimulate sensory receptors or of the adaptations that result from these changes. These natural reflexes, processed in the brainstem or portions of the spinal cord, affect not only our physical response but also the behavior that may result. We can train ourselves to be aware of the stimuli and purposefully adapt our responses; this is another example of a *conditioned reflex*. These learned behaviors are present in our daily actions, such as tying our shoes, and are also highlighted in forms of sports training and conditioning. We can learn to shoot a basketball or throw a baseball or swing a golf club. After the basic skills have been mastered, we do not have to think about most of the actions; these are conditioned reflexive patterns. Personal habits such as nail biting or eating while watching television also are conditioned reflexive patterns, and these habits may be hard to break after they become reflexive.

When an appropriate stimulus stimulates a sensory receptor, the receptor sends an impulse to the CNS, where the information is processed. Sensory receptors adapt by becoming less sensitive to a stimulus, and they reduce the number of signals sent, or stop altogether, even if the stimulus is still present. If this did not happen, we would never get used to things such as clothing because the nervous system constantly would be aware of the sensations and would be unable to sort through what is important to respond to and what is not. Some forms of minimal brain damage or learning difficulties that involve difficulty focusing or attending to sensory input seem to be perpetuated by a reduced ability for sensory adaptation. Some of the receptors, especially those associated with pressure and touch, adapt quickly; such receptors play a major role in signaling changes in a particular sensation. Other receptors, such as those that detect pain and body position, adapt slowly and signal information about steady states of the body.

Each sensory receptor is specialized to convert one form of stimulus into action potentials in the sensory nerves. The sensation perceived and the ability to localize the part of the body from which it originated are determined by the particular part of the sensory cortex activated by the impulse. Changes in the frequency of action potentials transmission and the number of receptors stimulated determine the intensity of sensation.

Numerous sensory structures are classified as **mechanical receptors:**

- **Mechanoreceptors** These structures detect changes in pressure, movement, temperature, or other mechanical forces. Massage stimulates these sensory receptors.
- **Pacinian (Lamellated) Corpuscles** This type of corpuscle senses brief touch, pressure, and high-frequency vibrations. Located in the submucosal, subcutaneous, and connective tissue of the hands, feet, genitals, joints, and other structures, pacinian corpuscles respond to most forms of rapidly changing mechanical stimulation.
- **Meissner's Corpuscles** These corpuscles are touch receptors found in the hairless portions of the skin, mainly on the palms, fingertips, and soles of the feet, and on the eyelids, lips, tongue, and genitals. The corpuscles can identify the exact location and quality of touch (known as discriminative touch), the initial onset of touch, and low-frequency vibration. Meissner's corpuscles adapt quickly.
- **Hair Root (Root Hair) Plexuses** This type of plexus is a network of dendrites that surrounds hair follicles. Subtle hair movements such as those caused by light touch or a soft breeze stimulate hair root plexuses. They respond and adapt quickly.
- **Ruffini's End-Organs** These structures are touch and pressure receptors located in the deeper areas of hairy

portions of our skin and in our joints. They recognize heavy and continuous touch, pressure, steady position, and direction of movement.

- **Merkel's Disks** These disks are a type of mechanoreceptor and can be found in hairless portions of the skin. They function in discriminative touch.
- **Free Nerve Endings** Some free nerve endings detect temperature and are known as **thermal receptors** (thermoreceptors). One type detects warmth, and another type senses the lack of warmth, or coolness. The brain compares this information to help identify what we would perceive as hot, warm, cool, or cold. The dorsal side of the hand has many thermal receptors, is suited ideally for identifying temperature, and is used commonly by caregivers to check a child for fever. A clinician can use the dorsal side of the hand to assess for warm areas on the body. Other **free nerve endings** detect itch and tickle sensations.
- **Nociceptors** Nociceptors are specific free nerve endings that detect painful stimuli. Actually, overstimulation of any receptor can signal pain as a protective response.
- **Proprioceptors** Mechanical receptors that provide us with information about body position and movement are called **proprioceptors.**

Kinesthesia is the sense of movement of body parts including the ability to feel movements of the limbs and body and the sensation of moving in space.

Proprioception is the sense of position of body parts. Proprioceptors monitor and provided feedback about the position and movement of the body.

Proprioception and kinesthesia are often used interchangably But they are slightly different. Kinesthesia is more about movement and proprioception is more about position.

We maintain posture balance and movement with input from muscle tension, joint position, and the relative movement of each of our limbs and the movement of the whole body.

Because proprioceptors adapt slowly to sensations, they tend to signal the CNS over longer periods. The motor control centers in the brain receive these signals and coordinate normal muscle actions and patterns of movement.

- Proprioception is our "body sense".
- It enables us to unconsciously monitor the position of our body.
- It depends on receptors in the muscles, tendons, and joints.

The following are proprioceptors:
- Muscle Spindles (Neuromuscular Spindles). Muscle spindles are located primarily in the belly of the muscle. They are stretch receptors that monitor and respond to sudden and excessive lengthening. These same fibers send signals via the spinal cord to inhibit actions in the antagonist muscle (the muscle that creates the opposite movement of an action).
- Golgi Tendon Organs. These fibers, which are found in the tendons and musculotendinous junctions, respond to increases in tension. The signals they send out produce a slight stimulation to the antagonist muscle, which prevents return responses from reaching the signaling muscle, causing it to relax.

- Joint Kinesthetic Receptors The ligaments have receptors that respond to excessive strain or tension applied to a joint. They initiate a signal that results in inhibition of the adjacent muscle of muscles.

When proprioceptors are stimulated, the somatic reflex arcs process and interpret the signal as a spinal reflex (Activity 5-2). A feedback loop works to protect the muscles and joints from injury. If the demand on either could cause injury, the result often is pain, weakness, or muscle relaxation.

Practical Application

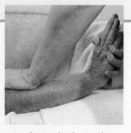

Massage introduces stimulation through touch, pressure, vibration, and movement, causing sensory receptors to respond. Input from the sensory systems plays a role in controlling motor functions by stimulating spinal reflex mechanisms. Almost all forms of bodywork use some aspect of touch that stimulates the various touch receptors found in the skin. Methods that use light touch stimulate root hair plexuses, free nerve endings, Merkel's disks, Meissner's corpuscles, and Ruffini's end-organs. Techniques such as compression; deep, gliding strokes; and joint movement stimulate the pressure receptors such as the pacinian corpuscles. The rapid, repetitive sensory signals of vibration and percussion techniques directly influence the pacinian corpuscles. Movement affects all the proprioceptors.

Reflex Arc

A reflex arc describes the pathway of a reflex. The nerve impulse travels from the receptor through sensory neurons to the spinal cord (or brain), then back through motor neurons to an effector. Association neurons between the sensory and motor neurons help connect the signal pathway for its most efficient routing. The effector is a muscle that contracts or a gland that secretes. A somatic reflex involves skeletal muscle contraction or relaxation, and an autonomic or visceral reflex results in glandular secretion or contraction of a smooth or cardiac muscle.

The somatic reflexes most often stimulated by massage are the *stretch reflex, tendon reflex, flexor reflex,* and *crossed extensor reflex.* These are discussed later in the chapter.

The simplest form of reflex results from a *monosynaptic* (one synapse) and *ipsilateral* (one-sided) reflex arc. The reflex begins with the stimulation of a receptor, which sends out a nerve impulse by way of an afferent (sensory) neuron. The signal travels to the brain or spinal cord and synapses with an efferent (motor) neuron.

The only true monosynaptic reflex is a deep tendon reflex, which involves just sensory and motor neurons. Deep tendon reflexes are important because they can be used to evaluate the sensory nerve, a portion of the spinal cord, the motor nerve, and the muscle or muscles supplied by the nerve. To evaluate the reflex, a physician or trained medical professional uses a device to tap the tendon, which stimulates the receptor in the tendon. The impulse travels along the sensory nerve to the spinal cord, where it synapses with motor neurons and continues along the motor axon, signaling the muscle to contract. A defect at any point in this arc interferes with the reflex contraction of the muscle.

The following are important deep tendon reflexes:
- The biceps and triceps reflexes help evaluate spinal cord levels C5 and C6, the brachial plexus, and the biceps and triceps muscles.
- The patellar reflex (the knee-jerk reflex) helps evaluate spinal cord level L4, the lumbar plexus, the femoral nerve, and the quadriceps muscle.
- The Achilles tendon reflex (the ankle-jerk reflex) helps evaluate spinal cord level S1, the sacral plexus, and the gastrocnemius and soleus muscles. The result of such an evaluation would be abnormal; for example, if low back pain that radiated to the leg and foot accompanied the stimulus (tendon tapping), this could indicate a disk problem at the level of L5 to S1.

Stretch Reflex

The stretch reflex is a protective contraction that results when a muscle is stretched suddenly or intensely. Not to be confused with the action of slow stretching or lengthening, the stretch reflex is a homeostatic mechanism that prevents muscle trauma in response to a stretch. The muscle spindles initiate a nerve impulse that travels to the posterior root of the spinal nerve and into the spinal cord. A nerve impulse then conducts back to the same muscle. The impulse reaches the muscle, generating the action potential and causing the muscle to contract. This contraction prevents the muscle spindle from initiating any more nerve impulses. The stretch reflex itself is monosynaptic (one synapse). However, the response becomes a polysynaptic (many synapses) reflex arc. Association neurons in the spinal cord cause synergist

muscles to contract and relay impulses. Other association neurons interrupt the signal to the antagonist muscles or muscle, allowing it to relax.

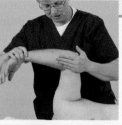

Practical Application

Reflex patterns can be used during massage to make muscles contract. This could be done to stimulate a weakened muscle or assist in lengthening and stretching by stimulating a muscle to contract, which would inhibit any action in its antagonist and thus allow the antagonist muscle to relax.

Reciprocal innervation prevents injury and creates coordinated actions by allowing the signal for contraction of one muscle while inhibiting the signal to its opposing muscle. This is why an antagonist relaxes when an agonist contracts, and vice versa. Reciprocal inhibition is named for this process. Because muscles operate in groups, this stretch reflex coordinates the various contractions and relaxation and the stabilization and balance we need to move effectively. During a massage the practitioner can use reciprocal inhibition as preparation for stretching to avoid stimulating the stretch reflex and thus prevent muscle spasm.

Tendon Reflex

Also known as the *inverse stretch reflex,* the tendon reflex is a feedback mechanism that controls muscle tension by allowing for muscle relaxation. Golgi tendon organs detect and respond to changes in muscle tension. As the tension increases, often because of an increase in a muscle contraction, these sensors initiate a signal that follows the sensory neuron to the spinal cord. Association neurons inhibit any signal from returning to the same muscle, whereas other neurons continue allowing a signal to reach the antagonist by way of the motor neurons. This causes a slight contraction in the antagonist, which allows the prime mover to relax because no impulse is available to generate the action potential.

In some medical texts the term *tendon reflex* is used to describe a reflex action initiated by tapping a tendon rather than by stretching the muscle belly (which may be called a *muscle reflex* even if the result is the same for both). Be aware that such references describe the stimulus and not the resulting reflex action.

The stretch reflex and tendon reflex are simple examples of the way our bodies are programmed to maintain homeostasis. In our normal actions, these reflexes usually are activated for full-body responses instead of isolated muscle groups. The flexor (withdrawal) reflex and the crossed extensor reflex are polysynaptic reflex arcs that work with larger areas and the whole body.

Flexor Reflex

The flexor reflex begins with stimulation of the sensory receptor, often by something painful such as stepping on a pin or

Practical Application

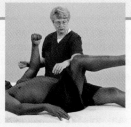

Massage methods can use the stretch reflex to normalize weakened muscle patterns by stretching the muscles just to the point of initiating the reflex. The response would be for the muscle to begin contracting. The result is restoration of a more normal strength pattern in the muscle. An awareness of this reflex response is important in all methods intended to lengthen and relax the muscles to their more normal resting length. In these instances the stretch reflex must be avoided. As a caution, for stretch reflexes to become hyperactive is not uncommon, resulting in increased muscle tension. Such hyperactivity may occur in the leg muscles after a fall when the muscles are quickly and extensively stretched. The stretch reflex may become more sensitive, and cramping may be more common in affected muscles.

Practical Application

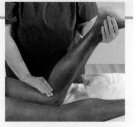

The most common massage technique used to stimulate the tendon reflex is postisometric relaxation. A muscle is contracted against a resisting force, which increases the tension in the tendon. If the load or stimulation is sufficiently strong, initiating the tendon reflex results in relaxation of the muscle. During the relaxation phase the muscle can be lengthened or stretched (or both) more easily. The tissue demonstrates an increased tolerance to stretch after contraction. This technique increases tension at the tendon by introducing contraction in the muscle, usually the result of the client's active participation.

contact with a noxious stimulus such as a hot flame. The signal travels to the spinal cord, crosses association neurons (as in the tendon reflex), and returns to the muscles involved. This muscle contracts to withdraw; simultaneously, signals have been sent to other muscles on the same limb to do likewise. For example, if you step on a pin with your left foot, your left anterior tibialis muscle, quadriceps (rectus femoris), and psoas contract. The antagonist muscles, including the gastrocnemius, soleus, hamstrings, and gluteus maximus, are inhibited from acting (remember the way in which the association neurons can block signals), thus allowing the entire leg to remove itself from the stimulus. The withdrawal reflexes are powerful, taking precedence over all other concurrent reflex actions.

Crossed Extensor Reflex

The crossed extensor reflex works in coordination with the flexor reflex. When the initial signal reaches the spinal cord, it not only travels to the flexor muscles on the same side of the body to allow the limb to withdraw but also crosses the spinal cord and travels to the extensor muscles to maintain balance. This action starts contraction of the right gastrocnemius, soleus, hamstrings, and gluteus maximus while inhibiting the action of the right anterior tibialis, quadriceps, and psoas. The muscles of the torso and arms also can be stimulated or inhibited through this reflex for complete balance if needed.

This reflex action explains why a tension pattern in one part of our body can be seen in other areas. The extensive pathways that the signals follow are called *contralateral reflex arcs*. The initial stimulus given in the previous example was pain, but the body can respond similarly to other stimuli. If you are standing and begin to walk by lifting your right foot off the floor, the signal of loss of balance begins this process, allowing the right leg and left arm to swing forward (flexing) and the left leg and right arm to keep the body steady (extending). This reflex interaction is known as *gait* (Activity 5-3).

✎ ACTIVITY 5-3

Try to determine three upper and lower body interactions based on the withdrawal and contralateral reflex arc. An example is provided to get you started. Pay attention to the patterns and movements, not the specific names and functions of muscles.

Example
Lower body situation: Tight calf on the left
Possible interactions:
Weak dorsiflexors on the left; tight dorsiflexors on the right
Weak calf on the right
Weak hip flexors on the left; tight hip flexors on the right
Tight hip extensors on the left; weak hip extensors on the right
Weak arm flexors on the left; tight arm flexors on the right
Tight arm extensors on the left; weak arm extensors on the right
Weak neck extensors; tight neck flexors

Weak abdominal muscles
Tight back extensors

Your Turn
1. _____
_____
_____
_____
2. _____
_____
_____
_____
3. _____
_____
_____
_____

Practical Application

The effects produced by massage depend heavily on the reflex mechanism. The effectiveness of the particular techniques depends on how efficiently one stimulates the receptors for these reflexes. The practitioner must reach the targeted receptor with the appropriate technique and level of intensity so that the reflex stimulated is allowed to function in the appropriate manner. Fast- and slow-acting receptors, light- and deep-touch receptors, and others are stimulated by different durations and levels of intensity of touch and movement. The massage practitioner must understand what type of message to send to the CNS to be processed. Treatment methods do not produce the desired benefit if they send the wrong signal.

Most benefits derived from massage therapies result from resetting tension patterns caused by reflex actions, especially those that begin as a result of a fall or trauma, repetitive movement, or maintenance of a fixed position. The practitioner who understands the interactive patterns can use corrective massage procedures to resolve or support these actions.

Because of the crossed extensor reflex, the massage massage practitioner can deliberately stimulate limbs on one side of the body to affect the limbs on the opposite side of the body.

For example:

• If the goal is relaxation of the flexors of a lower limb, stimulating the extensors of the upper limb on the opposite side produces reciprocal innervation in the thigh flexors, resulting in this relaxation response.

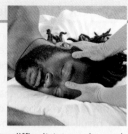

You can figure out many of these patterns by thinking in terms of reflex patterns. By effective application of these reflex arcs, a therapist can affect any neuromuscular area of the somatic system without even touching that area; this is beneficial for sensitive areas that are in pain or areas that are difficult to reach, such as the deep muscles of the axilla or groin.

Reflex patterns are also responsible for many compensatory body patterns found in relation to posture. Imagine that a person suddenly stumbles when walking. The crossed extensor reflexes, via contralateral reflex arcs, respond to restore balance. The attempt by the body to stay upright by avoiding the fall may result in a chain reaction of muscle tension and relaxation adjustments throughout the body, which can develop into postural distortion over time if the situation continues. The body may readjust muscle tension patterns, and neuromuscular feedback loops may become confused. The resulting skeletal muscle pathologic conditions can lead to discomfort and postural distortion from uneven muscle contraction and relaxation patterns. Therapeutic massage often resets these unproductive reflex patterns. Resetting of reflex communication patterns may result in a return of more efficient and coordinated movement patterns.

Proprioception: Gamma Motor Neurons and Muscle Tone

Gamma motor neurons innervate muscle spindles. If the gamma motor neuron is stimulated, contraction occurs at both ends of the spindles, resulting in stretching of the middle region of the spindle where the sensory nerves are located. The sensory nerve endings detect the stretch and produce action potentials that cause the muscle to be more sensitive to stretch. Gamma motor neurons are then responsible for the motor tone of muscle.

A muscle that offers little resistance to stretch is said to be *flaccid*. Flaccidity occurs if the nerve to the muscle is cut. A muscle is *hypotonic* when the gamma motor neuron discharge is low. A muscle that offers great resistance to stretch is said to be *hypertonic* or *spastic*. Spasticity occurs when hyperactive stretch reflexes exist and may be seen in individuals with spinal cord injury or stroke, in whom the inhibitory impulses to the gamma motor neurons from the brain have been removed.

Control of Gamma Motor Neuron Discharge

The gamma motor neurons regulate the sensitivity of the muscle spindles, and hence the stretch reflexes and motor tone of the muscle can be altered according to the change in posture. Many factors affect the gamma motor neuron discharge. For example, anxiety and stress increase its discharge, resulting in tensing of muscles and hyperactive tendon reflexes. If the skin of the hand on one side is stimulated by a painful stimulus, the result is increased discharge to the flexors and decreased discharge to the extensors of the same side, facilitating flexion and quick removal. At the same time, the opposite happens on the other side, adjusting posture and weight distribution.

Touch and movement are considered stimuli because they constitute a change in the environment. When the body is called on to restore homeostasis, problematic nerve transmission pathways often can be overridden and a more effective pattern can be established. Learning the receptor language of the body and exploring the reflex patterns initiated by the various forms of stimuli are worthwhile ways to override these nonproductive transmissions. The more this information is incorporated into practical applications, the more effective the therapeutic massage intervention will be.

Fascial Innervations

New to our understanding of somatic nervous system function is the extensive nerve supply to the fascia. Fascia is a form of connective tissue. Some of the functions of fascia are sliding, gliding and separation of muscle structures, transmission of movement cause from muscle contraction to the bone and joints, suspending organs in place, and providing a supportive and movable covering for nerves and blood vessels as they pass through and between muscles. Anatomists have known for a long time that fascia wraps nerves and nerves pass through fascia. Recent research has found that fascia— once thought to simply be passive connective tissue like a spider web is actually innervated and has its own smooth muscle tissue This means that the brain and the rest of the central nervous system has influencing of fascia through neural activity.

Both somatic and autonomic sensory receptors are imbedded in fascia. Typically the receptors are monitoring stability and movement. The smooth muscle bundles in fascia act as effectors and the nervous system can signal increase contraction which would tighten up the fascia. This is an appropriate response if there is instability. It is possible that various pain syndromes are due to an inappropriate response of the fascia to these types of nerve signals.

AUTONOMIC NERVOUS SYSTEM

SECTION OBJECTIVES

Chapter objectives covered in this section:

3. Explain the structure and function of the autonomic nervous system.
After completing this section, the student will be able to perform the following:
- Name the two divisions of the autonomic nervous system.
- List and compare the functions of the sympathetic and parasympathetic nervous systems.
- Describe the Eastern/Western connection as it relates to the functions of the autonomic nervous system.

Maintenance of the internal environment of the body is the responsibility of the ANS. The ANS controls the actions of the smooth muscles and glands. As in the somatic PNS, ANS information from sensory receptors goes to the brain, which in turn relays the most effective effector response to maintain homeostasis through motor nerves. The sensors are located in areas such as the smooth muscles, blood vessels, lungs, and glands. Motor neurons carry the signals to these same organs to prompt an increase or decrease in the rate of our heartbeat, breathing, or digestive processes or to initiate glandular secretion. The system is called *involuntary* because its actions normally are outside conscious control. A very interesting finding is that fascia is innervated by the ANS.

Divisions of the Autonomic Nervous System

The ANS is divided into the sympathetic and parasympathetic divisions. In general, the **sympathetic nervous system** tends to stimulate and functions primarily when the body is under stress. The **parasympathetic nervous system,** which usually diminishes or inhibits actions, tends to work most often under normal body conditions or to conserve energy (Figure 5-9). The enteric nervous system (ENS) is a third division of the autonomic nervous system that you do not hear much about. The enteric nervous system is a meshwork of nerve fibers that innervate gastrointestinal tract, pancreas, and gall bladder. The ENS is sometimes called the belly brain (Table 5-3).

Differences between the Somatic and Autonomic PNS

Our skeletal muscles are innervated by neurons that carry a signal to contract or carry no signal at all, which causes the

Table 5-3	Enteric ANS Neurotransmitters
Transmitter	Functions
Nitric oxide (NO)	Parasympathetic—important in erection and in gastric emptying
Vasoactive intestinal ploypeptide (VIP)	Parasympathetic—important throughout the body
Serotonin (5HT)	Important in enteric neurons (peristalsis)
Gamma-amino butyric acid (GABA)	Enteric
Substance P	Sympathetic ganglia, enteric neurones

muscles to relax. The ANS has a different form of control. Most of the organs contain neurons from the sympathetic and parasympathetic divisions; this is called *dual innervation.* By constantly receiving signals from both divisions, the body can maintain or quickly restore homeostasis because the organs can be stimulated or inhibited rapidly.

This form of autonomic antagonism is another example of the duality of wholeness discussed previously in this text. If sympathetic impulses tend to stimulate an effector, parasympathetic impulses tend to inhibit it, and vice versa. This type of antagonistic activity gives precise control, much like the accelerator and brake pedals of a car.

For example, moment-to-moment regulation of blood pressure involves continuously changing sympathetic and parasympathetic signals to the heart. The regulation comes from centers in the brainstem that "turn up" or "turn down" each type of input to keep blood pressure constant as the body changes position or activity.

Another major difference is that in the ANS, two neurons relay the signal from the brainstem or spinal cord to the organ, gland, or smooth muscle innervated. The first neuron synapses with the second, and the second synapses with the receptor.

In the sympathetic nervous system, the synapse, or ganglion, is located near the spinal cord. In the parasympathetic system the ganglion is near or at the receptor organ, gland, or muscle. The neurotransmitter released at the ganglion synapse near the spinal cord is acetylcholine, just as in the somatic nervous system. The sympathetic postganglionic synapse to the organs releases noradrenaline (norepinephrine), except in the adrenal medulla, which releases adrenaline (epinephrine) and only some noradrenaline. The benefit of adrenaline in the blood is that it reinforces and prolongs the effect of noradrenaline.

Sympathetic Structure and Function

The sympathetic nervous system begins in the spinal cord, where the neurons exit between the first thoracic vertebra and second lumbar vertebra. Because of the location, the system often is referred to as the *thoracolumbar division.*

The sympathetic ganglia found near the spinal cord are connected by collateral tissues and form a chain. This interconnected chain allows for many different sources of input of sympathetic activity to each of the effectors, thus producing more sympathetic activity with little input. The preganglionic neurons are short and end in this chain; the

Box 5-1   ANS Neurotransmitters and Receptors

Acetylcholine is found in the parasympathetic postganglionic synapse. Based on the neurotransmitter secreted, the ANS can be divided into cholinergic (acetylcholine-secreting) and adrenergic (adrenaline-secreting) divisions. All preganglionic and postganglionic fibers of the parasympathetic system belong to the cholinergic division. Postganglionic sympathetic fibers that supply sweat glands and blood vessels of skeletal muscles produce vasodilation and are cholinergic. The postganglionic fibers of the sympathetic system are adrenergic.

Other neurotransmitters such as dopamine are secreted by interneurons located in the ganglia. Stimulation of the sympathetic nervous system can excite or inhibit the smooth muscles, depending on the receptors in the organ involved. Receptors are divided into two major groups: alpha receptors, which respond to norepinephrine (noradrenaline) and certain blocking substances, and beta receptors, which respond to epinephrine (adrenaline) and similar blocking substances. Each of these groups can be divided again, into alpha-1 and alpha-2 and beta-1 and beta-2, which better classifies the generalized responses they produce.

When alpha receptors are stimulated, they cause dilation of the pupils and constriction of the smooth muscles and blood vessels. Stimulation of beta-1 receptors, which are found mainly in the heart, results in an increase in the force and rate of heart muscle contraction; beta-2 receptors, located in the lungs, cause relaxation of the bronchial muscles, resulting in bronchodilation.

As with sympathetic nerve fibers, the effect of the parasympathetic postganglionic fibers on a target organ depends on the type of receptors present in the cells.

Two types of receptors, nicotinic and muscarinic, have been identified. The nicotinic receptors are present in the parasympathetic and sympathetic ganglions and in the neuromuscular junction. The muscarinic receptors are located in target organs supplied by postganglionic parasympathetic fibers. The terms nicotinic and muscarinic are based on the effects of nicotine, a powerful toxin that can be obtained from a variety of sources including tobacco, and muscarine, a toxin present in poisonous mushrooms. Thus, if one ingests a large quantity of nicotine, it produces symptoms according to the presence of nicotinic receptors such as vomiting, diarrhea, sweating (parasympathetic effects), high blood pressure, rapid heart rate, and sweating. By stimulating skeletal muscles, convulsion also may occur.

The symptoms produced by muscarine poisoning are almost all caused by parasympathetic effects and include vomiting, diarrhea, constriction of bronchi, low blood pressure, and slow heart rate.

Knowledge of the receptors, actions, and distribution of parasympathetic and sympathetic nervous systems is important to all health professionals. Almost all drugs used in conditions such as asthma, hypertension, the common cold, constipation, diarrhea, and many other conditions have been developed and are being used based on this knowledge. Side effects of all these drugs can be derived logically if one knows which receptors they affect and whether the drug imitates or opposes the sympathetic and parasympathetic systems.

The effect the neurotransmitter has on a target organ depends on the type of receptor for the neurotransmitter the cells of the organ possess. For example, the effect of postganglionic parasympathetic fibers may be stimulatory or inhibitory depending on the receptor. In general, postganglionic sympathetic fibers are excitatory.

---

postganglionic neurons are much longer and end at the effector organs.

The major function of the sympathetic nervous system involves the emergency response. The signals sent out allow the body to be more prepared for an increase in the intensity of activities that require increased metabolism, higher blood sugar levels, a stronger heartbeat, and dilated bronchi, allowing for more oxygen to the lungs and faster exhalation of carbon dioxide. During this function the blood is rerouted from the digestive system to the muscles so that they can respond to the increased stress.

Whether the stimulus is physical or psychological or whether the threat is real or imagined, all our responses are set into action immediately. Walter B. Cannon described this group of sympathetic responses as the *fight-or-flight* reaction. These responses are normal and healthy in times of stress. However, chronic exposure to stress or perceived threats to our well-being can affect our health adversely, leading to dysfunction of sympathetic effectors and perhaps even to the dysfunction of the ANS itself. Excessive sympathetic output causes most of the stress-related diseases physicians encounter. Problems with headaches, gastrointestinal difficulties, high blood pressure, anxiety, muscle tension and aches, and sexual dysfunction can be related to excessive sympathetic stimulation.

We think of the previously mentioned sympathetic functions as life preserving because they can be used to remove us from dangerous situations and keep us active in self-preservation. However, the sympathetic system also is active during many of our normal daily functions. Dual innervation allows the sympathetic system to oppose the effects of the parasympathetic system, providing balance and maintaining homeostasis. Smooth muscles in the walls of the blood vessels are innervated only by sympathetic fibers. The fibers maintain the tone of the muscles of the arteries, resulting in proper blood pressure whether we are active or at rest. This is another example of general homeostatic balance (Box 5-1).

Parasympathetic Structure and Function

The parasympathic division of the ANS can be throught of as the *rest, digest,* and *restore* system.

The parasympathetic nervous system is referred to as the *craniosacral division* because of the location of its nerves. Parasympathetic fibers leave the CNS through cranial nerves, including the oculomotor, facial, glossopharyngeal, and vagus nerves and at the sacrum and some pelvic nerves. The three long preganglionic neurons that innervate the pupil and the salivary and lacrimal glands end outside the actual organs.

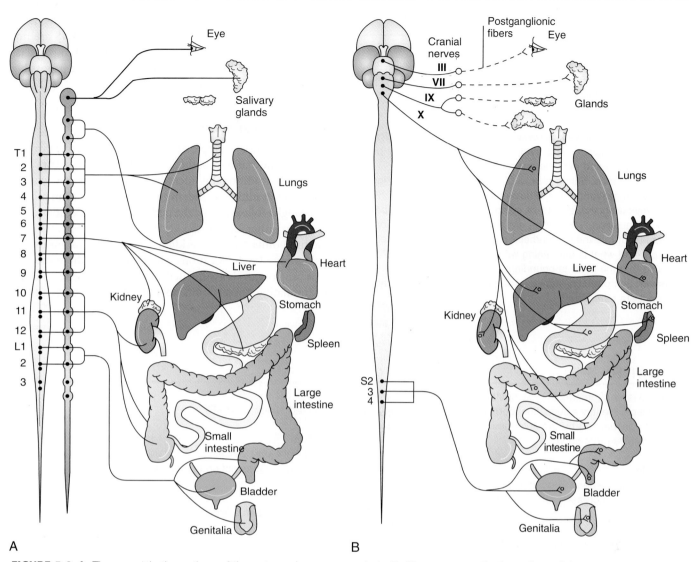

FIGURE 5-9 A, The sympathetic portions of the autonomic nervous system. **B,** The parasympathetic portions of the autonomic nervous system with the vagus nerve distribution to the enteric devices.

The rest of the preganglionic neurons end at the walls of the organs, with the short postganglionic fibers entering the organs. This configuration is the opposite of the sympathetic division, in which the neurons end just before the organ.

The parasympathetic system generally functions as the energy conservation system, which allows the body to rest and restore itself after emergency responses. The result is a relaxation response. To maintain balance with the sympathetic division, the parasympathetic system is dominant under nonstressful conditions; this means that during nonstressful times, more impulses to the effectors are received by parasympathetic fibers than by sympathetic fibers.

The parasympathetic system is active in regulating digestive processes, slowing the heart rate, and constricting eye muscles to focus on near vision. In addition, the parasympathetic system increases glandular secretions, constricts the bronchioles in the lungs, and slows breathing. Parasympathetic stimulation of the nerves to the internal and external genitalia in males and females causes vasodilation in the clitoris and labia minora and erection in the penis.

Reactions to parasympathetic stimulation are highly localized and tend to counteract the adrenergic effects of the sympathetic system (Activities 5-4 and 5-5; Table 5-4). Learning one system usually is simpler, because the other is the opposite. Memorizing the fight-or-flight response seems to be the more practical way. These responses make fighting or fleeing possible; for example, pupil dilation improves vision, faster heart rate increases cardiac output to supply muscles with blood, bronchodilation improves breathing, and slowing of digestive responses reduces interference with fight or flight.

Fascia and ANS

As mentioned, the fascia is rich in somatic proprioceptive nerve endings. Fascia is also innervated by autonomic nerves. These receptors are called interstitial type III & IV muscle receptors or. Functions include inhibition of sympathetic activity. Changes in vasodilation plus affects on plasma movement into the tissues (Schleip 2003). The implication of these findings expands the understanding of stress on soft tissue. Activities such as stretching and massage that stretches the

✎ ACTIVITY 5-4

Identify a control process you use to influence the sympathetic and parasympathetic divisions of the autonomic nervous system, and explain the way it works. An example is provided to get you started.

Example
Sympathetic: Brisk walking for 30 minutes in the morning. The fast pace activates the sympathetic functions and helps wake me up and give me energy for the day.
Parasympathetic: Eating a bowl of cereal before bed. Eating signals digestion and also helps make me sleepy.
After reviewing the effects of sympathetic and parasympathetic stimulation, you will be given a behavior or sensation. Determine if it is the sympathetic or parasympathetic system at work and what is happening within the body:
Feeling that the heart is pounding
Answer: Sympathetic: increased rate and strength of contraction (beta receptors).

tissues changes the shape of the soft tissue activating the nerve receptors in fascia. The potential effects on the ANS are not yet understood. However, since the interstitial myofascial tissue receptors inhibited sympathetic function, it is possible that these methods would support relaxation.

Eastern/Western Connection

The ANS is a clear example of the yin and yang concept. The ganglia of the parasympathetic system tend to occupy the same areas traditionally identified as chakras, or energy centers, by traditional Indian medicine. The sympathetic chain ganglia follow one of the paths of the bladder meridian, located on either side of the vertebral column. Specific acupuncture points on this meridian, called *back-shu* points, are considered to be the locations where the Qi of the respective yin or yang organs is assimilated. Practitioners use techniques for stimulating these points to relieve dysfunctions of the

✎ ACTIVITY 5-5

After reviewing the effects of sympathetic and parasympathetic stimulation, identify a sensation, body function, daily activity, or behavior influenced by the autonomic nervous system. Examples are given to help you.

Example
Feeling that the heart is pounding
Sympathetic: Increased rate and strength of contraction

Your Turn
Parasympathetic: Decreased rate of strength of contraction

Example
Possible lower blood pressure; may feel washed out or fatigued

Your Turn
Smooth muscle of blood vessels
Sympathetic: Skin, blood vessels: constriction (alpha receptors)

Example
Hands and feet get cold

Your Turn
Parasympathetic: No effect

Example
Hands and feet get warmer

Your Turn
Skeletal muscle blood vessels
Sympathetic: Dilation (beta receptors)

Example
Feels as if the body wants to move and is restless

Your Turn
Parasympathetic: No effect

Example
Increased ability to sit still

Your Turn
Abdominal blood vessels
Sympathetic: Constriction (alpha receptors)

Example
Stomach seems in a knot

Your Turn
Parasympathetic: No effect

Example
Stomach seems relaxed

Your Turn
Blood vessels of external genitals
Sympathetic: Constriction (alpha receptors)

Example
May not feel sexual

Your Turn
Parasympathetic: Dilation of blood vessels, causing erectile tissues to engorge

Example
May have sexual thoughts

Your Turn
Smooth muscle of hollow organs and sphincters
Bronchioles
Sympathetic: Dilation (beta receptors)

Example
May feel like not getting enough air

✏ ACTIVITY 5-5—cont'd

Your Turn
Parasympathetic: Constriction

Example
Breathing may get slower

Your Turn
Digestive tract, except sphincters
Sympathetic: Decreased peristalsis (beta receptors)

Example
May be constipated

Your Turn
Parasympathetic: Increased peristalsis

Example
May digest food better

Your Turn
Digestive tract sphincters
Sympathetic: Constriction (beta receptors)

Your Turn
Parasympathetic: Relaxation

Example
May leak urine when coughing

Your Turn
Eye
Iris
Sympathetic: Contraction of radial muscle; dilated pupil

Example
May need sunglasses even in moderate lighting

Your Turn
Parasympathetic: Contraction of circular muscle; constricted pupil

Example
Frequently finds lighting too dim

Your Turn
Ciliary body
Sympathetic: Relaxation; accommodation for far vision

Example
May find newspaper harder to read

Your Turn
Parasympathetic: Contraction; accommodation for near vision

Table 5-4 Sympathetic and Parasympathetic Effects on Structures and Systems of the Body

Structure/System	Parasympathetic System Response	Sympathetic System Response
Eye		
Radial muscle of iris	None	Contraction: results in pupil dilation
Sphincter muscles of iris	Contraction: results in pupil constriction	None yet identified
Ciliary muscle	Contraction: results in near sight	Reflex action: far sight
Tear glands	Secretion	None
Skin		
Sweat glands	None	Secretion increased
Arrector pili muscle	None	Contraction, erection of hairs
Cardiovascular System		
Blood vessels to skin	None	Constriction
Blood vessels to skeletal muscle	None	Dilation
Blood vessels to heart	None	Dilation
Blood vessels to intestines	None	Constriction
Heart	Heart rate and contraction force decreased	Heart rate and contraction force increased; vasodilation
Blood coagulation	None yet identified	Coagulation increased of coronary vessels
Digestive System		
Liver	Glycogen synthesis	Glycogen breakdown; glucose synthesis and release
Salivary glands	Mucus secretion	Watery, serous secretion
Intestinal peristalsis	Increased	Decreased
Sphincters	Relaxation	Contraction
Digestive secretions	Stimulation	Possible inhibition
Adipose tissue	None yet identified	Breakdown and release of fatty acid
Skeletal muscles	None	Contraction force increased
Urinary System		
Kidney	Urine production increased	Urine production decreased
Sphincter	Relaxation	Contraction
Respiratory System		
Bronchial muscles	Contraction	Relaxation
Mental Activity	Calm	Alertness increased

✎ ACTIVITY 5-6

Using basic massage methods, describe how you would design and implement a 45-minute massage that would result in the following:

A. Sympathetic dominance

B. Parasympathetic dominance

corresponding organs. One can see a correlation between sympathetic ANS function and these important organ points in the Asian meridian system.

It is now generally accepted that the traditional meridian system is connected with the fascia. Dr. Langevin and associates have completed multiple studies on the relationship of fascia to acupuncture points and meridians. They have found substantial overlap of acupuncture points and meridians to fascial planes in the body. The needle grasp effect found in acupuncture is also related to the fascia. We now know that the fascia is innervated with both somatic and autonomic sensors and receptors.

Research over the past 20 years has identified the crucial role that the ANS plays in stress-related disorders. This research also has validated the effectiveness of many ancient healing, cultural, and spiritual practices that serve to bring the ANS under voluntary control, bringing conscious control to homeostatic processes (Activity 5-6).

FIVE BASIC SENSES

SECTION OBJECTIVES

Chapter objectives covered in this section:

4. Describe the structure and function of the five basic senses of touch, hearing, vision, taste, and smell.

After completing this section, the student will be able to perform the following:

- List the five basic senses.
- Describe the five basic senses.
- Describe the relevance of the five basic senses to daily function.

With all the possibilities of sensory stimulation, compartmentalizing the types of stimuli and our responses makes studying and understanding the phenomena easier. More than 20 different senses have been identified (Box 5-2). For our purposes, we focus our study on the basic five special senses we encounter and use daily. The five basic senses are touch, hearing, vision, taste, and smell. Touch is covered in detail in the discussion of the integumentary system in Chapter 11. Research brings new information about the way senses work, the way they are processed in our brains, and the way they interact to enhance our lives.

Receptors for the general senses are scattered throughout the body and are relatively simple in structure. These receptors

Practical Application

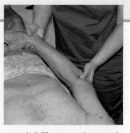

Massage modalities seem initially to stimulate sympathetic functions. Homeostatic mechanisms then work to increase restorative parasympathetic functions as needed. Point holding methods such as acupressure, reflexology, or the dry needling of acupuncture release the body's own painkillers and mood-altering chemicals from the entire endorphin class. These chemicals stimulate the parasympathetic responses of relaxation and contentment. Acupressure is specific pinpoint compression over motor points and other areas of neurovascular concentration. These specific points and areas are the focal meeting of superficial nerves in the sagittal plane, superficial nerves or plexuses, and muscle tendon junctions at the Golgi tendons. These areas, where nerves are close to the surface of the body, correspond with many of the traditional acupuncture points within the fascia. Acupressure produces sympathetic inhibition. Acupuncture probably works by taking advantage of the natural inhibitory influences in the body, such as endorphins and enkephalins, that normally block pain pathways. For example, researchers have established that sensory pain fibers release the neurotransmitter known as substance P, which increases the transmission of pain impulses. Endorphins and enkephalins block the release of substance P, inhibiting pain transmission to the brain. The effects of these and other neurotransmitters may validate the use of sensory stimulation methods to treat pain and anxiety.

Box 5-2 Our Many Senses

Balance or vestibular sense allows us to sense body movement, direction, and acceleration, and to attain and maintain postural equilibrium and balance. The vestibular labyrinthine system found in both of the inner ears is responsible for the senses of angular momentum, linear acceleration, and gravity.

Thermo sense is the sense of heat and the absence of heat which is the sensation of cold. There are specialized receptors for cold (declining temperature) and to heat. The thermoceptors in the skin are quite different from the homeostatic thermoceptors in the brain (hypothalamus), which provide feedback on internal body temperature.

Kinesthetic sense provides the brain with information on the relative positions of the parts of the body during movement. Doctors test this sense by telling patients to close their eyes and touch the tip of a finger to their nose.

Pain sense (nociception) signals near-damage or damage to tissue. The three types of pain receptors are cutaneous (skin), somatic (joints and bones), and visceral (body organs). Pain is a distinct phenomenon that intertwines with all the other senses, including touch.

Directional sense or magnetoreception is the ability to detect the direction one is facing based on the Earth's magnetic field. Directional awareness is most commonly observed in birds, although it is also present to a limited extent in humans.

Internal sense or interoception is the sense from within the body such as a full bladder or gastrointestinal sensation.

✏️ ACTIVITY 5-7

Describe how you could stimulate some of the senses during a massage session.

Your Turn

are classified according to the nature of the stimulus that excites them.

Important sensor classes include:
- Pain (nociceptors):
- Temperature (thermoreceptors
- Chemical stimuli (chemoreceptors):
- Touch/pressure/position (mechanoreceptors)

The processes involved in sensations are sensory receptors receiving mechanical, chemical, and thermal stimuli, transforming them into electrical signals, and sending that information to the brain to be processed and associated with previous experiences (Activity 5-7).

Touch

Touch, or mechanoreception, results from activation of neural receptors, generally in the skin, including hair follicles, but also in the tongue, throat, and mucous membranes. The sense of touch occurs when some sort of mechanical deformations of the skin and soft tissues of the body causing a change in the shape of the capsule surrounding the nerve ending. The nerve ending, called a mechanoreceptor, then detects this change in shape and produces an action potential sending nerve impulses. For a person to actually feel the sensation, the nerve impulses must make their way up to the brain.

Sensory nerve endings monitor what the body touches. The sense of touch is protective. Touch mechanoreceptors are also called tactile receptors and provide the sensations of touch, pressure, and vibration. A variety of sensory receptors are found in the skin; the six main ones are:
- Free nerve endings are sensitive to touch and pressure.
- Root hair plexus is made up of free nerve endings that detect hair movement.
- Merkel's discs are fine touch and pressure neurons located in the lower epidermal layer of the skin.
- Meissner's corpuscles are fine touch and pressure receptors located in the eyelids, lips, fingertips, nipples, and external genitalia.
- Pacinian corpuscles are large receptors sensitive to deep pressure and to pulsing or high-frequency vibrations.
- Ruffini corpuscles are located in the dermis of the skin and are sensitive to pressure and distortions of the skin.

When the tactile receptors are stimulated, the action potential codes for the touch's location on the skin, the amount of force, and its velocity so the central nervous system can interpret where the sensation is occurring and if it is safe or dangerous. Compared to the other senses, touch is very hard to isolate because tactile sensory information enters the nervous system from every single part of the body.

The physical characteristics of something you're touching can influence your feelings; this interpretation of touch has made its way into our language. Weight is metaphorically associated with concepts of seriousness and importance—for example, a "weighty matter" or "light reading." Roughness and smoothness are associated with difficulty and harshness; think of "a rough day" or "smooth sailing." Hardness and softness are associated with stability, rigidity, and strictness, as in being "hard-hearted" or "soft on someone." The study was supported by NIH and described in the June 25, 2010 edition of *Science* (Wein, 2010).

Affectionate touch lowers an individual's stress and anxiety levels. Physical contact affects oxytocin levels. Some studies, especially those done by Dr. Tiffany Field at the Touch Research Institute, have shown a decrease in stress hormones with massage, for both the person getting the massage and the one giving it.

Hearing

Sounds are vibrations created by mechanical methods that are turned into recognizable patterns of electrical energy in our nervous system. These vibrations can travel through air, water, or solid substances.

The brain can recognize immense variations in pitch, volume, and tone. When several sounds reach the ear, they are transferred to the hair cells in the ear. The lower-frequency signals are given priority when transmitted as electrical signals to the brain; thus a slow, deep, even voice is the best one to use when we really want to be heard.

Our sense of hearing is well-developed even at birth. Newborns can identify the direction of a voice and turn in response. Only in the past decade has investigation been conducted into the ability of the fetus to hear or sense sound carried through the amniotic fluid. Research indicates that the fetus does respond to sound.

The cochlea is the center of our hearing, named for its shape as a spiral shell, ("cochlea" from the Greek word for "snail"). The true organ of hearing is called the organ of Corti. This spiral structure within the cochlea contains hair cells that are stimulated by sound vibrations. The hair cells convert the vibrations into nerve impulses that are transmitted by the cochlear portion of the eighth cranial nerve to the brain.

Structures of the Ear

The ear is divided into three main parts: the external ear, the middle ear, and the inner ear.
- External Ear

The external ear is funnel-shaped to help guide sound waves into the ear. This part of the ear consists of the auricle,

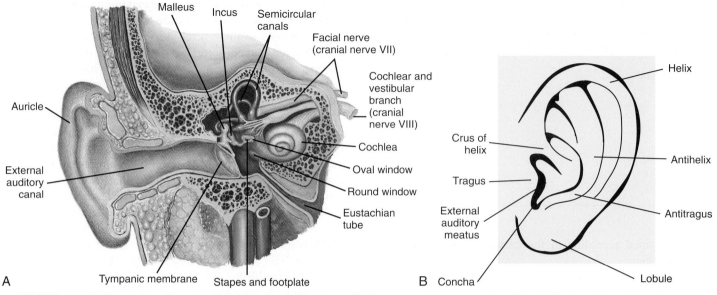

A

B

FIGURE 5-10 **A,** External auditory canal, middle ear, and inner ear. **B,** Structures of the external ear (pinna). (**A** from Barkauskas VH, et al: *Health and physical assessment,* ed 3, St Louis, 2002, Mosby.)

Practical Application

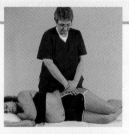

Any movement activity, especially those that cause head movements that affect the inner ear, shifts the perception of balance in the somatic system, thus altering muscle tension patterns. Many of the benefits of massage therapy are derived indirectly through the effect on the inner ear balance system.

Rhythmic rocking is used universally to calm infants, children, and adults because it interacts with balance mechanisms that influence the ANS to initiate parasympathetic functions. The rocking chair can be a lifelong calming companion in our hectic world.

sometimes referred to as the pinna, and the external acoustic meatus. The auricle is the part of the ear that is visible. The external acoustic meatus is the tubular structure that links the auricle to the tympanic membrane, commonly referred to as the ear drum
• The Middle Ear
This is a cavity linked to the eustachian tube. The eustachian (auditory) tube connects the middle ear with the throat and equalizes pressure between the middle ear and the outside air. Any imbalance in pressure can cause pain and distort or muffle sounds. Activities that open this tube (e.g., yawning, swallowing, chewing) often can relieve the pressure.

The middle ear has a layer of temporal bone that has two openings commonly known as the oval window and the round window. Three tiny bones known collectively as the auditory ossicles extend along the middle ear from the tympanic membrane to the oval window. They are known individually as the malleus, the incus, and the stapes.
• The Inner Ear

The inner ear is filled with fluid and is responsible for changing sound waves into nerve signals inside the cochlea.

This labyrinthine cavity is made up the bony labyrinth and the membranous labyrinth. The bony labyrinth consists of a vestibule, a cochlea, and three semi-circular canals. The vestibule expands into the middle ear and contains the round and oval windows. The vestibule contains two organs—the utricle and saccule—that are the organs of balance. The vestibular nerve carries signals from the balance organs into the brain.

The membranous labyrinth is separated from the bony labyrinth by fluid known as perilymph. It is the vibrations of the perilymph that stimulate the nerve impulses that deliver sound.

The Sequence of Hearing
• Vibrations in the air are taken in by the external ear, called the auricle or pinna.
• Vibrations are funneled into the external auditory meatus, which leads to the middle ear.
• Inside the middle ear, the sounds reach the tympanic membrane, or eardrum.
• As the eardrum vibrates in response to the sound vibration, it pulls on the tiny bones called ossicles to amplify the sounds.
• These three bones of the middle ear work together. The motion transfers to the hammer (malleus), which hits the anvil (incus), which pulls on the stirrup (stapes).
• The stapes rests on the oval window, a membrane at the beginning of the inner ear.
• Sound waves leave the middle ear and travel to the inner ear, to the cochlea.
• The sound waves travel through a thin membrane to the middle canal, and the organ of Corti. When sound is transmitted to the inner ear, the organ of Corti begins to vibrate up and down, which triggers the generation of nerve signals that are sent to the brain.

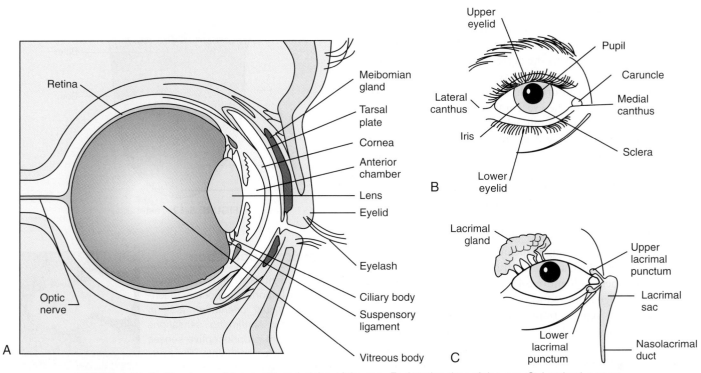

FIGURE 5-11 A, Structures of the eyelid and globe of the eye. **B,** Anterior view of the eye. **C,** Lacrimal system.

Balance and Equilibrium

The vestibular system is involved with maintaining body balance/equilibrium. Only the inner ear functions in the vestibular system. The inner ear consists of a group of fluid-filled tubes, running through the temporal bone of the skull. In this region of the inner ear, fluid-filled circular ducts are positioned at right angles to each other, and each duct contains hair cells embedded in a gelatinous substance. These specialized receptor cells respond to vibrations and motion. The semi-circular canals are three loops of fluid-filled tubes that are attached to the cochlea in the inner ear.

The semi-circular canals and vestibule function to sense movement and position. They help us maintain our sense of balance.

The three semi-circular canals lie perpendicular to each other, one to sense movement such as tilting, twisting, and bending. At the base of the canals are movement hair cells, (crista ampullaris). Depending on the movement, the fluid (endolymph) flowing within the semi-circular canals stimulates the appropriate movement hair cells. Static head position is sensed by the vestibule, specifically, its utricle and saccule, which contain the position hair cells. Different head positions produce different gravity effects on these hair cells. Small calcium carbonate particles (otoliths) are the ultimate stimulants for the position hair cells.

The maculae and the cristae are the sensory epithelium of the vestibular system (balance). There are two maculae (the saccule and the utricle), three cristae, and one organ of Corti on each side of the head.

The hair cells (stereocilia) of each macula are linked to an overlying structure whose movement causes them to bend. The stereocilia in a cristae are bent in response to movement of the fluid in a semicircular canal caused by changes in head position.

As we move, the directional hair cells transfer information about our head position and speed of movement. All this sensory information is transformed into electrical signals, which the auditory nerve conducts to the brain. Your brain interprets the incoming information and tells the muscles of the body what to do without your awareness.

For example:
- Tilting your head or slamming on your car's brakes causes the overlying mass in the maculae to move relative to the hair cells, bending the stereocilia bundle and activating the afferent nerve fibers connected to the hair cells.
- When watching a tennis match, you rotate your head to follow the ball. This causes the fluid in the "horizontal canal" to move relative to the crista, and the nerve fibers are stimulated. The end result is that the muscles of your eyes move (again, without your conscious attention) so as to stabilize the visual field.

If this proprioceptive balance mechanism is disrupted, the result often is vertigo, or balance problems. If the disruption goes undetected or untreated, the erroneous sensory information can contribute to anxiety and panic disorders.

Vision

The eyeball is a fluid-filled sphere composed of three layers of tissue (Figure 5-11). The outer layer comprises the sclera and the cornea. The sclera is a white, fibrous structure that maintains the shape of the eye and protects the inner structures. The cornea is the clear portion in the front that allows light to enter the eye.

In the middle layer of the eyeball are the ciliary body, choroid, and iris. The ciliary body, on the anterior portion, contains smooth muscles attached to the lens by ligaments. The choroid, which covers the posterior of the sclera, is filled with capillaries that nourish the eye. The cells of the choroid contain melanin and absorb light as it enters the eye. The iris, the colored portion of the eye, contains smooth muscles and controls the size of the pupil, which increases or decreases the amount of light allowed to enter the eye. Vision occurs when light rays enter through the lens and are focused onto the retina.

The inner layer of the eyeball is the retina, which contains photoreceptor cells and neurons. The rods, which are concentrated on the outer edges of the retina, take in information about the levels of lightness and darkness. The rods are responsible for recognizing shapes and patterns and providing contrast. Cones, which are concentrated at the fovea, or center, of the retina, help us identify color and brightness. We can see colors that range from red to purple. Rods and cones receive the mechanical signals, transform them into chemical substances, and create an electrical signal that is sent to the brain by way of the optic nerve. The optic nerve is created from association neurons in the retina. The point where the nerves exit the eye is called the *optic disk,* or *blind spot,* because it has no photoreceptors.

Vision signals are organized and processed in our cerebral cortex. Information received from the left and right eyes stays separate until it converges in the visual cortex. Signals received when we are not paying attention to any specific item are sent to the posterior parietal cortex for processing. Anything we focus on is sent to the visual cortex. Items that reflect a change in the environment cause a signal to be sent to the frontal lobe. These three areas of the brain (cerebral cortex, visual cortex, and parietal cortex) work to process and coordinate visual information.

The eyeball is protected by the skull within cavities known as *orbits.* Six muscles control movement of the eyeball. These muscles are highly sensitive and coordinate to control the position of the eye. Eyelids and eyelashes close over the eyes for protection and to block light and maintain distribution of fluid. The lacrimal glands produce tears, which keep our eyes moist, fight infections, and remove foreign particles. These glands, which are located supralaterally, release their product into the eye, where it evaporates or drains into the nasolacrimal duct alongside the nose, thus explaining why the nose becomes stuffed up and runs when we cry.

Taste

Taste is one of the more complex of our senses. Separating taste from smell is difficult. Specific areas on the tongue correspond to four distinct tastes: sweet, sour, salty, and bitter (Figure 5-12). Molecules of food bind to receptor sites on the tongue, cheeks, and floor of the mouth. The rest of our tasting is done through our nose and combines with the sense of smell. (You can confirm this by holding your nose and tasting something.)

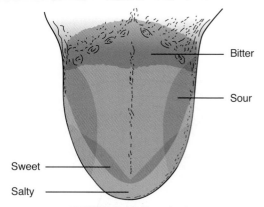

FIGURE 5-12 Tastebuds.

Practical Application

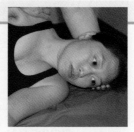

Visual orientation and eye movement are important in posture mechanisms. Visual orientation aids in posture by confirming sensations coming from proprioceptive senses in the muscles and joints. The body shifts positions as necessary to keep the eyes level with the horizontal plane. Position of the eyes is involved in righting reflexes that orient the body in gravity. The combination of proprioceptive, visual, and inner ear (vestibular) information activates various posture or righting reflexes that activate muscular responses to regain balance. Disturbance of the vestibular, visual, or proprioceptive impulses that initiate these reflexes may cause equilibrium disturbances, nausea, vomiting, muscle tension, and other symptoms. Some forms of movement methods use various eye positions as part of the intervention protocol. The effectiveness of these methods depends partly on the visual orientation aspects of posture. Because of the number of sensory receptors involved with the muscles of the eyes, coupled with the various posture reflexes, subtle movement activates muscle facilitation and inhibition of skeletal muscles, especially in the neck and shoulder area. A simple way to use this response therapeutically during massage is to have the client roll the eyes in slow circles as various massage methods are applied. Muscle groups that would turn the body in the direction of the eye position tense in preparation for movement while antagonist muscles begin to relax.

On average, an adult has more than 10,000 taste buds; however, as we age, our taste buds, which usually last about 10 days, are not replaced as frequently, which may explain why older adults are much less sensitive to taste than younger persons. Most of the nerve fibers that carry taste information to the brain can carry information about more than one taste, although they are mainly sensitive to just one and usually are classified as such.

Our individual preferences for certain tastes may be because of cultural differences or genetics. We can be much more or much less sensitive to certain tastes, making them something we love or something unpleasant. For most of us, bitter tastes are the most easily identified, which may be because most of the poisonous substances around us are bitter.

Smell

The sense of smell is a primitive sense that does not translate well to methods of human communication. For our ancestors, smell was a main lifesaving sense. Today smell still alerts us to dangers. The sense of smell is considered primitive because it deals with our unconscious, animal-like behaviors and experiences and elicits gut-level emotions. The nerves from the nose end in the olfactory bulb in the limbic area of the brain, the portion of the brain that also controls much of our autonomic, involuntary actions. The smell centers in the brain are connected with the limbic system and thus have an emotional and a behavioral effect.

Unlike our other senses, smells are hard to imagine. We can picture a scene, remember a soothing voice, and conjure up a taste that makes our mouth water, but most of us have difficulty imagining a smell. Smell also is the hardest sense to describe to another person.

The more civilized we become, the more we attempt to cover up our body smells and what they mean. Each of us has a unique body odor that changes in response to our emotions. It is true that we can smell fear, danger, anger, and sexual arousal and that we can smell a friend. Past memories, associated with déjà vu, are elicited most with our sense of smell. Much of the information we receive from smells helps integrate other information from the senses being processed at the same time.

The actual activity of olfaction, or smell, involves chemical receptors found in the roof of the nasal cavity Blocked nasal passages affect the senses of smell and taste. Figure 5-13 shows the structures of the nose. As an odor makes contact with the receptors, they transform chemical signals into electrical signals and transmit them to the temporal lobes of the brain.

The sense of smell is provided by paired olfactory organs located on either side of the nasal septum. Each is comprised of olfactory epithelium, which consists of olfactory receptors, supporting cells, and basal cells (stem cells). There is potential for the basal stem cells to be harvested and used to help treat various diseases and injuries.

Practical Application

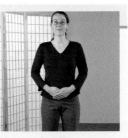

We can use smell therapies, such as aromatherapy, to deliberately influence our physiology and moods. Scents used as the trigger for conditioned learning can be helpful in establishing a method of reaching a more desirable state of homeostatic balance. Application involves connecting a smell to a particular state of consciousness, be it a relaxed state or a state of focused arousal. While the person is in the conscious state, he or she smells a chosen scent. If this is done consistently, the two become connected in the body. Eventually, the smell alone elicits the state of consciousness. This type of conditioned behavior is beneficial for managing pain and anxiety. With conditioning a pleasant scent is used to trigger responses such as reduced pain or increased activity. The scent of lavender has been shown to be calming. A person can carry drops of lavender or other pleasant aromas on a cotton ball and smell them as needed to support a calming effect.

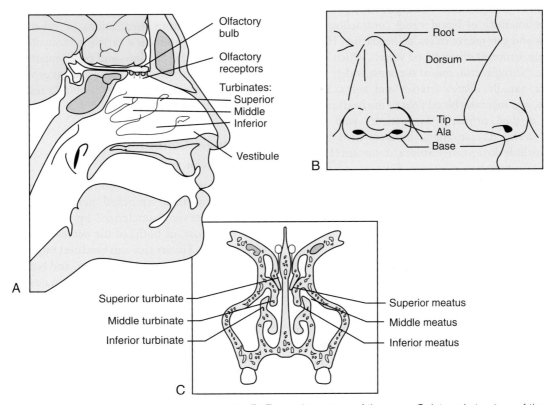

FIGURE 5-13 A, Lateral view of the right nasal cavity. **B,** External structure of the nose. **C,** Internal structure of the nose.

PATHOLOGIC CONDITIONS OF THE PERIPHERAL NERVOUS SYSTEM

SECTION OBJECTIVES

Chapter objectives covered in this section:

5. Describe pathologic conditions of the peripheral nervous system and the related indications/contraindications for massage.

After completing this section, the student will be able to perform the following:

- Describe the action of medication prescribed for pathologies of the peripheral nervous system.
- List the common pathologies of the peripheral nervous system.
- Discuss indications and contraindications, including cautions and adaptations, of massage therapy for pathologic conditions of the peripheral nervous system.
- Explain the way therapeutic massage supports health in the peripheral nervous system.

Medications That Affect the Autonomic Nervous System

Certain groups of medications bind to or join with alpha and beta receptors, thereby enhancing or blocking the receptor sites for the binding of norepinephrine (noradrenaline), acetylcholine, or other neurotransmitters and hormones. The effects determine the medication used to modify ANS function. The major problem with many of these medications is the side effects, which range from tachycardia to constipation.

Alpha-Adrenergic Blockers

Alpha-adrenergic blockers (alpha blockers) bind to receptors and thus prevent norepinephrine from binding, causing a decrease in blood vessel tone; this lowers blood pressure and increases circulation. Ergotamine (Cafergot, Ercaf, Wigraine) diminishes the intensity of blood vessel contraction in the cranial arteries and can relieve migraine headaches. Hydralazine (Apresoline, Unipres) dilates blood vessels, which reduces blood pressure. Nitroglycerin, one of the most widely known alpha blockers, rapidly dilates arteries and veins, reduces blood pressure, and increases blood flow to the heart muscles. Nitroglycerin is used primarily for patients with angina and coronary artery disease. Alpha blockers used to treat hypertension include doxazosin (Cardura), terazosin (Hytrin), and prazosin (Minipress).

Beta-Adrenergic Medications

Medications that include epinephrine (adrenaline, which is a beta-1– or beta-2–agonist) or that affect beta-2 receptors by enhancing the uptake of epinephrine (adrenaline) are used most commonly to treat respiratory disorders such as asthma, chronic bronchitis, and emphysema. Epinephrine-adrenaline inhalers (Bronkaid Mist, Primatene Mist) dilate bronchial tubes while causing the walls of the blood vessels to contract, increasing blood flow to the lungs. Other forms of this medication are used as eye drops for glaucoma to reduce internal eye pressure. Drugs that enhance epinephrine uptake without causing as many cardiac side effects include pirbuterol (Maxair), metaproterenol (Alupent, Metaprel), and albuterol (Proventil, Ventolin).

Beta-Adrenergic Blockers

Beta-adrenergic blockers (beta blockers) diminish the force and rate of heart muscle contractions and are used to treat hypertension, irregular heart rhythms, and angina. Commonly prescribed medications include metoprolol (Lopressor), penbutolol (Levatol), and atenolol (Tenormin). Propranolol (Inderal) and nadolol (Corgard) are beta blockers commonly used to treat hypertension and migraines.

Chemical substances that mimic the effect of or increase the uptake of norepinephrine (noradrenaline) are called sympathomimetics because they imitate sympathetic stimulation. Besides the bronchodilators used to treat asthma, bronchitis, and emphysema, these drugs include medications used during surgery to counteract the parasympathetic effects of anesthetics and maintain normal blood pressure. Ephedrine is used in many over-the-counter preparations for colds and sinus congestion.

Monoamine oxidase inhibitors are medications that reduce or stop the breakdown of norepinephrine and serotonin; they commonly are used to treat phobias, depression, migraines, and hypertension. The monoamine oxidase inhibitors interact with many other drugs, foods, and herbs, especially those containing the amino acid tyrosine.

Other drugs, such as codeine and opiates (e.g., codeine), also affect norepinephrine use by mimicking the sympathetic effect. A side effect is constipation.

Parasympathetic Blockers

Many of the alkaloid medications are anticholinergic and block the uptake of acetylcholine. Because of its bronchodilatory effect, the atropine-like drug ipratropium (Atrovent) is used to treat chronic bronchitis and emphysema, as well as some forms of asthma.

Withdrawal from medications or other substances that affect the ANS produces a variety of sympathetic effects (e.g., tachycardia, pupil dilation) and parasympathetic effects (e.g., increased tearing, diarrhea). The distress of withdrawal symptoms continues until the body is able to restore homeostatic balance without the substance.

Pathologic Conditions

Compression Syndromes

Compression syndromes, entrapment neuropathies, and nerve impingement (pinched nerve) are disorders of the peripheral nerves characterized by pain or loss of function (motor, sensory, or both) of the nerves as a result of chronic compression. Tissues that can bind and impinge on nerves are the skin, fasciae, muscles, ligaments, and bones.

The most common type of injury to a nerve is an impingement or "pinching" of the nerve. Nerve impingement often occurs at the spine and can be caused by being sandwiched between two spinal bones, pressed on by a bulging disk, or encroached on by bony overgrowth. In addition to impingement, nerves can also become "stuck" to surrounding soft tissues (muscles, ligaments, fascia), usually as a result of repetitive motion injuries. This is commonly referred to as a "trapped" nerve, or *nerve entrapment.*

Regardless of what is causing compression on the nerve, the symptoms are similar; however, the therapeutic intervention is different. Soft-tissue approaches are beneficial in entrapment but are less so with bony types of impingement.

Shortened muscles and connective tissue (fasciae) often impinge on major and minor nerves, causing discomfort. Because of the structural arrangement of the body, these impingements often occur at major nerve plexuses. The specific nerve root, trunk, or division affected determines the condition, producing disorders such as thoracic outlet syndrome, sciatica, and carpal tunnel syndrome.

If the cervical plexus is impinged, the person most likely will have headaches, neck pain, and breathing difficulties. The muscles most responsible for pressure on the cervical plexus are the suboccipital and sternocleidomastoid muscles. Shortened connective tissue at the cranial base also presses on these nerves. The cervical plexus is formed by the ventral rami of the upper four cervical nerves. The phrenic nerve is part of this plexus and innervates the diaphragm. Any disruption to this nerve affects breathing. Many cutaneous (skin) branches of the cervical plexus transmit sensory impulses from the skin of the neck, ear area, and shoulder. The motor branches innervate muscles of the anterior neck. Impingement causes pain in these areas.

The brachial plexus is situated partly in the neck and partly in the axilla and consists of virtually all the nerves that innervate the upper limb. Any imbalance that increases pressure on this complex of nerves can result in pain in the shoulder, chest, arm, wrist, and hand. The muscles most often responsible for impingement on the brachial plexus are the scalene, pectoralis minor, and subclavius muscles. The muscles of the arm also occasionally impinge on branches of the brachial plexus. Brachial plexus impingement is responsible for thoracic outlet symptoms, which often are misdiagnosed as carpal tunnel syndrome. Whiplash injury often causes impingement on the brachial plexus.

Carpal tunnel syndrome is caused by compression of the median nerve as it passes under the transverse carpal ligament at the palmar aspect of the wrist. The condition often occurs in postmenopausal women but also occurs in conditions in which fluid retention causes swelling of the hand and wrist. The syndrome is common in workers who use their hands in repetitive movements, usually because of inflammation that results in compression on the nerve. The symptoms are palmar pain and numbness in the first three digits. Surgically opening the transverse carpal ligament sometimes helps relieve the pain.

Impingement on the lumbar plexus gives rise to low back discomfort, which is marked by a beltlike distribution of pain and pain in the lower abdomen, genitals, thigh, and medial lower leg. The main muscles that impinge on the lumbar plexus are the quadratus lumborum and the psoas muscles. Shortening of the lumbar dorsal fascia exaggerates a lordosis and can cause vertebral impingement on the lumbar plexus.

The sacral plexus has about a dozen named branches. About half of these serve the buttock and lower limb; the others innervate pelvic structures. The main branch is the sciatic nerve. Impingement on this nerve by the piriformis muscle gives rise to sciatica. Shortened ligaments that stabilize the sacroiliac joint can affect the sacral plexus. Pressure on the sacral plexus can cause pain in the gluteal muscles, leg, genitals, and foot.

INDICATIONS/CONTRAINDICATIONS for Therapeutic Massage

Various forms of massage reduce muscle spasm, lengthen shortened muscles, and soften and stretch connective tissue, restoring a more normal space around the nerve and alleviating impingement and entrapment. When massage is combined with other appropriate methods, surgery is seldom necessary. If surgery is performed, the practitioner must manage adhesions appropriately to prevent reentrapment of the nerve by maintaining soft-tissue suppleness around the healing surgical area and, as healing progresses, using therapeutic massage to deal more directly with the forming scar. Before doing any work near the site of a recent incision, the practitioner must obtain the physician's approval. In general, work close to the surgical area can begin after the stitches have been removed and all inflammation abates. Direct work on a new scar usually is safe 8 to 12 weeks into healing.

Nerve Root Compression

Many different conditions can result in compression of the nerve root, including tumors, subluxation of vertebrae, and muscle spasms (entrapment) and shortening. Disk degeneration is a common cause. As the degeneration progresses and the fluid content of the disk decreases, the disk becomes narrower. As a result, the amount of space between vertebrae declines. Because spinal nerves exit and enter in the spaces between the vertebrae, this situation increases the likelihood of nerve root compression. The condition most commonly occurs in the areas where the spine moves the most: C6 to C7, T12 to L1, L3 to L4, and L5 to S1. The result is radiating nerve pain, often associated with protective and stabilizing muscle spasm, weakness, or both.

Disk Herniation

Disk herniation occurs when the fibrocartilage surrounding the intervertebral disk ruptures, releasing the nucleus pulposus, which cushions the vertebrae above and below. The resultant pressure on spinal nerve roots may cause pain and damage the surrounding nerves. This condition most often occurs in the lumbar region and involves the L4 or L5 disk and L5 or S1 nerve roots. This particular back pain radiates from the gluteal area down the lateral side or back of the thigh to the leg or foot. Back strain or injury often causes disk herniation, and coughing and sneezing occasionally precipitate the condition.

The symptoms of herniation are similar to those produced by a compressed disk but often are more severe. In extreme cases surgical intervention may be necessary; however, more conservative measures usually are attempted first. Conservative treatment consists of rest, exercise, and other methods, including massage to reduce spasm. Traction can be beneficial.

INDICATIONS/CONTRAINDICATIONS for Therapeutic Massage

Various forms of massage are important for managing the muscle spasm and pain associated with nerve root compression and disk herniation. Remember that the muscle spasms serve a stabilizing and protective function called *guarding*. Without some protective spasm, the nerve could be damaged further, but too much muscle spasm increases the discomfort. Therapeutic intervention seeks to reduce pain and excessive tension and restore moderate mobility while allowing for the resourceful compensation produced by the muscle tension pattern. Because low back pain is a common disorder, the massage practitioner must be familiar with its causes and treatment protocols.

Viral Infections

Bell's Palsy

Bell's palsy causes partial or total paralysis of the facial muscles on one side as the result of inflammation or injury to the seventh cranial nerve. The exact cause of the inflammation is unknown, but current research suggests a reactivation of the herpes simplex virus as one of the probable causes. Mechanical causes include bone spurs, tumors, or temporomandibular joint disorders. Bell's palsy also occurs in persons affected by diabetes and Lyme disease. The facial nerve swells and is compressed in its narrow course through the temporal bone. The primary method of treatment is oral administration of steroids. The condition usually resolves and normal functioning returns within 6 weeks.

Guillain-Barré Syndrome

Guillain-Barré syndrome, or infectious polyneuritis, may occur 1 or 2 months after a viral infection. Lymphocytes and macrophages invade the myelin sheath, causing partial demyelination. The person develops tingling in the hands or feet, motor weakness, and a decrease in deep tendon reflexes; mild sensory loss ensues. Paralysis usually begins in the legs and moves upward. Facial weakness is common and may appear as Bell's palsy. Sometimes respiratory support must be given. Most individuals recover in a few weeks.

Herpes

Herpes zoster, or shingles, is a self-limiting viral disease in which groups of vesicles (fluid-filled blisters) appear along a cutaneous nerve distribution, usually on one side of the trunk. Pain occurs before the rash is visible. The varicella-zoster virus, a member of the Herpesviridae family, is the same virus that causes chickenpox. Some researchers believe that after infection, the virus remains in the body in an inactive state in dorsal root ganglia. In a healthy person the immune system keeps the virus in check when it tries to flare up. If the immune system becomes compromised for any reason, it may not be able to contain the virus, and the result is shingles. Primary treatment consists of administration of an analgesic and the antiviral medication acyclovir (Zovirax).

The herpes simplex virus, which is categorized as type 1 or type 2, causes contagious, chronic viral infections that produce painful, fluid-filled blisters on the skin and mucous membranes. Outbreaks seem to be related to stress. Acyclovir can control the symptoms and accelerate healing but does not destroy the virus or cure the infection. Herpes virus lies dormant in the nerve between outbreaks.

Polio

Polio is a viral infection, first of the intestines and then (for about 1% of exposed persons) the anterior horn cells of the spinal cord. The destruction of CNS motor neurons leads to degeneration, atrophy, and finally paralysis of skeletal muscles.

INDICATIONS/CONTRAINDICATIONS for Therapeutic Massage

Massage approaches for infectious disease can be supportive and can reduce stress. Massage can help control the number of recurrent outbreaks by managing stress, especially in recurring viral conditions. The practitioner must follow universal precautions with any contagious disease. The patient's total stress load is an important factor. When a person is immunocompromised to the extent that he or she is susceptible to viral and bacterial disease, the stress load is greater. The practitioner should keep in mind that many forms of massage produce stress in a therapeutic sense. One must gauge the intensity and duration of any therapeutic intervention so that the demand on the body to adapt does not overtax an already stressed system, aggravating the condition. The less-is-more philosophy of intervention, which calls for shorter, more frequent interventions, often is indicated. Massage is beneficial for post-acute polio syndrome but only under a doctor's supervision.

Massage is beneficial for postacute polio syndrome but only under a doctor's supervision.

Multiple or Unknown Causes

Multiple Sclerosis

Multiple sclerosis is a disease of autoimmune or viral cause (or both) in which myelin degenerates in random areas of the CNS. Hard, plaquelike lesions replace the destroyed myelin, and inflammatory cells invade affected areas. The myelin around the axons is lost, impairing nerve conduction, and weakness, diminished coordination, gait difficulties, incontinence, vision problems, and speech disturbances occur. Multiple sclerosis is a chronic condition with periodic remissions, because the axon is preserved even though the myelin degenerates. Relapse shows some indication of the condition being responsive to stress. Multiple sclerosis should not be confused with amyotrophic lateral sclerosis, which involves degeneration of motor neurons.

Myasthenia Gravis

Myasthenia gravis is a disorder of neuromuscular transmission that usually affects muscles in the face, lips, tongue, neck, and throat, which are innervated by the cranial nerves; however, the condition can affect any muscle group. Eventually, muscle fibers may degenerate, and weakness, especially of the head, neck, trunk, and limb muscles, may become irreversible. When the disease involves the respiratory system, it may be life-threatening.

The disease follows an unpredictable course with periodic exacerbations and remissions. Spontaneous remissions occur in about 25% of patients. No cure exists, but thanks to drug therapy, patients may lead relatively normal lives except during exacerbations.

The cause of myasthenia gravis is unknown. The condition commonly accompanies autoimmune and thyroid disorders. Fifteen percent of patients with myasthenia gravis have thymoma.

INDICATIONS/CONTRAINDICATIONS for Therapeutic Massage

Massage can be an effective part of a comprehensive, long-term care program. Stress management also is an important component of an overall care program for any chronic disease. Massage and other forms of bodywork can help manage secondary muscle tension caused by the alteration of posture and the use of equipment such as wheelchairs, braces, and crutches. As previously mentioned, because therapeutic massage produces some stress, the practitioner must gauge the intensity and duration of any therapeutic intervention so as not to aggravate the condition.

Neurotransmitter-Based Disorders

Depression

Depression is one of the more common causes of physical complaints that are a manifestation of underlying psychiatric illness. Many forms of depression respond to medications that increase norepinephrine, dopamine, or serotonin in certain synapses in particular areas of the brain. Imipramine (Tofranil), amitriptyline (Elavil), fluoxetine (Prozac), and phenelzine (Nardil) are examples of these types of medications. Although primarily considered a CNS disease, dysfunction can be linked to synaptic transmission as the PNS delivers information to the CNS.

INDICATIONS/CONTRAINDICATIONS for Therapeutic Massage

Massage has the effect of increasing the availability of the aforementioned neurotransmitters and as such can play an important part in the care program for depression. Aerobic exercise is another important component in depression management. These methods use the PNS as the point of access.

Anxiety States

Anxiety states are classified into two basic types. The first type, endogenous anxiety, is a biochemical phenomenon usually unrelated to environmental stimuli. Panic disorder—involving hyperventilation syndrome and other breathing difficulties, heart palpitations, chest pain, dizziness, sweating, and feelings of impending doom—is an example of this type. An increase in the activity of the neurotransmitters gamma-aminobutyric acid, epinephrine, and norepinephrine is implicated. The medications imipramine, monoamine oxidase inhibitors, and alprazolam have proved moderately effective in treating panic disorder.

Breathing pattern disorder may be an underlying factor in anxiety, resulting in a change in body chemistry that alters the feedback loop mechanisms. Restrictions in the soft tissue or the bony structures of the thorax may interfere with appropriate breathing, predisposing a person to breathing in excess of physical need. Massage to the full body as well as specific focus to the thorax can be effective in restoring more balanced function and supporting appropriate breathing. Thus breathing restraint may be an important factor in managing anxiety. Chapter 12 presents additional information on hyperventilation syndrome.

The second basic anxiety type is reactive, or exogenous, anxiety, which is prompted by anxiety-provoking stimuli such as specific events, situations, relationships, and conflicts. Management of this type of anxiety requires dealing with the precipitating difficulties directly or improving mechanisms and skills for coping with environmental or social problems. Making changes in the stressful situation, resolving smoldering conflicts, using relaxation methods, and cognitive restructuring of the client's views of the situation are helpful. Professional counseling often is beneficial. Other helpful measures include avoiding caffeine, exercising regularly, eating a healthful diet, and generally gaining control over those things we can control ourselves. Diazepam-type medications such as Valium are useful in short-term management of this type of anxiety.

Both types of anxiety can be thought of as activation of the sympathetic ANS. With endogenous anxiety a faulty internal feedback system results in panic. With exogenous anxiety the tendency for responding with fight-or-flight behavior is present, but some sort of inhibition of those feelings is in place. What occurs is a fight-or-flight response without the appropriate expression; it therefore is internalized as anxiety.

INDICATIONS/CONTRAINDICATIONS for Therapeutic Massage

Massage and exercise are often effective as part of a comprehensive management strategy dealing with anxiety symptoms.

Neuropathy

Neuropathy is the inflammation or degeneration of the peripheral nerves. Neuralgia is severe nerve pain caused by a variety of noninflammatory disorders of the nervous system. Neuritis is the inflammation of a nerve.

Complex regional pain syndrome (reflex sympathetic dystrophy) is also called *causalgia syndrome.* The situation causes pain following soft-tissue or bone injury that does not follow a normal healing course. Instead, pain continues for no known reason after the healing process is complete.

Ketoacidosis and hypoglycemic reaction of diabetes cause diabetic neuropathy because they affect the myelin covering of the neuron. The condition is a painful and severe complication of diabetes for which effective control measures are limited. One such pain control measure is hyperstimulation analgesia, which interrupts the pain for a short period.

Trigeminal neuralgia (tic douloureux) causes sudden, severe pain in the jaw area on one side of the face. Often the pain is caused by chewing or simply by touching the face. The cause is unknown. One hypothesis is that the condition is related to a viral infection of the upper portion of the trigeminal nerve. The analgesic carbamazepine (Tegretol) can be effective in some cases, although surgical intervention sometimes is necessary. Extreme caution should be exercised if any form of therapy is to be performed in this area.

INDICATIONS/CONTRAINDICATIONS for Therapeutic Massage

> Nerve pain is difficult to manage, does not respond well to analgesics, and often is intractable. Massage, because of its interface with the nervous system, may provide short-term, symptomatic pain relief through shifts in neurotransmitters and stimulation of alternate nerve pathways, resulting in hyperstimulation analgesia and counterirritation. Any therapy that increases mood-elevating and pain-modulating mechanisms makes coping with nerve pain somewhat easier for short periods.

Headache

Headache is a common symptom with a multitude of causes. Because the brain has no sensory innervation, headaches do not originate in the brain. The pain of a headache is produced by pressure on the sensory nerves, vessels, meninges, or the muscle-tendon-bone unit.

A tension or muscle contraction headache is the most common type. Tension headaches are believed to be caused by a muscle-tendon strain at the origin of the trapezius and deep neck muscles at the occipital bone or at the origin of the frontalis muscle on the frontal bone (occipital or frontal headaches). Tension headache also can originate in the temporomandibular joint muscle complex. Connective tissue structures that support the head may be implicated in headache if they are shortened and pull the head into nerves, creating pain. Conversely, if connective tissue support structures are lax and fail to support the neck and head, nerve structures may be compressed as well.

The treatment for most headaches is nonsteroidal antiinflammatory drugs such as aspirin and ibuprofen.

INDICATIONS/CONTRAINDICATIONS for Therapeutic Massage

> Massage and other forms of soft-tissue therapy are effective in treating muscle tension headaches. Because stress often induces headaches, stress management in all forms usually is indicated in chronic headache conditions.

Vertigo

Vertigo is the sensation that the body or environment is spinning or swaying and can occur when disturbances occur in the inner ear balance mechanism or between the visual-vestibular balance mechanisms. The most common type of vertigo is called *benign paroxysmal positional vertigo*. This condition occurs when otolith particles in the inner ear stimulate movement sensations that do not actually exist. Muscle tension, nausea, and mood disturbances, particularly anxiety, can result.

INDICATIONS/CONTRAINDICATIONS for Therapeutic Massage

> Movement therapies can help or aggravate vertigo; therefore the practitioner must take care to design an individual therapeutic program based on the client's history. Massage methods can deal effectively with muscle tension and diminish anxiety and nausea, but the benefit is temporary because the symptoms return with a recurrence of vertigo.

SUMMARY

Understanding how the PNS works specifically influences the massage practitioner's ability to plan and arrange an effective massage session. Massage applications and outcomes experienced by the client from the massage session depend on the practitioner's knowledge of the physiologic effects of the massage manipulations and techniques. Understanding normal function and pathologic conditions of the PNS helps the massage professional make good decisions regarding indications and contraindications for massage.

In this chapter we studied the PNS, its components, and the names of its many parts. We presented important information about reflexes and sensory receptors because these portions of the PNS function directly with massage.

We reinforced the role of the ANS, the body/mind connection, and the perspectives of Eastern and Western thought as well.

We discussed the five basic senses briefly and related massage to specific functions of the PNS for four of the five. We will discuss touch much more in Chapter 11. A student of massage would do well to learn this particular material thoroughly because massage therapy works closely with the PNS. Such an understanding can only benefit the clients we strive to serve.

⟨e⟩volve

> http://evolve.elsevier.com/Fritz/essential
> Activity 5-1 Review the basics of the PNS by playing an
>   online bowling game.
> Activity 5-2 Complete a word chart on sensory receptors.
> Activity 5-3 Compare and contrast the sympathetic and
>   parasympathetic nervous systems.
> Activity 5-4 Answer questions following a brief case study
>   on nerve root compression.
> **Additional Resources:**
>   Peripheral Nervous System Scientific animations
>   Weblink: Additional reading on spinal cord injuries
>   Electronic Coloring Book
> *Remember to study for your certification and licensure
>   exams! Review questions for this chapter are located
>   on Evolve.*

REFERENCES

1. Schleip R: Fascial plasticity—a new neurobiological explanation, *J Bodywork Movement Ther* 7(1):11-19; 7(2):104-116, 2003.
2. Wein H: Touch affects impressions, decisions, *NIH Research Matters*, NIH, 2010. http://www.nih.gov/researchmatters.
3. http://www.fasciaresearch.con/innervationsexcerpt.pdf
4. http://www.somatics.de/somatics-07.html

Workbook Section

All Workbook activities can be done online as well as here in the book. Answers are located on ⊝volve.

Short Answer

1. Define the peripheral nervous system.

_____

2. List the components of the peripheral nervous system.

_____

3. List the cranial nerves, and describe the general function of each.

_____

_____

_____

_____

_____

4. List and describe the spinal nerves.

_____

_____

5. Identify the four nerve plexuses.

_____

_____

6. Compare and contrast a dermatome and a myotome.

_____

_____

_____

7. Explain reflex mechanisms and sensory receptor reflex arcs and their relationship to therapeutic massage and movement therapies.

_____

_____

_____

_____

8. Identify the two divisions of the autonomic nervous system.

_____

9. List and compare the functions of the sympathetic and parasympathetic nervous systems.

_____

_____

_____

_____

10. List the major drugs that affect the autonomic nervous system.

_____

_____

_____

_____

11. Describe the Eastern/Western connection as it relates to autonomic nervous system functions.

_____

_____

_____

_____

12. Describe the four basic senses discussed in this chapter.

_____

_____

_____

_____

13. List at least 12 of the various pathologic conditions of the peripheral nervous system.

1. _____
2. _____
3. _____
4. _____
5. _____
6. _____
7. _____
8. _____
9. _____
10. _____
11. _____
12. _____

14. Explain how therapeutic massage supports health in the peripheral nervous system.

_____

_____

_____

Fill in the Blank

The (1) _____ consists of neurons outside the central nervous system (CNS). The (2) _____ (sensory) division consists of nerves that link sensory receptors with the CNS. The efferent, or (3) _____, division consists of nerves that link the CNS to the effectors outside the CNS. The (4) _____ nervous system is made up of nerves that act to keep the body in balance with its external environment by transmitting impulses between the CNS and the skeletal muscles and skin. The (5) _____ nervous system connects the CNS to the glands, heart, and smooth muscles to maintain the (6) _____ body environment. The (7) _____ nervous system functions when the body is under stress, producing fight-or-flight responses. The (8) _____ nervous system functions under normal body conditions and is the energy conservation and restorative system, associated with what commonly is called the (9) _____ response.

A nerve is a group of (10) _____ nerve fibers, or axons, wrapped together. Twelve pairs of (11) _____ originate from the olfactory bulbs, thalamus, visual cortex, and brainstem. Thirty-one pairs of (12) _____ originate in the spinal cord and emerge from the vertebral column. (13) _____ nerves make sensation and movement possible.

A (14) _____ is a network of intertwining nerves that innervates a particular region of the body. The four nerve plexuses are the (15) _____ plexus, the (16) _____ plexus, the (17) _____ plexus, and the (18) _____ plexus.

A (19) _____ is a cutaneous (skin) section supplied by a single spinal nerve. A (20) _____ is a skeletal muscle or group of muscles that receives motor axons from a given spinal nerve. (21) _____ receptors are sensory receptors that detect changes in pressure, movement, or temperature or other mechanical forces.

(22) _____ receptors are sensory receptors that detect changes in temperature. (23) _____ are sensory receptors that detect painful stimuli.

(24) _____ are sensory receptors that provide the body with information about position, movement, muscle tension, joint activity, and equilibrium.

A reflex in the physiologic or functional unit of nerve function is a/an (25) _____ action. The (26) _____ reflex results when stretching of a muscle elicits a protective contraction of that same muscle. The tendon reflex operates as a feedback mechanism to control muscle (27) _____ by causing muscle relaxation. The flexor (withdrawal) and crossed extensor reflexes are (28) _____ reflex arcs. When these reflexes are stimulated, an entire area on one side of the body (29) (_____) or specific areas on both sides of the body (30) (_____) are affected.

The five basic senses discussed are
(31) _____, (32) _____,
(33) _____, and (34) _____ and
(35) _____.

Problem Solving

Read the problem presented. There is no correct answer; rather the exercise is intended to assist the student in developing the analytical and decision-making skills necessary in a professional practice. After reading the problem, follow the next six steps:
1. Identify the facts presented in the information.
2. Identify the possibilities presented ("what if" statements), or develop your own possibilities.

3. Evaluate each possibility in terms of the logical cause and effect and pros and cons.
4. Consider the effect on the persons involved.
5. Write each answer in the space provided.
6. Develop your solution by answering the question posed.

Problem

Most soft-tissue and movement therapies are beneficial because of a direct interaction with the peripheral nervous system. The sensory mechanisms of the peripheral nervous system are the communication link with the rest of the systems and functions of the body. Research is demonstrating the beneficial effects of these therapies on the somatic nervous system, primarily through reflex arcs and dermatome and myotome patterns, coupled with the interaction with the autonomic nervous system. Some difficulty may arise because various approaches have emerged within therapeutic massage and movement therapy based on specific protocols developed by gifted practitioners and teachers over the course of centuries. At the time the particular approach developed, science may not have been able to identify the underlying physiology. Consequently, many forms of therapeutic massage and movement therapy have developed along individual paths, and they work for the same physiologic reasons. This does not discount the uniqueness and value of any one particular approach. However, confusion results with many different methods working through the same basic anatomy and physiology with slight variations in style and different terminology bases. Professionals in therapeutic massage and movement therapies often may not realize that they are talking about the same thing. If we have some difficulty understanding one another, then how much more confusing is it for professionals outside the touch and movement therapy discipline? Explaining treatment methods in terms of anatomy and physiology may help because this language base is understood more universally. Such an effort could give rise to an agreement and understanding of the overlap of methods, especially in terms of the peripheral nervous system interaction.

Question

Examples are provided to get you started. Fill in at least two more statements.

Facts
1. Touch and movement therapies are not always explained in terms of anatomy and physiology.
2. _____
3. _____

Possibilities
1. Professionals may not be able to share information effectively.
2. _____
3. _____

Logical Cause and Effect

1. Appropriate referral between professionals would not happen because of a lack of information.
2. _____
3. _____

Effect

1. Professionals may feel frustrated when they discover that they were talking about the same thing all along.
2. _____
3. _____

How would you explain the benefit of touch and movement therapies in terms of the peripheral nervous system?

_____
_____
_____

Assess Your Competencies

Review the following objectives for Chapter 5:
1. Describe the peripheral nervous system.
   • Describe components of the peripheral nervous system.
   • List the cranial nerves, and describe the general function of each.
   • Explain the function of spinal nerves.
   • Identify the four nerve plexuses.
   • Compare and contrast dermatomes and myotomes.
2. Relate the reflex mechanisms of the peripheral nervous system to massage application.
   • Define a nerve reflex.
   • List the sensory receptors involved in reflex action.
   • Define a reflex arc.
   • Explain motor tone.
3. Explain the structure and function of the autonomic nervous system.
   • Name the two divisions of the autonomic nervous system.
   • List and compare the functions of the sympathetic and parasympathetic nervous systems.
   • Describe the Eastern/Western connection as it relates to the functions of the autonomic nervous system.
4. Describe the structure and function of the five basic senses of touch, hearing, vision, taste, and smell.
   • List the five basic senses.
   • Describe the five basic senses.
   • Describe the relevance of the five basic senses to daily function.
5. Describe pathologic conditions of the peripheral nervous system and the related indications/contraindications for massage.
   • Describe the action of medications prescribed for pathologies of the peripheral nervous system.
   • List the common pathologies of the peripheral nervous system.

   • Discuss indications and contraindications, including cautions and adaptations, of massage therapy, for pathologic conditions of the peripheral nervous system.
   • Explain the way therapeutic massage supports health in the peripheral nervous system.

Next, on a separate piece of paper or using an audio or video recorder, prepare a short narrative that reflects how you would explain this content to a client and how the information relates to how you would provide massage. See the example in Chapter 1 on p. 22. When read or listened to, the narrative should not take more than 5 to 10 minutes to complete. Simpler is better. Use examples, tell stories, and use metaphors. It is important to understand that there is no precisely correct way to complete this exercise. The intent is to help you identify how effectively you understand the content and how relevant your application is to massage therapy. An excellent learning activity is to work together with other students and share your narratives. Also share these narratives with a friend or family member who is not familiar with the content. If that person can understand what you have written or recorded, that indicates that you understand it. There are many different ways to complete this learning activity. Yes, it may be confusing to do this, but that's all right. Out of confusion comes clarity. By the time you do this 12 times, once for each chapter in this book, you will be much more competent.

Further Study

Using additional resource material (see the Works Consulted list at the back of this book), write a paragraph of additional information on each of the following:

Nerve distribution patterns for the four nerve plexuses

_____
_____
_____

Reflex mechanisms

_____
_____
_____

Autonomic nervous system and the body/mind influence

_____
_____
_____

Taste

_____
_____
_____

Smell

_____
_____
_____

Hearing

_____

_____

_____

Vision

_____

_____

_____

_____

Professional Application

Groups of individuals with a common need or interest sometimes are referred to as *populations*. When one considers touch and movement therapies, certain populations need different types of approaches. Working with an athlete on balancing reflex patterns is different from working with a person who has cerebral palsy who wants a similar outcome. Nerve entrapment in the elderly is common, but this condition also is common in repetitive work environments. Interaction with anxious clients is different from interaction with someone who is depressed, even though therapeutic intervention focuses on the autonomic nervous system. The approaches are similar, yet different. Identify a pathologic condition listed in this chapter, and develop two hypothetical treatment plans for the condition with two different populations. After you have done this, identify the differences and similarities in theories and the practical applications of the methods.

Endocrine System

http://evolve.elsevier.com/Fritz/essential

CHAPTER OBJECTIVES

After completing this chapter, the student will be able to perform the following:

1. Describe the physiologic processes of the endocrine system.
2. List the traditional endocrine glands.
3. Connect the endocrine system to the nervous system through the hypothalamus.
4. Define endocrine tissues, and give examples.
5. Describe the hypothalamic-pituitary-adrenal axis and its link to the general adaptation system.
6. Identify how the Eastern chakra system is related to the endocrine system.
7. List and describe the three main hormone types and their functions.
8. Identify the hormones produced by each endocrine gland and their associated functions.
9. Describe the hypersecretion and hyposecretion pathologic conditions of the endocrine system, and list the associated indications and contraindications for massage.

CHAPTER OUTLINE

OVERVIEW OF ENDOCRINE GLANDS AND TISSUES, 168
    Endocrine and Exocrine Glands, 168
    Other Endocrine Tissues, 169
    Endocrine Axis, 170
    Endocrine Glands and Chakras, 170
ENDOCRINE GLANDS, TISSUES, AND THEIR
    HORMONES, 171
    Hormones, 171
    Pituitary Gland, 173
    Other Hormones, 180
PATHOLOGIC CONDITIONS, 181
    Primary Mechanisms of Endocrine Disease, 181
    Nonglandular Disorders of the Endocrine System, 182
    Pituitary Pathologic Conditions, 182
    Thyroid Pathologic Conditions, 183
    Parathyroid Pathologic Conditions, 184
    Pancreatic Pathologic Conditions, 185
    Adrenal Pathologic Conditions, 186
    Pineal Pathology, 187
SUMMARY, 187

KEY TERMS

Axis Series of glands that signal each other in a sequence.
Endocrine glands (EN-doe-krin) Ductless glands that secrete hormones directly into the bloodstream.

Endorphins (en-DOR-finz) Peptide hormones that mainly work like morphine to suppress pain. They influence mood, producing a mild euphoric feeling such as is seen in runner's high.
Exocrine glands (EK-so-krin) Glands that secrete hormones through ducts directly into specific areas. Exocrine glands are part of the endocrine system.
Half-life The amount of time required for half of a hormone to be eliminated from the bloodstream.
Hypersecretion The excessive release of a hormone.
Hyposecretion The insufficient release of a hormone.
Hypothalamic-pituitary-adrenal (HPA) axis Complex set of direct influences and feedback interactions among the hypothalamus, the pituitary gland, and the adrenal glands.
Negative feedback system A control mechanism that provides a stimulus to decrease a function, such as a fire alarm, which causes a series of reactions that work to reduce the fire.
Neuroendocrine system Interactions between the nervous system and the endocrine system.
Tropic (or trophic) hormones Hormones produced by the endocrine glands that affect other endocrine glands.

LEARNING HOW TO LEARN

Repetition, repetition, and then more repetition. The key is that each repetition needs to be a little different so your brain remains interested. In the chapters of this textbook, novel repetition is built right in. The key terms are listed at the beginning of the chapter. Then, the key terms appear in the chapter. This activates reinforced information. The Evolve website has activities and links for more repetition. The online course is an excellent form of repetition. Finally, the workbook sections provide an opportunity for you to review the material again. Take advantage of repetition; your brain will pay attention.

As you have learned, the endocrine system and the nervous system control and regulate the body's response to events and return the body to homeostasis. The endocrine system works in partnership with other systems of the body, especially the nervous system, to maintain homeostasis in the body. In this capacity the endocrine system is involved primarily with physiologic function using chemicals called *hormones*. Not only are hormones of the endocrine system involved with maintaining homeostasis; they also direct the creation of our very form, such as our size, shape, and sexual characteristics. The following major physical form processes are controlled and integrated by hormones:

- Reproduction
- Growth
- Development

Therefore hormonal pathologic conditions affect function, as does the nervous system, and can also affect form. The endocrine system uses negative feedback to regulate physiologic functions. Negative feedback regulates the secretion of almost every hormone.

The key functions of the endocrine system are as follows:
- Regulation of metabolic functions
- Regulation of chemical reactions
- Regulation of transport of substances through cell membranes

In the previous chapters, we learned that a chemical found in the synapse is called a *neurotransmitter*. When the same chemical is found in the bloodstream or tissue, it is a hormone. Neurotransmitters act on adjacent cells, whereas hormones may travel long distances in the body before they reach their target cells. The main differences between the endocrine system and the nervous system control are speed and duration of effect:
- The nervous system is fast acting, with a short duration of effect.
- The endocrine system is slow acting, with a long duration of effect.

This offers a balance of control, with the nervous system responding quickly and the endocrine system taking over to sustain a response (Activity 6-1).

OVERVIEW OF ENDOCRINE GLANDS AND TISSUES

SECTION OBJECTIVES

Chapter objectives covered in this section:
2. List the traditional endocrine glands.
3. Connect the endocrine system to the nervous system through the hypothalamus.
4. Define endocrine tissues, and give examples.
5. Describe the hypothalamic-pituitary-adrenal axis and its link to the general adaptation system.
6. Identify how the Eastern chakra system is related to the endocrine system.

After completing this section, the student will be able to perform the following:
- Explain the difference between endocrine and exocrine glands.
- List the endocrine glands of the body.
- Explain why the hypothalamus is considered a neuroendocrine organ.
- Describe the body/mind and nerve/endocrine function.
- List the functions of the hypothalamus.
- Describe the hypothalamic-pituitary-adrenal axis and the relationship to stress.
- Compare the endocrine system to the chakra system.

Endocrine and Exocrine Glands

The **endocrine glands** are ductless glands that secrete hormones directly into the bloodstream or diffuse into nearby tissues (Figure 6-1). In contrast, **exocrine glands,** or glands with ducts, such as salivary and sweat glands, secrete their products directly into ducts that open to specific areas.

✏ ACTIVITY 6-1

List three situations in which you believe that nervous system control is most effective, and explain why. An example is given.

Example
While we are driving, a car stops suddenly in front of us. Normal reflexes activate our muscles to step on the brake. The quick response of the nervous system and short duration of response is sufficient to handle this situation.

1. _____
   _____
   _____
2. _____
   _____
   _____
3. _____
   _____
   _____

List three situations in which you believe endocrine system control would be most effective, and explain why. An example is given.

Example
Sledding in the cold for a couple of hours: The longer effect of hormones better supports the increase in heat production required to maintain body temperature.

1. _____
   _____
   _____
2. _____
   _____
   _____
3. _____
   _____
   _____

The endocrine glands of the body include the following:
- Pituitary gland
- Hypothalamus
- Thymus
- Pineal gland
- Testes
- Ovaries
- Thyroid
- Adrenal glands
- Parathyroid glands
- Pancreas

Hypothalamus

The hypothalamus is considered part of the nervous system, but it also produces and releases hormones and thus can be considered a **neuroendocrine** organ. Pathologic conditions are found mainly with **hyposecretion** (not enough) and **hypersecretion** (too much). This pattern now should seem familiar as the elegance of the body shows itself in the repetition of basic patterns (Figure 6-2).

The hypothalamus is the link in the body/mind and nerve/endocrine function. The main purpose of the hypothalamus

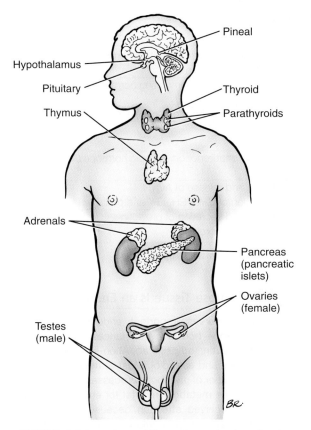

FIGURE 6-1 Locations of the major endocrine glands.

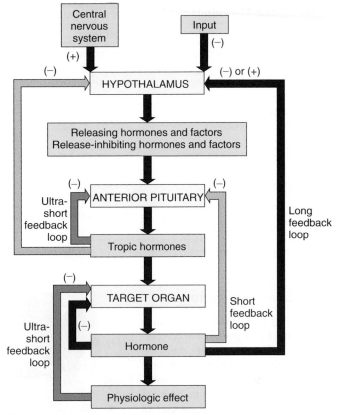

FIGURE 6-2 Feedback loops. General model for control and negative feedback to hypothalamic-pituitary target organ systems. Negative-feedback regulation is possible at three levels: target organ (ultrashort feedback), anterior pituitary gland (short feedback), and hypothalamus (long feedback). (From McCance KL, Huether SE: *Pathophysiology: the biologic basis for disease in adults and children,* ed 6, St Louis, 2010, Mosby.)

is homeostasis: for example, its effects on blood pressure, body temperature, and fluid and electrolyte balance. The hypothalamus has the following functions:

- To control blood pressure and electrolyte balance through thirst and salt craving
- To regulate body temperature through the influence of both the autonomic nervous system and behavior that seeks a warmer or cooler environment
- To regulate energy metabolism through influence on feeding behavior, digestion efficiency, and metabolic rate
- To regulate reproduction through hormonal control of sexual and mating behavior, pregnancy, and lactation
- To direct responses to stress by altering blood flow to specific tissues and stimulating adrenal gland to secrete stress hormones

During stress the hypothalamus translates nerve impulses into hormone secretions by endocrine glands. The hypothalamus plays a role in the following:

- Awareness of pleasure and pain
- Expression of emotions, such as fear and rage
- Sexual behaviors

The hypothalamus exerts its primary influence over the pituitary gland, which in turn controls other endocrine glands with tropic hormones. **Tropic hormones** cause secretion of other hormones. The hypothalamus secretes releasing or inhibiting hormones that affect the secretion of pituitary hormones.

Psychosocial dwarfism, failure-to-thrive syndrome, and delayed tissue healing, which result from stress, emotional

disorders, and deprivation, are the consequences of suppression of the hypothalamic release of growth hormone–releasing hormone. This hormone signals the secretion of growth hormone from the pituitary gland (Table 6-1).

Other Endocrine Tissues

Endocrine glands are not the only tissues that secrete hormones. Numerous cells and tissues throughout the brain, gut, and cardiovascular system produce hormones as well. New research in endocrinology continues to discover endocrine tissues that are separate from the traditional endocrine glands. The heart and intestinal mucous membranes are now known to secrete hormones. The concept of tissue hormones or hormone-like substances such as the prostaglandins has altered and expanded the idea of hormones being carried throughout the blood to distant sites in the body. Prostaglandins not only have a local effect in surrounding tissue, but because they are carried by blood, they also affect distant sites in the body.

The following are examples:

- Placenta
- Heart
- Kidney
- Brain

Table 6-1   Hypothalamic Hormones (Hypophysiotropic Hormones)

Hormone	Target Tissue	Action
Thyrotropin-releasing hormone (TRH)	Anterior pituitary	Stimulates release of thyroid-stimulating hormone (TSH) Modulates prolactin secretion
Gonadotropin-releasing hormone (GnRH)	Anterior pituitary	Stimulates release of follicle-stimulating hormone (FSH) and luteinizing hormone (LH)
Somatostatin	Anterior pituitary	Inhibits release of growth hormone (GH) and TSH
Growth hormone–releasing factor (GHRF)	Anterior pituitary	Stimulates release of GH
Corticotropin-releasing hormone (CRH)	Anterior pituitary	Stimulates release of adrenocorticotropic hormone (ACTH) and beta β-endorphin
Substance P	Anterior pituitary	Inhibits synthesis and release of ACTH Stimulates secretion of GH, FSH, LH, and prolactin
Dopamine	Anterior pituitary	Inhibits synthesis and secretion of prolactin
Prolactin-releasing factor (PRF)	Anterior pituitary	Stimulates secretion of prolactin

From McCance KL, Huether SE: *Pathophysiology: the biologic basis for disease in adults and children,* ed 6, St Louis, 2010, Mosby.

Practical Application

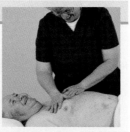

According to the National Institutes of Health, many people use complementary and alternative medicine (CAM), which is a group of diverse medical and health care systems, practices, and products that are not presently considered to be part of conventional medicine. Complementary medicine is used in conjunction with conventional medicine, and alternative medicine is used in place of conventional medicine in pursuit of health and well-being.

Mind/body practices focus on the interactions among the brain, mind, body, and behavior, with the intent to use the mind to affect physical functioning and promote health.

The term *massage therapy* means pressing, rubbing, and moving muscles and other soft tissues of the body, primarily by using the hands and fingers. The aim is to increase the flow of blood and oxygen to the massaged area. Therapy encompasses many different techniques. In general, therapists press, rub, and otherwise manipulate the muscles and other soft tissues of the body. People use massage for a variety of health-related purposes, including to relieve pain, rehabilitate sports injuries, reduce stress, increase relaxation, address anxiety and depression, and aid general well-being.

Modified from NCCAM, National Institutes of Health: What Is Complementary and Alternative Medicine? Accessed May 6, 2011, at http://nccam.nih.gov/health/whatiscam/.

- Intestine
- Adipose tissue (Box 6-1)

Endocrine Axis

When a series of glands signal each other in a sequence, it is called an *axis.* For example, the **hypothalamic-pituitary-adrenal axis,** or **HPA axis,** is a complex set of direct influences and feedback interactions among the hypothalamus, the pituitary gland, and the adrenal glands. This communication network between the nervous system and the endocrine system is now considered the neuroendocrine system. The

Box 6-1   Adipose Tissue Is an Endocrine Tissue

Adipose tissue serves important endocrine functions. It secretes numerous hormone substances, including leptin, resistin, adiponectin, adipsin, acylation-stimulating protein, angiotensinogen, and estradiol. Most of these hormones are involved in a number of metabolic processes, such as glucose regulation and the metabolism of fat for energy production.

Leptin has received attention because it is involved in appetite and obesity. Leptin acts on receptors in the hypothalamus to inhibit appetite. This system is more sensitive to starvation than to overfeeding. Leptin circulates at levels proportional to body fat.

A condition called *leptin resistance* may be a factor in some types of obesity. This hormone signals the brain that our appetites are satisfied and we can stop eating. Leptin resistance is similar to insulin resistance in diabetics. Leptin resistance occurs when the body fails to transport leptin past the blood-brain barrier to the hypothalamus. For leptin to control body weight and metabolism, it must do so from the hypothalamic centers in the brain. When levels of leptin in the hypothalamus are low as a result of leptin resistance, food cravings and weight gain occur because the body believes that it is hungry and goes into a state of continued fat storage. Recent work from Harvard researchers has tied leptin to a crucial pathway in fat metabolism in muscle. This pathway suggests a role for leptin in clearing fat out of cells and sheds light on the connection between diabetes and obesity.

Leptin's legacy: *HHMI Bulletin,* March 2003, vol. 16, no. 1. Chin-Chance C, Polonsky K, Schoeller D: Twenty-four hour leptin levels respond to cumulative short-term energy imbalances and predict subsequent intake, *J Clin Endocrinol Metabol* 85(8): 2685-2691, 2000.

HPA axis controls the general adaptation syndrome (GAS) described by Dr. Selye (Box 6-2).

Endocrine Glands and Chakras

The endocrine glands have important implications in the Eastern chakra system. The chakra system is a mapping of energy centers with interesting anatomic correlations to the autonomic nervous system plexus and functional aspects interrelated with the endocrine gland functions. Many Eastern

Box 6-2 General Adaptation Syndrome

Dr. Hans Selye's research into the effects of stress describes a universal response of the human body to stressors, which he termed the *general adaptation syndrome.* There are three stages: alarm, resistance, and exhaustion.

1. **Alarm:** When the stressor is identified, the body's stress response is a state of alarm. The HPA axis is activated. Adrenaline is produced, setting off the fight-or-flight response.

2. **Resistance:** If the stressor persists, it becomes necessary to attempt some means of coping with the stress. The adrenal glands begin producing cortisol. The resistance stage can be thought of as enduring. Although the body tries to adapt to demands, it cannot keep this up indefinitely, and functioning reserves become depleted. The ability to maintain homeostasis is strained.

3. **Exhaustion:** The body's resources are depleted, and the body is unable to sustain normal function. The ability to maintain homeostasis is lost. Long-term damage may result as the capacity of glands, especially the adrenal gland, and the immune system is exhausted and function is impaired, resulting in illness.

Table 6-2 Categories of Hormones

Structural Category	Examples
Water Soluble	
Peptides	Growth hormone
	Insulin
	Leptin
	Parathyroid hormone
	Prolactin
Glycoproteins	Follicle-stimulating hormone
	Luteinizing hormone
	Thyroid-stimulating hormone
Polypeptides	Adrenocorticotropic hormone
	Antidiuretic hormone
	Calcitonin
	Endorphins
	Glucagon
	Hypothalamic hormones
	Lipotropins
	Melanocyte-stimulating hormone
	Oxytocin
	Somatostatin
	Thymosin
	Thyrotropin-releasing hormone
Amines	Epinephrine
	Norepinephrine
Lipid Soluble	
Thyroxine (an amine but lipid soluble)	Thyroxine (both thyroxine [T_4] and triiodothyronine [T_3])
Steroids (cholesterol is a precursor for all steroids)	Estrogens
	Glucocorticoids (cortisol)
	Mineralocorticoids (aldosterone)
	Progestins (progesterone)
	Testosterone
Derivatives of arachidonic acid (autocrine or paracrine action)	Leukotrienes
	Prostacyclins
	Prostaglandins
	Thromboxanes

From McCance KL, Huether SE: *Pathophysiology: the biologic basis for disease in adults and children,* ed 6, St Louis, 2010, Mosby.

healing traditions (e.g., Ayurvedic, Tibetan) work from this knowledge base, just as many Asian healing philosophies were developed around the meridian system.

The body of knowledge of the chakra system is expansive and consistent with Western scientific thought. Just as the meridian system sees anatomy and physiology as an interrelated system encompassing emotional and spiritual energy conjoined with the major organs, the chakra system represents similar patterns in relationship to the endocrine functions. As we describe various endocrine functions, we also present the related chakra pattern (Figure 6-3).

ENDOCRINE GLANDS, TISSUES, AND THEIR HORMONES

SECTION OBJECTIVES

Chapter objectives covered in this section:

7. List and describe the three main hormone types and their functions.
8. Identify the hormones produced by each endocrine gland and their associated functions.

After completing this section, the student will be able to perform the following:

• List and describe three main hormone types.
• Describe endocrine glands and hormone functions.
• Relate the two main categories of endocrine pathology to the negative feedback control.
• List various organs and tissues that have an endocrine function.

Hormones

Hormones are secreted from endocrine glands and tissues. Each hormone causes a response in a specific target organ or group of cells, rather than on the body as a whole. Exocrine hormones are secreted through a duct into the blood and usually affect a distant organ or tissue. Endocrine hormones are secreted within the tissue and enter the bloodstream through capillaries.

There are three main hormone types:

• *Amines* are simple molecules.
• *Proteins and peptides* are chains of amino acids.
• *Steroids* are derived from cholesterol. (see Table 6-2).

The hormones of the endocrine system maintain homeostasis as we respond life events and our real or perceived emotions and resulting mood. Functional aspects of hormone molecules include the mobilization of body defenses against stressors; maintenance of electrolyte, water, and nutrient balance of the blood; and regulation of cellular metabolism and energy balance.

Hormones exert their effect on target organs and cells at low blood concentrations. The concentration of a hormone in the blood is determined by the rate of release and the speed of inactivation and removal from the body. The influence of a hormone in the blood can range from seconds to 30 minutes.

The term **half-life** describes the time required for half of the hormone to be eliminated from the bloodstream. After

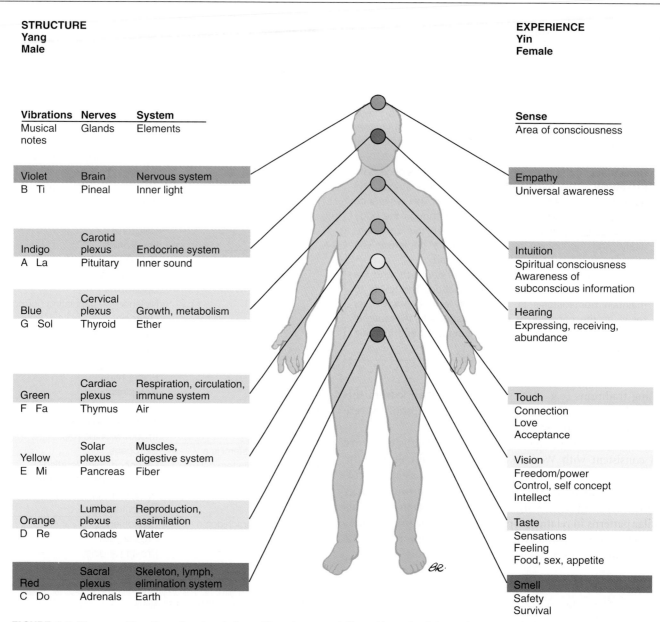

STRUCTURE
Yang
Male

EXPERIENCE
Yin
Female

Vibrations Musical notes	Nerves Glands	System Elements
Violet B Ti	Brain Pineal	Nervous system Inner light
Indigo A La	Carotid plexus Pituitary	Endocrine system Inner sound
Blue G Sol	Cervical plexus Thyroid	Growth, metabolism Ether
Green F Fa	Cardiac plexus Thymus	Respiration, circulation, immune system Air
Yellow E Mi	Solar plexus Pancreas	Muscles, digestive system Fiber
Orange D Re	Lumbar plexus Gonads	Reproduction, assimilation Water
Red C Do	Sacral plexus Adrenals	Skeleton, lymph, elimination system Earth

Sense
Area of consciousness

Empathy
Universal awareness

Intuition
Spiritual consciousness
Awareness of
subconscious information

Hearing
Expressing, receiving,
abundance

Touch
Connection
Love
Acceptance

Vision
Freedom/power
Control, self concept
Intellect

Taste
Sensations
Feeling
Food, sex, appetite

Smell
Safety
Survival

FIGURE 6-3 Name and location of major chakras. There is a correlation with each of the major chakras and the endocrine glands.

this occurs, the effect is slowed. Hormones require various amounts of time to generate noticeable influences in the body or on behavior. Some hormones promote target organ responses almost immediately, such as the effect of epinephrine on the heart. In contrast, steroid hormones such as testosterone and estrogen may require hours or days for their effects to be seen.

Endocrine glands release hormones in response to three types of stimuli:
- Hormones are released when a shift occurs in the concentration of a specific substance in the body fluids, such as when the parathyroid gland responds to a rise and fall in calcium levels in the blood.
- Hormones are released when the larger endocrine gland receives instructions from another endocrine organ. For example, the ovaries secrete estrogen under the influence of trophic hormones from the pituitary gland.

- Hormones are secreted when the nerves stimulate the gland, as when the adrenal gland releases adrenaline when stimulated by sympathetic nerves.

Endocrine glands and other specialized cells secrete hormones into the bloodstream to bind to specific receptors on or in their target cells. In a lock-and-key mechanism, hormones bind only to receptor molecules that "fit" them exactly. Any cell with one or more receptors for a particular hormone is said to be a *target* of that hormone. Cells usually have many different receptors, so they can be target cells for many different hormones (Figure 6-4).

A new concept of the lock-and-key mechanism is that molecular chains that form the various hormones actually change shape as necessary to stimulate the cell receptors. This theory represents a more dynamic quantum view of neurohormonal function than the more static Newtonian lock-and-key systems. As with most understanding, as knowledge

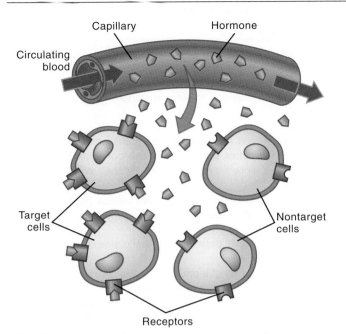

FIGURE 6-4 The target cell concept. A hormone acts only on cells that have receptors specific to that hormone because the shape of the receptor determines which hormones can react with it. This is an example of the lock-and-key model of biochemical reactions. (From Thibodeau GA, Patton KT: *Anatomy and physiology,* ed 6, St Louis, 2007, Mosby.)

evolves, the answer is most likely a combination of both ideas instead of an either/or pattern (Box 6-3).

Each hormone–receptor interaction produces different regulatory changes within the target cell. Hormones bring about their characteristic effects on the normal cellular processes of target cells by increasing or decreasing the rate of those cell processes. Even though the diffusion of a hormone is usually system-wide through the blood, the effects are more specific because of the specificity of the target cells in organs and tissues. Ancient healing practices speak often of internal communication mechanisms and identify the blood as an important life-giving force. Today, what science calls *hormones* seems to be representative of this ancient wisdom (Activity 6-2).

Pituitary Gland

The pituitary gland, or hypophysis, is located in the head at about eye level. The gland hangs down from the hypothalamus and sits in the sella turcica, a recessed area in the sphenoid bone. About the size of a peanut, the pituitary gland has an anterior lobe and a posterior lobe. The posterior lobe is not a true endocrine gland because it only stores and releases hormones but does not synthesize them. According to tradition, the pituitary gland and its regulating counterpart, the hypothalamus, are related to the crown or brow chakra, with primary functions of integration of energetic patterns and realization of the total self.

The pituitary gland secretes hormones that regulate growth, fluid balance, lactation, and childbirth. The gland is the main source of tropic hormones, hormones that have a stimulating

Box 6-3 Newtonian or Quantum or Both

The Newtonian view involves a logical, step-by-step linear view with a beginning, middle, and end. Boundaries are solid. Life runs through a filter of the past and includes traditions and rules. Newtonian thinking embraces "either/or" and "status quo" concepts.

The quantum view does not involve beginning, middle, or end. It is limitless. Processes create multiple possibilities, and every single action holds breakthrough potential. New ideas cause change; processes create multiple possibilities. Quantum thinking can be confusing, disrupts the status quo, and creates uncertainty.

Our bodies are both. Anatomy is more Newtonian, whereas physiology is more quantum. Physiology is an ever-changing stream of information and energy. Our physical form changes. Most of the atoms in our body were not there a year ago. The skin renews every month, the stomach lining renews every 4 days, liver every 6 weeks, and brain cells every year. The endocrine system is definitely quantum in function.

The Newtonian world is like a well-worn path, and it feels safe. The quantum world is an unknown maze with multiple pathways.

Frost R: Change in world view; From Newtonian concepts to quantum mechanics and chaos theory. In *Applied kinesiology: a training manual and reference book of basic principles and practice,* Berkeley, Calif., 2002, North Atlantic Books.

✐ ACTIVITY **6-2**

Before we go any further in this chapter, do the following. In 1 minute, list as many physiologic processes influenced by hormones as you can. Come back at the end of the chapter, and compare your before and after knowledge.

Example
Pregnancy

Your Turn

effect on other endocrine glands. The hypothalamus regulates the pituitary gland through releasing and inhibiting hormones. The negative feedback mechanism affects the pituitary gland by acting on the hypothalamus. (A **negative feedback system** provides a stimulus to decrease a function.) The terms *primary* and *secondary* refer to target organ problems as opposed to problems in other organs that affect the target gland. For example, *primary hyperthyroidism* means that the cause is in the thyroid gland. *Secondary hyperthyroidism* refers to the pituitary gland and its influence on the thyroid gland.

The large anterior lobe secretes seven major hormones, and the posterior lobe secretes two major hormones.

Practical Application

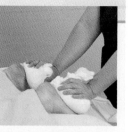

It is important for the body to be able to deal with its individual stress load systems. That is why stress management systems are so important. If we analyze ancient healing practices and spiritual wisdom made concrete through ritual practices, we can easily see similarities to current recommendations for stress management programs.

Because isolation is a recognized problem for many, even within social groups ("lonely in a crowd"), many types of professionals are concerned about the quality of physical, emotional, and spiritual health for those without touch interactions. Psychosocial influences on hypothalamic function reflect the importance of resourceful contact with fellow human beings or loving pets. Even caring for plants has been shown to increase the sense of well-being for some. We seem to be preconditioned to need others to be healthy. On a professional level, practitioners using a primary modality of touch can offer important health-restoring interventions and act in a preventive mode for those at risk from touch deprivation (Activity 6-3).

Anterior Pituitary Hormones

Growth Hormone or Somatotropin

Growth hormone, or somatotropin, stimulates most body cells to increase in size and divide. The major target organs are bones and muscles. In the adult the response of growth hormone is the repair and rebuilding of tissues. Growth hormone follows a circadian cycle, with the highest levels occurring during evening sleep, primarily delta-wave sleep. Growth hormone releases stored fat and raises blood glucose concentrations to provide us with energy. Growth hormone also is triggered for release during exercise and periods of hurt, tension, and stress. As we age, the total amount of growth hormone secreted declines.

Growth hormone release can be inhibited by emotional deprivation, excessive blood sugar, and high blood fat levels. Disruption in the sleep pattern interferes with growth hormone functions as well. Growth hormone disturbances often are implicated in chronic pain disorders such as fibromyalgia.

Thyroid-Stimulating Hormone

Thyroid-stimulating hormone (TSH) is a tropic hormone that promotes and maintains the growth and development of the thyroid gland and controls the release of thyroid hormones in a negative feedback system. Production of TSH often increases in response to cold temperature.

A licensed medical professional may recommend hydrotherapy (the use of water) for therapeutic intervention to encourage the production of TSH if hyposecretion is a concern. Cold has an effect on the hypothalamus, resulting in the release of TSH. Typical applications include standing in cold water or alternating hot and cold water baths or showers. Whenever one uses cold therapeutically, the client's body needs to be warm first. Before the client stands in cold water,

ACTIVITY 6-3

First, identify a current stress management program, and briefly describe the process. Then describe a ritual process with which you are familiar. Compare the two processes. Two examples are provided to get you started.

Example
1. Current stress management programs often use a combined method of sitting quietly and concentrating on the number 1 while repeating the word "one" slowly over and over.
   Ancient meditative practices used seated positions while chanting a mantra, sound, or phrase slowly over and over.
Comparison
Both use repetitive patterns and static positions to reduce stress responses.
2. Current practices of therapeutic massage use oil lubricants to rub the soft tissues of the body.
   Many ancient religious practices use anointing or rubbing with oil as part of a healing or purification ritual.
Comparison
Both use the application of oil and rubbing.

Your Turn
Current practice

Ancient practice

Comparison

Practical Application

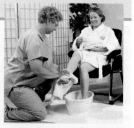

Growth hormone stimulates the production of fibroblasts, mast cells, ground substance, and collagen fibers and is essential in healing wounds. Because growth hormone is most active during delta-wave sleep and the sleep pattern usually is disrupted in fibromyalgia and other pain and fatigue syndromes, the body may have problems with cellular repair. Given this premise, a disrupted sleep pattern has been suggested as one of the primary causes of fatigue and pain syndromes.

Therapeutic massage has been shown through research to have a beneficial influence on the development of a restful sleep pattern, thus enabling the body to better restore and heal itself.

his or her feet should be warmed in a foot bath. The client then alternates hot and cold baths or showers, beginning with a warm water application for 5 to 15 minutes, then adding cold applications, starting with 15 to 30 seconds, gradually increasing to up to 5 minutes. The entire cold process starts with tepid water, and gradually over days or even weeks, the practitioner reduces the temperature and increases the duration of the cold water application. These methods are contraindicated in conditions in which a hypersensitivity to cold, such as Raynaud's disease, exists.

Adrenocorticotropic Hormone

Adrenocorticotropic hormone (ACTH) is a tropic hormone that promotes and maintains normal growth and development of the adrenal cortex by stimulating the release of glucocorticoids and androgens. Androgens are hormones such as testosterone that produce secondary male characteristics. Stress, mild to moderate fevers, and hypoglycemia can increase the amount of ACTH secreted.

Practical Application

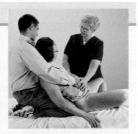

Stress encountered over a long period generates abnormal glucocorticoid effects on the body that are responsible for some diseases. Glucocorticoids are known to suppress the immune system. Any modality that reduces the effects of stress, including therapeutic massage, promotes appropriate levels of ACTH and thus brings the immune system back in balance.

Research has shown that giving and receiving massage reduces sympathetic arousal. This enhances the effects of oxytocin, supporting lactation and bonding between infants and parents. Research also has shown that pleasurable rhythmic skin stimulation increases levels of oxytocin. This could explain some of the feelings of connectedness that occur between the client and massage practitioner when these types of methods are used.

Follicle-Stimulating Hormone

Follicle-stimulating hormone is a tropic hormone in the female that stimulates the growth and maturation of ovarian follicles, which contain eggs. Follicle-stimulating hormone also stimulates the secretion of estrogen; in the male it stimulates sperm production.

Luteinizing Hormone

In women luteinizing hormone is a tropic hormone that causes ovulation (the release of the mature egg) and stimulates progesterone production in the ovaries. In men luteinizing hormone stimulates the production and secretion of testosterone in the testes.

Prolactin

Although found in men and women, prolactin primarily works in two areas of a woman's body. First, in combination with other hormones, prolactin plays a part in breast development. Second, prolactin initiates milk production when stimulated by the central nervous system. Receptors for prolactin in lymphocytes suggest that prolactin is involved in immune function.

Melanocyte-Stimulating Hormone

Melanocyte-stimulating hormone acts on the pigment cells in the skin and the adrenal glands. The exact function is uncertain. One theory suggests that melanocyte-stimulating hormone, ACTH, and other hormones that darken the skin control pigmentation of normal skin.

Posterior Pituitary Hormones

Posterior pituitary hormones are made by hypothalamic neurons and stored in the posterior pituitary gland.

Oxytocin

Oxytocin stimulates smooth muscle contraction, especially in the uterus. Oxytocin is released in large quantities just before a woman gives birth. This is part of a positive feedback cycle that ends when the child is born. Pitocin is synthetic oxytocin used mainly to induce labor in women. Oxytocin stimulates the milk letdown response, which causes the breast ducts to contract and release milk. Oxytocin also may be implicated in bonding behavior or feelings of belonging to another, as occurs between a parent and child. When increased sympathetic activity releases epinephrine, which inhibits oxytocin, problems in lactation and bonding may occur. Oxytocin is found in men and nonpregnant women and pregnant and postpartal women. The role of this hormone in men has been suggested to be to support pair bonding in couples and enhance parental behavior.

Antidiuretic Hormone

Also known as *vasopressin*, antidiuretic hormone (ADH) stimulates the kidneys to remove water from urine and release it into the bloodstream. Release of ADH is stimulated by pain, anxiety, nicotine, tranquilizers, and low blood pressure. Release of ADH is inhibited by alcohol, so the amount of urine produced increases. Because ADH can cause arterioles to contract, it increases blood pressure, which is beneficial during hemorrhaging because of the rerouting of blood to the internal organs. ADH can decrease the rate of perspiration, thus helping a person who is dehydrated (Figure 6-5).

Practical Application

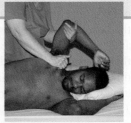

Therapeutic massage reduces the perception of pain and anxiety and indirectly interacts with the release of ADH, possibly supporting a more effective homeostatic function (Activity 6-4).

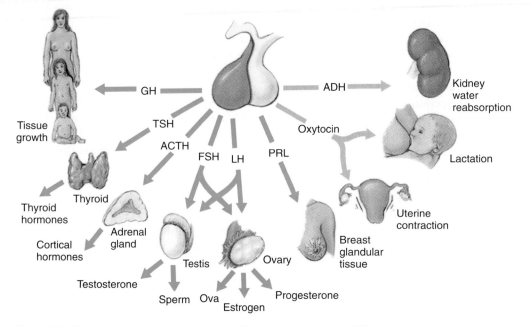

FIGURE 6-5 The effect of pituitary hormones on target tissues. *GH*, Growth hormone; *TSH*, thyroid-stimulating hormone; *ACTH*, adrenocorticotropic hormone; *FSH*, follicle-stimulating hormone; *LH*, luteinizing hormone; *PRL*, prolactin; *ADH*, antidiuretic hormone. (From Applegate E: *The anatomy and physiology learning system*, ed 4, Philadelphia, 2011, Saunders.)

✎ ACTIVITY 6-4

If the pituitary hormones were represented by cartoon characters, what would each one be? On a separate sheet of paper, create and draw a cartoon character or other figure or find a picture of one and paste it on the paper to represent each pituitary hormone.
Growth hormone
Thyroid-stimulating hormone
Adrenocorticotropic hormone
Follicle-stimulating hormone
Luteinizing hormone
Prolactin
Oxytocin
Antidiuretic hormone

Thyroid Gland

The thyroid gland lies on the trachea below the thyroid cartilage and consists of a right and left lobe connected by a bridge (isthmus), resulting in a butterfly shape. The gland is heavier in women than in men. The thyroid and parathyroid glands are related to the Eastern energy chakra of the throat, the function of which is communication and creativity in a balanced function.

The thyroid gland regulates metabolism in the body by maintaining an adequate amount of oxygen consumption at the cellular level. The two principal hormones are thyroxine and triiodothyronine. TSH from the pituitary gland stimulates these hormones, and iodine is necessary for their synthesis. A third hormone, calcitonin, inhibits bone reabsorption by limiting the rate at which bone tissue releases calcium to plasma. This in turn reduces the blood calcium level and counters the effect of the parathyroid hormones.

Parathyroid Glands

The parathyroid glands are made up of four round, pea-sized bodies located on the posterior surface of the thyroid lobes. Their hormone, parathormone, when combined with vitamin D, decreases the amount of calcium excreted, causes the release of calcium from bone, and absorbs more calcium from the gastrointestinal tract, resulting in an increase in blood levels of calcium and phosphorus.

Pancreas

The pancreas is a long, slender gland located behind the stomach. In Eastern philosophies the pancreas is related to the solar plexus chakra located at the thoracolumbar junction and navel. This chakra functions with willpower and awareness of emotion.

The pancreas is an exocrine and endocrine gland. Although the enzymes of the pancreas aid in digestion, our focus is on its hormone production. Islands of cells called the *islets of Langerhans* are interspersed within the exocrine gland tissues. These islets produce the hormones insulin and glucagon. The pancreas secretes two other hormones in small amounts: Somatostatin inhibits the release of all islet hormones, and amylin acts as an antagonist to insulin.

The beta cells of the islets of Langerhans secrete the hormone insulin, which lowers blood glucose levels by transporting glucose into cells to be used for energy. Insulin binds to the cells and allows glucose and potassium to be transported across the cell membrane. Although insulin receptors are present on most cell membranes, only our muscle, connective tissue, and white blood cells need it for glucose transport. However, glucose is readily available to the liver, brain, and kidneys no matter what our blood insulin levels. Insulin removes glucose from blood, making it available for cellular activity.

Insulin

The pancreas releases insulin when levels of blood sugar, amino acids, and fatty acids rise. Other hormones, including ACTH, growth hormone, epinephrine, thyroxine, and glucocorticoids, also affect insulin secretion. Because these hormones necessitate a response from muscles, the demand for energy increases; thus insulin secretion supplies energy. Fluctuations in blood sugar during experiences of stress put additional strain on the body because the body often actually does not need increased amounts of energy.

Glucagon

Alpha cells of the islets of Langerhans secrete the hormone glucagon, which increases blood glucose, the opposite of the insulin response. Growth hormone stimulates these cells, which are a part of the feedback loop in hypoglycemia. High protein intake and exercise raise the amount of amino acids in the blood, which also increases glucagon secretion. This happens by requiring the liver to speed up the conversion of glycogen to glucose, as well as creating glucose from fatty acids, lactic acid, and amino acids. Blood levels of glucose increase but do not enter the cells, so cellular levels of glucose decrease.

Adrenal Glands

We have two adrenal glands, one on top of each of our kidneys. Each gland consists of an inner portion called the *medulla* and an outer layer called the *cortex*. The adrenal glands are related to the root or basic chakra center located at the base of the spine and focused on functions of survival and grounding.

Adrenal Medulla

The tissue structure of the adrenal medulla is similar to nerve tissue and functions as part of the sympathetic nervous system. The adrenal medulla secretes two catecholamines, epinephrine (sometimes called *adrenaline)* and norepinephrine (or *noradrenaline)*. These hormones are active in the sympathetic fight-or-flight or alarm response to stress. Epinephrine has its primary influence on the heart, causing an increase in heart rate, whereas norepinephrine has a greater effect on peripheral vasoconstriction, which raises blood pressure. The hormones produced by the adrenal medulla prolong and intensify the activity begun by the sympathetic nervous system neurons. The hypothalamus, the adrenal medulla, and the adrenal cortex are linked and interdependent in the management of the stress response. When stress-producing events are unresolved within about 15 minutes (Selye's alarm phase), these symptoms activate a more prolonged stress-coping pattern of the adrenocortical responses (Selye's resistance phase). Over the long term, if epinephrine and norepinephrine remain elevated, they perpetuate predisposing factors for stress-related disease.

Adrenal Cortex

The adrenal cortex secretes three major glucocorticoid (glucose-producing steroid) hormones that are derived from cholesterol. ACTH from the pituitary gland, which receives its messages from the hypothalamus, stimulates the release of these hormones: cortisol, aldosterone, and the gonadocorticoids. The adrenal cortex hormones are involved with metabolism of most body cells. Without a functioning adrenal cortex, a person could die from excessive stress and its effects.

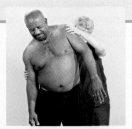

Practical Application

Therapeutic massage methods have been shown to help dissipate the concentration of adrenal medulla hormones, reducing their detrimental effects in the body. Because the effects of catecholamines dissipate within a short time, the usual goal for therapeutic massage is to support the body in a return to homeostasis and prevent a recurrence of the excessive alarm response so that the body can remain in a state of homeostasis. The general application in a typical 1-hour session is to work with more vigorous methods for the first 15 minutes to use the catecholamines and then begin the transition to trigger and support the relaxation response of parasympathetic function over the next 45 minutes.

Because the major repair and energy-restoring mechanisms of the body are supported most effectively in the parasympathetic pattern and because most energy is expended and tissue damage created during fight-or-flight activity, we can begin to see the wisdom in supporting parasympathetic function to allow sufficient time for restoration and repair of the body. A general rule of thumb is that for every 15 minutes of catecholamine-generated sympathetic activity, the body requires about 45 minutes of parasympathetic balancing time. In a healthy, well-balanced person, sympathetic activities account for 25% of daily actions, with parasympathetic restorative actions making up another 25%. The other 50% of the time is taken up with activities that use sympathetic and parasympathetic functions together. However, this seldom happens, and the ratio often is reversed. Dysfunction occurs when sympathetic activity dominates, often because of lifestyle demands. Over time the body cannot provide enough restorative action, and homeostatic balance is disrupted. Again, many of the healing rituals of old seem to be based on supporting parasympathetic activity and providing effective outlets for the fight-or-flight hormones of the adrenal glands. The use of sweat lodges, ceremonial bathing, quiet reflection, chanting, dancing, feasting, and other such activities are seen as effective ways to dissipate the fight-or-flight hormones while promoting restorative functions (Activity 6-5).

Cortisol

Cortisol is secreted in minute amounts. If the body does not have sufficient supplies of fat or glycogen stored to use for energy, cortisol synthesizes certain amino acids into glucose (gluconeogenesis), causing a rise in blood sugar. Cortisol also converts starches into glycogen in the liver if the body does not acquire enough carbohydrates to use.

Eating and activity stimulate cortisol secretion, which seems to follow daily biologic rhythms. Peak cortisol levels occur shortly after waking, whereas the lowest levels are reached just as the sleep cycle begins. High levels of cortisol in the blood may disrupt the sleep cycle. Any situation that

🖉 ACTIVITY 6-5

Design a personal 15-minute sympathetic activity sequence. Then design a personal 45-minute parasympathetic relaxation sequence. Remember that the idea of balance is important. The body needs glucocorticoids for normal function to achieve homeostasis. Excessive stress and use of steroids, such as pharmacologic agents, may lead to the disruption of this homeostasis.

Example

15-minute sympathetic activity sequence: I will go to the recreation center and spend 5 minutes on the track and 10 minutes on the stair-climbing machine.

45-minute parasympathetic relaxation sequence: I will spend 15 minutes doing slow stretching combined with coordinated breathing. I will take a 15-minute hot bath, and I will read inspirational and heart-warming stories for 15 minutes.

Your Turn

produces acute stress increases blood levels of cortisol, and the sympathetic nervous system overrides any inhibitory effects in feedback loop regulation. This results in a rise in blood levels of glucose, fatty acids, and amino acids, all because of cortisol. Levels of stress often are measured by cortisol levels, and research in stress-management methods often uses cortisol as a measurement criterion, with a drop indicating a reduction in the stress response. Cortisol contains antiinflammatory agents that limit the amount of substances released during the inflammatory response. Cortisol slows wound healing because of a decreased rate of connective tissue regeneration. Excessively high levels of cortisol, especially over a long period, can cause symptoms such as a decrease in cartilage and bone formation; inhibition of the inflammatory response, which reduces normal signals for tissue repair; depression of the activity of the immune system; increase in fat storage in adipose tissue; depression of brain activity; and promotion of detrimental changes in cardiovascular, neural, and gastrointestinal function.

Aldosterone

Aldosterone is a mineralocorticoid, a sodium- and potassium-regulating steroid. Aldosterone causes the kidneys to reabsorb more sodium and water and excrete more potassium and hydrogen. Although aldosterone is necessary for our survival, excessive amounts of the hormone lead to sodium and water retention accompanied by elevation of potassium ions and, in some instances, alteration of the acid-base balance of blood. Under excessive stress the hypothalamus secretes

Practical Application

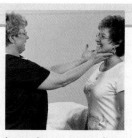

Studies show that massage reduces cortisol levels and therefore promotes activities such as improved sleep, better digestion, increased immune function, and improved tissue repair. Other forms of relaxation, including moderate aerobic exercise and slow stretching methods such as yoga, show similar results. The most effective interventions seem to be rhythmic, with a duration of 15 to 60 minutes producing the best results. Because the effects wear off within a 24-hour period, some sort of relaxation method needs to be done every day to best support well-being.

corticotropin-releasing hormone. ACTH blood levels rise and trigger an increase in aldosterone secretion. The resulting increase in blood volume and blood pressure helps ensure adequate delivery of nutrients and respiratory gases during the stressful period.

Practical Application

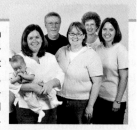

The release of aldosterone, although effective when the body is expending physical energy such as that required in actual fighting behavior, increases the likelihood of stress-induced disease such as high blood pressure when the energy expenditure is less than the physiologic response. This happens often as persons try to deal with increased emotional and mental stress without physical activity. Aerobic activity and moderate weight-resistance exercises are helpful in managing this situation, balancing emotional and mental activity (Activity 6-6).

Gonadocorticoids

Although the ovaries and testes produce most of the sex hormones, the adrenal glands also produce similar male and female sex steroids called *gonadocorticoids*. Both sexes secrete estrogen, progesterone, and the male androgens, with androgens predominating. This hormone secretion is significant in the fetus and during early puberty. The effect of the adrenal sex hormones increases as we age, and hormone production in the gonads decreases. For this reason postmenopausal women may use adrenal estrogen when ovarian function decreases.

Testes and Ovaries

The male and female gonads are located in the pelvic cavity and produce sex hormones identical to those of the adrenal cortex. Because this is the primary function of the gonads, they secrete larger amounts than the adrenal cortex and, in the female, secrete them in a cyclic manner to regulate the menstrual cycle, support pregnancy, and prepare for lactation.

📝 ACTIVITY 6-6

On a separate piece of paper, outline the progression of the adrenal hormone patterns in response to a stress that lasts 24 hours. Imagine a situation and identify the
- Emotion accompanying the stressor
- Possible duration of effect
- Hormones involved
- Possible results

Example

Situation: Parent worried about adolescent child who comes home 2 hours late.

1. Anger; first 15 minutes; epinephrine and norepinephrine; results in increase in fight-or-flight response and increased sympathetic activity.
2. Worry; next 30 minutes; with increase in anxiety still supporting continuance of catecholamine response.
3. Increased worry; next 60 minutes; shift to cortisol release, resulting in inability to sleep.
4. Recurring anger; 15 minutes; epinephrine and norepinephrine with aldosterone increase; results in increased fight-or-flight response and increased sympathetic activity with rise in blood pressure because of increasing fluid levels of blood.
5. Child comes home and is met by an angry and worried parent.
6. Inability of parent to sleep the rest of the night because of increased cortisol levels.
7. Fatigue the next day with irritability and a dull headache caused by effects of increased cortisol and aldosterone levels.
8. Because of increased cortisol and aldosterone levels, parent has suppressed immune function and catches a cold 3 days later.

The testes and ovaries are related to the root chakra located at the base of the lumbar vertebrae in the lower abdomen near the genitals and uterus. The function of this chakra is desire, pleasure, sexuality, and procreation, with the attraction of opposites.

The two primary female sex hormones are estrogen and progesterone. Male sex hormones are called *androgens*. The main male sex hormone is testosterone. These hormones help develop and maintain primary sexual characteristics. Sexual behavior, male and female brain development, and gender behavior have been linked directly to concentrations of these hormones. Testosterone has an effect on the sex drive (libido) for men and women. Sex hormones influence biologic function and behavior throughout life. Males and females are most similar in the beginning and end of life, with the greatest differences from puberty to midlife (the reproductive years), when these hormones are more active.

These sex hormones have other effects on the body. Estrogen, progesterone, and androgens affect epithelial and connective tissue and circulation. Continuing research concerning the sex hormones secreted by the adrenal glands indicates functions of these hormones other than reproduction.

Testosterone, along with other androgens, is known to influence hair growth and distribution of hair in men and women. Androgens also affect the skin and are a factor in acne development.

Androgens and estrogens exert their major influence at puberty. Androgens in particular stimulate growth and maturation of bone, cartilage, and muscle. Low levels of estrogens promote growth, whereas high levels inhibit growth. Beyond puberty, androgens increase hemoglobin levels, whereas estrogen protects against bone loss and epidermal tissue atrophy. Estrogen also can be synthesized by adipose tissue, which converts naturally occurring androgens.

Besides the primary sex hormones, the ovaries produce relaxin, a hormone that relaxes and dilates the cervix near the end of pregnancy and relaxes pelvic and pubic ligaments to prepare for delivery. The ovaries also produce inhibin, the hormone that inhibits follicle-stimulating hormone and luteinizing hormone after ovulation and during pregnancy. The testes produce inhibin, which controls sperm production.

Pineal Gland

The pineal is a tiny gland inside the brain within the diencephalon and surrounded by pia mater. All the functions of this gland have not been identified. To add to the mystery of the gland, it is located in the position of the third eye in many Eastern philosophies and is related to the crown or brow chakra, depending on the Eastern discipline. The functions of this chakra area involve inner sight or awareness.

Serotonin, norepinephrine, dopamine, histamine, and other neurotransmitters and hormones have been identified from this gland, but its major function seems to be to secrete melatonin. The gland is light-sensitive and is involved with regulating the rhythmic patterns of the body. The pineal gland also produces a hormone that stimulates secretion of aldosterone by the adrenal cortex.

Many body rhythms have long been known to move in step with one another or to be entrained. Body temperature, pulse, hormone concentrations, and the sleep-wake cycles seem to follow the same beat over a 24-hour period. The influences of light on the biologic clock of the hypothalamus activate many of these rhythms. Melatonin secretion is inhibited when light reaches the eyes and is enhanced during darkness. Light produces melatonin-mediated effects on reproductive, eating, and sleeping patterns. Light intensity, spectrum (color mixture), and timing (day/night or seasonal changes) influence individuals.

People have worshiped the sun since prehistoric times. Many ancient healing rituals were timed with the rising or setting of the sun. The cycles of the moon are also important in biologic rhythm regulation. Some native traditions refer to the menstrual cycle as the "moon time" because women would usually menstruate during the full moon. The word *lunatic* is derived from *lunar* (i.e., of or relating to the moon) because the moon is traditionally associated with increased emotional behavior.

Not only are we deficient in natural light; we are also starved of the dark. Exposure to artificial light well beyond the

ACTIVITY 6-7

Develop a daily schedule that supports biologic rhythms, particularly those mediated by the pineal gland. Carry this schedule from awakening to bedtime.

Example

5:30 AM: Wake up
5:45 AM: Quiet meditation
6:00 AM: Exercise outside in rising sun
7:30 AM: Breakfast

Your Turn

natural cycle has influenced the drastic increase in insomnia and disruptive sleep patterns. Our bodies are out of touch with the natural rhythms they were designed to follow, which puts more stress on our systems. Artificial lights do not provide the full spectrum of sunlight. The incandescent bulbs commonly used in homes primarily provide red wavelengths, whereas the fluorescent bulbs used in many businesses and schools provide yellow-green wavelengths. Animals exposed for long periods to artificial lighting exhibit reproductive abnormalities and an enhanced susceptibility to cancer. Could it be that some of us are unknowingly experiencing the same effects?

Scientists are just now beginning to understand the reasons for these effects, and as they do, they are increasingly concerned about windowless offices, restricted and artificial illumination of work areas, and the growing number of institutionalized and isolated individuals who rarely feel the energy of the sun, the natural rhythm of the moon, or the quieting enveloping of the dark (Activity 6-7).

Thymus

The thymus is a gland located deep to the sternum and mediastinum of the thorax and between the lungs at the level of the fourth and fifth thoracic vertebrae. Often considered part of the lymphatic system and identified as the master gland of the immune system, the thymus does have endocrine secretions. Thymus hormones are thymopoietin, thymic humoral factor, thymic factor, and thymosin. These hormones function in the growth and development of T cell lymphocytes of the immune system. The thymus is large in children, providing some evidence that its production of hormones may slow down with aging.

The thymus is located in the general region of the heart and is related to the heart chakras, with the functions of love, compassion, and transformation in Eastern doctrine.

Other Hormones

Endorphins

Endorphins belong to a family of peptide hormones that have many different effects, most notably suppressing pain in a manner similar to that of morphine. Endorphins are synthesized in the brain, primarily in the anterior lobe of the pituitary gland, and bind to receptors in the brain that increase pain thresholds. Endorphins appear to enhance the release of thyroid-releasing hormone from the hypothalamus and also influence the neurosecretion of vasopressin, ACTH, and growth hormone. Endorphins influence mood, producing a mild euphoric feeling such as that seen in runner's high. They also help control body temperature; assist with memory and learning; and help regulate the sex hormones that control the onset of puberty, sex drive, and reproduction. Endorphins are a factor in mental illness, especially schizophrenia and depression.

Atrial Natriuretic Factor

Besides pumping blood, the heart secretes an important hormone. Specific cells located in the right atrium produce atrial natriuretic hormone when blood entering the heart stretches cardiac muscle fibers. Atrial natriuretic hormone works like a calcium channel blocker, inhibiting aldosterone secretion and thereby lowering blood pressure by increasing the amount of water excreted, and it also inhibits the release of ADH, resulting in the same effect.

Erythropoietin

When oxygen levels in the body decrease, the kidneys produce erythropoietin to stimulate the production of red blood cells in the bone marrow.

Insulin-Like Growth Factor

Insulin-like growth factor is produced primarily in the liver and looks like the insulin molecule. The factor is released in response to growth hormone and stimulates the growth in target cells of insulin, matrix production in cartilage, and growth of fibroblasts in connective tissue. Insulin-like growth factor also synthesizes lipids and glycogen in adipose tissue.

Gastrointestinal Hormones

The mucosa of the gastrointestinal tract produces gastrointestinal hormones and releases them when food is present to help regulate digestion. Three of the most prominent are gastrin, secretin, and cholecystokinin.

Gastrin is produced in the mucosal cells of the stomach and duodenum and stimulates the release of hydrochloric acid and pepsin from the stomach. These are needed to digest proteins. *Secretin,* produced by the small intestine, stimulates the release of pancreatic enzymes that digest proteins, lipids, and carbohydrates. *Cholecystokinin* is produced in the mucosa of the intestine and secreted into the bloodstream. Cholecystokinin causes the release of bile from the gallbladder (bile is needed for efficient lipid digestion), stimulates the pancreas to release its digestive enzymes, and inhibits the secretion of stomach enzymes.

Tissue Hormones

Unlike most hormones that travel to distant target cells, most of the tissue hormones work in the vicinity of or on the exact organs where they are found. These local hormones are called *prostaglandins* and are a group of about 14 unsaturated fatty acid hormones. Prostaglandins are important and powerful substances found in a variety of tissues. They play an important role in communication and control of many body functions but do not meet the definition of a typical hormone. Prostaglandins are specific, highly concentrated, and the shortest acting of the naturally occurring biologic compounds. Prostaglandins are important in overall endocrine regulation and vascular, metabolic, gastrointestinal, reproductive, respiratory, and inflammatory functions.

Inflammation causes release of prostaglandins and histamines, resulting in vasodilation and pain. Aspirin and other antiinflammatory agents act as analgesics by inhibiting the synthesis of prostaglandins. Aspirin also acts as an anticoagulant by preventing the release of the prostaglandins that cause platelet clumping (Activity 6-8).

✎ ACTIVITY **6-8**

Review all the hormone functions described in this chapter, and make an intuitive choice by picking the one gland you believe needs the most consideration in support of your personal homeostasis and endocrine health. Justify the choice. After this choice, design a support program for yourself that includes a form of therapeutic massage and movement therapy.

Example

Thyroid gland: The idea that the thyroid gland is linked to communication and creativity intrigues me because a large part of my day is involved in communicating to teach others. Also, the link to metabolism and oxygen consumption seems relevant to my busy lifestyle. Because osteoporosis is a concern and healthy thyroid function supports proper bone density, it would serve me to support my thyroid function.

Program: The hypothalamus stimulates thyroid function in response to cold. As a program to support thyroid function, I could first take a warm shower in the morning and then turn the water to a cold shower. I could seek out a polarity practitioner and work on balancing my throat chakra. I could also increase my exercise walking pace to support oxygen delivery to the cells. Investigation of nutritional support for the thyroid gland along with a sound diet would be appropriate.

Your Turn

Gland:

Program:

PATHOLOGIC CONDITIONS

SECTION OBJECTIVES

Chapter objective covered in this section:

9. Describe the hypersecretion and hyposecretion pathologic conditions of the endocrine system, and list the associated indications and contraindications for massage.

After completing this section, the student will be able to perform the following:

- Explain endocrine hyper- and hyposecretion.
- Describe nonglandular disorders of the endocrine system.
- Determine indications and contraindications for specific endocrine pathology.

Primary Mechanisms of Endocrine Disease

Diseases of the endocrine system are numerous. They generally take the form of tumors or other abnormalities and frequently are caused when the glands secrete too much or too little of their hormones. Production of too much hormone by a diseased gland is called **hypersecretion.** If too little hormone is produced, the condition is called **hyposecretion.**

Hypersecretion

Any of several different mechanisms may be responsible for a given case of hypersecretion. Tumors are often responsible for an abnormal proliferation of endocrine cells and the resulting increase in hormone secretion. Another cause of hypersecretion is autoimmunity resulting from abnormal functioning of the immune system. Another possible cause of hypersecretion of a hormone is a failure of the feedback mechanisms that regulate secretion of a particular hormone.

Hyposecretion

Various mechanisms have been shown to cause hyposecretion of hormones. Although most tumors cause oversecretion of a hormone, they also can cause a gland to undersecrete its hormone(s). Tissue death, caused by a blockage or failure of blood supply, can cause a gland to reduce its hormonal output. Still another way in which a gland may reduce its secretion below normal levels is through abnormal operation of regulatory feedback loops. An example of this is hyposecretion of testosterone and gonadotropic hormones in men who abuse anabolic steroids. Men who take testosterone steroids increase their blood concentration of this hormone above set-point levels. The body responds to this high concentration by reducing its own output of testosterone and gonadotropins, which may lead to sterility and other complications.

Abnormalities of immune function also may cause hyposecretion. An autoimmune attack on glandular tissue sometimes has the effect of reducing hormone output. Some endocrinologists theorize that autoimmune destruction of pancreatic islet cells, perhaps in combination with viral and genetic mechanisms, is a culprit in many cases of diabetes mellitus (type I, insulin dependent).

Recent research has shown many types of hyposecretion disorders to be caused by insensitivity of the target cells to pituitary tropic hormones rather than by actual hyposecretion. Tropic (or trophic) hormones target other endocrine

List three causes of hypersecretion.
1. _____
2. _____
3. _____

List three causes of hyposecretion.
1. _____
2. _____
3. _____

Develop a list of at least three indications and contraindications for integrating therapeutic massage in combination with synthetic pharmacologic steroid use.

Example
Indications: Beneficial to sleep
Contraindications: Heavy compressive force on bones

Your Turn
Indications:
1. _____
2. _____
3. _____
Contraindications:
1. _____
2. _____
3. _____

glands, stimulate their growth, and promote their function (Activity 6-9).

Nonglandular Disorders of the Endocrine System

Some endocrine disorders are not caused by the glands themselves. The following are other possible causes of endocrine disorders:

- Some cancers can produce hormone-like substances that cause endocrine syndromes.
- An abnormal decrease in the number of hormone receptors on target cells can occur, thus blocking hormonal action.
- Target cells may have abnormal metabolic responses to the hormone-receptor complex.

Pharmacologic Use of Synthetic Adrenocorticosteroids

Synthetic steroids (corticosteroids and steroids) are used primarily to decrease the effects of inflammation by reducing capillary dilation and permeability. Steroids also prevent the release of vasoactive substances such as histamine and kinins. Allergic disorders such as asthma, reactions to bee stings, contact dermatitis, drug reactions, hay fever, and hives are treated with steroids. Steroids also are used to treat arthritis, bursitis, and autoimmune disorders such as lupus erythematosus and rheumatoid arthritis. Steroids have been shown to be useful in treating leukemia, multiple myeloma, Crohn's disease, ulcerative colitis, kidney failure, infections, and skin disorders.

Common side effects of synthetic steroid use include symptoms as diverse as mood changes, insomnia, high blood pressure, increased susceptibility to infection, glaucoma, headache, reduced wound healing, sweating, fragile skin, vertigo, stunted growth in children, osteoporosis, and an increased risk of bone breakage.

Using steroids for extended periods without reevaluation is dangerous. Periodic decreases in dosage are often necessary, but dosages must never be altered or stopped except by licensed medical practitioners. Weaning gradually from large doses of steroids is necessary because they suppress the pituitary gland and ACTH by negative feedback. When ACTH is suppressed, the adrenal glands do not function. When steroid treatment stops, sometimes the adrenal glands do not rebound to a functioning mode, and the person may lapse into Addison's disease. A side effect of oral steroid therapy is gastrointestinal bleeding. Protection of the stomach lining with

cimetidine (Tagamet) is often necessary when one uses oral steroids.

INDICATIONS/CONTRAINDICATIONS for Therapeutic Massage

Some forms of massage may be used to manage some of the side effects of synthetic steroids. However, the practitioner should avoid massage methods such as frictioning that may cause inflammation when a person is taking synthetic adrenocorticosteroids. Massage also is contraindicated directly over areas where steroids were injected to treat localized inflammation such as bursitis because it is important for the steroid to remain localized in the tissues (Activity 6-10).

Pituitary Pathologic Conditions
Gigantism

In gigantism and acromegaly, the pituitary gland produces excessive growth hormone. The term *gigantism* refers to the condition if it begins in infancy or early childhood. The condition results in excessive growth of the entire body. Acromegaly is an abnormality that occurs in adults in whom the excessive hormone thickens bones and enlarges organs. In secondary Cushing's disease the pituitary gland produces excessive ACTH, resulting in increased production of steroids by the adrenal gland. The symptoms include increased fat on the face and between the shoulder blades, thinning of bones and skin, and bruising. Treatment of gigantism, acromegaly, and secondary Cushing's disease includes surgery or radiation therapy. If a pituitary tumor is present, drug therapy with somatostatin is usually the treatment of choice.

Dwarfism

Decreased growth hormone production and insufficient tropic hormones may cause height deficiencies. In pituitary deficiency all pituitary hormones are decreased, which leads to the loss of target organ hormones, specifically adrenal steroids, thyroxine, and the gonadotropins. Dwarfism may result.

Dwarfism in children is treated by administration of synthetic growth hormone and, if necessary, replacement of thyroid, adrenal, and sex steroid hormones.

Diabetes Insipidus

In diabetes insipidus (not to be confused with diabetes mellitus), the pituitary gland releases less vasopressin than it should. Scarring or damage from head injuries often causes the condition. The ability of the water in urine to be reabsorbed decreases, and urine output increases, sometimes by as much as 20 L per day. Maintaining an adequate fluid intake may control mild cases, but in others treatment with a synthetic form of vasopressin has proved effective. If the inability of the kidney to respond to vasopressin causes diabetes insipidus, the normal treatment is reducing salt intake and taking medications focused on kidney function. Radiation therapy, surgery, or both are indicated in those rare cases in which a tumor causes diabetes insipidus.

Thyroid Pathologic Conditions

Hyperthyroidism

Hyperthyroidism, or thyrotoxicosis, is the second most common endocrine disorder after diabetes mellitus and mostly affects women. The most common cause is autoimmune dysfunction. Symptoms include increased metabolic rate, excessive sweating, weight loss even with increased food intake, fatigue, nervousness, loose stools, tachycardia, warm and moist skin, hand tremor, and hyperactivity. Hyperthyroidism mimics bipolar disorder psychosis and almost always is accompanied by a goiter. (A goiter, which is an enlarged thyroid gland, may be found in hyperfunction, hypofunction, or normal thyroid function.) Plummer's disease, or toxic nodular goiter, is another form of hyperthyroidism.

The symptoms of Graves' disease, also a form of hyperthyroidism, include an enlarged thyroid gland and abnormal eyeball protrusion, called *exophthalmos*, which results from excess fluid behind the eye and may not diminish even after treatment. Graves' disease runs in families, is associated with autoimmune problems, and is most common in women between the ages of 20 and 40. Treatments include thyroidectomy; the use of antithyroid medications such as propylthiouracil (which blocks iodine from being incorporated into thyroxine), or the use of radioactive iodine, which shrinks (destroys) the thyroid gland without affecting other tissues (Figure 6-6).

Hypothyroidism

Hypothyroidism can result from treatment for hyperthyroidism by radioactive iodine, overdose of antithyroid medication, or partial or complete thyroidectomy. The next most common causes are autoimmune dysfunction and a decrease in thyroid-releasing hormone from the hypothalamus. Symptoms include weakness, fatigue, lower metabolic rate, constipation, hoarseness, bradycardia, skin dryness, weight gain (often resulting in obesity), sluggishness, and slowed mental function (sometimes with psychotic behavior). Again, a goiter is often present. Mild hypothyroidism is common in perimenopausal women

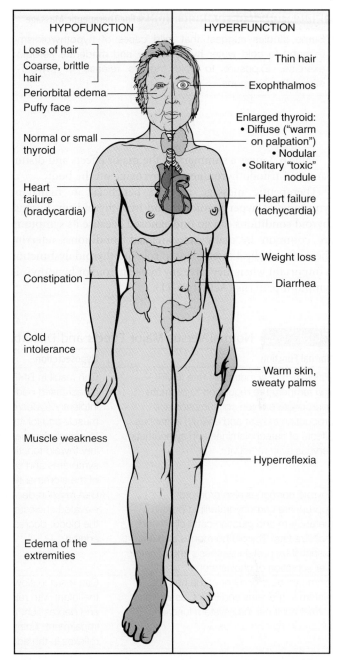

FIGURE 6-6 Comparison of hyperthyroidism and hypothyroidism. (From Damjanov I: *Pathology for the health professions,* ed 4, Philadelphia, 2012, Saunders.)

between the ages of 35 and 45. Because of this, thyroid function should be checked as part of the routine health care of women. Hypothyroidism responds well to oral medication.

If thyroid hormones are absent in the fetus or during infancy, the result can be cretinism, a condition that results in mental retardation and dwarfism. Hashimoto's disease is an autoimmune hypothyroid disorder that is hereditary, is found mainly in women between 30 and 50 years of age, and causes tissue changes in the thyroid gland itself. Myxedema is the most severe form of hypothyroidism, causing many of the previously mentioned symptoms and swelling of the face, hands, and feet (see Figure 6-6).

Some studies suggest that mild cases of hypothyroidism respond to cold water hydrotherapy and moderate aerobic exercise. Exposure to cold triggers release of thyroid-stimulating hormone.

Table 6-3 gives a summary of the major effects and disturbances of triiodothyronine and thyroxine on the body.

Therapeutic massage may be beneficial in managing symptoms of hyperthyroidism and hypothyroidism. Because thyroid conditions can go undiagnosed because its symptoms are common in many stress-related conditions, referring clients for medical assessment to rule out thyroid dysfunction is important when they have any hyperthyroid or hypothyroid symptom patterns (Activity 6-11).

Parathyroid Pathologic Conditions

An excess of parathormone causes too much calcium to be removed from bone, resulting in weak bones. A deficiency of parathormone can cause hypocalcemic tetany, the symptoms

ACTIVITY 6-11

List three thyroid dysfunction symptoms that may cause a client to seek bodywork modalities. Examples are provided to get you started.

Examples
Nervousness, fatigue, constipation

Your Turn
1. _____
2. _____
3. _____

Table 6-3 Normal Versus Major Effects and Disturbances of Triiodothyronine and Thyroxine on the Body

Normal Function	Hyposecretion	Hypersecretion
Maintains basal metabolic rate (BMR) and temperature regulation to promote appropriate oxygen consumption and production of heat and energy; enhances effects of catecholamines and sympathetic nervous system activity.	Can result in BMR less than normal with a decreased body temperature, cold intolerance, decreased appetite, weight gain, muscle and joint pain, decreased sensitivity to catecholamines, and general slowed state; low thyroid function mimics many disease symptoms and should be checked when any of the aforementioned symptoms are present.	Can result in BMR greater than normal with an increase in body temperature; heat intolerance; decreased appetite; weight loss; sensitivity to catecholamines, which may lead to hypertension (high blood pressure); mood changes; and anxiety-type symptoms.
Thyroid hormones also promote appropriate carbohydrate/lipid/protein metabolism and glucose catabolism and mobilize fats. Thyroid hormones also are essential for protein synthesis and enhance liver secretion of cholesterol.	Can result in decreased glucose metabolism, elevated cholesterol and triglyceride levels in the blood, decreased protein synthesis, and edema.	Can result in enhanced catabolism of glucose and fats, weight loss, increased protein catabolism, and loss of muscle mass.
Promotes development of the nervous system in the fetus and infant, as well as normal adult nervous system function.	Can result in slowed brain development in the infant with retardation and mental dulling, and depression, paresthesias, memory impairment, listlessness, and hypoactive reflexes in the adult.	Can result in irritability, restlessness, insomnia, overresponsiveness to environmental stimuli, bulging eyes (exophthalmos), and personality changes.
Promotes functioning of the heart.	Can result in decreased efficiency of the pumping action of the heart, slow heart rate, and lower blood pressure.	Can result in rapid heart rate and high blood pressure and, if prolonged, can lead to heart failure.
Promotes normal muscular development, tone, and function.	Can result in sluggish muscle action, muscle cramps, and myalgia.	Can result in muscle atrophy and weakness.
Promotes growth and maturation of the skeleton.	Can result in growth retardation, skeletal malabsorption, retention of child's body proportions in adults, and joint pain in the adult.	Can result in excessive skeletal growth initially, followed by early epiphyseal closure and short stature in children; adults experience demineralization of skeleton.
Promotes gastrointestinal motility and tone and increases secretion of digestive juices.	Can result in depressed gastrointestinal motility and tone and increased secretion of digestive juices.	Can result in excessive gastrointestinal motility, diarrhea, and loss of appetite.
Promotes female reproductive ability and normal lactation.	Can result in depressed ovarian function, sterility, and depressed lactation.	Can result in depressed ovarian function in females and impotence in males.
Promotes secretory activity of skin.	Can result in skin that is pale, thick, and dry; facial edema; coarse and thin hair; and hard, thick nails.	Can result in skin that is flushed, thin, and moist; may produce thin and soft hair and nails.

of which include loss of sensation, muscle twitches, uncontrolled spasm, and convulsion.

In hypoparathyroidism the levels of calcium in blood and urine are less than normal, frequently resulting in spasms of skeletal muscles. Moderate to mild deficiency can result in neuromuscular excitability that could be misdiagnosed as simple muscle tension. Anxiety may result as well. Ruling out hypoparathyroidism in cases of unresolved anxiety and muscle tension is important. Emergency treatment of tetany caused by hypoparathyroidism is an injection of calcium chloride. Calcium and vitamin D supplements are used for maintenance therapy.

INDICATIONS/CONTRAINDICATIONS For Therapeutic Massage

The symptoms of hyperparathyroidism include mild to severe skeletal pain and possibly osteoporosis. The client may seek body therapies for these conditions, and the massage therapist must take care to provide the appropriate referral to determine the underlying cause of the problem.

In primary hyperparathyroidism, which usually results from a benign tumor, levels of calcium increase in blood and urine. In secondary hyperparathyroidism, which mostly results from kidney disease, blood calcium decreases and urine calcium increases. The frequency of hyperparathyroidism is much more common than hypoparathyroidism and is increasing.

Pancreatic Pathologic Conditions
Hyperfunction

A benign tumor occasionally causes high insulin levels. More commonly, high insulin levels occur in diabetic clients who take insulin without eating properly. The result is what is known as an *insulin reaction,* which means the body is flooded with insulin. Glucose enters the cells at an increased rate, and the blood glucose level falls, causing hypoglycemia (low blood sugar). When the brain is deprived of glucose, confusion and weakness result. A deficient production of glucagon may cause hypoglycemia.

True hypoglycemia is rare. More common is reactive hypoglycemia, a diet-induced condition that can be corrected by eating a balanced diet on a regular schedule.

Hypofunction

The disorder known as *diabetes mellitus* results from the pancreas not producing enough insulin or totally stopping insulin production. Because cells do not absorb glucose, the amount in the bloodstream increases (hyperglycemia). Glucose is a powerful diuretic, so glucose entering the urine is accompanied by water. As glucose flows through the kidneys, some of the excess is released in the urine (glycosuria). This causes many of the first symptoms of diabetes, such as dehydration, increased thirst (polydipsia), increased urination (polyuria), and an increased appetite (polyphagia).

When the body is unable to use glucose, it uses fats for energy. The breakdown in fats results in the formation of ketones (ketoacids) as by-products, increasing body acidity and causing ketoacidosis. In severe instances the combination of dehydration, high blood sugar, and acidosis may depress the cerebral cortex to the point of coma. This metabolic acidosis stimulates the respiratory center to increase the breathing rate.

Two types of diabetes mellitus exist. Type I, or insulin-dependent diabetes, is usually severe and occurs at a young age. Symptoms develop quickly, with ketoacidosis often being the first manifestation. Ketoacidosis is treatable with saline, bicarbonate, potassium, and insulin. A controlled diet and the daily use of insulin are the most common long-term treatments.

Type II, or non–insulin-dependent diabetes, is usually milder and in most cases begins in adults. However, type II diabetes is occurring in younger persons. Heredity and obesity are important contributing factors. Symptoms include dehydration, increased thirst and appetite, frequent urination, reduced resistance to infection, blurred vision, and fatigue. These symptoms usually develop over a period of years. Treatment generally begins with dietary changes, such as those recommended by the American Diabetes Association. An exercise program is implemented to control weight and increase general fitness. Weight loss is an important first step because fewer insulin receptors are present and they become less sensitive to insulin in an overweight person. Oral medications, including chlorpropamide (Diabinese) or tolbutamide (Orinase), reduce blood sugar levels. Insulin may be used if blood sugar levels remain high, but it is not necessarily a permanent form of treatment.

Complications of diabetes sometimes include vascular disease because diabetes increases the development of arteriosclerosis. High glucose levels also raise the chances of infection because they provide a good medium for bacterial growth. Other complications include kidney disease, heart attacks (diabetic persons have twice the average rate), eye problems (diabetic retinopathy), impotence in men, and loss of menstrual cycles in women. Gangrene of the feet in diabetic clients accounts for more amputations of the feet than any other condition, including trauma. Treatment for the complications of diabetes includes meticulous attention to the hygiene of the feet and an exercise program for weight loss and fitness. Diabetic neuropathy, a painful and difficult-to-manage condition resulting from peripheral nerve damage, is more severe with type I diabetes because nerve damage results from the ketoacidosis (ketoacidosis is not seen as often in those with type II diabetes) (Figure 6-7).

INDICATIONS/CONTRAINDICATIONS for Therapeutic Massage

A general stress management program supports the management of diabetes. Therapeutic massage can be an integral part of such a program. An important part of working with the diabetic client is that bodywork be a part of an overall treatment program with medical supervision. Careful observation of the feet during massage supports a hygiene program. The practitioner should refer the client for immediate medical care of any noted tissue changes.

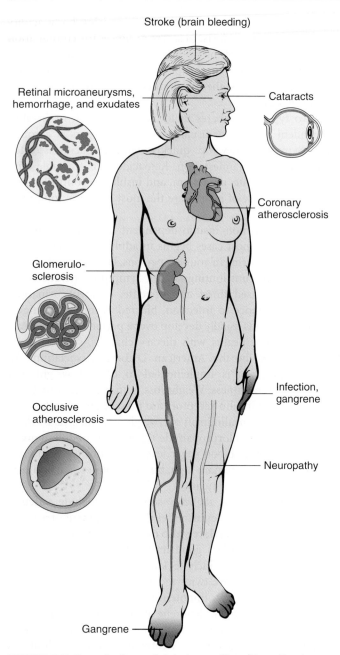

Stroke (brain bleeding)

Retinal microaneurysms, hemorrhage, and exudates

Cataracts

Coronary atherosclerosis

Glomerulo-sclerosis

Occlusive atherosclerosis

Infection, gangrene

Neuropathy

Gangrene

FIGURE 6-7 Complications of diabetes mellitus. (From Damjanov I: *Pathology for the health professions,* ed 4, Philadelphia, 2012, Saunders.)

In pain management of diabetic neuropathy, using massage approaches as part of a supervised program can prove beneficial for short-term reduction of pain symptoms (Activity 6-12).

Adrenal Pathologic Conditions

In *Cushing's syndrome,* corticosteroid levels in the blood and urine are elevated, specifically cortisol and urinary 17-hydroxycorticosteroid, both of which are excretory products of cortisol. The usual cause of Cushing's disease is taking large doses of corticosteroid drugs for long periods. ACTH is low in primary Cushing's disease. ACTH is high in secondary Cushing's disease. Usually caused by a pituitary tumor, the

ACTIVITY 6-12

Identify a reason why therapeutic massage can be beneficial as part of a total diabetes management program. Justify your position using the clinical reasoning model.

Example
Statement: Therapeutic massage supports weight management programs.
1. What are the facts?
Weight loss and changes in diet result in chemical changes in the body. Mood-elevating chemicals that are generated from high-sugar, high-fat foods are reduced substantially in a diabetic diet.
Therapeutic massage increases the feel-good chemicals in the body.
2. What are the possibilities?
Therapeutic massage can act as a substitute for food to provide stimulation for mood elevation.
3. What are the pros and cons? What are the consequences of not acting (not doing bodywork)? What are the consequences of acting (doing bodywork)?
Positive consequences include pleasure sensations that do not contribute to the diabetic problem. Negative consequences include the cost and inconvenience that may prevent easy implementation of these methods into a person's lifestyle.
4. What would be the effect on the persons involved: client, practitioner, and other professionals working with the client?
The person would feel cared for and supported as part of the weight management program by receiving the personal attention from a professional during a time in which he or she may feel deprived.

Your Turn
Statement:
1. What are the facts?

2. What are the possibilities?

3. What are the pros and cons? What are the consequences of not acting? What are the consequences of acting?

4. What would be the effect on the persons involved: client, practitioner, and other professionals working with the client?

secondary condition is referred to as *Cushing's disease* instead of *Cushing's syndrome.* In both cases, symptoms include fat accumulation, edema, hyperglycemia, muscle weakness, suppressed immunity, osteoporosis, acne, and increased facial hair. Diabetes mellitus can be brought on during Cushing's disease and can develop into a chronic condition.

Conn's syndrome, caused by an adrenal tumor, is primary hyperaldosteronism. In rare cases, if caused by a nonspecific enlargement of the adrenal glands, the syndrome is referred to as *aldosteronism.* Levels of aldosterone and sodium are elevated in plasma and urine, and potassium is decreased. Symptoms include headache; tingling and weakness in the limbs; increased thirst; fatigue; hypertension; and increase in urine volume, especially at night.

Addison's disease shows low plasma cortisol, low sodium, and high potassium levels (all opposite of Cushing's disease). Urinary 17-hydroxycorticosteroid and blood glucose levels are low. Primary Addison's disease shows a high ACTH level (with no cortisol to oppose ACTH). Secondary Addison's disease shows a low ACTH level because of nonstimulation of the adrenal gland by the pituitary gland. Symptoms include weakness, decreased endurance, increased pigmentation of the skin and mucous membranes, anorexia, dehydration, weight loss, intestinal disturbances, anxiety, depression (or similar emotional distress), and decreased tolerance to cold. The onset is usually gradual and may be mistaken as general stress symptoms. The condition can be life-threatening, and proper diagnosis is essential for appropriate treatment. After these conditions are diagnosed, stress management can be an important part of ongoing therapeutic management.

Pineal Pathology

Conditions such as illness, drug use, jet travel, alteration of eating pattern, weather changes, a change in work schedule to the night shift, or other disruptions in the sleep-wake cycle can throw these rhythms out of synchronization. Disruptions in these rhythms cause mood changes, affect the immune function, alter digestion, and unsettle the entire homeostatic balance. Researchers have identified a common emotional disorder called *seasonal affective disorder* in which mood swings are exaggerated grossly. As the days grow shorter each fall, persons with seasonal affective disorder become irritable, anxious, sleepy, and socially withdrawn. Their appetite becomes insatiable; they crave carbohydrates and gain weight readily. Phototherapy, the use of bright lights, for up to 2 hours daily reversed these symptoms in nearly 90% of persons studied and was more effective than the use of antidepressant drugs in the research. When the subjects stopped receiving phototherapy or were given melatonin, their symptoms returned as quickly as they had lifted, indicating that melatonin may be a key to seasonal mood changes as well.

Symptoms of seasonal affective disorder are virtually identical to those of individuals with carbohydrate-craving obesity and premenstrual syndrome, except that carbohydrate-craving obesity affects sufferers daily and premenstrual syndrome affects sufferers monthly. Phototherapy relieves premenstrual syndrome symptoms in some women, according to some research.

Night-shift workers exhibit reversed melatonin secretion patterns. When it is exposed to light during the night, the pineal gland releases no hormone; during daytime sleeping hours, the gland releases high levels of melatonin. If these individuals are awakened from sleep and exposed to bright light, their melatonin levels drop. The same sort of melatonin

inversion occurs in those who fly from coast to coast. The reversal disrupts sleep patterns. Anything that disrupts sleep eventually causes widespread stress in the body.

INDICATIONS/CONTRAINDICATIONS for Therapeutic Massage

Relaxation methods, including therapeutic massage, can support effective sleep patterns. Adhering to a bedtime and wake-time schedule can reestablish sleep patterns. Sleeping in the dark and experiencing adequate natural light during the day seem to be important. Engaging in moderate exercise during the day and a gentle stretching program before retiring is beneficial. Eating on a regular schedule also reinforces the rhythm.

SUMMARY

The ability to integrate knowledge into practical application, including effective clinical reasoning and decision making, is the foundation of competent practice. Regardless of whether we provide informed consent, the foundation of the work is taking a history, doing a physical assessment, determining outcome goals for the client, charting, maintaining appropriate scope of practice, supporting interdisciplinary teams, and understanding anatomy and physiology. The endocrine system may seem removed from the therapeutic application of massage, but it is not. Massage powerfully interacts with the endocrine system, a major system of control.

Endocrine functions coordinate most body functions with the nervous system. The nervous system functions as the yang portion, working quickly, expending energy, and responding to demand, whereas the endocrine system functions as the yin, sustaining, coordinating, and restoring physiologic function. The wisdom of ancient healing arts combines with the concreteness of scientific understanding to validate the wonder of human form and function.

These two systems of control (the nervous system and the endocrine system) provide the organic basis for the healing mysteries. As our understanding increases, more of the knowledge found in Eastern and Western healing traditions; ancient and future thought; and body, mind, and spirit likely will blend into our understanding.

⊝volve

http://evolve.elsevier.com/Fritz/essential

Activity 6-1 Complete a matching exercise by identifying which hormone corresponds to which function.

Activity 6-2 Answer True/False questions about the Endocrine System.

Additional Resources:

Endocrine System scientific animations

Weblinks: Access weblinks that give detail on how to prevent and/or manage diabetes

Electronic Coloring Book

Remember to study for your certification and licensure exams! Review questions for this chapter are located on Evolve.

Workbook Section

All Workbook activities can be done online as well as here in the book. Answers are located on ⊝volve.

Short Answer

1. What are the traditional endocrine glands?

_____
_____
_____
_____

2. What are endocrine tissues? Give examples.

_____
_____
_____
_____

3. What are the functions of hormones?

_____
_____
_____
_____

4. What is the difference between hormones and neurotransmitters?

_____
_____
_____
_____

5. Briefly describe hypersecretion and its causes.

_____
_____
_____
_____

6. Briefly describe hyposecretion and its causes.

_____
_____
_____
_____

Fill in the Blank

The main differences between endocrine system and nervous system control are speed and duration of effect. The nervous system is (1) _____ with a (2) _____ duration of effect, whereas the endocrine system is (3) _____ with a (4) _____ duration of effect.

The concentration of a (5) _____ in the blood is determined by the rate of release and the speed of inactivation and removal from the body. The term (6) _____ describes the time required for half of the hormone to be eliminated from the bloodstream. Hormones are secreted by endocrine glands and other specialized cells into the bloodstream to bind to specific (7) _____ on or in their (8) _____. In a (9) _____ mechanism, hormones bind only to receptor molecules that fit them exactly.

The (10) _____ is the link between the body/mind and the nerve/endocrine function. During stress, it translates nerve impulses into hormone secretions by endocrine glands. The (11) _____, or hypophysis, is located in the head at about eye level. It sits in a recessed area in the sphenoid bone and secretes hormones that regulate growth, fluid balance, lactation, and childbirth.

The (12) _____ gland lies on the trachea below the thyroid cartilage. It consists of a right and left lobe connected by a bridge (isthmus), resulting in a butterfly shape. It regulates metabolism in the body by maintaining an adequate amount of oxygen consumption at the cellular level.

The (13) _____ glands are made up of four round, pea-sized bodies located on the posterior surface of the thyroid lobes. Their hormone, parathormone, when combined with vitamin D, decreases the amount of calcium excreted, causes the release of calcium from bone, and absorbs more calcium from the gastrointestinal tract, resulting in an increase in blood levels of calcium and phosphorus.

The (14) _____ is a long, slender gland located behind the stomach. It is both an exocrine and endocrine gland.

We have two (15) _____ glands, one on top of each of our kidneys. Each gland consists of an outer layer called the *cortex* and an inner portion called the *medulla*.

The (16) _____ are the male and female gonads. They are located in the pelvic cavity and produce sex hormones identical to those of the adrenal cortex.

The (17) _____ gland is a tiny gland inside the brain within the diencephalon and is surrounded by pia mater. The complete functions of this gland have not been identified. Serotonin, norepinephrine, dopamine, histamine, and other neurotransmitters and hormones have been identified from this gland, but its major function seems to be to secrete melatonin. The gland is light-sensitive and is involved with regulating the rhythmic patterns of the body.

The (18) _____ gland is located deep to the sternum and mediastinum of the thorax and between the lungs at the level of the fourth and fifth thoracic vertebrae. Often considered part of the lymphatic system and identified as the master gland of the immune system, it does have endocrine secretions.

Problem Solving

Read the problem presented. There is no correct answer; rather the exercise is intended to assist the student in developing the analytical and decision-making skills necessary in professional practice. After reading the problem, follow the next six steps:

1. Identify the facts presented in the information.
2. Identify the possibilities ("what if" statements) presented, or develop your own possibilities that relate to the facts.
3. Evaluate each possibility in terms of the logical cause and effect and pros and cons.
4. Consider the effect on the persons involved.
5. Write each answer in the space provided.
6. Develop your solution by answering the question posed.

Problem

In the subclinical or early-onset stages of many endocrine dysfunctions, the symptoms are vague and may be mistaken easily for stress-related disease. More than in any other area of pathology, persons may seek therapeutic massage and movement therapists to deal with what seem to be simple stress-related symptoms. In reality, many forms of stress-induced disease are endocrine related and actually can be managed by stress management and lifestyle changes. Who is to know that a heavy stress load is not causing a substantial amount of endocrine dysfunction? Could it be possible that some early-stage endocrine dysfunction resolves itself when the body is better able to handle the stress load? Would the client be best served if stress management and a healthful lifestyle were the first intervention?

Of concern is the need to refer those with endocrine symptoms for proper diagnosis and the willingness of the medical community to take a look at symptoms of early-onset endocrine dysfunction. Changes in lifestyle and more generalized health approaches that support homeostasis can be used successfully after a thorough medical workup.

On the other side of this issue, even if a referral for diagnosis is made, we sometimes feel that we have to be really sick before the condition can be identified by standard laboratory tests. What do low or high normals mean?

Are these ends of the normal spectrum the beginning of dysfunction? What is normal anyway? Endocrine function is so variable, depending on so many physiologic factors, that the results of medical tests are often questionable. Maybe running the same test on different days would give a more reliable norm for a particular person. Therapeutic massage therapists need to observe subtle symptoms that could indicate endocrine dysfunction and refer clients to other health care professionals.

Question

What is the responsibility for referral by the massage therapist, and what type of education is necessary to support educated decisions in these matters? Analyze the information to formulate your response to the question posed. An example is provided as a guide to get you started. You will fill in at least two more statements.

Facts

1. In the subclinical or early-onset stages of many endocrine dysfunctions, the symptoms are vague and may be mistaken easily for stress-related disease.
2. _____
3. _____

Possibilities

1. Bodywork therapists may not be trained adequately to recognize these symptoms.
2. _____
3. _____

Logical Cause and Effect

1. Because the symptoms are not recognized, the massage practitioner may not refer clients.
2. _____
3. _____

Effect

1. Clients may be confused by the symptoms and not understand the referral.
2. _____
3. _____

What is the responsibility for referral of the massage therapist, and what type of education is necessary to support educated decisions in these matters?

_____
_____
_____
_____
_____
_____
_____
_____
_____
_____

Assess Your Competencies

Review the following objectives for Chapter 6:

1. Describe the physiologic processes of the endocrine system.
2. List the traditional endocrine glands.

3. Connect the endocrine system to the nervous system through the hypothalamus.

4. Define endocrine tissues and give examples.

5. Describe the hypothalamic-pituitary-adrenal axis and its link to the general adaptation syndrome.

6. Identify how the Eastern chakra system is related to the endocrine system.
   - Explain the difference between endocrine and exocrine glands.
   - List the endocrine glands of the body.
   - Explain why the hypothalamus is considered a neuroendocrine organ.
   - Describe the body/mind and nerve/endocrine function.
   - List the functions of the hypothalamus.
   - Describe the hypothalamic-pituitary-adrenal axis and the relationship to stress.
   - Compare the endocrine system to the chakra system.

7. List and describe the three main hormone types and their functions.

8. Identify the hormones produced by each endocrine gland and their associated functions.
   - List and describe three main hormone types.
   - Describe endocrine glands and hormone functions.
   - Relate the two main categories of endocrine pathology to the negative feedback control.
   - List various organs and tissues that have an endocrine function.

9. Describe the hypersecretion and hyposecretion pathologic conditions of the endocrine system, and list the associated indications and contraindications for massage.
   - Explain endocrine hyper- and hyposecretion.
   - Describe nonglandular disorders of the endocrine system.
   - Determine indications and contraindications for specific endocrine pathology.

Next, on a separate piece of paper or using an audio or video recorder, prepare a short narrative that reflects how you would explain this content to a client and how the information relates to how you would provide massage. See the example in Chapter 1 on p. 22. When read or listened to, the narrative should not take more than 5 to 10 minutes to complete. Simpler is better. Use examples, tell stories, and use metaphors. It is important to understand that there is no precisely correct way to complete this exercise. The intent is to help you identify how effectively you understand the content and how relevant your application is to massage therapy. An excellent learning activity is to work together with other students and share your narratives. Also share these narratives with a friend or family member who is not familiar with the content. If that person can understand what you have written or recorded, that indicates that you understand it. There are many different ways to complete this learning activity. Yes, it may be confusing to do this, but that's all right. Out of confusion comes clarity. By the time you do this 12 times, once for each chapter in this book, you will be much more competent.

Further Study

Using additional resource material (see the Works Consulted list at the back of this book), identify chapters pertaining to the information presented in this chapter. Locate the information presented in this text, and then elaborate by writing a paragraph of additional information on each of the following:

Hypothalamus

_____
_____
_____
_____
_____
_____
_____

Growth hormone

_____
_____
_____
_____
_____
_____
_____

Type II, or non–insulin-dependent, diabetes

_____
_____
_____
_____
_____
_____
_____

Aldosterone

_____
_____
_____
_____
_____
_____
_____

Pineal gland

_____
_____
_____
_____
_____
_____
_____

Thymus

_____
_____
_____

_____

_____

_____

_____

Prostaglandins

_____

_____

_____

_____

_____

_____

_____

Professional Application

Refer to Chapter 2 of this text to review negative feedback loops. Remember, if a stimulus (stress) disrupts homeostasis in a controlled condition monitored by receptors, afferent receptors send the input to a control center. The signal is interpreted, and output responses to effectors are sent to bring about a change or response that alters the controlled condition, returning it to balance.

If the response reverses the original stimulus, the system is a negative feedback system. Negative feedback systems stabilize physiologic function and are responsible for maintaining a constant internal environment. Most feedback systems are of this type.

Identify a hyposecretion and hypersecretion pathologic condition resulting from a failure of the negative feedback loop control. Then develop a plan for using therapeutic massage and movement therapy to support the care received by the primary physician. Justify each recommendation.

Complete the following:
1. Identify the hormone and gland.
2. Identify the pathologic condition.
3. List possible medical interventions.
4. Develop the support care plan.
5. Justify the plan.

Hypersecretion

1. _____
2. _____
3. _____
4. _____
5. _____

Hyposecretion

1. _____
2. _____
3. _____
4. _____
5. _____

CHAPTER 7

Skeletal System

http://evolve.elsevier.com/Fritz/essential

CHAPTER OBJECTIVES

After completing this chapter, the student will be able to perform the following:

1. List the components and seven main functions of the skeletal system.
2. Describe the structure, classification, and development of bone.
3. Identify bony landmarks.
4. Describe the two divisions of the skeleton.
5. List and describe the individual bones of the axial skeleton.
6. Describe the pathology of the skeletal system and the related indications/contraindications for massage.

CHAPTER OUTLINE

SKELETAL SYSTEM BASICS, 193
  Main Functions of the Skeletal System, 193
BONES, 194
  Bone Structure, 194
  Bone Development, 195
  Articular Cartilage, 195
  Ligaments, 197
  Classification of Bones, 197
  Bone Growth and Repair, 197
  Skeletal Changes Caused by Aging, 197
BONY LANDMARKS, 197
  Depressions and Openings, 198
  Processes That Form Joints, 198
  Processes to Which Tendons and Ligaments Attach, 199
DIVISIONS OF THE SKELETON, 199
INDIVIDUAL BONY FRAMEWORK BY REGION, 202
  Bones of the Axial Skeleton, 202
  Bones of the Appendicular Skeleton, 209
PATHOLOGIC CONDITIONS, 214
  Disorders Caused by Trauma, 214
  Developmental Conditions, 223
  Bone Demineralization Disorders, 224
  Disorders Caused by Radiation Therapy, 225
  Necrosis (Tissue Death), 225
  Infectious Diseases, 225
  Tumors, 225
  Nutritional Disorders, 226
SUMMARY, 226

KEY TERMS

Appendicular skeleton (ap-en-DIK-u-lar) The part of the skeleton composed of the limbs and their attachments.

Articulation (ar-tik-u-LAY-shun) Another word for joint, the structure created when bones connect to each other.

Axial skeleton (AK-see-al) The axis of the body; the axial skeleton consists of the head, vertebral column, ribs, and sternum.

Biomechanics The application of mechanical principles and engineering to human movement.

Cartilage (car-TI-lage) A tough, flexible connective tissue with a high water content that makes it softer than bone.

Compact (dense) bone The hard portion of bone that surrounds spongy bone and helps provide the firm framework of the body.

Endoskeleton The bony support structure found inside the human body; it accommodates growth.

Endosteum (en-DOSS-tee-um) A thin membrane of connective tissue that lines the marrow cavity of a bone.

Kinesiology (ki·ne·si·OL·o·gy) The study of movement that combines the fields of anatomy, physiology, physics, and geometry and relates them to human movement.

Periosteum (PAIR-ee-OSS-tee-um) The thin membrane of connective tissue that covers bones except at articulations.

Piezoelectric (PIE-eh-zoh-ee-LEK-trik) Ability to produce electrical current when deformed or compressed, especially in a crystalline substance such as bone matrix. When electric currents pass through them, these substances deform slightly and vibrate.

Sesamoid bones (SES-ah-moyd) Round bones that often are embedded in tendons and joint capsules. The largest of these is the patella.

Spongy (cancellous) bone The lighter-weight portion of bone, which is made up of trabeculae.

Trabeculae (tra·BEK-u-lee) An irregular meshing of small, bony plates that makes up spongy bone; its spaces are filled with red marrow.

LEARNING HOW TO LEARN

Learning the names of structures such as bones requires persistent and ongoing review, or else you will forget. Visualize all the people in your massage class or at your workplace. How do you remember their names? Association is one way. Association is when you compare two things. For example, one of the names you will learn is *scapula*. This is your shoulder blade. The association could be as follows: The word *scapula* reminds you of scraping, and you scrape with a blade. Singing the words enhances remembering.

A mnemonic is another memory tool. For example, the first letter of each word you are trying to remember might become the first letter in the word of a sentence. This is a remembering strategy described in this chapter.

Often, the words *kinesiology* and *biomechanics* are used interchangeably, which can be confusing. These have similarities and differences, including that they can be defined several ways. Definitions are as follows:

Kinesiology:
- The study of movement that blends anatomy, physiology, physics, and geometry and relates them to human movement.
- The science dealing with the interrelationship of anatomy and the physiology of the body with respect to movement.
- The study of human movement.

Biomechanics:
- Application of the mechanical principles in the study of living organism.
- The science of movement of a living body, including how muscles, bones, tendons, and ligaments work together to produce movement.
- The study of mechanical principles and actions applied to living bodies. This may involve looking at the static (nonmoving) or dynamic (moving) systems associated with various activities.
- The application of mechanical principles such as engineering to human movement.

From these definitions, you can see how the topics are similar but not identical. Consider how the following descriptions support the content of this unit:
- Kinesiology is the study of body movement. It involves anatomy and physiology.
- Developing a treatment plan requires an understanding of kinesiology.
- Biomechanics is the study of the effects of movement on the body. It involves math and measurement.
- Understanding the effects of the mechanical forces applied to the body during massage requires an understanding of biomechanics.

Chapters 7, 8, and 9 are about kinesiology. Chapter 10 is about biomechanics. These four chapters combined will help you understand why, how, and what happens when we move (Box 7-1).

| Box 7-1 | Kinesiology and Biomechanics |

Kinesiology is the study of human movement. There are two aspects of studying kinesiology: the anatomy and the process of movement.

Biomechanics is the study of mechanical principles of function and structure of the human body.

Though the terms are sometimes used interchangeably, this text follows the most current trend in which the term *kinesiology* is used for the broader meaning: the study of human movement with the study of anatomic kinesiology and how the anatomy works to produce movement. The term *biomechanics* refers to the mechanical principles of function, which includes information about how the body uses concepts of simple machines, center of gravity, force production, coordination of movement, and so forth.

SKELETAL SYSTEM BASICS

SECTION OBJECTIVES

Chapter objectives covered in this section:
1. List the components and seven main functions of the skeletal system.

After completing this section, the student will be able to perform the following:
- Define endoskeleton and exoskeleton.
- List the components of the skeletal system.
- Describe the seven functions of the skeletal system.

What would we look like if we did not have bones? Picture yourself as a mass of soft tissue with little form. Managing the forces of gravity would be almost impossible without the structure supplied by our skeletons. Getting from one place to another would be difficult. We would also be more susceptible to injury. As we explore the most concrete aspect of our anatomy—the skeletal system—the knowledge gives us an understanding of its functions.

Human beings have an **endoskeleton,** which means that our support structure is inside us and we grow around it. Some animals, such as lobsters, have an exoskeleton, a support structure that is on the outside of the body. Although an exoskeleton is appropriate for a lobster, it is not appropriate for a human being. Because an exoskeleton does not grow at the same rate as the rest of the body, it can become too small; also, it needs to be shed as a new one is grown. With an endoskeleton, growth is accommodated easily.

The skeletal system comprises the bones, joints, and related connective tissues. The connective tissue component is important to the functioning of the system. Bones connect at a joint, which is also known as an **articulation.** Bones are held together at joints by ligaments and other connective tissues, or both. Muscle contractions produce the forces that move the joints. The actions of skeletal muscles are voluntary, coordinated by the nervous system. When the structures of the muscles and bones are combined, they form the functional unit known as the *musculoskeletal system.*

Because the bones do not have enough room for all the muscles to attach, the membranes between the bones and the ligaments at the joints function to expand the skeletal structure, allowing adequate space for muscle attachments.

Because muscles attach to bones, learning the names, functions, and various landmarks of the bones first helps in locating the muscles studied later in this section. Other chapters focus on the joints, on biomechanics, and on kinesiology. Carefully studying each illustration in this chapter will be helpful when learning about the skeleton. The labeling of the illustrations is often more specific than the major features of the bones discussed in the text.

Main Functions of the Skeletal System

Besides the obvious functions of support and motion, bones have other important roles.

The seven major roles of bones are as follows:
1. Supporting soft tissues and serving as a framework for the entire body

2. Providing attachment points for muscles and ligaments
3. Protecting delicate internal organs such as the brain, spinal cord, heart, and lungs
4. Serving as levers to provide movement created by the attached muscles
5. Storing calcium, phosphorus, and other minerals for release to the body as needed
6. Storing lipids in bone marrow for use as energy
7. Producing blood cells in the red marrow

BONES

SECTION OBJECTIVES

Chapter objectives covered in this section:
2. Describe the structure, classification, and development of bone.
After completing this section, the student will be able to perform the following:
- Explain the structure of bone.
- Describe the structure/function relationship to bone structure.
- Define *compact* and *spongy bone.*
- Define *trabeculae.*
- Describe two kinds of marrow and their functions.
- List and describe the connective tissue coverings of bone.
- Describe the process of bone development.
- List and describe the five shapes of bone.
- Describe the classification system of bones.
- List the three stages of bone healing.
- Describe age-related changes in bone.

Bones are hard, dense, and slightly elastic organs of the skeleton. Bones have their own system of blood vessels, lymphatic vessels, and nerves. No matter their size, shape, or location, all bones are made of the same fundamental cells and matrix and are covered with the same sheets of connective tissue.

Bones develop into different shapes that serve specific functions. The location and shape of a bone determine its function. The protective bones of the skull differ in shape from the supportive long bones of the limbs. Disease, injury, and aging can all affect the structure and function of bones. The function of a bone can change its structure through a remodeling process, supporting once again the theme of form following function and function determining form.

During infancy humans have 270 to 300 bones. By the time adulthood is reached, some of the bones have fused together. The adult body has 206 bones, with some individual variations; for example, some individuals have more or fewer **sesamoid bones** (a type of bone that develops within a tendon or joint capsule), and others may have an extra rib.

Although all bones support the body, store calcium and other minerals, and house marrow for the production of red blood cells, some bones also play other, more specific roles. For example, the skull and the vertebral column protect the brain and spinal cord.

Bones are composed chiefly of bone tissue, called *osseous tissue.* Bones are not lifeless, but rather are ever-changing. The spaces between the cells of bone tissue are permeated with

Many cultural and healing traditions assert that certain kinds of stones and other crystalline substances, in particular quartz, have healing qualities. Some spiritual places reputed to have healing qualities are located in areas of stony form, particularly granite, or structures constructed of stone (often granite), or they contain statues made of stone. Quartz is considered a piezoelectric material, and granite, often used in building and sculpture, has a high concentration of quartz. We do know that very small electric currents can accelerate the healing of broken bones. Does this show a connection? In what way do the very small electric currents generated by bone affect homeostasis? Could a physiologic connection exist between the healing disciplines that use stones and these qualities of bone? These traditions are cross-cultural, which suggests the existence of some underlying, physiologically unified thread. The questions are interesting; the connection is plausible.

deposits of inorganic mineral salts of calcium and phosphorus, along with small amounts of magnesium, potassium, and sodium and carbonate ions. Two thirds of bone tissue is made up of these inorganic minerals, which provide rigidity, and one third of bone tissue is composed of organic material, which provides elasticity. Without this elasticity bone would break readily.

Bones are subject to considerable mechanical strain. Bones must support the weight of the body; disperse the impact shock of activities such as walking, running, and jumping; and withstand the force of muscle contractions.

Bones have a piezoelectric quality. **Piezoelectric** substances, such as the collagen in bones, deform slightly and vibrate when electric currents pass through them. In reverse, when stretched, twisted, or compressed, bone produces minute electric currents; the strength and direction of these currents change with the direction of the stress load. Bone formation patterns follow lines of stress load directed by these piezoelectric currents (Box 7-2 and Activity 7-1).

Bone Structure

All bones share four features that allow them to work together as parts of the skeleton:
1. A rigid matrix gives bones strength and shape to sustain weight and movement.
2. Bones usually articulate with other bones, thereby transferring forces and movement through the skeleton.
3. A connective tissue structure, called the periosteum, covers every bone and provides vessels for nutrition, bone cells for growth, and attachments for tendons and ligaments.
4. Growth of new bone matrix and remodeling of existing bone matrix are responsible for shaping bones.

The structure and function of bones are intrinsically connected. Bones remodel themselves constantly, depending on the functional demand. Although it may seem static, the skeletal system is one of the more dynamic systems of the body.

ACTIVITY 7-1

If you were to speculate about the piezoelectric quality of bones and other collagen connective tissues, what do you think would be the effects of the compressive, stretching, and twisting action of massage? List three. An example is provided to get you started.

Example
The electric current produced by compression against bone during massage methods may stimulate energetic mechanism of meridians understood in traditional Chinese medicine because energy lines generally follow bones.

Your Turn
1. _____
_____
_____
2. _____
_____
3. _____
_____

Bone Tissue

The different areas of a bone contain one of two types of tissue, **compact bone** or **spongy bone** (Figure 7-1).

Compact Bone

Compact (dense) bone has a compact arrangement of hard inorganic matrix. This hard portion of the bone makes up the main shaft of the long bones and the outer layer of all bones.

Compact bone protects spongy bone and provides the firm framework of the bone and the body.

The osteocytes in this type of bone are located in concentric rings called lamellae around a central canal, called the Haversian canal, and form cylinder-shaped units that are called osteons. Blood vessels are located within the Haversian canals.

Within the hard layers of lamellae, osteocytes are located within spaces called lacunae.

Spongy Bone

The second type, **spongy (cancellous) bone,** has larger spaces within the bony matrix than does compact bone, which makes the bones lighter in weight.

Cancellous bone is made of an irregular meshing of small, bony plates called trabeculae and is found at the ends of the long bones or at the center of all bones except the shafts of long bones.

In some bones the trabecular spaces are filled with red marrow, which produces blood cells.

Spongy bone tissue forms a supporting grid that can be altered mechanically by construction, destruction, or reorganization of the trabecular network.

Piezoelectric current seems to be responsible for guiding these changes, which occur in response to postural change, muscle tension, and the stresses of weight.

Bone Marrow

Bones contain two kinds of marrow, red and yellow:
• Red marrow, which manufactures blood cells, is found at the end of long bones and at the center of other bones of the thorax and pelvis.
• Yellow marrow is largely fat and found mainly in the central cavities of the long bones.

Periosteum and Endosteum

Except for the ends that form joints, bones are covered with **periosteum.** On the inside of this membrane are osteoblasts, which are essential to bone formation during periods of growth and in the repair of bones. In addition to blood and lymph vessels, the periosteum has nerve fibers that alert the person to trauma, such as a blow to the shin or a fractured arm.

A thinner membrane of connective tissue called the **endosteum** lines the marrow cavity of a bone; it too contains cells that aid in the growth and repair of bone tissue.

Bone Development

In the embryo bone development begins near the end of the second month. The process that creates our skeleton is called *ossification*. Ossification is the process of building bone by depositing calcium salts into tissues. *Calcification* is another term to describe the bone-making process. Ossification is a two-part process:
1. Chondroblasts, or cartilage-forming cells, create the cartilage model of bones.
2. Osteoblasts, or bone-building cells, develop the bone tissue from the cartilage model.

This process does not create the hard bones with which we are familiar. Instead, these cells remain soft and pliable, allowing the fetus to remain flexible in order to exit the body more easily during birth.

Shortly after birth, hardening of the cartilage into bones, which is called *osteogenesis*, occurs as calcium salts are deposited in the gel-like matrix of the forming bones. *Osteocytes* are mature bone cells that maintain the bone throughout our lifetime.

Articular Cartilage

Cartilage is a tough, flexible connective tissue with a high water content, so it is softer than bone. Recall that cartilage forms the skeletal framework in the fetus. In the adult the only remaining cartilage in bone is called *articular* (or hyaline) cartilage. This cartilage is smooth, slippery, porous, and malleable. It contains no nerves or blood vessels and is found wherever bones come together at synovial or freely movable joints. It allows the bones to move against each other easily.

Synovial fluid is secreted by synovial joints and provides lubrication, oxygen, and nutrition to the joint. Articular cartilage is "massaged" by synovial fluid during joint movement.

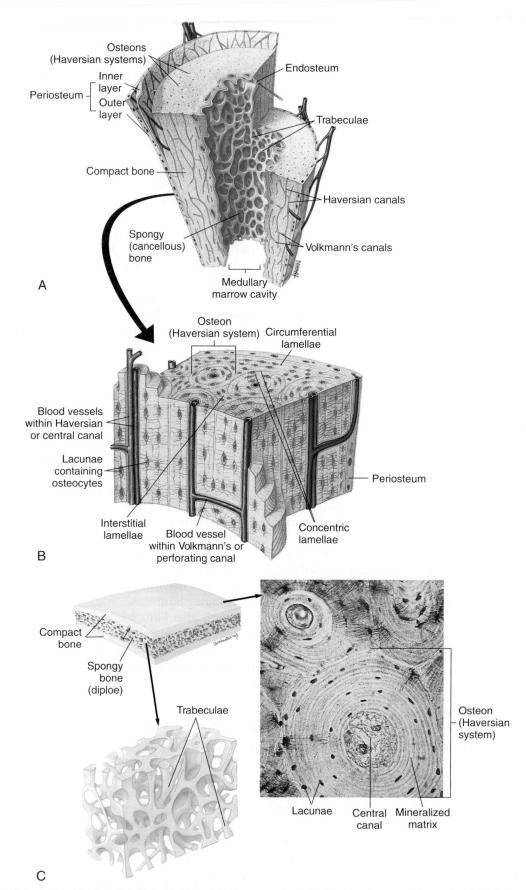

FIGURE 7-1 Structure of compact and cancellous bone. **A,** Longitudinal section of a long bone showing spongy (cancellous) and compact bone. **B,** Magnified view of compact bone. **C,** Section of a flat bone. Outer layers of compact bone surround cancellous bone. The fine structure of compact bone and cancellous bone is shown to the *right*. (From Patton KT, Thibodeau GA: *Anatomy and physiology,* ed 6, St Louis, 2007, Mosby.)

The degenerative process of arthritis involves the breakdown of articular cartilage.

Because cartilage is an integral component of the synovial joint, it is discussed in more detail in Chapter 8.

Ligaments

Ligaments are dense bundles of parallel connective tissue fibers, primarily collagen. Ligaments connect bones and stabilize the joints and can also serve as muscle attachment sites. Ligaments are not typically elastic, nor do they have much stretch. Some joint positions place ligaments under tension, whereas other positions slacken them. Because ligaments are specific to joint function, they also are discussed in more detail in Chapter 8. An important feature of ligaments is that they are poorly vascularized and consequently take longer to heal than do muscles.

Classification of Bones

The bones of the skeleton are identified by their different shapes. The common classifications are as follows:

- **Long Bones.** These are longer in one axis than another. Bones of this type are characterized by a medullary cavity; a hollow diaphysis, or shaft, of compact bone; and at least two epiphyses or ends, which are active in the growth of long bones. The hollow structure of the diaphysis gives strength with light weight. Most of the bones of the arms and legs are long bones. Examples: the femur and ulna.
- **Short Bones (sometimes classified as cube-shaped bones).** These are predominantly cancellous bone with a thin cortex of compact bone and no cavity. Examples: the wrist bones (carpals) and ankle bones (tarsals).
- **Flat Bones.** These are generally more flat than round. Examples: the ribs and skull bones.
- **Irregular Bones.** These have complex shapes that occur as two or more forms within the same bone structure. Examples: the vertebrae and scapulae.
- **Sesamoid Bones.** These are round bones often embedded in tendons and joint capsules. The patella is an example. Sesamoid bones are often considered to be a subdivision of irregular bones.

Bone Growth and Repair

Shortly after birth we begin the process of changing the pliable cartilage skeleton into the calcified hard bone. In a long bone the transformation of cartilage into bone begins at the center of the shaft. Later, secondary bone-forming centers develop at the epiphyses. The long bones continue to grow in length at these centers through childhood and into the late teens.

A growth spurt often is seen during puberty because of the influence of the sex hormones estrogen and testosterone. Both hormones promote the growth of long bones; testosterone also increases bone density. At higher levels of estrogen, long bone growth stops. This is the reason that women generally are shorter and have bones that are less dense than those of men (Activity 7-2).

Evolve Activity 7-3

ACTIVITY 7-2

Refer to Chapter 6, and explain the influence of the sex hormones on bone. Include the page number where you found the information.

An example is provided to get you started.

Example
High estrogen levels slow the growth of girls, including their bones, at puberty.

Provide two more explanatory statements.

Your Turn
1. _____
2. _____

Identify two other hormones that affect bone formation. (Hint: See the sections in Chapter 6 on the thyroid and parathyroid glands.)
1. _____
2. _____

By the late teens or early 20s, again through the influence of the sex hormones, the growth plate or epiphyseal disk of the long bones closes and the bones stop growing in length. The remnant of the growth plates harden and can be seen in radiographic films (x-rays) as a thin line across the end of the bone. Physicians can judge the future growth of the bone by the appearance of these lines on the radiographic film. As we grow, our bones widen and lengthen, and the central cavity follows this change in size. This all takes place because bone tissue is added in some areas of bone and reabsorbed in others.

As mentioned previously, children are more flexible because their bodies contain more cartilage and complete calcification has not yet taken place. In older adults this is reversed; bone cells outnumber cartilage cells, and bone is more brittle because it contains more minerals and fewer blood vessels. This makes bones prone to fracture and slower to heal.

Skeletal Changes Caused by Aging

As we age, various changes occur in the skeleton, such as loss of calcium and loss of protein. These changes can lead to brittle bones. Loss of calcium begins earlier in women than in men. Also, bone fractures heal more slowly in older persons. Beginning at approximately age 40, the vertebrae begin to thin, and the average person loses $\frac{1}{2}$ inch of height every 20 years. The cartilage on the ribs calcifies, leading to a decrease in the diameter of the rib cage and loss of flexibility.

BONY LANDMARKS

Evolve Activity 7-4

SECTION OBJECTIVES
Chapter objectives covered in this section:
3. Identify bony landmarks.
After completing this section, the student will be able to perform the following:
- Define bony landmarks.
- Explain the relationship of bony landmarks to muscles.
- Palpate bony landmarks.

Practical Application

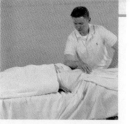

In the 1950s and 1960s, it was first recognized that bending bone creates a strain that results in electrical streaming potentials within the bone. This is a piezoelectric effect.

A bone stimulator is an external device that creates electromagnetic fields and is said to mimic the same electrical streaming potentials that the body produces; it therefore stimulates bone healing. Check out the research on the Evolve site for this chapter for more information. Another method of stimulating bone healing is by causing the bone to vibrate slightly a distance away from the fracture site. The vibration causes a frequency. Our bones heal best at a frequency between 20 and 50 Hz. Researchers have investigated the osteogenic (increasing bone cell production) effect of low-magnitude high-frequency vibration (LMHFV, 35 Hz, 0.3 g) on the enhancement of fracture healing in rats and it works. Some believe the frequency of a cat's purring has a healing influence. The frequency of the cat's purr falls within the range of 27 and 44 Hz.

A tuning fork is a two-pronged fork with the tines in the shape of a U. It is an acoustic resonator. When the tines vibrate, they create a sound. When tapped lightly, a tuning fork begins to vibrate at a specific frequency. There are tuning forks made for music as well as for engineering, physics, and medicine. When a vibrating tuning fork is placed near a break in a bone, a person's pain increases. If the vibrations do not increase the person's pain, it is a lot less likely that the person has suffered a bone fracture. The question then becomes, "If the vibration makes it hurt, might it also be possible to stimulate healing?"

The contour of bones varies and includes configurations such as flat areas, knobs, projections, spikes, dents, holes, and ridges. These landmarks often serve as regions for muscle or ligament attachment or provide passage or space for nerves and vessels. It is extremely important that you can identify and palpate the bony landmarks because this knowledge will assist you in learning muscle attachments later in this study.

The landmarks are categorized by shape and function (Activities 7-3 and 7-4).

Depressions and Openings

Canal. A tunnel or tube in bone. Example: the carotid canal in temporal bone.

Fissure. A groove or slit between two bones. Example: the orbital fissure of the sphenoid bone.

Foramen. An opening, or hole, in a bone. Example: the vertebral foramen of a vertebra through which the spinal cord passes.

Fossa. A shallow depression in the surface or at the end of a bone. Example: the infraspinous and supraspinous fossae of the scapula.

✎ ACTIVITY 7-3

For each of the landmarks listed, identify a metaphor that will help you remember what each represents. A few examples are provided to get you started.

Examples
Foramen: hula hoop
Groove: ditch
Sinus: cave

Your Turn
Canal:
Fissure:
Foramen:
Fossa:
Groove:
Meatus:
Notch:
Sinus:
Sulcus:
Condyle:
Head:
Facet:
Process:
Trochlea:
Crest:
Epicondyle:
Spinous process, or spine:
Trochanter:
Tubercle:
Tuberosity:

✎ ACTIVITY 7-4

Palpating the landmarks: Using the skeleton in your classroom, practice palpating the bony landmarks by feeling the bones with your eyes closed. When you find a dent, hole, point, knob, ridge and so forth, identify it as a type of bony landmark (e.g., meatus, tuberosity).

Groove. A depression in the bone that holds a blood vessel, nerve, or tendon. Example: the radial groove of the humerus.

Meatus. A tunnel or canal found in a bone. Example: the canal in the skull that extends from the external ear to the eardrum.

Notch. An indentation or large groove. Example: the greater and lesser sciatic notches of the ilium.

Sinus. An air cavity within a bone. Example: the frontal sinuses.

Processes That Form Joints

Condyle. A rounded projection at the end of a bone that articulates with other bones to form a joint. Example: the medial and lateral condyles of the femur.

Head. A rounded projection atop the neck of a bone. Example: the head of the femur.

Facet. A smooth, flat surface. Example: the facet of a rib or vertebra.

Process. Any prominent, bony growth that projects. Example: the olecranon process of the ulna.

Trochlea. A pulley-shaped structure. Example: the trochlea of the humerus.

Processes to Which Tendons and Ligaments Attach

Crest. A ridge on a bone. Example: the iliac crest.

Epicondyle. A projection on a condyle. Example: the medial epicondyle of the femur.

Line. A ridge that is smaller than a crest. Example: the linea aspera of the femur.

Spinous process, spine, or spina. A sharp, bony, or slender projection. Example: the spinous process of the vertebral column or spine of the scapula.

Trochanter. One of two large, bony processes found only on the femur. Example: the greater or lesser trochanter.

Tubercle. A small, rounded process. Example: the adductor tubercle of the femur.

Tuberosity. A large, rounded protuberance. Example: the tibial tuberosity.

DIVISIONS OF THE SKELETON

SECTION OBJECTIVES

Chapter objective covered in this section:

4. Describe the two divisions of the skeleton.

After completing this chapter, the student will be able to perform the following:

- Define axial skeleton and appendicular skeleton.
- Explain the differences between the axial and appendicular skeleton.
- Name the bones of the axial and appendicular skeleton.
- Compare the similarities and differences between the bones of the upper limb and lower limb.

✏ ACTIVITY 7-5

Match six similar sets of bones of the upper and lower appendicular skeleton. An example is provided.

Example
Femur/humerus

Your Turn
1. _____
2. _____
3. _____
4. _____
5. _____
6. _____

The skeleton is divided into two groups of bones: the axial skeleton and the appendicular skeleton.

The axial skeleton, which forms the center or axis of the body, consists of the head, vertebral column, ribs, and sternum. The axial skeleton provides the body with form and protection.

The appendicular skeleton is composed of the limbs (appendages) of the body and their attachments (Activity 7-5). The shoulder and hip girdles, which have similar structures, connect the appendicular skeleton to the axial skeleton.

The bones of our body, in combination with the muscles, provide our fine and gross motor movements. Long bones of the limbs allow for large movements. In the same manner, the short carpals and phalanges of the wrist and fingers and the tarsals and phalanges of the ankle and toes allow for the flexibility needed in the wrist, hands, ankles, and feet.

The more we study the basic construction of the skeletal system, the more we notice its elegant and simple pattern. Simplicity and repetition of form reflect this effective biomechanical design (Figure 7-2).

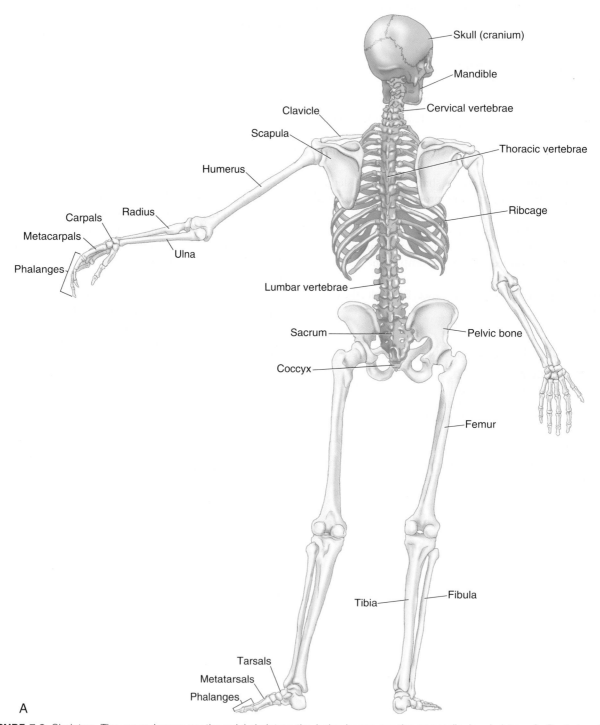

A

FIGURE 7-2 Skeleton. The *green* bones are the axial skeleton; the *beige* bones are the appendicular skeleton. **A,** Posterior view.

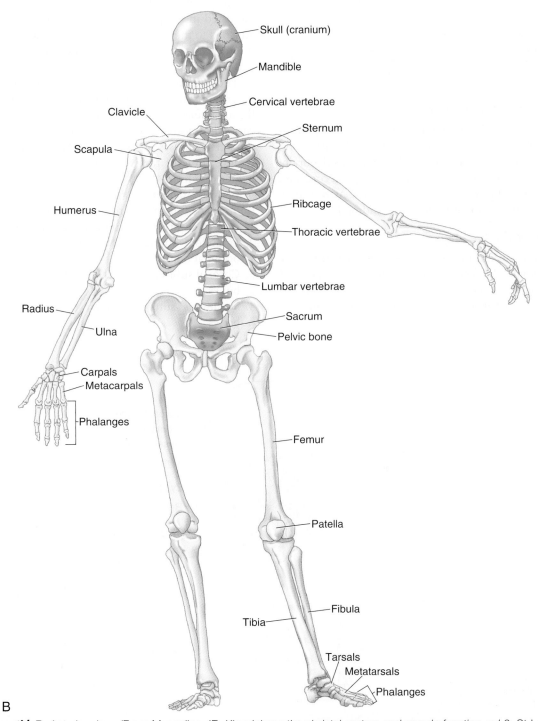

FIGURE 7-2, cont'd B, Anterior view. (From Muscolino JE: *Kinesiology: the skeletal system and muscle function, ed 2,* St Louis, 2011, Mosby.)

INDIVIDUAL BONY FRAMEWORK BY REGION

SECTION OBJECTIVES

Chapter objective covered in this section:

5. List and describe the individual bones of the axial skeleton.

After completing this section, the student will be able to perform the following:

- List and palpate the bones of the head, spine, and thorax.
- Describe major features of the bones of the axial skeleton.
- Explain the difference between the infant and adult skull.
- List and palpate the bones of the upper and lower limbs.
- Describe the major features of the bones of the upper and lower limbs.
- Describe the features of the shoulder and pelvic girdles.

Bones of the Axial Skeleton

The axial skeleton makes up the central and essential structures of the body. The structures contain vital organs and provide protection. For example, the skull contains the brain, the vertebral column houses and protects the spinal cord, and the ribs contain and protect the heart and lungs. As you study each figure in this section, find the bony landmarks.

Framework of the Head

The bony framework of the head, or skull, is made up of the cranial bones and the facial bones (Figure 7-3). Figure 7-3 labels the structure of the head in detail, and the text describes the most prominent areas. Be sure to study the diagram carefully (Box 7-3).

The bones of the face provide the framework for the appearance of the face. Facial bones provide protection for the eyeball, structure for the nose, and anchor for the teeth (Box 7-4).

In addition to the cranial and facial bones, other bones of the axial skeleton are found in the neck and head. The six auditory bones called *ossicles*, three in each middle ear, are discussed in Chapter 5. The hyoid bone is a U-shaped bone attached to the tongue. Although it is attached to other bones by muscles and ligaments, it does not form an articulation with any other bones.

The structure of the skull is important to the function of other systems. Nerves and blood vessels enter and exit the skull through holes, or foramina, in the base. Muscles attach to the various projections and prominences on the outside of the skull. The sinuses are air spaces that resonate the voice and remove some of the weight of the bones, making the head lighter (Figure 7-4).

Between the bones of the skull are specialized joints called *sutures*. The four most prominent sutures are as follows:

1. Sagittal suture, between the parietal bones
2. Lambdoid suture, between the parietal bones and the occipital bone
3. Coronal suture, between the parietal bones and the frontal bones
4. Squamous suture, between the temporal and parietal bones

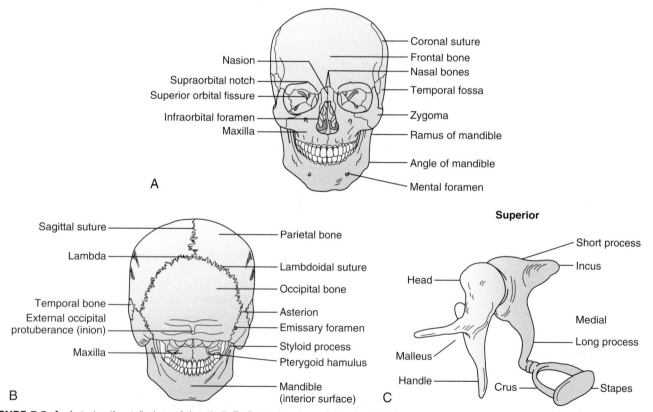

FIGURE 7-3 A, Anterior (frontal) view of the skull. **B,** Posterior view of the skull. **C,** The three auditory ossicles. The malleus attaches to the inner surface of the tympanic membrane (eardrum). The incus links the malleus to the stapes. The stapes is attached to the wall of the inner ear.

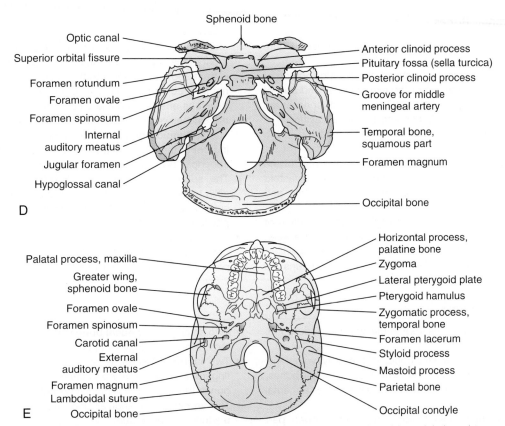

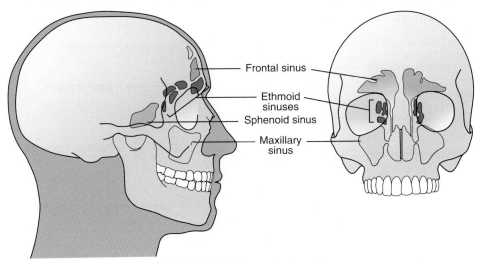

FIGURE 7-3, cont'd D, Detailed view of the internal surface of the base of the skull. The sphenoid, occipital, and temporal bones are presented as slightly separated to show that many of the important apertures traversing the floor of the skull are found within one of these bones or along their mutual borders. **E,** Basal view of the skull, showing several of the important foramina that convey nerves and vessels in and out of the cranial cavity.

FIGURE 7-4 Air sinuses in the nose.

The Infant Skull

In the skull of an infant, bone formation is incomplete in some areas; these soft spots are called *fontanelles*. Found between the cranial bones, fontanelles are formed from very dense connective tissue, which is replaced with bone as the infant grows. The fontanelles allow for compression of the skull as the infant travels through the birth canal and for expansion of the skull as the brain grows. The fontanelles close when the child is 18 to 24 months old. The largest of the fontanelles is the anterior fontanelle, found near the front of the head at the junction between the two parietal bones and the frontal bone (Figure 7-5).

Framework of the Trunk and Neck

The skeletal structure of the trunk and neck is made up of the vertebral column and the bones of the chest. A

Box 7-3 Cranial Bones

Eight cranial bones enclose and protect the brain (see Figure 7-3; Activity 7-6):

- The **frontal bone** forms the forehead, the anterior portion of the roof of the skull, the top of the eye sockets, and part of the floor of the cranium. The frontal sinuses (air spaces) are within the frontal bone and open into the nasal cavities.
- Two **parietal bones** form most of the sides and top of the cranium.
- Two **temporal bones** form part of the side and part of the floor of the skull. Each temporal bone contains mastoid sinuses, an ear canal, an eardrum, and the middle and inner ears.
- The **ethmoid bone,** which is part of the anterior portion of the cranial floor, is a very light, spongy bone located between the eyes. The ethmoid bone forms part of the medial wall of the eye sockets and most of the nasal roof and contains the ethmoid sinuses. An extension of the ethmoid bone forms most of the superior portion of the nasal septum. If this bone is fractured, its proximity to the brain means that cerebrospinal fluid could leak into the nasal cavity. A runny nose that develops after a head injury could be the result of trauma to the sinuses or an indication of a serious condition.
- The **sphenoid bone** is in the middle of the base of the skull in front of the temporal bones. When viewed from above, the sphenoid bone looks like a bat with its wings extended. The sphenoid sinuses are located within this bone. The sella turcica, or "Turkish saddle," is a cavity on the superior surface of the body of the sphenoid that supports the pituitary gland.
- The **occipital bone** forms the posterior portion and a large part of the base of the cranium. This large, curved bone provides attachments for muscles of the neck and trunk.

Box 7-4 Facial Bones

Fourteen facial bones form the front of the skull (see Figure 7-3; Activity 7-6):

- The **mandible,** or lower jaw bone, is the only voluntarily movable bone of the skull. The largest of the facial bones, the mandible forms the chin, which is classified as a mental prominence.
- Two **maxillary bones** unite to form the upper jawbone, part of the floor of the eye sockets, part of the roof of the mouth, including the anterior portion of the hard palate, and the outer walls and floor of the nasal cavity. Each maxilla contains the maxillary sinus, a large air space that empties into the nasal cavity.
- Two **zygomatic bones,** or cheek bones, form the prominences of the cheeks and a portion of the floor and outer wall of the eye sockets.
- Two small, oblong **nasal bones,** in the superior middle of the face, form the bridge of the nose.
- Two **lacrimal bones,** each about the size and shape of a fingernail, are posterior and lateral to the nasal bone. These bones form part of the medial wall of the eye sockets.
- The **vomer** is a triangular bone that forms the inferior and posterior nasal septum.
- Two L-shaped **palatine bones** form the posterior portion of the hard palate and part of the floor of the nasal cavity.
- Two inferior **nasal conchae bones** form a portion of the lateral wall of the nasal cavities. The inferior conchae work with the superior and middle conchae of the ethmoid bone to circulate and filter air that enters the nose.

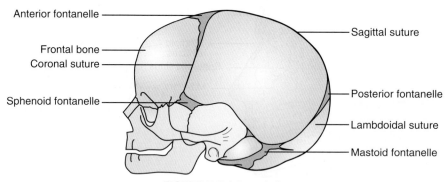

FIGURE 7-5 Infant skull.

child's vertebral column has 33 (or sometimes 34) irregularly shaped bones, which fuse in the lower portion to become 26 bones in the adult. Each of the vertebrae has two main sections, the anterior body and the posterior arch. All vertebrae, except the atlas and the axis, have the following characteristic features:

1. A drum-shaped body, or centrum, located toward the anterior, serves as the weight-bearing portion of the bone.
2. A vertebral arch, which encircles the spinal cord, is connected to the body by two pedicles (feet). Two lamina (part of vertebra) unite posteriorly to form the spinous process. The spinous process usually can be felt just under the skin of the back. The thickened junctions between the pedicles and the laminae have superior and inferior cartilaginous articular facets and a laterally projecting transverse process.
3. A large hole, or foramen, in the center of each vertebra. All the vertebrae are linked in a series by strong ligaments, and these spaces form the spinal canal, a bony cylinder that protects the spinal cord. As the vertebrae bodies stack upon one another, a space is created between the upper and lower pedicles, forming the intervertebral foramina, which allow passage of the spinal nerves.

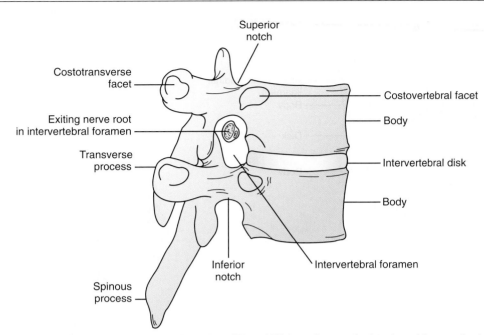

FIGURE 7-6 Lateral view of the intervertebral foramen. Vertebrae T5 and T6 have been articulated, and the resultant intervertebral foramen is shown with a segmental nerve in place. Blood vessels (not shown) also enter and leave the interior of the vertebral canal through the intervertebral foramen.

ACTIVITY 7-6

The names of the cranial bones start with various letters. To help you remember them, make up a sentence that uses the first letter of each in whatever order works for you. Get creative!

- Occipital
- Parietal
- Frontal
- Temporal
- Ethmoid
- Sphenoid

Example
Please Stop The Flying Ostrich Egg.

Your Turn
The facial bones are the following:
- Nasal

- Vomer

- Lacrimal

- Zygomatic

- Palatine

- Maxilla

- Mandible

- Inferior nasal concha

Make up a creative sentence that uses the first letter of each.

4. Vertebrae that are stacked one on the other. Each vertebra has three joint surfaces, two articular facets that provide the articulating surface for this stacking arrangement, and one intervertebral disk joint.

The vertebrae are named and numbered according to their location from the neck downward:
- 7 cervical vertebrae called C1-C7
- 12 thoracic vertebrae called T1 through T12
- 5 lumbar vertebrae called L1 through L5

The sacrum and coccyx form the base of the vertebral column. During childhood the sacrum consists of five individual bones and the coccyx is made up of three to five bones. The individual bones of the sacrum and coccyx fuse in the adult, becoming two solid bones.

Although not technically a part of the vertebrae, the intervertebral disks (or discs; both spellings are correct) between the vertebral bodies act as shock absorbers and spacers and provide flexibility (Figure 7-6). The disk consists of two components. The outer portion, or annulus fibrosus, is composed of concentric rings of fibrocartilage arranged like the layers of an onion. Internally, the center, or nucleus pulposus, is made of a gelatinous substance. If a disk ruptures, the fibrocartilage splits and the nucleus pulposus leaks. The disk becomes smaller and is less able to disperse pressure and maintain space between the vertebrae. In severe cases the ruptured disk vertebra can impinge on nerves.

The vertebral arteries heading toward the brainstem pass through the foramina of the transverse processes of the cervical vertebrae. These vessels are subject to stretching injuries with extreme cervical rotation of the extended neck.

Again, study all illustrations carefully because the labeling of the detail is more complete than what is provided in the discussion and major features of the bones in the text.

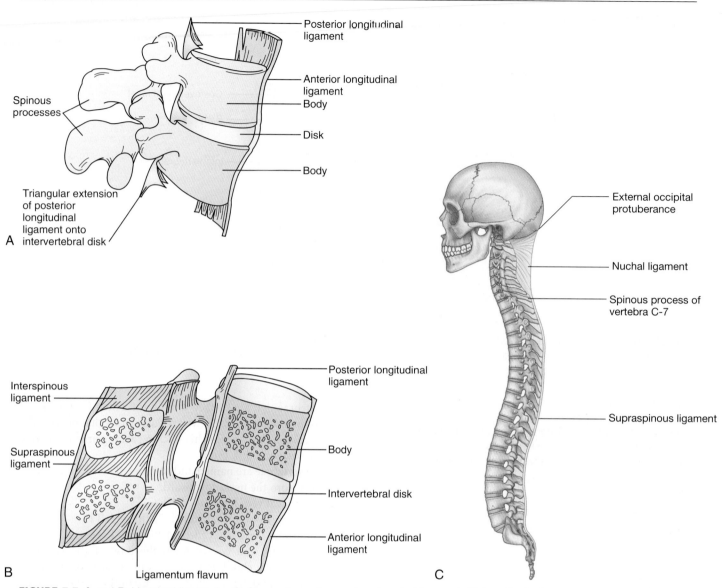

FIGURE 7-7 A and **B,** Vertebral ligaments. **C,** Supraspinous ligament and nuchal ligament. (**C** from Drake RL et al: *Gray's anatomy for students,* ed 2, Edinburgh, 2010, Elsevier.)

Ligaments

Three ligaments extend the length of the vertebral column:

1. The anterior longitudinal ligament attaches to the front of the vertebral bodies and acts to restrain extension.
2. The posterior longitudinal ligament attaches to the back of the vertebral bodies and acts to restrain flexion.
3. The supraspinous ligament runs along the tips of the spinous processes and restrains flexion.

A strong, fibrous band called the *nuchal ligament* (a thickening of the supraspinous ligament) runs along the notched spinous processes of C2 to C6 and helps support the weight of the head. Other vertebral ligaments are placed between individual vertebrae.

The ligamenta flava connects the laminae of each adjacent vertebra.

The interspinous ligaments connect the spinous processes.

The intertransverse ligaments connect the transverse processes (Figures 7-7 and 7-8).

Right-side lateral flexion stretches the left intertransverse ligaments, and left-side lateral flexion stretches the right intertransverse ligaments. Vertebral movement patterns are discussed in detail in Chapter 8 (Box 7-5).

Vertebral Curves

When viewed from the side, the vertebral column can be seen to have curves that correspond to the groups of vertebrae. In a newborn the entire column is a concave-forward shape; this is the primary kyphotic curve. When the infant begins to assume an erect posture, secondary lordotic curves, which are convex-forward in shape. For example, the cervical lordotic curve appears when the infant begins to hold up his or her head at about 3 months of age; the lumbar lordotic curve appears when the child begins to walk. The curves of the vertebral column provide some of the resilience and spring so essential to walking and running.

- The cervical region is convex forward, or has a *lordosis.*
- The thoracic region is concave forward, called a *kyphosis.*

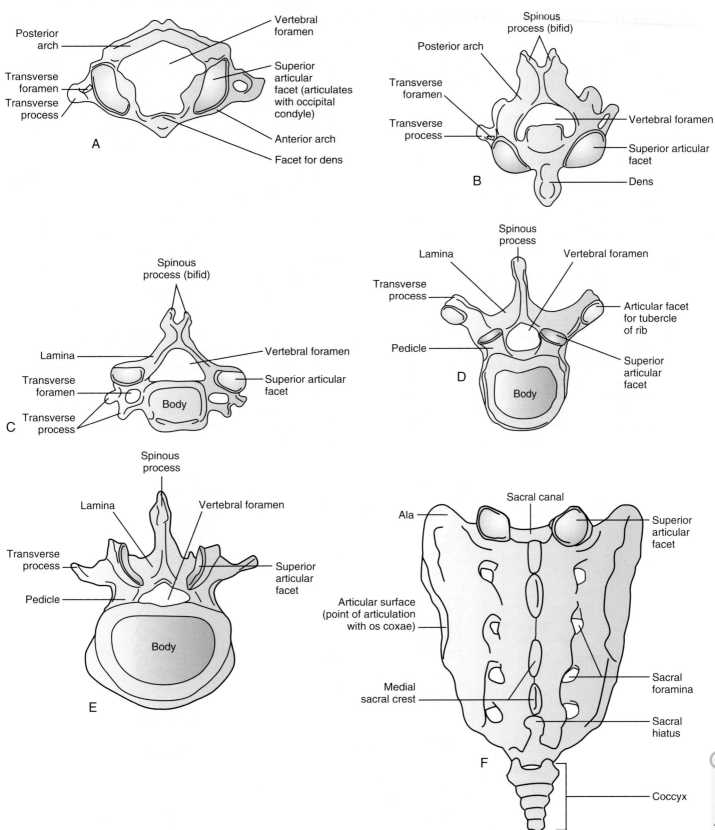

FIGURE 7-8 Six types of vertebrae: **A,** atlas, **B,** axis, **C,** cervical, **D,** thoracic, **E,** lumbar, **F,** sacrum.

Box 7-5   Bones and Structures of the Vertebral Column (see Figures 7-6 to 7-9)

The seven cervical vertebrae (C1 to C7) are located in the neck.
- The first vertebra (C1), called the *atlas,* supports the head. When you nod your head "yes," the occipital bone of the skull rocks on the atlas. The atlas is greatly modified for articulation within the occipital region of the skull. The atlas does not have a body or spinous process; rather, it essentially is a bony ring consisting of anterior and posterior arches and two lateral masses.
- The second cervical vertebra (C2), called the *axis,* serves as a pivot when the head is turned from side to side (as in the gesture "no"). The axis has a peglike dens, or odontoid process, projecting superiorly from its anterior side.
- The pivot joint of C1 to C2 consists of a ringlike structure (the atlas) that rotates around the dens. Considerable movement, especially as seen in rotation, is possible because of the design of this joint.

The 12 thoracic vertebrae (T1 to T12) are located in the thorax of the trunk (the body area between the neck and diaphragm). The main functions of the thoracic vertebrae are to provide spaces on which to build the rib cage, which protects the heart and lungs, and to house the spinal cord.
- The posterior ends of the 12 pairs of ribs are attached to these vertebrae at posterior facets and hemifacets (thought of as one half of a facet).
- T1 has a whole facet joint space for the first rib articulation and an inferior hemifacet, which works with the corresponding superior hemifacet of T2 for articulation with the second rib.
- T2 to T8 each has superior and inferior hemifacets, which together form the vertebral portion of the articulation with the ribs. T9 has one superior hemifacet, and T10 to T12 each has a whole facet to articulate with the ribs.
- The arrangement of the vertebrae in the thorax allows for a certain amount of flexion, extension, side bending, and rotation; but movements generally are limited, with most movement occurring at the thoracic-lumbar junction at T11, T12, and L1.

The five lumbar vertebrae (L1 to L5) are located in the abdomen of the trunk. They are larger and heavier than the other vertebrae, which allows them to support more weight.
- The interlocking shape of the lumbar vertebrae makes rotation difficult but facilitates flexion, extension, and side bending. L4 and L5 allow the most motion.
- Most disk injuries occur at L4 to L5 and L5 to S1 (the area of the lumbar-sacral junction).

The sacral vertebrae are five separate bones in a child; however, they eventually fuse to form a single bone, the sacrum, in an adult.
- Wedged between the two pelvic bones, the sacrum completes the posterior part of the bony pelvis. Four transverse ridges are the remnants of intervertebral disks. At the ends of each ridge are paired sacral foramina, through which the sacral nerves pass.

The coccyx, or tailbone, consists of four or five tiny bones in a child. As a person develops, these bones fuse to form a single bone in an adult

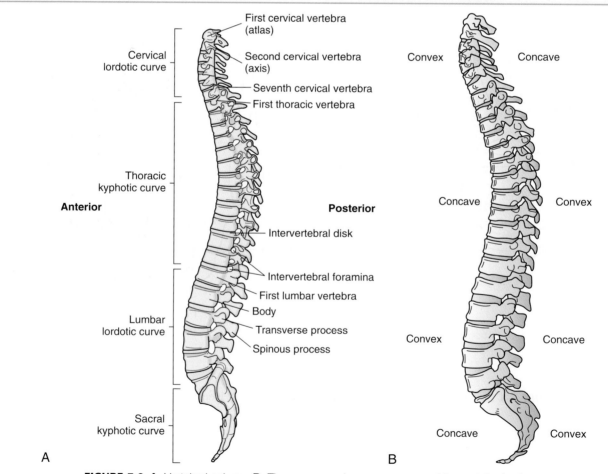

FIGURE 7-9 A, Vertebral column. **B,** The convex and concave curves of the vertebral column.

Box 7-6 Bones of the Thorax (See Figure 7-10)

- The sternum is fairly flat.
- The sternum consists of three parts:
  - The manubrium at the top
  - The body in the middle
  - The xiphoid process at the lower end
- The ribs are elongated, flattened, and twisted bones.
- Most ribs articulate with two thoracic vertebrae at three points:
  - The two facets on the head of the rib contact the hemi-facets of the vertebral bodies.
  - The tubercle contacts the transverse process.
- At the posterior end of each rib is a head, which has two facets for articulation with the body (or bodies) of the thoracic vertebra.
- The neck of the rib is a constricted portion next to the head.
- The tubercle has an articular part, which is connected to the transverse process of a thoracic vertebra, and a nonarticular part for ligament attachment.

- The body, or shaft, is long and curved.
- The shaft also has a sharp bend, called the *costal angle*.
- The anterior end is joined to the costal cartilage.
- Each of our ribs attaches to the posterior vertebrae. The intercostal spaces, between the ribs, contain muscles, blood vessels, and nerves.
- The 12 pairs of ribs are classified by their anterior attachments.
  - The first seven pairs are the true ribs; they attach directly to the sternum by way of their costal cartilages.
  - The next five pairs of ribs are known as *false ribs*. The first three (or the eighth, ninth, and tenth ribs) attach to the cartilage of the above rib.
  - The eleventh and twelfth false rib pairs are referred to as *floating ribs* because they have no anterior attachment.

- The lumbar region is also lordotic.
- The sacrum is also kyphotic.

Vertebral curvatures develop dysfunction generally from exaggerated posture, activity, obesity, pregnancy, trauma, and disease. These conditions have the same name as the normal curves but are considered abnormal if they are exaggerated enough to cause problems.

For example:
- Osteoporosis can lead to the development of a hump in the thoracic vertebrae, called *hyperkyphosis* or *dowager's hump.*
- A swayback of the lower back is a hyperlordosis.
- A different type of abnormal curvature is called scoliosis. It is a lateral curvature of the spine.

Any exaggerated curve puts a strain on the musculoskeletal posture mechanisms and may predispose a person to pain and impaired movement (see Figure 7-9).

Bones of the Thorax

The thorax is the region of the trunk between the base of the neck and top of the abdomen (where the diaphragm muscle is located). The bones of the thorax form a cone-shaped cage that protects the heart, the lungs, and other thoracic cavity structures. Twelve pairs of ribs form the ribcage. The ribcage attaches posteriorly to the spinal column and anteriorly to the sternum, or breast bone. The xiphoid process is the inferior portion of the sternum and is used as a landmark in cardiopulmonary resuscitation (CPR) for chest compressions. Chest compressions are performed above the xiphoid process to avoid breaking it off (Box 7-6; Figure 7-10).

Bones of the Appendicular Skeleton

The appendicular skeleton may be considered as having two divisions, the upper extremity and the lower extremity.

The upper extremity includes the shoulders or pectoral girdles; the arms between the shoulders and the elbows; the forearms between the elbows and the wrists; and the wrists and hands, including the fingers. In everyday conversation we refer to the arm as the whole appendage from the shoulder joint to the wrist joint. In anatomic terms the arm is the portion from shoulder joint to elbow joint. The only bony attachment of the upper extremity to the axial skeleton occurs at the sternoclavicular joint, the articulation of the clavicle and the manubrium of the sternum.

The lower extremity includes the hips or pelvic girdles; the thighs between the hips and knees; the legs between the knees and ankles; and the ankles and feet, including the toes. Note that in anatomic terms, the leg is only the portion from the knee joint to the ankle joint.

Bones of the Upper Extremity

The bones of the upper extremity can be divided into two groups. One group consists of the bones of the pectoral girdle, which include the clavicle, and the scapula (some references include the manubrium, upper thoracic vertebrae, and first two ribs as functional units of the pectoral girdle). The other group includes the bones of the arm, forearm, and hand (Box 7-7; Figures 7-11 and 7-12; Activity 7-7).

The Humerus, Radius, Ulna, and Bones of the Wrist and Hand

The second group of bones of the upper division consists of the bones of the upper extremity, which are the humerus, radius, ulna, and bones of the wrist and hand. The medial and lateral epicondyles of the humerus are attachment points for muscles and are prone to problems from repetitive use (Figure 7-13).

The head of the radius, at the proximal end, articulates with the capitulum of the humerus during flexion and extension. During flexion and extension, the radial head slides on the

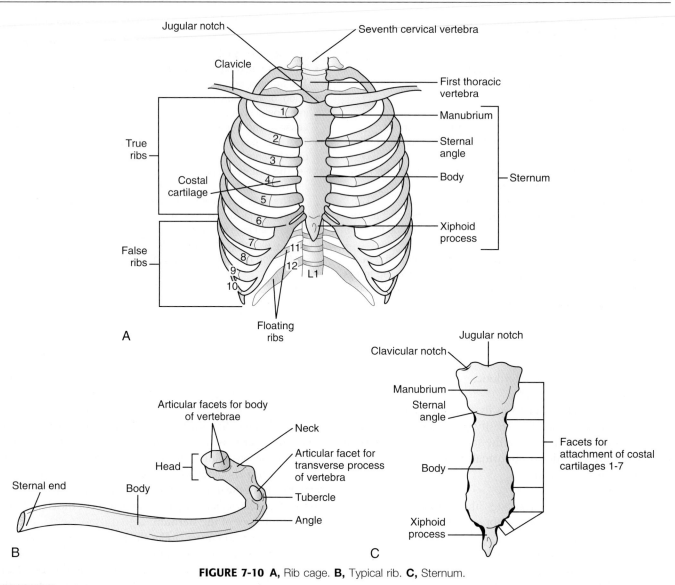

FIGURE 7-10 A, Rib cage. **B,** Typical rib. **C,** Sternum.

Box 7-7 **Bones of the Pectoral Girdle** (See Figures 7-11, 7-12)

Clavicle. The clavicle, or collar bone, is long and flat and has two bends, which gives it an S shape. This fragile bone transmits force from the arms to the thorax. For this reason, when a person falls with arms outstretched, this bone often breaks or the joint separates when the clavicle hits the acromion.
- The lateral clavicle articulates with the acromion of the scapula, and together they form the upper portion of the shoulder.
- This structure functions as a strut by keeping the scapula posterior, which maintains the position of the glenoid fossa (the point of articulation of the humerus on the scapula).
- The clavicle articulates medially with the manubrium to form the sternoclavicular joint.

Scapula. The scapula, or shoulder blade, is an irregular, triangular bone with a flat anterior surface. The edges of the bone are also landmarks and attachment points for muscles; these are the medial, superior, and lateral borders.
- The posterior surface has a large spine and two major processes, all easy to palpate.
  - At the lateral end of the scapular spine is the acromion process, the highest point of the bony portion of the shoulder.

- The coracoid process is a fingerlike projection from the anterior portion of the superior border.
- The three corners of this triangular-shaped bone are referred to as the *inferior, superior,* and *lateral angles.*
- The scapula has three borders referred to as the *medial, superior,* and *lateral borders.*
  - The medial border is also known as the *vertebral border.*
  - The superior border is the hardest to palpate because it lies under the shoulder muscles.
  - The lateral (or axillary) border is the thickest of the three. The lateral border contains the glenoid cavity, a shallow depression that articulates with the head of the humerus to form the shoulder joint.
- The scapula has three fossae that are attachment points for muscles that connect the scapula to the humerus
  - Supraspinous fossa on the posterior and upper portion of the scapula
  - Infraspinous fossa on the posterior and upper portion of the scapula
  - Subscapular fossa on the anterior portion of the scapula

capitulum, and the trochlear notch of the ulna slides over the trochlea of the humerus.

In full flexion the radial head and the ulnar coronoid process fit into the radial and coronoid fossae of the humerus. At full extension the olecranon process of the ulna moves into the olecranon fossa of the humerus, which prevents extension beyond 180 degrees. During full flexion the radius slides into the radial fossa of the humerus. At the distal end of the radius, the articular surface combines with the proximal carpals to form the wrist joint.

The styloid process of the radius is a bony projection at the distal end, just proximal to the thumb. The radius and ulna articulate with each other in three places: proximally near the elbow, in the middle between the shafts, and distally near the wrist. Motion between the radius and ulna is important for orienting the placement of the hand. It is important to remember that all anatomic references are made when the forearm and hand are in anatomic position.

The actions of the joints of the shoulder girdle, arm, and forearm are discussed in more detail in Chapter 8 (Box 7-8; Figure 7-14).

The two bones of the lower arm—the radius and the ulna—meet at the hand to form the wrist. Technically, the wrist is part of the hand and considered a joint that consists of eight bones forming the proximal skeletal segment of the hand. The hand is made up of the wrist, palm, and fingers. The bones of the hand are the carpals (wrist bones), metacarpals (in the palm), and phalanges (finger bones). Many skeletal injuries occur with falls on the hand, especially when it is forced into extreme hyperextension. Fractures of the scaphoid and radius are common because forces produced by a fall on the hand are transmitted through the scaphoid and lunate and are absorbed by the radius (Box 7-9; Activity 7-8).

Bones of the Lower Extremity

The bones of the lower extremity are grouped together in a manner similar to that of the upper extremity. The two primary groups of the lower extremity are the bones of the pelvic girdle and the bones of the thigh, leg, and foot. The pelvis supports the trunk and the organs in the pelvic cavity. The pelvis also absorbs stress from the lower limbs when we are moving, whether walking or jumping. The female pelvis is adapted for pregnancy and childbirth and is wider and lighter than the male pelvis. The second group of bones of the lower extremity are structured for weight bearing during walking and standing and therefore are larger that the bones of the upper limb.

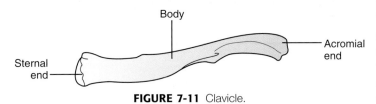

FIGURE 7-11 Clavicle.

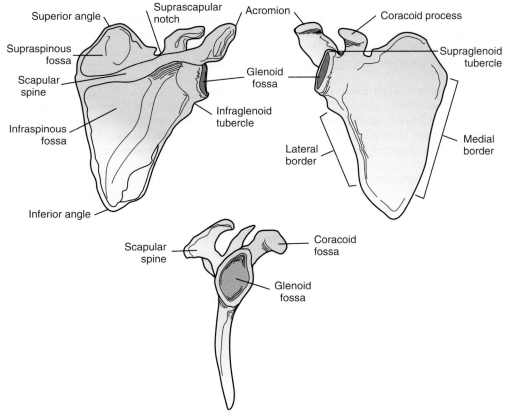

FIGURE 7-12 Scapula (three views).

Box 7-8   Features of the Humerus, Radius, and Ulna (See Figures 7-13, 7-14)

The Humerus

The humerus, or arm bone, is a long bone. The head of the humerus, at the proximal end, articulates with the glenoid fossa of the scapula, forming the glenohumeral (shoulder) joint.

- The distal end of the humerus articulates with the radius and ulna to form the elbow joint.
- On the lateral edge of the distal end of the humerus is a rounded surface called the *capitulum*.
- The medial edge of the distal end of the humerus forms a pulley-shaped surface, the *trochlea*.
- Just above these projections on the anterior surface are the radial and coronoid (ulnar) fossae.
- The *olecranon fossa* is on the posterior surface.

  The lower part of the upper limb is called the *forearm*. It is composed of two bones: the **radius** and the **ulna**. The radius and ulna lie parallel to each other when the forearm is supinated.

The Radius

- The radius is bigger and longer than the ulna.
- The radius is the bone on the lateral (thumb) side of the arm.
- The *radius* is narrow at the elbow and widens just above the wrist.
- During pronation radius crosses ulna.

- The radius takes most of the strain when weight is placed on the wrist.
- The radius is a common site of fractures.

The Ulna

- The ulna provides most of the stability of the forearm.
- Opposite in shape to the radius, the ulna is wider at the elbow and narrower at the wrist.
- At the proximal end of the ulna is the trochlear notch, which articulates with the trochlea of the humerus.
- The olecranon process is the large projection on the posterior side that is easily palpable. Most individuals refer to it as their *elbow*. This process slides into the olecranon fossa of the humerus during extension.
- The coronoid process is located on the ulna, which moves into the coronoid fossa of the humerus during full flexion.
- At the distal end of the ulna is the head. The head of a bone usually is found at the proximal end.
- The styloid process of the ulna is a bony landmark found proximal to the wrist.
- Just beyond the proximal end is an articular disk, which articulates with the carpals to provide some of the movements of the wrist.

Box 7-9   The Bones of the Wrist and Hand (see Figure 7-15)

The Wrist

The wrist is the joint between the hand and the forearm. The structure of the wrist allows movement of the hand. The hand is an elegant and versatile structure that allows the digits (fingers and thumb) to move independently and form an effective grip.

- The wrist contains the carpals—eight small, cube-shaped bones arranged in two rows of four.
- In the proximal row are the scaphoid, lunate, and triquetrum, which articulate with the radius to form the wrist joint.
- The pisiform is also in the proximal row but does not articulate with the radius.
- The distal row contains the trapezium, trapezoid, capitate, and hamate.
- The transverse arch of the wrist, formed by the carpals, is anteriorly concave.
- A wide, thick ligament, the flexor retinaculum, connects the pisiform and hamate to the scaphoid and trapezium or the anterior side.
- The posterior (dorsal) side of the wrist has six tunnels for the extensor tendons.
- The palmar side of the wrist has two tunnels to carry nerves, arteries, and flexor tendons.

- The carpal tunnel, the largest of the two palmar tunnels, is the most commonly traumatized. The carpal tunnel contains the median nerve, which can become compressed, especially when repetitive movements of the hand and fingers cause friction and inflammation.

The Hand

The human hand has 27 bones: The carpus or wrist accounts for eight; the metacarpals or palm contains five; the remaining fourteen are digital bones, fingers, and thumb. In the palm of the hand are five metacarpal bones, long bones that form the framework of each hand.

- Knuckles are the rounded distal ends of the metacarpals.
- Fourteen phalanges, or finger bones, are found in each hand, two for the thumb and three for each finger.
- Each of these long bones is called a *phalanx*.
- The first, or proximal phalanx, articulates with a metacarpal.
- The second and third are referred to as the *middle* and *distal phalanges*.
- The thumb has only a proximal phalanx and a distal phalanx (Figures 7-15 and 7-16; Activity 7-8).

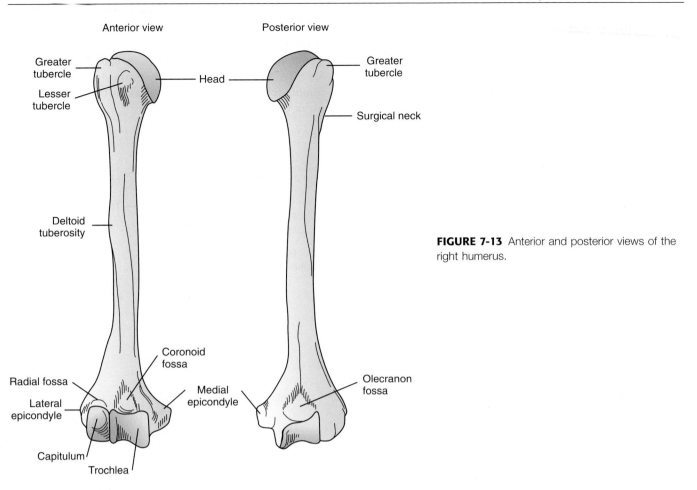

Anterior view — Posterior view

Greater tubercle
Lesser tubercle
Head
Deltoid tuberosity
Radial fossa
Lateral epicondyle
Capitulum
Trochlea
Coronoid fossa
Medial epicondyle
Greater tubercle
Surgical neck
Olecranon fossa

FIGURE 7-13 Anterior and posterior views of the right humerus.

✎ ACTIVITY 7-7

Draw the posterior view of the scapula, and label the following:
Acromion process
Scapular spine
Inferior angle
Superior angle
Lateral border
Medial border
Superior border
Glenoid fossa
Supraspinous fossa
Infraspinous fossa

Bones of the Thigh, Leg, Ankle, and Foot

The second group of bones of the lower division consists of the bones of the lower extremity, which are the femur of the thigh, patella or knee cap, tibia, fibula of the leg, and bones of the ankle and foot. The bones of the ankle and foot pair with the bones of the wrist and hand. Whereas the hand is adapted for mobility and dexterity with the opposable thumb, the foot is much less mobile and provides a platform for us to walk on.

The bones and joints of the foot form the arches of the foot. The *transverse arch* of the foot is also known as the *instep*. The transverse arch is concave from the medial to lateral aspect of the foot. The *medial longitudinal arch* is the longest and highest arch. This arch is made up of the calcaneus and talus and the navicular, cuneiform, and first metatarsal bones. The *lateral longitudinal arch* is made up of the calcaneus and cuboid and fifth metatarsal bones.

The *plantar aponeurosis* is a large band of connective tissue that begins at the inferior calcaneus and runs along the plantar surface of the foot, attaching at the toes. The plantar aponeurosis adds stability to the arches of the foot but can shorten if the person often wears improperly fitting shoes. Plantar fasciitis is a painful condition caused by this shortening. Inflammation from repetitive use is common in track athletes, dancers, airport workers, and members of many other professions (Boxes 7-10 through 7-12; Figures 7-17 through 7-23; Activity 7-9). For a complete review of the bones, try Activity 7-10 on p. 222.

✎ ACTIVITY **7-8**

The following list names the bones of the upper extremity:
Clavicle
Scapula
Humerus
Radius
Ulna
Carpals
Metacarpals
Phalanges

Make up a silly sentence to help you remember these bones by using the first letter of each name.

PATHOLOGIC CONDITIONS

SECTION OBJECTIVES

Chapter objective covered in this section:
6. Describe the pathology of the skeletal system and the related indications/contraindications for massage.
After completing this section, the student will be able to perform the following:
• List common disease conditions of the skeletal system.
• Determine indications and contraindications for massage based on skeletal pathology.

The most common skeletal system pathologic conditions are due to trauma. Other pathologies include developmental conditions and spinal curve abnormalities. Bone demineralization disorders are common, especially in the elderly. Disorders caused by necrosis (tissue death), infectious disease, tumors, and nutritional deficiencies are less common.

Disorders Caused by Trauma

Fractures

Severe force can fracture almost any bone. The term *fracture* means a break or rupture in a bone (see Figure 7-24 on p. 223). Fractures may be classified as follows:

• *Avulsion fracture:* A fragment of bone tears away from the main mass of a bone.
• *Compound (open) fracture:* The skin and other soft tissues are torn, and the bone protrudes through the skin.
• *Simple (closed) fracture:* The break in the bone does not break the skin or injure soft tissue.

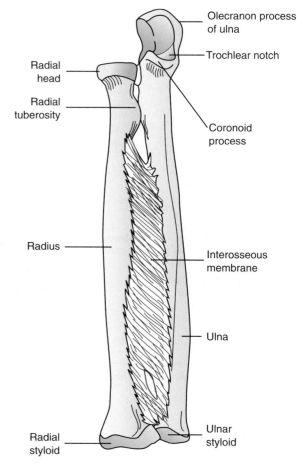

FIGURE 7-14 Anterior view of the forearm bones.

Box 7-10 **Bones of the Pelvic Girdle (see Figure 7-17)**

The pelvic girdle is a strong, bony ring composed of the pelvic (coxal) bones and the sacrum. Unlike the shoulder girdle, the pelvis is attached anteriorly at the symphysis pubis and posteriorly at the sacroiliac joints.
• Three bones fuse as we grow to create the pelvic bones, which form the front and sides of the pelvic girdle. These three bones are as follows:
  • The ilium, which forms the superior flared portion
  • The ischium, which is the inferior portion and the strongest
  • The pubis, which forms the anterior portion of the pelvic bone
• In the middle of the pubis is the symphysis pubis, which is the anterior connection of the pelvis. The fibrocartilaginous disk at the symphysis pubis allows this joint to function as a shock absorber.
• The posterior portion of the pelvic girdle is created from the sacrum, which is discussed along with the spine.

• The lateral portion of the pelvis, where the ilium, ischium, and pubis fuse, creates a deep socket called the *acetabulum.*
• The acetabulum articulates with the head of the femur to form the hip joint.
• At the superior portion is the iliac crest. On the anterior end of the crest is the anterior superior iliac spine (ASIS), which often is used as a bony landmark, especially in assessment and treatment.
• The posterior superior iliac spine (PSIS) is a bony prominence at the posterior end of the iliac crest.
• Just below the posterior superior iliac spine on each side is the posterior joint of the pelvis, the sacroiliac joint.
• On the surface of the body is a small dimple or depression over the sacroiliac joint; the posterior superior iliac spine lies just above it.

Box 7-11 Features of the Femur and Patella, Tibia, and Fibula (See Figures 7-18 to 7-20)

Femur

The femur, or thigh bone, is the longest, strongest, and heaviest bone in the body.

- At the proximal end is the head, which has a smooth, spherical surface that fits into the acetabulum to form the hip joint.
- A depression in the center of the head, called the *fovea capitis,* serves as an attachment for the ligamentum teres.
- All areas of the head except the fovea are covered with articular cartilage.
- The neck of the femur, distal to the head, is a common site of fracture in the elderly.
- The greater and lesser trochanters are projections that serve as muscle attachments.
- The shaft of the femur, as in most long bones, is triangular in cross-section.
- On the posterior shaft is a prominent ridge, called the *linea aspera,* to which the adductor and vastus muscles attach.
- The lateral and medial condyles are smooth surfaces that articulate with the proximal tibia.
- Between the condyles on the anterior side is the trochlear (patellar) groove.
- The lateral and medial epicondyles, which are on the condyles, are points of muscle attachment.
- The intercondylar fossa is a depression on the posterior surface between the condyles that articulates with the intercondylar eminence of the tibia.
- The menisci are cartilaginous cushions (lateral and medial) that lie between the femur and tibia.

Patella

The patella, or kneecap, is a sesamoid bone encased within the tendons of the quadriceps femoris group, where it crosses the knee joint.

- The patella is triangular; the broad superior edge is called the *base,* and the more pointed inferior edge is called the *apex.*
- The patella sits in the trochlear groove of the femur.

- The two articular facets on its posterior surface fit against the medial and lateral condyles of the femur.

Bones of the Leg

The leg comprises two bones, the tibia and the fibula.

Tibia

- The tibia, or shin bone, is on the medial, big-toe side of the leg.
- The tibia is the longer and stronger of the two bones and is a weight-bearing bone.
- At the proximal end are the *lateral* and *medial condyles,* which fit against the identically named surfaces of the femur.
- The medial condyle is larger than the lateral condyle.
- The *intercondylar eminence,* a ridge that separates the two condyles, moves into the intercondylar fossa of the femur during knee extension.
- The *tibial tuberosity,* at the proximal anterior tibia, is the attachment point for the patellar ligament.
- The distal end forms the *medial malleolus,* a prominent bony landmark of the ankle.
- The tibia articulates with the fibula at the proximal end (the proximal tibiofibular joint) and at the distal end (the distal tibiofibular joint). The tibia also articulates the tarsal (ankle) bone, called the *talus.*

Fibula

The fibula is on the lateral little-toe side of the leg. This slender bone does not reach the knee joint and so does not bear weight. The main function of the fibula is to serve as an attachment for muscles and fascia.

- The head of the fibula articulates with the tibia.
- The distal end of the fibula, which forms the *lateral malleolus* (another prominent bony landmark of the ankle), articulates with the talus.
- Despite its small size, the fibula can withstand more tensile pull and strain than any other bone in the body.
- As with the forearm, an interosseous membrane connects the tibia and fibula.

- *Greenstick fracture:* The break in the bone is incomplete, producing a split such as might occur in a green piece of wood. This type is most common in children.
- *Impacted fracture:* The broken ends of the bones are jammed into each other.
- *Comminuted fracture:* The break involves more than one fracture line, with several fragments resulting, often with much soft-tissue damage.
- *Complete fracture:* The break goes across the entire bone.
- *Incomplete fracture:* The break does not go across the entire bone.
- *Compression fracture:* The bone is squeezed or crushed (this type most often occurs in the spinal column).
- *Depressed fracture:* Bone in the skull is driven inward.
- *Stress fracture:* This type of fracture actually is a crack in the bone, often caused by repeated mechanical stress and strain. Stress fractures may not be readily detected. Referral is indicated if the history would point toward a mechanical

✎ ACTIVITY 7-9

The list below names the bones of the lower limb:

Pelvic bone: ilium, ischium, pubis

Femur

Patella

Tibia

Fibula

Tarsals

Metatarsals

Phalanges

Make up a silly sentence to help you remember these bones by using the first letter of each name.

---

stress condition such as a participation in a recent athletic event.

- *Spiral fracture:* A break in which the bone is twisted apart. These fractures are common in skiing accidents.

The signs and symptoms of fractures include local swelling; pain; loss of function or abnormal movement of the affected

Text continued on page 220.

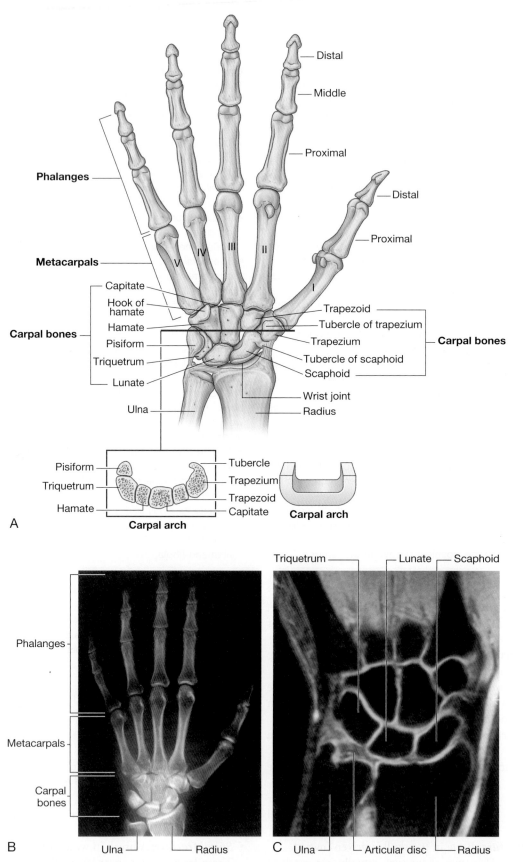

FIGURE 7-15 A, Anterior view of the bones of the hand. **B** and **C,** Radiographs of the bones of the hand. (From Drake RL et al: *Gray's anatomy for students,* ed 2, Edinburgh, 2010, Churchill Livingstone.)

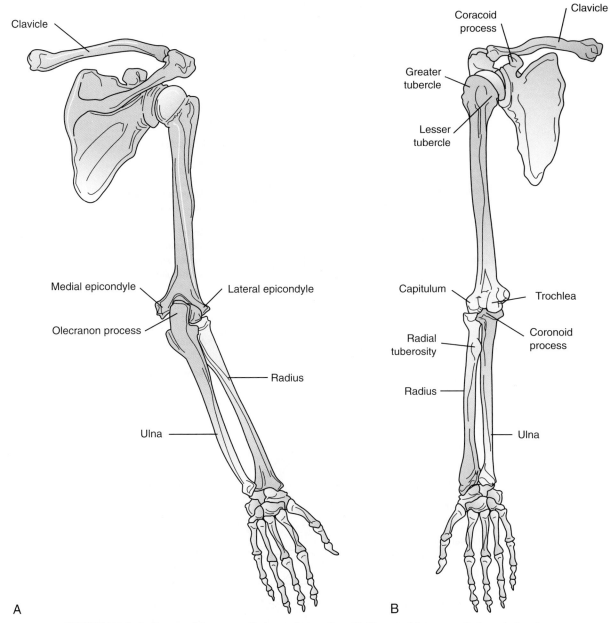

Clavicle

Medial epicondyle

Olecranon process

Lateral epicondyle

Radius

Ulna

A

Coracoid process

Clavicle

Greater tubercle

Lesser tubercle

Capitulum

Trochlea

Radial tuberosity

Coronoid process

Radius

Ulna

B

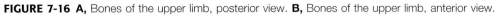

FIGURE 7-16 A, Bones of the upper limb, posterior view. **B,** Bones of the upper limb, anterior view.

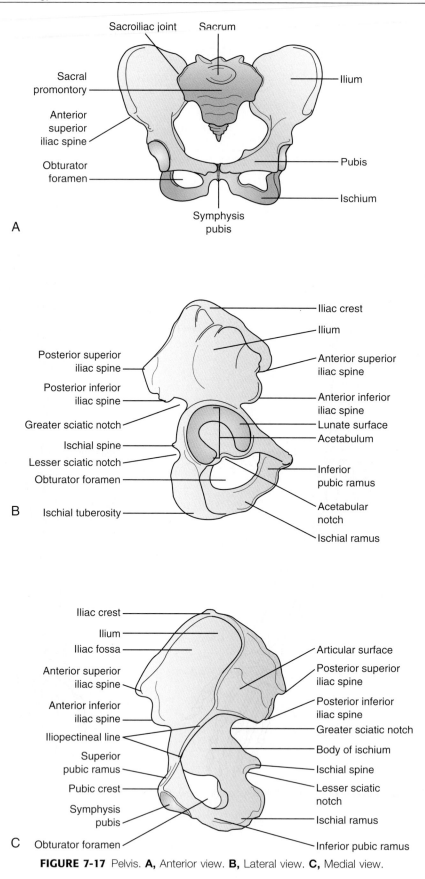

FIGURE 7-17 Pelvis. **A,** Anterior view. **B,** Lateral view. **C,** Medial view.

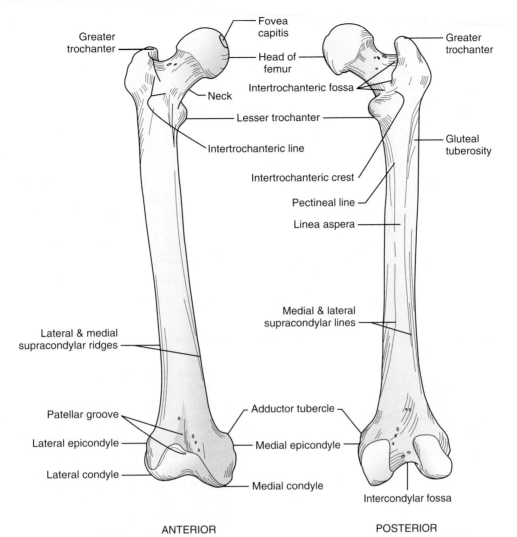

Greater trochanter

Fovea capitis

Head of femur

Neck

Lesser trochanter

Intertrochanteric line

Greater trochanter

Intertrochanteric fossa

Gluteal tuberosity

Intertrochanteric crest

Pectineal line

Linea aspera

Lateral & medial supracondylar ridges

Medial & lateral supracondylar lines

Patellar groove

Lateral epicondyle

Lateral condyle

Adductor tubercle

Medial epicondyle

Medial condyle

Intercondylar fossa

ANTERIOR   POSTERIOR

FIGURE 7-18 Anterior and posterior views of the right femur.

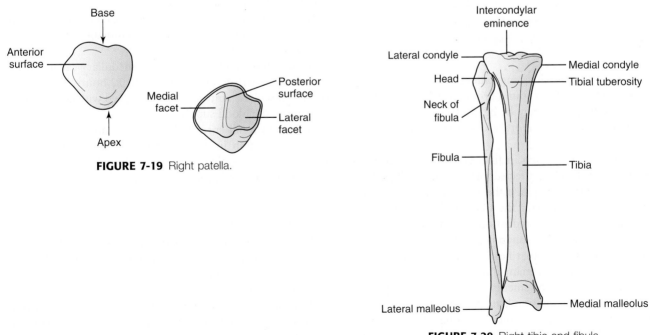

Base

Anterior surface

Apex

Medial facet

Posterior surface

Lateral facet

FIGURE 7-19 Right patella.

Intercondylar eminence

Lateral condyle

Head

Neck of fibula

Fibula

Lateral malleolus

Medial condyle

Tibial tuberosity

Tibia

Medial malleolus

FIGURE 7-20 Right tibia and fibula.

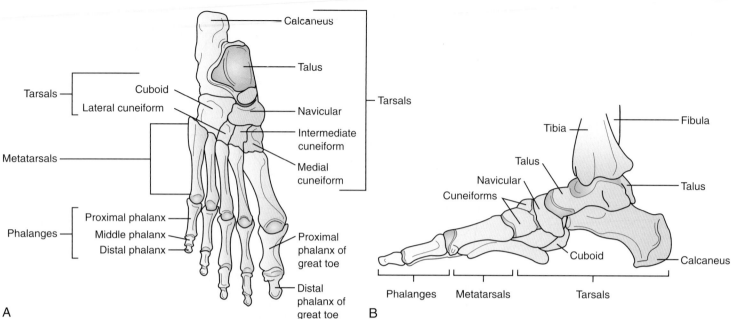

FIGURE 7-21 A, Dorsal view of the bones of the foot. **B,** Medial view of the bones of the foot and ankle.

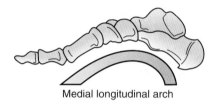

Medial longitudinal arch

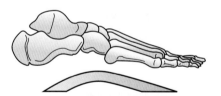

Lateral longitudinal arch

FIGURE 7-22 Arches of the foot.

part; and deformities such as angulation, shortening, or rotation. *Crepitation*, a grating sound produced when bone fragments rub together, also may be heard. Pain may not occur immediately because of temporary loss of nerve function and shock.

The most important step in first aid for a fracture is to prevent movement of the affected parts. Expert help should be summoned immediately, and the area should be protected to prevent movement, leaving the area "as is" if possible.

A fracture is treated by reduction, which means that the broken ends are pulled into alignment and the continuity of the bone is established so that healing can take place. Closed reduction is performed by manual manipulation of the fractured bone so that the fragments are brought into proper alignment; no surgical incision is made. Open fractures occur when the end of a broken bone pushes through the skin. Open fractures are highly contaminated and must be débrided

(scraped and cleaned) and irrigated in the operating room to flush out debris.

A fracture may also require internal fixation with pins, nails, metal plates, or screws to stabilize the alignment. Once reduction is accomplished, the bone is immobilized by application of a cast or by an apparatus exerting traction on the distal end of the bone (Gelfand, 2007).

Acute fracture healing follows the same phases that soft-tissue healing does, but it is more complex. Fracture healing involves cell and tissue proliferation and differentiation, bone breakdown by osteoclasts, and bone-building by osteoblasts. In general, acute fracture healing has three main stages: fracture hematoma formation, reparative phase, and remodeling phase.

Fracture Hematoma Formation

When a bone fractures, there is trauma to the periosteum and surrounding soft tissue. Acute inflammation usually lasts approximately 4 days.

A hematoma accumulates in the medullary canal and surrounding soft tissue in the first 48 to 72 hours. The exposed ends of vascular channels become blocked with clotted blood, disrupting the blood supply.

The hematoma surrounding the fracture site provides a loose fibrin mesh in which fibroblasts and capillaries form granulation tissue that replaces the blood clot. Osteoblasts and chondroblasts become active in forming new bone and cartilage.

Reparative Phase

Within approximately 7 days the hematoma becomes a soft-tissue callus. This temporary bony union is called a *procallus*. Eventually, the procallus is replaced by bone, and a rigid, bony callus is formed.

With adequate immobilization and compression, the bone ends become crossed with new Haversian systems that eventually lead to the laying down of primary bone.

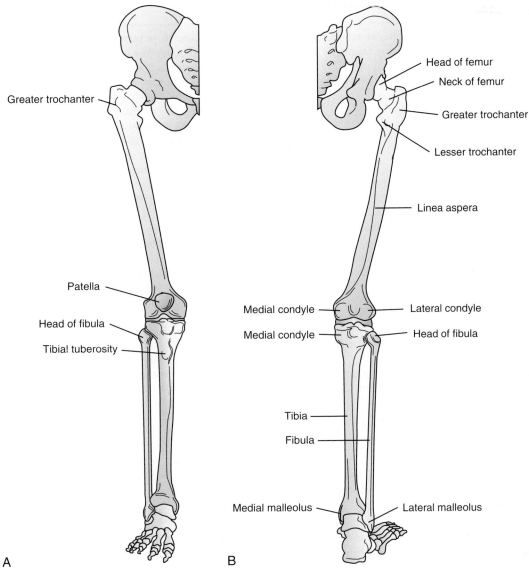

Greater trochanter

Patella

Head of fibula

Tibial tuberosity

A

Head of femur

Neck of femur

Greater trochanter

Lesser trochanter

Linea aspera

Medial condyle — Lateral condyle

Medial condyle — Head of fibula

Tibia

Fibula

Medial malleolus — Lateral malleolus

B

FIGURE 7-23 A, Bones of the lower limb, anterior view. **B,** Bones of the lower limb, posterior view.

Box 7-12 **Bones of the Ankle and Foot (See Figure 7-21)**

Ankle
Ankle structure is similar to wrist structure. Seven *tarsal (ankle) bones* connect the foot to the leg.
- The largest is the *calcaneus,* or heel bone.
- The *talus* is the major weight-bearing bone of the foot during upright motions; it is next in size to the calcaneus.
- The talus and calcaneus are the most posterior of the tarsal bones; they articulate anteriorly with the other tarsals.
- The talus articulates with the tibia and fibula on its superior side and with the calcaneus inferiorly.
- Because no muscles insert on the talus, motion occurs by the movement of the bone and soft-tissue structures around it.
- The other tarsals are cube-shaped and lie between the talus, calcaneus, and the metatarsals; they are the anterior tarsals.
- The navicular bone articulates with the talus, cuneiform bones, and the cuboid bone.

- The cuboid bone articulates with the calcaneus, navicular, third cuneiform, and metatarsals.

Foot
The structure of the foot is similar to that of the hand. The difference lies in the fact that, because the foot supports the weight of the body, it must be stronger and does not have to be as mobile as the hand. The foot has 26 bones.
- Five short metatarsal bones form the instep.
- The heads of these bones form the ball of the foot.
- These bones articulate proximally with the three cuneiforms and the cuboid and distally with the phalanges.
- The phalanges are organized in the same way as in the hand.
- Each toe has three phalanges.
- The great toe has two phalanges.
- The phalanges are identified in the same manner as in the hand: the *proximal, middle,* and *distal phalanges.*

✎ ACTIVITY 7-10

Locate each of the following bony landmarks on yourself. You may need to refer to the illustrations in this chapter.

Zygomatic bone (cheek bone)

Seventh cervical vertebra (the most pronounced of the cervical vertebrae, especially with the neck flexed)

Mastoid process of the temporal bone

Clavicle (collar bone)

Coracoid process of the scapula

Sternum (breast bone) between the ribs

Jugular notch of the manubrium

Xiphoid process (at the inferior end of the sternum; it has a pointed tip)

Scapula

Acromion of the scapula (the highest point of the shoulder)

Spine of the scapula

Medial or vertebral border

Lateral or axillary border

Inferior angle

Superior angle

Humerus

Greater and lesser tubercles

Bicipital or intertubercular groove (runs between the two tubercles)

Anatomic neck (just below the head of the humerus)

Deltoid tuberosity (the distal attachment point for the deltoid muscle)

Lateral epicondyle (a bump at the distal end)

Medial epicondyle (a bump at the distal end)

Olecranon process (the point of the elbow)

Head of the radius (the bony knob just distal to the lateral epicondyle; you can feel it rolling during supination and pronation)

Pisiform bone (the medial carpal bone on the anterior wrist)

Iliac crest (near the level of the waist)

Anterior superior iliac spine (ASIS)

Posterior superior iliac spine (PSIS)

Sacrum (the curved, triangular bone beneath the lumbar spine)

Coccyx (the caudal tip of the vertebral column, deep between the gluteal muscle masses)

Ischial tuberosity (the "sit bones" in the middle of the lower gluteal muscles)

Pubic symphysis (the anterior midline joint of the pelvic girdle)

Femur

Greater trochanter (large protuberance on the lateral side)

Lesser trochanter (small elevation; on the medial side near the top of the inner thigh)

Medial condyle

Lateral condyle

Patella

Head of the fibula (the bump at the lateral proximal leg)

Tibial tuberosity (the large bump just distal to the patella)

Lateral malleolus

Medial malleolus

Calcaneus

Remodeling Phase

In this new phase bone has been completely laid down. The fracture has been bridged and firmly united. Excess callus has been resorbed by osteoclasts.

Remodeling or reshaping of the new bone occurs after the callus has been resorbed and trabecular bone is laid down along the lines of stress. Complete remodeling sometimes takes many years.

Often, the site of a break is stronger than surrounding bone because of the increased activity of the osteoblasts and remodelling process, which essentially creates bone-scar tissue.

The healing process for a fractured bone usually takes 6 weeks, and it is essential that this process not be interrupted. This is why immobilization and casting often are required. Extensive soft-tissue damage, including nerve damage and infection, can result from the fracture. These conditions can continue to cause difficulties long after the bone itself has healed.

INDICATIONS/CONTRAINDICATIONS for Therapeutic Massage

Massage and bodywork are contraindicated locally over a trauma area until healing is complete. Very light, subtle methods of touch therapies (e.g., a gentle laying on of hands) may be beneficial in diminishing pain. The process usually is calming and soothing, which encourages healing through stress management. Bodywork methods are beneficial in supporting the rest of the body during the healing process, especially in managing compensation patterns caused by immobilization of an area and in helping the client learn the use of crutches and canes.

Shin Splints

Shin splints involve muscle strain and potential hairline fractures of the tibia.

Plantar Fasciitis

Plantar fasciitis develops from strain or injury to the plantar fascia of the foot. The signs and symptoms include acute pain when assuming activity after a period of rest. The pain lessens as the tissue warms and then begins to hurt again with continued use. A deep sharp and bruised sensation is felt at the arch and at the attachment at the heel.

INDICATIONS/CONTRAINDICATIONS for Therapeutic Massage

Massage is beneficial for plantar fasciitis and shin splints as long as it does not cause an increase in pain and inflammation. Tibial fractures are contraindicated and need to be ruled out before massage is applied.

Developmental Conditions

Spina Bifida

If the vertebral arches in a growing fetus do not fuse into the spinous processes, the result is spina bifida. Instead of being protected by bone, the nerves of the dorsal spinal cord may be covered by a thin membrane, skin, muscle, or spinal meninges. This condition may range from a mild case, with the child showing no symptoms, to severe spinal cord damage and paraplegia. The most common site of the defect is the lumbosacral region.

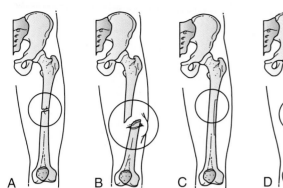

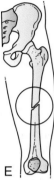
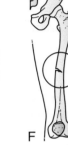
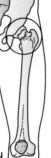
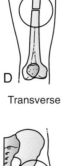

A	B	C	D
Closed or simple	Open or compound	Longitudinal	Transverse

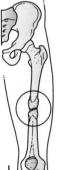
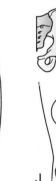
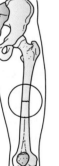

E	F	G	H
Oblique	Greenstick	Comminuted	Impacted

I	J	K	L
Pathologic	Nondisplaced	Displaced	Spiral

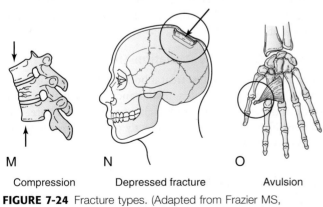
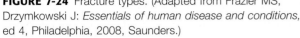

M	N	O
Compression	Depressed fracture	Avulsion

FIGURE 7-24 Fracture types. (Adapted from Frazier MS, Drzymkowski J: *Essentials of human disease and conditions,* ed 4, Philadelphia, 2008, Saunders.)

Cleft Palate

Cleft palate is a congenital deformity involving a gap in the roof of the mouth from behind the teeth to the back of the mouth. Newborns with this defect may have difficulty nursing or swallowing because their mouths are open to the nasal cavities above. Newborns suck in air rather than milk, or the milk may enter the nose instead of the throat. The condition is corrected surgically.

Osteogenesis Imperfecta

Osteogenesis imperfecta comprises a group of hereditary disorders that appear in newborns or young children. The bones are deformed and fragile as a result of demineralization and defective formation of connective tissue.

Clubfoot (Talipes)

Clubfoot is the most common of the lower extremity congenital deformities. In most cases one or both feet are bent downward and inverted; in other cases the feet are pointed upward and everted. Mild cases respond to splinting and stretching, but severe cases require surgical correction. Clubfoot is more prominent in boys and may be the result of genetic predisposition or of the position of the fetus in the uterus.

Spinal Curve Abnormalities

Abnormal curvatures of the spine (Figure 7-25) may be congenital, may result from paralysis or weakness or tension in spinal muscles, or may be the result of asymmetry in the length of the lower extremities. Bad posture habits, especially during periods of accelerated growth, can contribute to the problem. As discussed previously, exaggeration of the thoracic curve is known as *hyperkyphosis* (or hunchback), and excessive lumbar curvature is referred to as *hyperlordosis*. Scoliosis is most often found in young girls, especially during or just after puberty. When discovered and treated early, good results are often seen. One of the major problems caused by any extreme spinal curve is compression of the internal organs.

INDICATIONS/CONTRAINDICATIONS for Therapeutic Massage

If skeletal problems create or are part of a permanent condition, supportive care is required. Any type of aggressive compressive force or joint movement methods are contraindicated for a fragile skeletal structure, regardless of the cause. Light, superficial methods, such as the gentle laying on of hands used in some forms of touch methods, might be indicated. Always consult with the client's physician when conditions indicate extreme caution. Back pain is one of the most common complaints. Most back pain is caused by soft-tissue problems and not skeletal changes, and massage can be indicated and very beneficial to the client. Massage methods are helpful in managing compensatory muscle spasms and connective tissue changes when actual vertebral pathology is present.

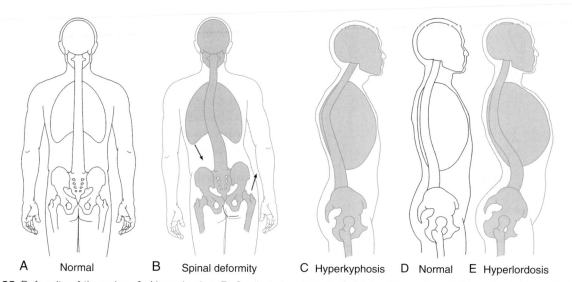

FIGURE 7-25 Deformity of the spine. **A,** Normal spine. **B,** Scoliosis is a lateral deviation of the spine. **C,** Hyperkyphosis, a flexion deformity of the spine. **D,** Normal spine. **E,** Hyperlordosis, an extension deformity of the spine. (Modified from Barkauskas VH, Baumann LC, Darling-Fisher CS: *Health and physical assessment,* ed 3, St Louis, 2002, Mosby.)

Osgood-Schlatter Disease

Osgood-Schlatter disease, which affects the tibial tuberosity, most often occurs in boys between 10 and 15 years of age. The tuberosity becomes inflamed or separates from the tibia because of irritation caused when the patellar tendon pulls on the tuberosity during periods of rapid growth or overuse of the quadriceps femoris group.

General Growing Pains

One of the many causes of growing pains occurs during growth spurts in children and adolescents when the bone grows faster than the attached muscles and other soft tissues. The pain results when the soft tissues pull on the pain-sensitive periosteum.

INDICATIONS / CONTRAINDICATIONS for Therapeutic Massage

Treatment of local areas may be contraindicated if inflammation is present. General growing pains often are soothed by methods that do not introduce any sort of therapeutic inflammation, such as intense stretching and frictioning methods, which should be avoided. Methods that relax and lengthen the muscle and soften the connective tissue are appropriate.

Bone Demineralization Disorders

Osteoporosis

Osteoporosis is a disorder of the bone in which calcium and other minerals are lacking and bone protein is diminished. Under normal conditions, osteoblasts replace bone. In osteoporosis this happens much more slowly, leaving the bones soft, fragile, and more likely to break. Osteoporosis primarily affects the spine and pelvis. The condition is seen most often in postmenopausal women as a result of the decrease in estrogen levels. Other causes include deficiencies in the nutritional intake, absorption, or assimilation of protein and minerals; cigarette smoking; and inactivity. Treatments include implementing hormone therapy (primarily estrogen, progesterone, and calcitonin); increasing exercise; and including more sources of calcium, magnesium, boron, and vitamin D in the daily diet.

Paget Disease

Paget disease, or osteitis deformans, occurs when the bones undergo normal periods of calcium loss followed by periods of excessive new cell growth. Bone cells are replaced with fibrous tissue and blood vessels. As a result, the bones harden, deform, and become susceptible to fracture. Currently, neither the cause nor the cure is known. The condition is most commonly found in men older than 40 years of age.

Osteitis Fibrosa Cystica

In osteitis fibrosa cystica, bone tissue is replaced by fibrous tissue and cysts, making the bones weak and prone to fracture. This disorder is seen in long-standing hyperparathyroidism.

Disorders Caused by Radiation Therapy

When radiation is used to treat a bone disorder or is given as part of the treatment of a malignancy, bone may become brittle and fragile because of the changes in its structure. This happens if the bone is treated directly or if the treatment site involves bony structures.

Necrosis (Tissue Death)

Osteonecrosis (Ischemic Necrosis)

Various pathologic changes occur in the bone when its blood supply is diminished or cut off, or when infection, malignancy, or trauma occurs, leading to tissue death or necrosis. These conditions are among the common causes of hip pain and

INDICATIONS/CONTRAINDICATIONS for Therapeutic Massage

Caution is necessary before any massage and bodywork requiring any amount of compressive force is used on a client with a condition that causes demineralization of bone or that results in brittle, fragile bones. A fragile skeletal structure, regardless of the cause, is a contraindication for any type of compressive force or joint movement methods unless these are carefully supervised by the appropriate medical professionals. Light, superficial methods, such as the gentle laying on of hands used in some forms of touch methods, might be indicated with supervision. Bone involvement may be localized, such as with radiation treatment. In these cases, bodywork methods can be used on the unaffected areas and avoided over the involved area.

disability. The changes usually occur subsequent to a primary disease such as lupus, especially when the disease is treated with glucocorticoids. Symptoms include pain during active motion and at night. Because of the slow, progressive deterioration, necrosis may go undiagnosed.

Legg-Calvé-Perthes Disease

More commonly known as *Perthes disease*, Legg-Calvé-Perthes disease involves degeneration and necrosis at the head of the femur, followed by recalcification. The disorder, most often seen in young boys, occurs when the vascular supply to the head of the femur is compromised, resulting in developmental deformity. The condition lasts about 3 years and may predispose the child to arthritis in the area as an adult. Symptoms include hip pain and gait abnormalities.

Scheuermann Disease

Scheuermann disease is most commonly caused by necrosis or inflammation in bone or in a thoracic disk. The disease begins during puberty, is the result of genetic predisposition or trauma (or both), and leads to back pain and hyperkyphosis. The excessive curvature is caused by the changes in the structure of the vertebrae, from columnar to wedge-shaped.

Osteochondritis Dissecans

In osteochondritis dissecans the cartilage and adjacent bone separate from the bone itself. This disorder is most common in adults and is caused by inflammation and necrosis of the particular area. At the affected joint, portions of dead tissue may break away and lodge in the joint capsule, restricting movement and causing pain. The condition is most often seen in the knee joint.

INDICATIONS/CONTRAINDICATIONS for Therapeutic Massage

Necrosis usually is a localized condition that requires regional avoidance of the involved bone area. Because massage provides the generalized effect of enhanced local circulation, indirect benefits might occur with careful use of these methods. However, because these disorders are pathologic conditions, massage must be done with the permission and supervision of the primary health care provider.

Infectious Diseases

Osteomyelitis

Osteomyelitis is an inflammation in the bone, bone marrow, or periosteum usually caused by pyogenic (pus-producing) bacteria. The bacteria reach the bone through the bloodstream or by way of an injury in which the skin is broken. Osteomyelitis is most often seen in children, near the joints in the upper or lower extremities. When osteomyelitis is promptly treated medically, the chance of a full recovery is excellent.

Tuberculosis

Tuberculosis is a systemic disease caused by the tubercular bacillus. Involvement in the skeletal system causes destruction of the bone tissue and necrosis. Tuberculosis of the spine, known as *Pott's disease*, affects mostly children. The onset of skeletal tuberculosis is insidious, usually marked by vague complaints of pain.

INDICATIONS/CONTRAINDICATIONS for Therapeutic Massage

Massage is contraindicated in infectious disease unless carefully supervised by medical personnel. The therapist must always refer clients with vague pain symptoms for proper diagnosis.

Tumors

Tumors in the skeletal system can be primary or secondary. Primary tumors such as cysts or osteomas (bony knobs in or on a bone) are rare and usually benign. Some tumors are malignant, such as *osteosarcomas*, which often arise in the femur or tibia of a young person. Some of the signs of malignancy are pain, unexplained swelling over a bone, a feeling of warmth on the skin, and prominent veins over the area.

Secondary tumors develop from primary sites, most often in the breast, lungs, or prostate. In older individuals metastases from epithelial tumors or carcinomas of various organs can spread to the bones.

Tumors also can be found in cartilage. Osteochondroma is a benign tumor of the cartilage and bone tissue of long bones. *Chondrosarcomas* are malignant tumors of the cartilage.

INDICATIONS/CONTRAINDICATIONS for Therapeutic Massage

Prompt referral for diagnosis is a must for any sign that may indicate the growth of a tumor. Benign tumors are a local contraindication for massage. These therapies are contraindicated for individuals with malignant tumors unless the therapist is supervised directly and carefully by the medical team.

Nutritional Disorders

Rickets

Rickets is a childhood disease that is rare in the Western world but still occurs with conditions of extreme nutritional deficiency. Rickets is characterized by numerous bone deformities. Deficiency of the active form of vitamin D prevents the

✎ ACTIVITY 7-11

List three benefits of massage in dealing with pathologic conditions of the skeletal system.

Example
Stress management promotes healing.

Your Turn
1. _____
2. _____
3. _____

List three contraindications for the use of massage in dealing with pathologic conditions of the skeletal system.

Example
Necrosis is locally contraindicated.

Your Turn
1. _____
2. _____
3. _____

absorption of calcium and phosphorus through the intestine; these minerals, then, are not available for deposit in the bones, which remain soft and become distorted. The deformity patterns may be noticeable in older clients who had rickets as children.

Scurvy

Scurvy is a vitamin C deficiency. Vitamin C is necessary for the production of collagen of the fibrous tissue and bone matrix. With scurvy, bone density is lost. Treatment involves increasing the vitamin intake, but some damage may be permanent. As with rickets, this disease is rare in the Western world, but it can occur under conditions of inadequate nutrition, such as with eating disorders.

INDICATIONS/CONTRAINDICATIONS for Therapeutic Massage

Regardless of the cause, a fragile skeletal structure is a contraindication for any type of compressive force or joint movement methods unless these methods are carefully supervised by the appropriate medical professionals. Light, superficial methods, such as the gentle laying on of hands used in some forms of touch methods, might be indicated, with supervision (Activity 7-11).

SUMMARY

This chapter has focused on the general structure of the skeletal system and the specific anatomy of the bones of the body. The various activities have reviewed and integrated the data so that the names, shapes, and functions of bones are familiar. Information about the skeleton is important to our study of the way the body moves, which continues in later chapters.

The author would like to thank Joseph E. Muscolino for his special contributions to this chapter.

℮volve

http://evolve.elsevier.com/Fritz/essential
Activity 7-1 Sound it out: study skeletal-related pronunciations.
Activity 7-2 Complete a Word Search to study bone structure.
Activity 7-3 Place the five classifications of bones into their appropriate category.
Activity 7-4 Go on a skeletal system research webquest!
Activity 7-5 Label the bones of the head.
Activity 7-6 Label the 6 types of vertebrae.
Activity 7-7 Label the bones and bony landmarks of the ribcage and sternum.
Activity 7-8 Drag and drop the names of the bones of the scapula and the arm into their correct locations.
Activity 7-9 Did you know you could study the bones of the body while playing Tetris? Give it a try on the Evolve website!
Additional Resources:
Skeletal System scientific animations and cadaver dissection video.
Weblinks: Access weblinks that lead to enhanced learning activities, descriptions of biomechanics classes, and an in-depth look at the textbook *Gray's Anatomy*.
Remember to study for your certification and licensure exams! Review questions for this chapter are located on Evolve.

REFERENCE

Gelfand JL: Health Center: Understanding osteoporosis-treatment (website): www.webmd.com/osteoporosis/understanding-osteoporosis-treatment. Accessed 10/19/2007.

Workbook Section

All Workbook activities can be done electronically online as well as here in the book. Answers are located on ⊖volve.

Short Answer

1. List the seven main functions of the skeletal system.

_____
_____
_____

2. Describe the structure and development of bone.

_____
_____
_____
_____
_____
_____
_____

3. List and describe the five shapes of bone.

_____
_____
_____

4. List and describe bony landmarks, and give an example of each type.

_____
_____
_____
_____
_____
_____
_____
_____
_____

5. Describe the two divisions of the skeleton and list the bones in each division.

_____
_____
_____
_____
_____
_____
_____
_____

Fill in the Blank

The appendicular skeleton is composed of the
(1) _____ of the body and their attachments.
Another name for a joint is a/an (2) _____.
   The (3) _____ skeleton consists of
the head, the vertebral column (spine), and the ribs and
sternum. It provides the body with form and protection.

Compact bone is the (4) _____
portion of bone that protects spongy bone and provides the
firm framework of the bone and the body. The osteocytes in
this type of bone are located in concentric rings called
(5) _____ around a central (6) _____
canal, through which nerves and blood vessels pass.
   The (7) _____ is a thin membrane of
connective tissue that lines the marrow cavity of a bone.
   An endoskeleton is found (8) _____
the human body; it accommodates growth.
   The (9) _____ is a thin membrane of
connective tissue that covers bones except at the
articulations.
   The (10) _____ quality of bones allows
them to deform slightly and vibrate when electric currents
pass through them.
   Sesamoid bones are round bones that often are
embedded in tendons and joint capsules. The largest of these
is the (11) _____.
   Spongy bone is also known as (12)
_____ bone.
   (13) _____ are an irregular meshing
of small, bony plates that make up spongy bone. Their
spaces are filled with (14) _____
marrow.
   A bone fracture is treated by (15) _____,
which means that the broken ends are pulled into alignment.
In general, acute fracture healing has three main stages:
fracture hematoma formation, (16) _____
phase, and remodeling phase. A (17) _____
accumulates in the (18) _____ canal and
surrounding soft tissue in the first 48 to 72 hours.

Exercise

Identify each bone in the following figure on p. 228 by filling
in the blanks with the appropriate name.
   Carpals
   Clavicle
   Costal cartilage
   Cranium
   Femur
   Fibula
   Humerus
   Ilium
   Innominate bone
   Ischium
   Mandible
   Maxilla
   Metacarpals
   Metatarsals
   Nasal bone

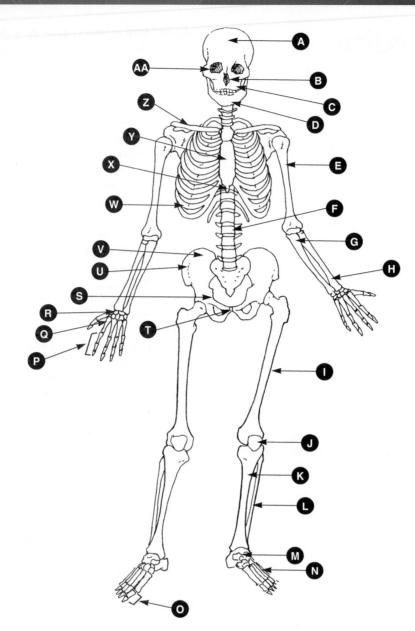

Orbit
Patella
Phalanges (use twice)
Pubis
Radis
Sternum
Tarsals
Tibia
Ulna
Vertebral column
Xiphoid process

A. _____
B. _____
C. _____
D. _____
E. _____
F. _____
G. _____

H. _____
I. _____
J. _____
K. _____
L. _____
M. _____
N. _____
O. _____
P. _____
Q. _____
R. _____
S. _____
T. _____
U. _____
V. _____
W. _____
X. _____
Y. _____

Z. _____

AA. _____

Now identify each part of the vertebral column, shown in the following figure, by filling in the blanks with the appropriate name.

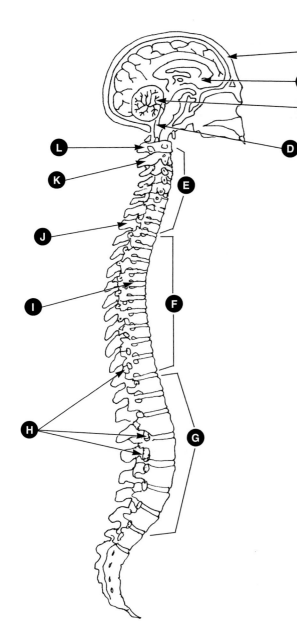

Brain
Brainstem
Cerebellum
Cervical curve
First cervical vertebra (atlas)
Intervertebral disk
Intervertebral foramina
Lumbar curve
Second cervical vertebra (axis)
Seventh cervical vertebra
Skull
Thoracic curve

A. _____
B. _____
C. _____
D. _____
E. _____
F. _____
G. _____
H. _____
I. _____
J. _____
K. _____
L. _____

ACTIVITY

Draw a thoracic or lumbar vertebra from the superior view, and label the following areas. Be as accurate as you can without worrying about artistic ability. Looking at an anatomy picture or diagram will help (see Figures 7-6, 7-7, and 7-8).
Body (centrum)
Vertebral arch
Vertebral foramen
Pedicles
Laminae
Spinous process
Transverse processes
Articular facets
Hemifacets for ribs
Now draw two stacked vertebrae from a side view, and label the following:
Intervertebral disk
Intervertebral foramen
Anterior longitudinal ligament
Posterior longitudinal ligament
Supraspinous ligament
Ligamenta flava
Interspinous ligaments
Intertransverse ligaments

ACTIVITY

Draw the vertebral column, and label the structures in the list below. Include the vertebral curve pattern, and label the curves. Again, be accurate in your drawing, but do not worry about artistic ability. Using diagrams or pictures from this text is helpful.
Atlas
Axis
Cervical vertebrae (C1 to C7)
Nuchal ligament
Thoracic vertebrae (T1 to T12)
Thoracic-lumbar junction at T11, T12, and L1
Lumbar vertebrae (L1 to L5)
Lumbar-sacral junction at L4 to L5 and S1
Sacrum
Coccyx

ACTIVITY

Draw the sternum, and label the following:
Manubrium
Body
Xiphoid process

✎ ACTIVITY

Draw a typical rib, and label the following:
Head (with two facets for articulation)
Neck
Tubercle
Body (shaft)
Costal angle

✎ ACTIVITY

Draw the clavicle, and label the following:
Articulation with the manubrium at the sternal end
Articulation with the acromion at the acromial end
Body

✎ ACTIVITY

Draw the anterior and posterior views of the humerus, and label the following:
Head
Greater tubercle
Lesser tubercle
Deltoid tuberosity
Capitulum
Trochlea
Radial fossa
Coronoid fossa
Olecranon fossa
Medial epicondyle
Lateral epicondyle
Diaphysis (shaft)

✎ ACTIVITY

Draw the anterior view of the radius and ulna in the supinated position as they are connected by the interosseous membrane, and label the following:
Ulna
Radius
Radial tuberosity
Trochlear notch
Olecranon process
Ulna head
Ulnar styloid
Radial styloid
Interosseous membrane

✎ ACTIVITY

Draw the wrist and hand, and label the following:
Scaphoid
Lunate
Triquetrum
Pisiform
Trapezium
Trapezoid
Capitate
Hamate
Five metacarpal (metacarpus) bones
Fourteen phalanges

✎ ACTIVITY

Draw the anterior and lateral views of the pelvis, and label the following:
Sacrum
Sacroiliac joint
Ilium
Ischium
Pubis
Symphysis pubis
Acetabulum
Iliac crest
Obturator foramen
Anterior superior iliac spine (ASIS)
Anterior inferior iliac spine (AIIS)
Posterior superior iliac spine (PSIS)
Posterior inferior iliac spine (PIIS)
Ischial tuberosity
Greater sciatic notch

✎ ACTIVITY

Draw the anterior and posterior views of the femur, and label the following:
Head of the femur
Fovea capitis
Neck
Greater trochanter
Lesser trochanter
Lateral condyle
Medial condyle
Lateral epicondyle
Medial epicondyle
Linea aspera
Intercondylar fossa
Trochlear (patellar) groove

✎ ACTIVITY

Draw the anterior view of the tibia and fibula, and label the following:
Tibia
Fibula
Lateral condyle of the tibia
Medial condyle of the tibia
Intercondylar eminence
Tibial tuberosity
Medial malleolus
Head of the fibula
Neck of the fibula
Lateral malleolus

✎ ACTIVITY

Draw the dorsal view of the bones of the foot, and label the following:
Calcaneus
Talus
Cuboid
Navicular
Cuneiforms
Metatarsals
Phalange (Figure 7-22; see Activities 7-20 and 7-21).

Problem Solving

Read the problem presented. There is no correct answer; rather, the exercise is intended to assist the student in developing the analytical and decision-making skills necessary in a professional practice. The following six steps can help you with this exercise:
1. Identify the facts presented in the information.
2. Identify the possibilities ("what if" statements), or develop your own possibilities from a careful reading of the facts.
3. Evaluate each possibility in terms of the logical cause and effect and the pros and cons.
4. Consider the effect on the persons involved.
5. Write down each in the space provided.
6. Develop your solution by answering the question posed.

Problem

The bones are not thought of as soft tissue. For this reason direct work with the bones could be considered outside the scope of practice of the soft-tissue or movement therapist. However, because muscles attach to bone and movement is related directly to bones, it seems logical that bones would be part of the anatomy and physiology affected by massage. Any approach that promotes general well-being affects the entire body, including the bones.

Question

In what way would you justify a scope of practice that included the bones as part of the body affected by soft-tissue and movement therapies? The first response is provided as a guide to get you started. Fill in at least two more statements.

Facts

1. Muscles attach to bones.
2. _____
3. _____

Possibilities

1. Direct work with bones could be considered outside the scope of practice for soft-tissue and movement therapists.
2. _____
3. _____

Logical Cause and Effect

1. Logically, soft-tissue and movement therapies will affect bone; therefore bones should be part of the scope of practice.
2. _____
3. _____

Effect

1. Clients may be uncertain as to who can address certain situations if the scope of practice line is not clear.
2. _____
3. _____

How would you justify a scope of practice that includes the bones as part of the body affected by soft-tissue and movement therapies?

Assess Your Competencies

Review the following objectives for Chapter 7:

1. List the seven main components and functions of the skeletal system.
   - Define *endoskeleton* and *exoskeleton*.
   - List the components of the skeletal system.
   - Describe the seven functions of the skeletal system.
2. Describe the structure, classification, and development of bone.
   - Explain the structure of bone.
   - Describe the structure/function relationship to bone structure.
   - Define *compact* and *spongy bone*.
   - Define *trabeculae*.
   - Describe two kinds of marrow and their functions.
   - List and describe the connective tissue coverings of bone.
   - Describe the process of bone development.
   - List and describe the five shapes of bone.
   - Describe the classification system of bones.
   - List the five stages of bone healing.
   - Describe age-related changes in bone.
3. Identify bony landmarks.
   - Define bony landmarks.
   - Explain the relationship of bony landmarks to muscles.
   - Palpate bony landmarks.
4. Describe the two divisions of the skeleton.
   - Define *axial skeleton* and *appendicular skeleton*.
   - Explain the differences between the axial and appendicular skeleton.
   - Name the bones of the axial and appendicular skeleton.
   - Compare the similarities and differences between the bones of the upper limb and lower limb.
5. List and describe the individual bones of the axial skeleton.
   - List and palpate the bones of the head, spine, and thorax.
   - Describe major features of the bones of the axial skeleton.
   - Explain the difference between the infant and adult skull.
   - List and palpate the bones of the upper and lower limbs.
   - Describe the major features of the bones of the upper and lower limbs.
   - Describe the features of the shoulder and pelvic girdles.
6. Describe the pathology of the skeletal system and the related indications/contraindications for massage.
   - List common disease conditions of the skeletal system.
   - Determine indications and contraindications for massage on the basis of skeletal pathology.

Next, on a separate piece of paper or using an audio or video recorder, prepare a short narrative that reflects how you would explain this content to a client and how the information relates to how you would provide massage. See the example in Chapter 1 on p. 22. When read or listened to, the narrative should not take more than 5 to 10 minutes to complete. Simpler is better. Use examples, tell stories, and use metaphors. It is important to understand that there is no precisely correct way to complete this exercise. The intent is to help you identify how effectively you understand the content and how relevant your application is to massage therapy. An excellent learning activity is to work together with other students and share your narratives. Also share these narratives with a friend or family member who is not familiar with the content. If that person can understand what you have written or recorded, that indicates that you understand it. There are many different ways to complete this learning activity. Yes, it may be confusing to do this, but that's all right. Out of confusion comes clarity. By the time you do this 12 times, once for each chapter in this book, you will be much more competent.

Further Study

Learn more by using additional resources and writing a paragraph of additional information on each of the following topics.

Piezoelectric quality of bones

_____
_____
_____
_____
_____
_____
_____
_____
_____

Remodeling process of bone

_____
_____
_____
_____
_____
_____
_____
_____

Degenerative process of articular cartilage

_____
_____
_____
_____
_____
_____
_____
_____

Bone growth and repair

_____
_____
_____
_____
_____
_____
_____
_____
_____

The foot

_____
_____
_____
_____
_____
_____
_____
_____
_____
_____

Skeletal changes caused by aging

_____
_____
_____
_____
_____
_____
_____
_____
_____

Spinal curve abnormalities

_____
_____
_____
_____
_____
_____
_____
_____

Sinuses

_____
_____
_____
_____
_____
_____
_____
_____

Osteoporosis

_____
_____
_____
_____
_____
_____
_____

CHAPTER

8 Joints

http://evolve.elsevier.com/Fritz/essential

CHAPTER OBJECTIVES

After completing this chapter, the student will be able to perform the following:

1. Describe the basic principles of joint design.
2. List the mechanical forces that act on the body.
3. Identify and describe three categories of joints.
4. Demonstrate the principles of joint motion.
5. Identify and palpate individual joints of the skull, shoulder, elbow, wrist, and hand.
6. Identify and palpate individual joints of the pelvis and hip, knee, ankle and foot, spine, and thorax.
7. Design a joint movement sequence for the body.
8. Identify pathologic conditions of joints, and describe general treatment protocols used for intervention.

CHAPTER OUTLINE

JOINT OVERVIEW, 235
    The Balance between Joint Stability and Joint Mobility, 236
    Connective Tissue and Joint Structure, 236
    Mechanical Forces That Act on the Body, 240
    Joint Categories, 242
JOINT MOTION, 244
    Categories of Joint Movement, 244
    Joint Positions and Stability, 246
    Movements of Joints, 247
    Classification of Synovial Joints by Movements, 248
    Kinematic Chains, 250
IDENTIFICATION AND PALPATION OF SPECIFIC JOINTS, 253
    Joints of the Skull, 254
    Joints of the Shoulder, 255
    Joints of the Elbow, 257
    Joints of the Wrist and Hand, 258
    Joints of the Pelvis and Hip, 259
    Joints of the Knee, 262
    Joints of the Ankle and Foot, 264
    Joints of the Spine and Thorax, 266
INTEGRATING JOINT MOVEMENT INTO MASSAGE, 270
    Determining Range of Motion, 271
    Elements That Can Cause Joint Dysfunction, 271
    Types of Joint Movement Methods, 272
PATHOLOGIC CONDITIONS OF JOINTS, 273
    Conditions Caused by Movement, 273
    Inflammatory Joint Disease (Arthritis), 273
    Conditions Caused by Injury, 275
    Conditions Caused by Structural Deviations, 277
    Other Conditions of the Joints, 277
SUMMARY, 277

KEY TERMS

Anatomic range of motion The amount of motion available to a joint based on the structure of the joint and determined by the shape of the joint surfaces, joint capsule, ligaments, muscle bulk, and surrounding musculotendinous and bony structures. The anatomic range of motion is the limit of passive range of motion.

Arthrokinematics (AR-thro-ki-ne-MA-tiks) Movement of bone surface in the joint capsule, including roll, spin, and slide.

Articulation (ar-tik-u-LAY-shun) A place where two or more bones meet to connect parts and allow for movement in the body.

Ball-and-socket joint Joint that allows movement in three planes around a central point. Ball-and-socket joints are ball-shaped convex surfaces fitted into concave sockets. This type of joint gives the greatest freedom of movement but also is the most easily dislocated.

Bursa (BER-sah) A flat sac of synovial membrane in which the inner sides of the sac are separated by a fluid film. Bursae are located where moving structures rub over each other and are considered high-friction areas.

Closed kinematic chain The positioning of joints in such a way that motion at one of the joints is accompanied by motion at an adjacent joint.

Close-packed position The position of a synovial joint in which the surfaces fit precisely together and maximal contact between the opposing surfaces occurs. The compression of joint surfaces permits no movement, and the joint possesses its greatest stability.

Condyloid (condylar) joint Joint that allows movement in two planes, but one motion predominates. The joint resembles a condyle, which is a rounded protuberance at the end of a bone forming an articulation.

Diarthrosis (dye-ar-THRO-sis) A freely movable synovial joint.

Fibrocartilage (fye-bro-KAR-ti-lij) A connective tissue that permits little motion in joints and structures. It is found in places such as the intervertebral disks and the menisci of the knees.

Gliding joints Known also as *synovial plane joints,* gliding joints allow only a gliding motion in various planes.

Hinge joint Joint that allows flexion and extension in one plane, changing the angle of the bones at the joint, like a door hinge.

Hyaline cartilage (HYE-ah-lin) The thin covering of articular connective tissue on the ends of the bones in freely movable joints in the adult skeleton. Hyaline cartilage forms a smooth, resilient, low-friction surface for the articulation of one bone with another; distributes forces; and helps absorb some of the pressure imposed on the joint surfaces.

Hypermobility A range of motion of a joint greater than would be permitted normally by the structure. Hypermobility may result in instability. Some hypermobility may be present without instability if sufficient dynamic stabilization is present.

Hypomobility A range of motion of a joint less than what would be permitted normally by the structure. Hypomobility results in restricted range of motion.

Joint capsule A connective tissue structure that connects the bony components of a freely movable joint.

Joint play The involuntary movement that occurs between articular surfaces that is separate from the axial range of motion of a joint produced by muscles. Joint play is an essential component of joint motion and must occur for normal functioning of the joint.

Least-packed position Joint capsule is at its most lax. Joints assume least-packed position when they are inflamed.

Loose-packed position The position of a synovial joint in which the joint capsule is most lax and the joint is least stable. Joints tend to assume this position to accommodate the increased volume of synovial fluid when inflammation occurs.

Open kinematic chain A position in which the ends of the limbs or parts of the body are free to move without causing motion at another joint.

Pathologic range of motion The amount of motion at a joint that fails to reach the normal physiologic range or exceeds normal anatomic limits of motion of that joint.

Physiologic range of motion The amount of motion available to a joint determined by the nervous system from information provided by joint sensory receptors. This information usually prevents a joint from being positioned such that injury could occur.

Pivot joint A bony projection from one bone fits into a ring formed by another bone and ligament structure to allow rotations around its own axis in one plane.

Saddle joint Joint that is convex in one plane and concave in the other with the surfaces fitting together like a rider on a saddle.

Suture A synarthrotic joint in which two bony components are united by a thin layer of dense fibrous tissue.

Symphysis (SIM-fi-sis) A cartilaginous joint in which the two bony components are joined directly by fibrocartilage in the form of a disk or plate.

Synarthrosis (sin-ar-THRO-sis) A limited-movement, nonsynovial joint.

Synchondrosis (SIN-kond-ROE-sis) A joint in which the material used for connecting the two components is hyaline cartilage.

Syndesmosis (SIN-dez-mo-sis) A fibrous joint in which two bony components are joined directly by a ligament, cord, or aponeurotic membrane.

Synovial fluid (si-NO-vee-al) A thick, colorless, lubricating fluid secreted by the joint cavity membrane.

Synovial joints Freely moving joints allowing motion in one or more planes of action.

Viscoelasticity The combination of resistance offered by a fluid to a change of form and the ability of material to return to its original state after deformation.

Yellow elastic cartilage Cartilage that is more opaque, flexible, and elastic than hyaline cartilage and is distinguished further by its yellow color. The ground substance is penetrated in all directions by frequently branching fibers.

LEARNING HOW TO LEARN

Kinesthetic learning is about using your body to learn to do something. This chapter is perfect for kinesthetic learning. There are activities that ask you to move and to palpate. These activities reinforce learning. You cannot understand this information by reading alone; you have to do it. In addition, you can visualize the actions in your mind and read the words out loud. If you do all three—do, see, hear—you will remember better.

Chapter 8 is the second chapter in the specific study of kinesiology and biomechanics. Chapter 7 described the bones. Bones are a combination of structure and function, as with the rest of the human body. As mentioned in Chapter 7, the study of the skeletal system involves the study of joints. The purpose of most joints is to allow movement. Connective tissue that connects bones to create joints is an essential part of joint structure and function. Without connective tissue the structural integrity of joints would not be maintained. Joints allow movement but require the contraction of muscle tissue to actually create movement. The human body is highly specialized. The individual cells have specific jobs and can no longer function effectively outside of the community of the whole body. Each part needs another.

JOINT OVERVIEW

SECTION OBJECTIVES

Chapter objective covered in this section:
1. Describe the basic principles of joint design.
2. List the mechanical forces that act on the body.
3. Identify and describe three categories of joints.

After completing this section, the student will be able to perform the following:
- Define *articulation*.
- Explain the functions of stability and mobility.
- Discuss the role of connective tissue in joint function.
- Describe collagen and elastin.
- Define and locate bursae.
- Describe three types of cartilage.
- Explain the properties of connective tissue.
- List the mechanical forces that act on the body.
- Relate the five mechanical forces to the process of joint injury.
- List and explain three joint categories.

Move. Wiggle. Put on some music and dance. Hug someone. Scratch your nose. Touch your toes. Joints are where we bend and twist. Body movement depends on joints. Many systemic body functions such as respiration and movement of blood and lymph also depend on the mechanical pumping action of joint movement or muscle contraction alone. For example, lymph nodes often are located at jointed areas so that with every movement, the body massages the lymph system. The mechanical actions of breathing in and out depend on movement of the ribs.

A firm understanding of the anatomy and physiology of jointed areas is necessary because massage therapists interact directly with the somatic structures of the body wall—muscles, connective tissue, joint structure, bones—as the entry point to the entire body.

Metaphorically, joints are interdependent relationships.

- A joint cannot exist with only one bone; at least two must work together.
- Joints seldom operate independently of other joints. Instead, an orchestrated, synchronized network of links develops similar to relationships within a family, friends, and work teams.
- Joints are passive and unable to function without the muscles. They can do nothing alone and depend on others to get the job done; again, this resembles the interactions of families, friends, and work teams.
- Joints and muscles need one another. Joints must move to be healthy and function best only in the way they are designed to move. Muscles need to function effectively to produce the joint movement. (Chapter 9 provides additional information relating to muscle structure and function.)

The same can be said of us. Human beings need to be active and do best when they work with their unique assortment of personal gifts. An elbow cannot operate as a knee, but an elbow is essential and no less important than the knee in the function of the body.

A joint or **articulation** connects parts of a structure. In the body the structures joined are, of course, the bones. Joints illustrate the strong relationship between structure and function. The design of a joint depends on its function, and vice versa. Structure, such as bone shape and the way the bones attach at the joint, determines joint function in the body. For example, joints that require stability or are weight-bearing are structured differently from joints that provide greater mobility. Also, each part of a joint has one or more specific functions essential for the overall performance of the joint. Any disruption or change in any of the parts affects the function of the whole joint.

The Balance between Joint Stability and Joint Mobility

Joints connect approximately 200 bones of various sizes and shapes in the human skeleton. Effective functioning of the total structure depends on the integrated action of many joints, some providing greater stability with less mobility and some providing mobility with less stability. Most joints serve a dual function of allowing mobility but maintaining stability. However, in general, stability must be achieved before mobility. As will be seen, structures associated with joints such as joint capsules, ligaments, and tendons stabilize joints.

Joint designs in the human body vary from simple to complex.

- The simplest human joints usually are less mobile and more stable.
- The more complex joints usually allow greater mobility and are less stable.

Complex joints are more likely to be affected by injury, disease, or aging than are simple joints because the complex joints have more parts and are subject to more wear and tear than simple joints (Box 8-1 and Activity 8-1).

Connective Tissue and Joint Structure

Whereas Chapter 1 first discussed connective tissue, this chapter provides more specific detail relating to joint function.

Connective tissue is used in the construction of human joints in the form of bones, ligaments, tendons, bursae, disks, plates, menisci, fat pads, and membranes. As discussed in Chapter 1, the structure of the connective tissue is characterized by a large extracellular matrix and a wide dispersion of cells. The extracellular matrix located between cells has a nonfibrous component, referred to as the *ground substance,* and a fibrous component.

| Box 8-1 | Form and Force Stability

Stability and Mobility
- Form closure/stability is dependent on the shape of the bones of the joint and the way everything fits together.
- Force closure/stability is the action of muscle contraction to stabilize the joint.

- Excessive form stability results in a stuck or fixed joint.
- Excessive force stability can result in excess form stability by jamming the joint surfaces.
- Decreased form stability results in increased muscle contraction to produce force stability.
- Decreased force stability results in strain on the joint capsule.

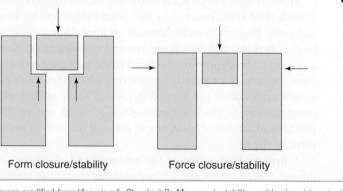

Form closure/stability   Force closure/stability

Figures modified from Vleeming A, Stoeckart R: *Movement, stability, and lumbopelvic pain: integration of research and therapy,* 2007, with permission from Elsevier.

✎ ACTIVITY 8-1

Consider the following principles and characteristics of joint design. Write down a social interaction that is similar. Some examples are provided to get you started.

Example
Some joints provide greater stability than other joints.
Having my grandmother over to talk stabilizes my connection with my family and my past.
Some joints provide greater mobility than other joints.
Relationships with my teachers move my knowledge forward.
The structure of the joint determines the function of the joint.
The relationship I have with my dog is one of companionship, and the relationship I have with my chickens is one of a caretaker.
A breakdown or change of any joint structure affects the entire joint function.
My son's divorce affected our entire immediate family, and the holidays were particularly difficult the first year.

Your Turn
Joints connect two or more bones together.
The design of a joint depends on its function.
Some joints provide greater stability than other joints.
Some joints provide greater mobility than other joints.
The structure of the joint determines the function of the joint.
Each part of the joint has a specific function that is essential to the whole function of the joint.
The breakdown of any joint structure affects the entire joint function.
Complex joints are more likely to malfunction than simple joints.
Effective functioning of the whole body depends on the integrated action of many joints working together.
Generally, stability must be achieved before mobility.
Most joints serve a dual function of allowing mobility and maintaining stability.
Simple joints provide more stability.
Complex joints provide more mobility.

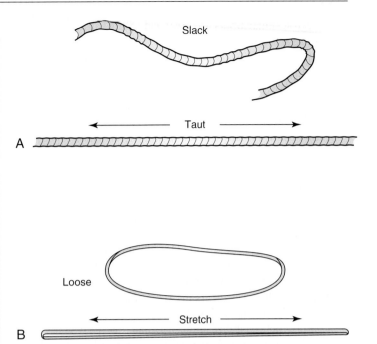

FIGURE 8-1 A, Collagen: like a rope. **B,** Elastin: like a rubber band.

The ground substance consists of proteins responsible for attracting and binding water. The concentration of these proteins in the extracellular matrix of bone, cartilage, membranes, tendons, or ligaments affects the water content and therefore the pliability of these structures. The nonfibrous component also plays an important role in protecting the connective tissue structure and strengthening it.

The fibrous component of the extracellular matrix contains two types of fibers: collagen and elastin.

Collagen

- The primary fibrous component of the extracellular matrix in dense fibrous tissue is **collagen** (white fibrous tissue). Collagen has a tensile strength similar to steel and is responsible for the functional stability of connective tissue structures.
- Collagen fibers are nonelastic but still provide limited mobility. In the relaxed position of some structures, collagen fibers assume a wavy configuration called *crimp*. The crimp or wave can be straightened out, allowing for some flexibility in the structure.
- Collagen has piezoelectric properties that generate small electric currents when it is deformed, and collagen oscillates or vibrates if electric currents travel through it (Figure 8-1, *A*).

Elastin

- **Elastin,** or yellow fibrous tissue, has elastic properties that allow fibers to return to their original condition after a stretching force has been applied (Figure 8-1, *B*).
- The arrangement of the collagen fibers along with the collagen-to-elastin fiber ratio in various ligaments and tendons determines the ability of these structures to provide stability and mobility for a particular joint.

The fibrous component of the extracellular matrix in ligaments contains a greater collagen content than elastin content. However, the ratio of collagen to elastin fibers and their arrangement vary considerably among different ligaments.

Joint Capsule

The joint capsule is a dense fibrous connective tissue that is attached to the bone and forms a sleeve around the joint, sealing the joint space. It also provides passive stability by limiting movements. The capsule varies in thickness, is locally thickened to form capsular ligaments, and may also incorporate tendons. See the discussion of diarthroses (synovial joints) later in this section for more detailed information on the joint capsule.

Ligaments

The cells within ligaments are fibroblasts. Ligaments consist of 70% to 80% collagen, which gives the tissue tensile strength. Elastin fibers in the extracellular matrix provide some flexibility.

- The extracellular fibers are arranged in the same direction, forming a regular arrangement.
- Ligaments are avascular, meaning they do not have a blood supply like skin or organs. Ligaments obtain nourishment from the blood vessels in the membranes around the joint.
- Extrinsic ligaments are found on the outside of the joint capsule and physically separate from the capsule. Intrinsic ligaments are actually thickenings of the articular capsule.

Tendons

A tendon, like a ligament, is composed of dense regular connective tissue, and it connects bone to muscle. In addition to the usual connective tissue components associated with tendons, loose areolar connective tissue forms complete or partial sheaths around them. Double layers of connective tissue around the tendons at the wrist and hand form complete sheaths; these tendons sometimes are called *sheathed tendons*. The sheath protects the tendon and produces synovial fluid, which helps reduce friction.

Tendons help stabilize joints in that they pass across or around a joint to provide mechanical support; however, they can limit the range of movement in a joint.

Bursae

A **bursa** is a flat sac of synovial membrane in which the inner sides of the sac are separated by a fluid film. Bursae are located where moving structures are apt to rub against each other. Subcutaneous bursae are located between the skin and bones. Subtendinous bursae are located between tendons and bones. Submuscular bursae are located between muscles and bones. Although most of us have bursae in the same places, bursae can form as a response to demand if the body needs additional cushioning.

Cartilage

Cartilage is usually divided into three types: white fibrocartilage, yellow elastic cartilage, and hyaline cartilage.
- *White fibrocartilage.* White **fibrocartilage** consists primarily of collagen fibers and forms the cement in joints that permit little motion. This type of cartilage also forms the intervertebral disks and the menisci in the knees.
- *Yellow Elastic Cartilage.* Yellow **elastic cartilage** is found in the ears and epiglottis and differs from white fibrocartilage in that it has a higher ratio of elastin to collagen fibers. Yellow elastic cartilage is more opaque, flexible, and elastic than hyaline cartilage and is distinguished further by its yellow color. The ground substance is penetrated in all directions by frequently branching fibers.
- *Hyaline Cartilage.* **Hyaline cartilage** forms a thin covering of articular cartilage on the ends of the bones in freely movable joints in the adult skeleton. Hyaline cartilage forms a smooth, resilient, low-friction surface for the articulation of one bone with another and disperses joint pressure over a wider area. Hyaline cartilage distributes any additional stresses applied to a joint and helps absorb some of the pressure imposed on the joint surfaces. These cartilaginous surfaces are capable of bearing and distributing weight over the lifetime of a person, assuming the individual has normal

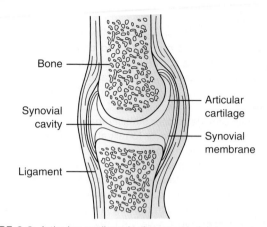

FIGURE 8-2 Articular cartilage in the generic joint capsule. (Adapted from Barkauskas VH et al: *Health and physical assessment,* ed 3, St Louis, 2002, Mosby.)

biomechanics, no injury, and no habits that wear down the cartilage. Water is the most abundant component of hyaline cartilage and, when combined with protein substances in the ground substance, forms a stiff gel (Figure 8-2).

Synovial fluid is distributed during joint motion or when the cartilage is compressed. The fluid flows back into the cartilage after motion or compression stops. Because hyaline cartilage in the adult is devoid of blood vessels and nerves, its nourishment is derived solely from this back-and-forth flow of fluid. The free flow of fluid is essential for the survival of cartilage and as an aid to reducing friction.

The effects of immobilization, in which compression of joint surfaces is absent or diminished, can cause hyaline cartilage to degenerate.

Bone

Bone is the hardest of all connective tissues found in the body. As with other forms of connective tissue, bone consists of a cellular component, a ground substance, and a fibrous component.

Viscoelasticity of Connective Tissue

Although connective tissue appears in many forms throughout the body, all connective tissue exhibits the common property of **viscoelasticity.** The behavior of viscoelastic materials is a combination of the properties of elasticity and viscosity.
- *Elasticity* refers to the ability of a material to return to its original state after being stretched.
- *Viscosity* refers to the resistance to a change of form offered by a fluid.

When a constant compressive or tensile force deforms connective tissue, the tissue moves in the direction of the force and then attempts to return to its original state. Under normal conditions viscoelastic materials initially modify in the direction of the force applied and then slowly return to their original state; this is called *creep*. If a connective tissue structure is held in a deformed position for an extended period, over days or weeks, the viscous creep pattern may become permanent, thus altering the structure and therefore the function of a joint.

Practical Application

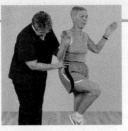

Movement is essential to joint health. Therapeutic massage can support joint function and, in some instances, replace movement to encourage the production and distribution of synovial fluid in the joint. Methods that use passive and active forms of movement are the modalities of choice in these instances.

Plastic Range

Connective tissue subjected to sudden, prolonged, or excessive mechanical forces may exceed its elastic limits, and the tissue may enter the plastic range. In the plastic range the tissue is permanently deformed and is no longer able to return to its original state after the removal of the deforming mechanical force. When the plastic range of connective tissue is exceeded by a mechanical force, a failure, such as a break or tear of the tissue, occurs.

- In the case of a ligament or tendon, the failure may occur in the middle of the structures, through tearing and disruption of the connective tissue fibers, and is called a *rupture*.
- Failure that occurs through a pulling off of part of the bone attached to the ligament is called *avulsion*; there is no injury to the ligament because it is still attached to a bony fragment.
- Failure that occurs in bony tissue is called a *fracture*.

Each type of connective tissue can undergo a certain percentage of deformation before failure. This percentage varies not only among the types of connective tissue but also within the various types. Generally, tendons can deform more than ligaments, ligaments can deform more than cartilage, and cartilage can deform more than bone.

Two types of general pathologic conditions develop with changes in elasticity and viscosity of connective tissue: laxity and shortening.

Laxity

Laxity occurs when connective tissue is too long and usually happens with prolonged overstretching of joint structures or a sudden trauma. The ligaments are no longer capable of returning to their original length after being elongated and remain in a partial state of elongation. Ligament laxity places a joint at risk for injury because it compromises an important source of joint support and protection. Gymnastics, dancing, figure skating, and excessive use of stretching systems such as yoga can produce this condition. Too much flexibility results in instability. Remember that stability is established before mobility. When connective tissue is unstable around a joint, the muscles of the jointed area increase contraction to provide the necessary joint stability. This action pulls the bones of a joint together, decreasing joint space, which may result in increased compression upon the bones of the joint. Although this is a good short-term strategy, other problems with joint function, such as predisposition to osteoarthritis, develop over the long term.

Massage approaches can be used to manage the muscle contractions around the joint and support the compensation pattern by keeping the muscle contractions appropriate to the need for stabilization and minimizing the excessive pulling together of the bones of the joint. The use of certain types of frictioning techniques on individual connective tissue structures such as ligaments can create a therapeutic inflammation process. Because inflammation triggers the formation of connective tissue, the massage practitioner possibly can encourage the development of additional ligament structure. This procedure is combined with moderate immobilization, which is necessary to allow the connective tissues to form, as well as rehabilitative exercise to prevent adhesions from developing during the restructuring process. Therefore a combination of purposeful therapeutic inflammation, external stability in the form of moderate immobilization (e.g., wrapping the area with elastic bandages or soft supports), and appropriate rehabilitative exercise that includes range of motion without resistance creates a broadening of the muscles or connective tissue structures of the area. A series of active joint movement using a pulsing action may increase stability in lax ligaments. These movements do not stretch the tissues but instead mobilize the area through a gentle range of motion. The rehabilitation progresses to resistance exercises used to challenge dynamic stabilizers of the joint in order to provide improved strength and ultimately stability of the joint. This form of intervention for lax ligaments is a slow and deliberate process.

Shortening

Connective tissue also tends to shorten and dehydrate, pulling structures together and stiffening the area, thereby decreasing mobility. This situation provides too much stability and tends to develop to compensate for form alteration in response to a change in function. Should the body need to alter position for an extended period, such as a static position while working at a computer for hours at a time every day, connective tissue slowly alters to support that position. Connective tissue can also thicken and shorten if any inflammatory process does not resolve itself effectively.

In these situations the plastic component of connective tissue must be elongated in the direction of the shortening to restore the pliability and redirect the creep pattern. When a massage therapist stretches a shortened connective tissue structure to elongate it, the tissue should be warm. An appropriately intense but slow pulling or pushing force is applied to the connective tissue area and sustains it to produce creep and increase pliability. The goal is to extend the elastic range of connective tissue structures by altering the plastic range of shortened connective tissue. Myofascial massage therapy methods incorporate these principles. Movement methods such as yoga and other forms of slow, sustained stretching are based on similar principles.

To access the plastic range of connective tissue, it is necessary to avoid the protective muscle contraction initiated by the stretch-reflex response. Lengthening all muscle components to their available resting length is important before increasing the force to stretch beyond the elastic range to elongate the plastic component of connective tissue. As already mentioned, an adequate intake of water is essential for the success of these methods.

Some restricted joint function develops from the tissues surrounding the joint instead of within and directly around the capsule itself. Because of this, it is necessary to assess the entire area for shortening. For example, shortening in the lumbodorsal fascia or pectoral fascia can limit the range of motion of the shoulder joint. Over time the reduction in movement causes pathologic immobilization in the joint. Therefore any therapeutic massage or movement methods affecting joint function should address the entire body broadly. Working with connective tissue is a slow process. Allowing time for the form to change gently and integrate effectively into the entire function of the jointed area and surrounding tissue is essential (Activities 8-2 and 8-3).

Mechanical Forces That Act on the Body

Mechanical forces are actions that involve pushing, pulling, friction, or sudden loading, such as a direct blow. Every time we take a step, push against an object with our arms, or bend and twist, our bones and joints have to dissipate the stress of the mechanical forces imposed on them. When these forces meet an obstacle such as a bend or curve in a bone, the bone absorbs some forces and reflects others. Absorbed forces are transmitted to the soft tissues outside the bone, which helps dissipate excessive stress on joint surfaces. Five different kinds of force act on the body tissues. Tissue types respond differently to different forces. Bending forces seldom harm the soft tissues but will break bone. Tensile forces seldom injure bone but often damage soft tissues. Massage therapists can use these same mechanical forces therapeutically during massage application.

The following paragraphs describe the types of mechanical forces and the potential injury and therapeutic application pertinent to therapeutic massage.

Compression

Compression forces occur when two structures are pressed together (Figure 8-3). Compression is a common way that tissues become injured. Ligaments and tendons resist compressive injury. Muscle tissue, because of its extensive vascular

structure, is not as resistant to compressive forces. Excessive compression force ruptures or tears the integrity of the muscle tissue, causing bruising and connective tissue damage. Compression is a major mechanical force used in the application of massage to support circulation, stimulate nerve function, and restore connective tissue pliability. The massage therapist applies compression in such a way as to achieve benefits without damaging tissue, usually with the broad-based application of compressive force.

Tension

Tension forces, also called *tensile forces*, occur when two ends of a structure are pulled away from each other (Figure 8-4).

Bone resists tensile forces. However, tensile stress injuries are the most common way soft tissues are damaged. Examples of tensile stress injuries include avulsion (complete tearing of attachment), muscle strains, ligament sprains, tendinitis, fascial pulling or tearing, and nerve traction injuries (sudden nerve stretching such as that which occurs in stingers). Tensile stress injuries are described as first degree (mild), second degree (moderate), and third degree (severe). Tensile force is applied during massage, particularly during gliding and traction. Therapeutically, tensile force supports proper alignment of fiber structures and can increase pliability in connective tissue.

Bending

Bending forces are a combination of compression and tension (Figure 8-5). One side of a structure is exposed to compressive forces, whereas the other side is exposed to tensile forces. Bending forces are a common cause of bone fractures and ligament injuries but seldom harm other soft tissues. Bending is used during massage when kneading methods are applied. The proprioceptors in muscles and tendons respond to these

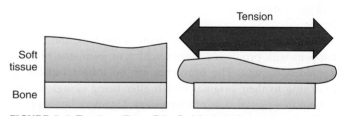

FIGURE 8-4 Tension. (From Fritz S: *Mosby's fundamentals of therapeutic massage,* ed 5, St Louis, 2013, Mosby.)

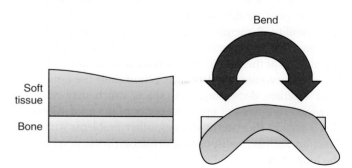

FIGURE 8-5 Bend. (From Fritz S: *Mosby's fundamentals of therapeutic massage,* ed 5, St Louis, 2013, Mosby.)

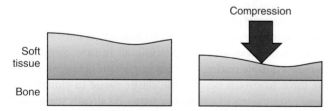

FIGURE 8-3 Compression. (From Fritz S: *Mosby's fundamentals of therapeutic massage,* ed 5, St Louis, 2013, Mosby.)

✏ ACTIVITY 8-3

Develop a therapeutic intervention for a hypothetical connective tissue dysfunction. First, define and describe the assessment procedures you would use. Then develop a therapeutic goal for the area. Finally, develop treatments based on the listed principles. Make plans for a hypermobile and hypomobile situation. Use therapy modalities you are studying presently in your technique classes. Remember that the actual implementation of such a plan often would be supervised by the appropriate health care professional, who would approve the plan before it is implemented. The principles are listed next, followed by an example.

Assessment Principles
Hypermobility
- Connective tissue becomes lax.
- Too much flexibility results in instability.
- Muscle splinting develops to stabilize the area.

Hypomobility
- The entire area must be assessed for shortening.
- Over time, the reduction in movement causes pathologic immobilization in the joint itself.
- Any therapeutic massage methods affecting joint function need to address the body broadly.

Therapeutic Goals
Hypermobility
- Restore stability to connective tissue structures.
- Reduce muscle spasms surrounding the jointed area.

Hypomobility
- Extend the elastic range of connective tissue structures by altering the plastic range.
- Elongate the plastic component of connective tissue to reverse the shortening.
- Restore pliability.
- Redirect the creep pattern.

Treatment Principles
Hypermobility
- Manage the muscle contraction around the joint to support the compensation pattern by keeping the muscle contraction appropriate to the need for stabilization and minimizing the excessive pulling together of the joint cavity.
- Apply frictioning techniques to individual connective tissue structures such as ligaments to create a therapeutic inflammation process.
- Combine this procedure with moderate immobilization.
- Use rehabilitative exercise to prevent adhesions from developing.

Hypomobility
- Avoid the protective muscle contraction initiated by the stretch reflex response to access the plastic range of connective tissue.

- Lengthen all muscle components to their available resting length before increasing the force to stretch beyond the elastic range to elongate the plastic component of shortened connective tissue.

To stretch out (elongate) a connective tissue structure:
1. Warm the tissue.
2. Use an appropriately intense but slow pulling or pushing force.
3. Sustain the force for a time to produce creep and increase pliability.
4. Work toward the goal of extending the elastic range of connective tissue by altering the plastic range.
5. Make sure the person has an adequate intake of water.

Example
Situation: Hypermobile ankle from a bad sprain 3 years ago.
   Assessment:
- Assess ankle for laxity in ligaments and other connective tissue structures by studying range of motion.
- Assess for muscle splinting and spasm with palpation.

   Therapeutic goal:
- Increase stability of the ankle to prevent future ankle sprains.
   Treatment principles:
- Manage the muscle contraction around the joint with therapeutic massage.
- Create a therapeutic inflammation process by use of frictioning on the appropriate lax ligaments.
- Suggest that the client wrap the ankle for moderate immobilization.
- Teach client ways to move the frictioned area through a series of pulsing activities that do not stretch the tissues but instead mobilize the area through a gentle range of motion to prevent adhesions from developing. Encourage more specific rehab protocols, including proprioception; active exercises are the only evidence-based approach to prevent reinjury. These activities include standing on one foot, using wobble boards, and walking on soft surfaces such as a mat.

Your Turn
Hypermobility
Situation:
Assessment:
Therapeutic goal:
Treatment principles:
Hypomobility
Situation:
Assessment:
Therapeutic goal:
Treatment principles:

forces. Bending forces also affect connective tissues, especially the viscosity of the ground substance.

Shear

Shear is a sliding mechanical force with friction created between structures that are sliding against each other (Figure 8-6). Excessive shearing force at a ligament or tendon creates an inflammatory irritation that leads to adhesion and fibrosis. Shear and friction, called *cross-fiber friction,* is a massage method that uses specific force to create therapeutic inflammation to reverse fibrotic connective tissue changes.

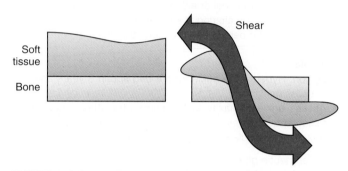

FIGURE 8-6 Shear. (From Fritz S: *Mosby's fundamentals of therapeutic massage,* ed 5, St Louis, 2013, Mosby.)

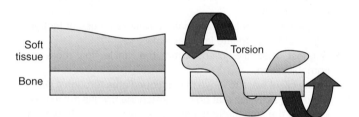

FIGURE 8-7 Torsion. (From Fritz S: *Mosby's fundamentals of therapeutic massage,* ed 5, St Louis, 2013, Mosby.)

Torsion

Torsion forces are twisting forces (Figure 8-7). Torsion occurs with other forces, such as tension and shear. Torsion stress applied to a joint is likely to cause significant injury. Kneading massage methods introduce torsion force into tissue and are especially effective in increasing pliability of connective tissue.

Joint Categories

The joints of the human body are divided into three categories according to the type of motion allowed at the joint and the material connecting the joint. The three categories of joints (arthroses) are as follows:

1. **Synarthrosis:** Nonsynovial, *fibrous,* limited-movement joint
2. **Amphiarthrosis**: Nonsynovial *cartilaginous* joint that is slightly movable
3. **Diarthrosis:** *Synovial,* freely movable joint (most of our joints are diarthrosis joints)

Synarthroses (Fibrous Joints)

In fibrous joints the fibrous connective tissue directly connects bone to bone in a solid configuration that allows either an extremely small amount or no movement (Figure 8-8). The material used to connect the bony components in synarthrodial joints is interosseous fibrous and cartilaginous connective tissues.

Three different types of fibrous joints are found in the human body: sutures, gomphoses, and syndesmoses.

- A **suture** is a joint in which two articulating bones are held together by a thin layer of dense fibrous tissue that is continuous with the periosteum. The ends of the bony components are grooved so that the edges interlock or overlap. This type of joint is found only in the skull. Early in life these

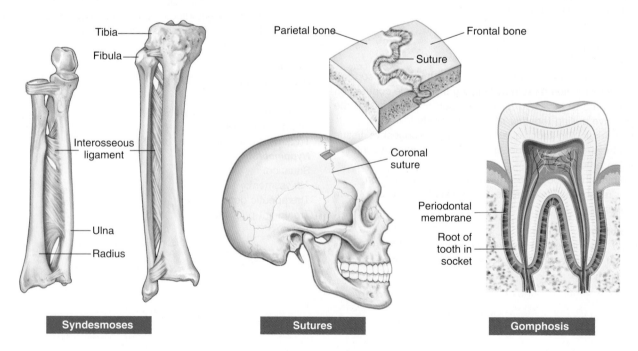

FIGURE 8-8 Examples of the types of fibrous joints. (From Thibodeau GA, Patton KT: *Anatomy and physiology,* ed 6, St Louis, 2007, Mosby.)

sutures allow a small amount of movement. In adulthood the bones slowly grow together to form a synostosis, or bony union, in which little or no motion is possible. The coronal suture is an example of a suture.

- A **gomphosis** is a joint in which the bony components fit together like a peg in a hole. The only gomphosis joint that exists in the human body is found between a tooth and the mandible or maxilla. In most adults the loss of teeth mainly results from disease processes that affect the connective tissue cementing or holding the teeth. Under normal conditions in the adult, these joints do not permit motion.
- A **syndesmosis** is a fibrous joint in a ligament, cord, or aponeurotic membrane that joins the articulating bones. For example, a membrane joins the shaft of the tibia directly to the shaft of the fibula. A slight amount of motion at this joint accompanies movement at the knee and ankle joints.

Practical Application

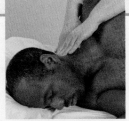

One particular method of therapeutic massage deals with the slight movements of the cranial sutures and works to normalize the gentle cranial/sacral rhythm, of which movement of the cranial sutures is a part. Experts disagree about the mechanisms involved in the cranial rhythm and whether the cranial sutures do indeed move in the adult skull. Many theories exist, none of which has solid validation. However, the methods that work with the cranial sutures seem to have clinical validity, even without agreed-on scientific justification. The massage practitioner uses gentle pressure, and the client experiences more of an intent or thought of movement.

Amphiarthroses (Cartilaginous Joints)

An amphiarthrosis is a slightly movable joint (Figure 8-9). Fibrocartilage or hyaline growth cartilage holds the bony surfaces together. The two types of cartilaginous joints are symphyses and synchondroses.

- A **symphysis** is a joint in which thin layers of hyaline cartilage over each bone are separated from each other by fibrocartilage in the form of disks or plates. The symphysis pubis is the articulation of the two pubic bones. The structure of the symphysis pubis is quite stable, with the thick fibrocartilage providing a secure union between the two bones.
- A **synchondrosis** is a joint in which a thin layer of hyaline growth cartilage connects the two bones. The cartilage forms a bond between the two ossifying centers of bone. This type of joint permits bone growth while providing stability and allowing a small amount of movement. When bone growth is complete, these joints ossify and convert to bony unions. Sternocostal joints are synchondroses. Articular cartilage directly connects the adjacent surfaces of the rib and sternum.

Diarthroses (Synovial Joints)

Most of our joints are **synovial joints,** which are freely movable. A smooth layer of articular cartilage protects the bone surfaces in freely movable joints (Figure 8-10). All synovial joints are constructed similarly, with the following features:

- A joint capsule formed of fibrous tissue surrounds the joint.
- The joint capsule encloses a joint cavity.
- A synovial membrane lines and forms the inner surface of the joint capsule.

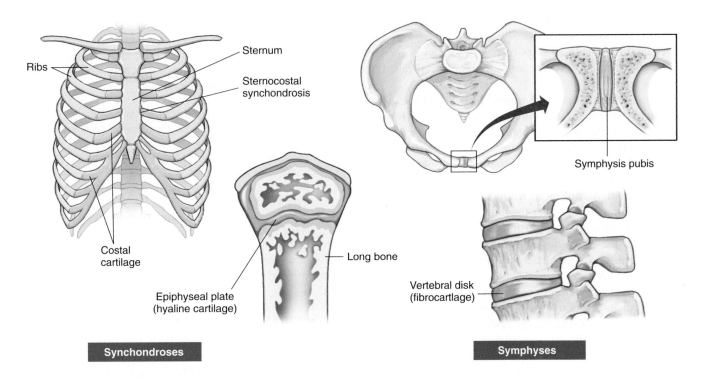

FIGURE 8-9 Examples of the types of cartilaginous joints. (From Thibodeau GA, Patton KT: *Anatomy and physiology,* ed 6, St Louis, 2007, Mosby.)

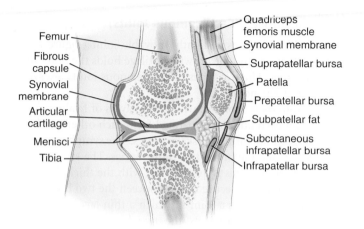

FIGURE 8-10 Structures of the knee as a representation of a synovial joint. (From Muscolino JE: *Kinesiology: the skeletal system and muscle function,* ed 2, St Louis, 2011, Mosby.)

- Synovial fluid is secreted by the synovial membrane into the joint cavity; it forms a lubricating film over the joint surfaces.
- Hyaline cartilage covers the joint surfaces.

In synovial joints the ends of the bony components move freely in relation to one another because no fibrous or cartilaginous tissue directly connects the bones. The bones in this type of joint have a space between them called the *joint* or *synovial cavity,* and the bony components connect indirectly to one another by means of a joint capsule, ligaments, and tendons. Ligaments and tendons play an important role in keeping joint surfaces connected and often assist in guiding motion. While the bones are connected, some separation is necessary for the bones to be able to move. Separation of joint surfaces is limited by passive tension in ligaments, the joint capsule, and tendons. Active tension in muscles also limits the separation of joint surfaces.

The **joint capsule** consists of two layers: an outer layer called the *stratum fibrosum* and an inner layer called the *stratum synovium.*

The stratum fibrosum, composed of dense fibrous tissue, completely surrounds the joint and is continuous with the periosteum of the adjoining bones. The outer layer is poorly vascularized but richly innervated by joint receptors. The receptors located in and around the joint capsule can detect the rate and direction of motion, compression, tension, vibration, and pain. According to Hilton's law, a nerve trunk that supplies a joint also supplies the muscles of the joint and the skin over the attachment of the muscles. Therefore the stratum fibrosum is the source for extensive sensory data that affect the joint, muscles, and skin in the area.

The inner layer, or stratum synovium, of the joint capsule is highly vascularized but poorly innervated and is insensitive to pain but undergoes vasodilation in response to heat and vasoconstriction in response to cold. The stratum synovium produces matrix collagen synovial fluid and serves as an entry point for nutrients and an exit point for waste materials. **Synovial fluid** is a thick, colorless fluid that resembles uncooked egg white. Synovial fluid lubricates the joint and provides nutrition to the tissues within the synovial cavity.

Practical Application

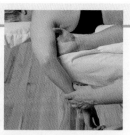

The joint design of our body not only helps provide stability for the joint but also permits motion. Small sacs called *bursae* are filled with synovial fluid and are located near some joints. As discussed before, bursae lie in areas subject to stress and help ease movement over and around the joints. In addition, synovial joints often have accessory structures such as fibrocartilaginous disks and plates or menisci. Menisci, disks, and the synovial fluid help prevent excessive compression of opposing joint surfaces.

The same structures that hold joints together also serve to maintain joint space or hold joints apart. When these structures weaken and become worn, the joint cavity is not maintained as effectively, and the ends of bones begin to contact each other and rub together. Friction develops, and production of synovial fluid increases in an attempt to reduce friction and maintain joint space. The end result of the deterioration most often is called "osteoarthritis" but more accurately is called *degenerative joint disease.* Massage application can be used to improve movement and decrease the pain in the diseased joint.

JOINT MOTION

SECTION OBJECTIVES

Chapter objective covered in this section:
4. Demonstrate the principles of joint motion.
After completing this chapter, the student will be able to perform the following:
- Define arthrokinematics.
- Describe joint play.
- Define osteokinematics.
- Demonstrate and explain joint movement to identify range of motion.
- Explain three categories of osteokinematic movement.
- Explain hypomobility and hypermobility.
- Define *end feel.*
- Describe the structures that contribute to joint stability.
- Describe joint movement in the three planes of movement of the body
- Demonstrate and name the general joint movements.
- Demonstrate and name joint movement specific to the forearm, wrist, thumb, ankle, and foot.
- Demonstrate and name joint movement specific to the shoulder girdle and shoulder joint.
- Demonstrate and name joint movement specific to the spine and pelvis.
- Describe the classification of synovial joint movement.
- Define *kinematic chains.*

Categories of Joint Movement

Joints are designed to permit body movement. The specifics of the design, including the size and shapes of the bones and the connective structure, influence the two types of movement of joints.

There are two categories of joint movement.

- *Arthrokinematic movement:* Arthrokinematic movements are small, involuntary movements that occur inside the joint capsule at the joint surfaces.
- *Osteokinematic movement:* This term describes the actual direction the bones move and includes extension, flexion, adduction, abduction, and internal and external rotation.

Arthrokinematics

The term **arthrokinematics** refers to movements of the articulating surfaces of the bones at joint surfaces. Most often, one of the joint surfaces is more stable than the other and serves as a base for the motion, whereas the other surface moves on this relatively fixed base.

The terms *roll, slide,* and *spin* describe the type of motion that the moving part performs (Figure 8-11).

- A *roll* refers to the rolling of one joint surface on another, similar to a bowling ball rolling down an alley. In the knee the femoral condyles roll on the fixed tibial surface.
- *Sliding* refers to the gliding of one component over another, as when you slide on ice. When the scapula elevates and depresses, it slides on the underlying rib cage.
- *Spin* refers to a rotation of the movable component, as when a top spins. The head of the radius spins on the capitulum of the humerus during supination and pronation of the forearm.

Combinations of rolling, sliding, and spinning occur during the process of joint motion. A large amount of motion can occur in a confined space by combining motions. When a moving component in a joint alternately rolls in one direction while sliding in the opposite direction, the range of motion available to the joint increases and opposing joint surfaces remain in contact with each other. Another method of increasing the range of available motion is by permitting both components to move at the same time. The humerus and the scapula move together during flexion and extension and during abduction and adduction at the glenohumeral joint.

Joint Play

The involuntary movements that occur between articular surfaces, which have nothing to do with the range of motion of a joint produced by muscles, are an essential component of joint motion and must occur for the joint to function normally. Called **joint play,** these small movements are essential for proper joint function.

The rolling and sliding movements of the articular surfaces are not usually visible or under voluntary control. An externally applied force, such as that applied by a therapist or physician, can produce movement of one articular surface on another, and the amount of joint play present can be assessed.

A door hinge is an excellent example. If you examine a door hinge, you will find that there are two plates, one attached to the door frame and one attached to the door. Between the two plates is a cylinder, and inside the cylinder is a pin. The pin fits inside the cylinder with just enough space around it so that the pin is free to rotate in the cylinder, allowing the door to swing. The distance the door swings is comparable to the range of motion of a joint, whereas the amount of space in the cylinder that allows the pin to roll is comparable to joint play.

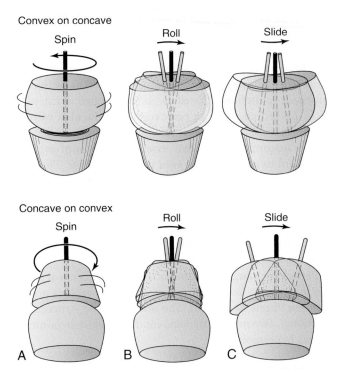

FIGURE 8-11 Arthrokinematic movements. **A,** Spin. **B,** Roll. **C,** Slide. (From Malone TR, McPoil T, Nitz AJ: *Orthopedic and sports physical therapy,* ed 3, St Louis, 1997, Mosby.)

In an optimal situation a joint has a sufficient amount of play to allow normal motion. For the human body the amount of joint play is almost always approximately $\frac{1}{8}$ inch, no matter which synovial joint is being examined or the amount of range of motion of that joint. If the supporting joint structures are lax, the joint may have too much play and become unstable. If the joint structures are tight or if inflammation or degeneration is present, the joint has too little movement between the articular surfaces, the amount of joint play is reduced, and range of motion may be restricted.

Osteokinematics

Osteokinematics refers to the movement of the bones by action of the muscles rather than the movement of the articular surfaces. The amount of movement available through which a joint can be moved is called the **range of motion (ROM)** of the joint. ROM is a measurement. ROM measurements determine the amount of movement allowed at a joint. Not everyone has the same ROM. Aging, disease, obesity, trauma, and injury all may affect a person's ROM. ROM is measured by active or passive movement of the joint. The anatomic position is considered the 0-degree point for measurement purposes.

Three categories of osteokinematic movement are anatomic, physiologic, and pathologic.

Anatomic osteokinematic movement refers to the amount of motion available to a joint within its structural limits. A number of factors determine the extent of the anatomic range, including the shape of the joint surfaces, the joint capsule, ligaments, muscle bulk, and surrounding musculotendinous and bony structures. Some joints have no bony joint limitations to motion, and the movement is limited only by soft-tissue structures. For example, the knee joint has no bony limitations to motion. Flexion is limited by soft tissues, often muscles, whereas extension stops with ligament stretch. Other joints have definite bony restrictions to motion in addition to soft-tissue limitations. The elbow joint is limited in extension (close-packed position) by bony contact of the ulna with the olecranon fossa of the humerus.

The anatomic motion may extend the limits of available movement to a point where joint injury can occur. Therefore many joints have an established **physiologic range of motion** set by the nervous system from information provided by joint sensory receptors. Physiologic ROM is defined as "active ROM" (i.e., what the client can do). Usually, this physiologic ROM is less than the anatomic ROM, preventing a joint from being positioned where injury could occur.

Pathologic range of motion occurs when motion at a joint fails to reach the normal physiologic range or exceeds normal anatomic limits of motion. The limits may be structural or functional. Two main pathologic conditions exist: hypomobility and hypermobility.

Hypomobility

When the ROM is less than what normally would be permitted by the structure, the joint is hypomobile. **Hypomobility** may be caused by bony or cartilaginous blocks to motion or by the inability of the capsule, ligaments, or surrounding tissues to elongate sufficiently to allow a normal ROM. Contracture, which describes the shortening of soft-tissue structures around a joint, is one cause of hypomobility.

An increased sensitivity and reactivity of joint receptors can cause the nervous system to increase muscle tension patterns, which in turn would limit ROM because muscles would not return to their normal resting length. The result would be hypomobility of joint movement even though nothing is dysfunctional in the joint itself. If this limited range is maintained, the joint capsule often alters tissue structure and becomes dysfunctional itself. These conditions are much more difficult to manage because of the complexities of dysfunctional patterns and compensation throughout the body.

Hypermobility

Hypermobility may be caused by a failure to limit motion by the bony or soft tissues and results in instability. Weak or flaccid muscles can contribute to hypermobility because they are less able to provide a stabilizing force to the joints. The joint may be subject to more trauma or damage because of excessive ROM, instability of the surrounding structures, or inability to withstand stresses.

End Feel

The ability to palpate normal end feel and to distinguish changes from normal end feel is important in protecting joints during ROM assessment and massage application. The three major types of end feel are soft, hard or bony, and capsular. Soft end feel of a joint is the normal sensation for most physiologic limits of ROM. The joint moves in a normal arc and, when the range limit is reached, a small, pliable give remains

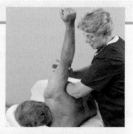
if slightly more pressure is given. The space identified is the range between the physiologic and anatomic barriers. Bony or hard end feel is characterized by a hard and abrupt limit to joint movement. This occurs when bone contacts bone at the end of the ROM. An example would be normal elbow extension. Usually, a hard end feel indicates a pathologic condition. Capsular end feel is characterized by a hard, leatherlike limitation of motion that has a slight give and occurs in full normal joint motion of the shoulder; otherwise, this type of end feel indicates dysfunction and is related to capsular restriction.

There are two additional characteristics to quantify the limitation of joint motion. A rebound, or spring-back, movement at the end of the ROM is characteristic of springy block. This sensation occurs with internal derangement of a joint, such as when cartilage is torn or connective tissue structures are binding. Asymptomatic limited ROM results from soft-tissue approximation and occurs when the soft tissue of body segments prevents further motion, such as at normal terminal elbow flexion when the arm and forearm meet and the muscles touch.

Joint Positions and Stability

In most of our synovial joints, the ends of the articulating surfaces of the bones are opposite in shape to each other, usually convex and concave. All synovial joints have only one position where the surfaces fit together and in which maximal

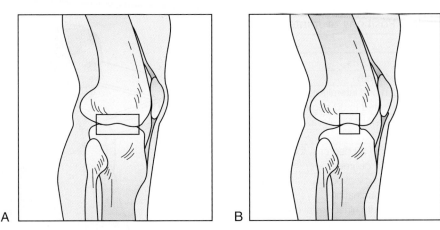

FIGURE 8-12 The congruence of articular surfaces. **A,** Close-packed position. **B,** Loose-packed position.

contact between the opposing surfaces occurs. This is called the **close-packed position,** or locked position, and it allows no movement. The close-packed position is usually at the extreme end of the ROM, where the joint surfaces are compressed and the joint exhibits its greatest stability. The position of extension is the close-packed position for the elbow, knee, and interphalangeal joints. When not in this position, the joint is said to be in the **loose-packed position,** or unlocked, where the amount of contact is reduced and movements of spin, roll, and glide may occur (Figure 8-12). Each joint also has a **least-packed position** in which the capsule is at its most lax. Joints tend to assume this position when inflammation occurs to accommodate the increased volume of synovial fluid. In an injured joint that has swelling, the close-packed position is a position of discomfort. In the least-packed position the joint cavity has a greater volume, and therefore the position is one of comfort.

Movement in and out of the close-packed position is likely to have a beneficial effect on joint nutrition because the movement squeezes out the synovial fluid during each compression against the cartilage, and the fluid is reabsorbed when the compression is removed (Tables 8-1 and 8-2).

Movements of Joints

Cardinal Planes

Joint movement is named for the plane in which the movement occurs. Defining joint and segment motions and recording the location in space of specific points on the body both require a reference point (Figure 8-13). In kinesiology the three-dimensional, rectangular coordinate system is used to describe anatomic relationships of the body. Three imaginary planes are arranged perpendicular to each other through the body. These planes are called *cardinal planes* of the body.

- The *frontal (coronal) plane* divides the body into front and back parts. Motions that occur in this plane are defined as right and left lateral flexion or as *abduction* and *adduction*. Right and left lateral flexions are side-bending at the head, neck, or trunk. Abduction is a position or motion of the segment away from the midline, regardless of which segment moves. Abduction of the hip occurs when the thigh segment moves away from the midline or the pelvic segment

Table 8-1	Least-Packed Positions of Joints
Joint(s)	**Position**
Spine	Midway between flexion and extension
Temporomandibular	Mouth slightly open
Glenohumeral	55 degrees abduction, 30 degrees horizontal adduction
Acromioclavicular	Arm resting by side in normal physiologic position
Sternoclavicular	Arm resting by side in normal physiologic position
Elbow	70 degrees flexion, 10 degrees supination
Radiohumeral	Full extension and full supination
Proximal radioulnar	70 degrees flexion, 35 degrees supination
Distal radioulnar	10 degrees supination
Wrist	Neutral with slight ulnar deviation
Carpometacarpal	Midway between abduction/adduction and flexion/extension
Thumb	Slight flexion
Interphalangeal	Slight flexion
Hip	30 degrees flexion, 30 degrees abduction, and slight lateral rotation
Knee	25 degrees flexion
Ankle	10 degrees plantar flexion, midway between maximum inversion or eversion
Subtalar	Midway between extremes of range of movement
Midtarsal	Midway between extremes of range of movement
Tarsometatarsal	Midway between extremes of range of movement
Metatarsophalangeal	Neutral
Interphalangeal	Slight flexion

From Magee DJ: *Orthopedic physical assessment,* ed 5, Philadelphia, 2008, Saunders.

approaches the thigh, as in tilting to the side while standing on one leg. Adduction is a position or motion toward the midline.

- The *sagittal plane* divides the body into right and left sides. Joint motions occurring in the sagittal plane are defined as *flexion* and *extension*. Flexion indicates that two segments

Table 8-2   Close-Packed Positions of Joints

Joint(s)	Position
Spine	Extension
Temporomandibular	Clenched teeth
Glenohumeral	Abduction and lateral rotation
Acromioclavicular	Arm abducted to 30 degrees
Sternoclavicular	Maximum shoulder elevation
Elbow	Extension
Radiohumeral	Elbow flexed 90 degrees, forearm supinated 5 degrees
Proximal radioulnar	5 degrees supination
Distal radioulnar	5 degrees supination
Wrist	Extension with ulnar deviation
Carpometacarpal	Full flexion
Thumb	Full opposition
Interphalangeal	Full extension
Hip	Full extension and medial rotation*
Knee	Full extension and lateral rotation of tibia
Ankle	Maximum dorsiflexion
Subtalar	Supination
Midtarsal	Supination
Tarsometatarsal	Supination
Metatarsophalangeal	Full extension
Interphalangeal	Full extension

From Magee DJ: *Orthopedic physical assessment,* ed 5, Philadelphia, 2008, Saunders.
*Some authors include abduction.

approach each other; for example, flexion of the elbow may be accomplished by flexion of the forearm on the arm or by flexion of the arm on the forearm, as in a pull-up. Extension occurs when two segments move away from each other.

• The *horizontal/transverse plane* divides the body into upper and lower parts and is like a view from above. Rotations occur in this plane. Medial rotation, inward or internal rotation, is transverse rotation oriented to the anterior surface of the body. Medial rotation of the hip brings points marked on the anterior surface of the pelvis and femur closer together regardless of which of the segments moves. *Pronation* is the term for medial rotation of the forearm. Lateral rotation, outward or external rotation, is in the opposite direction and is oriented to the posterior surface of the body. *Supination* is a term used at the forearm and is the reference point for the anatomic position.

Sagittal, frontal, and transverse planes may be laid through any point of the body. For example, laying three planes through the center of a joint, such as the hip joint, may be convenient for determining body points in relation to such a joint. In the hand the sagittal plane is centered through the third segment; in the foot the sagittal plane is centered through the second segment.

Motion or position away from the reference segment is called *abduction,* and motion toward the segment is called *adduction.* At the wrist the motion of abduction frequently is referred to as *radial deviation* (toward the radius), and adduction is called *ulnar deviation.* In the anatomic position the foot is at a right angle to the dorsal aspect of the leg in the sagittal plane. Movement of the foot toward the tibia is called *dorsiflexion,* and movement of the sole of the foot away from the tibia is called *plantar flexion.*

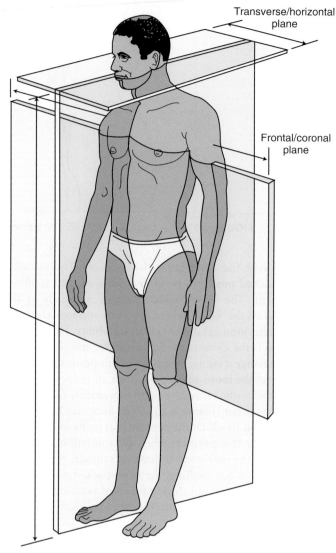

Transverse/horizontal plane

Frontal/coronal plane

Sagittal plane

FIGURE 8-13 The three imaginary planes of the body are called *cardinal planes.* (From Fritz S: *Mosby's fundamentals of therapeutic massage,* ed 5, St Louis, 2013, Mosby.)

The thumb is also a special case because it normally rotates 90 degrees from the plane of the hand. Thus motions of flexion and extension occur in the frontal plane, and abduction and adduction occur in the sagittal plane.

Joint design permits many different types of movement. Some joints permit only flexion and extension. Others permit a wide range of movements, depending largely on the joint structure. Some movement terms may be used to describe motion at several joints throughout the body, whereas other terms are specific to a joint or group of joints. Motions or positions of flexion, abduction, and medial and lateral rotation are recorded as they move toward 180 degrees (Box 8-2; Figures 8-14 and 8-15; and Activity 8-4).

Classification of Synovial Joints by Movements

Traditionally, synovial joints have been divided into three main categories based on the number of axes around which motion occurs. The three main categories are uniaxial, biaxial,

Box 8-2 Terms Describing Joint Movements

The following terms describe joint movements in general:
- **Flexion.** Bending movement that results in a decrease of the angle in a joint by bringing bones together. An example is the elbow joint when the hand is drawn to the shoulder.
- **Extension.** Straightening movement that results in an increase of the angle in a joint by moving bones apart. An example occurs when the hand is on the shoulder and moves away from the shoulder.
- **Abduction.** Lateral movement away from the midline of the trunk. An example is moving the arms or thighs out to the side.
- **Adduction.** Movement medially toward the midline of the trunk. An example is moving the arms to the side of the body or the thighs back to the anatomic position.
- **Diagonal Abduction.** Movement by a limb through a diagonal plane directly across and away from the midline of the body. An example is moving the right arm from in front of the left hip to in front of the right shoulder.
- **Diagonal Adduction.** Movement by a limb through a diagonal plane toward and across the midline of the body. An example is the return of the right arm from a flexed position to in front of the left hip.
- **Horizontal Abduction.** Movement of the humerus in the horizontal plane away from the midline of the body. The movement also is known as horizontal extension or transverse abduction.
- **Horizontal Adduction.** Movement of the humerus in the horizontal plane toward the midline of the body. The movement also is known as horizontal flexion or transverse adduction.
- **Circumduction.** Circular movement of a limb, combining the movements of flexion, extension, abduction, and adduction, to create a cone shape. An example is the shoulder joint moving in a circular fashion around a fixed point, as in doing arm circles.
- **Rotation.** Twisting or turning of a bone on its own axis. An example is turning the head from side to side to indicate "no."
- **Medial Rotation.** Rotary movement around the longitudinal axis of a bone toward the midline of the body. The movement also is known as inward rotation or internal rotation. An example is turning the palms of the hands from the anatomic position to facing backward.
- **Lateral Rotation.** Rotary movement around the longitudinal axis of a bone away from the midline of the body. The movement also is known as outward rotation or external rotation. An example is returning the palms from facing backward to the anatomic position so that they face forward.

The following terms describe movements specific to one of the following body parts: forearm, wrist, thumb, ankle, and foot:
- **Pronation.** Medial rotation of the radius where it lies diagonally across the ulna, resulting in the palm-down position of the forearm.
- **Supination.** Lateral rotation of the radius where it lies parallel to the ulna, resulting in the palm-up position of the forearm.
- **Radial Deviation or Wrist Abduction.** Abduction movement at the wrist joint of the thumb side of the hand toward the forearm.

- **Ulnar Deviation or Wrist Adduction.** Adduction movement at the wrist joint of the little finger side of the hand toward the forearm.
- **Opposition of the Thumb.** Diagonal movement of the thumb across the palmar surface of the hand to make contact with the fingers.
- **Eversion.** Turning of the sole of the foot outward or laterally. An example is moving the body weight to the inner edge of the foot.
- **Inversion.** Turning of the sole of the foot inward or medially. An example is moving our body weight to the outer edge of the foot.
- **Dorsiflexion (or Dorsal Flexion).** Movement of the ankle that results in the top of the foot moving toward the anterior tibia. An example of this is pointing the toes up.
- **Plantar Flexion.** Movement of the ankle that results in the foot or toes moving away from the anterior fibia. An example of this is pointing the toes down.

The following terms describe movements of the shoulder girdle and shoulder joint:
- **Elevation.** Movement of the shoulder girdle to become closer to the ears. Such movement occurs in shrugging of the shoulders.
- **Depression.** Inferior movement of the shoulder girdle. An example is returning to the normal position from a shoulder shrug.
- **Protraction.** Forward movement of the shoulder girdle away from the spine, also known as *abduction*.
- **Retraction.** Backward movement of the shoulder girdle toward the spine, also known as *adduction*.
- **Downward Rotation.** Rotary movement of the scapula such that the glenoid fossa orients downward (the inferior angle of the scapula moves medially). The movement occurs when the acromion process moves down.
- **Upward Rotation.** Rotary movement of the scapula such that the glenoid fossa orients upward (the inferior angle of the scapula moves laterally). The movement occurs when the acromion process moves up.

The following terms describe movements of the spinal and pelvic girdle joints:
- **Lateral Flexion (side bending).** Movement of the head, neck, or trunk laterally to the side.
- **Nutation (posterior pelvic tilt).** Forward motion of the base of the sacrum into the pelvis (tuck your tail) or the backward rotation of the ilium on the sacrum (see Figure B on p. 250).
- **Counternutation (anterior pelvic tilt).** Backward motion of the base of the sacrum out of the pelvis (wag your tail) or forward rotation of ilium on the sacrum (see Figure A on p. 250).
- **Iliosacral motion.** This is ilium movement on the sacrum. Movements of the ilium include anterior/posterior rotation, superior/inferior movement, and medial/lateral flaring.
- **Sacroilial motion.** This is sacral movement on the ilium. Movements of the sacrum include flexion/extension and rotation.

Continued

Box 8-2 Terms Describing Joint Movements—cont'd

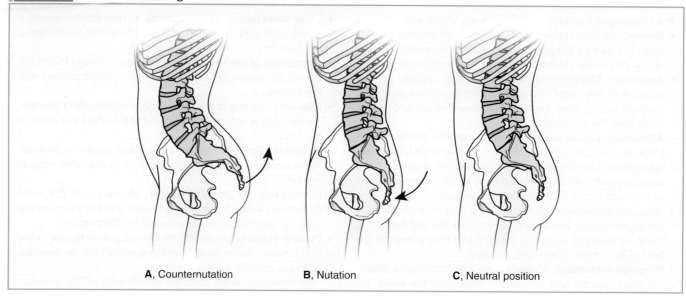

A, Counternutation   **B,** Nutation   **C,** Neutral position

and triaxial. A further subdivision of the joints is made according to the shape and configuration of the ends of the bony components.

A **uniaxial** joint is constructed so that motion of the bony components is allowed in only one of the planes around a single axis. The two types of joints in this category are hinge joints and pivot joints.

- A **hinge joint** allows flexion and extension in one direction, changing the angle of the bones at the joint, as in a door hinge. Examples include the elbow and interphalangeal joints.
- A **pivot joint** allows rotation around the length of the bone. A pivot (trochoid) joint is a type of joint constructed so that one component is shaped like a ring and the other component is shaped such that it can rotate within the ring. Examples include the joint between the first and second cervical vertebrae and the joint at the proximal ends of the radius and the ulna.

Biaxial joints allow movement in two planes around two axes. The two types of joints in this category are condyloid joints and saddle joints.

- A **condyloid joint,** also called an *ellipsoid joint,* allows movement in two directions, but one motion dominates. The joint surfaces in a condyloid joint are shaped such that one bony surface is concave and the other is convex. Movements allowed are flexion, extension, abduction, and adduction. Examples include the wrist joint, metacarpophalangeal joints, metatarsophalangeal joints, and the atlantooccipital joint.
- In a **saddle joint,** each joint surface is convex in one plane and concave in the other, and these surfaces fit together similar to a rider on a saddle. Movements allowed are flexion, extension, abduction, adduction, and a small degree of axial rotation. Examples include the joint between the wrist and the metacarpal bone of the thumb (first carpometacarpal joint) and the sternoclavicular joint.

Triaxial joints are joints in which the bony components are free to move in three planes around three axes. Motion at these joints may also occur in oblique planes. The two types of joints in this category are ball-and-socket joints and plane or gliding joints.

- A **ball-and-socket joint** allows movement in many directions around a central point. Ball-and-socket joints are formed when a ball-shaped convex surface is fitted into a concave socket. Movements allowed are flexion, extension, abduction, adduction, and rotation. This type of joint gives the greatest freedom of movement but also is the easiest to dislocate. Examples are the hip and shoulder joints.
- A **gliding joint,** also called *synovial plane joint,* permits gliding between two or more bones. These joints allow only a gliding motion in various planes. Examples include the superior tibiofibular joint, acromioclavicular joint, costovertebral joints, and zygapophyseal joints between the vertebral arches (Figure 8-16).

Kinematic Chains

A **kinematic chain** is a system of rigid bodies, or bones, connected together by joints. Kinematic chains describe the association between joints as they operate in relation to one another. The concept of kinematic chains is useful for analyzing human motion and the effects of injury and disease on the joints of the body. Two types are closed kinematic chains and open kinematic chains.

Closed Kinematic Chain

Some joints of the human body are linked together into a series in which motion at one of the joints is accompanied by motion at an adjacent joint. This is called a **closed kinematic chain.** For instance, when a person is standing erect and bends both knees, simultaneous motion must occur at the ankle and hip joints. The interaction between joints in the chain is

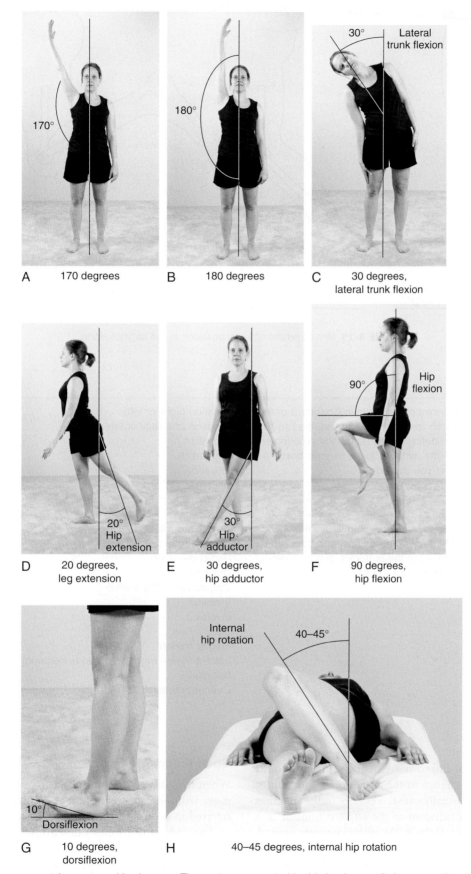

A 170 degrees

B 180 degrees

C 30 degrees, lateral trunk flexion

D 20 degrees, leg extension

E 30 degrees, hip adductor

F 90 degrees, hip flexion

G 10 degrees, dorsiflexion

H 40–45 degrees, internal hip rotation

FIGURE 8-14 Joint movement is measured in degrees. The system presented in this book uses 0 degree as the reference point for the standard anatomic position. Motions or position of flexion, extension, abduction, and medial and lateral rotation are recorded as they move toward 180 degrees.

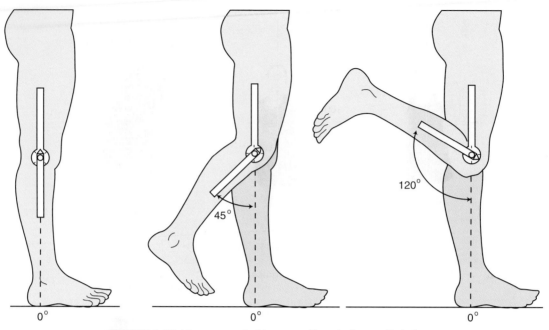

FIGURE 8-15 Measurement of knee positions in the sagittal plane.

✏ ACTIVITY 8-4

Find the definitions of the joint movements in Chapter 3 of this text, and compare them to the ones you just studied in this chapter. Then, using both definitions, design a joint movement sequence that moves all the synovial joints in your body. An example is provided to get you started.

Example

Flexion

Drop chin to chest, make a fist, bend elbows so that hands touch the shoulders, bring a knee to the chest and then repeat with other knee, bring the heel to the buttocks, and then repeat with other heel, curling toes toward the sole of the feet.

Your Turn

Abduction
Adduction
Extension
Horizontal abduction
Horizontal adduction
Circumduction

Rotation (right or left)
Rotation (medially or laterally)
Pronation
Supination
Elevation
Depression
Protraction
Retraction
Downward rotation
Upward rotation
Radial deviation
Ulnar deviation
Opposition of the thumb
Eversion
Inversion
Dorsiflexion
Plantar flexion
Lateral flexion (right or left; side bending)
Nutation
Counternutation

---

predictable in terms of linked movement because the joints are interdependent. A change in the structure or function of one joint in the chain usually causes a change in the function of a joint immediately adjacent to the affected joint or at a distal joint. For example, if the ROM at the knee was limited, the hip and ankle joints would have to compensate so that the foot could clear the floor to avoid stumbling when a person walks. A closed kinematic chain occurs when the foot is on the floor or the hand grasps an immovable object. If the hand applies a compressive force to a fixed object, a closed kinematic chain is created.

Open Kinematic Chain

When the ends of the limbs or parts of the body are free to move without causing motion at another joint, the system is referred to as an **open kinematic chain.**

The ends of our limbs often are not fixed but are free to move without necessarily causing motion at another joint. When a person lifts the lower limb from the ground, the knee is free to bend without causing or changing motion at the hip or ankle. The motion of waving the hand may occur at the wrist without causing motion of the elbow or shoulder. In an open kinematic chain, motion does not occur in a predictable

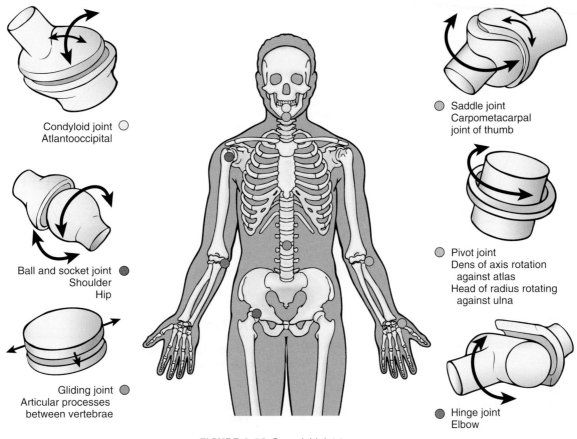

FIGURE 8-16 Synovial joint types.

fashion because joints may function independently (i.e., in unison). For example, you can wave your whole upper limb by moving your arm at the shoulder or by moving only at the wrist.

Closed and open kinematic chains influence ergonomics, exercise, rehabilitation, and robot design.

Practical Application

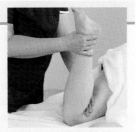

An understanding of joint movement is fundamental to any therapeutic massage system. Many systems, particularly movement modalities, are based on body movement patterns provided by joints. A comparison of these systems, such as yoga, tai chi, or Feldenkrais, reveals the intricate and interactive interplay of the joint moved alone or in a dynamic combination of movement.

All types of athletes depend on proper functioning of their joints, as do dancers and others who purposefully move their bodies, including massage therapists. These people often seek out therapeutic massage to enhance their performance and maintain or restore optimal functioning. Especially when working with closed kinematic chains, the practitioner must address all joints in the pattern for proper function to be restored in any particular area.

IDENTIFICATION AND PALPATION OF SPECIFIC JOINTS

SECTION OBJECTIVES

Chapter objective covered in this section:

5. Identify and palpate individual joints of the skull, shoulder, elbow, wrist, and hand.
6. Identify and palpate individual joints of the pelvis and hip, knee, ankle and foot, spine, and thorax.

After completing this section, the student will be able to perform the following:

- Palpate and describe the following jointed areas:
  - Joints of the skull
  - Joints of the shoulder
  - Joints of the elbow
  - Joints of the wrist and hand
  - Joints of the pelvis and hip
  - Joints of the knee
  - Joints of the ankle and foot
  - Joints of the spine and thorax

As massage therapists, we touch and move the body during massage for both assessment and massage intervention. When we are touching the body to gather assessment information, we are palpating, which is an essential assessment skill. Joint movement is also an assessment skill that is necessary to learn. The information and activities in this section will help you develop palpation and joint movement assessment skills.

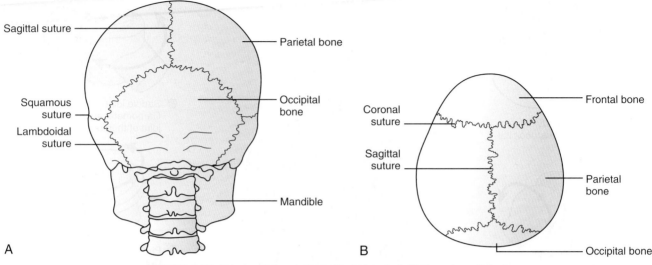

FIGURE 8-17 Sutures of the skull. **A,** Posterior skull. **B,** Top view of skull.

Joints of the Skull

The joints of the skull are the cranial sutures and the temporomandibular joint.

Cranial Sutures

Recall from Chapter 7 that the four cranial sutures are as follows:

1. Coronal: between the frontal and parietal bones
2. Sagittal: between the two parietal bones
3. Squamous: between the parietal and temporal bones
4. Lambdoidal: between the occipital and parietal bones

Palpation

Palpate the sutures of the skull as follows:

- Place your fingertips on your eyebrows and slide them firmly up your forehead to the top of your skull to where you feel the first indentation; this is the coronal suture.
- Pressing your finger firmly into the suture, follow the indentation down on either side to where the suture ends, about midway between the top of the ear and the eye.
- Move posteriorly along the next indentation that arcs over your ear; this is the squamous suture.
- Behind the ear, just above the mastoid process, palpate the indentation that moves in an arc superiorly and posteriorly; this is the lambdoidal suture.
- At the midway point of the lambdoidal suture, find the indentation that travels superiorly and anteriorly along the middle of the skull to join with the coronal suture; this is the sagittal suture (Figure 8-17).

Temporomandibular Joint

The temporomandibular joint (TMJ) consists of the following structures:

- **Articulating Bones.** Temporal bone and mandible
- **Joint Type.** Synovial modified hinge joint
- **Ligaments.** Lateral temporomandibular ligament from the zygomatic arch to the mandible; sphenomandibular ligament from the sphenoid to the mandible (not pictured in

✎ ACTIVITY 8-5

Move your temporomandibular joint through each of the five movement patterns.

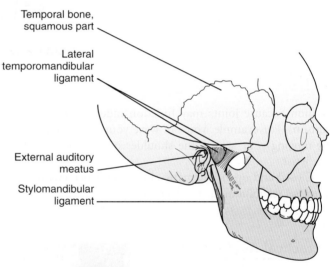

FIGURE 8-18 Temporomandibular joint.

Figure 8-18); and the stylomandibular ligament from the styloid process to the mandible

The temporomandibular joint is one of the strongest joints in the body and is the only biarticular joint in the body. This means that the joint has two separate cavities. This construction requires a balanced action in the joint so that both jointed areas work freely. When this is not the case, the result is temporomandibular joint dysfunction.

The temporomandibular joint allows the following five movements: depression, elevation, protraction, retraction, and lateral deviation to the left and right.

Palpation

- Palpate the joint just in front of each ear while opening and closing the jaw (Figure 8-18 and Activity 8-5).

Joints of the Shoulder

The shoulder joints include the glenohumeral, sternoclavicular, and acromioclavicular joints and the scapulocostal junction.

Glenohumeral Joint

The glenohumeral joint consists of the following structures:
- **Articulating Bones.** Humerus and scapula
- **Joint Type.** Synovial ball and socket
- **Ligaments.** Glenohumeral: inferior, middle, and superior, from the glenoid cavity of the scapula to the head of humerus; coracohumeral ligament from coracoid process to the greater and lesser tuberosity of humerus (not pictured in Figure 8-19). The glenohumeral joint is the main joint of the shoulder and the most mobile joint in the body. The joint is shallow, which allows for its high degree of mobility, but also accounts for its decreased stability. Because of this decrease in stability, it can be easily injured. Most of the support for this joint is provided by the muscles of the joint (especially the rotator cuff muscles, which are discussed in Chapter 9). The shoulder joint does get considerable stability from the glenoid labrum, which acts as a lip to the shallow fossa, deepening it. Some further support is provided by the ligaments and a loose joint capsule, with little support by the bony structures themselves. The tendons of the rotator cuff muscles provide additional stability (Figure 8-19).

The glenohumeral joint allows the following movements: flexion, extension, abduction, adduction, medial (internal) rotation, and lateral (external) rotation.

Sternoclavicular Joint

The sternoclavicular joint consists of the following structures:

- **Articulating Bones.** Clavicle and manubrium of sternum
- **Joint Type.** Synovial saddle joint
- **Ligaments.** Anterior and posterior sternoclavicular ligament from clavicle to sternum; interclavicular ligament joining both clavicles; costoclavicular ligament from clavicle to first rib; and a fibrocartilaginous (articular) disk located within the joint

The movements of the sternoclavicular joint follow the movements of the scapula and clavicle because no muscle works directly on this joint. A decrease or loss of mobility in this joint directly affects shoulder movement. This joint is the only direct connection between the axial skeleton and the shoulder girdle and arm (Figure 8-20).

The sternoclavicular joint allows the following movements: elevation, depression, protraction, retraction, upward rotation, and downward rotation.

Acromioclavicular Joint

The acromioclavicular joint consists of the following structures:
- **Articulating Bones.** Clavicle and scapula
- **Joint Type.** Synovial gliding joint
- **Ligaments.** Acromioclavicular ligament from the acromion process to the clavicle and coracoclavicular ligament from the coracoid process to the clavicle

The acromioclavicular joint may contain a fibrocartilaginous disk. Note that some people do not have an acromioclavicular joint because the bones have fused.

Although a small joint, the acromioclavicular joint is important for shoulder movements (Figure 8-21).

The acromioclavicular joint allows the following movements: anterior and posterior gliding, upward and downward rotation, and elevation and depression. Movements that separate the joint are also possible (Box 8-3).

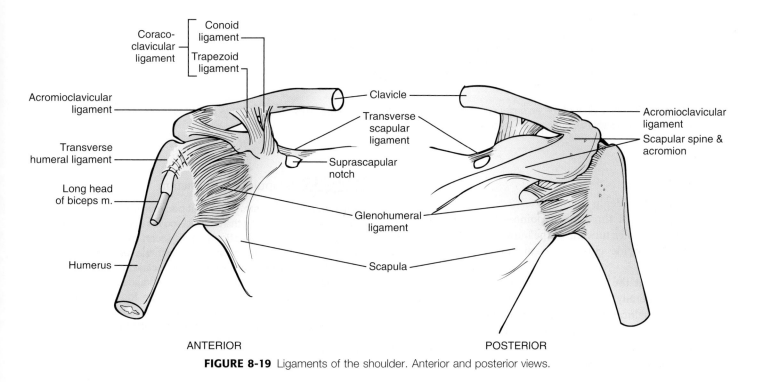

FIGURE 8-19 Ligaments of the shoulder. Anterior and posterior views.

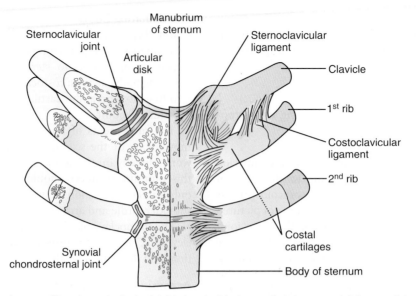

FIGURE 8-20 Joints of the sternum. The sternoclavicular joint is located between the sternum and the medial end of the clavicle. The sternoclavicular joint contains an articular disk.

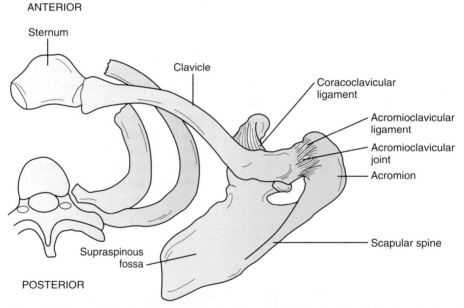

FIGURE 8-21 Superior view of the acromial clavicular joint of the shoulder girdle. This view illustrates the attachments of the lateral end of the clavicle, especially to the acromion and coracoid process.

Palpation

Palpate the shoulder as follows:

- The position of three major points—the tip of the acromion, the greater tubercle of the humerus, and the coracoid process—provide clues as to the exact position of the shoulder.
- Beginning at the jugular notch of the manubrium, move slightly laterally to locate the sternoclavicular joint. To confirm the location of the joint, hold lightly while moving the same side arm into flexion and extension. Compare this joint movement with the direction of the scapular movements.

| Box 8-3 | Scapulocostal Junction |

Although not a true structural joint because it does not involve bone-to-bone contact, the scapula moves across the rib cage (thorax), creating a functional joint. Much of the movement results from sternoclavicular action, with the rest of the action provided by movement in the acromioclavicular joint. If the scapula is limited in its movement, all shoulder movement is restricted, although one can compensate for restrictions in retraction most easily. The movements of the scapulocostal junction include elevation, depression, protraction, retraction, and upward and downward rotation.

- Continue along the clavicle, following the convex curve of the medial two thirds and the concave curve of the lateral third.
- Reach back to the spine of the scapula and follow it laterally; at its end move superiorly and anteriorly, where it becomes the acromion (the high point of the shoulder). This is a large flat area, with a slight concavity.
- Find the anterior tip of the acromion and move slightly medially; the elevated ridge marks the start of the acromioclavicular joint.
- Move back to the top of the acromion, then laterally and inferiorly to the outer edge of the greater tubercle of the humerus.
- Moving anteriorly and medially, locate the lesser tubercle.
- Continuing medially on to the soft tissues of the anterior chest, press in to locate the coracoid process of the scapula just below the concave portion of the lateral clavicle.
- The glenohumeral joint, where the arm connects to the body, is easiest to palpate when the arm is in passive extension or actively moving through circumduction.
- The fibrous capsule of the rotator cuff (muscles and tendons that surround the joint) often makes feeling the bony structures difficult.
- Of the four muscles of the rotator cuff, three—the supraspinatus, infraspinatus, and teres minor—attach together on the greater tubercle of the humerus, and their attachments are easiest to palpate.
- The fourth, the subscapularis, inserts on the lesser tubercle and is not palpated easily (Activity 8-6).

Joints of the Elbow

The joints of the elbow joint region are the ulnohumeral, radiohumeral, and proximal radioulnar joints.

Move your shoulder joints, individually and (if possible) together, through the ranges of motion.

Ulnohumeral and Radiohumeral Joints

The ulnohumeral and radiohumeral joints consist of the following structures:
- **Articulating Bones.** Humerus with the ulna and humerus with the radius
- **Joint Type.** Synovial hinge (ulnohumeral)
- **Ligaments.** Medial (ulnar) collateral: anterior, posterior, transverse fibers from the medial epicondyle of the humerus and olecranon process of the ulna to the coronoid process of the ulna; radial collateral from the lateral epicondyle of the humerus to the annular ligament; and annular ligament from the anterior portion of radial notch around to the posterior margin of radial notch

Because of the bony structure and the support of muscles and ligaments, the elbow is a stable joint. Most elbow action involves the ulnohumeral joint, even though the radius also interacts with the humerus. During flexion the trochlear notch of the ulna slides on the humeral trochlea, while the head of the radius slides on the capitulum. In extension the movements are reversed and stop when the olecranon process reaches its anatomic barrier at the olecranon fossa. The elbow is one of the few areas in the body where a hard end feel and anatomic barrier occurs. Hyperextension is possible in those individuals who have a small olecranon process or a large olecranon fossa (Figure 8-22).

The ulnohumeral and radiohumeral joints allow the following movements: flexion and extension

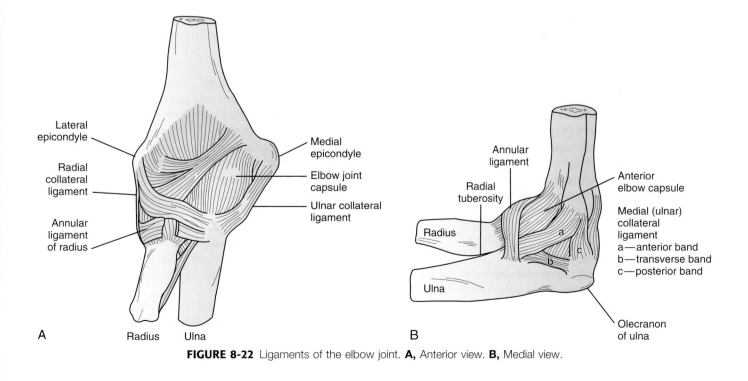

FIGURE 8-22 Ligaments of the elbow joint. **A,** Anterior view. **B,** Medial view.

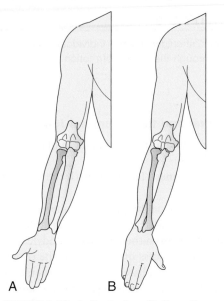

FIGURE 8-23   A, Supination. **B,** Pronation.

Radioulnar Joints

The three radioulnar joints are the proximal, middle, and distal radioulnar joints.

The proximal radioulnar joints consist of the following structures:
- **Articulating Bones.** Radius and ulna
- **Joint Type.** Synovial pivot (proximal radioulnar joint)
- **Ligaments.** Annular ligament (see the previous joint)

The proximal radioulnar joint articulates at the proximal ends of the radius and ulna and is listed as part of the elbow complex because it has the same soft-tissue support as the elbow joint and most of the actions occur in this area (see Figure 8-22). The head of the radius moves clockwise and counterclockwise around the ulna at the proximal end. During pronation the distal cut of the radius crosses the ulna and ends diagonal to the ulna, allowing the palm to face down. Supination returns the radius and ulna to parallel positions, with the palm facing up, as in holding a bowl of soup (soup = supination, or up as in sUPination—a clue to remembering the position).

The interosseous membrane forms the middle radioulnar joint and connects the shafts of the ulna and radius; its fibers run in a diagonal pattern perpendicular to one another. This membrane is taut during supination and relaxed in pronation. The distal radioulnar joint is located between the distal ends of the radius and ulna (Figure 8-23).

The proximal radioulnar joint allows the following movements: pronation and supination.

Palpation

Palpate the elbow as follows:
- Locate the medial and lateral epicondyles of the humerus and the olecranon process of the ulna.
- A bursa lies between the olecranon process and the skin. The bursa will feel like a small bubble.
- The synovial membrane is most accessible to examination between the olecranon and the epicondyles. You can trace

Move your elbow joint through the range of motion positions.

the ulna by following the bony ridge toward the wrist from the olecranon.
- The area between the medial epicondyle and olecranon may be sensitive because of the proximity of the ulnar nerve.
- Supinate and pronate the forearm at the radioulnar joints, and feel the radius rotate on the ulna (Activity 8-7).

Joints of the Wrist and Hand

The joints of the wrist and hand include the radiocarpal and carpometacarpal joints.

Radiocarpal (Wrist) Joint

The radiocarpal joint consists of the following structures:
- **Articulating Bones.** Radius, scaphoid, and lunate, with some triquetral bone involvement
- **Joint Type.** Synovial condyloid
- **Ligaments.** Palmar radiocarpal ligament from the radius to the scaphoid, lunate, and triquetral bones; palmar ulnocarpal ligament from the ulna to the scaphoid, lunate, and triquetral bones; and dorsal radiocarpal ligament from the radius to the scaphoid, lunate, and triquetral bones

The wrist is called the *radiocarpal joint* because the radius alone articulates with the carpal bones. The ulna joins the wrist indirectly by a disk that articulates with the carpal bones. This allows forearm pronation and supination to take place without affecting any wrist movements. The joint capsule of the wrist is loose in the anterior and posterior directions, allowing easy flexion and extension, but tight laterally and medially, allowing for minimal ulnar deviation and radial deviation

The radiocarpal joint allows the following movements: flexion, extension, and radial and ulnar deviation.

Hand Joints

This intricate pattern of hand joints is where all the movements involving the fingers take place. The hand is capable of a variety of functions that vary from the precise handling of objects to acts of great strength. The opposable thumb allows us to grasp and manipulate objects. Because the thumb in the resting position is rotated relative to the rest of the fingers, the thumb faces the other fingers.

The first carpometacarpal joint of the thumb consists of the following structures:
- **Articulating Bones.** First metacarpal with trapezium
- **Joint Type.** Synovial saddle
- **Ligaments.** Radial and ulnar collateral and anterior and posterior oblique ligaments of the thumb, with assistance from the articular capsule

The first carpometacarpal joint allows the following movements: opposition (abduction, flexion, and medial rotation) and reposition (adduction, extension, and lateral rotation).

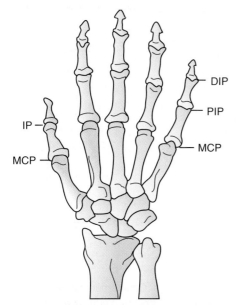

FIGURE 8-24 Hand joints. *DIP,* Distal interphalangeal joints; *IP,* interphalangeal joints; *MCP,* metacarpophalangeal joints; *PIP,* proximal interphalangeal joints.

The metacarpophalangeal (MCP) joints between the metacarpals of the palm and the phalanges of the fingers form condyloid joints that allow flexion, extension, abduction, and adduction of the fingers.

Joints between phalanges are hinge joints that permit flexion and extension. These joints are called *proximal interphalangeal (PIP) joints* and *distal interphalangeal (DIP) joints* (Figure 8-24).

Palpation

Palpate the wrist and hand as follows:
- At the wrist, locate the bony tips of the radius (laterally) and the ulna (medially).
- On the dorsum of the wrist, palpate the groove of the radiocarpal or wrist joint.
- Each carpal bone within the hand cannot be identified readily, so instead palpate the carpal structure while moving the wrist. Palpate each of the five metacarpals and the proximal, middle, and distal phalanges and connecting joints.
- Remember that the thumb lacks a middle phalanx.
- Partially flex your fingers, and find the groove marking the MCP joint of each finger. The joint is located at the first knuckle and is palpated best on either side of the extensor tendon (Activity 8-8).

Joints of the Pelvis and Hip

The joints of the hip and pelvis include the sacroiliac joints, symphysis pubis, and hip joints (Box 8-4).

Sacroiliac Joint

The sacroiliac joint consists of the following structures:
- **Articulating Bones.** Sacrum and the two ilia
- **Joint Type.** The joint is part synovial (anterior half) and part fibrous.

ACTIVITY 8-8

Move your hand and fingers through the ranges of motion.

- **Ligaments.** The anterior sacroiliac ligament covers the anterior and inferior aspects of the joint; the interosseous sacroiliac ligament links the sacrum and the ilium; and the dorsal sacroiliac ligament covers the posterior aspect of the joint. The sacrotuberous ligament connects the sacrum with the ischial tuberosity, and the sacrospinous ligament connects the sacrum to the ischial spine.

The sacroiliac joints connect the ilia to the spine, transfer the weight of the body to the hip, and work as shock absorbers during walking and running. Ligaments provide much support. They are more relaxed in the female. This laxity increases with hormones released during menstrual cycles and especially during pregnancy.

The movement allowed is a small but important anterior, posterior, lateral, and medial rotation in a side-lying, figure-of-eight pattern. This rotary movement of the pelvis allows the vertebral column to remain relatively still as we walk. When the sacroiliac joint does not move, the sacral lumbar junction compensates for the lack of rotation, putting strain on the spine. No direct muscle action occurs at the sacroiliac joint. Instead, the sacroiliac joint moves as a result of other joint movements in the area.

Symphysis Pubis

The symphysis pubis (also called *pubic symphysis*) consists of the following structures:
- **Articulating Bones.** The two pubic bones
- **Joint Type.** Cartilaginous
- **Ligaments.** The superior pubic ligament supports the anterior, posterior, and superior aspects, and the arcuate (inferior) pubic ligament supports the inferior aspect (these ligaments are not shown in Figure 8-25).

Stability of this joint is important. The joint connects the left and right coxal or hip bones anteriorly. Should this joint become misaligned, which can happen during childbirth or trauma such as a fall, the stability of the pelvis is compromised and many postural and soft-tissue problems can result (Figure 8-25).

The symphysis pubis allows for independent motion of each side of the pelvis, which is important when walking, for example. Symphysis pubis motion is especially important during pregnancy and delivery.

Hip Joint

The hip joint consists of the following structures:
- **Articulating Bones.** Acetabulum of the pelvic bone (formed by the ilium, pubis, and ischium) and the femur
- **Joint Type.** Synovial ball and socket
- **Ligaments.** Iliofemoral ligament from the anterior superior iliac spine to the intertrochanteric line of the femur; ischiofemoral ligament from the ischium to the femur on the posterior side; pubofemoral ligament from the pubis to the intertrochanteric line of the femur; and the ligamentum

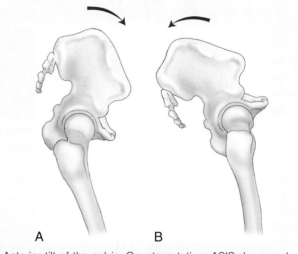

| Box 8-4 | The Complex Pelvis |

The pelvis comprises three bones arranged in a ring. The pelvis has three important functions:
1. Transmits weight from the axial skeleton to the lower limbs in the standing position or to the ischial tuberosities when sitting
2. Provides proximal attachments for muscles that insert onto and move the legs
3. Protects the lower structures of the digestive and urinary tracts and the reproductive systems of males and females
During the birth of a baby, the head of the infant must pass through the ring (pelvic outlet) of the pelvic girdle.

The pelvis is connected to the skeleton of the upper body at the sacroiliac joint. The sacrum and the coccyx also have a connection to the pelvis.

The joints of the pelvis are capable of tiny movement. Much of this movement occurs at the sacroiliac (SI) joint.
- Nutation/Counternutation describes sacral movement in relationship to the movement of the ilium.
  - Nutation is the forward motion of the base of the sacrum into the pelvis (tuck your tail) or the backward rotation of the ilium on the sacrum.
  - Counternutation is the opposite movement of nutation. A lordotic position or anterior pelvic tilt is created by the rotation of ilium on the sacrum or backward motion of the base of the sacrum out of the pelvis (wag your tail).
- Iliosacral movement is ilium movement on the sacrum—anterior/posterior rotation, superior/inferior movement, and medial/lateral flaring.
- Sacroiliac motion is sacral movement on the ilium—flexion/extension and rotation.
- Symphysis pubis joint motion may be either superior or inferior. There is only approximately 2 mm of motion possible at this joint.
- **Outflare** is the external [outward] rotation of the ilium on the sacrum. This movement closes the SI joints and opens the pubis.

A, Anterior tilt of the pelvis. Counternutation: ASIS down and PSIS up. This rotation closes or compresses the sacral iliac joint. **B,** Posterior tilt of the pelvis nutation. ASIS up and the PSIS down. This rotation opens or gaps the SI joint. *ASIS,* Anterior superior iliac spine, *PSIS,* posterior superior iliac spine. (From Muscolino JE. *Kinesiology: the skeletal system and muscle function,* ed 2, St Louis, 2011, Mosby.)

- **Inflare** is the internal rotation of the ilium on the sacrum. This will open the SI joint in the back and close the pubis joint in the front.

All these tiny movements can become very confusing. They all relate to the sacral iliac joint movement and the way the symphysis pubis moves. When these integrated but independent movements are disrupted, many pain patterns result.

teres, also known as the *ligament of the head of the femur,* from the head of the femur to the acetabulum (Figure 8-26).

A fibrocartilaginous ring called the *labrum* attaches around the edge of the acetabulum and is reinforced by the transverse acetabular ligament. This ring helps hold the femoral head in place by increasing the depth of the acetabulum (not shown).

The hip joint is a massive joint. Although a mobile ball-and-socket joint, the hip joint is less mobile than the shoulder joint because of the round head of the femur fitting into the deep socket of the acetabulum of the pelvis. This structure provides stability. Therefore the hip joint is less susceptible to injury than the shoulder joint. In anatomic position the femoral head is not fully in the hip socket. A better fit is when the femur is flexed to 90 degrees, slightly abducted, and laterally rotated. The most relaxed position is flexion, abduction, and lateral rotation (e.g., such as when sitting in a relaxed position with the leg falling to the side).

The joint capsule is large. The capsule is looser in flexion than in extension.

Usually the thigh moves on the pelvis, but the pelvis can move on the thigh if the thigh is fixed. The pelvis can move forward. This motion is called *anterior tilt* and tends to increase the lordosis of the lumbar spine. Posterior tilt, the opposite movement, decreases lumbar lordosis. The pelvis can also elevate, depress, and rotate to the right or left.

The hip joint allows the following movements: flexion, extension, abduction, adduction, medial rotation, and lateral rotation.

Palpation

Palpate the pelvic and hip joint region as follows:
- The hip joint itself lies deep within the body and is not directly palpable.
- The posterior edge of the greater trochanter of the femur is easiest to locate and can be felt about a palm's width below the iliac crest.
- The superficial trochanteric bursa lies on the posterolateral surface of the greater trochanter.
- At the same level as the greater trochanter, locate the pubic tubercles.

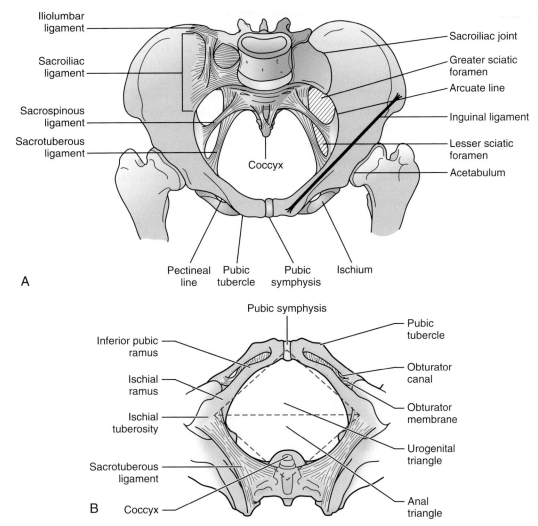

A

B

FIGURE 8-25 A, Pelvic ligaments, anterior view. These important ligaments give the pelvis its strength. **B,** Ligaments of the symphysis pubis.

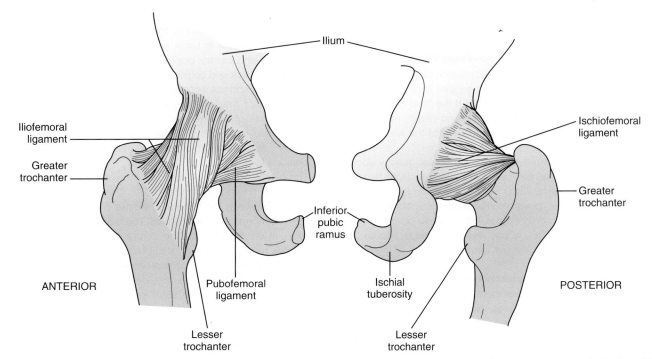

FIGURE 8-26 Ligaments of the hip joint. The three principal hip joint ligaments are arranged in a continuum that surrounds the joint. The iliofemoral ligament is especially important in limiting extension of the hip.

ACTIVITY 8-9

Move your pelvis and hip through the ranges of motion.

- The symphysis pubis can be palpated at the anterior midline of the body.
- The sacroiliac joint is located just inferior to the posterior superior iliac spine near the dimples of the gluteal area. It is not directly palpable because it is covered with ligaments, but movements can be felt there. A small degree of motion can be felt if the finger or thumb is held in this area while a person is walking or marching in place. You may also feel nutation/counternutation (Activity 8-9).

Joints of the Knee

The tibiofemoral joint is located between the femur and tibia. The patellofemoral joint is found between the patella and the trochlear groove of the femur. These two joints consist of the following structures:

- **Articulating Bones.** Femur, tibia, and patella
- **Joint Type.** Synovial modified hinge
- **Ligaments.** The patellar ligament runs from the patella to the tibial tuberosity (the quadriceps femoris tendon also provides stability to the patella); the oblique popliteal ligament joins the lateral aspect of the fibrous capsule to the lateral condyle of the femur; the tibial (medial) collateral ligament joins the medial epicondyle of the femur to the medial condyle of the tibia; the fibular (lateral) collateral ligament joins the lateral epicondyle of the femur to the

fibula; the anterior cruciate ligament joins the anterior medial intercondylar area of the tibia to the posteromedial surface of the lateral condyle of the femur; the posterior cruciate ligament joins the posterior intercondylar area of the tibia to the anteromedial condyle of the femur; the posterior meniscofemoral ligament attaches the lateral meniscus to the posterior surface at the femur; the transverse ligament joins the medial meniscus to the lateral meniscus (Box 8-5 and Figure 8-27).

The knee joints allow the following movements: flexion, extension, medial rotation, and lateral rotation.

Palpation

Palpate the knee joint as follows:
- Landmarks in and around the knee help orient you to this complicated joint.
- Locate the flat medial surface of the tibia, the shin.
- Follow its anterior border upward to the tibial tuberosity.
- Move medially and follow the medial border of the tibia upward until it merges into a bony prominence, the medial tibial condyle, which is higher than the tibial tuberosity.
- In a comparable location on the other side of the knee, find a similar prominence, the lateral condyle of the tibia.
- Just below the level of the lateral tibial condyle, find the head of the fibula.
- Now identify three parts of the distal femur. Bring your fingertips firmly down the medial surface of the thigh along a line where the inner seam of your pant leg would be.
- Your fingers will run up against an abrupt bony prominence, the adductor tubercle.

Box 8-5 The Complex Knee

The knee joint is the most complicated joint in the body, is not as stable as other joints, and yet is one of the most frequently used joints. Prolonged standing while the knee is in a slightly flexed position, instead of the normal locked extension position, puts stress on the articular surfaces of the condyles and can damage the cartilage.

- The medial condyle is more curved than the lateral condyle, which contributes to the automatic rotation of the knee during flexion and extension when the knee joint is near full extension. The femoral condyle first rolls off the tibial condyle and then glides, producing a combined rolling-gliding movement. The opposite action occurs in extension of the knee: first a glide and then rolling.
- In the male the acetabulum is located almost directly above the knee, which allows for even distribution of weight-bearing forces during movement. In contrast, the wider female pelvis results in the knee being medial to the acetabulum. This arrangement puts strain on the female knee during movement. Female knees are not as well equipped to handle the strain of running and repetitive impact activities of the lower extremities.
- The fibrocartilaginous menisci provide more surface contact on the tibia for the femur, which allows for stability between the rounded femoral condyles, which sit on an almost flat tibia. The menisci are attached to muscles and connected by ligaments to each other and to the bones. These shock absorbers protect bone and cartilage and increase the

movement of synovial fluid. The menisci move in the joint capsule, depending on the forces imposed on them. If the movement against the menisci is too abrupt or quickly changes direction such that they cannot shift position, the menisci can be crushed or torn.

- The joint capsule is slack anteriorly and taut posteriorly in extension and just the opposite in flexion. The posterior knee capsule is thick and consists of two strong bands connecting the femoral and tibial condyles. These ligaments resist hyperextension of the joint and provide stability in the standing position in normal extension. In normal extension all the ligaments are taut, and one can stabilize the joint passively without any muscular action. Extension is the most stable position for the knee.
- The patella protects the knee joint from external impact, such as falling forward onto the knees. The patella moves in a groove between the femoral condyles by the contraction of the quadriceps femoris muscles. The more flexion, the greater the pull on the patella. The contraction of the quadriceps femoris tends to pull the patella laterally during active extension. The position of the patella becomes somewhat unstable in this position. The patella provides an increased mechanical advantage for the quadriceps femoris muscles when contracting to move the knee into extension. The knee is prone to injury because it relies on soft tissue for much of its support when in a flexed position.

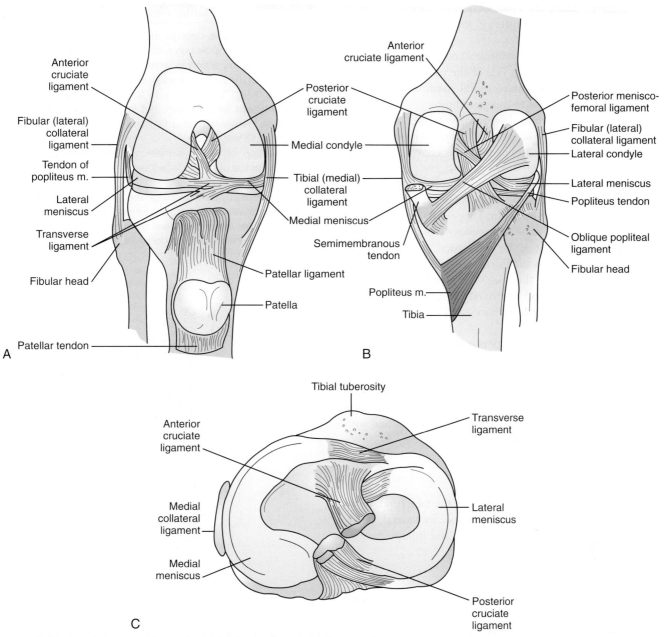

FIGURE 8-27 Knee joint opened, anterior, posterior, and proximal views. **A,** Anterior view of the knee joint, opened by folding the patella and patellar ligament inferiorly. On the lateral side is the fibular collateral ligament, separated by the popliteal tendon from the lateral meniscus. On the medial side, the tibial collateral ligament is attached to the medial meniscus. The anterior and posterior cruciate ligaments are seen between the femoral condyles. **B,** Posterior view of the opened knee joint, with a more complete view of the posterior cruciate ligament. **C,** The femur is removed, showing the proximal (articular) end of the right tibia. On the medial side is the gently curved medial meniscus; on the lateral side is the more tightly curved lateral meniscus. The anterior end of the medial meniscus is anchored to the surface of the tibia by the transverse ligament. The cut ends of the anterior and posterior cruciate ligaments are shown, as well as the meniscofemoral ligament.

- Just below this is the medial epicondyle.
- The lateral epicondyle of the femur is found in a similar area on the other side.
- The patella rests on the anterior articulating surface of the femur, roughly midway between the epicondyles, and lies within the tendon of the quadriceps femoris muscles.
- This structure continues below the knee joint as the patellar ligament and attaches on the tibial tuberosity.

- Two collateral ligaments, one on each side of the knee, give medial and lateral stability to the joint.
- To feel the lateral collateral ligament, cross one leg so that your ankle rests on the opposite knee.
- Find the firm cord that runs from the lateral epicondyle of the femur to the head of the fibula.
- The medial collateral ligament can usually be palpated on the medial side.

- Two cruciate ligaments cross obliquely within the knee joint and give it anteroposterior stability and cannot be palpated.
- With the knee joint flexed to about 90 degrees, you can press your thumbs—one on each side of the patellar ligament—into the groove of the tibiofemoral joint. Note that the patella lies just proximal to this joint line.
- As you press your thumbs downward, you can feel the edge of the proximal surface of the tibia. Follow it medially, then laterally until you are stopped by the converging femur and tibia.
- The medial and lateral menisci, crescent-shaped fibrocartilaginous pads that lie on the tibial plateaus, form cushions between the tibia and femur. They can be palpated in the space between the tibia and femur either side of the midline.
- The soft tissue in front of the joint space, on either side of the patellar ligament, is the infrapatellar fat pad.
- Several bursae lie near the knee. The prepatellar bursa lies between the patella and the overlying skin, whereas the superficial infrapatellar bursa lies anterior to the patellar ligament.
- Observe the concavities that are usually evident at each side and above the patella. In these areas is the synovial cavity of the knee joint. Although the synovium is not normally detectable, these areas may become swollen and tender when the joint is inflamed. You may also see the swelling from protrusion of the fat pad, which is often confused with effusion (fluid in the capsule) (Activity 8-10).

Joints of the Ankle and Foot

The joints of the ankle and foot include the talocrural, distal tibiofibular, subtalar (talocalcaneal joints), intertarsal, tarsometatarsal, metatarsophalangeal (MTP), and interphalangeal joints (Figure 8-28).

Talocrural Joint

The talocrural joint (the ankle joint) consists of the following structures (Box 8-6):
- **Articulating Bones.** Tibia, fibula, and talus
- **Joint Type.** Synovial hinge joint
- **Ligaments.** Medial collateral or deltoid from the medial malleolus to the navicular, calcaneus, and talus; talofibular ligaments from the lateral malleolus to the talus; and calcaneofibular from the fibula to the lateral calcaneus

The metatarsals make up the body of the foot, and the phalanges make up the toes (Figures 8-28 and 8-29).

The talocrural joint allows the following movements: dorsiflexion (extension) and plantar flexion (flexion).

Distal Tibiofibular Joint and Subtalor/Talocalcaneal Joint

The distal tibiofibular joint is a fibrous syndesmosis joint that holds the tibia and fibula together. The ankle (talocrural)

ACTIVITY 8-10

Move your knee joint through the range of motion positions.

| Box 8-6 | Why Plantar Flexion and Dorsiflexion? |

- A transverse axis through the ankle joint allows a pair of actions similar to flexion and extension at the wrist joint.
- The analogous action to wrist flexion is one that would tip the sole of the foot downward, increasing the angle between foot and leg. The usual term for the increase in such an angle would be *extension,* but in order to emphasize the relation between foot and hand, this action is instead termed *plantar flexion.*
- The action similar to extension at the wrist would be a tipping of the upper surface (dorsum) of the foot toward the anterior surface of the leg.
- However, this would decrease the angle between the body segments, an action usually termed *flexion.* Because the term *plantar flexion* has been used for the opposite action, this is now referred to as *dorsiflexion.*

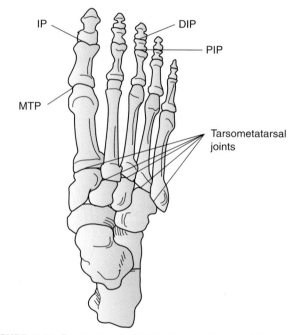

FIGURE 8-28 Foot joints. *DIP,* Distal interphalangeal joints; *IP,* interphalangeal joints; *MTP,* metatarsophalangeal joints; *PIP,* proximal interphalangeal joints.

joint is formed by the distal ends of tibia and fibula meeting the talus.

Immediately distal to the ankle joint is the talocalcaneal joint, or the articulation of the talus with the calcaneus. This joint is often referred to as the *subtalar joint.* It is reinforced by the joint capsule and interosseous ligaments. No muscles attach on the talus, which is moved indirectly by the structures surrounding it. The subtalar joint is most stable when in a supinated position (the major component of supination is inversion). It is least stable when pronated (the major component of pronation is eversion).

Motions of the ankle joint itself are limited to dorsiflexion and plantar flexion, as previously stated. Inversion and

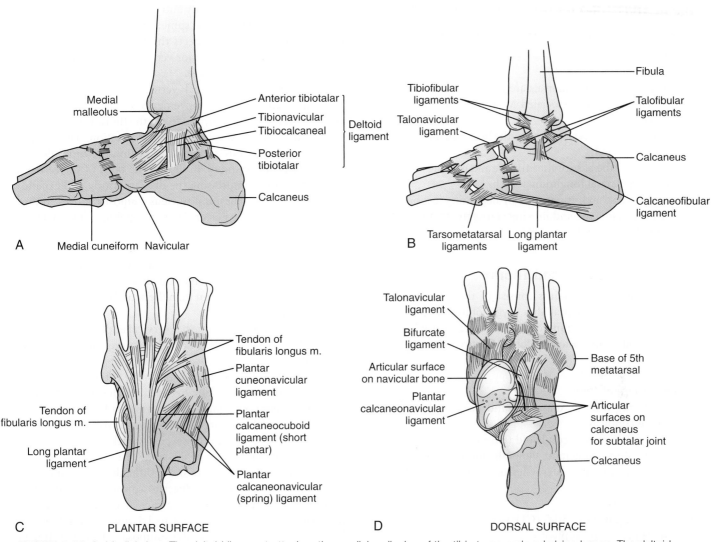

FIGURE 8-29 A, Medial view. The deltoid ligament attaches the medial malleolus of the tibia to several underlying bones. The deltoid ligament consists of anterior tibiotalar, tibionavicular, tibiocalcaneal, and posterior tibiotalar portions. **B,** Lateral view of ligaments of the ankle. **C,** Plantar view of plantar ligaments of the foot, including the long plantar, short plantar, and spring ligaments. **D,** Dorsal view with the talus removed, showing the rounded socket in which it articulates (the talocalcaneonavicular joint). The bifurcate and talonavicular ligaments help stabilize the bones forming this articulation.

eversion of the foot are functions of the subtalar and transverse tarsal joints (Figure 8-29).

Foot Joints

The joints of the foot are as follows:
- *Intertarsa:* between the tarsal bones
- *Tarsometatarsal:* between the tarsals and the metatarsals
- *Metatarsophalangeal:* between the metatarsals and the phalanges
- *Interphalangeal:* between the proximal, middle, and distal phalanges

The MTP joints are condyloid joints. The great toe has one interphalangeal joint. The remaining toes have two interphalangeal joints each. The more proximal joint is the PIP joint, and the distal joint is the DIP joint. The interphalangeal joints are hinge joints. The design of the foot bones and joints creates curved structures called *arches.* The foot has three

arches: a medial arch, a lateral longitudinal arch, and a transverse arch.

The medial longitudinal arch is the highest and composed of the calcaneus, talus, navicular, cuneiforms, and the first three metatarsals. The lateral longitudinal arch is lower and flatter than the medial arch. It is composed of the calcaneus, cuboid, and the fourth and fifth metatarsals. The *transverse arch* is composed of the cuneiforms, the cuboid, and metatarsals.

Palpation

Palpate the ankle and foot joint as follows:
- Identify the landmarks of the ankle, which are the medial malleolus, the bony prominence at the distal end of the tibia, and the lateral malleolus, at the distal end of the fibula.
- Ligaments extend from each malleolus into the foot.

Move your ankles and feet through the ranges of motion.

- The heads of the metatarsals are palpable in the ball of the foot. These and the associated MTP joints are proximal to the webs of the toes.
- From the base of the large toe to the heel, palpate the medial longitudinal arch.
- Beginning at the base of the little toe and moving to the heel, palpate the lateral longitudinal arch.
- The transverse arch is palpated by beginning just below the base of the large toe and moving across the foot to the base of the little toe (Activity 8-11).

Joints of the Spine and Thorax

The spine and thorax joints consist of the atlantooccipital, atlantoaxial, intervertebral disk, zygopophyseal, costospinal (costovertebral, costotransverse), and sternocostal (costochondral and chondrosternal) joints (Figure 8-30).

Joints of the Spine
Atlantooccipital Joint
- **Articulating Bones.** Atlas (C1) and occipital bone at the occipital condyles
- **Joint Type.** Synovial condyloid (ellipsoid) joint
   The atlantooccipital joint allows the following movements: flexion, extension, right lateral flexion, and left lateral flexion.

Atlantoaxial Joint
- **Articulating Bones.** Atlas (C1) and axis (C2)
- **Joint Type.** Synovial pivot
   The atlantoaxial joint allows right and left rotation.

Intervertebral Disk Joints
- **Articulating Bones.** Adjacent vertebrae
- **Joint Type.** Cartilaginous symphysis
   Individual intervertebral disk joints allow minimal movement; movement of the spine as a whole unit is much larger.

Zygapophyseal (Facet) Joints
- **Articulating Bones.** Superior and inferior articulating facets of adjacent vertebrae
- **Joint Type.** Synovial gliding joints
   The zygapophyseal joints allow the following movements: flexion, extension, right and left lateral flexion, right and left rotation, and gliding.

Ligaments
The supraspinous ligament and interspinous ligaments run along the ends of the spinous processes of each vertebra; the supraspinous ligament enlarges in the cervical region and becomes the ligamentum nuchae in the cervical area; intertransverse ligaments connect the transverse processes; ligamenta flava connect adjacent laminae; the anterior longitudinal ligament, which connects the anterior vertebral body and disk to the anterior vertebral body and disk located directly above, runs the entire length of the spine; and the posterior longitudinal ligament, which connects the posterior vertebral body and disk to the above posterior vertebral body and disk, runs the entire length of the spine.

Movements of individual vertebrae are slight, but the cumulative effect of main movements occurs at C7 to T1, the cervical thoracic junction; T12 to L1, the thoracolumbar junction; and L5 to S1, the sacral lumbar junction. These areas, where one curve ends and another begins, are more flexible and more prone to injury. In flexion the body of the vertebra moves forward, compressing the disk anteriorly and expanding it posteriorly. The fluid nucleus pulposus moves toward the back, and the posterior ligaments stabilize. In extension the opposite occurs.

Lateral flexion creates a similar pattern. Compression on the side of the lateral flexion increases pressure in the disk on the opposite side. The action of the disks and the ligaments is more involved in movement than the actual bony components of the spine.

Viewed laterally, the spine has cervical and lumbar lordoses and a thoracic kyphosis. The sacral curve forms a second kyphosis.

The most mobile portion of the spine is the neck. Flexion and extension occur chiefly between the head and the first cervical vertebra, rotation occurs primarily between the first and second vertebrae, and lateral bending involves the cervical spine from the second to the seventh vertebra.

Movements of the rest of the spine (i.e., from the sacrum to the base of the neck) are more difficult to measure than those in the neck and are subject to considerable individual variation. The most mobile areas are at the thoracolumbar junction of T11 to T12, L1, L4 to L5, and the lumbosacral joint (L5-S1). The angle at the lumbosacral joint is tipped anteriorly so that when the lumbar vertebra wants to slide forward, contact between the superior articular processes of S1 and the inferior articular process of L5 prevents the movement. What looks like spinal flexion takes place partly at the hip joints. For this reason, and because the length of the limbs varies so much among individuals, flexion cannot be estimated accurately by noting the distance of our fingertips from the floor when we bend over. On forward flexion, watch the lumbar area; its normal lordosis should flatten (Figures 8-31 to 8-33).

Palpation
Palpate the spinal joints as follows:
- Beginning just below the skull, palpate the spinous processes of the cervical vertebrae.
- The spinous processes of C2, C7, and often T1 are usually larger and more prominent.
- Continue along the thoracic spine, noticing the bony prominences of each vertebra.
- A line drawn between the iliac crests runs between the spinous processes of L4 and L5. This point is used often as a reference to locate the other vertebrae.
- Palpate each of the vertebrae, locating each spinous process.

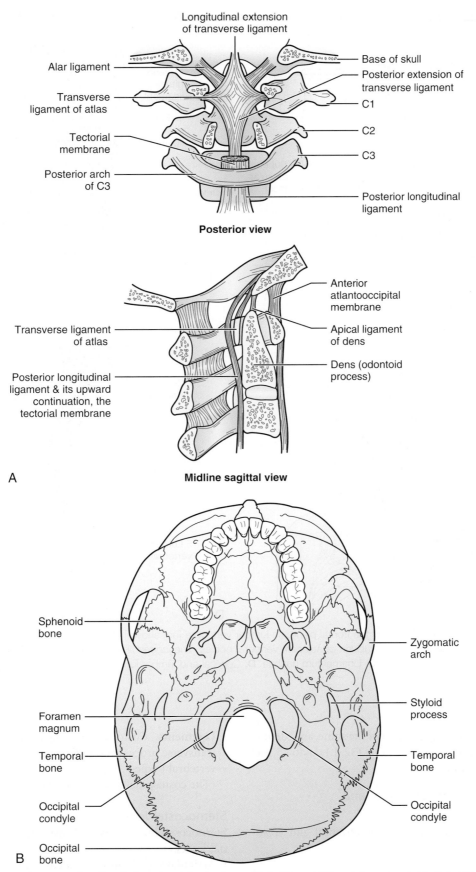

FIGURE 8-30 A, Ligaments connecting the skull and vertebral column. Both C1 and C2 vertebrae are separately attached to the base of the skull to ensure maximal stability. The transverse ligament of the atlas prevents the dens from moving posteriorly and crushing the spinal cord as it passes through the foramen of the C1 vertebra. With its upward and downward extensions, the transverse ligament forms the cruciform ligament. **B,** Base of the skull. On this view the large occipital condyles are shown. These are the surfaces at which the skull articulates with the C1 vertebra, the atlas.

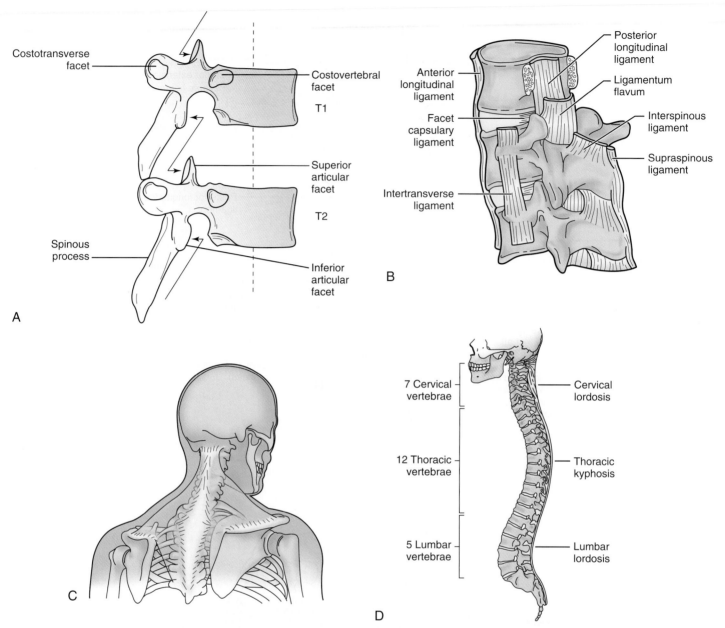

FIGURE 8-31 A, Vertebral articulations in the frontal plane. (In lumbar vertebrae [not shown] the articular facets are in the sagittal plane.) The *vertical dashed line* indicates the articulation of adjacent vertebral bodies. The *jagged lines* indicate the way articular facets align with one another. **B,** Ligaments of the spine. **C,** Ligamentum nuchae. **D,** Cervical and lumbar lordoses and a thoracic kyphosis. The sacral curve forms a second kyphosis.

- Then palpate again during rotation of the spine, and identify the thoracolumbar junction of T11 to T12, L1, L4 to L5, and the lumbosacral joint.

Joints of the Thorax: Costospinal and Sternocostal

The costospinal joints consist of costovertebral and costotransverse joints.

Costospinal Joints
- **Articulating Bones.** Rib with facets and hemifacets on adjoining vertebrae
- **Joint Type.** Synovial plane joints

- **Ligaments.** Costotransverse ligaments from the rib to the transverse process and radiate ligaments from the rib to the vertebral bodies

  The costospinal joints allow gliding (Figure 8-34).

Sternocostal Joints
Sternocostal joints consist of costochondral and chondrosternal joints.
- **Articulating Bones.** Costochondral joints: The first through the seventh ribs articulate with a costal cartilage. Chondrosternal joints: The cartilage articulates with the sternum.
- **Joint Type.** Cartilaginous and synovial

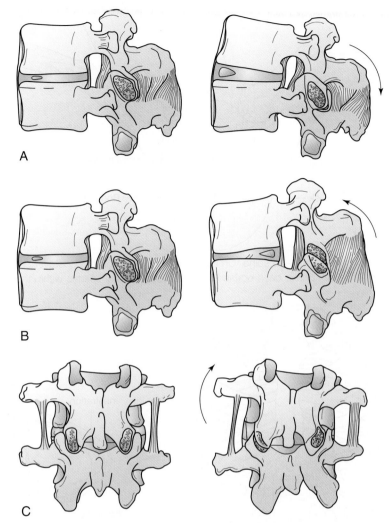

A

B

C

FIGURE 8-32 Motion between adjacent vertebrae. **A** to **C,** *Left,* Vertebrae in their neutral positions. **A,** *Right,* Vertebra in extension. The anterior longitudinal ligament is becoming taut. **B,** *Right,* Vertebra in flexion. Notice that the interspinous and supraspinous ligaments, as well as the ligamentum flavum, are being stretched. **C,** *Right,* Vertebra in right lateral flexion. The left intertransverse ligament is becoming taut.

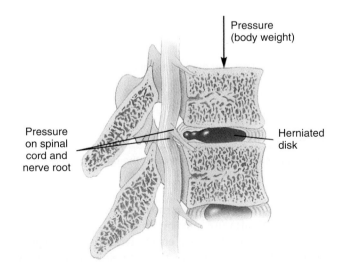

Pressure (body weight)

Herniated disk

Pressure on spinal cord and nerve root

FIGURE 8-33 Herniated disk. (From Thibodeau GA, Patton KT: *Anatomy & physiology,* ed 6, St Louis, 2007, Mosby.)

- **Ligaments.** Costochondral joints are synchondroses and have no ligaments for support; chondrosternal joints are synovial and are supported by an intraarticular ligament and a thin capsule.

  The sternocostal and costospinal joints allow the following movement: similar to the movement of a handle on a bucket, movement of the thoracic cage occurs during respiration. Small movement of the ribs at the costospinal joints produce large movements anteriorly of the sternum and laterally of the rib shafts. The result is a change in diameter of the thoracic cage that shifts intrathoracic pressure and enables inspiration to occur (Figure 8-35).

Palpation

Palpate the joints of the thorax as follows:

- In the thoracic region, follow each rib from its costospinal joints to the costal cartilage.
- Feel for the bucket-handle motion of the ribs during breathing (Activity 8-12).

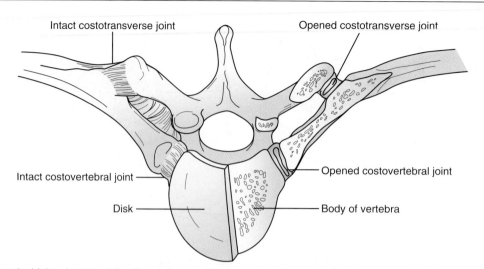

FIGURE 8-34 Costospinal joints between the ribs and spine. On the *left* are shown the intact costovertebral and costotransverse joints, reinforced by ligaments. On the *right* the joints have been opened, revealing the synovial spaces within them.

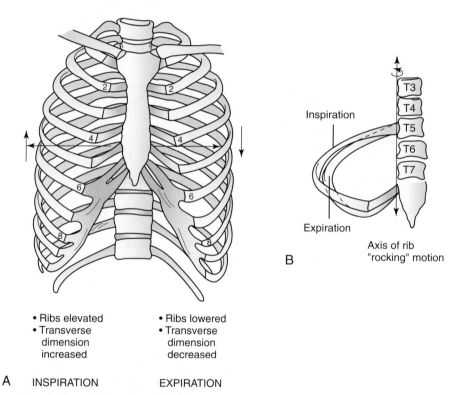

FIGURE 8-35 Rib cage and respirations. **A,** The rib cage in inspiration and expiration, illustrating the upward and lateral excursion that takes place at inspiration. This results in an increase in intrathoracic volume and the movement of air into the tracheobronchial tree. **B,** The "bucket handle" motion of a sample single rib during inspiration and expiration.

INTEGRATING JOINT MOVEMENT INTO MASSAGE

SECTION OBJECTIVES

Chapter objective covered in this section:

7. Design a joint movement sequence for the body.

After completing this section, the student will be able to perform the following:

- Describe why joint movement is important to massage application.
- Use joint movement to assess for normal and abnormal range of motion of a joint.
- Demonstrate two types of joint movement: active and passive.

ACTIVITY 8-12

Move your spine and thorax through the ranges of motion.

Joint movement is how we move an area to measure the joint ROM. We also use joint movement to position an area for the application of muscle energy techniques to lengthen muscles and for stretching methods to elongate connective tissues. For this reason the massage professional should concentrate on developing the ability to use joint movement efficiently and effectively.

Evolve Activity 8-2

Joint movement is effective because it provides a means of controlled stimulation to the joint mechanoreceptors. Movement initiates muscle tension readjustment through the reflex center of the spinal cord and lower brain centers. As positions change, the supported movement gives the nervous system an entirely different set of signals to process. The joint sensory receptors can learn not to be so hypersensitive. As a result, any protective spasms and movement restrictions may lessen.

Joint movement also encourages lubrication of the enhanced joint and contributes an important addition to the lymphatic and venous circulations. Much of the pumping action that moves these fluids in the vessels results from compression against the lymph and blood vessels during joint movement and muscle contraction.

The tendons, ligaments, and joint capsule are warmed from the movement. This mechanical effect helps keep these tissues pliable.

Determining Range of Motion

The most important aspect of joint movement is that it is used to assess whether a jointed area is functioning effectively. Recall that ROM is the angle through which a joint moves from the anatomic position to the ends of its motion in a particular direction. It is measured in degrees. There is a normal ROM for each joint. Assessment methods that move a joint can determine if a joint is able to move within a normal ROM. If the joint moves less than the normal range or more than the normal range, a problem may exist. Remember that individuals may vary from "normal or average" without having a problem. Compare each individual ROM to the other side if there is a paired joint. The findings should be similar. If there is a discrepancy from side to side, this is a more accurate assessment than a comparison to "normal."

By comparing what is considered normal ROM for a joint to what the massage client is able to do, the massage therapist may be able to determine indications for massage intervention or possible referral (Box 8-7).

The range or amount of movement at a joint is determined by the following factors:
- The shape of the bones that form the joint
- The tautness or laxness of the ligament and capsule structure of the joint
- The length of the soft tissue structure that supports and moves the joint
- Whether the joint is moving independently of other joints (open chain) or links to other joints in a combined movement (closed chain)

Box 8-8 reviews joint movement.

Elements That Can Cause Joint Dysfunction

Joints have various degrees of ROM. There are anatomic, physiologic, and pathologic barriers to motion. A barrier is a point of resistance and can feel hard, such as when bone contacts bone or during binding, when soft tissue is short.

Anatomic barriers are determined by the shape and fit of the bones at the joint. The anatomic barrier is seldom reached

---

| **Box 8-7** | Normal Range of Motion for Each Joint |

Remember that each person is unique, and many factors influence available range of motion. Just because a joint does not have the textbook range of motion does not mean that what is displayed is abnormal. Abnormality is indicated by nonoptimal function. This can be either a limit or an exaggeration in the "textbook normal" range of motion.

Available range of motion is measured from the neutral anatomic position (0). Note: If 0 is listed first, this means movement is away from neutral; if 0 is listed second, it means the joint is moving toward neutral.

Normal Values (in degrees):
- Hip flexion 0-125
- Hip extension 115-0
- Hip hyperextension 0-15
- Hip abduction 0-45
- Hip adduction 45-0
- Hip lateral (external) rotation 0-45
- Hip medial (internal) rotation 0-45
- Knee flexion 0-130
- Knee extension 120-0
- Ankle plantar flexion (movement downward) 0-50
- Ankle dorsiflexion (movement upward) 0-20
- Foot inversion (turned inward) 0-35
- Foot eversion (turned outward) 0-25
- Shoulder flexion 0-90
- Shoulder extension 0-50
- Shoulder abduction 0-90
- Shoulder adduction 90-0
- Shoulder lateral (external) rotation 0-90
- Shoulder medial (internal) rotation 0-90
- Elbow flexion 0-160
- Elbow extension 145-0
- Elbow pronation 0-90
- Elbow supination 0-90
- Wrist flexion 0-90
- Wrist extension 0-70
- Wrist abduction 0-25
- Wrist adduction 0-65

---

because the possibility of injury is greatest in this position. Instead, the body protects the joint by establishing physiologic barriers.

Physiologic barriers are the result of the limits in ROM imposed by protective nerve and sensory function to support optimal function. The sensation at the barrier is soft and pliable.

An adaptation in a physiologic barrier that causes the protective function to limit instead of support optimal functioning is called a **pathologic barrier.** Pathologic barriers often are manifested as stiffness, pain, or a "catch."

Factors that contribute to the pathologic condition can occur as follows:
- If the ligaments and connective tissue that make up the joint capsule are not firm enough to maintain joint space, the joint play is lost.
- If the capsule is too tight, joint play is lost as well. Muscles around a joint can shorten, pulling the bone ends together and affecting joint play.

Box 8-8   Review of Joint Movement

- Joints allow us to move. Joint position and velocity receptors inform the central nervous system where and how the body is positioned in gravity and how fast it is moving. These sensory data are the major determining factors for muscle motor tone patterns.
- Joint movement techniques focus on the *synovial,* or freely movable, joints in the body. To a lesser extent, these methods can address the joints of the vertebral column, hand, and foot as well as the facet joints of the ribs, the sacroiliac joint, and the sternoclavicular joint. These joints are not directly influenced by muscles but rather move through indirect muscle action.
- We can control some joint movements voluntarily; we can move our limbs through various motions, such as flexion, extension, abduction, adduction, and rotation. These are referred to as *physiologic movements,* or **osteokinematic movements.**
- For normal physiologic movement, other types of movements *(accessory movements,* or **arthrokinematic movements**) must occur as a result of the inherent laxity, or **joint play,** that exists in each joint. This laxity allows the ends of the bones to slide, roll, or spin smoothly on each other inside the joint capsule. These essential movements occur during movement of the joint and are not under voluntary control.

    A good example of joint motion is found on a door.
    - The hinge holds the door both to the casing and away from the casing.
    - For the door to open and close efficiently *(osteokinematic movement),* the space between the door and the door casing must be maintained and the fit must be correct.
    - If the fit of the door in the door casing is incorrect or if the space is not maintained, the door will not open and close correctly.
    - Ligaments act as the hinges in the body.
    - The door hinge must be oiled. In the joint the synovial membrane secretes synovial fluid, produced on demand by joint movement.
    - If a joint does not move or is not moved, it will lock up like a rusty door hinge, and movement will be restricted or lost.
    - If you look closely at a door hinge, you will notice the space around the pin in the hinge.
    - If you move the hinge back and forth (not swing the door), the hinge and pin mechanism moves a little *(arthrokinematic movement).*
    - This little movement can be likened to joint play.

- If the ligaments and joint capsule are not pliable, flexibility is lost.
- If the ligaments and joint capsule do not support the joint, the fit is disrupted.
- Muscle contraction may pull the joint out of alignment. Muscle groups that flex and adduct the joints are about 30% stronger and have more mass than the extensors and abductors.
- If the body uses muscle contraction to stabilize a joint, the uneven pull between flexors and extensors and adductors and abductors disturbs the fit of the bones at the joint.

Box 8-9   Variations for Joint Movement

Active Joint Movement

In **active joint movement,** the client moves the area without any type of interaction by the massage practitioner. This is a good assessment method and should be used before and after any type of soft-tissue work, because it provides information about the limits of range of motion and the improvement after the work is complete. Active joint movement is also great to teach as a self-help tool.

There are two variations of active joint movement methods: active assisted and active resistive.

- **Active Assisted Joint Movement.** In active assisted joint movement, the client moves the joint through the range of motion and the massage practitioner helps or assists the movement. This approach is very useful in cases of weakness or pain with movement. The action remains within the comfortable limits of movement for the client. The focus is to create movement within the joint capsule, encouraging synovial fluid lubrication to warm and soften connective tissue and support muscle function.
- **Active Resistive Joint Movement.** In active resistive joint movement, the massage practitioner firmly grasps and holds the end of the bone just distal to the affected joint. The massage practitioner leans back slightly to place a small traction on the limb to take up the slack in the tissue. Then the practitioner instructs the client to push slowly against a stabilizing hand or arm while moving the joint through its entire range of motion. A tap or light slap against the limb to begin the movement works well to focus the client's attention. The counterforce applied by the massage practitioner does not exceed the pushing or pulling action of the client, but rather matches it and then allows movement.
- **Passive Joint Movement.** If a client is paralyzed or very ill, only passive joint movement may be possible. Some clients do not wish to participate in active joint movement and prefer to take a very passive role during the massage. Client participation is not necessary.

Types of Joint Movement Methods

Joint movement involves moving the jointed areas within the client's physiologic limits of ROM.

The two types of joint movement are active joint movement and passive joint movement.

- In **active joint movement** the client moves the joint by active contraction of muscle groups. The two variations of active joint movement are **active assisted movement**, which occurs when both the client and the massage practitioner move the area, and **active resistive movement**, which occurs when the client actively moves the joint against resistance provided by the massage practitioner.
- In **passive joint movement** the client's muscles remain relaxed and the massage practitioner moves the joint with no assistance from the client. When doing passive joint movement, the massage practitioner should feel for the soft or hard end feel of the joint ROM (Box 8-9).

Whether active or passive, joint movements are always done within the comfortable limits of the client's ROM. The client's body must always be stabilized; only the joint being addressed should be allowed to move. Occasionally, the entire limb is moved to allow for coordinated interaction among all the joints of the area, but the rest of the body is stabilized. It is essential to move slowly, because quick changes or abrupt moves may cause the muscles to initiate protective contractions.

Joint-specific work, including any type of high-velocity thrust manipulation, is beyond the scope of practice of the beginning massage professional. Because of the interplay among the joint proprioceptors, muscle tone, innervation of the joint, and surrounding muscles by the same nerve pattern, any damage to a joint can cause long-term problems. Working within the physiologic ranges of motion for the particular client is within the scope of practice of the massage professional. Specific corrective procedures for pathologic range of motion are best applied in a supervised health care setting.

Applying Joint Movement Methods

When massage therapists use joint movement techniques, they must remain within the physiologic barriers. If a pathologic barrier exists that limits motion, techniques are used to gently and slowly encourage the joint structures to increase the limits of the ROM to the physiologic barrier. If a pathologic barrier exists where there is excessive joint motion, techniques are used to gently and slowly encourage the joint structures to decrease the limits of the ROM to the physiologic barrier.

Hand placement with joint movement is very important. Make sure the area is not squeezed, pinched, or restricted in its movement pattern. One hand should be placed close to the joint to act as a stabilizer and allow evaluation. As an alternative method of positioning the stabilizing hand, the jointed area can be moved without stabilization while the massage practitioner observes where the client's body moves most in response to the ROM action. The stabilizing hand then is placed at this point. The other hand is placed at the distal end of the bone; this is the hand that actually provides the movement. The stabilizing hand must remain in contact with the client and must be placed near the affected joint.

The movements are rhythmic, smooth, slow, and controlled. It is neither necessary nor desirable to have the client's limbs flailing about. During a massage session, strive to move every joint. Joint movement should be incorporated into every massage when possible.

PATHOLOGIC CONDITIONS OF JOINTS

SECTION OBJECTIVES

Chapter objective covered in this section:

8. Identify pathologic conditions of joints, and describe general treatment protocols used for intervention.

After completing this section, the student will be able to perform the following:

- Categorize joint pathology into the similar causal factors.
- Explain the role of inflammation in joint pathology.
- Describe the mechanisms of joint injury.
- Explain the effect of immobilization on joint function.
- Define seven types of abnormal spinal curvatures.
- Describe how joint pathology relates to backache.
- Apply recommendations from indications and contraindications to massage treatment plans.

Any process or event that disturbs the normal function of a specific joint usually sets up a chain of events that eventually affects every part of a joint and its surrounding structures. Joint conditions can result from repetitive overuse; inflammatory joint disease; injuries; and structural deviations such as kyphosis, lordosis, and scoliosis.

Conditions Caused by Movement
Repetitive Overuse

Constant static stress on the joints, such as occurs in prolonged standing, sitting, or squatting, can damage joint structures. Ligaments subjected to constant tensile loads creep and can undergo excessive lengthening.

Cartilage subjected to constant compressive loading also can creep and may undergo excessive deformation. Joints and their supporting structures subjected to repetitive loading can be injured and fail because they do not have time to recover their original dimensions before they are subjected to another loading cycle. These types of injuries are common in massage therapists, athletes, dancers, musicians, and factory and office workers.

Bursitis

Bursitis is one of the most common causes of joint pain. Inflammation of the bursae—especially those located between the bony prominences and a muscle or tendon, such as in the shoulder, elbow, hip, or knee—usually results from trauma. Repetitive overuse or rheumatoid or gouty arthritis also may cause bursitis. A common treatment includes the use of rest during the acute phase but only for a short time to avoid pathologic immobilization. Analgesics and local injections of antiinflammatory medications also can be helpful. Ice can reduce inflammation and pain. Massage that reduces any muscle tension contributing to the development of inflammation and a readjustment of activities to reduce strain on the bursa are beneficial. Often, a postural deviation changes the angle of function at a joint, resulting in irritation at an area of a bursa. Restoring normal postural alignment alleviates the irritation, and the bursitis may resolve itself.

Lateral Epicondylitis (Epicondylosis)

Lateral epicondylitis (tennis elbow) follows repetitive extension of the wrist or pronation-supination of the forearm. Pain and tenderness develop at the lateral epicondyle and possibly in the proximal extensor muscles. When the wrist is extended against resistance, pain increases. Treatment is as for bursitis.

Medial Epicondylitis (Epicondylosis)

Medial epicondylitis (golfer's or pitcher's elbow) follows repetitive wrist flexion, as in throwing. Tenderness is maximal at the medial epicondyle. Wrist flexion against resistance increases the pain. Again, treatment is as for bursitis.

Inflammatory Joint Disease (Arthritis)

The most common type of joint disorder is termed *arthritis,* which means "inflammation of the joint." Several different kinds of arthritis occur (Figure 8-36). The four types of inflammatory joint disease (arthritis) are physical stress-induced, immune-related, crystal-induced, and infectious.

Physical Stress Induced: Degenerative Joint Disease (Osteoarthritis)

Osteoarthritis, or degenerative joint disease, usually first occurs in middle age and progresses with the aging process as a result of normal wear and tear. Although osteoarthritis appears to be a natural result of aging, factors such as obesity, repeated physical stressors, and previous injury without restoring area to normal function can help bring it about earlier and more intensely. Osteoarthritis may be a genetic disorder. Although some inflammation may be present, it results from the degenerative process. The disease process involves the growth of new bone (called *spurs* or *osteophytes*) at the edges of the articular surfaces, thickening of the synovial

membrane, atrophy of the cartilage, and calcification of the ligaments. Friction increases between the joint surfaces, further increasing the degenerative process. Pain is usually less intense in the morning and steadily worsens throughout the day. Osteoarthritis occurs mostly in joints used in weight bearing, such as the hips, knees, and spinal column, but it can occur in any joint. Previously injured joints tend to develop some arthritis later in life.

In the hands nodules on the dorsal lateral aspects of the DIP joints, called *Heberden's nodes,* result from the bony overgrowth of osteoarthritis. Flexion and deviation deformities may develop. Usually hard and painless, Heberden's nodes affect the middle-aged or elderly and often are associated with arthritic changes in other joints.

Methods of treatment include the use of nonsteroidal antiinflammatory and pain medications. Nonpharmaceutical interventions include moderate exercise that does not cause pain, the use of ice, and topical counterirritant ointments such as capsicum-based preparations.

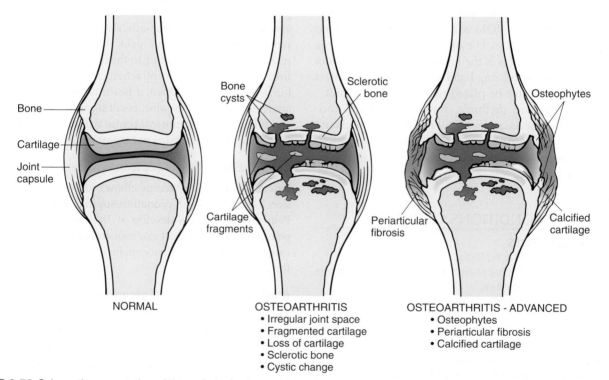

NORMAL

OSTEOARTHRITIS
• Irregular joint space
• Fragmented cartilage
• Loss of cartilage
• Sclerotic bone
• Cystic change

OSTEOARTHRITIS - ADVANCED
• Osteophytes
• Periarticular fibrosis
• Calcified cartilage

FIGURE 8-36 Schematic presentation of the pathologic changes in osteoarthritis. Fragmentation and loss of cartilage denude the subchondral bone, which undergoes sclerosis and cystic change. Osteophytes form on the lateral sides and protrude into the adjacent soft tissues, causing irritation, inflammation, and fibrosis. (From Damjanov I: *Pathology for the health professions,* ed 4, Philadelphia, 2012, Saunders.)

Immune-Related: Rheumatoid Arthritis

Rheumatoid arthritis is the most common immune-related form of inflammatory joint disease. Rheumatoid arthritis has many characteristics similar to other autoimmune disorders in which antibodies attack normal body tissues. The disease is a crippling condition characterized by swelling of the joints in the hands, feet, and other parts of the body as a result of inflammation and overgrowth of the synovial membranes and other joint tissues. The disease process changes the composition and quantity of the synovial fluid, altering the lubrication of the joint. The articular cartilage gradually is destroyed, the joint cavity develops adhesions, and the surfaces become stuck together. The joints stiffen and may eventually become useless. The cause of rheumatoid arthritis is uncertain, and the interaction of multiple agents is probable. Genetic factors may influence susceptibility.

Treatment includes the use of various nonsteroidal anti-inflammatory drugs (disease-modifying antirheumatic drugs, or DMARDs, are the standard of care in rhematoid arthritis and should be used very early in the process). The administration of steroids and gold salts may provide some relief in severe conditions. Localized injection of steroids can reduce severe acute localized symptoms. The use of steroids is controversial, and benefits do not always outweigh the risks of long-term use.

> **INDICATIONS/CONTRAINDICATIONS** for Therapeutic Massage
>
> Because the progression and flare-ups of the disease are often stress related, the generalized gentle stress-reduction methods provided by massage therapy may be beneficial in long-term management of the condition, if supervised as part of a total care program. The practitioner should refrain from performing frictioning techniques or any other forms of massage therapy that cause inflammation. General systemic changes in the neurotransmitters and hormones that accompany exercise and many forms of massage therapy can elevate mood and thereby reduce pain perception.

Crystal-Induced Arthritis

Gout is a form of arthritis caused by a disturbance of metabolism or underexcretion of uric acid in patients with a relatively normal serum concentration. One of the by-products of metabolism is uric acid, which normally is excreted in the urine. If an overproduction of uric acid occurs or for some reason an insufficient quantity is excreted, the accumulated uric acid forms crystals, which are deposited as masses around the joints and other parts of the body. Gout is characterized by a painful and tender, hot, dusky-red swelling that extends beyond the margin of the joint. Gout is easily mistaken for cellulitis. Any joint can be involved, but the one most commonly affected is the MTP joint of the great toe. Most victims of gout are men past middle age. Treatment includes dietary modifications and several medications to increase excretion of uric acid by the kidneys.

> **INDICATIONS/CONTRAINDICATIONS** for Therapeutic Massage
>
> Massage therapy is regionally contraindicated.

Infectious Arthritis

Infectious arthritis can be brought on by infections such as rheumatic fever, gonorrhea, and tuberculosis. Gonorrheal arthritis is becoming widespread because of the tremendous increase in the number of cases of gonorrhea.

The joints and bones themselves are subject to attack by the tuberculosis organism, and the result may be gradual destruction of parts of the bone near the joint. The organism is carried by the bloodstream, usually from the lungs or lymph nodes, and may cause considerable damage before being discovered. Several vertebrae sometimes are affected, or one hip or other single joint may be diseased. The client may complain only of difficulty in walking, and diagnosis is difficult unless an accompanying lung tuberculosis has been found. This disorder is most common in children. Referral for proper diagnosis is important.

> **INDICATIONS/CONTRAINDICATIONS** for Therapeutic Massage
>
> Infectious disease is a contraindication for massage unless the massage practitioner is directly supervised by appropriate health care professionals.

Conditions Caused by Injury

Joint injuries usually are classified as dislocations and sprains. A dislocation is a dislodging of the joint parts. A sprain is the wrenching of a joint with rupture or tearing of the ligaments, the joint capsule, or both.

Injury such as the tearing of a ligament or joint capsule results in a lack of support for the joint (Figure 8-37). Instability causes the separation of the articulating bones, with wobbling or deviation from the normal alignment of the bones of the joint. These changes in alignment create an abnormal joint distraction on the side where a ligament is torn. As a result, the other ligaments, tendons, and the joint capsule may become excessively stretched in the area of the injury.

Injury on one side of the joint also can affect the other side by subjecting it to abnormal compression during weight bearing or movement. Compensation in movement patterns, from instability and pain, can result in uneven pressure on the joint. Protective muscle spasms develop, which limit movement. In the short-term acute phase of injury, this action provides effective splinting of the area, but if the restriction in ROM continues, immobilization can result.

Joint injury usually is measured as follows:

- **First Degree.** A partial tear (5%) with pain and swelling but with the ability to bear weight and move through the normal ROM
- **Second Degree.** Larger tearing of structures with pain and swelling and inability to bear weight without pain and weakness that compromises ROM. Assessment reveals increased laxity compared with other side, but still firm end point.
- **Third Degree.** Extensive injury to joint structures, including full ligament tears and the inability to bear weight and loss of normal ROM; no obvious end point with increased laxity

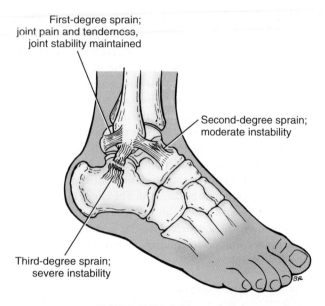

First-degree sprain;
joint pain and tenderness,
joint stability maintained

Second-degree sprain;
moderate instability

Third-degree sprain;
severe instability

FIGURE 8-37 Ankle sprains.

Immobilization

Immobilization is detrimental to joint structure and function and can be caused by a cast or other form of external restraining mechanism, by muscle splinting, as a reaction to pain and inflammation, or by paralysis. Immobilization affects the surrounding soft tissues, the articular surfaces of the joint, and the underlying bone. The detrimental effects of immobilization include development of fibrofatty connective tissue within the joint space; adhesions between the folds of the synovium; atrophy of cartilage; regional osteoporosis; weakening of ligaments at attachment sites; and a decrease in the water content of articular cartilage, tendons, ligaments, and the joint capsule. Swelling or immobilization of a joint also inhibits and weakens the muscles surrounding the joint; therefore the joint is unable to function normally and is at high risk for additional injury.

An injured joint subjected to inflammation and swelling assumes a least-packed position of comfort to minimize the pressure within the joint space. Pain decreases in this position. If the joint movement is restricted for a few weeks in the position of comfort, contractures can develop in the surrounding soft tissues and the joint capsule. As a result, normal range of joint motion is compromised.

Casts and Splints

Immobilization, such as from casts and splints, is more difficult to handle. Physicians recognize that prolonged immobilization is undesirable and have developed forms of external stabilization that allow mobility. Dynamic movable splinting devices such as air casts and continuous passive motion devices that are capable of moving joints passively and repeatedly through a specified ROM have been beneficial in reducing immobilization in joints.

Paralysis

In conditions involving paralysis, therapeutic massage helps maintain and in some instances restore pliability of connective

Practical Application

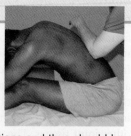

Management and rehabilitation of joint problems are part of a long-term process that often requires a multidisciplinary approach. Ice, massage, and rehabilitative exercise are usually methods of choice because they are drugless therapies. Ice is contraindicated in some conditions and thus should be used with caution. All three methods require active participation by the client, and the methods are not always pleasant. Compliance can be a problem, and the client needs to be motivated toward healing for the best results.

The pain and swelling of joint injury can be alleviated with the judicious and short-term use of pain medication, ice, and appropriate rehabilitative exercise. Soft-tissue methods such as massage, myofascial release, and trigger point work are often effective after the acute phase (approximately 2 to 3 days). The application of ice along with rehabilitative exercise is beneficial. The practitioner needs to give attention to the scope of practice and appropriate training to deal with rehabilitation programs.

INDICATIONS/CONTRAINDICATIONS for Therapeutic Massage

Therapeutic massage can be used to maintain pliability in accessible musculature and connective tissue structures. Therapeutic massage methods and movement approaches are beneficial in assisting a return to normal function after removal of the splinting.

Massage therapy also can aid management of compensatory patterns that develop because of casting and other forms of immobilization. Although direct work over an area that is actively healing is contraindicated unless the massage practitioner is supervised, massage and other forms of soft-tissue work, coupled with movement therapies, can manage the tension and possible pain that the rest of the body may develop from the changes in movement; sleeping positions; and other issues caused by the casting, immobilization process, gait changes, and compensation patterns.

tissues. Joint movement applications can passively replace lost joint movement and mimic compressive forces on the bones and jointed areas, helping prevent contracture and any other detrimental effects of immobilization. Massage intervention for those with paralysis must be supervised as part of a total treatment program. The practitioner must exercise caution when applying pressure and intensity because normal feedback mechanisms are disrupted.

Adhesive Capsulitis (Frozen Shoulder)

Adhesive capsulitis refers to a mysterious fibrosis of the glenohumeral joint capsule, manifested by diffuse, dull, aching pain in the shoulder and progressive restriction of motion but usually no localized tenderness. The condition is usually unilateral and most often occurs in those 50 to 70 years of age, specifically people with diabetes. Onset often is preceded by some sort of pathologic condition, resulting in the joint being immobilized. Pathologic immobilization sets in. The course is chronic, lasting months to years, but the disorder often resolves itself spontaneously, at least partially. Treatment is with physical therapy, including ROM exercises.

Conditions Caused by Structural Deviations

Abnormal Spinal Curvatures

Abnormal spinal curvatures result from postural deviation. Several types occur:

- Flattening of the lumbar curve (hypolordosis) accompanied by muscle spasm in the lumbar area and decreased spinal mobility is a combination of signs suggesting the possibility of a herniated lumbar disk or, especially in men, *ankylosing spondylitis*.
- *Hyperlordosis* is an accentuation of the normal lumbar lordotic curve that develops as a result of an excessively anteriorly tilted pelvis. Hyperlordosis also may compensate for a thoracic hyperkyphosis or flexion deformities of the hips.
- *Hyperkyphosis*, a rounded thoracic convexity, is common in aging and occurs especially in women.
- *Gibbus* is an angular deformity of a collapsed vertebra. Causes include metastatic cancer and tuberculosis of the spine.
- *List* is a lateral tilt of the spine. When a plumb line dropped from the spinous process of T1 falls to one side of the gluteal cleft, a list is present. Causes include a herniated disk and painful spasms of the paravertebral muscles.
- *Scoliosis* is a lateral S or C curvature of the spine and is associated with lateral flexion and rotation of the vertebrae on one another, and the rib cage is deformed accordingly. Structural scoliosis is seen best when the client bends forward. On the side of the thoracic convexity, the ribs bulge posteriorly and are separated widely. On the opposite side, the ribs are displaced anteriorly and are close together.
- *Functional scoliosis* compensates for other abnormalities such as unequal lower limb lengths. The scoliosis disappears with forward flexion.

Other Conditions of the Joints

Backache

Backache is a common complaint. Although lower back pain is the most common complaint, neck or cervical pain is also common. The usual cause is muscular and is discussed later. A list of some joint causes of backache follows.

In disorders of the intervertebral disks, pain may be severe, with muscle spasms and the resulting nerve impingement extending symptoms along the course of the nerve to the legs and groin. The condition can degenerate to a ruptured disk, which is most commonly a posterior or posterolateral protrusion of the nucleus pulposus through a tear in the annulus fibrosus, placing pressure on nerves.

Abnormalities of the vertebrae or ligaments and other supporting structures include the following:

- Strains on the lumbosacral joint (where the lumbar region joins the sacrum) or strains on the sacroiliac joint (where the sacrum joins the ilium)

- Spondylolisthesis, or the moving forward of one vertebra on another, which usually occurs at the L5/S1 junction
- Spondylitis, or inflammation of more than one vertebra
- Ankylosing spondylitis, or rheumatoid inflammatory disorder, in which the articular hyaline cartilage is destroyed, the bones fuse, and the spinal ligaments ossify. The disease tends to begin in the sacroiliac joints and progress up the spine.
- Spondylosis, or degenerative joint disease (osteoarthritis) of the spine, induces the formation of bony spurs at the disk margin of the vertebral bodies. The disease causes degenerative changes in the intervertebral disks.

INDICATIONS/CONTRAINDICATIONS for Therapeutic Massage

Most backaches are preventable. The back muscles should not be used for lifting. Instead, you should bring the weight close to the body, above the hips if possible, and allow the legs to do the actual lifting. An adequate exercise program is also important.

Massage therapy modalities are effective in managing backache. The benefits derive from a reduction in protective muscle spasm compensation (guarding) and generalized pain-modulating effects. The practitioner should be aware that protective spasm provides stabilization. The goal is not to eliminate protective spasm totally but rather to support the body in managing dysfunctional patterns. Complex backache involving the joint structures requires that therapeutic massage be incorporated into a total treatment program with supervision by the appropriate health care professional.

Therapeutic massage can be a beneficial adjunct treatment, especially with the symptomatic management of pain in supporting an increase in ROM.

Ganglia

Ganglia are cystic, round, usually nontender swellings located along tendon sheaths or joint capsules. The dorsum of the hand and wrist is a frequent site of involvement. Flexion of the wrist makes ganglia more prominent, whereas extension tends to obscure them. Ganglia also may develop elsewhere on the hands, wrists, ankles, and feet.

INDICATIONS/CONTRAINDICATIONS for Therapeutic Massage

Massage methods are regionally contraindicated.

SUMMARY

A comprehensive understanding of joint structure and function is necessary for the effective practice of therapeutic massage for the joints. The massage practitioner can use methods to support joint health and provide benefits in managing joint dysfunction.

The health and strength of joint structures depend on a certain amount of stress and strain. Cartilage and bone nutrition and growth depend on joint movement and muscle contraction. Cartilage nutrition depends on joint movement through a full ROM to ensure that all the articular cartilage receives the nutrients necessary for health. Ligaments and muscles (and their tendons) depend on a normal amount of stress and strain to maintain and increase strength. Bone density and strength increase after the stress and strain created by muscle and joint activity. Bone density and strength decrease when stress and strain are absent.

Without stress and strain the joints do not function well, but with too much stress and strain a pathologic condition may develop. Human beings are similar in that we need to be exposed to challenges in life, but attempting to deal with too much can be overwhelming. The concept of balance is illustrated again in joint health and personal well-being.

The author would like to thank Joseph E. Muscolino for his special contributions to this chapter.

Θvolve

http://evolve.elsevier.com/Fritz/essential

Activity 8-1 Fill in a crossword puzzle testing your knowledge of joint terminology.

Activity 8-2 Take a matching quiz to identify joints based on their illustrations.

Activity 8-3 View a video of range of motion techniques used in massage.

Additional Resources:

Scientific animations and cadaver dissection video

Weblinks: Access weblinks that lead to research articles and an anatomy lesson from a Georgetown University instructor

Electronic Coloring Book

Remember to study for your certification and licensure exams! Review questions for this chapter are located on Evolve.

Workbook Section

All Workbook activities can be done online as well as here in the book. Answers are located on ⊖volve.

Short Answer

1. Describe the elementary principles of joint design.

_____
_____
_____
_____
_____
_____
_____
_____
_____
_____
_____
_____

2. Define the three main types of joints.

_____
_____
_____
_____
_____
_____
_____
_____
_____

3. Define arthrokinematics and osteokinematics and the three categories of joint movement.

_____
_____
_____
_____
_____
_____
_____
_____
_____
_____
_____
_____
_____

4. Describe joint play.

_____
_____
_____

_____
_____

5. List the structures that contribute to joint stability.

_____
_____
_____
_____

6. Identify the generalized joint disorders, and describe a treatment protocol used for each.

_____
_____
_____
_____
_____
_____
_____
_____
_____

Fill in the Blank

(1) _____ refers to the amount of motion available to a joint within the anatomic limits of the joint structure. An articulation, or (2) _____, is where two or more bones meet to connect parts and allow for movement in the body.

(3) _____ are flat sacs of synovial membrane in which the inner sides of the sacs are separated by a fluid film. Bursae are located where moving structures are apt to (4) _____.

A (5) _____ occurs when joints of the human body are linked together into a series in such a way that motion at one of the joints is accompanied by motion at an adjacent joint.

The (6) _____ is the only position in a synovial joint in which the surfaces fit precisely together and maximal contact occurs between the opposing surfaces. Because the joint surfaces are (7) _____, they permit the least movement, and the joint possesses its greatest stability.

Collagen is a fibrous tissue that provides stability to (8) _____ tissue structures.

(9) _____ is a fibrous tissue that has elastic properties and allows flexibility of connective tissue structures. A diarthrosis is a freely movable (10) _____ joint. (11) _____ is a connective tissue that permits little motion in joints and structures. It is found in places such as the intervertebral disks and forms our ears. Hyaline cartilage is the thin

covering of (12) _____ connective tissue on the ends of the bones in freely movable joints in the adult skeleton.

Hypermobility occurs when the range of motion (ROM) of a joint is (13) _____ than normally would be permitted by the structure. It results in (14) _____. (15) _____ occurs when the ROM of a joint is less than what normally would be permitted by the structure. It results in (16) _____ ROM. The joint (17) _____ is a connective tissue structure that indirectly connects the bony components of a joint. Joint play is the (18) _____ movement that occurs between articular surfaces, which has nothing to do with the ROM of a joint produced by (19) _____. It is an essential component of joint motion and must occur for normal functioning of the joint.

The least-packed position is the position of a synovial joint where the joint capsule is at its most (20) _____. Joints tend to assume this position when (21) _____ occurs to accommodate the increased volume of synovial fluid.

Open kinematic chain occurs when the ends of the limbs or parts of the body are free to move without causing (22) _____ at another joint.

(23) _____ ROM is the amount of motion at a joint that fails to reach the normal physiologic range or exceeds normal anatomic limits of motion of that joint.

Physiologic ROM is the amount of motion available to a joint determined by the nervous system from information provided by joint (24) _____ receptors. This information usually prevents a joint from being positioned where (25) _____ could occur.

A (26) _____ is a limited-movement, nonsynovial joint.

A suture is a (27) _____ joint in which two bony components are united by a thin layer of dense fibrous tissue.

A symphysis is a (28) _____ joint in which the two bony components are joined directly by fibrocartilage in the form of a disk or plate.

A synchondrosis is a joint in which the material used for connecting the two components is (29) _____ growth cartilage.

A syndesmosis is a (30) _____ joint in which two bony components are joined directly by a ligament, cord, or aponeurotic membrane.

(31) _____ fluid is a thick, colorless, lubricating fluid secreted by the membrane of the joint cavity.

Types of (32) _____ joints include the following:

Hinge joints allow flexion and extension movements in (33) _____ direction, changing the angle of the bones at the joint, similar to a door hinge.

(34) _____ joints allow rotation around the length of the bone.

Condyloid (condylar) joints allow movement in (35) _____ directions, but one motion predominates.

A saddle joint is (36) _____ in one plane and concave in the other, and these surfaces fit together like a rider on a saddle.

A (37) _____ joint allows movement in many directions around a central point.

Gliding joints, also known as synovial (38) _____ joints, allow only a gliding motion in various planes.

(39) _____ is the combination of resistance offered by a fluid to a change of form and the ability of material to return to its original state after deformation. This term is used to describe (40)_____ tissue.

Problem Solving

Read the problem presented. There is no correct answer; rather the exercise is intended to assist the student in developing the analytical and decision-making skills necessary in a professional practice. After reading the problem, follow the next six steps.
1. Identify the facts presented in the information.
2. Identify the possibilities ("what if" statements) presented, or develop your own possibilities that relate to the facts.
3. Evaluate each possibility in terms of the logical cause and effect and pros and cons.
4. Consider the effect on the persons involved.
5. Write each answer in the space provided.
6. Develop your solution by answering the question posed.

Problem

All movement involves joints. Individuals who move for a living, such as professional athletes and dancers, are particularly susceptible to joint dysfunction. Injury is more than an inconvenience; it can end a career. Many of those affected continue to work in pain. They do not allow proper healing time, and additional damage may result. Young children who begin to train for competition before puberty develop a more pliable joint structure. Hypermobility may result. As these children age, joint structure is compromised by laxity in the joints, and pain and various degrees of disability can result.

Question

In what ways can a massage therapist use the information presented in this chapter to educate the vulnerable client about the need for support of the joints so that accumulating damage does not continue?

Facts
1. Persons who move professionally are susceptible to joint injury.
2. _____
3. _____

Possibilities

1. Persons may work with joint injury.
2. _____
3. _____

Logical Cause and Effect

1. Performance would not be as good.
2. _____
3. _____

Effect

1. The massage professional may feel frustrated working with someone who will not or cannot take time off for appropriate healing.
2. _____
3. _____

In what ways can a massage therapist use the information presented in this chapter to educate the vulnerable client about the need for support of the joints so that accumulating damage does not continue?

_____
_____
_____
_____
_____
_____
_____
_____

Professional Application

Connective tissue plays an important role in joint health. What are the specific massage applications to affect connective tissue function? What other knowledge would you require to work more effectively with connective tissues? What referral base would be necessary to best support a client with connective tissue dysfunction affecting the joints?

_____
_____
_____
_____
_____
_____
_____
_____
_____
_____
_____

Assess Your Competencies

Review the following objectives for Chapter 8:

1. Describe the basic principles of joint design.
2. Define *articulation*.
3. Explain the functions of stability and mobility.
4. Discuss the role of connective tissue in joint function.
5. Describe collagen and elastin.
6. Define and locate bursae.
7. Describe three types of cartilage.
8. Explain the properties of connective tissue.
9. List the mechanical forces that act on the body.
10. Relate the five mechanical forces to the process of joint injury.
11. List and explain three joint categories.
12. Demonstrate the principles of joint motion.
13. Define arthrokinematics.
14. Describe joint play.
15. Define osteokinematics.
16. Demonstrate and explain joint movement to identify range of motion.
17. Explain three categories of osteokinematic movement.
18. Explain hypomobility and hypermobility.
19. Define end feel.
20. Describe the structures that contribute to joint stability.
21. Describe joint movement in the three planes of movement of the body.
22. Demonstrate and name the general joint movements.
23. Demonstrate and name joint movement specific to the forearm, wrist, thumb, ankle, and foot.
24. Demonstrate and name joint movement specific to the shoulder girdle and shoulder joint.
25. Demonstrate and name joint movement specific to the spine and pelvis.
26. Describe the classification of synovial joint movement.
27. Define kinematic chains.
28. Identify and palpate individual joints of the body.
29. Palpate and describe the following jointed areas:
    • Joints of the skull
    • Joints of the shoulder
    • Joints of the elbow
    • Joints of the wrist and hand
    • Joints of the pelvis and hip
    • Joints of the knee
    • Joints of the ankle and foot
    • Joints of the spine and thorax
30. Design a joint movement sequence for the body.
31. Describe why joint movement is important to massage application.
32. Use joint movement to assess for normal and abnormal range of motion of a joint.
33. Demonstrate two types of joint movement: active and passive.
34. Identify pathologic conditions of joints, and describe general treatment protocols used for intervention.
35. Categorize joint pathology into the similar causal factors.
36. Explain the role of inflammation in joint pathology.
37. Describe the mechanisms of joint injury.
38. Explain the effect of immobilization on joint function.
39. Define seven types of abnormal spinal curvatures.
40. Describe how joint pathology relates to backache.
41. Apply recommendations from indications and contraindications to massage treatment plans.

Next, on a separate piece of paper or using an audio or video recorder, prepare a short narrative that reflects how you would explain this content to a client and how the information relates to how you would provide massage. See the example in Chapter 1 on p. 22. When read or listened to, the narrative should not take more than 5 to 10 minutes to complete. Simpler is better. Use examples, tell stories, and use metaphors. It is important to understand that there is no precisely correct way to complete this exercise. The intent is to help you identify how effectively you understand the content and how relevant your application is to massage therapy. An excellent learning activity is to work together with other students and share your narratives. Also share these narratives with a friend or family member who is not familiar with the content. If that person can understand what you have written or recorded, that indicates that you understand it. There are many different ways to complete this learning activity. Yes, it may be confusing to do this, but that's all right. Out of confusion comes clarity. By the time you do this 12 times, once for each chapter in this book, you will be much more competent.

Further Study

Using additional resource material (see the Works Consulted list at the back of this book), elaborate on the following topics:

Connective tissue

_____

_____

_____

_____

_____

_____

Cartilage

_____

_____

_____

_____

_____

Kinematic chains

_____

_____

_____

_____

_____

_____

_____

Immobilization pathology

_____

_____

_____

_____

_____

Repetitive overuse syndrome

_____

_____

_____

_____

Ergonomics

_____

_____

_____

_____

Muscles

ⓔ http://evolve.elsevier.com/Fritz/essential

CHAPTER OBJECTIVES

After completing this chapter, the student will be able to perform the following:

1. Explain the various terminologies used to describe muscles.
2. Describe the relationship between structure and function of muscles.
3. Describe the anatomy and physiology of skeletal muscle fibers.
4. List the components of myotatic units.
5. Identify the different muscle shapes and fiber arrangements.
6. Describe the response of proprioceptors to stimuli and the most common reflexes.
7. Describe the process of muscle firing patterns/muscle activation sequences.
8. Describe the integrated connective tissue structure of muscle.
9. Explain and demonstrate the three types of muscle actions.
10. Describe how muscles are named.
11. Learn how to palpate individual muscles.
12. Identify the attachments, actions, synergist, antagonist, and common trigger points of individual muscles.
13. Identify common pathology related to muscles and explain indications and contraindications for massage.

CHAPTER OUTLINE

TERMINOLOGY, 284
 International Anatomic Terminology, 285
 Muscle Attachment Terminology, 285
MUSCLE STRUCTURE AND FUNCTION, 286
 Muscle Tissue and the Whole Body, 286
 Anatomy and Physiology of Muscle Fibers, 289
 Myotatic Units (Functional Muscle Groups), 294
 Proprioceptors and Reflexes, 295
 Muscle Firing Patterns/Muscle Activation Sequences, 297
CONNECTIVE TISSUE COMPONENT OF MUSCLE, 298
 Pathologic Connective Tissue Changes, 303
INDIVIDUAL MUSCLES, 304
 How Muscles Are Named, 304
 Muscle Attachment Terminology, 307
 How to Palpate Muscles, 307
 Organization of This Section, 307
 Muscles of the Face and Head, 307
 Muscles of the Neck, 323
 Deep Muscles of the Back and Posterior Neck, 335
 Muscles of the Torso, 350
 Muscles of the Gluteal Region, 369
 Muscles of the Anterior and Lateral Leg, 393
 Muscles of the Posterior Leg, 400

 Intrinsic Muscles of the Foot, 406
 Muscles of Scapular Stabilization, 415
 Muscles of the Musculotendinous (Rotator) Cuff, 422
 Muscles of the Shoulder Joint, 426
 Muscles of the Elbow and Radioulnar Joints, 433
 Muscles of the Wrist and Hand Joints, 439
 Intrinsic Muscles of the Hand, 451
PATHOLOGIC CONDITIONS, 458
 Mechanisms of Disease, 458
 Specific Disorders, 460
SUMMARY, 463

KEY TERMS

Agonist (AG-on-ist) A muscle that causes or controls joint motion through a specified plane of motion; also known as a *mover*.

All-or-none response The property of a muscle fiber (cell) which, when stimulated to contract, contracts to its full ability or does not contract at all.

Antagonist (an-TAG-a-nist) A muscle usually located on the opposite side of a joint from the mover (agonist) and having the opposite action. The antagonist must lengthen when the mover contracts and shortens.

Aponeurosis (AP-o-nu-RO-sis) A broad, flat sheet of fibrous connective tissue.

Concentric action (kon-SEN-trik) A contraction in which the muscle shortens with tone because its contractile force is greater than the opposing force at the attachments of the muscle. Concentric contractions are contractions of a mover (agonist) wherein it creates the movement of a body part.

Contractility (kon-trak-TIL-i-tee) The ability of a muscle to shorten forcibly with adequate stimulation. This property sets muscle apart from all other types of tissue.

Deep fascia (FASH-ea) A coarse sheet of fibrous connective tissue that binds muscles into functional groups and forms partitions, called *intermuscular septa,* between muscle groups.

Dynamic force Force applied to an object that produces movement in or of the object.

Eccentric action (ek-SEN-trik) A contraction in which the muscle lengthens with tone because its contractile force is less than the opposing force at the attachments of the muscle. Eccentric contractions are contractions of an antagonist that usually restrain or control the action of the prime mover. Eccentric contractions sometimes are described as *negative contractions.*

Elasticity The ability of a muscle to recoil and resume its original resting length after being stretched.

Excitability The ability of a muscle to receive and respond to a stimulus.

Extensibility (eks-ten-si-BIL-i-tee) The ability of a muscle to be stretched or extended.

Fascia (FASH-ea) A fibrous or loose type of connective tissue; a fibrous membrane covering, supporting, and separating muscles; the subcutaneous tissue that connects the skin to the muscles.

Fixator (fik-SAY-tor) A stabilizing muscle located at a joint or body part that contracts to fix, or stabilize, the area, enabling another limb or body segment to exert force and move. The fixator also may be described as a muscle (or other force) that stops one attachment of a muscle from moving so that the other attachment of the muscle must move.

Insertion The attachment of a muscle that moves (or usually moves) when the muscle contracts. The insertion of a muscle is usually the distal attachment of the muscle. For muscles located on the axial body, the insertion is usually the superior attachment of the muscle or the part of the muscle that attaches farthest from the midline, or center, of the body.

Isometric action (i-so-MET-rik) A contraction in which the muscle stays the same length with tone because its contractile force equals that of the opposing force at the attachments of the muscle. The muscle tenses but does not produce movement. Isometric contractions are usually contractions of a fixator/stabilizer muscle (or neutralizer muscle) that acts to stabilize or fix a body part in position while another joint action is occurring.

Isotonic action (i-so-TON-ik) The action of the muscle that occurs when tension develops in the muscle while it shortens or lengthens.

Maximal stimulus The point at which all motor units of a muscle have been recruited and the muscle is unable to increase in strength.

Motor unit A motor neuron and all of the muscle fibers it controls.

Myogloblin (MI-eh-GLO-ben) A red pigment similar to hemoglobin that stores oxygen within the muscle cells.

Origin The attachment of a muscle that does not move (or usually does not move) when the muscle contracts. The origin of a muscle is usually the proximal attachment of the muscle. For muscles located on the axial body, the origin is usually the inferior attachment of the muscle or the part of the muscle that attaches closest to the midline, or center, of the body.

Oxygen debt The extra amount of oxygen that must be taken in to remove the buildup of lactic acid from anaerobic respiration of glucose (to convert lactic acid to glucose or glycogen).

Resting tone The state of tension in resting muscles.

Reverse action When a muscle contracts and the attachment that normally stays fixed (the origin) moves, and the attachment that usually moves (the insertion) stays fixed.

Sliding filament mechanism The process describing skeletal muscle contraction in which the thick and thin filaments slide past one another.

Static force Force applied to an object in such a way that it does not produce movement.

Synergist (SIN-er-jist) Movers of a joint other than the prime mover(s); that is, assistant, secondary, or emergency movers. A *synergist* may be more broadly defined as any muscle that helps the action occur (i.e., also may be a fixator, neutralizer, or support muscle, as well as other movers).

Threshold stimulus The stimulus at which the first observable muscle contraction occurs.

Trigger points A hyperirritable locus within a taut band of skeletal muscle, located in the muscular tissue or its associated fascia. The spot is painful on compression and can evoke characteristic referred pain and autonomic phenomena.

LEARNING HOW TO LEARN

Volumes have been written about the intricacies of soft-tissue structure and function. This text, by necessity, limits itself to the most functionally practical information related to the methods used by massage therapists. It will also be helpful to continue formal study and self-study of this material.

According to the learning theory of Bloom's Taxonomy, we go through a learning process. The process is as follows:

- First we learn to remember.
- Next we learn the same information to understand.
- Once we understand, then we can apply what we have learned.
- Understanding allows us to analyze, evaluate, and create.

It is necessary to be patient while learning about muscles. Repetition is the key, and each time we repeat the content, we move closer to understanding and applying the information.

Muscles and their associated connective tissue make up the soft tissues of our bodies. Using artistic terms, you could say that muscles and connective tissue are the media of massage practitioners. Just as a sculptor needs to understand clay, the massage therapist needs to understand muscles. Because soft tissue accounts for about half the tissue mass of the body and most pain patterns find themselves connected to soft-tissue dysfunctions of various types, the careful study of this area of anatomy and physiology is obviously important.

When studying anatomy and physiology, we must continue to see the body as a whole, in structure and function, and this is especially true in the study of the muscles. Physiologically, one muscle does not operate independently of others. Structural design knits together the muscles, bones, and connective tissue structures into intertwining spans that are necessary for stability and mobility. To assist you in learning about muscles, this chapter breaks the anatomy into isolated segments. Chapter 10 then puts all these pieces back together so that you can better understand how to apply the information in massage therapy treatments.

The body has three types of muscle tissue: skeletal muscle, cardiac muscle, and smooth muscle. This chapter focuses on skeletal muscle tissue and provides a brief overview of cardiac and smooth muscle.

TERMINOLOGY

SECTION OBJECTIVES

Chapter objective covered in this section:

1. Explain the various terminologies used to describe muscles.

After completing this section, the student will be able to perform the following:

- Identify areas of terminology confusion.
- Explain the importance of the Terminologia Anatomica.
- Use muscle attachment terminology based on both anatomy and physiology.

Why It Is Confusing

The following are just a few examples showing how terminology can become confusing:

Muscle Name Variations
Musculus deltoideus (derived from Latin and German)
Deltoid (English)
Which is correct: deltoideus or deltoid?

Multiple Names for the Very Same Muscles
Peronealis (derived from Latin and German)
Fibularis (derived from Latin and German)
Peroneal (English)
Fibular (English)
Which is correct: peronealis, peroneal, fibularis, or fibular?
Venter frontalis musculus occipitofrontalis (derived from Latin and German)
Venter frontalis musculi occipitofrontalis (derived from Latin and German)
Frontal belly of occipitofrontalis (English)
Frontalis (English)
Frontal part of occipitofrontalis
Which is correct? There are five different names.

Word Sequence Issues
Musculus serratus posterior inferior (derived from Latin and German)
Serratus posterior inferior (English)
Inferior serratus posterior (English)
Which is correct: inferior at the beginning or at the end, and posterior in the middle or at the end?

Muscle Attachment Terminology
Origin/Insertion
Proximal/Distal
Arises from/Attaches to
From/To
Which is correct? Consultation with anatomy experts yielded the following response: "It depends." All the terms are correct, even if confusing.

Anatomic terminology for muscle names and attachments is sometimes confusing. Terminology used for the muscular system is not always consistent. Multiple names and spellings for muscle names, and duplicate terminology to describe the location of muscles, exist. Additionally, muscular terminology can vary from country to country depending on language (Box 9-1).

International Anatomic Terminology

Terminologia Anatomica (TA) is the international standard on human anatomic terminology. The revision of modern anatomic terminology was initiated in 1887. More than 100 years later, the new *Terminologia Anatomica: International Anatomical Terminology* was finally accepted by the International Federation of Associations of Anatomists in 1997. This means that all medical practitioners (traditional and complementary) in every country around the world now have a common terminology. The problem is that the common terminology is not used consistently. Anatomic terminology is the foundation of medical terminology, and Latin is the international anatomic language. Only Latin is the international basis for creating equivalent terms in other languages. English is not the basis for terminology in other languages, yet many terms commonly used are English.

Muscle Attachment Terminology

Muscles have to be attached to bone in order to function. The terms most commonly used in the past to describe muscle attachments to the bone or other tissue are **origin** and **insertion.** Classically, the origin of a muscle has been defined as the attachment that does not move when the muscle contracts; the origin is usually the proximal attachment or the attachment closer to the midline or center of the body. The insertion has been defined as the attachment that does move when the muscle contracts; the insertion is usually the distal attachment or the attachment farther from the midline or center of the body. Origin and insertion terminology is a *physiologic description* of a muscle's attachments because it names an attachment on the basis of whether or not it moves (Muscolino, 2007).

However, this terminology can lead to confusion regarding the structural locations of muscles and the ways in which muscles really function. The problem with this terminology is that it can create an impression that one attachment of a muscle is always fixed and that the other attachment always moves. Origins and insertions of a muscle often switch—that is, the insertion could stay fixed while the origin moves. When this situation occurs, the movement is called a **reverse action.** Simple examples of reverse actions are when the biceps brachii contracts and causes the arm to move toward the forearm (instead of the forearm moving toward the arm) when doing a chin-up or when the quadriceps femoris group contracts and causes the thigh to move toward the leg (instead of the leg moving toward the thigh) when standing up from a seated position (Muscolino, 2007).

In an effort to simplify the learning and understanding of muscles and their attachment and actions, a simpler terminology is becoming more widespread and accepted, which is to name the attachments of a muscle by the locations of the attachments. This system would be an *anatomical naming system.* For example, the attachments of the biceps brachii on to the scapula would be called the *proximal attachments* and the attachment onto the forearm would be called the *distal attachment.* There has also been an attempt to use "arises from" and "attaches to" or, even more simply, *from* and *to.*

On the basis of this information, muscle attachments can be stated as follows:
- Origin/Insertion: based on physiology or function
- Proximal/Distal: based on anatomy or structure
- Arises from/Attaches to: based on anatomy or structure
- From/To: based on anatomy or structure

This textbook includes all the ways that attachments can be stated. It may be cumbersome, but it is the only way to be accurate. The most proximal (origin) attachment is typically listed first. Here is how the attachment terminology will appear in the individual muscle sections that follow:
- Origin, proximal attachment, arises from:
- Insertion, distal attachment, attaches to:

MUSCLE STRUCTURE AND FUNCTION

SECTION OBJECTIVES

Chapter objective covered in this section:

2. Describe the relationship between structure and function of muscles.
3. Describe the types of skeletal muscle fiber.
4. List the components of myotatic units.
5. Identify the different muscle shapes and fiber arrangements.
6. Describe the response of proprioceptors to stimuli and the most common reflexes.
7. Describe the process of muscle firing patterns/muscle activation sequences.

After completing this section, the student will be able to perform the following:

- Explain the function of muscles.
- List the three types of muscles.
- List and describe four functional characteristics of muscle.
- Define and demonstrate two types of muscle actions and the variations of each.
- Describe a muscle as an organ and the structural and functional components.
- Explain the length-tension relationship.
- Define *resting muscle tone.*
- Identify the energy source for muscle contraction.
- Explain the difference between red slow-twitch and white fast-twitch muscle fibers.
- Describe the connective tissue component of muscle.
- Explain how muscles attach to bone or related tissue.
- List the components of myotatic units.
- List and draw four distinct muscle shapes.
- Describe the nervous system functions of proprioception and reflexes related to muscle function.
- Define *muscle activation sequences.*

A prominent functional characteristic of muscle is its ability to transform chemical energy from adenosine triphosphate (ATP) into mechanical energy. When this happens, muscle can exert force. Recall that force is energy applied in such a way that it initiates motion, changes the speed or direction of a motion, or alters the size and shape of an object.

Energy is defined technically as the capacity to do work. Many cultures use the words *force* and *energy* in referring to esoteric concepts. We find it in Eastern philosophy as Qi or prana and in the *Star Wars* movies as "The Force." All these words translate to energy, vital force, life force. One does not have to stretch the imagination very far to see the metaphor of muscles in these more expansive concepts.

When a muscle contracts, muscle tissue transforms one form of energy into another and is able to produce force. **Dynamic force** creates movement and change; **static force** produces no movement or noticeable change but still expends energy. If therapeutic interaction can help transform static force into dynamic force, the energy to achieve therapeutic goals can be released; this often is the objective that massage professionals seek to achieve with their clients.

Muscle Tissue and the Whole Body
The Three Types of Muscle and Their Functions

The functions of the three muscle types—smooth, cardiac and skeletal—are integral to the maintenance of homeostasis of the whole body. Skeletal, cardiac, and smooth muscles produce movement, such as that involved in breathing, the heartbeat, digestion, and elimination. All three types of muscle tissue produce the movement necessary for survival. Skeletal muscle moves the skeleton at the joints so that we can seek shelter, gather food, and protect ourselves.

Function of Skeletal Muscle

The four major functions of skeletal muscle are as follows:

1. To produce movement
2. To stabilize joints
3. To maintain posture
4. To generate heat

Stabilization of joint structures is an often overlooked function of muscle. The dynamic and static contraction of muscles surrounding the joint provides external stability, supporting the structures of the joint. This is especially true of the more mobile joints, which by nature have a loose structural design. To maintain stable body posture, the dynamic tension of muscle contraction opposes the force of gravity. The relative constancy of the internal temperature of the body is maintained in a cool external environment by the heat generated as a by-product of muscle tissue contraction.

Function of Cardiac and Smooth Muscle Tissue

Cardiac and smooth muscle tissues operate by mechanisms similar to those in skeletal muscle tissues.

Cardiac Muscle

Cardiac muscle (Figure 9-1, *A*), also known as *striated involuntary* muscle, is found in only one organ of the body, the heart. Forming the bulk of the wall of each heart chamber, cardiac muscle contracts rhythmically and continuously to provide the pumping action necessary to maintain a consistent blood flow through our internal environment.

The functional anatomy of cardiac muscle tissue resembles that of skeletal muscle but has specialized features related to the role of pumping blood continuously. Each cardiac muscle fiber contains parallel myofibrils composed of sarcomeres that give the whole fiber a striated appearance. However, the cardiac muscle fiber does not taper like a skeletal muscle fiber; rather, it forms strong, electrically coupled junctions (intercalated disks) with other fibers.

Cardiac muscle forms a continuous contractile band around the heart that conducts a single impulse across a continuous sarcolemma, allowing for an efficient, coordinated pumping action. This means that even though many adjacent cardiac muscle cells contract simultaneously, they have a prolonged contraction rather than a rapid twitch. Cardiac muscle does not normally run low on ATP and thus does not experience fatigue. Obviously, this characteristic of cardiac muscle is vital for keeping the heart pumping continuously.

Unlike skeletal muscle, in which a nervous impulse is necessary to excite the sarcolemma to produce its own impulse, cardiac muscle can be self-exciting. Cardiac muscle cells can have a continuing rhythm of excitation and contraction on their own, although the rate of self-induced impulses is usually

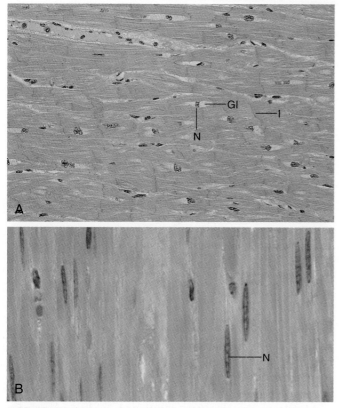

FIGURE 9-1 A, Micrograph of cardiac muscle. The intercalated disks *(I)* are characteristic of cardiac muscle. *N,* Nuclei. *GI,* glycogen deposits. **B,** Micrograph of smooth muscle. The central placement of nuclei *(N)* in the spindle-shaped smooth muscle fibers is notable. (From Gartner LP, Hiutt JL: *Color textbook of histology,* ed 3, Philadelphia, 2007, Saunders.)

too slow to allow for strenuous activity. Central nervous system control of the heart is normal and is necessary for strenuous activity and for generally altering the rate of the heart contractions to meet the demands placed on the heart.

Smooth Muscle

Smooth muscle comprises small, tapered cells with single nuclei (Figure 9-1, *B*). Smooth muscle fibers lack striations because the thick and thin myofilaments are arranged differently from skeletal or cardiac muscle fibers. These arrangements of myofilaments crisscross the cell and attach at their ends to the plasma membrane of the cell.

When cross-bridges pull the thin filaments together, the muscle balls up and thus contracts the cell. Because the myofilaments are not organized into sarcomeres, they have more freedom of movement and can contract a smooth muscle fiber to shorter lengths than in skeletal and cardiac muscle.

The two types of smooth muscle tissue are visceral muscle and multiunit muscle. In visceral or single-unit muscles, gap junctions join individual smooth muscles into large, continuous sheets, much like the fibers observed in cardiac muscle. Visceral muscle is the most common type of smooth muscle and forms the muscular layer in the walls of many hollow structures such as in the digestive, urinary, and reproductive tracts.

Similar to cardiac muscle, visceral smooth muscle commonly has a rhythmic self-excitation, or autorhythmicity (meaning self-rhythm), that spreads across the entire tissue. When these rhythmic, spreading waves of contraction become strong enough, they can push the contents of a hollow organ progressively along its lumen (the interior of a tubular structure). This type of contraction, called *peristalsis,* moves food along the digestive tract, assists the flow of urine to the bladder, and pushes a baby out of the uterus during labor. Such contractions also can be coordinated to produce mixing movements in the stomach and other organs.

Multiunit smooth muscle tissue does not act as a single unit as does visceral muscle; instead, it is composed of many independent, single-cell units. Each independent fiber does not generate its own impulse but rather responds only to nervous input. Although this type of smooth muscle can form thin sheets, as in the walls of large blood vessels, it more often is found in bundles (e.g., the erector pili muscles of the skin) or as single fibers, such as those surrounding small blood and lymph vessels.

Functional Characteristics of Muscles

Muscles have the following four functional characteristics (Activity 9-1):

1. **Excitability** is the ability to receive and respond to a stimulus. A stimulus is a change in the internal or external environment. One of the major reasons massage applications are beneficial is that they provide specific forms of stimulus to the muscles through the application of mechanical forces and with movement, which help maintain homeostasis.

2. **Contractility** is the ability to shorten forcibly with adequate stimulation. This property sets muscle apart from all other types of tissue. As mentioned before, muscle tissue interacts with all body systems, but it makes a unique contribution. The ability to contract allows the entire body to move, as well as certain parts of the body, such as the digestive tract.

3. **Extensibility** is the ability to be stretched or extended. In a typical movement pattern, one group of muscles contracts (concentrically shortens) while the group that has opposing actions lengthens. Because of this, the integrated functions of stability, balance, and the ability to return to the neutral position occur.

4. **Elasticity** is the ability to recoil and resume the original resting length after being stretched.

A number of systems support muscle tissue functions:

- The nervous system directly controls the contraction of skeletal muscle and smooth muscle and also influences the rate of rhythmic contraction in cardiac muscle and visceral smooth muscle.

- The endocrine system produces hormones that promote repair of muscle tissue and assist the nervous system in regulating muscle contraction throughout the body.

- The blood delivers nutrients and carries away waste products.

- Nutrients for the muscles come from the digestive system. For example, the energy for muscle contraction is ATP;

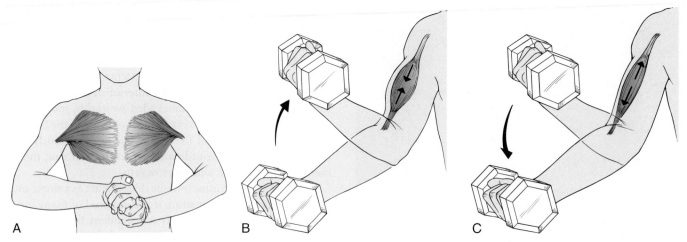

FIGURE 9-2 A, Isometric exercise is muscle activity with no change in length. No work is performed. **B,** Concentric muscle activity. Muscle shortens during tension production. **C,** Eccentric muscle activity. Muscle lengthens during tension production. (From Greenstein GM: *Clinical assessment of neuromusculoskeletal disorders,* St Louis, 1997, Mosby.)

✎ ACTIVITY 9-1

On a separate piece of paper, using the functional characteristics of muscle as a metaphor, provide examples of the ways in which your learning thus far has functioned like a muscle. Examples are provided to get you started.

Example

Excitability: The ability to receive and respond to a stimulus. *Learning the names of the muscles is a new stimulus.*

Contractility: The ability to shorten forcibly and produce movement when adequately stimulated. *Using the information about the endocrine system has helped me better understand mood so that I can move more deliberately from one mood to another.*

Extensibility: The ability to be stretched or extended. *Seeking to understand the Eastern concepts in this text has stretched my belief system.*

Elasticity: The ability to recoil and resume the original resting length after being stretched. *My self-awareness has been reinforced by acquiring knowledge about my body.*

Your Turn

Excitability: The ability to receive and respond to a stimulus.

Contractility: The ability to shorten forcibly and produce movement when adequately stimulated.

Extensibility: The ability to be stretched or extended.

Elasticity: The ability to recoil and resume the original resting length after being stretched.

---

glucose is the fuel for the manufacture of ATP. Potassium and insulin are required for glucose to enter the muscle cell.

• The digestive, respiratory, and urinary systems eliminate the waste products of muscle metabolism. Lactic acid can be an end product of muscle work and can be broken down within the muscle cell by the Krebs cycle or can be transported by the bloodstream to the liver to be converted back to glucose. These processes use oxygen.

• The immune system helps defend muscle tissue against infection and cancer, as it does for all body tissues.

Types of Muscle Actions

As with changes in attachment terminology, a change is occurring in descriptive terms for muscle function. The word *action* is replacing *contraction*. Muscles can contract, or produce actions, in different ways depending on the demand.

Muscle tension is often mentioned in discussions of a "tight" muscle. However, a muscle can be "tight" for several reasons: because it is shortened, because it is lengthened and taut, or because it has increased fluid (hydrostatic pressure). With regard to muscle action, tension occurs because the muscle fibers are shortening.

Isometric and Isotonic Actions

Muscle actions are classified as isometric or isotonic.

Isometric

An isometric action (contraction) occurs when tension develops within a muscle but no appreciable change occurs in the joint angle or the length of the muscle. In other words, muscle tension increases but no movement occurs. Isometric actions are static actions because large amounts of tension develop in the muscle to maintain the joint angle in a static or stable position, such as upright posture. Fixing or stabilizing a proximal joint so that a distal joint can move is an example of the way the body uses isometric functions (Figure 9-2, *A*).

Isotonic

Isotonic action occurs when tension develops in the muscle while it shortens or lengthens. Isotonic actions are dynamic contractions because the varying degrees of tension in the muscle cause the joint angles to change. Isotonic contractions produce movement. Isotonic muscle actions can be classified as concentric or eccentric depending on whether shortening or lengthening occurs.

In a **concentric action** the muscle develops tension as it shortens, and the contraction develops enough force to overcome any applied resistance. Concentric actions cause movement against gravity or resistance and are described as being positive contractions. Concentric actions occur as the angle of the joint decreases. An example is the biceps brachii curl, in

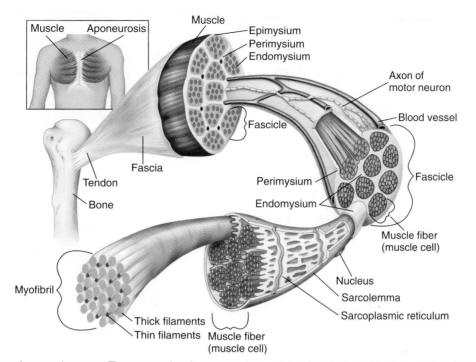

FIGURE 9-3 Structure of a muscle organ. The connective tissue coverings—the epimysium, perimysium, and endomysium—are continuous with each other and with the tendon. Muscle fibers are held together by the perimysium in groups called *fascicles*. (From Thibodeau GA, Patton KT: *Anatomy and physiology,* ed 5, St Louis, 2003, Mosby.)

which one lifts a weight toward the shoulder by moving the forearm toward the arm by bending the elbow (Figure 9-2, *B*).

Eccentric actions take place when the muscle lengthens while under tension and changes in tension to control the descent of the resistance. Eccentric actions control movement with gravity or resistance. Typically, eccentric actions happen as an **antagonist** lengthens in a controlled fashion in response to a force (usually a force external to the body) that is moving a body part at the joint in the opposite direction. The muscle slowly yields to resistance, allowing it to be lengthened. Eccentric actions occur as the angle of joint increases. An example is the reverse of the biceps curl, such as when one lowers a weight from the shoulder by extending the forearm at the elbow joint (Figure 9-2, *C*). Gravity, which is the prime mover, creates the action while the eccentric action of the biceps brachii keeps the movement under control. The amount of tension in the muscle may increase or decrease, depending on the weight of the object providing the resistance to gravity. Using the previous example, if the object is light, the biceps brachii decreases in tension as it lengthens. If the weight is substantial, the biceps brachii increases in tension.

Anatomy and Physiology of Muscle Fibers

Each skeletal muscle is an individual organ made of hundreds or thousands of muscle fibers (or cells), large amounts of connective tissue and nerve fibers, and many blood vessels (Figure 9-3).
- Skeletal muscle fibers are long, cylindric, tapered cells that have cross-striations created by the contractile structure inside.

- The sarcolemma is the plasma membrane that covers muscle cells. Numerous nuclei lie beneath the sarcolemma.
- The sarcoplasm of a muscle fiber is similar to the cytoplasm of other cells but contains large amounts of stored glycogen and a unique oxygen-binding protein called *myoglobin.*
- **Myoglobin** is a red pigment similar to hemoglobin that stores oxygen within the muscle cells.
- Sarcomeres are the structural units of contraction in skeletal muscle fibers.
- Myofibrils, which are chains of sarcomeres, are packed side by side within the sarcoplasm.

The functional units of skeletal muscles are small portions of the myofibrils, and each myofibril is a chain of sarcomere units laid end to end. These structures are held together by various layers of connective tissue. When a muscle cell contracts, its individual sarcomeres shorten. Within a neuromuscular unit, once a contraction has been initiated, it cannot be stopped, and the muscle fibers contract to their full ability or do not contract at all. This is called the **all-or-none response.**

In muscle contraction, shortening of a sarcomere occurs because of the two types of filaments found within the myofibril. The thick filaments are myosin, and the thin filaments are actin. The actin and myosin filaments slide over one another, shortening the myofibrils. This is called the **sliding filament mechanism.** The contraction sequence is as follows:
- The nervous system activates muscle fibers by stimulating the motor neuron.
- The neurotransmitter acetylcholine crosses the synapse between the motor neuron and the muscle cell.
- Myosin attaches to active sites on the actin subunits of the filaments, forming cross-bridges, and the sliding begins.

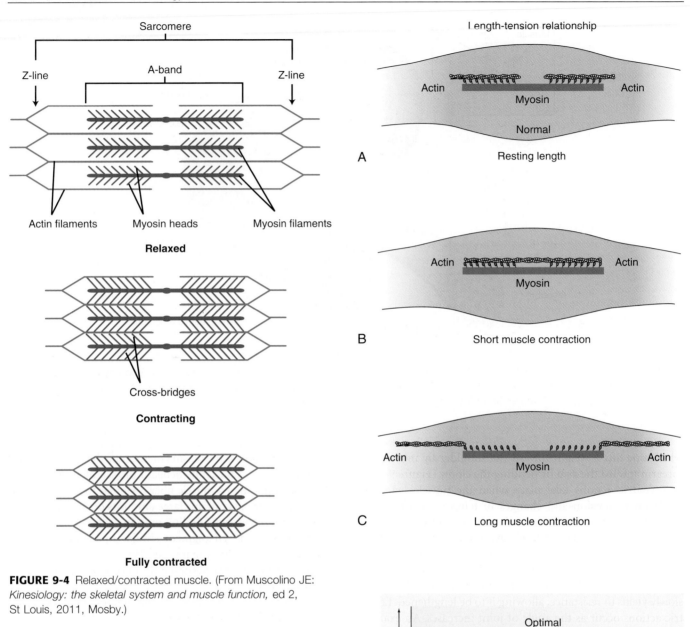

FIGURE 9-4 Relaxed/contracted muscle. (From Muscolino JE: *Kinesiology: the skeletal system and muscle function,* ed 2, St Louis, 2011, Mosby.)

- Each cross-bridge attaches and detaches several times during a contraction, working like a tiny ratchet to generate tension and pull the thin actin filaments toward the center of the sarcomere. In this way the actin "crawls" along the myosin.
- As this event occurs simultaneously in the sarcomeres throughout the cell, the muscle cell shortens (Figure 9-4).

The attachment of myosin cross-bridges to actin requires calcium, and the nerve impulse leading to contraction causes an increase in calcium ions within the muscle cell. Sliding of these filaments continues as long as the calcium signal and ATP are present. Relaxation occurs when the nerve impulse no longer stimulates calcium release and the myosin can no longer grip the actin, and so the sliding reverses.

Length-Tension Relationship

A direct relationship exists between tension development in a muscle and the length of the muscle (Figure 9-5). An optimum length exists at which the muscle is capable of developing

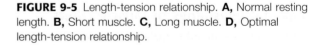

FIGURE 9-5 Length-tension relationship. **A,** Normal resting length. **B,** Short muscle. **C,** Long muscle. **D,** Optimal length-tension relationship.

maximal tension. Muscles can develop maximal tension because the actin and myosin filaments are positioned to form the maximum number of cross-bridges. If the muscles are shortened or lengthened beyond the optimum length, the amount of tension that the muscle is able to generate decreases.

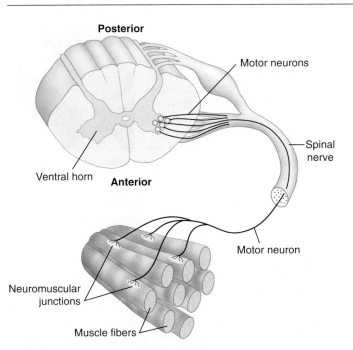

FIGURE 9-6 Motor unit. (From Muscolino JE: *Kinesiology: the skeletal system and muscle function,* ed 2, St Louis, 2011, Mosby.)

A muscle that is too short cannot create a pulling force because there is little or no "crawl" space for the actin and myosin. If the muscle is too long, it cannot contract much because the actin and myosin are positioned too far apart to create an effective "crawl" action for muscle contraction.

In addition to the contractile components of the actin and myosin cross-bridge structures, elastic connective tissue elements of muscles influence the length-tension relationship. The elastic component of the muscle connective tissue coverings (i.e., epimyosium, perimyosium, or endomyosium) and the tendon limit the length of the muscle structure.

Innervation

The autonomic division of the peripheral nervous system innervates the cardiac and smooth muscles. The somatic division of the peripheral nervous system innervates the skeletal muscles. Motor nerves stimulate the skeletal muscles to contract. The area of contact between the motor nerve and the muscle is the motor end plate, or myoneural (neuromuscular) junction. The motor end plate is a modified synapse consisting of a terminal bud of a nerve cell axon and a muscle fiber. When the nerve is stimulated, the terminal bud releases acetylcholine, and contraction follows (Figure 9-6).

A motor point is the location at which the motor neuron enters the muscle and a visible contraction can be elicited with a minimal amount of stimulation. Motor points most often are located in the belly of the muscle. Muscles with a large belly may have more than one motor point. The motor point works in the same way a pilot light does in a gas furnace. Even though all the burners in the furnace are not on (much as with a muscle at rest), because of the pilot light, the furnace can respond quickly to the signal of the thermostat for more heat, causing more burners to light.

A single motor neuron innervates many muscle fibers, delivering stimuli to each one and making them all contract as a group; such a group is called a **motor unit.** The muscle fibers in a single motor unit are not clustered together but are spread throughout the muscle; thus the stimulation of a single motor unit causes a weak contraction of the entire muscle. The more strength that is needed, the more motor units are recruited. The size of the motor units determines whether a muscle contracts forcefully or minimally. Large motor units with 700 fibers are found in the quadriceps femoris and other large, strong muscles that participate in running and walking. At the other extreme, 5 to 10 fibers per motor unit provide the extrinsic muscles of the eyeball with the ability to produce fine eye motions.

Resting Muscle Tone

When the synapses in normal muscles stop firing, the muscles relax. Even so, they maintain a certain amount of contraction that keeps them ready to respond; this minimal amount of tautness is known as **resting tone.** Resting tone maintains the natural firmness of our muscles and their state of ready responsiveness. Appropriate amounts of resting tone help stabilize our joints and maintain our posture. Resting muscle tone is controlled by small signals from the spinal cord, brain, and spindles of the individual muscles. Because the stimulation occurs alternately to different sets of motor units within the muscle itself, some parts of the muscle contract while others relax. This keeps the muscle, especially postural muscles, from fatiguing.

This changeover in the signaling, which maintains resting muscle tone, can easily be demonstrated. Hold a heavy book in your hand as you slowly start to flex your forearm at the elbow joint. The small twitch in the muscle occurs with a changeover in motor units. Sometimes it feels like a small loss of strength that quickly returns.

Threshold Stimulus and Treppe

The stimulus at which the first noticeable muscle contraction occurs is called the **threshold stimulus.** Beyond this point the muscle contracts more vigorously as the intensity of the stimulus increases. The stimulus intensity beyond which the muscle fails to increase in strength is called the **maximal stimulus,** or the point at which all the motor units of the muscle have been recruited. Thus the same muscle can apply a gentle stroke or a firm slap depending on the intensity of the stimulus.

The first contraction of a muscle unit may be as little as one half the strength of those that occur in succession after it; this is called **treppe.** Many factors cause this stair-step effect; for example, as the muscle begins work and produces heat, the muscle enzyme systems become more efficient, releasing more calcium ions, and this produces a stronger contraction with each successive twitch during the beginning phase of muscle activity. Treppe is one reason that warming up before exercise is important.

Energy Source for Muscle Contraction

The energy required for muscular contraction comes from ATP. Efficient contraction of muscle fibers requires glucose

Practical Application

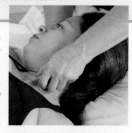

Because the motor point is always "on the alert," it quickly can trigger the rest of the muscle to respond if needed. The increased activity in these areas logically could lead to localized hyperstates in the muscle called **trigger points**. The classic definition of a trigger point, from the master of trigger point knowledge, Janet Travell, is this: "A myofascial trigger point is a hyperirritable locus within a taut band of skeletal muscle, located in the muscular tissue and/or its associated fascia. The spot is painful on compression and can evoke characteristic referred pain and autonomic phenomena." Trigger points occur for many reasons, including motor end plate dysfunction, ATP and calcium imbalance, and ischemia (lack of oxygen because of decreased blood flow).

Most massage applications manage trigger points effectively. First, the practitioner introduces some sort of sensory stimulation to the trigger point area that interrupts the existing neurologic signal and calcium flow; myosin releases from the actin. Then the practitioner lengthens the muscle to restore the normal resting length. Lengthening is different than stretching. Lengthening involves neurochemical responses of the muscle fiber. Stretching is a mechanical force directed to altering a connective tissue structure.

The traditional approach, called *ischemic compression,* involves compressing the trigger point with direct pressure or pinching the point. The pressure is held for as long as 30 seconds. After the application of pressure, the practitioner lengthens the area of the trigger point in a muscle to reestablish an optimal length-tension relationship. More recently, the recommended approach has been to use a series of deep strokes across the trigger point. Muscle energy methods that use

various types of muscle contraction, directed to the muscle or its antagonist, assist in the lengthening process.

This theme has many variations. For example, applying ice over the trigger point instead of compression, followed by lengthening, is often successful. Methods that position the muscle fiber, holding the trigger point in an eased, nonpainful position and then gently lengthening it, are effective for tender trigger points. If fibrotic tissue changes have occurred around the trigger point, connective tissue stretching is necessary to elongate the connective tissue structures in the area.

A strong correlation exists among the locations of motor points, acupuncture points, and trigger points. However, researchers disagree about the differences and similarities of these areas. Acupuncture points correspond to motor point locations and the locations of the Golgi tendon organs; this explains why trigger and acupuncture points can be found in the belly and near the attachment ends of a muscle. Some agreement has been reached that these points correspond to neurovascular bundles in the muscles; this supports the idea of a neurologic and a vascular component of pathologic conditions of these points and the benefits of acupuncture and trigger point methods. Acupuncture points may be the nervous system aspect of the point phenomenon, and the trigger point may be the myofascial aspect of the same phenomenon. In this chicken-and-egg situation, the logical step is to follow the teaching of an old, wise, and experienced Russian physician, who said, "Where is pain, I rub" (Activity 9-2).

✐ ACTIVITY 9-2

Do you think the statement "Where is pain, I rub" is a valid therapeutic approach? Use the clinical reasoning model to formulate your position.
What are the facts?
What is considered normal or balanced function?
What has happened?
What caused the imbalance?
What was done or is being done?
What has worked or not worked?
What are the possibilities?
What does my intuition suggest?
What are the possible patterns of dysfunction?
What are the possible contributing factors?
What are possible interventions?
What might work?
What are other ways to look at the situation?
What do the data suggest?

What is the logical progression of the symptom pattern, contributing factors, and current behaviors?
What are the logical consequences of each intervention identified as a possibility?
What are the pros and cons of each intervention suggested?
What are the consequences of not acting?
What are the consequences of acting?
In terms of each intervention considered, what would be the impact on the persons involved: client, practitioner, and other professionals working with the client?
How does each person involved feel about the possible interventions?
Does the practitioner feel qualified to work with such situations?
Does a feeling of cooperation and agreement exist among all parties involved?
Summarize your reasons for determining the validity or invalidity of the statement "Where is pain, I rub."

and oxygen. Some muscle fibers store glucose in the form of glycogen, which is then broken down into glucose as the muscle fiber needs it. Glucose is a nutrient molecule that contains many chemical bonds. The potential energy stored in these chemical bonds is released during catabolic reactions in the sarcoplasm and mitochondria. Oxygen is needed for the catabolic process known as *aerobic respiration.* Myoglobin

contains iron groups that attract oxygen molecules and hold them temporarily. When the oxygen concentration inside a muscle fiber decreases rapidly, such as occurs during exercise, myoglobin can resupply it quickly. Muscle fibers that contain large amounts of myoglobin are deep red and are called *red fibers* (slow twitch). Muscle fibers with little myoglobin in them are light pink and are called *white fibers* (fast twitch).

Most muscle tissues contain a mixture of red and white fibers. These are discussed in more detail in the section on the types of muscle fibers.

When the oxygen concentration is low, muscle fibers can shift use to another catabolic process called *anaerobic respiration,* which does not require the immediate use of oxygen. Muscle fibers having difficulty getting oxygen or fibers that generate a great deal of force quickly may rely on anaerobic respiration. Anaerobic respiration results in the formation of lactic acid, which may accumulate in muscle tissue during activity in which insufficient oxygen is available. The lactic acid then can be broken down by way of aerobic respiration if oxygen becomes present or can diffuse into the blood and be taken to the liver, where it is converted back to glucose.

These processes require oxygen. After heavy exercise the lack of oxygen in some tissues is called *oxygen debt.* **Oxygen debt** is defined as the extra amount of oxygen that must be taken in to break down or convert the lactic acid. A person may continue to breathe heavily to repay the oxygen debt and process the lactic acid by way of aerobic respiration in the muscle cell or in the liver. Lower levels of oxygen in the blood and the correspondingly higher levels of carbon dioxide and lactic acid (by-products of metabolism from muscle action) signal the brainstem to increase the rate of breath in order to compensate for the oxygen debt. When the oxygen debt has been paid, lactic acid has been converted, and oxygen levels rise back to normal levels, breathing returns to normal.

Heat is a by-product of muscle activity. Several homeostatic mechanisms, such as radiation of heat from the skin surface and sweating, prevent heat buildup from reaching dangerous levels. When the external environment is cold, shivering causes muscle contraction, which produces more heat.

Muscle Fatigue

Muscle fatigue is a state of exhaustion (a loss of strength or endurance) produced by strenuous muscular activity. Two types of muscle fatigue are physiologic and psychological. Low levels of ATP cause physiologic muscle fatigue, and the myosin cross-bridges become incapable of producing the force required for further muscle contractions. The lack of ATP that produces fatigue may result from a depletion of oxygen or glucose in muscle fibers or from the inability to regenerate ATP quickly enough. Acidic metabolic waste products alter the normal ph balance and also contribute to physiologic fatigue. Complete physiologic fatigue seldom occurs. Usually, psychological fatigue is what produces the exhausted feeling that stops us from continuing a muscular activity. We feel tired and do not want to continue an activity. The mechanism is protective and keeps the body from continually functioning at maximal levels and producing physiologic fatigue that is stressful and draining on the whole body.

Blood Supply

Contracting muscle fibers use tremendous amounts of oxygen and nutrients and give off large amounts of metabolic waste. The blood delivers oxygen and nutrients and takes away waste products. Muscle tissue is highly vascularized, and the structure of capillaries in muscle has been modified so that they are long and winding. Thus when a muscle stretches, the capillaries can easily accommodate the change in shape.

Types of Muscle Fibers

Muscles contain fast-, slow-, and intermediate-twitch fibers, which contract at different rates and with different characteristics, allowing muscles a wide range of action.

- **Fast-twitch (white) fibers** contract more rapidly and forcefully, are larger than red fibers, and belong to larger motor units that activate when the nervous system demands rapid, powerful motion. They fatigue quickly and are considered anaerobic because they do not require much oxygen to contract. Muscles that need to respond quickly for short range of motion movements predominantly have fast-twitch fibers. Because white fibers are anaerobic, they fatigue more easily because the lactic acid accumulates and interferes with contractions. As previously mentioned, the liver needs oxygen to convert the lactic acid to glucose or glycogen.
- **Slow-twitch (red) fibers** are smaller; contract more slowly and with less intensity; and belong to smaller motor units that respond during slower, more fine movements. These fibers contain much larger quantities of myoglobin and are classified as aerobic because they require oxygen for contraction. Some texts divide red fibers into fast and slow types. Because of their aerobic quality, red fibers do not produce lactic acid. For this reason postural muscles, which are composed mainly of red fibers, can sustain a contraction longer without fatiguing.
- **Intermediate-twitch fibers** combine the qualities of red and white fibers to provide a rapid, moderately forceful contraction with moderate fatigue resistance. Muscles of the limbs are an example.

Although the fiber composition varies from muscle to muscle, on average 50% of the fibers in a muscle are red, 35% are intermediate, and 15% are white. As many as 90% of the fibers in postural muscles are red, whereas leg muscles contain a higher proportion of white and intermediate fibers.

Genetics greatly determines the fiber configuration, but this can change as a result of demands made on the muscles. For example, the most successful sprinters are born with more white fibers in their leg muscles. To a certain extent, sometimes others can be trained to be sprinters because their fiber configuration adjusts to the demands of sprinting.

Practical Application

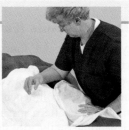

The primary type of fiber in a muscle can affect the length of application of pressure methods (e.g., compression, direct pressure, acupressure) and tension methods (e.g., tensing, relaxing) that are used in progressive relaxation and muscle energy approaches. Red fibers often take longer to respond to these methods than white fibers.

Practical Application

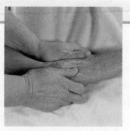

The massage application influences the muscle fibers most if it affects the nervous system proprioceptors. The proprioceptors respond to shortening and lengthening of the fibers; therefore massage methods that passively or actively move the muscle will cause changes.

The connective tissue network is influenced more by a mechanical approach that affects the components of this tissue. As described in Chapter 8 and again in this chapter, sustained, slow elongation of connective tissue at an intensity sufficient to cause a change in the plastic properties is necessary to affect these structures therapeutically. If too much force is applied too quickly to the tissue, the gel matrix responds with increased resistance. If not enough force is applied, the intensity will not be sufficient to cause change. As one stretches the fascia and applies manipulative mechanical force, the matrix becomes softer and more pliable.

Most researchers agree that connective tissue changes are part of a degenerative process. Restoration of function helps reverse degenerative processes, supporting a return to homeostasis and an increase in well-being. Myofascial shortening in one area affects alignment of the tensegrity structure. The myofascial tracts, or *meridians,* as Tom Myers, author of **Anatomy Trains: Myofascial Meridians for Manual and Movement Therapists** calls them, are integral in myofascial performance. Appropriate massage intervention helps restore the balance of the myofascial spans interconnected with the bone and joint structure.

Practical Application

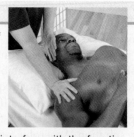

The goals for supporting healing of the skeletal muscle injury are to promote satellite cell repair processes and manage the development of scar tissue. This process allows the connective tissue that develops to be as normal as possible and to stay pliable so it does not interfere with the function of the muscles. Stimulation of muscle function seems to encourage the satellite cells and support muscle regeneration. Movement therapies can support these activities. Massage methods can encourage appropriate mobile connective tissue development so that adhesions do not develop. Because connective tissue originates along the direction of tension, scar tissue can be encouraged to form along lines of external pressure provided by methods that orient by stroking and pulling the tissue in the direction of the desired connective tissue formation.

Areas of muscle healing formed primarily from connective tissue with adhesion and random directional formation can be encouraged to reheal through the use of massage methods that introduce therapeutic inflammation. These methods must be followed with appropriate rehabilitation processes, including broadening contractions to encourage mobility in the scar and decrease adhesion formation. Techniques are applied to small areas. Friction, which is a massage method that moves muscle tissue against the muscle fiber configuration pattern, is the approach most commonly used. Stretching methods that exceed the elastic range of connective tissue to alter the plastic range can pull apart adhesions and can be used to create the controlled area of inflammation.

Repair of Muscle

Most of an adult's muscle cells are already in place at birth. As we grow, existing muscle fibers enlarge (hypertrophy) by as much as 30% of their original size. An injured muscle often is repaired with connective tissue. The body has a specific repair process for regenerating muscle cells. Within hours of an injury, enzymes in the body begin to digest the damaged cell portion. Satellite cells, which are inactive during normal muscle activity, begin to form the new fibers by creating myotubes, which combine to form myofibrils. These new cells take on the characteristics of muscle fibers. Exercise influences the growth of satellite cells and aids in maintaining plasticity of connective tissue. Cardiac muscle has no satellite cells, and its damaged cells are replaced with fibrous connective tissue. Smooth muscle is able to regenerate itself throughout life.

Myotatic Units (Functional Muscle Groups)

Myotatic units are functional muscle groups. They are interconnected neurologically so that movement occurs smoothly, sequentially, and in a coordinated manner. Only rarely does any muscle act independently. Most muscles play a part in a movement pattern, just as actors do in a play. Roles can change, depending on the response required. A muscle can be the star, or prime mover, and in the next instant become one of the supporting cast. A moment later the same muscle can assume the opposite role. As previously described, three types of muscle actions exist: concentric, in which the muscle shortens (acceleration) and the joint angle decreases; eccentric, in which the muscle maintains a controlled lengthening (deceleration) response as the joint angle increases; and isometric, in which the muscle shortens but produces no movement. The terms *mover (**agonist**), prime mover, antagonist, **fixator** (stabilizer), neutralizer, support,* and **synergist** describe the function of muscles in a complete movement pattern.

Because the central nervous system processes movement patterns, understanding the interaction of muscles in functional units is important. This integrated function often is called the *kinetic chain* and is explained in depth in Chapter 10 (Box 9-2).

The mover/antagonist interaction is easy to visualize in muscle pairs such as the biceps brachii, which flexes the elbow joint, and triceps brachii, which extends the elbow joint. However, the interaction becomes more complex when we consider that the deltoid and quadriceps femoris and the adductors and hamstrings form a functional unit because of our gait, or walking pattern. The various functional units that require muscles to cooperate in producing bodywide movements (e.g., walking, maintaining balance) need sophisticated reflex control by the nervous system. Recall that reflex arcs are covered in Chapter 4; it may be helpful to review this information. When the role of stabilization is factored into a

Box 9-2 Names of Muscles by Function

Mover (agonist) A muscle or muscles using concentric contractions that are the main force causing a joint motion through a specified plane of motion; the mover or movers most responsible for the action can be called the *prime mover(s)*.

Antagonist A muscle that has the opposite action to the mover and usually is located on the opposite side of the joint and eccentrically contracts and lengthens, restraining and controlling an opposite force (usually a force external to the body such as gravity).

Fixator (stabilizer) A muscle that surrounds the joint or body segment and isometrically contracts to support or stabilize one attachment of the mover (or antagonist), enabling the other attachment of the mover (or antagonist) to work effectively. Usually, the fixator establishes a firm base for the more distal attachment to carry out movements.

Neutralizer A muscle that stops an unwanted action of the mover (or antagonist) at the attachment of the mover (or antagonist) that is moving. Like fixators, neutralizers work by way of isometric contractions.

Support muscle A muscle that acts at a joint other than where the action in question is occurring to hold a body part in position while the action in question is occurring. Support muscles generally work by way of isometric contractions.

Synergist A helper mover (assistant mover or emergency mover) of the action that is occurring, more broadly defined as any muscle that helps an action occur. Synergists are sometimes known as *guiding muscles.*

Mover and antagonist muscles can contract at the same time in what is called a *co-contraction.* The result is no movement because the forces generated resist each other. Isometric contraction occurs, providing stability.

movement pattern, the functional (or myotatic) muscle group interaction becomes quite complex. Whenever maintaining posture is part of the pattern, a bodywide process is involved. Chapter 10 presents more information on biomechanics.

Practical Application

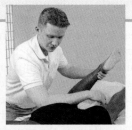

When considering myotatic units and the development of patterns of compensation to any change in the body, one may assume logically that any alteration in musculoskeletal function has a bodywide effect. For example, the arm and thigh muscles are connected in agonist/antagonist patterns through the gait reflex, and the neck and trunk muscles interact together through the ocular/pelvic and righting reflexes that keep us upright with eyes forward. Because the components of the body are interdependent, everything affects everything else. Often, effective applications of massage depend on unravelling complex functional groups of muscles. In many cases, addressing the entire body during each session in what is called a *general constitutional approach* is just as effective. Spot work, or addressing an isolated area and excluding the rest of the body, is less effective.

Muscle Shapes

The bundles of muscle fibers known as *fascicles* form different patterns in muscles, resulting in the different shapes of muscles (Figure 9-7). These fascicle forms affect function, primarily the strength and direction of movement. The following are the more common patterns of fascicle arrangement:

Parallel

The fascicles are long and oriented parallel with the longitudinal axis of the muscle. Some of these muscles are straplike (e.g., the sartorius), and others are fusiform with an expanded belly (e.g., the biceps brachii).

Convergent

The fascicle pattern begins with a broad origin and converges to blend with a much smaller tendon. The result is a triangular muscle (e.g., the pectoralis major).

Pennate

The fascicles are short, lie at an angle to the muscle, and attach to one or more tendons running the length of the muscles. A unipennate muscle (e.g., the extensor digitorum longus) has fascicles that insert on only one side of the tendon. A bipennate muscle (e.g., the rectus femoris) has fascicles that insert into the tendon from both sides; the result looks like a feather. A muscle resembling many feathers, all inserted into one large tendon, is called a *multipennate muscle.*

Circular

The fascicles are arranged in concentric rings around external body openings. These muscles, which contract to close the openings, are called *sphincters.*

The various patterns of fascicle arrangement determine the strength and amount of movement a muscle provides. Skeletal muscles can shorten to about 50% of their resting length when contracted. The longer and more parallel the muscle fibers to the long axis of the muscle, the greater the muscle shortening. Parallel muscles shorten as a direct result of the shortening of their fibers; these muscles produce the greatest amount of shortening. The fibers do this at the expense of strength; parallel muscles are not powerful. The fibers of pennate muscles rotate around their tendon attachments. Pennate muscles can pack more fibers into the same amount of space as parallel fibers and thus can produce the stronger contraction, albeit over a shorter range of motion (Activity 9-3).

Proprioceptors and Reflexes

The central nervous system coordinates motion by being constantly aware of any muscle action. Recall from Chapter 5 that proprioceptors are sensory receptors that provide the central nervous system with information about position, movement, muscle tension, joint activity, and equilibrium. Methods that move, stretch, and apply tension to the muscles and joints stimulate the following receptors:

1. Muscle spindles: Respond to sudden and prolonged stretch.
2. Tendon organs: Respond to tension in the muscle that is relayed to the tendon. Ligaments contain receptors that respond to strain at the joint and feed back information to adjust the tension patterns of associated muscles.

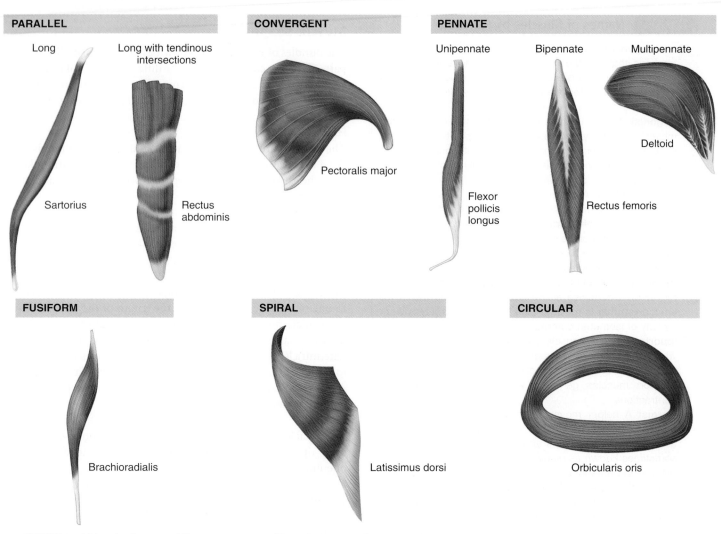

FIGURE 9-7 Muscle shape and fiber arrangement. (From Patton KT, Thibodeau GA: *Anatomy and physiology,* ed 7, St Louis, 2010, Mosby.)

✎ ACTIVITY 9-3

Draw the following muscle shapes on a separate sheet of paper:
  Parallel
  Pennate
  Convergent
  Circular

---

3. Joint kinesthetic receptors in the joint capsule: Respond to pressure, acceleration, and deceleration of joint movement. The two main types of joint kinesthetic receptors are type II cutaneous mechanoreceptors and pacinian (lamellated) corpuscles.

Somatic reflex arcs interpret and process stimulation of nervous system receptors (Figure 9-8). The reflexes most often stimulated are the stretch reflex, tendon reflex, flexor reflex, and crossed extensor reflex.

Stretch Reflex

The sensitivity of muscle spindles to stretching sets the level of muscle tone throughout the body. The muscle spindles activate the stretch reflex when a muscle is subjected to sudden or prolonged stretching. This activation causes a reflexive contraction of the same muscle. As was explained in Chapter 5, a muscle spindle produces nerve impulses that it sends by way of a sensory neuron to the dorsal root of the spinal cord, where an impulse synapses with a motor neuron. The motor neuron carries the impulse to the stretched muscle, generating a muscle action potential and causing the muscle and its synergists to contract. Muscle contraction stops spindle cell discharge unless the muscle is held in a lengthened state, and a small amount of stretch reflex continues to be generated. The effect of the muscle fiber length stimulates the stretch reflex, resulting in facilitation and concentric shortening of the muscle.

The principle of reciprocal inhibition comes into play during the stretch reflex. At the same time the original muscle is stimulated to contract, sensory signals synapse with association neurons to its antagonist(s), inhibiting any signal through the motor neurons to the antagonists; this results in relaxation of the antagonist. To simplify, when one muscle contracts, its antagonist or opposing muscle group must relax. The massage practitioner can initiate the pathway of this

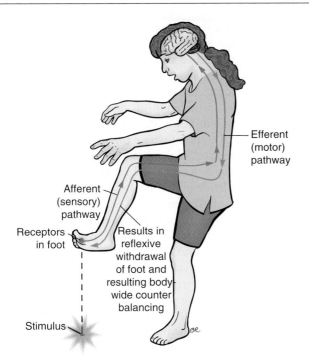

FIGURE 9-8 Reflex response. Local stimulation of a few specific receptors leads to a large number of outgoing impulses, which affect many muscles. (From Fritz S: *Mosby's fundamentals of therapeutic massage,* ed 5, St Louis, 2013, Mosby.)

inhibition circuitry (reciprocal innervation) therapeutically to assist in muscle relaxation.

Tendon Reflex

The tendon reflex operates as a feedback mechanism that monitors and controls muscle tension by inducing muscle relaxation. This reflex is mediated by the tendon organs that detect and respond to changes in muscle tension caused by a sudden or intense muscle contraction. When the tendon organ is stimulated, it sends a signal along a sensory neuron to the spinal cord, where it synapses with an inhibitory association neuron, which inhibits the motor neurons that innervate the original muscle. This inhibition causes the muscle to relax.

At the same time the original muscle is inhibited from acting, a small increase occurs in the signal sent to the antagonist. The opposite of reciprocal inhibition, this signal causes a small contraction to take place in the antagonist. It is possible to initiate this signal therapeutically to assist in relaxing a tense muscle and in stimulating its antagonist.

Practical Application

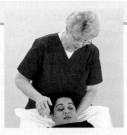

The most common technique used to stimulate the tendon reflex is an isometric (or isotonic) contraction, followed by postisometric relaxation. This technique increases tension at the tendon to elicit relaxation. This method of stretching may be called *proprio-neuro-facilitation stretching.* These methods work, but possibly not because of the reflex affect but instead an increased tolerance to the stretching sensation.

Flexor Reflex and Crossed Extensor Reflex

The flexor (withdrawal) and crossed extensor reflexes are polysynaptic reflex arcs. A single sensory neuron, most likely located in the skin, can activate several motor neurons. Stimulation of these reflexes affects both sides of the body through intersegmental reflex arcs. The flexor reflex withdraws the limb from an unpleasant or painful stimulus, whereas the crossed extensor reflex extends the limb on the opposite side of the spinal cord to maintain balance. The circuitry of contralateral reflex arcs synchronizes control over the contracting and inhibited muscles. These reflexes also explain why tension patterns are seldom found on only one side of the body. As with the stretch reflex, the principle of reciprocal inhibition is active in flexor and extensor reflexes.

Postural Reflexes

In addition, a series of reflexes maintain posture and the position of the head so that the eyes remain in the horizontal plane and oriented forward. These righting and tonic neck reflexes, together with oculopelvic reflexes, coordinate position and function of the neck, trunk, and pelvic muscles. Looking back over the head or tipping the head back activates the extensors and inhibits the flexors. Looking down toward the navel or tipping the head down activates the flexors and inhibits the extensors. Looking left or turning the head to the left activates muscles that would rotate the body left and inhibits those that would rotate the body right. Losing postural balance during eye and head movement causes the opposite reaction, returning the body to an upright position in gravity.

Practical Application

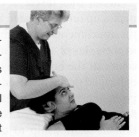

The withdrawal response can stimulate opposite-side patterns of tension or weakness. The response is powerful because flexor or withdrawal reflexes take priority over all other reflex activity taking place simultaneously. Massage can reset reflex patterns that are unproductive or that lead to discomfort and postural distortion from uneven contraction and relaxation muscle patterns. The effectiveness of the techniques depends on how efficiently the receptors are stimulated for these reflexes. The practitioner must stimulate the targeted receptor with the appropriate technique and intensity to allow the stimulated reflex to function appropriately. The positioning of the eyes and head can be used to influence muscle interaction and during muscle energy methods to initiate contraction or inhibition of muscle.

Muscle Firing Patterns/Muscle Activation Sequences

Reflex patterns also regulate the order in which muscles contract to produce movement. The prime movers contract first. Then stabilization occurs so that fixators or co-contractors (mover and antagonist) contract next. Fixators often are located in the deep layers of muscles. Muscles that are shorter and cross only one joint have the best mechanical advantage to start or initiate and guide a joint movement contract third in the sequence. These muscles are often the middle layer of muscles and may be classified as synergists. This pattern is general, and exceptions occur, but the pattern provides a framework for understanding muscle interaction. Disruption of the activation sequence causes labored movement, and muscle fatigue often occurs. Chapter 10 provides more discussion on muscle firing patterns, but considering the firing sequence when learning about reflex patterns and the coordination of muscle movement is helpful.

CONNECTIVE TISSUE COMPONENT OF MUSCLE

SECTION OBJECTIVES

Chapter objective covered in this section:
8. Describe the integrated connective tissue structure of muscle.
After completing this section, the student will be able to perform the following:
- Describe the biochemical activities of connective tissue.
- Define fascia.
- Define biomechanical terms relating to fascia.
- Describe the concept of myofascial continuity.
- Explain pathologic connective tissue changes.

Recall from Chapter 1 that the connective tissue **matrix, which consists of the ground substance and the fibers,** ranges from a fluid to a semisolid or gel and is composed mostly of polysaccharides (protein and sugar). Aside from cells and fibers, matrix also contains many blood vessels and nerves.

Recall that **fascia** is one form of connective tissue and makes up one integrated and totally connected network, from the attachments on the inner aspects of the skull to the fascia in the soles of the feet, and from the skin to the innermost center of the body. If any part of a fascial structure becomes deformed or distorted, adverse effects can occur on any of the interconnected structures within the network. Chapters 1 and 8 previously discussed connective tissue structure and function in relationship to tissue types and joint structure and function. Fascia will now be discussed in relationship to muscles.

The fascial network surrounds and permeates muscles (Figure 9-9):
- Each muscle fiber is surrounded by a fine sheath of collagenic connective tissue called the *endomysium.*
- Several muscle fibers are wrapped together in side-by-side bundles, called *fascicles.*
- Fascicles are wrapped in a collagenic sheath called the *perimysium.*
- The fascicles are bound together with more dense, fibrous connective tissue called the *epimysium.*
- The epimysium surrounds the entire muscle.
- External to the epimysium is the deep fascia, an even coarser sheet of fibrous connective tissue that binds muscles into functional groups.
- The deep fascia forms partitions between muscle groups called *intermuscular septa.*

All these connective tissue sheaths are continuous with one another. Near the ends of muscles, the actual muscle fiber ends, but the connective tissue continues and converges to become the tendons and aponeuroses that join muscles to bones or other connective tissue structures. Tendons and aponeuroses are the continuation of the endomysium, perimysium, and epimysium minus the muscle fibers, which attach muscle to bone. The point where the muscle fiber ends and the tendon begins is called the *musculotendinous junction.* The difference between a tendon and an aponeurosis is one of shape. A tendon by definition is round and cordlike; an **aponeurosis** is a broad, flat sheet.

The tendon or aponeurosis blends and wraps into the connective tissue coverings and structures, including ligaments and other tendons, or into a seam of fibrous connective tissue, called a *raphe,* at the attachment site. Muscle attachments do not stick on bone but wrap around the bone such that the muscles can lift the bone when they contract. The middle of the muscle or the area with the largest and broadest concentration of muscle fibers is the belly of the muscle (Figure 9-10).

When muscle fibers contract, they pull on the connective tissue sheaths, which transmit the force to the bone to be moved. Because the individual skeletal muscle fibers are fragile, the connective tissue supports each cell, reinforces the muscle as a whole, and gives muscle tissue its natural elasticity. These sheaths also provide entry and exit routes for the blood vessels and nerve fibers that serve the muscles, as well as a vast surface area for muscular attachment.

The entire connective tissue network is one structure. Nerve and blood vessels do not just pass through holes in the connective tissue; rather, they are contained and supported in wrappings of connective tissue that intertwine into the entire fascial network. Movement of any one body part creates a force that can be transmitted along fascial planes far and away in the body. Pulling on your big toe could transmit a force all the way to your head and every other structure in your body. No dysfunction is isolated; everything is connected.

Fascia is involved in numerous complex biochemical activities:
- Connective tissue provides a supporting matrix for more highly organized structures and attaches extensively to and invests into muscles.
- The superficial fascia, which forms the adipose tissue, allows for the storage of fat and also provides a surface covering that aids in the conservation of body heat.
- **Deep fascia** ensheaths and preserves the characteristic contour of the limbs and promotes circulation in the veins and lymphatic vessels.
- Connective tissue sheaths cover muscle structures.
- The ensheathing layer of deep fascia, as well as intermuscular septa and interosseous membranes, provides vast surface areas used for muscular attachment.
- Fascia supplies restraining mechanisms in the form of retention bands and fibrous pulleys, thereby assisting in the coordination of movement.
- Where connective tissue has a loose texture, it allows movement between adjacent structures and, by the formation of bursal sacs, reduces the effects of pressure and friction.

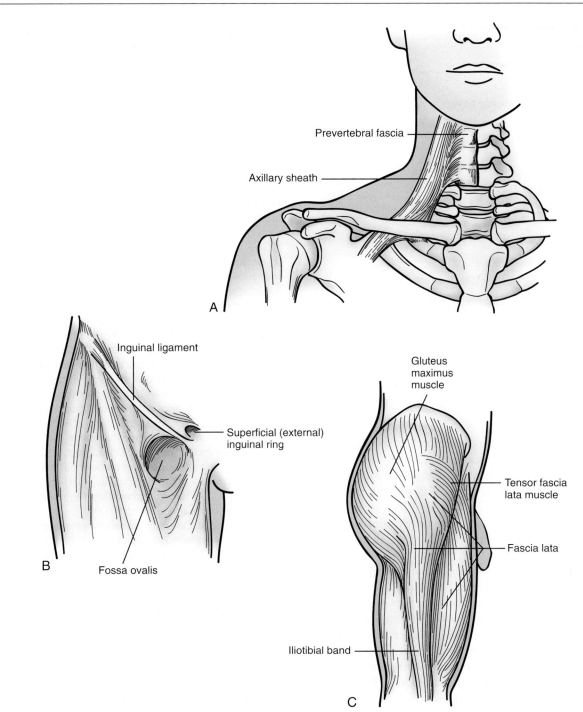

FIGURE 9-9 A, Cervical fascia and the axillary sheath. **B,** Fascia of the upper anterior thigh. **C,** Deep fascia of the lateral thigh. On the lateral side of the thigh, the fascia lata thickens to form the elongated iliotibial band. (Adapted from Mathers LH, Chase RA, Dolph J et al: *Clinical anatomy principles,* St Louis, 1995, Mosby.)

- Fascia is able to contract in a smooth, musclelike manner because of the presence of myofibroblasts.
- Because connective tissue contains embryonic-like mesenchymal cells, it is capable of developing into more specialized elements.
- Connective tissue provides (by its fascial planes) pathways for nerves and blood and lymphatic vessels and structures.
- Many of the neural structures in fascia are sensory.

- Fascia has the ability to convert mechanical force into neurochemical signals forming a bodywide communication network.
- The mesh of loose connective tissue contains the tissue fluid and provides an essential medium through which to bring the cellular elements of other tissues into functional contact with blood and lymph.
- Connective tissue has a nutritive function and contains about a quarter of all body fluids.

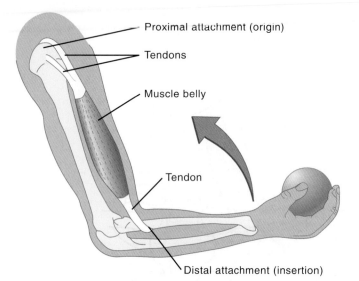

Proximal attachment (origin)

Tendons

Muscle belly

Tendon

Distal attachment (insertion)

FIGURE 9-10 Attachments of a skeletal muscle. A muscle attaches at a relatively stable part of the skeleton (proximal attachment—origin) and inserts at the skeletal part that is moved when the muscle contracts (distal attachment—insertion). (Modified from Thibodeau GA, Patton KT: *Anatomy and physiology,* ed 6, St Louis, 2007, Mosby.)

- Chemical (nutritional) factors influence the strength of connective tissue coverings of muscles and bones.
- Because of its fibroblastic activity, connective tissue aids in the repair of injuries by generating collagenous fibers, creating scar tissue.
- Fascia is a major location of inflammatory processes.
- Fluids and infectious processes often travel along fascial planes.
- A histiocyte is a type of immune cell that eats foreign substances in an effort to protect the body from infection. The histiocytes of connective tissue comprise part of an important defense mechanism against bacterial invasion by their phagocytic activity. Histiocytes also play a part as scavengers in removing cell debris and foreign material.
- Connective tissue represents an important neutralizer or detoxifier to endogenous toxins (those produced in the body from physiologic processes) and exogenous toxins (from outside the body).
- The mechanical barrier presented by fascia has important defensive functions in cases of infectious pathogen invasion.

Fascia is involved deeply in almost all of the fundamental processes of the structure, function, and metabolism of the body. In therapeutic terms trying to consider muscle as a separate structure from fascia is illogical because the two are related so intimately. Without connective tissue, muscle would be a jellylike structure without form or functional ability (Boxes 9-3 and 9-4).

Mechanical forces are important regulators of connective tissue homeostasis. This tissue is designed to move, and lack of movement creates dysfunction. Fibroblasts sense force-induced deformations (strains) in the extracellular

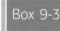

Box 9-3 Biomechanical Laws: The Influence on the Fascia and Muscle Unit

Basic laws govern the mechanical principles influencing the body neurologically and anatomically.

Wolff's law states that biologic systems (including soft and hard tissues) deform in relation to the lines of force imposed on them.

Hooke's law states that deformation (resulting from strain) imposed on an elastic body is in proportion to the stress (force load) placed on it.

Newton's third law states that when two bodies interact, the force exerted by the first on the second is equal in magnitude and opposite in direction to the force exerted by the second on the first.

The Ardnt-Schultz law states that weak stimuli excite physiologic activity, moderately strong ones favor it, strong ones retard it, and very strong ones arrest it.

Hilton's law states that the nerve supplying a joint also supplies the muscles that move the joint and the skin covering the articular insertion of those muscles.

These biomechanical laws influence the behavior of the fascia/muscle fiber unit: the myofascial complex. Application of massage must respect these laws for massage to be effective. Appropriate application of force introduced into the tissue by massage is the key. Depth of pressure and direction coupled with drag and duration are qualities of massage application that determine the type of force introduced. Wolff's law, Hooke's law, and Newton's law in particular describe how forces interact. For example, if a client shows a connective tissue shortening in a diagonal pattern from the top of the shoulder at the acromioclavicular joint to the lumbar dorsal fascia, the forces imposed by the massage have to interact with that same directional line.

Muscle and fascia are anatomically inseparable. Therefore fascia moves during muscular activities acting on bone, joints, ligaments, and tendons. Sensory receptors of the nervous system exist in fascia and relate to proprioception and pain reception.

Fascia is colloidal, as is most of the soft tissue of the body. A colloid consists of particles of solid material suspended in fluid like wallpaper paste; the colloid conforms to the shape of the container it is in and responds to pressure in predictable ways. The amount of resistance colloids offer to pressure applied to the tissues increases proportionally to the velocity (how fast) of force applied to them. This response makes a slow touch a fundamental requirement of massage application; it is necessary to avoid resistance when attempting to produce a change in, or release of, restricted fascial structures.

Adapted from Chaitow L, DeLany J: *Clinical applications of neuromuscular technique,* vol 2, New York, 2008, Churchill Livingstone.

matrix. Changes in cell shape are well-established factors regulating a wide range of cellular functions, including signal transduction, gene expression, and matrix adhesion The extracellular matrix plays a key role in the transmission of mechanical forces generated by muscle contraction or externally applied mechanical forces such as are applied during massage application.

Creep Continued deformation (increasing strain) of a viscoelastic material under constant load (traction, compression, twist).

Hysteresis Process of energy loss caused by friction when tissues are loaded and unloaded.

Load The degree of force (stress) applied to an area.

Strain Change in shape as a result of stress.

Stress Force (load) normalized over the area on which it acts (all tissues exhibit stress-strain responses).

Thixotropy A quality of colloids in which the more rapidly force is applied (load), the more rigid is the tissue response.

Viscoelastic The potential to deform elastically when load is applied and to return to the original nondeformed state when load is removed.

Viscoplastic A permanent deformation resulting from the elastic potential having been exceeded or pressure forces sustained.

Adapted from Chaitow L, DeLany J: *Clinical applications of neuromuscular technique,* vol 2, New York, 2008, Churchill Livingstone.

Muscle tissue has elasticity that allows it to withstand deformation when force or pressure is applied, but fascia is more plastic, and therefore these forces can be detrimental. Massage can introduce various mechanical forces to reverse the detrimental changes. Applying force is called *loading,* and releasing force is called *unloading.* Theoretically, when a mechanical force is gradually applied to fascia, it has an elastic reaction in which a degree of slack is allowed to be taken up, and then the tissue begins to creep because of its viscoelastic nature. Recall from Chapter 8 that creep is the term for the slow, delayed, and continuous deformation that occurs in response to a sustained, slowly applied load. Therapeutically, the goal is to produce creep to elongate shortened and binding tissue to a more healthy position. The mechanical forces created by massage application may produce creep and must be applied with slow and appropriate pressure with sustained drag and without causing injury. Many soft-tissue methods, including massage, operate from this premise. However, the available research does not totally support the premise. Another theory is that the loading and unloading of fascia changes the water content of the tissue; according to yet another theory, myofibroblast contraction produces fascial tone as a reason for fascial changes due to manual force application.

Thixotropy relates to the quality of gelatinous substances called colloids in which the more rapidly the force is applied (load), the more rigid and the less pliable the tissue response will be. Muscle tissue that is rigid or feels dense may have undergone thixotropic changes. If the practitioner gradually applies force, as described previously, the tissues absorb and store energy. To increase connective tissue pliability, massage application must not be abrupt or the tissue will respond by becoming more rigid.

Hysteresis describes the process of energy loss because of friction and tiny structural damage that occurs when tissues are loaded and unloaded repetitively. The tissues produce heat as they are loaded and unloaded, which occurs with on-and-off pressure application. Creating hysteresis reduces stiffness and improves the way the tissue responds to subsequent application of a load. The properties of hysteresis and creep provide the basis for myofascial release techniques, but again, new research is questioning these theories and offering new possibilities. One of the most plausible is that loading and unloading fascia changes the water content of the tissue, which in turn would change the pliability. Still another is that the fascia is a communication network wherein loading and unloading the tissue changes the shape of the cells, resulting in a chemical change.

If the elastic potential of fascia has been exceeded or pressure forces are sustained for an extended period, a viscoplastic response develops and deformation can become permanent. This response results in a dysfunctional change. The same process can be used to create a therapeutic change to reverse dysfunction. Elastic recoil occurs when the application of force ceases to prevent recoil, especially if released quickly. Therefore mechanical force introduced during massage gradually should be released gradually. A viscoplastic permanent deformation change depends on the uptake of water by the tissues. Subclinical dehydration contributes to dysfunctional changes. Therefore drinking water for proper hydration is essential to support therapeutic change.

Myofascial Integration

As explained by Tom Myers in his text *Anatomy Trains: Myofascial Meridians for Manual and Movement Therapists,* muscles operate across functionally integrated bodywide continuities within the fascial network. These sheets and lines follow the network of the connective tissue system, weaving a pattern of interconnected myofascial structures (Figure 9-11). Strain, tension, fixation, compensations, and most movement are distributed along these lines.

The term *myofascial continuity* describes the connection between two adjacent and aligned structures within the structural webbing. These structures create lines of pull, which transmit strain and movement through the myofascia around the skeleton (Figure 9-12). According to Myers, *tensegrity* was coined from the phrase "tension integrity" by the designer R. Buckminster Fuller (working from original structures developed by artist Kenneth Snelson). The term refers to structures that maintain their integrity primarily because of a balance of continuous tensile forces through the structure (see Figure 9-12). Although every structure ultimately is held together by a balance between tension and compression, tensegrity structures, are characterized by continuous tension and local compression. Tension forces naturally transmit the shortest distance between two points, so the components of tensegrity structures are positioned to best withstand stress (Figure 9-13).

In the body the bones, muscle, and fascia create a tensegric structure. The bones are the compression members and the myofascia is the surrounding tension member of a tensegrity system of the body. Soft-tissue balance is necessary to hold the

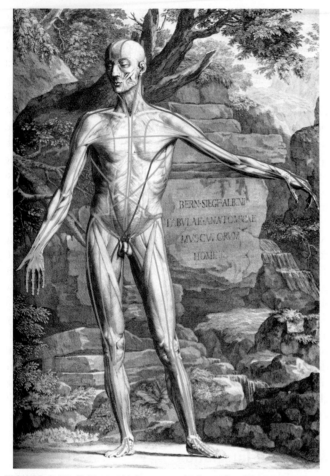

FIGURE 9-11 Pattern of interconnected myofascial structures. (Reprinted with permission of Dover Publications.)

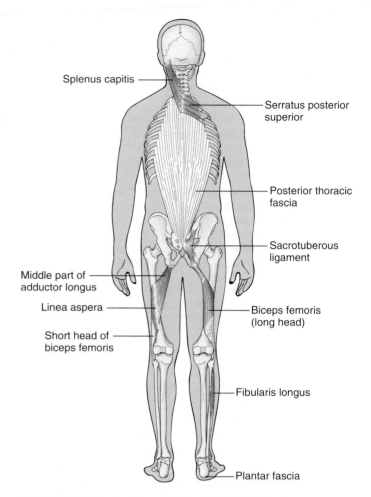

FIGURE 9-12 Myofascial continuity. The body is an interconnected system. This example shows an anatomic connection from the skull to the bottom of the foot. This muscle/fascia joining is necessary for the body to function as an integrated unit. (Adapted from Myers T: *Anatomy trains: myofascial meridians for manual and movement therapists,* London, 2002, Churchill Livingstone.)

skeleton upright. The bones are "spacers" pushing out into the soft tissue, and balanced structure is determined by the tone of the tensile myofascia. A tent made of canvas, poles, and tension supplied by ropes is a good example.

The stability of a tensegrity structure is less stiff and more resilient than the continuous compression structure where one structure is piled on another like a brick wall. Load one "corner" of a tensegrity structure, and the whole structure gives a little to accommodate. Load the structure too much, and the structure ultimately breaks, but not necessarily anywhere near the load. Because the structure distributes strain throughout the structure along the lines of tension, the tensegrity structure may give at some weak point away from the area of applied strain. A principle of massage application that supports this process is to identify the symptoms (the weak part) and look elsewhere for the cause (origin of the strain).

All the interconnected structural elements of a tensegrity model rearrange themselves in response to a local stress. As the applied stress increases, more of the components come to lie in the direction of the applied stress, resulting in a linear stiffening of the material.

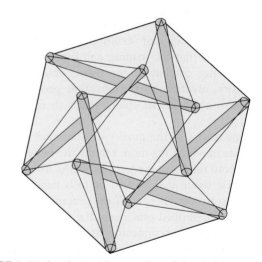

FIGURE 9-13 An abstract image of a cell that is kept together by tensegrity.

In other words, tensegrity structures show resiliency, becoming more stable as the load increases, up to a certain point. Through response to piezoelectric charges, as well as to simple pull, the fibrous body reacts as a tensegrity structure when confronted with extra strain. A simple way to see this is to take a wad of loose cotton batten and gently pull on the ends to see the multidirectional fibers suddenly line up in a similar way.

Myers further indicates that tensegrity concepts create a system or interconnected view of body structure and function, with the body construed as an integrated system. An injury at any given site often can be caused by long-term strain in other parts. Discovering these pathways and easing chronic strain at some point removes the painful portion and then becomes a natural part of restoring systemic ease and preventing future injuries. Full-body massage applications best address the tensegric nature of the body. Full-body massage that addresses these areas of strain creates ease in the tensegrity system. Spot work often is directed at the symptom and not the cause and therefore is less effective.

Specific Properties of Water

The ground substance of fascia consists mainly of water, but not ordinary water as we think of it. This water is stabilized by a complex of **glycosaminoglycans (GAGs), proteoglycans,** and **glycoproteins.** The effect of GAGs in water is very similar to that of gelatin. Mixing a package of gelatin in water transforms the water from a flowing liquid into a solid mass, or gel. Because of the presence of proteins bound to the water, water in our bodies is in more of a gel-like state. The concept of a liquid crystalline, or gel-like, state of water is not new. The leading researcher in this field, Dr. Gerald Pollack, University of Washington professor of bioengineering, has shown that water can at times demonstrate a tendency to behave in a crystalline manner (Chaitow, 2005; Pollack, 2006). It is likely that changes in connective tissues may relate to sponge-like squeezing and refilling effects in the semi-liquid ground substance, with its water-binding glycosaminoglycans and proteoglycans. The water content of fascia partially determines its stiffness, and that stretching, or compression, of fascia (as occurs during almost all manual therapies), causes water to be extruded (like a sponge), making the tissues more pliable. As water in the fascia is squeezed out during tissue compression and stretching, tissues can be mobilized and stretched more effectively and comfortably than if they were still densely packed with water. The change in water content of fascia increases the tolerance to the uncomfortable stretching sensation in muscle tissues. Because the client is more comfortable, the myofascial unit can be elongated more effectively.

Pathologic Connective Tissue Changes

Pathologic changes in connective tissue result in alterations such as thickening, shortening, calcification, and erosion.

These changes may result from sudden or sustained torsion, tension, compression, and bend and shear mechanical forces as well as lack of proper movement. Sustained inappropriate forces cause the fascia to adapt and result in reduced pliability and may lead to varying degrees of fascial entrapment of nerve structures and consequently a wide range of symptoms and dysfunctions. Nerve receptors within the fascia report to the central nervous system as part of any adaptation process. The pacinian corpuscles are particularly important because they inform the central nervous system about the rate of acceleration of movement taking place in the area. This involvement can affect reflex responses. Other sensing input in response to biomechanical stress involves fascial structures, such as tendons and ligaments, which contain highly specialized and sensitive mechanoreceptor and proprioceptor reporting stations. Fascial changes adversely influence many of these sensing receptors, which are implicated in pain syndromes.

Apparently, fascial tone might be influenced and regulated by the state of the autonomic nervous system. Intervention in the fascial system might have an effect on the autonomic nervous system in general and on the organs that are affected directly by it. For example, increased breathing rate can cause an increase in fascial tone, which in turn can stabilize the low back.

Recall that in ground substance collagen molecules bind together and orient along the lines of tension and piezoelectric charge. This adaptive process can be beneficial or dysfunctional. If dysfunction occurs, the muscles become overworked and undernourished and may develop trigger point pain, weakness, increased density in the surrounding ground substance, and increased metabolite toxicity. As previously mentioned, counterforces introduced by methods such as massage, exercise, and stretching can reduce strain. The fascia remodels, and the muscles can be restored to full function. Two elements, however, are necessary for successful resolution of these situations, whether achieved through movement or soft-tissue manipulation:

1. Restoring healthy structure of the tissue. This helps restore fluid content, muscle function, and connection with the sensory-motor system
2. Easing of the force that caused the increased stress on that tissue in the first place

Either of these alone produces temporary or unsatisfactory results. Both the cause and the effect need to be addressed in the therapeutic intervention.

Pathologic and therapeutic viscoplastic changes are not absolutely permanent because collagen has a limited half-life (300 to 500 days) and then is replaced by new tissue formation. Negative stresses (e.g., poor posture and use) can be changed, therapeutic forces can be applied through appropriate massage methods, and appropriate exercise can be used for positive results. Dysfunctional connective tissue changes usually improve in about a year with ongoing therapeutic intervention. However, the client often requires long-term maintenance to support the therapeutic changes.

INDIVIDUAL MUSCLES

SECTION OBJECTIVES

Chapter objectives covered in this section:

9. Explain and demonstrate the three types of muscle actions.
10. Describe how muscles are named.
11. Learn how to palpate individual muscles.
12. Identify the attachments, actions, synergist, antagonist, and common trigger points of individual muscles.

After completing this section the student will be able to perform the following:

- Explain and demonstrate the three types of muscle actions
- Describe how muscles are named
- Learn how to palpate individual muscles
- Draw muscles, identifying location, fiber direction, attachments, and common trigger point location
- Apply knowledge of the muscular system to therapeutic massage application

Although we understand that the body operates as a unit, the massage practitioner must know the individual parts making up that unit. The following section describes the individual muscles most often discussed by massage professionals. We discuss their primary function or functions; attachments; innervation; synergists; antagonists; and, if applicable, common trigger point areas and referred pain patterns.

This section contains a great deal of information. One way to study it is to get to know the muscles as you would a new friend. Knowing where to find them, what they do, who their friends are, and what bothers them is helpful. Activities such as palpation and movement; coloring, drawing, and labeling the attachment points; and locating common trigger points reinforce your knowledge of the structure and function of individual muscles or groups of muscles.

To appreciate friends as individuals, you do not need to know every detail of their lives. If you need to know more about a muscle, you can always ask questions and look up additional material in reference texts as needed (one such reference is Joseph Muscolino's *The Muscular System Manual: The Skeletal Muscles of the Human Body,* ed 3, St Louis, 2010, Mosby). Note that not all authors agree about specific details, and different references list slightly different attachment sites, functions, and so forth. As with most differing opinions, the answer is not always black or white, but somewhere in between.

Muscles are arranged in layers, and most body areas have three to five layers of muscles. Those muscles considered deep lie closest to the bone, and those considered superficial lie closest to the skin (Figure 9-14). Muscles with similar function are bundled together by deep fascia into compartments (e.g., the anterior, medial, and posterior compartments of the thigh).

Muscles have three main actions:

- **Concentric action,** when the muscle fibers shorten as a result of the neurologic and chemical response of actin and myocin. The muscle contraction pulls and moves a bone that is part of a joint and the joint moves. This movement is typically considered the muscle's primary function. When a muscle is functioning during concentric action, it is called the **prime mover** or **agonist.** The muscle is producing acceleration (increase of motion or action).

- **Eccentric action** restrains and controls movement produced by the agonist by lengthening while at the same time maintaining muscle fiber shortening. The eccentric action is as important as the concentric action and even more important in terms of muscle dysfunction. When a muscle is functioning eccentrically, it is usually called the **antagonist.** The muscle is producing deceleration (decrease of motion or action).

- **Isometric action** occurs when the muscle fibers shorten and attempt to pull on a bone but the actual movement is prevented at the joint. The tissue stiffens and become contracted when the muscle is acting as **stabilizers (fixators)** and **neutralizers.** Stabilization and guiding of movement are essential for proper function.

Each muscle can perform these three actions, and they are all important. However, a muscle can efficiently perform only one action at a time. Dysfunction can occur when these muscle actions are not used efficiently (e.g., if a muscle tries to produce movement when what is really needed is stabilization, or the muscle attempts to create a movement but at the same time is opposing the movement). Remember that muscles work in functional units, never alone. Functional units consist of three or more muscles, bundled into compartments, alternating among concentric, eccentric, and isometric actions and integrated within myofacial continuity.

When these functions of muscles are specifically important to the massage profession, we discuss them as well. When studying the individual muscles, pay attention to all elements provided for each muscle. Also pay attention to referred pain patterns because these are the symptoms clients will complain about if dysfunction with the muscle occurs (see Appendix B).

How Muscles Are Named

Muscle names seem more logical and easier to learn when the reasons for the names are clear. Many of the muscles of the body are named using one or more of the following features:

- *Location:* Many muscles are named for their location using medical terminology. The brachialis (arm muscle) and gluteus (buttock) muscles are examples.

- *Function:* The function of a muscle is frequently a part of its name. The adductor muscles of the thigh adduct or move the thigh at the hip joint toward the midline of the body.

- *Shape:* Shape is a descriptive feature used for naming many muscles. The deltoid (triangular) muscle covering the shoulder is shaped like a delta or triangle.

- *Direction of fibers:* Muscles may be named according to the orientation of their fibers. The term *rectus* means "straight." The fibers of the rectus abdominis muscle run straight up and down (vertically) and are parallel to one another.

- *Number of heads or divisions:* The number of divisions or heads (points of attachment) may be used to name a muscle. The word part *-cep* means "head." The biceps (two), triceps (three), and quadriceps (four) refer to multiple heads or points of attachment. The biceps brachii is a muscle having two heads located in the arm.

- *Points of attachment:* A muscle attaches from one site to another site. These attachment sites may be used to name a

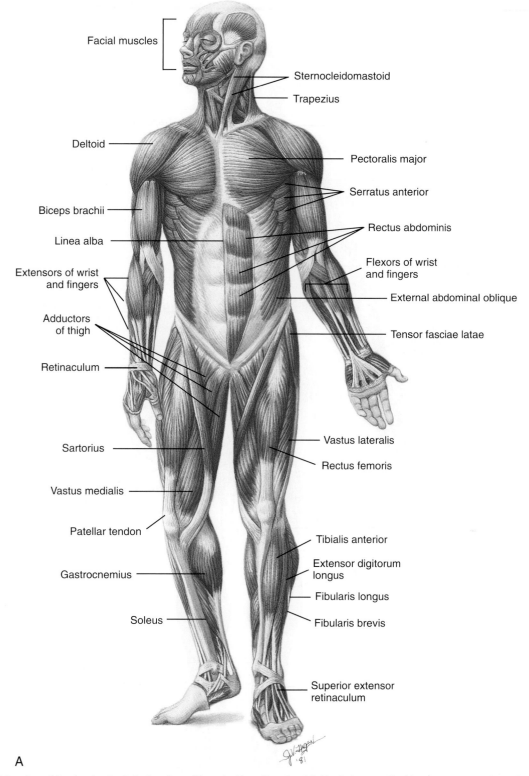

Facial muscles

Sternocleidomastoid

Trapezius

Deltoid

Pectoralis major

Serratus anterior

Biceps brachii

Rectus abdominis

Linea alba

Flexors of wrist
and fingers

Extensors of wrist
and fingers

External abdominal oblique

Adductors
of thigh

Tensor fasciae latae

Retinaculum

Sartorius

Vastus lateralis

Rectus femoris

Vastus medialis

Patellar tendon

Tibialis anterior

Extensor digitorum
longus

Gastrocnemius

Fibularis longus

Soleus

Fibularis brevis

Superior extensor
retinaculum

A

FIGURE 9-14 Muscles of the body. **A,** Anterior view. (From LaFleur Brooks, M: *Exploring medical language: a student-directed approach,*
ed 8, St Louis, 2012, Mosby.)

Continued

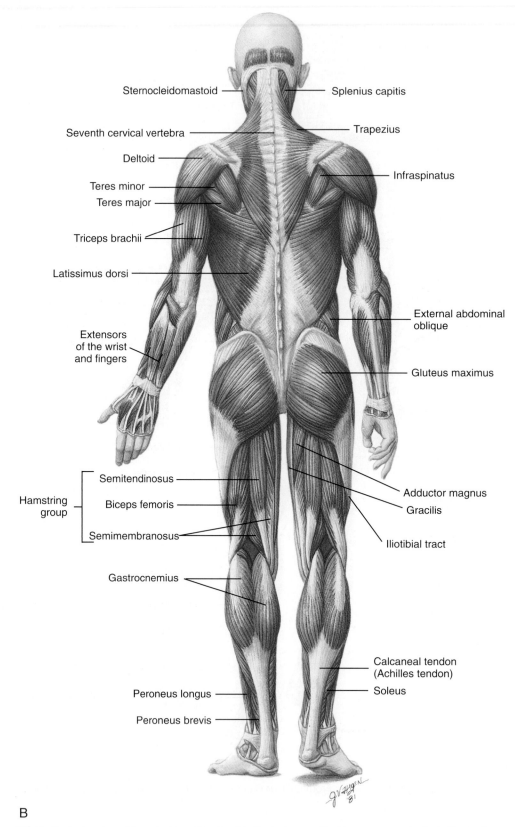

B

muscle. For example, the sternocleidomastoid has an attachment on the sternum and clavicle and another attachment on the mastoid process of the temporal bone.

- *Size of muscle:* The size of a muscle can be used to name a muscle, especially if it is compared with the size of nearby muscles. For example, the gluteus maximus is the largest muscle of the gluteal (Greek *glautos*, meaning "buttock") region. Nearby is a small gluteal muscle, gluteus minimus, and a midsize gluteal muscle, gluteus medius.

Muscle Attachment Terminology

As discussed previously, unless terminology is consistent, it can be confusing. Terminology used for the muscular system is not consistent. There are multiple names and spellings for muscle names and duplicate terminology to describe the location of muscles. The attachment terminology will appear as follows in the following individual muscle sections:

- Origin, proximal attachment, arises from:
- Insertion, distal attachment, attaches to:

The repetition of attachment terminology variations will prepare you to understand information presented in other textbooks and various exams.

How to Palpate Muscles

Massage is palpation, and palpation is assessment; both are part of an intervention process. It is essential that you feel the muscle and associated connective tissues during massage. It is essential to understand the tissue you massage. Practice, practice, and practice palpation.

You can palpate muscles that are relaxed or contracted as follows:

- Distinguishing whether you are touching the correct muscle is difficult at times because many structures such as tendons, fascia, and ligaments can attach in the same place.
- With relaxed muscles, locating the muscle depends on anatomic knowledge and the ability to identify bony landmarks.
- To palpate muscles when they are relaxed, read the attachment descriptions carefully and place your hand on the location described. Then trace the path of the muscle between the attachments.
- Notice the fiber direction, which determines the angle of pull when the muscle shortens.
- The largest area of the muscle is usually near the middle of the muscle and is called the *belly*.
- To identify a specific muscle, first identify the attachments and belly of the muscle while the muscle is relaxed, and then have the client actively contract the muscle.
- You can do this by placing the muscle in the concentric action position and then having the client hold that position or move the muscle a bit between concentric and eccentric patterns.
- While the client holds the position or slightly contracts the specific muscle, you should be able to feel the muscle tensing, bunching up, or pushing out.
- Remember that three or more layers of muscles cover each area and are bundled into compartments.

- A compartment is easiest to palpate. The more superficial muscles in a compartment are easier to palpate than the deeper muscles.
- Identifying the deeper muscle layers is more difficult. The deeper muscles usually have smaller movement patterns, so using a slight contraction to initiate a tiny movement to differentiate the smaller deeper layers is helpful.
- Then initiate a larger or stronger contraction to identify the more superficial layers of the muscle.
- Palpation of deeper muscles requires more pressure but should not feel painful or abrupt to the massage client.

Organization of This Section

Before each specific body section, a series of illustrations borrowed from *Gray's Anatomy for Students* is provided. The intent of each mini atlas is to provide visual orientation of muscle locations and relationships to one another. The mini atlas provides a visual orientation for references when studying each of the individual muscles in that section. The more realistic illustration provided by each mini atlas is coupled with the more graphic view of individual muscle. Although the mini atlases can provide excellent overview and orientation, it is not possible to display each muscle because of the overlapping structure of muscle layers. Much more learning material is located on the Evolve website. The accompanying online course for this textbook also offers an excellent learning aid.

Individual Muscle Drawing Activities

Skeletal pictures are provided in this chapter to be used as coloring/drawing activities. Use these pictures to draw individual muscles or muscle groups. If the activity requires more than one muscle to be drawn on the same picture, you should make each muscle a different color. Label the attachment sites with different colors, and use those colors consistently throughout all the activities. Mark the trigger point or points in yet another color, again being consistent throughout the activities. Fine-point colored pencils work best for these activities. This type of kinesthetic learning activity is very effective for memory retention. Do not become overly concerned with your artistic ability. The learning occurs in the doing, not the result. You can also use the coloring book program on the Evolve site as a review tool in learning about the individual muscles.

Muscles of the Face and Head

The superficial muscles of the head, including those of the scalp and face, produce movement for facial expressions, which are vital to nonverbal communication (Figure 9-15). The muscles vary in shape and strength. Many adjacent muscles tend to be fused together. Unlike most skeletal muscles, which attach onto bones of the skeleton, many muscles of facial expression attach into skin or other muscles. Muscles of the head and face lift our eyebrows, flare our nostrils, and open and close our eyes and mouth. Many of these muscles are implicated in headaches and tend to tense when a person is stressed, especially if he or she is in pain. Careful massage to the area can be soothing and effective in managing tension headaches.

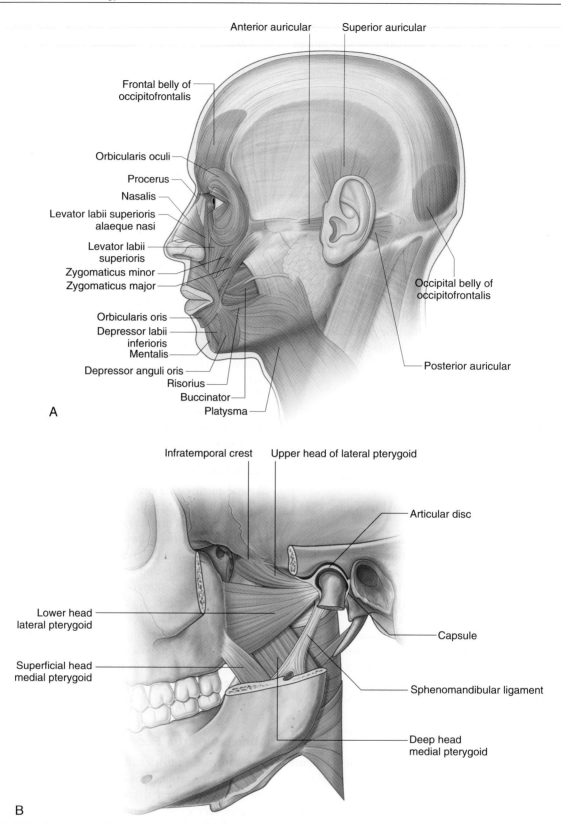

FIGURE 9-15 A, Facial muscles. **B,** Lateral pterygoid muscle. (From Drake RL, Vogl W, Mitchell WM: *Gray's anatomy for students,* ed 2, Edinburgh, 2010, Churchill Livingstone.)

Facial Expression Muscles

Occipitofrontalis (ok-SIP-ih-toe-fron-TAL-iss)

Also called the *epicranius, occipitofrontalis* means "back of the head and related to the forehead." The muscle sometimes is described as separate muscles, the occipitalis and the frontalis.

Lateral

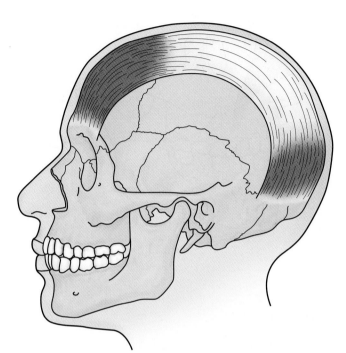

Concentric action:

Draws the scalp anteriorly and posteriorly, elevates the eyebrows, and wrinkles the forehead

Origin, proximal attachment, arises from:

Occipital belly—lateral two thirds of the highest nuchal line of the occipital bone and the mastoid area of the temporal bone

Frontal belly—galea aponeurotica near the coronal suture

Insertion, distal attachment, attaches to:

Occipital belly—galea aponeurotica

Frontal belly—fascia and skin superior to the eye and nose

Innervation:

Occipitalis—posterior auricular branch of the facial nerve (cranial nerve VII)

Frontalis—temporal branches of the facial nerve (cranial nerve VII)

Major synergists:

Occipitalis—no major synergists

Frontalis—no major synergists

Major antagonists:

Occipitalis—frontalis

Frontalis—occipitalis, corrugator supercilii, and procerus

Trigger points:

Occipitalis—near attachment at the galea aponeurotica

Frontalis—belly of the muscle superior to the eyebrow

Referred pain patterns:

Eye, ear, and the scalp superior to the ear and deep occipital pain

Procerus (pro-SEHR-us)

Procerus means "tall."

Anterior

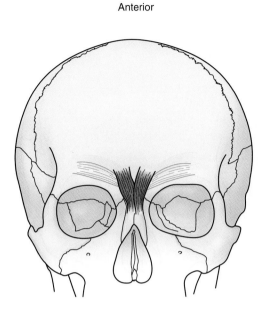

Concentric action:

Draws medial angle of the eyebrow downward and produces transverse wrinkles over the bridge of the nose

Origin, proximal attachment, arises from:

Fascia covering the inferior part of the nasal bone and the superior part of the lateral nasal cartilage

Insertion, distal attachment, attaches to:

Skin over the lower forehead between the eyebrows

Innervation:

Superior buccal branch of the facial nerve (cranial nerve VII)

Major synergist:

Corrugator supercilii

Major antagonist:

Occipitofrontalis

Trigger point:

No common trigger point identified. Trigger points that form are likely located in the belly of the muscles.

▌*Corrugator supercilii* (kor-u-GA-tor su-per-SIL-ee-eye)

Corrugator supercilii means "to wrinkle the eyebrows."

Anterior

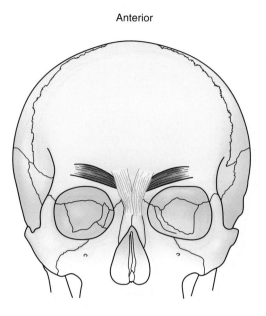

Concentric action:
Draws the eyebrow inferiorly and medially
Origin, proximal attachment, arises from:
Medial end of the superciliary arch of the frontal bone
Insertion, distal attachment, attaches to:
Skin deep to the medial portion of the eyebrow
Innervation:
Temporal branch of the facial nerve (cranial nerve VII)
Major synergist:
Procerus
Major antagonist:
Occipitofrontalis
Trigger point:
No common trigger point identified. Trigger points that form
are likely located in the belly of the muscles.

▌*Nasalis* (nay-SAL-iss)

Nasalis means "related to the nose."

Lateral

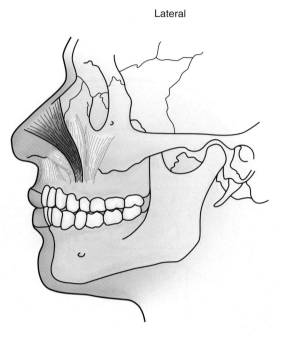

Concentric action:
Flares the nasal aperture
Origin, proximal attachment, arises from:
Transverse part—maxilla, lateral to the nose
Alar part—nasal notch of the maxilla and lesser alar
cartilage
Insertion, distal attachment, attaches to:
Aponeurosis of the procerus and the same muscle on the
opposite side and cartilage of the nose
Innervation:
Superior buccal branch of the facial nerve (cranial nerve VII)
Major synergist:
Levator labii superioris alaeque nasi
Major antagonist:
Depressor septi nasi
Trigger point:
No common trigger point identified. Trigger points that form
are likely located in the belly of the muscles.

⬭ ACTIVITY 9-4

Draw and color the **facial expression muscles** in the spaces provided. For each muscle, do the following:

1. Label the origin and insertion attachment points: *O* for origin; *I* for insertion.

2. Place an X on the trigger points.
3. Palpate these muscles; identify the attachment points and the bellies of the muscles.
4. Move these muscles on yourself.

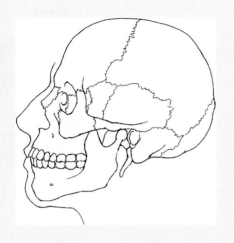

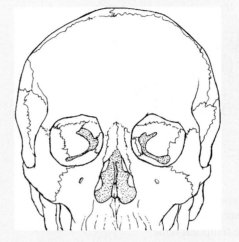

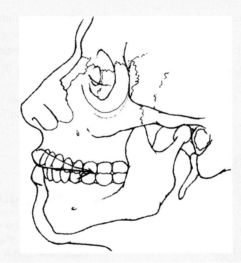

Ear Muscles

Auricularis posterior

Lateral

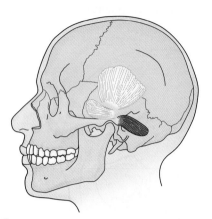

Concentric action:
Draws the ear posteriorly
Origin, proximal attachment, arises from:
Mastoid area of the temporal bone
Insertion, distal attachment, attaches to:
Inferior part of the cranial part of the conchae of the ear
Innervation:
Posterior auricular branches of the facial nerve (cranial nerve VII)

Auricularis superior

Lateral

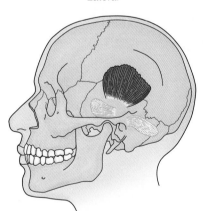

Concentric action:
Elevates the ear and tightens and moves the scalp
Origin, proximal attachment, arises from:
Galea aponeurotica
Insertion, distal attachment, attaches to:
Superior part of the cranial surface of the ear
Innervation:
Temporal branches of the facial nerve (cranial nerve VII)
Major synergist:
Temporoparietalis
Major antagonists:
Auricularis anterior and auricularis posterior
Trigger point:
No common trigger point identified. Trigger points that form are likely located in the belly of the muscles.

Auricularis (aw-RIK-u-lar-iss) anterior

The auricularis muscles, as a group, move the ear. *Auricularis* means "belonging to the ear."
Concentric action:
Draws the ear anteriorly and tightens and moves the scalp

Lateral

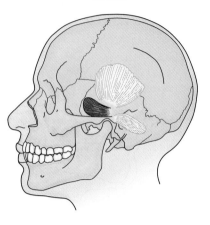

Origin, proximal attachment, arises from:
Lateral edge of the galea aponeurotica
Insertion, distal attachment, attaches to:
Spine of the helix of the ear
Innervation:
Temporal branches of the facial nerve (cranial nerve VII)
Trigger points that form are likely located in the belly of the muscles.

✏ ACTIVITY 9-5

Draw and color the **ear muscles** in the spaces provided. For each muscle, do the following:
1. Label the origin and insertion attachment points: *O* for origin; *I* for insertion.
2. Palpate these muscles; identify the attachment points and the bellies of the muscles.
3. Move these muscles on yourself.

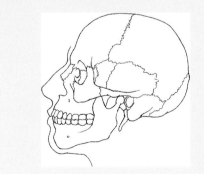

Eye Muscle

Orbicularis oculi (or-BIK-you-LAR-iss OK-you-li)

Orbicularis oculi means "a small disk belonging to the eye." This muscle is a sphincter muscle of the eye and has three parts: orbital, palpebral, and lacrimal.

Anterior

Concentric action:
Closes and squints the eye, depresses the upper eyelid, and elevates the lower eyelid

Origin, proximal attachment, arises from:
Orbital portion—medial orbital margin
Palpebral (eyelid) portion—medial palpebral ligament
Lacrimal portion—lacrimal bone

Insertion, distal attachment, attaches to:
Orbital portion—medial orbital margin (this muscle returns to attach to the same place from which it originated)

Palpebral portion—lateral palpebral ligament
Lacrimal portion—medial palpebral raphe

Innervation:
Temporal and zygomatic branches of the facial nerve (cranial nerve VII)

Major synergists:
No major synergists

Major antagonist:
Levator palpebrae superioris

Trigger point:
Orbital area superior to the eyelid

Referred pain pattern:
To the nose

✎ ACTIVITY 9-6

Draw and color the **eye muscle** in the space provided. Do the following:

1. Label the origin and insertion attachment points: *O* for origin; *I* for insertion.
2. Place an X on the trigger point.
3. Palpate this muscle; identify the attachment points and the belly of the muscle.
4. Move this muscle on yourself.

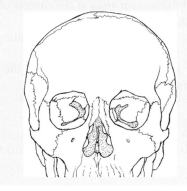

Muscles that Move the Mouth
Orbicularis oris (or-BIK-you-LAR-iss OR-iss)

Orbicularis oris means "a small disk belonging to the mouth."

Anterior

Depressor anguli oris (de PRESS-or ANG-you-li OR-iss)

Depressor anguli oris means "to press down the corner belonging to the mouth."

Lateral

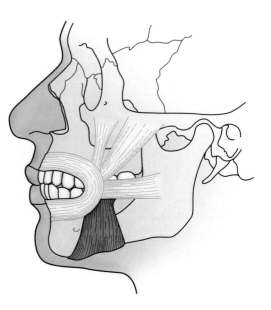

Concentric action:

Closes the mouth, protracts the lips (causes the lips to protrude anteriorly), and draws the angle of the mouth medially

Origin, proximal attachment, arises from:

Modiolus, a fibromuscular mass at the corners of the mouth

Insertion, distal attachment, attaches to:

Skin and fascia of the lips and tissue surrounding the lips

Innervation:

Lower buccal and mandibular branches of the facial nerve (cranial nerve VII)

Major synergist:

Mentalis

Major antagonists:

Depressor labii inferioris, platysma, and levators of the upper lip

Trigger points:

No common trigger points identified

Concentric action:

Draws the angle of the mouth downward and laterally (This muscle is involved in opening the mouth and in expressions of sadness.)

Origin, proximal attachment, arises from:

Oblique line of the mandible, inferior and lateral to the depressor labii inferioris

Insertion, distal attachment, attaches to:

Angle of the mouth

Innervation:

Mandibular branch of the facial nerve (cranial nerve VII)

Major synergists:

Risorius and zygomaticus major

Major antagonists:

Levator anguli oris and zygomaticus major

Trigger points:

No common trigger points identified. Trigger points that form likely are located in the belly of the muscle.

Risorius (rih-ZOR-ee-us)

Risorius means "to cause one to laugh."

Lateral

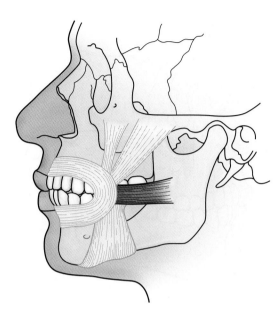

Concentric action:
Draws the angle of the mouth laterally
Origin, proximal attachment, arises from:
Parotid fascia superficial to the masseter muscle
Insertion, distal attachment, attaches to:
Fascia at the lateral angle of the mouth
Innervation:
Mandibular branches of the facial nerve (cranial nerve VII)
Major synergists:
Zygomaticus major and depressor anguli oris
Major antagonist:
Orbicularis oris
Trigger points:
No common trigger points identified. Trigger points that form
likely are located in the belly of the muscle.

Zygomaticus major (ZYE-go-MAT-ik-us)

Zygomaticus means "connected to the yoke or connector"; *major* means "larger."

Lateral

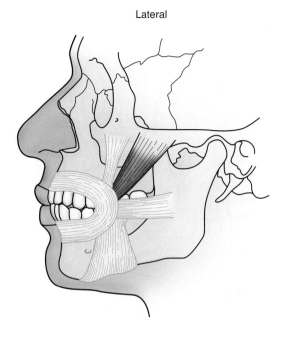

Concentric action:
Elevates and draws the angle of the mouth laterally (as in
laughing)
Origin, proximal attachment, arises from:
Zygomatic bone anterior to the zygomaticotemporal suture
Insertion, distal attachment, attaches to:
Angle of the mouth, blending with the levator anguli oris and
the orbicularis oris
Innervation:
Buccal branches of the facial nerve (cranial nerve VII)
Major synergist:
Levator anguli oris
Major antagonist:
Depressor anguli oris
Trigger points:
No common trigger points identified. Trigger points that form
likely are located in the belly of the muscle.

Zygomaticus minor (ZYE-go-MAT-ik-us)

Zygomaticus means "connected to the yoke or connector"; *minor* means "smaller."

Lateral

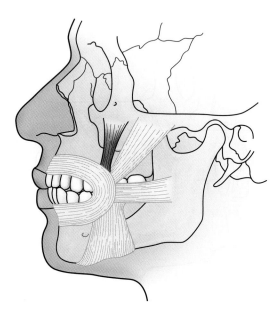

Levator labii superioris (le-VAY-tor LAY-bee-eye su-PEER-ee-OR-iss)

Levator labii means "one that raises the lip"; *superioris* means "above" or "upper."

Lateral

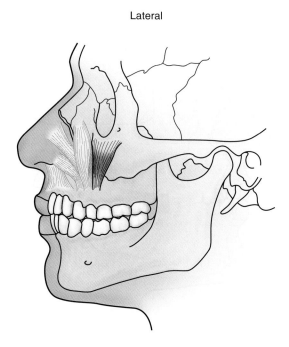

Concentric action:
Elevates and everts the upper lip and produces the nasolabial sulcus
Origin, proximal attachment, arises from:
Lateral surface of the zygomatic bone, immediately posterior to the zygomaticomaxillary suture
Insertion, distal attachment, attaches to:
Angle of the mouth, blending with the levator labii superioris
Innervation:
Buccal branches of the facial nerve (cranial nerve VII)
Major synergists:
Levator labii superioris and levator labii superioris alaeque nasi
Major antagonist:
Orbicularis oris
Trigger points:
No common trigger points identified. Trigger points that form likely are located in the belly of the muscle.

Concentric action:
Elevates and everts the upper lip
Origin, proximal attachment, arises from:
Maxilla and zygomatic bone, from the lower margin of the orbital opening immediately superior to the infraorbital foramen
Insertion, distal attachment, attaches to:
Muscular substance of the lateral part of the upper lip
Innervation:
Buccal branches of the facial nerve (cranial nerve VII)
Major synergists:
Levator labii superioris alaeque nasi and zygomaticus minor
Major antagonist:
Orbicularis oris
Trigger points:
No common trigger points identified. Trigger points that form likely are located in the belly of the muscle.

Levator labii superioris alaeque nasi (le-VAY-tor LAY-bee-eye su-PEER-ee-OR-iss AL-ek-wee NAY-see)

Levator labii and *alaeque nasi* mean "one that raises the lip" and "belonging to the wing of the nose," respectively; *superioris* means "above" or "upper."

Lateral

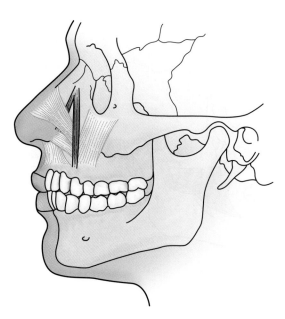

Concentric action:
Elevates and everts the upper lip and flares the nostril
Origin, proximal attachment, arises from:
Frontal process of the maxilla
Insertion, distal attachment, attaches to:
The muscle divides into the lateral slip, which inserts into the lateral part of the upper lip, and the medial slip, which inserts into the greater alar cartilage and the skin of the nose.
Innervation:
Buccal branches of the facial nerve (cranial nerve VII)
Major synergists:
Levator labii superioris and zygomaticus minor
Major antagonists:
Orbicularis oris and depressor septi nasi
Trigger points:
No common trigger points identified. Trigger points that form likely are located in the belly of the muscle.

Depressor labii inferioris (de-PRESS-or LAY-bee-eye in-FEAR-ee-or-iss)

Depressor labii means "to press down the lip"; *inferioris* means "lower" or "beneath."

Anterior

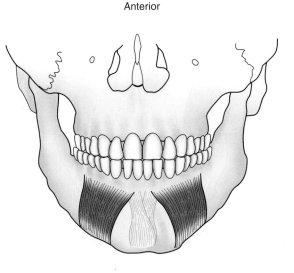

Concentric action:
Depresses, everts, and draws the lower lip laterally
Origin, proximal attachment, arises from:
Oblique line of the mandible, between the symphysis menti and the mental foramen
Insertion, distal attachment, attaches to:
Skin of the lower lip, blending with the orbicularis oris
Innervation:
Buccal branches of the facial nerve (cranial nerve VII)
Major synergist:
Platysma
Major antagonists:
Mentalis and orbicularis oris
Trigger points:
No common trigger points identified. Trigger points that form likely are located in the belly of the muscle.

Levator anguli oris (le-VAY-tor ANG-you-li OR-iss)

Levator anguli oris means "one that raises the corner of the mouth."

Anterior

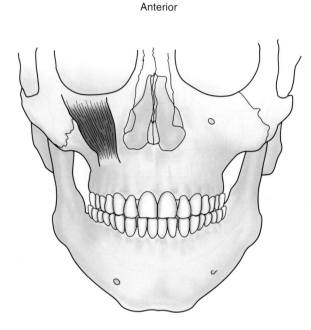

Concentric action:
Elevates the angle of the mouth and produces the nasolabial sulcus

Origin, proximal attachment, arises from:
Canine fossa of the maxilla, just inferior to the infraorbital foramen

Insertion, distal attachment, attaches to:
Angle of the mouth, blending with the zygomaticus major, depressor anguli oris, and orbicularis oris

Innervation:
Buccal branches of the facial nerve (cranial nerve VII)

Major synergist:
Zygomaticus major

Major antagonist:
Depressor anguli oris

Trigger points:
No common trigger points identified. Trigger points that form likely are located in the belly of the muscle.

Buccinator (BUK-sin-ate-or)

Buccinator means "trumpeter."

Lateral

Concentric action:
Compresses the cheek against the teeth (This muscle aids in mastication and forcing air out between the lips.)

Origin, proximal attachment, arises from:
Alveolar processes of the maxilla and mandible and the pterygomandibular raphe

Insertion, distal attachment, attaches to:
Angle of the mouth

Innervation:
Lower buccal branches of the facial nerve (cranial nerve VII)

Major synergists:
No major synergist

Major antagonists:
No major antagonist

Trigger points:
No common trigger points identified. Trigger points that form likely are located in the belly of the muscle.

Platysma (PLAH-tiz-ma)

Platysma means "a flat plate."

Anterior

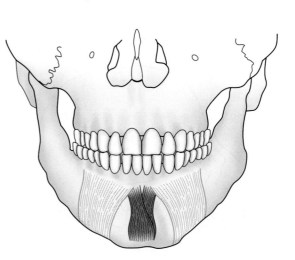

Concentric action:

Draws up the skin of the superior chest and neck, creating ridges of skin in the neck; depresses and draws the lower lip laterally; and depresses the mandible at the temporomandibular joint

Origin, proximal attachment, arises from:

Fascia covering the superior parts of the pectoralis major and deltoid

Insertion, distal attachment, attaches to:

Mandible and the fascia of the lower face (blending with the contralateral platysma and many other muscles of facial expression)

Innervation:

Cervical branch of the facial nerve (cranial nerve VII)

Major synergists:

Depressor labii inferioris and depressors of the mandible

Major antagonists:

Mentalis, orbicularis oris, and elevators of the mandible

Trigger points:

No common trigger points identified. Trigger points that form likely are located in the belly of the muscle.

Mentalis (men-TAL-iss)

Mentalis means "related to the chin."

Anterior

Concentric action:

Elevates, everts, and protracts the lower lip and wrinkles the skin of the chin

Origin, proximal attachment, arises from:

Incisive fossa of the mandible

Insertion, distal attachment, attaches to:

Skin of the chin

Innervation:

Mandibular marginal branch of the facial nerve (cranial nerve VII)

Major synergists:

Orbicularis oris and depressor labii inferioris

Major antagonists:

Platysma and depressor labii inferioris

Trigger points:

No common trigger points identified. Trigger points that form likely are located in the belly of the muscle.

ACTIVITY 9-7

Draw and color the **muscles that move the mouth** in the spaces provided. For each muscle, do the following:
1. Label the origin and insertion attachment points: *O* for origin; *I* for insertion.
2. Palpate these muscles; identify the attachment points and the bellies of the muscles.
3. Move these muscles on yourself.
    Note: Levators help us smile. Depressors help us frown.

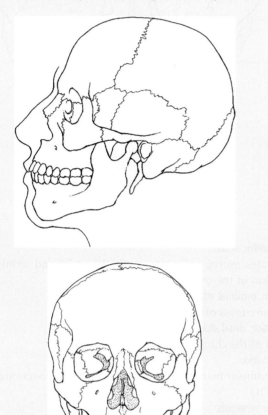

Muscles of Mastication (Chewing)

Four main pairs of muscles are involved in mastication (chewing) because they move the temporomandibular joint (TMJ). These muscles are powerful. The masseter and temporalis muscles are the prime movers of jaw closure (elevation of the mandible at the TMJ). The medial and lateral pterygoid muscles provide side-to-side grinding movements. Tension and tone imbalance in these groups of muscles are common causes of TMJ dysfunction. The buccinator muscles keep the cheeks close to the teeth to help us chew. The tongue is composed of specialized muscle fibers that curl, squeeze, and fold the tongue.

Masseter (MAS-sit-er)

Masseter means "one who chews."

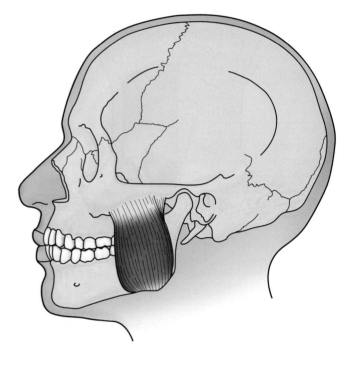

Lateral

Concentric action:
Elevates the mandible at the TMJ
Eccentric action:
Restrains depression of the mandible
Origin, proximal attachment, arises from:
Superficial portion—anterior two thirds of the inferior border of the zygomatic arch
Deep portion—medial surface of the zygomatic arch
Insertion, distal attachment, attaches to:
Coronoid process, ramus, and angle of the mandible
Innervation:
Mandibular division of the trigeminal nerve (cranial nerve V)
Major synergists:
Temporalis and medial pterygoid
Major antagonists:
Suprahyoid muscles
Trigger points:
Superior at the tendinous junction near the zygomatic arch and in the belly of the muscle
Referred pain patterns:
Upper jaw (maxillary region) and lower jaw (mandibular region), the ear, and the eyebrow

Temporalis (temp-or-AL-iss)

Temporalis means "related to the temple of the head."

Lateral

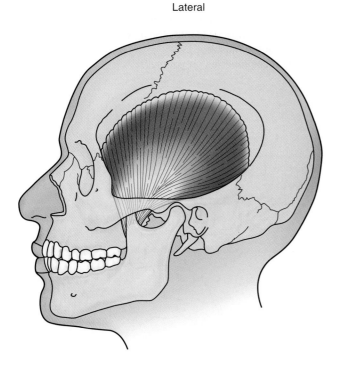

Lateral (external) pterygoid (TER-ih-goyd) (pterygoideus lateralis)

Pterygoid means "wing shaped"; *lateral* means "to the side."

Lateral

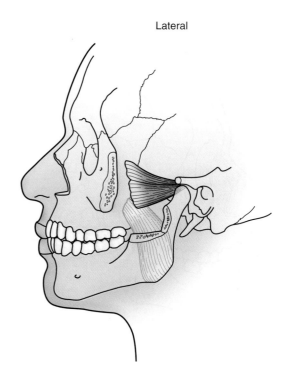

Concentric action:
Elevates the mandible at the TMJ
Eccentric action:
Restrains depression of the mandible
Origin, proximal attachment, arises from:
Temporal fossa and deep surface of the temporal fascia
Insertion, distal attachment, attaches to:
Ramus of the mandible and medial surface and anterior border of the coronoid process
Innervation:
Anterior and posterior deep temporal nerve from the mandibular portion of the trigeminal nerve (cranial nerve V)
Major synergists:
Masseter and medial pterygoid
Major antagonists:
Suprahyoid muscles
Trigger points:
Anterior, medial, and posterior along the inferior aspect of the muscle near the tendinous junction at the coronoid process of the mandible
Referred pain patterns:
Temporal region, eyebrow, and upper teeth

Concentric actions:
Protraction and contralateral deviation (movement to the opposite side) of the mandible at the TMJ
Origin, proximal attachment, arises from:
Superior head—greater wing of the sphenoid bone
Inferior head—lateral surface of the lateral pterygoid plate of the sphenoid bone
Insertion, distal attachment, attaches to:
Anterior surface of the neck of the mandible and articular capsule and disk of the TMJ
Innervation:
Mandibular division of the trigeminal nerve (cranial nerve V)
Major synergist:
Medial pterygoid
Major antagonists:
Opposite-sided lateral and medial pterygoid muscles
Trigger points:
Belly of both divisions of the muscle
Referred pain pattern:
Cheek and TMJ
The student should note that the lateral pterygoid is palpated from inside the mouth.

Medial (internal) pterygoid (TER-ih-goyd)
(pterygoideus medialis)

Pterygoid means "wing shaped"; *medial* means "related to the middle."

Lateral

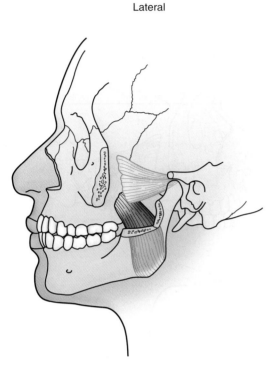

Concentric action:
Elevation, protraction, and contralateral deviation (movement to the opposite side) of the mandible at the TMJ
Origin, proximal attachment, arises from:
Medial surface of the lateral pterygoid plate of the sphenoid bone, pyramidal surface of the palatine bone, and tuberosity of the maxilla
Insertion, distal attachment, attaches to:
Internal surface of the angle and inferior ramus of the mandible
Innervation:
Mandibular division of the trigeminal nerve (cranial nerve V)
Major synergists:
Lateral pterygoid, temporalis, and masseter
Major antagonists:
Suprahyoid muscles and opposite-sided lateral and medial pterygoid muscles
Trigger points:
Belly of the muscle, with best access from inside the mouth
Referred pain pattern:
Back of the throat and into the ear

✎ ACTIVITY 9-8

Draw and color the **mastication muscles** in the spaces provided. For each muscle, do the following:
1. Label the origin and insertion attachment points: *O* for origin; *I* for insertion.
2. Place an X on the trigger points.
3. Palpate this muscle; identify the attachment points and the bellies of the muscles.
4. Move these muscles on yourself.

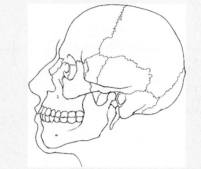

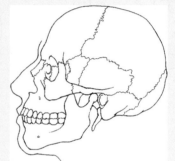

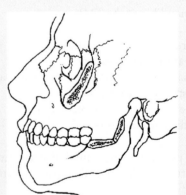

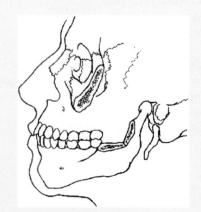

Muscles of the Neck

The sternocleidomastoid muscles divide the neck into the anterior and posterior triangles. Muscles of the neck move the neck at the cervical spinal joints. Most of the muscles of the anterior neck also assist in swallowing. Muscles of the neck that attach to the head provide movements of the head on the neck at the atlantooccipital joint. The sternocleidomastoid muscles are the major neck flexors. The sternocleidomastoid and deeper neck muscles, including the scalenes, and several straplike muscles of the vertebral column at the back of the neck provide lateral flexion of the neck. The posterior muscles of the neck, including the upper trapezius and other deeper musculature, provide extension of the neck. The sternocleidomastoid assists in head extension if the neck is stabilized. Tension and muscle imbalances of the neck muscles are a major cause of headaches and arm and shoulder pain and

dysfunction because of impingement of the cervical and brachial plexuses of nerves. These muscles do more than just provide head movement. These muscles isometrically act to stabilize and balance the head in an upright, eyes-forward position and therefore are involved in righting and postural reflexes. These muscles often act in sequence with trunk flexors and extensors. Therefore neck muscle problems are a common finding with low back pain and with hamstring and quadriceps dysfunction. Because the head is so heavy, these muscles often become short and increase in tension, especially with a postural imbalance. Because many of these muscles attach to the upper ribs, they function as accessory breathing muscles and can become dysfunctional if these muscles are used excessively during breathing. In massage that targets this area, the practitioner must address muscles of the region effectively while being cautious of underlying nerves and vessels (Figure 9-16).

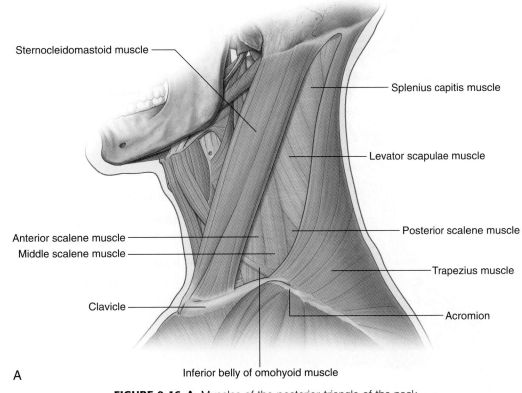

Sternocleidomastoid muscle

Splenius capitis muscle

Levator scapulae muscle

Anterior scalene muscle
Middle scalene muscle

Posterior scalene muscle

Trapezius muscle

Clavicle

Acromion

A

Inferior belly of omohyoid muscle

FIGURE 9-16 A, Muscles of the posterior triangle of the neck.

Continued

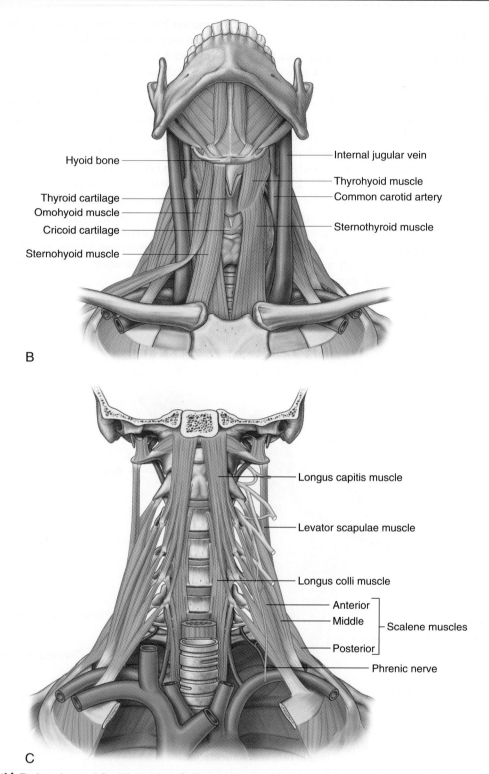

Hyoid bone

Thyroid cartilage
Omohyoid muscle
Cricoid cartilage

Sternohyoid muscle

Internal jugular vein

Thyrohyoid muscle
Common carotid artery

Sternothyroid muscle

B

Longus capitis muscle

Levator scapulae muscle

Longus colli muscle

Anterior
Middle   Scalene muscles
Posterior

Phrenic nerve

C

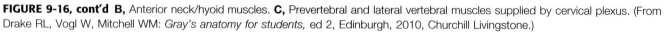

FIGURE 9-16, cont'd B, Anterior neck/hyoid muscles. **C,** Prevertebral and lateral vertebral muscles supplied by cervical plexus. (From Drake RL, Vogl W, Mitchell WM: *Gray's anatomy for students,* ed 2, Edinburgh, 2010, Churchill Livingstone.)

Sternocleidomastoid (STER-no-CLY-do-mas-toyd) (sternocleidomastoideus)

Sternocleidomastoid means "connecting to the sternum, clavicle, and mastoid process of the skull."

Anterior

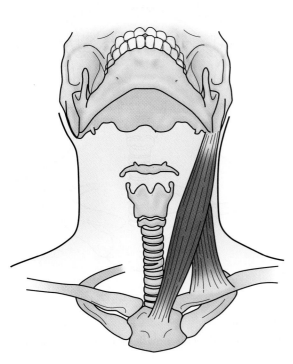

Concentric action:

Flexion of the neck at the spinal joints, lateral flexion and contralateral rotation of the neck and the head at the spinal joints, and extension of the head at the atlantooccipital joint

Eccentric action:

Restrains extension of the neck, contralateral lateral flexion of the neck and head, ipsilateral rotation of the neck and head, and flexion of the head

Isometric action:

Assists in stabilizing the head in space when the mandible moves

Origin, proximal attachment, arises from:

Sternal head—superior aspect of anterior surface of manubrium of the sternum

Clavicular head—superior border of the anterior surface of the medial third of the clavicle

Insertion, distal attachment, attaches to:

Superior surface of the mastoid process and lateral half of the superior nuchal line of occiput

Innervation:

Spinal accessory nerve (cranial nerve XI) and ventral rami of second and third cervical spinal nerves

Major synergists:

Scalenes, opposite-sided splenius capitis, and suboccipital muscles

Major antagonists:

Upper trapezius and semispinalis capitis (opposite-sided sternocleidomastoid)

Trigger points:

Several points along the entire length of both divisions of the muscle

Referred pain pattern:

Head and face, particularly the occipital region, ear, and forehead. Autonomic nervous system phenomena and proprioceptive disturbances are common.

✎ ACTIVITY 9-9

Draw and color the **sternocleidomastoid muscle** in the space provided. Do the following:

1. Label the origin and insertion attachment points: *O* for origin; *I* for insertion.
2. Place an X on the trigger point.
3. Palpate this muscle; identify the attachment points and the belly of the muscle.
4. Move this muscle on yourself.

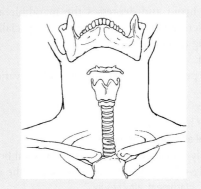

Anterior Triangle of the Neck

As a group, the suprahyoid muscles are located superior to the hyoid bone. These muscles can elevate the hyoid bone, which affects the movement of the tongue and other movements necessary for swallowing. If the mandible and hyoid bone are stabilized, this group of muscles can act as weak accessory flexors of the neck at the spinal joints.

Digastric (dye-GAS-trik) *(digastricus)*

Digastric means "two bellies."

Anterior

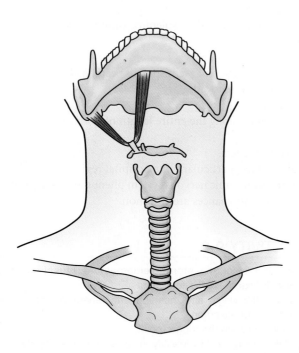

Stylohyoid (STY-low-HY-oyd) *(stylohyoideus)*

Stylohyoid means "pen" and "U shaped."

Anterior

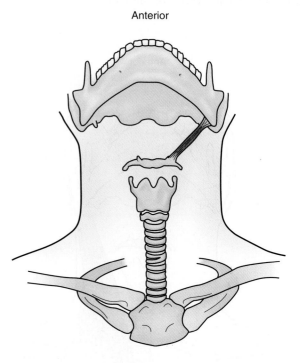

Concentric action:
Elevates the hyoid and depresses the mandible at the TMJ (The posterior belly of this muscle is especially active in swallowing and chewing.)
Eccentric action:
Restrains depression of the hyoid and elevation of the mandible
Isometric action:
Stabilizes the hyoid bone
Origin, proximal attachment, arises from:
Posterior belly—mastoid notch of the temporal bone
Anterior belly—digastric fossa on the base of the mandible
Insertion, distal attachment, attaches to:
Body of the greater cornu of the hyoid bone by way of a fibrous sling of tissue
Innervation:
Trigeminal (cranial nerve V) and facial (cranial nerve VII) nerves
Major synergists:
Other suprahyoid muscles
Major antagonists:
Infrahyoid muscles, temporalis, and masseter
Trigger points:
Belly of each division of the muscle
Referred pain pattern:
Sternocleidomastoid area and bottom front teeth

Concentric action:
Elevates the hyoid (This muscle is effective at elevating the tongue.)
Eccentric action:
Restrains depression of the hyoid
Isometric action:
Stabilizes the hyoid bone
Origin, proximal attachment, arises from:
Posterior surface of the styloid process
Insertion, distal attachment, attaches to:
Body of the hyoid bone, at the junction with the greater cornu
Innervation:
Facial nerve (cranial nerve VII, stylohyoid branch)
Major synergists:
Other suprahyoid muscles
Major antagonists:
Infrahyoid muscles, temporalis, and masseter
Trigger points:
Likely to form in the belly

▍*Mylohyoid* (MY-lo-HY-oyd) *(mylohyoideus)*

Mylohyoid means "molar" and "U shaped."

Anterior

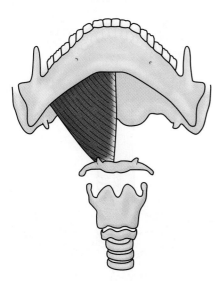

Concentric action:
Elevates the hyoid and depresses the mandible at the TMJ (This muscle is important in elevating the floor of the mouth during the first stage of swallowing.)

Eccentric action:
Restrains depression of the hyoid and elevation of the mandible

Isometric action:
Stabilizes the hyoid bone

Origin, proximal attachment, arises from:
Mylohyoid line of the mandible

Insertion, distal attachment, attaches to:
Posterior fibers—anterior surface of the body of the hyoid bone near the inferior border
Middle and anterior fibers—median fibrous raphe stretching from the symphysis menti to the hyoid bone

Innervation:
Mylohyoid branch of the inferior alveolar nerve of the trigeminal nerve (cranial nerve V)

Major synergists:
Other suprahyoid muscles

Major antagonists:
Infrahyoid muscles, temporalis, and masseter

Trigger points:
Likely to form in the belly

▍*Geniohyoid* (JEEN-ee-oh-HY-oyd) *(geniohyoideus)*

Geniohyoid means "chin" and "U shaped."

Anterior

Concentric action:
Elevates the hyoid (this muscle elevates the tongue and draws it forward) and depresses the mandible at the TMJ

Eccentric action:
Restrains depression of the hyoid and elevation of the mandible

Isometric action:
Stabilizes the hyoid bone

Origin, proximal attachment, arises from:
Inferior mental spine on the posterior surface of the symphysis of the mandible

Insertion, distal attachment, attaches to:
Anterior surface of the body of the hyoid bone

Innervation:
Hypoglossal nerve (cranial nerve XII)

Major synergists:
Other suprahyoid muscles

Major antagonists:
Infrahyoid muscles, temporalis, and masseter

Trigger points:
Likely to form in the belly

✎ ACTIVITY 9-10

Draw and color the **muscles in the anterior triangle of the neck** in the spaces provided. For each muscle, do the following:

1. Label the origin and insertion attachment points: *O* for origin; *I* for insertion.
2. Place an X on the trigger points.
3. Palpate this muscle; identify the attachment points and the bellies of the muscles.
4. Move these muscles on yourself.

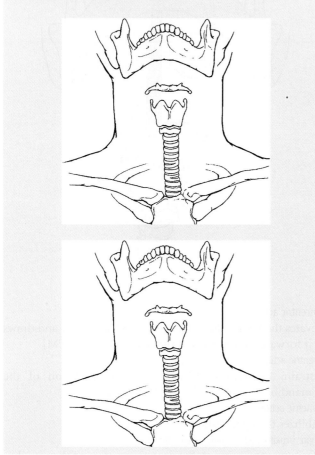

Infrahyoid muscles

These muscles are located inferior to the hyoid bone. As a group, they depress the hyoid bone and influence swallowing and the production of sound.

▌ *Sternohyoid* (STERN-oh-HY-oyd) *(sternohyoideus)*

Sternohyoid means "chest" and "U shaped."

Anterior

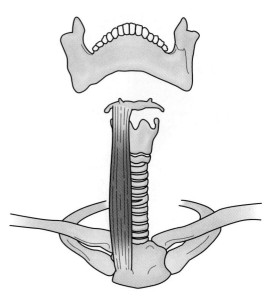

Concentric action:
Depresses the hyoid (This muscle plays a part in speech and mastication.)
Eccentric action:
Restrains elevation of the hyoid
Isometric action:
Stabilizes the hyoid bone
Origin, proximal attachment, arises from:
Posterior surface of the medial end of the clavicle, posterior sternoclavicular ligament, and superior and posterior parts of the manubrium
Insertion, distal attachment, attaches to:
Inferior border of the body of the hyoid bone
Innervation:
Branches from the ansa cervicalis of the cervical plexus
Major synergists:
Thyrohyoid and omohyoid
Major antagonists:
Suprahyoid muscles
Trigger points:
Likely to form in the belly

▌*Sternothyroid* (STERN-oh-THY-royd) *(sternothyroideus)*

Sternothyroid means "chest" and "shaped like a shield."

Anterior

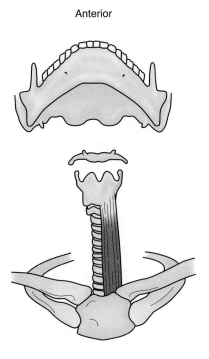

Concentric action:
Depresses the thyroid cartilage
Eccentric action:
Restrains elevation of the thyroid cartilage
Isometric action:
Assists stabilization of the hyoid bone through its pull on the thyroid cartilage
Origin, proximal attachment, arises from:
Posterior surface of the manubrium and cartilage of the first rib
Insertion, distal attachment, attaches to:
Oblique line on the lamina of the thyroid cartilage
Innervation:
Branches from the ansa cervicalis of the cervical plexus
Major synergists:
Sternohyoid and omohyoid (if the thyroid cartilage is fixed to the hyoid bone)
Major antagonist:
Thyrohyoid
Trigger points:
Likely to form in the belly

▌*Omohyoid* (OH-mo-HY-oyd) *(omohyoideus)*

Omohyoid means "shoulder" and "U shaped."

Anterior

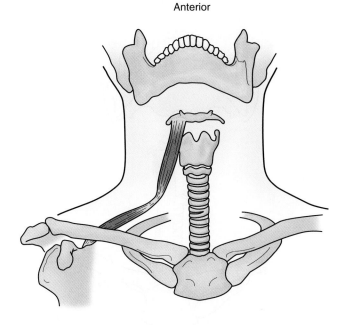

Concentric action:
Depresses the hyoid
Eccentric action:
Restrains elevation of the hyoid
Isometric action:
Stabilizes the hyoid bone
Origin, proximal attachment, arises from:
Inferior belly—superior border of the scapula near the scapular notch and suprascapular ligament (ends at its central tendon attaching to the clavicle by a fibrous sling of tissue deep to the sternocleidomastoid)
Superior belly—from its central tendon at the clavicle
Insertion, distal attachment, attaches to:
Inferior border of the body of the hyoid bone
Innervation:
Branches from the ansa cervicalis of the cervical plexus
Major synergists:
Sternohyoid and thyrohyoid
Major antagonists:
Suprahyoid muscles
Trigger points:
Likely to form in the belly

❙ *Thyrohyoid* (THY-ro-HY-oyd) *(thyrohyoideus)*

Thyrohyoid means "shaped like a shield" and "U shaped."

Anterior

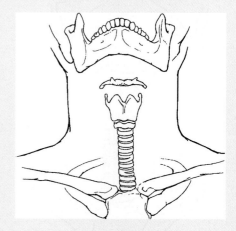

Concentric action:
Depresses the hyoid and elevates the thyroid cartilage
Eccentric action:
Restrains elevation of the hyoid and depression of the thyroid cartilage
Isometric action:
Stabilizes the hyoid bone and the thyroid cartilage
Origin, proximal attachment, arises from:
Lamina of the thyroid cartilage at the oblique line
Insertion, distal attachment, attaches to:
Inferior border of the greater cornu and the body of the hyoid bone
Innervation:
First cervical spinal nerve via the hypoglossal nerve (cranial nerve XII)
Major synergists:
Infrahyoid muscles for depression of the hyoid and suprahyoid muscles for elevation of the thyroid cartilage (if the thyroid cartilage is fixed to the hyoid bone)
Major antagonists:
Suprahyoid muscles for elevation of the hyoid and sternothyroid for depression of the thyroid cartilage
Trigger points:
Likely to form in the belly

✐ ACTIVITY 9-11

Draw and color the **infrahyoid muscles** in the spaces provided. For each muscle, do the following:
1. Label the origin and insertion attachment points: *O* for origin; *I* for insertion.
2. Swallow to identify the hyoid bone and the action of these muscles.
3. Identify the attachment points and the bellies of the muscles.

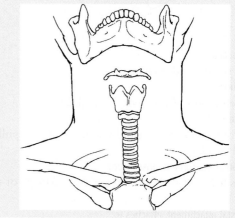

Longus colli (LONG-us KOAL-ee)

Longus colli means "long" and "belonging to the neck."

Anterior

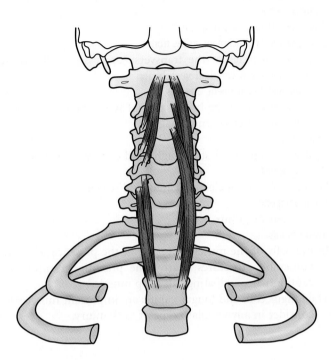

Concentric action:

Flexion, lateral flexion, and contralateral rotation of the neck at the spinal joints

Eccentric action:

Restrains extension, contralateral lateral flexion, and ipsilateral rotation of the neck

Isometric action:

Stabilizes the cervical spine and can be compared with the psoas major and psoas minor in the lumbar region

Origin, proximal attachment, arises from:

Superior oblique portion—anterior tubercles of the transverse processes of the third, fourth, and fifth cervical vertebrae

Inferior oblique portion—anterior bodies of the first three thoracic vertebrae

Vertical portion—anterior bodies of the lower three cervical vertebrae and the upper three thoracic vertebrae

Insertion, distal attachment, attaches to:

Superior—anterior arch of the atlas

Inferior—anterior tubercles of the transverse processes of the fifth and sixth cervical vertebrae

Vertical—anterior bodies of the second, third, and fourth cervical vertebrae

Innervation:

Ventral rami of the second through sixth cervical spinal nerves

Major synergists:

Longus capitis, sternocleidomastoid, and scalenes

Major antagonists:

Neck extensor group

Trigger points:

In the belly of the muscle (Because of the presence of many vulnerable structures nearby, the practitioner must use caution when palpating this deep muscle.)

The longus colli and longus capitis are important muscles to consider in any whiplash type of neck injury.

Longus capitis (LONG-us KAP-ih-tiss)

Longus capitis means "long" and "belonging to the head."

Anterior

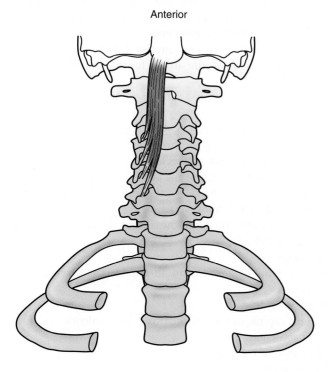

Concentric action:

Flexion and lateral flexion of the head and the neck at the spinal joints

Eccentric action:

Restrains extension and contralateral lateral flexion of the head and neck

Isometric action:

Stabilizes the cervical spine

Origin, proximal attachment, arises from:

Anterior tubercles of the transverse processes of the third through sixth cervical vertebrae

Insertion, distal attachment, attaches to:

Inferior surface of the basilar part of the occipital bone just anterior to the foramen magnum

Innervation:

Ventral rami of the first through third cervical spinal nerves

Major synergists:

Longus colli, sternocleidomastoid, and scalenes

Major antagonists:

Neck extensor group

Trigger points:

In the belly of the muscle (Because of the presence of many vulnerable structures nearby, the practitioner must use caution when palpating this deep muscle.)

The longus colli and longus capitis are important muscles to consider in any whiplash type of neck injury.

✎ ACTIVITY 9-12

Draw and color the **muscles of the deep anterior triangle of the neck** in the spaces provided. For each muscle, do the following:

1. Label the origin and insertion attachment points: *O* for origin; *I* for insertion.
2. Move these muscles on yourself.

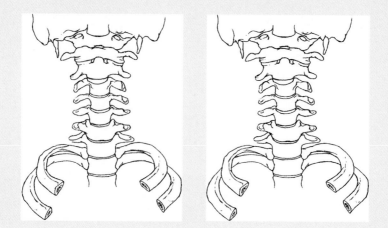

Scalene Group

Anterior scalene (scalenus anterior) (skay-LEE-nus)

Scalenus means "triangular with unequal sides"; *anterior* means "before" or "in front."

Anterior

Middle scalene (scalenus medius) (skay-LEE-nus)

Scalenus means "triangular with unequal sides"; *medius* means "middle."

Anterior

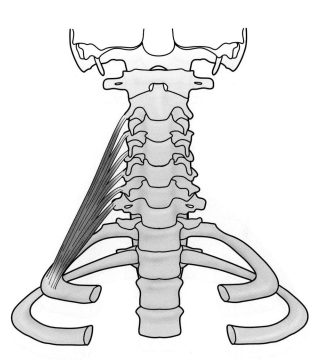

Concentric action:

Flexion and lateral flexion of the neck at the spinal joints; elevation of the first rib at the sternocostal and costovertebral joints (thus functioning as an accessory muscle of respiration)

Eccentric action:

Restrains extension and contralateral lateral flexion of the neck and depression of the first rib

Isometric action:

Stabilizes the cervical spine

Origin, proximal attachment, arises from:

Anterior tubercles of the transverse processes of the third through sixth cervical vertebrae

Insertion, distal attachment, attaches to:

Scalene tubercle on the inner border of the first rib and superior surface of the first rib

Innervation:

Ventral rami of the fourth through sixth cervical spinal nerves

Major synergists:

Middle and posterior scalenes and sternocleidomastoid

Major antagonists:

Neck extensors and lateral flexors on the opposite side of the neck

Trigger points:

Belly of the muscle near the rib attachment

Referred pain pattern:

Pectoral region, rhomboid region, and the entire length of the arm into the hand

Concentric action:

Flexion and lateral flexion of the neck at the spinal joints and elevation of the first rib at the sternocostal and costovertebral joints (thus functioning as an accessory muscle of respiration)

Eccentric action:

Restrains extension and contralateral lateral flexion of the neck and depression of the first rib

Isometric action:

Stabilizes the cervical spine

Origin, proximal attachment, arises from:

Posterior tubercles of the transverse processes of the second through seventh cervical vertebrae

Insertion, distal attachment, attaches to:

Superior surface of the first rib

Innervation:

Ventral rami of the third through eighth cervical spinal nerves

Major synergists:

Anterior and posterior scalenes and sternocleidomastoid

Major antagonists:

Neck extensors and lateral flexors on the opposite side of the neck

Trigger points:

Belly of the muscle near the rib attachment

Referred pain pattern:

Pectoral region, rhomboid region, and the entire length of the arm into the hand

| *Posterior scalene (scalenus posterior)* (skay-LEE-nus)

Scalenus means "triangular with unequal sides"; *posterior* means "behind."

Anterior

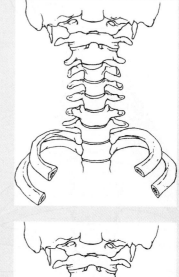

Concentric action:
Lateral flexion of the neck at the spinal joints and elevation of the second rib at the sternocostal and costovertebral joints (thus functioning as an accessory muscle of respiration)

Eccentric action:
Restrains contralateral lateral flexion of the neck and depression of the second rib

Isometric action:
Stabilizes the cervical spine

Origin, proximal attachment, arises from:
Posterior tubercles of the transverse processes of the fifth through seventh cervical vertebrae

Insertion, distal attachment, attaches to:
Outer surface of the second rib

Innervation:
Ventral rami of the sixth through eighth cervical spinal nerves

Major synergists:
Anterior and middle scalenes and sternocleidomastoid

Major antagonists:
Lateral flexors on the opposite side of the neck

Trigger points:
Belly of the muscle near the rib attachment

Referred pain pattern:
Pectoral region, rhomboid region, and the entire length of the arm into the hand

✎ ACTIVITY 9-13

Draw and color the **muscles of the scalene group** in the spaces provided. For each muscle, do the following:
1. Label the origin and insertion attachment points: *O* for origin; *I* for insertion.
2. Place an X on the trigger points.
3. Palpate this muscle; identify the attachment points and the bellies of the muscles.
4. Move these muscles on yourself.

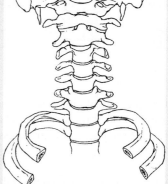

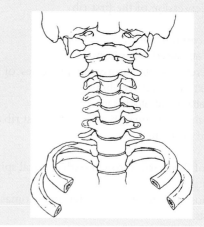

Deep Muscles of the Back and Posterior Neck

When concentrically contracted, the splenius muscles are responsible for neck and head extension, lateral flexion, and rotation. The deep, or intrinsic, back muscles associated with the vertebral column affect trunk movements. Isometrically, these muscles also play an important role in maintaining the normal curvature of the spine. The deep muscles of the back form a complex column that extends from the sacrum to the skull. Thinking of each of the individual deep back muscles as a string that, when pulled, causes one or more vertebrae to move on the vertebrae below is helpful. Because the attachments of the different muscle groups overlap extensively, entire regions of the vertebral column can move simultaneously and smoothly. Concentrically acting together, the deep back muscles can extend the trunk, neck, or head. Contraction of muscles on only one side causes extension, lateral flexion, and rotation of the trunk, neck, or head. Eccentric contraction restrains the opposite actions, primarily flexion, lateral flexion to the opposite side, and perhaps rotation.

The largest deep back muscle group is the erector spinae group. Assisting the long muscles of the back are a number of short muscles that extend from one vertebra to the next; these small intrinsic muscles act primarily as stabilizers for the spine. Postural deviation of any type—including forward head position or scoliosis, excessive kyphosis, and excessive lordosis or any rotational adaptation of the shoulder girdle and pelvic girdle—strains the deep postural muscles. These muscles are more involved in stabilization than mobility; therefore, when dysfunctional patterns exist, these muscles tend to shorten because of sustained isometric functioning. Massage affecting these muscles must be deep enough to access them without causing protective tensing (guarding) of the more superficial muscles. Massage is most effective when applied with a slow, sustained, broad-based compressive force that penetrates the superficial layers to affect the deep muscles (Figure 9-17).

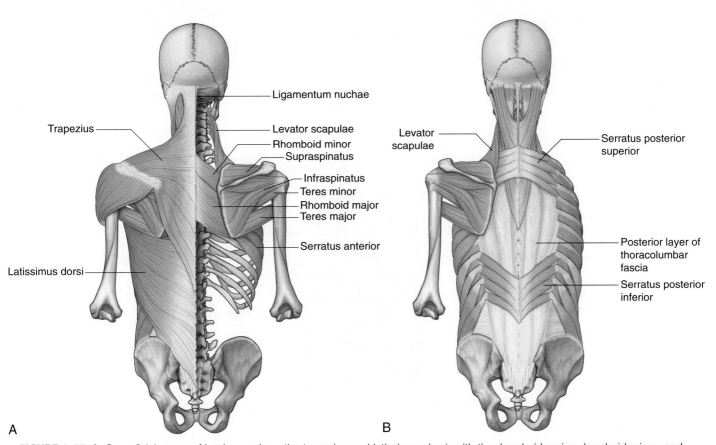

FIGURE 9-17 A, Superficial group of back muscles—the trapezius and latissimus dorsi, with the rhomboid major, rhomboid minor, and levator scapulae located deep to the trapezius in the superior part of the back. **B,** Intermediate group of back muscles—serratus posterior muscles.

Continued

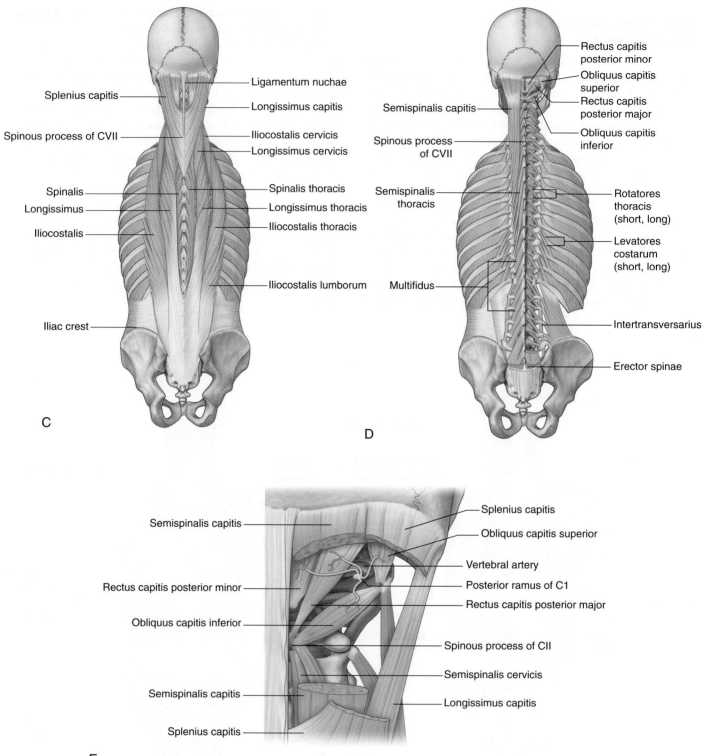

FIGURE 9-17, cont'd C, Deep group of back muscles—erector spinae muscles. **D,** Deep group of back muscles—transversospinales and segmental muscles. **E,** Deep group of back muscles—suboccipital muscles. This also shows the borders of the suboccipital triangle. (From Drake RL, Vogl W, Mitchell WM: *Gray's anatomy for students,* ed 2, Edinburgh, 2010, Churchill Livingstone.)

Deep Posterior Cervical Muscles

Splenius capitis and splenius cervicis (SPLEEN-ee-us KAP-ih-tiss, SIR-vih-siss)

Splenius means "bandage," *capitis* means "head," and *cervicis* means "belonging to the neck."

Posterior

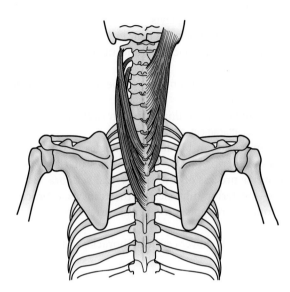

Concentric action:
Extension, lateral flexion, and ipsilateral rotation of the head and the neck at the spinal joints

Eccentric action:
Restrains flexion, contralateral lateral flexion, and contralateral rotation of the neck and the head

Isometric action:
Stabilizes the cervical spine

Origin, proximal attachment, arises from:
Capitis—nuchal ligament and the spinous processes of the seventh cervical and first four thoracic vertebrae
Cervicis—spinous processes of the third through sixth thoracic vertebrae

Insertion, distal attachment, attaches to:
Capitis—lateral one third of the superior nuchal line of the occipital bone deep to the attachment of the sternocleidomastoid and the mastoid process of the temporal bone
Cervicis—posterior tubercles of the transverse processes of the upper three cervical vertebrae

Innervation:
Capitis—dorsal rami of the middle cervical spinal nerves
Cervicis—dorsal rami of the lower cervical spinal nerves

Major synergists:
Posterior cervical extensors, opposite-sided upper trapezius, and opposite-sided sternocleidomastoid

Major antagonists:
Anterior cervical flexors, same-sided upper trapezius, and same-sided sternocleidomastoid

Trigger points:
Belly of the muscles closer to the head

Referred pain patterns:
To the top of the skull (the pain often feels as though it is inside the head), to the eye, and into the shoulder

✎ ACTIVITY 9-14

Draw and color the **deep posterior cervical muscles** in the spaces provided. For each muscle, do the following:
1. Label the origin and insertion attachment points: *O* for origin; *I* for insertion.
2. Place an X on the trigger points.
3. Palpate this muscle; identify the attachment points and the bellies of the muscles.
4. Move these muscles on yourself.

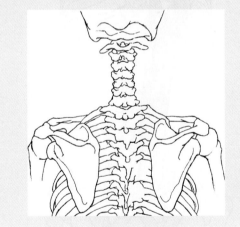

Vertical Muscles, Erector Spinae Group

Also called the *sacrospinalis muscles,* the muscles in the erector spinae (ee-REK-tor SPIN-aye) group are the principal extensors of the spinal joints.

> **Iliocostalis lumborum, iliocostalis thoracis, and iliocostalis cervicis** (ILL-ee-oh-kos-TAL-iss lum-BOR-um, thor-AH-siss, SIR-vih-siss)

Iliocostalis means "connecting the ilium" to the loins (lumborum), ribs (costa), chest (thoracis), and neck (cervicis).

Posterior

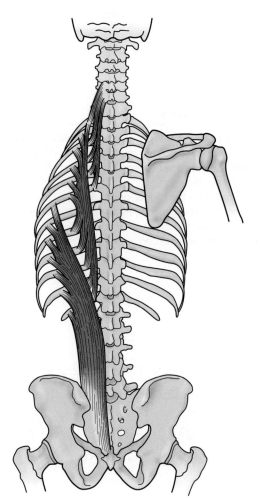

Concentric action:

Extension, lateral flexion, and ipsilateral rotation of the trunk and neck at the spinal joints and anterior tilt of the pelvis at the lumbosacral joint

Eccentric action:

Restrains flexion, contralateral lateral flexion, and contralateral rotation of the trunk and neck and allows posterior tilt of the pelvis

Isometric action:

Stabilizes the spine and pelvis

Origin, proximal attachment, arises from:

Lumborum—medial iliac crest and medial and lateral sacral crests

Thoracis—lower six ribs medial to the tendons of the iliocostalis lumborum

Cervicis—angles of the third through sixth ribs

Insertion, distal attachment, attaches to:

Lumborum—inferior border at the angles of ribs 7 to 12

Thoracis—superior border at the angles of ribs 1 to 6 and transverse process of seventh cervical vertebra

Cervicis—posterior tubercles of the transverse processes of the fourth through sixth cervical vertebrae

Innervation:

Dorsal rami of the lower cervical, thoracic, and lumbar spinal nerves

Longissimus thoracis, longissimus cervicis, and longissimus capitis (lon-GISS-ih-mus thor-AH-siss, SIR-vih-siss, KAP-ih-tiss)

Longissimus means "the longest"; these muscles relate to the thorax, neck, and head, respectively.

Posterior

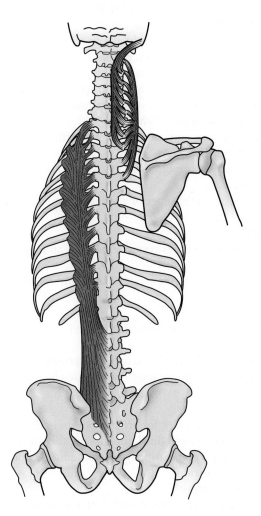

Concentric action:
Extension, lateral flexion, and ipsilateral rotation of the trunk, neck, and head at the spinal joints and anterior tilt of the pelvis at the lumbosacral joint

Eccentric action:
Restrains flexion, contralateral lateral flexion, and contralateral rotation of the trunk, neck, and head and allows posterior tilt of the pelvis

Isometric action:
Stabilizes the spine and pelvis

Origin, proximal attachment, arises from:
Thoracis—transverse processes of the lumbar vertebrae, lumbocostal aponeurosis, and medial iliac crest and posterior sacrum

Cervicis—transverse processes of the upper five thoracic vertebrae

Capitis—transverse processes of the upper four or five thoracic vertebrae and articular processes of the lower three or four cervical vertebrae

Insertion, distal attachment, attaches to:
Thoracis—transverse processes of all thoracic vertebrae and lower 9 or 10 ribs

Cervicis—posterior tubercles of the transverse processes of the second through sixth cervical vertebrae

Capitis—mastoid process of the temporal bone

Innervation:
Dorsal rami of the lower cervical, thoracic, and lumbar spinal nerves

Spinalis thoracis, spinalis cervicis, and spinalis capitis
(spy-NAL-iss thor-AH-siss, SIR-vih-ciss, KAP-ih-tiss)

Spinalis means "related to the spine"; these muscles relate to the chest, neck, and head, respectively.

Posterior

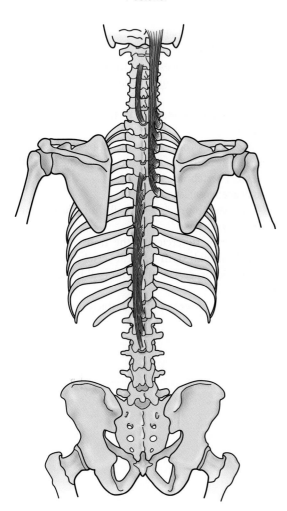

Concentric action:

Extension, lateral flexion, and ipsilateral rotation of the trunk, neck, and head at the spinal joints

Eccentric action:

Restrains flexion, contralateral lateral flexion, and contralateral rotation of the trunk, neck, and head

Isometric action:

Stabilizes the spine

Origin, proximal attachment, arises from:

Thoracis—spinous processes of the first two lumbar and the last two thoracic vertebrae

Cervicis—spinous processes of the first and second thoracic and the seventh cervical vertebrae

Capitis—transverse processes of the upper seven thoracic and the seventh cervical vertebrae and articular processes of the fourth through sixth cervical vertebrae

Insertion, distal attachment, attaches to:

Thoracis—spinous processes of the fourth through eighth thoracic vertebrae

Cervicis—spinous processes of the second and third cervical vertebrae

Capitis—between the superior and inferior nuchal lines of the occipital bone

Innervation:

Dorsal rami of the lower cervical, thoracic, and lumbar spinal nerves

Elements common to the erector spinae and transversospinalis group

Major antagonists:

Flexors of the trunk (abdominal muscles)

Major synergists:

Extension is assisted by the serratus posterior inferior and the quadratus lumborum; rotation is assisted by the abdominal obliques.

Trigger points:

The most common site for trigger points is the superficial long-fibered, longitudinal muscles in the erector spinae group; trigger points usually are found in the midscapular and lumbar regions.

Referred pain patterns:

Scapular, lumbar, abdominal, and gluteal areas; also local area and adjacent spinal segment

ACTIVITY 9-15

Draw and color the **vertical muscles (erector spinae group)** in the spaces provided. For each muscle, do the following:
1. Label the origin and insertion attachment points: *O* for origin; *I* for insertion.
2. Place an X on the trigger points.
3. Palpate this muscle; identify the attachment points and the bellies of the muscles.
4. Move these muscles on yourself.

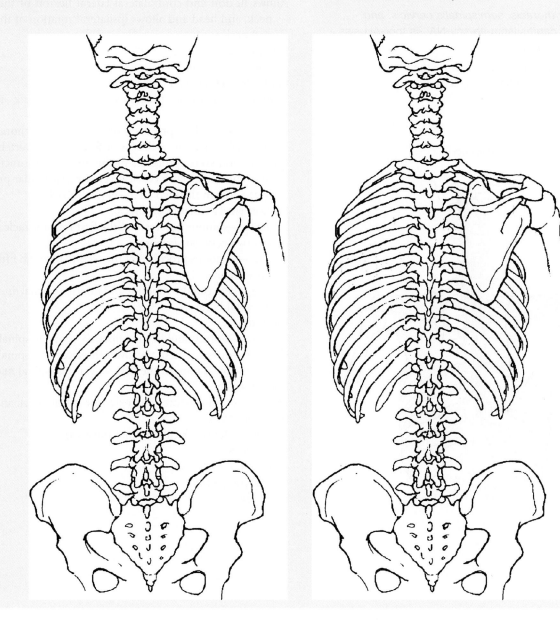

Oblique Muscles, Transversospinales Group

The transversospinales group of muscles extends, laterally flexes, and contralaterally rotates the spinal joints and also functions to move and stabilize the pelvis.

> **Semispinalis thoracis, semispinalis cervicis, and semispinalis capitis** (sem-ee-spy-NAL-is thor-AH-siss, SIR-vih-siss, KAP-ih-tiss)

Semispinalis means "half" and "spine"; these muscles relate to the chest, neck, and head, respectively.

Posterior

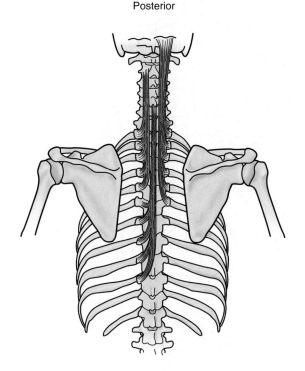

Concentric action:

Extension and lateral flexion of the trunk, neck, and head at the spinal joints and contralateral rotation of the trunk and neck at the spinal joints

Eccentric action:

Allows flexion and contralateral lateral flexion of the trunk, neck, and head and allows ipsilateral rotation of the trunk and neck

Isometric action:

Stabilizes the spine

Origin, proximal attachment, arises from:

Thoracis—transverse processes of the last six thoracic vertebrae

Cervicis—transverse processes of the upper six thoracic and articular processes of the lower four cervical vertebrae

Capitis—transverse processes of the upper six thoracic vertebrae and the seventh cervical vertebrae; articular processes of the fourth through sixth cervical vertebrae

Insertion, distal attachment, attaches to:

Thoracis—spinous processes of the first four thoracic and the last two cervical vertebrae

Cervicis—spinous processes of the second through fifth cervical vertebrae

Capitis—between the superior and inferior nuchal lines of the occipital bone

Innervation:

Thoracis—dorsal rami of the upper six thoracic spinal nerves

Cervicis—dorsal rami of the lower three cervical spinal nerves

Capitis—dorsal rami of the first six cervical spinal nerves

Major synergists:

Multifidus and rotatores and extensors of the neck and head

Major antagonists:

Flexors of the trunk (abdominal muscles)

Trigger points:

Belly of the muscles

Referred pain patterns:

Local area

▌*Multifidus* (mul-tih-FYE-dus) *(musculi multifidi)*

Multifidus means "many split parts."

Posterior

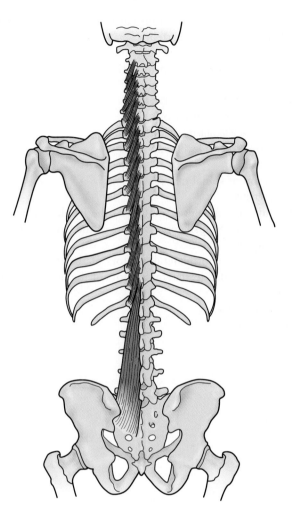

Concentric action:

Contralateral rotation, lateral flexion, and extension of the trunk and neck at the spinal joints and anterior tilt and elevation of the pelvis at the lumbosacral joint

Eccentric action:

Allows ipsilateral rotation, contralateral lateral flexion, and flexion of the trunk and neck and allows posterior tilt and depression of the pelvis

Isometric action:

Stabilizes the spine and pelvis

This muscle group provides proprioceptive input about posture and movement.

Origin, proximal attachment, arises from:

Articular processes of the last four cervical vertebrae, transverse processes of all thoracic vertebrae, mammillary processes of the lumbar vertebrae, posterior superior iliac spine, posterior sacroiliac ligaments, and posterior surface of the sacrum

Insertion, distal attachment, attaches to:

Spinous processes of the vertebrae two to four levels superior to the vertebrae of origin

Innervation:

Dorsal rami of the spinal nerves

Major synergists:

Semispinalis and rotatores

Major antagonists:

Flexors of the trunk (abdominal muscles)

Trigger points:

Belly of the muscles

Referred pain patterns:

Local area and sacroiliac joint

Rotatores (ro-TA-to-reez)

Rotatores means "one that rotates."

Posterior

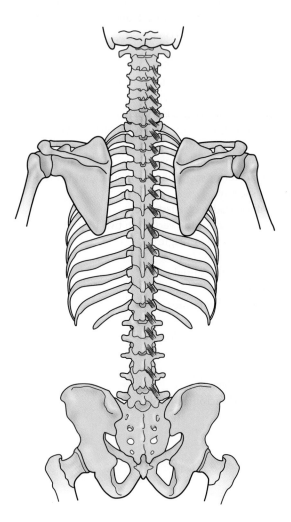

Concentric action:

Contralateral rotation and extension of the trunk and neck at the spinal joints

Eccentric action:

Restrains ipsilateral rotation and flexion of the trunk and neck

Isometric action:

Stabilizes the vertebral column particularly on the transverse plane between each vertebra

The rotatores are an important muscle group (with the multifidi) in providing proprioceptive posture information to the central nervous system.

Origin, proximal attachment, arises from:

Transverse process (inferiorly)

Insertion, distal attachment, attaches to:

Lamina one to two levels superior

Innervation:

Dorsal rami of spinal nerves

Major synergists:

Same-sided contralateral rotators of the trunk and neck and opposite-sided ipsilateral rotators of the trunk and neck

Major antagonists:

Opposite-sided contralateral rotators of the trunk and neck and same-sided ipsilateral rotators of the trunk and neck

Trigger points:

Belly of the muscles

Referred pain patterns:

Local area

Intertransversarii lumborum, intertransversarii thoracis, and intertransversarii cervicis (IN-ter-TRANS-ver-SAIR-ee-eye lum-BOR-um, thor-AH-siss, SIR-vih-siss)

Intertransversarii means "between or among the transverse processes of the vertebrae"; these muscles relate to the loins, thorax, and neck, respectively.

Posterior

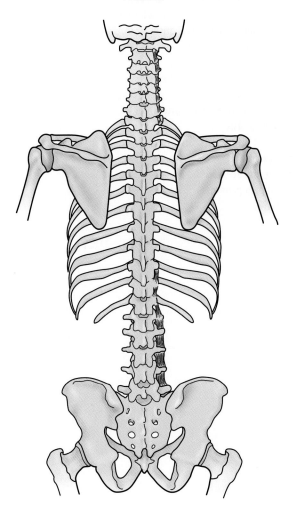

Concentric action:
Lateral flexion of the trunk and neck at the spinal joints
Eccentric action:
Restrains contralateral lateral flexion of the trunk and neck
Isometric action:
Provides intersegmental stability of the spine in the frontal plane
The intertransversarii muscles are active in proprioceptive input to the central nervous system.
Origin, proximal attachment, arises from:
Between transverse processes of the cervical, thoracic, and lumbar vertebrae (best developed in the cervical and lumbar regions)
Insertion, distal attachment, attaches to:
Between transverse processes of the cervical, thoracic, and lumbar vertebrae (best developed in the cervical and lumbar regions)
Innervation:
Ventral and dorsal rami of the spinal nerves
Major synergists:
Ipsilateral lateral flexors of the trunk and neck
Major antagonists:
Contralateral lateral flexors of the trunk and neck
Trigger points:
Belly of the muscles
Referred pain patterns:
Local area

Interspinales lumborum, interspinales thoracis, and interspinales cervicis (in-ter-spy-NAL-eez lum-BOR-um, thor-AH-siss, SIR-vih-siss)

Interspinales means "between or among the parts of the spine"; these muscles relate to the loins, chest, and neck, respectively.

Posterior

Concentric action:
Extension of the trunk and neck at the spinal joints
Eccentric action:
Restrains vertebral flexion
Isometric action:
Provides intersegmental stability of the spine in the sagittal plane
Interspinales muscles provide proprioceptive input concerning spinal stabilization and neuromuscular control.
Insertion, distal attachment, attaches to:
Between the spinous processes of the vertebrae
Origin, proximal attachment, arises from:
Between the spinous processes of the vertebrae
Innervation:
Dorsal rami of the spinal nerves
Major synergists:
Extensors of the trunk and neck
Major antagonists:
Flexors of the trunk and neck
Trigger points:
Belly of the muscle
Referred pain patterns:
Local area

✎ ACTIVITY 9-16

Draw and color the **oblique muscles (transversospinales group)** in the spaces provided. For each muscle, do the following:

1. Label the origin and insertion attachment points: *O* for origin; *I* for insertion.

2. Place an X on the trigger points.
3. Palpate this muscle; identify the attachment points and the bellies of the muscles.
4. Move these muscles on yourself.

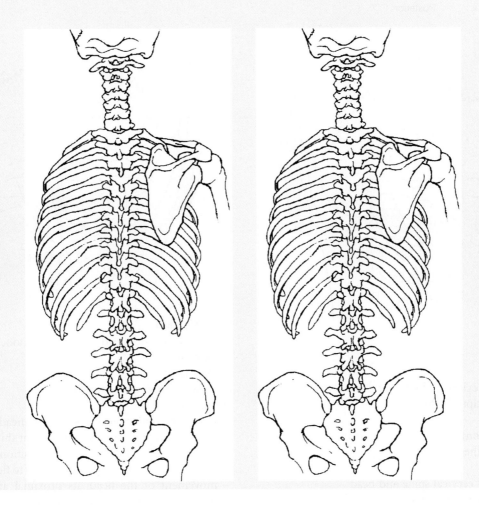

Suboccipital Muscles

As a group, the suboccipital muscles extend and rotate the head at the atlantooccipital joint in small and precise movements. More often, these muscles isometrically function as stabilizers of the head. These muscles are also important postural muscles and are neurologic reporting stations on balance and proprioceptive monitors of cervical spine and head position.

▌*Rectus capitis posterior major* (REK-tus KAP-ih-tiss)

Rectus means "straight," *capitis* means "belonging to the head," *posterior* means "behind," and *major* means "larger."

▌*Rectus capitis posterior minor* (REK-tus KAP-ih-tiss)

Rectus means "straight," *capitis* means "belonging to the head," *posterior* means "behind," and *minor* means "smaller."

Posterior

Posterior

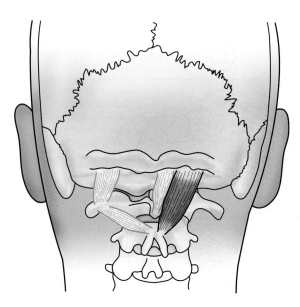

Concentric action:

Extension, lateral flexion, and ipsilateral rotation of the head at the atlantooccipital joint

Eccentric action:

Restrains flexion, contralateral lateral flexion, and contralateral rotation of the head

Isometric action:

Stabilizes the upper cervical spine and head

Origin, proximal attachment, arises from:

Spinous process of the axis

Insertion, distal attachment, attaches to:

Lateral aspect of the inferior nuchal line of the occipital bone lateral to the rectus capitis posterior minor

Innervation:

Dorsal ramus of the first cervical spinal nerve (the suboccipital nerve)

Major synergists:

Semispinalis capitis, rectus capitis posterior minor, and the splenius capitis on the same side

Major antagonists:

Rectus capitis anterior and the sternocleidomastoid on the same side

Trigger points:

Belly of the muscle, located with deep palpation at the base of the skull

Referred pain pattern:

Around the ear on the same side, sensation of compressed junction of skull and neck, and bandlike headache

Concentric action:

Extension of the head at the atlantooccipital joint (see Isometric)

Eccentric action:

Restrains flexion of the head

Isometric action:

Stabilizes the upper cervical spine and head

Recent myographic studies indicate that this muscle does not act in extension beyond neutral position, but rather functions more importantly as a restraint to flexion and forward movement of the head; its proximal attachment weaves into the dura through the foramen magnum (Greenman, 2003). This muscle actively provides proprioceptive input on positioning and posture to the central nervous system.

Origin, proximal attachment, arises from:

Posterior tubercle of the atlas

Insertion, distal attachment, attaches to:

Medial aspect of the inferior nuchal line of the occipital bone just superior to the foramen magnum

Innervation:

Dorsal ramus of the first cervical spinal nerve (the suboccipital nerve)

Major synergists:

Semispinalis capitis and rectus capitis posterior major

Major antagonists:

Rectus capitis anterior and longus capitis on the opposite side

Trigger points:

Belly of the muscle, located with deep palpation at the base of the skull

Referred pain pattern:

Around the ear on the same side, sensation of compressed junction of skull and neck, and bandlike headache

Oblique capitis superior (obliquus capitis superior) (oh-BLI-kwus KAP-ih-tiss)

Obliquus means "slanting," *capitis* means "head," and *superior* means "above" or "higher."

Posterior

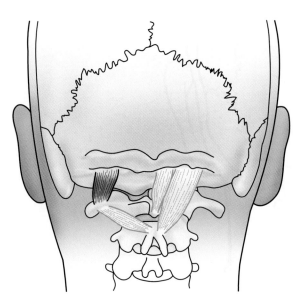

Concentric action:

Extension and lateral flexion of the head at the atlantooccipital joint

Eccentric action:

Restrains flexion and contralateral lateral flexion of the head

Isometric action:

Stabilizes the upper cervical spine and head

Origin, proximal attachment, arises from:

Superior surface of the transverse process of the atlas

Insertion, distal attachment, attaches to:

Between the superior and inferior nuchal lines of the occipital bone and lateral to the semispinalis capitis

Innervation:

Dorsal ramus of the first cervical spinal nerve (the suboccipital nerve)

Oblique capitis inferior (obliquus capitis inferior) (oh-BLI-kwus KAP-ih-tiss)

Obliquus means "slanting," *capitis* means "head," and *inferior* means "lower" or "beneath."

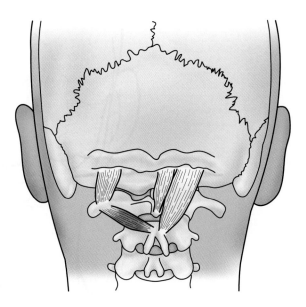

Concentric action:

Ipsilateral rotation of the atlas at the atlantoaxial joint

Eccentric action:

Restrains contralateral rotation of the atlas

Isometric action:

Stabilizes the upper cervical spine

Origin, proximal attachment, arises from:

Superior part of the spinous process of the axis

Insertion, distal attachment, attaches to:

Inferior and posterior aspect of the transverse process of the atlas

Innervation:

Dorsal ramus of the first cervical spinal nerve (the suboccipital nerve)

Major synergists:

Semispinalis capitis and the rectus capitis posterior major and rectus capitis posterior minor

Major antagonists:

Rectus capitis anterior and rectus capitis lateralis on the opposite side

Trigger points:

Belly of the muscle, located with deep palpation at the base of the skull

Referred pain pattern:

Around the ear on the same side, sensation of compressed junction of skull and neck, and bandlike headache

✎ ACTIVITY 9-17

Draw and color the **suboccipital muscles** in the spaces provided. For each muscle, do the following:

1. Label the origin and insertion attachment points: *O* for origin; *I* for insertion.

2. Place an X on the trigger points.
3. Palpate this muscle; identify the attachment points and the bellies of the muscles.
4. Move these muscles on yourself.

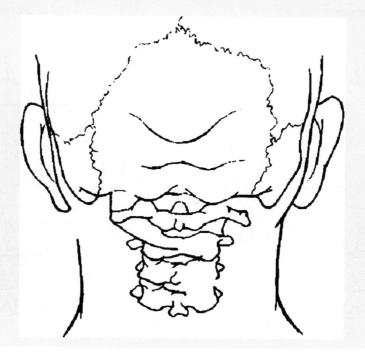

Muscles of the Torso

The primary function of the deep muscles of the thorax is to create movements necessary for breathing. Contraction of the diaphragm creates relaxed, quiet inspiration. Relaxed, quiet expiration requires no muscular contractions at all; rather, expiration is caused by the elastic recoil of the lungs themselves and the abdominal viscera that were stretched during inspiration. Forced inspiration and forced expiration result from the contraction of accessory muscles of respiration in addition to the diaphragm (Figures 9-18 and 9-19).

Some anatomists have considered the abdominal and thorax muscle groups as one group. However, unlike the abdominal muscles, the thoracic muscles are short, extending between the ribs. When they contract, they elevate or depress the ribs. The external intercostal muscles (the most superficial layer) generally are accepted as elevating the ribs for inspiration, whereas the internal intercostal muscles (from the intermediate layer) depress the ribs for expiration. The transversus thoracis (the deepest layer) is also involved in depression of ribs.

The diaphragm is the most important muscle of inspiration and forms a muscular partition between the thoracic and abdominopelvic cavities. When relaxed, the diaphragm is dome shaped, but when it is contracted, its central dome moves inferiorly and flattens, increasing the volume of the thoracic cavity. The alternating contraction and relaxation of the diaphragm cause pressure changes in the abdominopelvic cavity that assist the return of lymph fluid to the venous blood and to the heart. We can contract the diaphragm to increase the intraabdominal pressure voluntarily to help evacuate urine or feces or to deliver a baby.

An increase in intraabdominal pressure also aids in lifting weight. When we take a deep breath to fixate our diaphragm, we can increase the abdominal pressure enough to support the spine while lifting a heavy weight. Fibers from the quadratus lumborum and psoas muscles weave into the diaphragm. With this direct relationship, we can see how low back function and breathing function are interrelated.

Forced breathing involves a number of other muscles that insert into the ribs. During forced inspiration the scalenes and sternocleidomastoid muscles may assist in lifting the ribs. Contraction of the abdominal wall muscles assists respiration. Massage in this area can positively influence effective breathing.

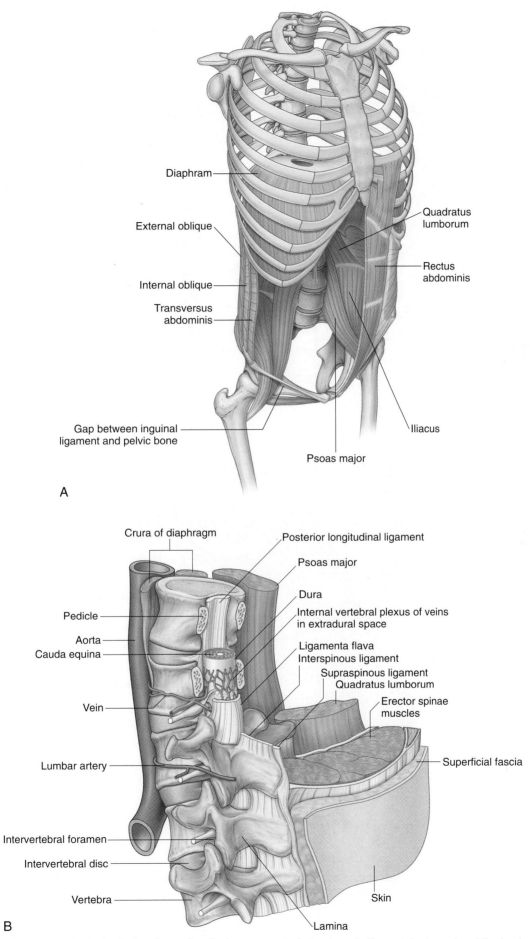

FIGURE 9-18 A, Abdominal wall muscles. **B,** Arrangement of structures in the vertebral canal and the back.

Continued

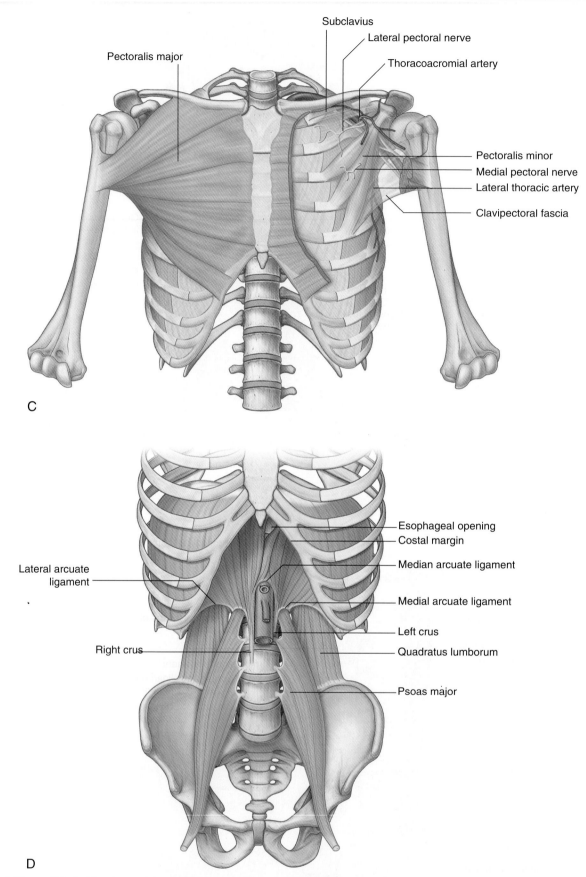

C

Subclavius
Lateral pectoral nerve
Thoracoacromial artery
Pectoralis major
Pectoralis minor
Medial pectoral nerve
Lateral thoracic artery
Clavipectoral fascia

D

Esophageal opening
Costal margin
Median arcuate ligament
Lateral arcuate ligament
Medial arcuate ligament
Left crus
Right crus
Quadratus lumborum
Psoas major

FIGURE 9-18, cont'd C, Muscles and fascia of the pectoral region. **D,** Anterior view of deep muscles. (From Drake RL, Vogl W, Mitchell WM: *Gray's anatomy for students,* ed 2, Edinburgh, 2010, Churchill Livingstone.)

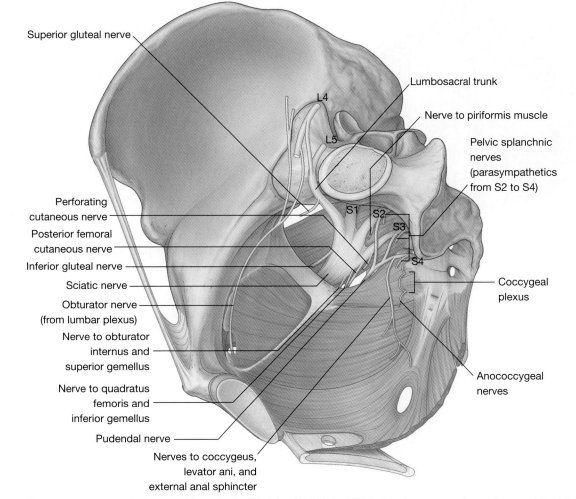

FIGURE 9-19 Sacral and coccygeal plexuses. (From Drake RL, Vogl W, Mitchell WM: *Gray's anatomy for students,* ed 2, Edinburgh, 2010, Churchill Livingstone.)

Muscles of the Thorax and Posterior Abdominal Wall

Diaphragm (DYE-ah-fram)

Diaphragm means "a partition or wall" (between the thoracic and abdominal cavities).

Anterior-Inferior

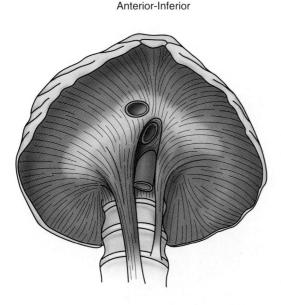

Concentric action:

Inspiration (breathing in); diaphragmatic contractions increase the volume of the thoracic cavity

Eccentric action:

Restrains expiration as the diaphragm relaxes (eccentrically contracts)

Isometric action:

Stabilizes the thoracic and abdominopelvic cavities during breath holding and stabilizes the thoracic and lumbar spine

Origin, proximal attachment, arises from:

First three lumbar vertebrae, the lower six costal cartilages, and the inner surface of the xiphoid process

Insertion, distal attachment, attaches to:

Muscle fibers arch superiorly and inward to end in tendinous fibers, which form the central tendon; the central tendon is a large aponeurosis.

The diaphragm is a broad, thin muscle that spans the thoracoabdominal cavity, separating the thorax from the abdomen. It can be visualized as plastic wrap around the edges of a bowl. The central tendon (the insertion) is not attached to any solid structure; rather, the middle of the plastic wrap becomes a thickened fascial structure. When the muscle component of the diaphragm contracts, it pulls and flattens the central tendon, which increases the volume of the thoracic cavity.

Innervation:

Phrenic nerve (C3 to C5)

Major synergists:

Accessory muscles of inspiration: external intercostal muscles, scalenes, and sternocleidomastoids

Major antagonists:

Accessory muscles of expiration: internal intercostal muscles and anterior and anterolateral muscles of the abdominal wall. The elastic recoil of the soft tissues of the thoracic and abdominal cavities also provides an opposing force. The pelvic floor muscles may act as antagonists as well.

▍*Serratus posterior superior* (suhr-RATE-us)

Serratus means "saw shaped," *posterior* means "behind," and *superior* means "above."

Posterior

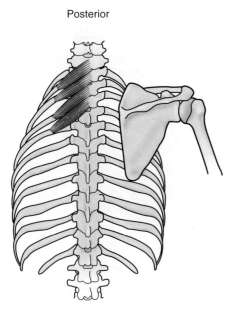

Concentric action:
Elevates ribs 2 to 5 at the sternocostal and costovertebral joints during inspiration

Eccentric action:
Restrains depression of ribs 2 to 5

Isometric action:
Stabilizes the rib cage

Origin, proximal attachment, arises from:
Lower portion of the nuchal ligament and spinous processes of vertebrae C7 to T3

Insertion, distal attachment, attaches to:
Superior borders and external surfaces of the second through fifth ribs, just lateral to their angles
This muscle lies deep to the rhomboid muscles.

Innervation:
Second through fifth intercostal nerves

Major synergists:
Diaphragm and other muscles of inspiration

Major antagonists:
Muscles of expiration, including the serratus posterior inferior

Trigger points:
Deep to the scapula near the insertion of the muscle on the ribs

Referred pain pattern:
Deep to the superior portion of the scapula into the posterior deltoid, elbow, wrist, and ulnar portion of the hand

▍*Serratus posterior inferior* (suhr-RATE-us)

Serratus means "saw shaped," *posterior* means "behind," and *inferior* means "below."

Posterior

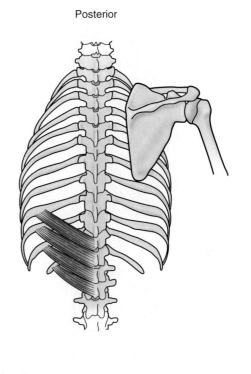

Concentric action:
Depresses ribs 9 to 12 at the sternocostal and costovertebral joints during expiration

Eccentric action:
Restrains elevation of ribs 9 to 12

Isometric action:
Stabilizes the rib cage

Some studies disagree that depression of ribs 9 to 12 for expiration is the function, finding no electromyographic activity of this muscle during respiration. Perhaps the serratus posterior inferior acts as a stabilizer during forced expirations such as coughing, which would be a concentric function.

Origin, proximal attachment, arises from:
Spines of T11, T12, and L1 to L3; supraspinous ligament; and thoracolumbar fascia

Insertion, distal attachment, attaches to:
Inferior borders and outer surfaces of the lower four ribs (9 to 12) just lateral to the angles

Innervation:
Subcostal nerve and intercostal nerves 9 to 11

Major synergists:
Other muscles of expiration

Major antagonists:
Diaphragm and serratus posterior superior

Trigger points:
Belly of the muscle near the eleventh rib

Referred pain pattern:
Nagging ache in the area of the muscle

External intercostal muscles (in-ter-KOS-tal)
(musculi intercostales externi)

Intercostal means "between or among the ribs"; *external* means "on the outside."

Lateral

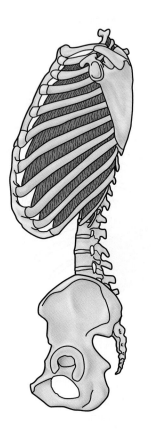

Concentric action:

Elevates the ribs at the sternocostal and costovertebral joints, increasing the volume of the thoracic cavity for inspiration

The external intercostal muscles also may contribute to contralateral rotation of the trunk.

Eccentric action:

Restrains depression of ribs

Isometric action:

Stabilizes the rib cage

Origin, proximal attachment, arises from:

Eleven total, each arising from the inferior border of a rib

Insertion, distal attachment, attaches to:

Superior border of the inferior rib

Innervation:

Adjacent intercostal nerves

Major synergists:

Diaphragm and other muscles of inspiration

Major antagonists:

Muscles of expiration

Trigger points:

The external intercostal muscles can develop trigger points, which can be located by palpating the muscles between the ribs.

Referred pain pattern:

Spans the intercostal segment, especially noticeable with deep breathing or rotational movement

---

Internal intercostal muscles (in-ter-KOS-tal)
(musculi intercostales interni)

Intercostal means "between or among the ribs"; *internal* means "on the inside."

Lateral

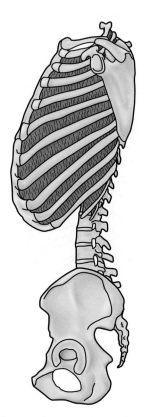

Concentric action:

Depresses the ribs at the sternocostal and costovertebral joints, decreasing the volume of the thoracic cavity for expiration

The internal intercostal muscles also may contribute to ipsilateral rotation of the trunk.

Eccentric action:

Restrains elevation of ribs

Isometric action:

Stabilizes the rib cage

Origin, proximal attachment, arises from:

Eleven total, each arising from the ridge of the inner surface of a rib and corresponding costal cartilage

Insertion, distal attachment, attaches to:

Inferior border of the superior rib

Innervation:

Adjacent intercostal nerves

Major synergists:

Muscles of expiration

Major antagonists:

Diaphragm and other muscles of inspiration

Trigger points:

The internal intercostal muscles can develop trigger points, which can be located by palpating the muscles between the ribs.

Referred pain pattern:

Spans the intercostal segment, especially noticeable with deep breathing or rotational movement

Innermost intercostal muscles (in-ter-KOS-tal) (musculi intercostales intimi)

Intercostal means "between or among the ribs."

The muscles of this small group attach to the internal aspects of two adjoining ribs. They are believed to act with the internal intercostal muscles.

Lateral

Transversus thoracis (trans-VER-sus thor-AH-siss)

Transversus means "lying crosswise," and *thoracis* means "related to the chest."

Posterior

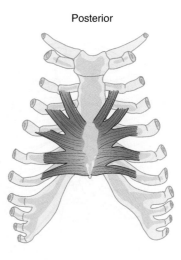

Concentric action:

Depresses ribs 2 to 6 at the sternocostal and costovertebral joints

Eccentric action:

Restrains elevation of ribs 2 to 6

Isometric action:

Stabilizes the rib cage

Origin, proximal attachment, arises from:

Inner surface of the body of the sternum (caudal one third), xiphoid process, and sternal ends of the costal cartilages of ribs 4 to 7

Insertion, distal attachment, attaches to:

Costal cartilages of the second through sixth ribs

Innervation:

Adjacent intercostal nerves

This muscle is on the inside of the rib cage.

Major synergists:

Muscles of expiration

Major antagonists:

Diaphragm and other muscles of inspiration

Trigger points:

Because of its location, this muscle is difficult to palpate for trigger points.

Referred pain pattern:

Spans the intercostal segment, especially noticeable with deep breathing or rotational movement

Quadratus lumborum (kwad-RATE-us lum-BOR-um)

Quadratus means "square shaped," and *lumborum* means "of the loins."

Anterior

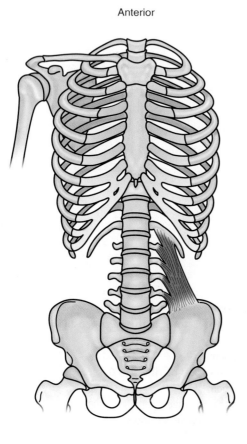

Concentric action:

Elevation and anterior tilt of the pelvis at the lumbosacral joint, lateral flexion and extension of the trunk at the spinal joints, and depression of the twelfth rib at the costovertebral joints

Eccentric action:

Allows depression and posterior tilt of the pelvis and allows contralateral lateral flexion and flexion of the trunk and elevation of the twelfth rib

Isometric action:

Assists normal inspiration by stabilizing the twelfth rib against the pull of the diaphragm and also stabilizes the lumbar spine and pelvis

Origin, proximal attachment, arises from:

Iliolumbar ligament and posterior portion of the iliac crest

Insertion, distal attachment, attaches to:

Inferior border of the last rib and transverse processes of the first four lumbar vertebrae

Innervation:

Ventral rami of the twelfth thoracic and upper three lumbar spinal nerves

Major synergists:

Erector spinae group

The quadratus lumborum also functions with the gluteus medius, fascia lata, and adductors to stabilize the body in the frontal plane.

Major antagonists:

Posterior fibers of gluteus medius and the anterior and contralateral anterolateral abdominal wall muscles

Trigger points:

Laterally near the rib or iliac attachment and medially near the iliac attachment at the transverse processes of the lumbar vertebra

Referred pain pattern:

Gluteal and groin area, sacroiliac joint, and greater trochanter; these points are implicated in most low back pain. The dual function of lumbar stabilization (isometric function) and respiration (concentric function) can cause severe pain in the low back with a cough or sneeze if these trigger points are active. Low back pain often is related more to maintenance of posture than to trigger point activity; therefore finding corresponding pain patterns in the muscles that laterally flex the head and neck, such as the scalenes, is common.

Psoas major (SO-as)

Psoas means "of the loins"; *major* means "larger."

Anterior

Concentric action:

Flexion and lateral rotation of the thigh at the hip joint, flexion and lateral flexion of the trunk at the spinal joints, and anterior tilt of the pelvis at the hip joint

Eccentric action:

Allows extension and medial rotation of the thigh and allows extension and contralateral lateral flexion of the trunk and posterior tilt of the pelvis

Isometric action:

Stabilizes the lumbar spine and the lumbosacral and hip joints

Origin, proximal attachment, arises from:

Bodies and corresponding intervertebral disks of last thoracic and all lumbar vertebrae, anterior surface of transverse processes of all lumbar vertebrae, and tendinous arches extending across the sides of the bodies of the lumbar vertebrae

Insertion, distal attachment, attaches to:

Lesser trochanter of the femur

Innervation:

Ventral rami of lumbar plexus nerves (L1 to L3)

Major synergists:

Iliacus, sartorius, rectus femoris, and anterior and anterolateral abdominal wall muscles

Major antagonists:

Extensors of the thigh, extensors of the trunk, and posterior tilters of the pelvis

Trigger points:

Near both attachment points

Referred pain pattern:

Entire lumbar area into the superior gluteal region and to the anterior thigh; may be associated with menstrual aching and can mimic appendicitis. Shortening of this muscle is a major cause of low back pain and often occurs during the isometric stabilization function. If tension or trigger point activity is located at the distal attachment, pain can mimic a groin pull. Because of postural reflexes, muscles that flex the head and neck are facilitated with psoas major activation. A common correlation exists between neck pain and stiffness to psoas major pain and low back stiffness. The massage therapist often must address both areas in sequence to be effective.

The psoas major and psoas minor are located on the anterior spine posterior to the abdominal muscles and viscera.

Psoas minor (SO-as)

Psoas means "of the loins"; *minor* means "smaller."

Anterior

Iliacus (ILL-ee-AK-us)

Iliacus means "of the hip."

Anterior

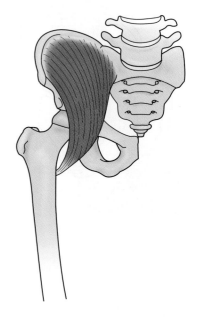

Concentric action:
Flexion of the trunk at the spinal joints and posterior tilt of the pelvis at the lumbosacral joint

Eccentric action:
Restrains extension of the trunk and anterior tilt of the pelvis
This muscle is absent in approximately half of all human beings.

Origin, proximal attachment, arises from:
Sides of the bodies of the twelfth thoracic and first lumbar vertebrae and from the intervertebral disk between them

Insertion, distal attachment, attaches to:
Pectineal line of the pubis and the iliopectineal eminence of the ilium and pubis

Innervation:
Branch from L1 spinal nerve
The psoas major and psoas minor are located on the anterior spine posterior to the abdominal muscles and viscera.

Major synergists:
Anterior and anterolateral abdominal wall muscles

Major antagonists:
Erector spinae group

Trigger points:
Belly of the muscle

Referred pain pattern:
Lumbar

Concentric action:
Flexion and lateral rotation of the thigh at the hip joint and anterior tilt of the pelvis at the lumbosacral joint

Eccentric action:
Allows extension and medial rotation of the thigh and allows posterior tilt of the pelvis

Isometric action:
Stabilizes the pelvis and the hip joint

Origin, proximal attachment, arises from:
Internal lip of the iliac crest; anterior sacroiliac, lumbosacral, and iliolumbar ligaments; superior two thirds of the iliac fossa; and ala of the sacrum

Insertion, distal attachment, attaches to:
Lesser trochanter of the femur, into the posterior side of the psoas major tendon

Innervation:
Femoral nerve (L2 to L3)

Major synergist:
Psoas major

Major antagonists:
Gluteus maximus and hamstrings

Trigger points:
Inner border of the ilium posterior to the anterior superior iliac spine

Referred pain pattern:
Hip and groin

✏ ACTIVITY **9-18**

Draw and color the **muscles of the thorax and posterior abdominal wall** in the spaces provided. For each muscle, do the following:

1. Label the origin and insertion attachment points: *O* for origin; *I* for insertion.

2. Place an X on the trigger points.
3. Palpate this muscle; identify the attachment points and the bellies of the muscles.
4. Move these muscles on yourself.

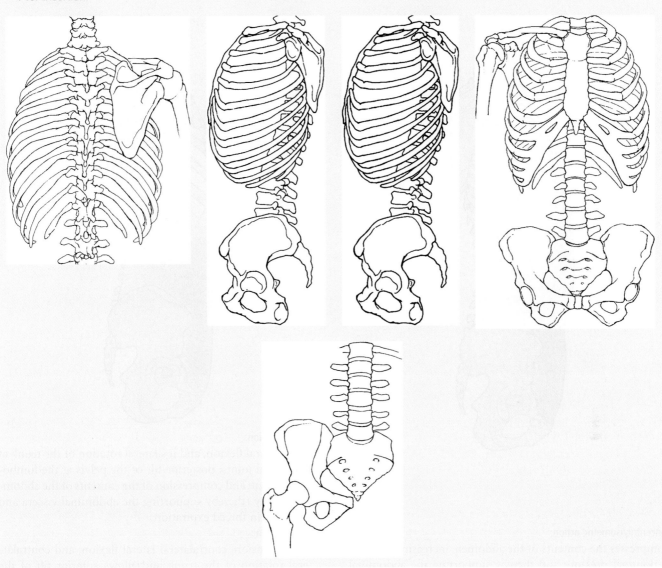

Muscles of the Anterior and Anterolateral Abdominal Wall

The abdominal muscles and extensive fascia form the anterior and anterolateral abdominal wall. The muscle fiber arrangement produces a crisscross fiber pattern similar to plywood, with vertical support provided by the rectus abdominis and the pyramidalis. These muscles attach directly or indirectly to a strong, fibrous cord in the midline of the abdomen called the *linea alba,* which is formed from the fusion of the two anterior abdominal aponeuroses (each abdominal aponeurosis is formed from the fusion of the aponeuroses of the external abdominal oblique and the transversus abdominis). The linea alba extends from the xiphoid process to the symphysis pubis and contains the umbilicus.

As a group, these muscles act to compress the abdominal contents during expiration, urination, and defecation. They help maintain pressure on the curve of the low back, resisting excessive lumbar lordosis. Isometric stabilization is an important function of this group. Along with the deep muscles of the back, the abdominal muscles provide stability for the entire trunk of the body. The muscles also work with the adductors of the thighs at the hip joint to maintain upright posture. Massage application to this area is important because the muscles are involved in posture and breathing. The fascial aponeuroses may shorten, and the muscles are frequently weak and long. Methods to encourage normal muscle tone are effective. These exercises are usually called *core training.*

Transversus abdominis (trans-VER-sus ab-DAHM-in-iss)

Transversus means "lying crosswise," and *abdominis* means "of the abdomen."

The transversus abdominis is the innermost layer of the abdominal wall just superficial to the peritoneum.

Lateral

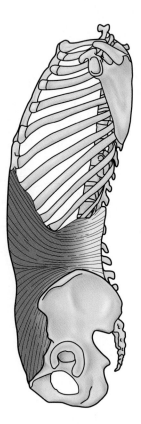

Internal obliques (ab-DAHM-in-al oh-BLEEK) (obliquus internus abdominis)

The internal oblique muscle is located within the anterolateral abdominal wall, deep to the external abdominal oblique and superficial to the transversus abdominis. The muscle is positioned at a slant.

Lateral

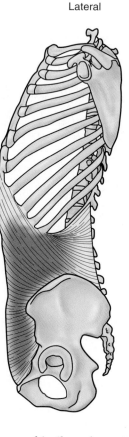

Concentric action:

Flexion, lateral flexion, and ipsilateral rotation of the trunk at the spinal joints; posterior tilt of the pelvis at the lumbosacral joint; and compression of the contents of the abdominal cavity (thereby supporting the abdominal viscera and assisting in forced expiration)

Eccentric action:

Allows extension, contralateral lateral flexion, and contralateral rotation of the trunk and allows anterior tilt of the pelvis

Origin, proximal attachment, arises from:

Inguinal ligament, iliac fascia, anterior two thirds of the middle lip of the iliac crest, and lumbar fascia

Insertion, distal attachment, attaches to:

Upper fibers into cartilages of last three ribs; the remainder into the aponeurosis extending from the tenth costal cartilage to the pubic bone into the linea alba

Innervation:

Ventral rami of the lower six thoracic and first lumbar spinal nerves

Major synergists:

Opposite-sided external abdominal oblique and the rectus abdominis

Major antagonists:

Extensors of the spine and opposite-sided internal abdominal oblique

Concentric/isometric action:

Compresses the contents of the abdomen, increasing intraabdominal pressure and thereby supporting the abdominal viscera and assisting in forced expiration

Origin, proximal attachment, arises from:

Inner surfaces of the cartilages of the last six ribs, anterior three fourths of the iliac crest, lateral one third of the inguinal ligament, and thoracolumbar fascia

Insertion, distal attachment, attaches to:

Linea alba, abdominal aponeurosis, and pubis

Innervation:

Ventral rami of the lower six thoracic and first lumbar spinal nerves

Major synergists:

Rectus abdominis and external and internal abdominal obliques

Major antagonists:

Not clearly defined

External oblique (ab-DAHM-in-al oh-BLEEK)
(obliquus externus abdominis)

This muscle is located within the abdominal wall, superficial to the internal abdominal oblique; its fibers are slanted like pockets of a coat.

Lateral

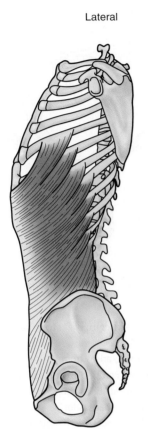

Rectus abdominis (REK-tus ab-DAHM-in-iss)

Rectus means "straight," and *abdominis* means "of the abdomen."

Anterior

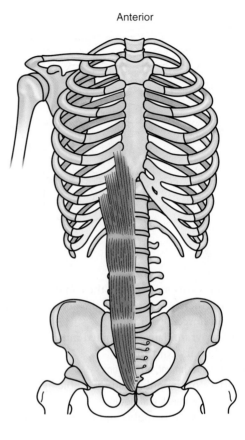

Concentric action:
Flexion, lateral flexion, and contralateral rotation of the trunk at the spinal joints; posterior tilt of the pelvis at the lumbosacral joint; and compression of the contents of the abdominal cavity (thereby supporting the abdominal viscera and assisting in forced expiration)
Eccentric action:
Allows extension, contralateral lateral flexion, and ipsilateral rotation of the trunk and allows anterior tilt of the pelvis
Origin, proximal attachment, arises from:
Outer lip of the iliac crest, pubic bone, and linea alba
Insertion, distal attachment, attaches to:
External surface of the lower eight ribs by interdigital slips
Innervation:
Ventral rami of the lower six thoracic spinal nerves
Major synergists:
Opposite-sided internal abdominal oblique and the rectus abdominis
Major antagonists:
Extensors of the spine and opposite-sided external abdominal oblique

Concentric action:
Flexion and lateral flexion of the trunk at the spinal joints, posterior tilt of the pelvis at the lumbosacral joint, and compression of the contents of the abdominal cavity (thereby supporting the abdominal viscera and assisting in forced expiration)
Eccentric action:
Allows extension and contralateral lateral flexion of the trunk and allows anterior tilt of the pelvis
Origin, proximal attachment, arises from:
Pubis and the pubic symphysis
Insertion, distal attachment, attaches to:
Cartilages of the fifth, sixth, and seventh ribs and the xiphoid process of the sternum
Major synergists:
External and internal abdominal obliques
Major antagonists:
Extensors of the spine
Innervation:
Anterior primary rami of the lower six intercostal nerves

Pyramidalis (peer-AM-id-al-iss)

Pyramidalis means "pyramid shaped."

Anterior

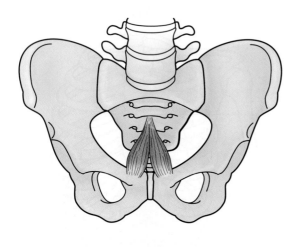

Action:

Tenses the linea alba to compress the contents of the abdominal cavity (thereby supporting the abdominal viscera and assisting in forced expiration)

Although the pyramidalis is a striated muscle, it usually is not under voluntary control.

Origin, proximal attachment, arises from:

Ventral surface of the pubis and the pubic ligament

Insertion, distal attachment, attaches to:

Linea alba (between the pubis and the umbilicus)

Innervation:

Subcostal nerve (ventral ramus of T12)

Cremaster (KREE-mast-er)

Cremaster means a "suspender."

Anterior/Superior

Action:

Pulls the testes superiorly (to help regulate their temperature)

Origin, proximal attachment, arises from:

Lower edge of the internal oblique muscle and the middle aspect of the inguinal ligament

Insertion, distal attachment, attaches to:

Pubic tubercle and the crest of the pubis

Innervation:

Genital branch of the genitofemoral nerve (L1 to L2)

Synergists:

Quadratus lumborum and diaphragm; rotation—lower serratus anterior and posterior, latissimus dorsi, iliocostalis

Antagonists:

Flexion—paraspinal extensor group; rotation—contralateral muscles

Trigger points:

Located throughout the area but concentrated more in the external circle of the abdominal wall, rather than toward the middle near the umbilicus; the exceptions are points often found in the rectus abdominis just below the umbilicus on either side of the linea alba.

Referred pain pattern:

Pain likely to appear in the same quadrant and in the back; these trigger points are capable of causing somatovisceral responses (e.g., vomiting, nausea, intestinal problems, diarrhea, bladder symptoms, pain).

ACTIVITY **9-19**

Draw and color the **muscles of the anterior and anterolateral abdominal wall** in the spaces provided. For each muscle, do the following:

1. Label the origin and insertion attachment points: *O* for origin; *I* for insertion.

2. Place an X on the trigger points.
3. Palpate this muscle; identify the attachment points and the bellies of the muscles.
4. Move these muscles on yourself.

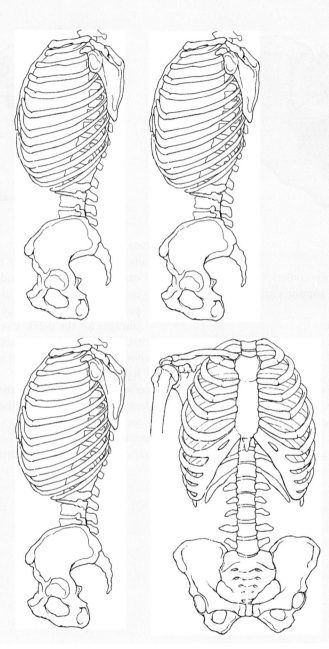

Pelvic and Perineal Muscles

The levator ani and the coccygeus muscles form the pelvic floor (also called the *pelvic diaphragm*) (see Figure 9-19). These muscles close the inferior outlet of the pelvis; support and elevate the pelvic floor; and counterbalance increased intraabdominal pressure, which would expel the contents of

the bladder, rectum, and uterus. The pelvic diaphragm has openings for the rectum, urethra, and vagina. The massage therapist usually does not massage this area with direct methods; however, attention to antagonistic and synergistic muscles that are accessed more easily is indicated. Isometric stabilization is a major function of these muscles.

Levator ani (le-VAY-tor AIN-eye)

Levator means "one that raises"; *ani* means "belonging to the anus or rectum."

Superior

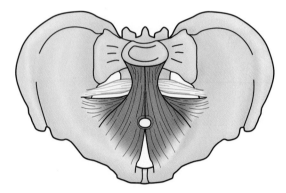

Action:

Forms the floor of the pelvic cavity, constricts the lower end of the rectum and vagina, and supports and slightly raises the pelvic floor

Origin, proximal attachment, arises from:

Pelvic surfaces of the pubis, inner surface of the ischial spine, and the obturator fascia

Insertion, distal attachment, attaches to:

Last two segments of the coccyx, anococcygeal raphe uniting with fibers from the opposite side, and the sides of the rectum anterior into the perineal body

Innervation:

Muscular branches of the perineal division of the pudendal nerve

Coccygeus (kok-SIH-jee-us)

Coccygeus means "related to the coccyx or tail bone."

Superior

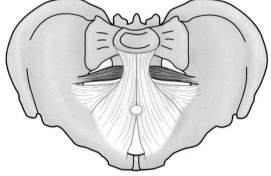

Action:

Pulls forward and supports the coccyx; exerts rotary tension on the sacroiliac joint; and with the levator ani and piriformis muscles, assists in closing the posterior part of the pelvic outlet and forms the supporting muscular diaphragm for the pelvic viscera

Origin, proximal attachment, arises from:

Pelvic surface of the spine of the ischium and the sacrospinous ligament

Insertion, distal attachment, attaches to:

Margin of the coccyx and the side of the fifth segment of the sacrum

Innervation:

Branch of the fourth and fifth sacral nerves

External anal sphincter (SFINK-tur AIN-eye)
(sphincter ani externus)

External means "on the outside," *sphincter* means "band," and *ani* means "related to the anus or rectum."

Inferior

Action:
Closes the anal orifice
Origin, proximal attachment, arises from:
Superficial fibers from the anococcygeal raphe; deeper fibers surround the anal canal
Insertion, distal attachment, attaches to:
Superficial fibers surround the anus, meeting posteriorly at the coccyx and anteriorly at the central point of the perineum.
Innervation:
Perineal branch of the fourth sacral nerve and the inferior rectal branch of the pudendal nerve

Deep transverse perineals (pair-i-NEE-als)
(transversus perinei)

Transverse means "crossing" or "around"; *perineal* means "to empty or defecate."

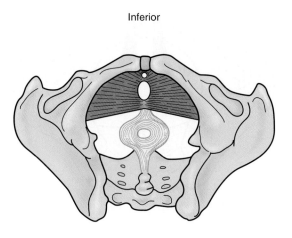

Inferior

Action:
Simultaneous contraction of both muscles helps to fix the perineal body.
Origin, proximal attachment, arises from:
Medial and anterior part of the ischial tuberosity
Insertion, distal attachment, attaches to:
Central tendinous point of the perineum
Innervation:
Perineal branches of the pudendal nerve

Ischiocavernosus (ISS-she-oh-KAV-ern-oh-sus)

Ischiocavernosus means "hip" and "cavernlike."

Inferior

Action:

Compresses the crus penis, which obstructs venous return and therefore is believed to play a part in maintaining erection of the penis or clitoris

Origin, proximal attachment, arises from:

Inner surface of the ischial tuberosity behind the crus penis or clitoris and the ramus of the ischium on both sides of the crus

Insertion, distal attachment, attaches to:

Aponeuroses on the sides and undersurface of the crus penis or clitoris

Innervation:

Perineal branch of the pudendal nerve (S2 to S4)

Bulbospongiosus (BUL-bo-SPON-jee-oh-sus)

Bulbospongiosus means "bulb" and "spongy."

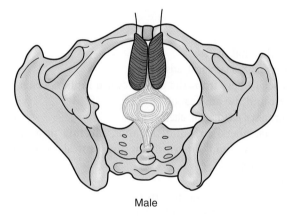

Inferior

Female

Male

Action:

Aids in emptying the urethra; the muscle is relaxed during the greater part of micturition, coming into action only at the end of the process, and can be used to assist urination; it constricts the orifice of the vagina and contributes to erection of the penis and clitoris.

Origin, proximal attachment, arises from:

Central tendinous point of the perineum, with fibers surrounding the vaginal orifice and vestibular bulbs (female)

Insertion, distal attachment, attaches to:

Lower surface of the perineal membrane, dorsal surface of the corpus spongiosum, deep fascia on the dorsum of the penis, and corpora cavernosa clitoris (female)

Innervation:

Perineal branch of the pudendal nerve (S2 to S4)

The following elements are common to the pelvic and perineal muscles:

Synergists:

All muscles are synergistic; the gluteus maximus supports the closure of the anus.

Antagonists:

No direct antagonist pattern to the pelvic floor has been identified in the literature; however, because the gluteus

ACTIVITY **9-20**

Draw and color the **pelvic and perineal muscles** in the spaces provided. For each muscle, do the following:
1. Label the origin and insertion attachment points: *O* for origin; *I* for insertion.
2. Move these muscles on yourself.

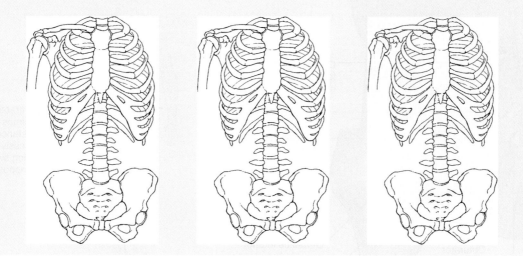

maximus is powerfully synergistic with these muscles, one could assume that antagonist patterns to the gluteus maximus, such as the psoas, would have an antagonistic influence on the pelvic floor muscles. The diaphragm muscle also may act as an antagonist to this muscle group.

Trigger points:
Trigger points do develop in these muscles; These trigger points usually can be palpated internally, rectally, or vaginally.

Referred pain patterns:
To the pelvic floor itself and to the coccyx region

Muscles of the Gluteal Region

The muscles of the gluteal region are some of the most powerful muscles of the body. The more superficial muscles, especially the large gluteus maximus, extend the thigh during forceful extension. The gluteus maximus also stabilizes the iliotibial band and thoracolumbar fascia. The gluteus medius and gluteus minimus are especially strong at abduction and medial (internal) rotation of the thigh. The deep lateral (external) rotators of the thigh at the hip joint are six small, deep muscles of the gluteal region that oppose medial rotation. As a group, the gluteal muscles are related to shoulder extensors and flexors and arm medial and lateral rotators because of gait (walking) reflex patterns to promote the appropriate counterbalancing arm swing. Facilitation between muscles of the arms that flex and extend along with thigh muscles in contralateral patterns occurs. The massage therapist usually needs to consider the muscles of the shoulder joint with muscles of the hip joint and apply massage in a correlated pattern. Although not listed with synergists and antagonists, the flexors of the thigh at the hip joint work with flexors of the arm at the shoulder joint on the opposite side (i.e., right with left and left with right). These muscles also display inhibitory patterns with each other. For example, right extensors of the thigh at the hip joint are inhibitory to left flexors of the arm at the shoulder joint. On the same side (right arm with right thigh, left arm with left thigh), flexors and extensors work with each other. Adductors and medial rotators of the shoulder joint work with adductors and medial rotators of the hip joint on the opposite side. This same concept is true for abductors and lateral rotators. Conversely, same-side adductors of the shoulder and hip are inhibitory to each other, as are same-side abductors and lateral rotators. Although these patterns may seem confusing, the connection becomes apparent if you take a step and analyze the patterns of the muscles that are working together (Figure 9-20).

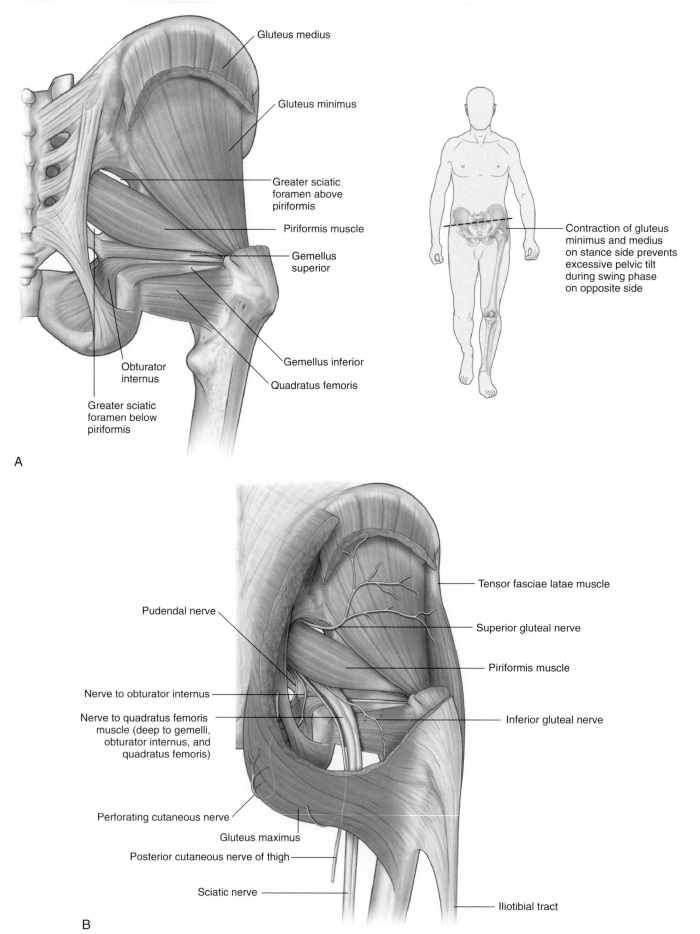

A

B

FIGURE 9-20 A, Deep muscles in the gluteal region. **B,** Nerves of the gluteal region. Posterior view. (From Drake RL, Vogl W, Mitchell WM: *Gray's anatomy for students,* ed 2, Edinburgh, 2010, Churchill Livingstone.)

▌*Gluteus maximus* (GLUE-tee-us MAX-uh-mus)

Gluteus means "buttocks"; *maximus* means "greatest or largest."

Posterior

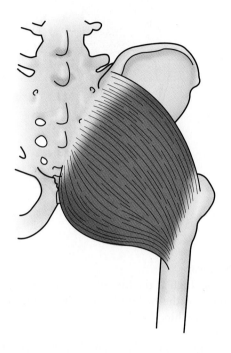

Concentric action:

Extends and laterally rotates the thigh at the hip joint—the upper fibers abduct the thigh at the hip joint, and the lower fibers adduct the thigh at the hip joint—and provides posterior tilt of the pelvis at the hip joint (The gluteus maximus is active primarily during strenuous activity, such as running, jumping, and climbing stairs.)

Eccentric action:

Restrains flexion and medial rotation of the thigh and anterior tilt of the pelvis (The upper fibers restrain adduction of the thigh, and the lower fibers restrain abduction of the thigh.)

Isometric action:

These muscles are important postural muscles that help maintain the upright posture, stabilize the pelvis, and provide tension to the iliotibial band to keep the fascial band taut.

Origin, proximal attachment, arises from:

Posterior gluteal line of the ilium, dorsal surface of the lower aspect of the sacrum and the side of the coccyx, sacrotuberous ligament and gluteal aponeurosis, and aponeurosis of the erector spinae

Insertion, distal attachment, attaches to:

Iliotibial band of the fascia lata and gluteal tuberosity of the femur

Innervation:

Inferior gluteal nerve (L5 to S2)

Major synergists:

Hamstring muscles and piriformis

Major antagonists:

Iliopsoas, tensor fasciae latae, and gluteus medius (anterior fibers)

Trigger points:

Three main areas—near the sacrum at the musculotendinous junction midway down from the iliac crest, near the ischial tuberosity, and in the belly of the muscle closer to the lower fibers

Referred pain pattern:

Regionally into the gluteal area, especially to the ischial tuberosity, the tip of the greater trochanter, and the sacrum. A shortened and tight gluteus maximus can be responsible for tightness of the iliotibial band and thoracolumbar fascia. These superficial muscles are thick and require firm massage application to be effective. The smaller deeper muscle layers have to be accessed by pressure that penetrates through the gluteus maximus. Positioning the client so that this muscle is in a passive contraction by propping the client such that the attachments of the muscle are closer together is helpful. If no active contraction is taking place, the area becomes softer and it is easier for compressive forces of massage to reach the underlying muscle layers.

Gluteus medius (GLUE-tee-us MEED-ee-us)

Gluteus means "buttocks"; *medius* means "middle."

Lateral

Gluteus minimus (GLUE-tee-us MIN-ih-mus)

Gluteus means "buttocks"; *minimus* means "smallest."

Lateral

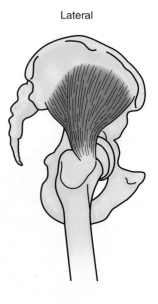

Concentric action:
Abducts the thigh at the hip joint. Anterior fibers medially rotate and flex the thigh at the hip joint and allow anterior tilt of the pelvis at the hip joint; posterior fibers laterally rotate and extend the thigh at the hip joint and allow posterior tilt of the pelvis at the hip joint.

Eccentric action:
Restrains adduction of the thigh. The anterior fibers restrain extension and lateral rotation of the thigh and posterior tilt of the pelvis; the posterior fibers restrain flexion and medial rotation of the thigh and anterior tilt of the pelvis.

Isometric action:
Stabilizes the pelvis (especially when a person is standing on one foot)

Origin, proximal attachment, arises from:
External surface of the ilium inferior to the iliac crest, between the anterior and posterior gluteal lines, and the gluteal aponeurosis

Insertion, distal attachment, attaches to:
Lateral surface of the greater trochanter of the femur

Innervation:
Superior gluteal nerve (L4 to S1)

Major synergists:
Gluteus minimus, tensor fasciae latae, and piriformis

Major antagonists:
The adductors of the thigh

Trigger points:
Along the musculotendinous junction at the iliac crest

Referred pain pattern:
Low back, posterior crest of the ilium to the sacrum, and to the posterior and lateral areas of the buttock into the upper thigh

Concentric action:
Abducts the thigh at the hip joint, medially rotates and flexes the thigh at the hip joint, and allows anterior tilt of the pelvis at the hip joint

Eccentric action:
Restrains adduction of the thigh. The anterior fibers restrain extension and lateral rotation of the thigh and posterior tilt of the pelvis.

Isometric action:
Stabilizes the pelvis (especially when a person is standing on one foot)

Origin, proximal attachment, arises from:
External surface of the ilium inferior to the iliac crest, between the anterior and inferior gluteal lines

Insertion, distal attachment, attaches to:
Anterior border of the greater trochanter of the femur

Innervation:
Superior gluteal nerve (L4 to S1)

Major synergist:
Gluteus medius

Major antagonists:
Adductors of the thigh

Trigger points:
Belly of the muscle

Referred pain pattern:
Lower lateral buttock and down the lateral to posterior aspect of the thigh, knee, and leg to the ankle

Tensor fasciae latae (TEN-sore FAH-she-a LAT-uh)

Tensor means "one that stretches," *fasciae* means "bands or bandages," and *latae* means "wide."

Anterior

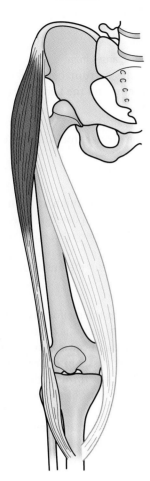

Concentric action:

Flexion, medial rotation, and abduction of the thigh at the hip joint; anterior tilt of the pelvis at the hip joint; and extension of the leg at the knee joint

Eccentric action:

Restrains extension, lateral rotation, and adduction of the thigh and allows posterior tilt of the pelvis and flexion of the leg

Isometric action:

Tenses the iliotibial band, counterbalancing the backward pull of the gluteus maximus on the iliotibial band, and stabilizes the pelvis and the knee

Origin, proximal attachment, arises from:

Anterior aspect of the outer lip of the iliac crest and outer surface of the anterior superior iliac spine

Insertion, distal attachment, attaches to:

Iliotibial band, one third of the way down the thigh

Innervation:

Superior gluteal nerve (L4 to S1)

Major synergists:

Gluteus medius (anterior fibers) and iliopsoas

Major antagonists:

Gluteus medius (posterior fibers), adductors of the thigh group, gluteus maximus, and hamstrings

Trigger points:

In the belly of the muscle and near the distal attachment

Referred pain pattern:

Localized in the hip and down the lateral side of the thigh to the knee

ACTIVITY 9-21

Draw and color the **gluteal muscles and tensor fasciae latae** in the spaces provided. For each muscle, do the following:

1. Label the origin and insertion attachment points: *O* for origin; *I* for insertion.
2. Place an X on the trigger points.
3. Palpate this muscle; identify the attachment points and the bellies of the muscles.
4. Move these muscles on yourself.

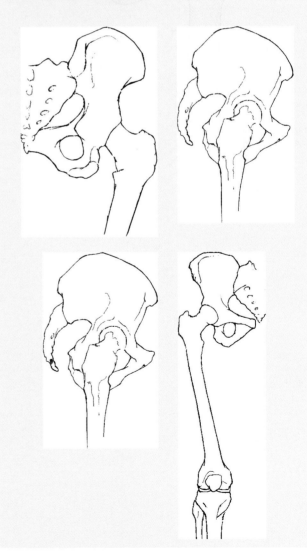

Deep Lateral Rotators of the Thigh at the Hip Joint

▎*Piriformis* (PEER-ih-FOR-miss)

Piriformis means "pear shaped."

Posterior

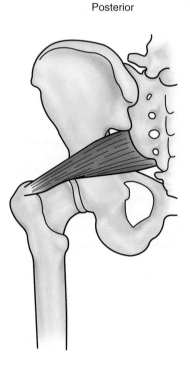

Concentric action:

Lateral rotation of the thigh at the hip joint and abduction and medial rotation of the thigh at the hip joint if the thigh is first in a position of flexion at the hip joint

Eccentric action:

Restrains medial rotation of the thigh and also may restrain adduction and lateral rotation of the thigh (if the thigh is in a position of flexion)

Isometric action:

Stabilizes the hip joint

Origin, proximal attachment, arises from:

Anterior surface of the sacrum between the first through fourth sacral foramina and the pelvic surface of the sacrotuberous ligament

Insertion, distal attachment, attaches to:

Superior border of the greater trochanter of the femur

Innervation:

Lumbosacral plexus (L5 to S2)

Major synergists:

All deep lateral rotators of the thigh at the hip joint are synergistic with one another; posterior fibers of the gluteus medius are also major synergists.

Major antagonists:

Anterior fibers of the gluteus medius, gluteus minimus, and the tensor fasciae latae

Trigger points:

The main trigger points in the piriformis muscle are near the attachments. The belly may have trigger points as well. Tension in this muscle can cause entrapment of the sciatic nerve, which normally passes inferior to the piriformis but in some individuals passes through the muscle, predisposing the person to symptoms of sciatica.

Referred pain pattern:

Sacroiliac region, entire buttock, and down the posterior thigh to just proximal to the knee

Obturator internus (OB-tur-ATE-or in-TER-nus)

Obturator means "one that covers an opening"; *internus* means "interior."

Posterior

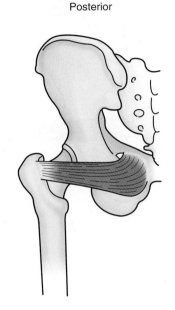

Concentric action:

Lateral rotation of the thigh at the hip joint and abduction of the thigh at the hip joint if the thigh is first in a position of flexion at the hip joint

Eccentric action:

Restrains medial rotation of the thigh and also may restrain adduction of the thigh (if the thigh is in a position of flexion)

Isometric action:

Stabilizes the hip joint

Origin, proximal attachment, arises from:

Internal surface of the obturator membrane and the margins of the obturator foramen (on the ilium, ischium, and pubis)

Insertion, distal attachment, attaches to:

Medial surface of the greater trochanter of the femur

Innervation:

Nerve to obturator internus from the lumbosacral plexus (L5 to S1)

Major synergists:

All deep lateral rotators of the thigh at the hip joint are synergistic with one another; posterior fibers of the gluteus medius are also major synergists.

Major antagonists:

Anterior fibers of the gluteus medius, gluteus minimus, and the tensor fasciae latae

Trigger points:

The belly of the muscle

Referred pain pattern:

Sacroiliac region, entire buttock, and down the posterior thigh to just proximal to the knee joint

Obturator externus (OB-tur-ATE-or ex-STIR-nus)

Obturator means "one that covers an opening"; *externus* means "exterior."

Anterior

Concentric action:

Lateral rotation of the thigh at the hip joint

Eccentric action:

Restrains medial rotation of the thigh

Isometric action:

Stabilizes the hip joint

Origin, proximal attachment, arises from:

External surface of the obturator membrane and the margins of the obturator foramen (on the ischium and pubis)

Insertion, distal attachment, attaches to:

Trochanteric fossa of the femur

Innervation:

Obturator nerve (L3 to L4)

Major synergists:

All deep lateral rotators of the thigh at the hip joint are synergistic with one another; posterior fibers of the gluteus medius are also major synergists.

Major antagonists:

Anterior fibers of the gluteus medius, gluteus minimus, and the tensor fasciae latae

Trigger points:

The belly of the muscle

Referred pain pattern:

Sacroiliac region, entire buttock, and down the posterior thigh to just proximal to the knee joint

Quadratus femoris (kwad-RATE-us FEM-or-iss)

Quadratus means "square shaped"; *femoris* means "related to the thigh."

Posterior

Gemellus superior (JEM-ell-us)

Gemellus means "twin"; *superior* means "above."

Posterior

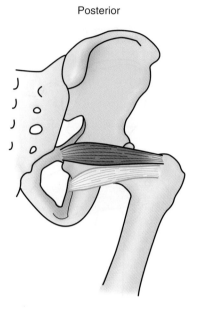

Concentric action:
Lateral rotation and adduction of the thigh at the hip joint (if the thigh is in a position of flexion)
Eccentric action:
Restrains medial rotation of the thigh and also may restrain abduction of the thigh
Isometric action:
Stabilizes the hip joint
Origin, proximal attachment, arises from:
Lateral border of the ischial tuberosity
Insertion, distal attachment, attaches to:
Small tubercle on the upper part of the intertrochanteric crest of the femur
Innervation:
Nerve to quadratus femoris from the lumbosacral plexus (L5 and S1)
Major synergists:
All deep lateral rotators of the thigh at the hip joint are synergistic with one another; posterior fibers of the gluteus medius are also synergistic.
Major antagonists:
Anterior fibers of the gluteus medius, gluteus minimus, and the tensor fasciae latae
Trigger points:
The belly of the muscle
Referred pain pattern:
Sacroiliac region, entire buttock, and down the posterior thigh to just proximal to the knee joint

Concentric action:
Lateral rotation of the thigh at the hip joint and abduction of the thigh at the hip joint if the thigh is first in a position of flexion at the hip joint
Eccentric action:
Restrains medial rotation of the thigh and also may restrain adduction of the thigh (if the thigh is in a position of flexion)
Isometric action:
Stabilizes the hip joint
Origin, proximal attachment, arises from:
Dorsal surface of the ischial spine
Insertion, distal attachment, attaches to:
Medial surface of the greater trochanter of the femur
Innervation:
Nerve to obturator internus (L5 to S1)
Major synergists:
All deep lateral rotators of the thigh at the hip joint are synergistic with one another; posterior fibers of the gluteus medius are also synergistic.
Major antagonists:
Anterior fibers of the gluteus medius, gluteus minimus, and the tensor fasciae latae
Trigger points:
The belly of the muscle
Referred pain pattern:
Sacroiliac region, entire buttock, and down the posterior thigh to just proximal to the knee joint

Gemellus inferior (JEM-ell-us)

Gemellus means "twin"; *inferior* means "below."

Posterior

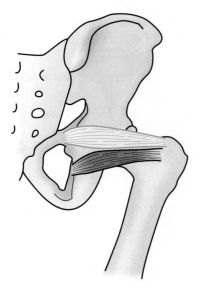

Concentric action:

Lateral rotation of the thigh at the hip joint and abduction of the thigh at the hip joint if the thigh is first in a position of flexion at the hip joint

Eccentric action:

Restrains medial rotation of the thigh and also may restrain adduction of the thigh (if the thigh is in a position of flexion)

Isometric action:

Stabilizes the hip joint

Origin, proximal attachment, arises from:

Upper part of the ischial tuberosity

Insertion, distal attachment, attaches to:

Medial surface of the greater trochanter

Innervation:

Lumbosacral plexus

Major synergists:

All deep lateral rotators of the thigh at the hip joint are synergistic with one another; posterior fibers of the gluteus medius are synergistic.

Major antagonists:

Anterior fibers of the gluteus medius, gluteus minimus, and the tensor fasciae latae

Trigger points:

The belly of the muscle

Referred pain pattern:

Sacroiliac region, entire buttock, and down the posterior thigh to just proximal to the knee joint

ACTIVITY **9-22**

Draw and color the **deep lateral rotators of the thigh at the hip joint** in the spaces provided. For each muscle, do the following:

1. Label the origin and insertion attachment points: *O* for origin; *I* for insertion.
2. Place an X on the trigger points.
3. Palpate this muscle; identify the attachment points and the bellies of the muscles.
4. Move these muscles on yourself.

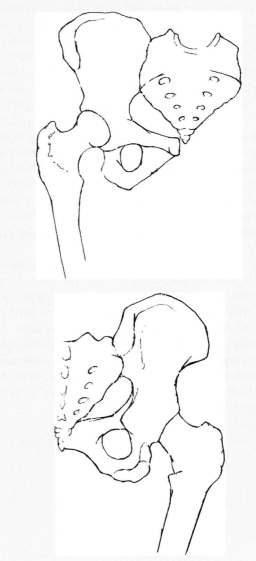

Muscles of the Posterior Thigh

The hamstring muscle group crosses two joints, the hip and the knee. These muscles posteriorly tilt the pelvis at the hip joint, extend the thigh at the hip joint, and flex the leg at the knee joint. The muscles of the massive hamstring group are the main extensors of the thigh. Because these muscles are active during walking, all gait reflexes are involved with the shoulder muscles to promote the appropriate counterbalancing arm swing. Facilitation between muscles of the arms that flex and extend occur along with thigh muscles in contralateral patterns. The massage therapist usually needs to consider the muscles of the shoulder joint with muscles of the hip and massage in a correlated pattern. Although not listed with synergists and antagonists, the flexors of the arm at the shoulder joint work with the flexors of the thigh at the hip joint on the opposite side (i.e., right with left and left with right). This concept is also true for the extensors of the arm and thigh. These muscles show patterns of inhibition as well; for example, right-side extensors of the thigh at the hip joint inhibit right-side extensors of the arm at the shoulder joint. Adductors and medial rotators of the arm at the shoulder joint work with adductors and medial rotators of the thigh at the hip joint on the opposite side. This concept holds true for abductors and lateral rotators as well. Of course, these muscles also exhibit inhibitory patterns.

These muscles are thick, and massage application must address the muscles adequately but not painfully compress them against the underlying bone. The side-lying position is most suitable for applying compressive force during the massage and moving the muscles away from the bone. These muscles have a tendency to adhere together, and although this may be a compensation pattern for repetitive movement in extension of the thigh at the hip joint or flexion of the leg at the knee joint, adhesion can reduce and interfere with range of motion of the associated joints (Figure 9-21).

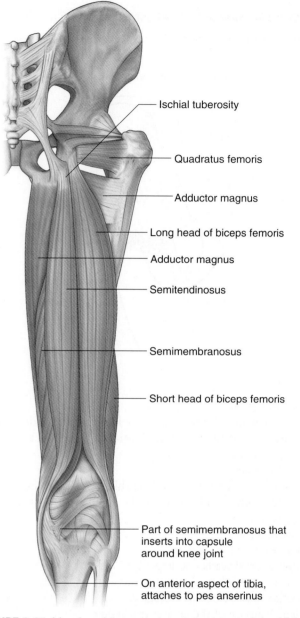

Ischial tuberosity

Quadratus femoris

Adductor magnus

Long head of biceps femoris

Adductor magnus

Semitendinosus

Semimembranosus

Short head of biceps femoris

Part of semimembranosus that inserts into capsule around knee joint

On anterior aspect of tibia, attaches to pes anserinus

FIGURE 9-21 Muscles of the posterior compartment of the thigh. Posterior view. (From Drake RL, Vogl W, Mitchell WM: *Gray's anatomy for students,* ed 2, Edinburgh, 2010, Churchill Livingstone.)

Semimembranosus (SEM-ee-MEM-bran-oh-sus)

Semimembranosus means "half membrane."

Posterior

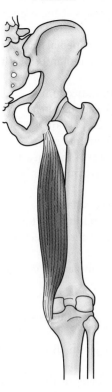

Concentric action:
Flexion and medial rotation of the leg at the knee joint (the knee joint must be semiflexed for medial rotation to occur), extension of the thigh at the hip joint, and posterior tilt of the pelvis at the hip joint. The semimembranosus also serves to move the medial meniscus posteriorly during knee flexion.
Eccentric action:
Restrains extension and lateral rotation of the leg and allows flexion of the thigh and anterior tilt of the pelvis
Isometric action:
Stabilizes the knee and hip joints
Origin, proximal attachment, arises from:
Upper lateral aspect of the ischial tuberosity
Insertion, distal attachment, attaches to:
Posteromedial surface of the medial condyle of the tibia; attaches to the medial meniscus
Innervation:
Tibial portion of the sciatic nerve (L5 to S2)
Major synergists:
Semitendinosus, biceps femoris, and gluteus maximus
Major antagonists:
Quadriceps femoris group, iliopsoas, and tensor fasciae latae
Trigger points:
Several areas in the belly of the muscle and at the musculotendinous junction near the knee joint
Referred pain pattern:
Ischial tuberosity, back of the knee, and the entire posterior thigh and leg to midcalf

Semitendinosus (SEM-ee-TEN-din-oh-sus)

Semitendinosus means "half tendon."

Posterior

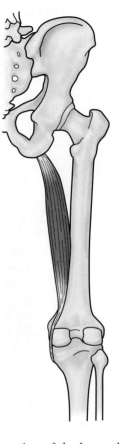

Concentric action:
Flexion and medial rotation of the leg at the knee joint (the knee joint must be semiflexed for medial rotation to occur), extension of the thigh at the hip joint, and posterior tilt of the pelvis at the hip joint
Eccentric action:
Restrains extension and lateral rotation of the leg and allows flexion of the thigh and anterior tilt of the pelvis
Isometric action:
Stabilizes the knee and hip joints
Origin, proximal attachment, arises from:
Distal part of the medial aspect of the ischial tuberosity
Insertion, distal attachment, attaches to:
Proximal anteromedial tibia at the pes anserinus tendon and deep fascia of the leg
Innervation:
Tibial portion of the sciatic nerve (L5 to S2)
Major synergists:
Semimembranosus, biceps femoris, and gluteus maximus
Major antagonists:
Quadriceps femoris group, iliopsoas, and tensor fasciae latae
Trigger points:
Several areas in the belly of the muscle and at the musculotendinous junction near the knee joint
Referred pain pattern:
Ischial tuberosity, back of the knee, and the entire posterior thigh and leg to midcalf

Biceps femoris (BI-seps FEM-or-iss)

Biceps means "two headed"; *femoris* means "related to the thigh."

Posterior

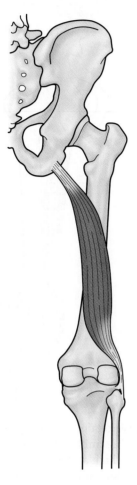

Concentric action:

Entire muscle—flexion and lateral rotation of the leg at the knee joint (The knee joint must be semiflexed for lateral rotation to occur.)

Long head—extension of the thigh at the hip joint and posterior tilt of the pelvis at the hip joint

Eccentric action:

Restrains extension and medial rotation of the leg and restrains flexion of the thigh and anterior tilt of the pelvis

Isometric action:

Stabilizes the hip and knee joints

Origin, proximal attachment, arises from:

Long head—posterior part of the ischial tuberosity and the sacrotuberous ligament

Short head—lateral lip of the linea aspera, lateral intermuscular septum, and proximal two thirds of the supracondylar line

Insertion, distal attachment, attaches to:

Lateral side of the fibular head, lateral condyle of the tibia, and deep fascia on the lateral aspect of the leg

Innervation:

Tibial and common fibular portions of the sciatic nerve (L5 to S2)

Major synergists:

Semitendinosus, semimembranosus, and gluteus maximus

Major antagonists:

Quadriceps femoris group, iliopsoas, and tensor fasciae latae

Trigger points:

Several areas in the belly of the muscle and at the musculotendinous junction near the knee joint

Referred pain pattern:

Ischial tuberosity, back of the knee, and the entire posterior thigh and leg to midcalf

Muscles of the Medial Thigh and Anterior Thigh

The medial thigh muscles, called the *adductor group of the thigh*, adduct the thigh at the hip joint. Interaction between abduction and adduction of the thighs (co-contraction) keeps the weight of the body balanced over the weight-bearing lower extremity when a person is walking. Because of gait reflexes, these muscles work with adductors of the arm at the shoulder joint and inhibit abductors of the arm at the shoulder joint on the opposite side. These muscles also work with the abdominal muscles to support the trunk and pelvis in an upright position. This muscle group is massive, and the massage therapist can manage it most easily with the client in the side-lying position with the top lower extremity bent and forward to expose the adductor muscles of the bottom thigh.

Muscles of the Anterior Thigh

The majority of the musculature of the anterior thigh is composed of the muscles of the quadriceps femoris group; the main action of this group is to extend the leg at the knee joint. The quadriceps femoris and hamstring muscle groups obviously are antagonistic, yet together they ensure the stability of the knee joint. The vastus lateralis and vastus medialis of the quadriceps femoris group also function together for proper tracking of the patella. The rectus femoris of the quadriceps

✎ ACTIVITY **9-23**

Draw and color the **muscles of the posterior thigh** in the spaces provided. For each muscle, do the following:
1. Label the origin and insertion attachment points: *O* for origin; *I* for insertion.

2. Place an X on the trigger points.
3. Palpate this muscle; identify the attachment points and the bellies of the muscles.
4. Move these muscles on yourself.

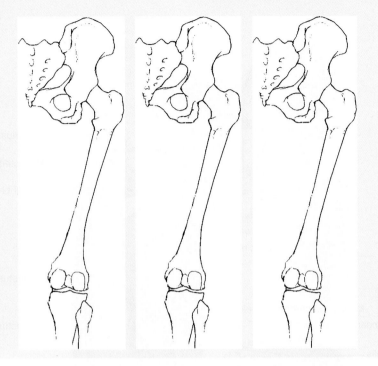

femoris group is the only one that also crosses the hip joint. Because the rectus femoris crosses the hip joint anteriorly, it can flex the thigh at the hip joint. Another muscle of the anterior thigh is the sartorius, which also flexes the thigh at the hip joint and flexes the leg at the knee joint. The rectus femoris and sartorius fall into gait patterns and reflexes with flexors and extensors of the arm at the shoulder joint. The remaining quadriceps femoris muscles work with muscles that flex and extend the forearm at the elbow joint, these patterns being synergistic on opposite sides and antagonistic on the same side. Muscles of the anterior thigh can adhere to each other, particularly the rectus femoris to the underlying vastus intermedius. Should this happen, the rectus femoris will not have the necessary functional range during flexion of the thigh at the hip joint and extension of the leg at the knee joint. Adhesion compromises range of motion, and pain occurs, usually in the knee.

A major function of the quadriceps femoris group is to move the thigh into extension at the knee; this is sometimes called a *reverse action* because the proximal attachment moves in this situation and the distal attachment stays fixed. Examples would be standing up from a seated position or coming up into a straight-leg position from a squat. This action requires moving the upper body and the thigh. Therefore the quadriceps femoris group is large and strong (Figure 9-22).

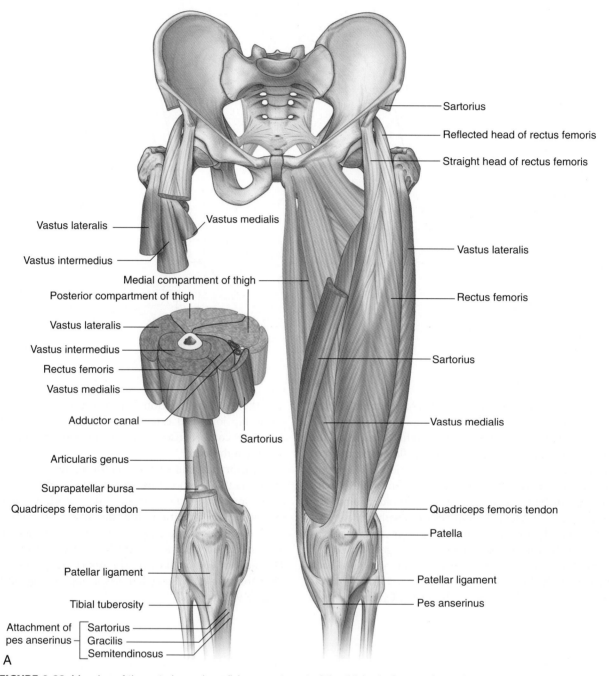

FIGURE 9-22 Muscles of the anterior and medial compartment of the thigh. **A,** Composite and cutaway view of the thigh.

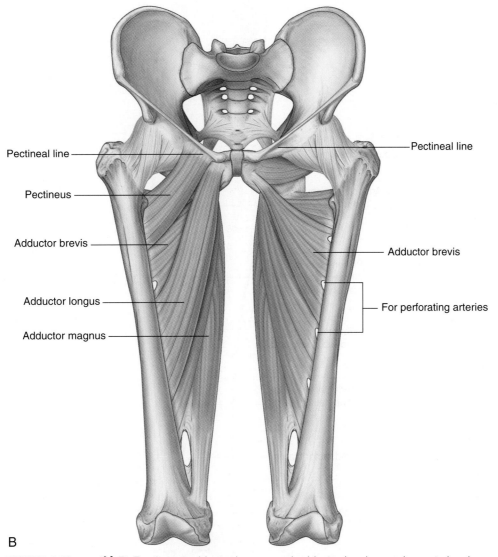

Pectineal line

Pectineus

Adductor brevis

Adductor longus

Adductor magnus

Pectineal line

Adductor brevis

For perforating arteries

B

FIGURE 9-22, cont'd B, Pectineus, adductor longus, and adductor brevis muscles, anterior view.

Continued

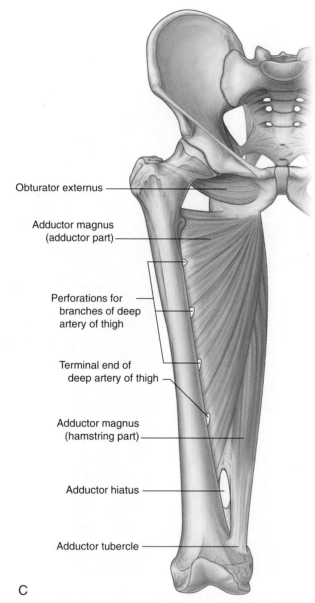

Obturator externus

Adductor magnus
(adductor part)

Perforations for
branches of deep
artery of thigh

Terminal end of
deep artery of thigh

Adductor magnus
(hamstring part)

Adductor hiatus

Adductor tubercle

C

FIGURE 9-22, cont'd C, Adductor magnus and obturator externus muscles, anterior view. (From Drake RL, Vogl W, Mitchell WM: *Gray's anatomy for students,* ed 2, Edinburgh, 2010, Churchill Livingstone.)

Muscles of the Medial Thigh
Pectineus (PEK-tih-NEE-us)

Pectineus means "related to the pubic bone."

Anterior

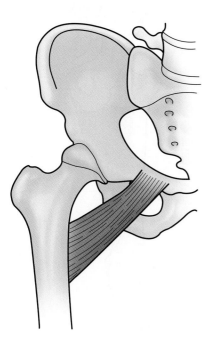

Adductor brevis (ad-DUCK-tur BREV-us)

Adductor means "to lead toward"; *brevis* means "short."

Anterior

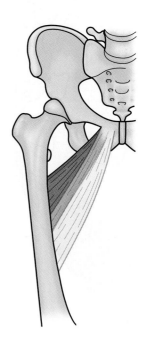

Concentric action:

Adduction and flexion of the thigh at the hip joint and anterior tilt of the pelvis at the hip joint

Eccentric action:

Restrains abduction and extension of the thigh and posterior tilt of the pelvis

Isometric action:

Stabilizes the pelvis at the hip joint

Origin, proximal attachment, arises from:

Pectineal line of the pubis (on the superior ramus of the pubis)

Insertion, distal attachment, attaches to:

Pectineal line of the femur (line extending from the lesser trochanter of the femur to the linea aspera)

Innervation:

Femoral nerve (L2 to L3)

Major synergists:

The adductor group of the thigh is synergistic, as is the iliopsoas.

Major antagonists:

Gluteus medius and gluteus minimus, tensor fasciae latae, and hamstrings

Trigger points:

Within the belly of each muscle and near the ischial tuberosity attachment

Referred pain pattern:

Deep in the groin, into the medial thigh and downward to the knee and leg; may mimic hamstring tension

Concentric action:

Adduction and flexion of the thigh at the hip joint and anterior tilt of the pelvis at the hip joint

Eccentric action:

Restrains abduction and extension of the thigh and posterior tilt of the pelvis

Isometric action:

Stabilizes the pelvis at the hip joint

Origin, proximal attachment, arises from:

Outer surface of the inferior ramus of the pubis between the gracilis and the obturator externus

Insertion, distal attachment, attaches to:

Linea aspera of the femur

Innervation:

Obturator nerve (L2 to L3)

Major synergists:

The adductor group of the thigh group is synergistic, as is the iliopsoas.

Major antagonists:

Gluteus medius and gluteus minimus, tensor fasciae latae, and hamstrings

Trigger points:

Within the belly of each muscle and near the ischial tuberosity attachment

Referred pain pattern:

Deep in the groin, into the medial thigh and downward to the knee and leg; may mimic hamstring tension

▎*Adductor longus* (ad-DUCK-tur LONG-us)

Adductor means "to lead toward"; *longus* means "long."

Posterior

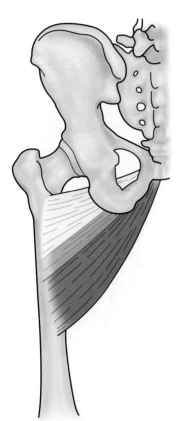

▎*Adductor magnus* (ad-DUCK-tur MAG-nus)

Adductor means "to lead toward"; *magnus* means "great."

Posterior

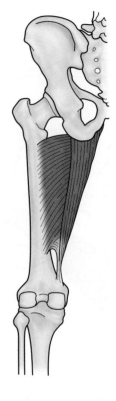

Concentric action:

Adduction and flexion of the thigh at the hip joint and anterior tilt of the pelvis at the hip joint

Eccentric action:

Restrains abduction and extension of the thigh and posterior tilt of the pelvis

Isometric action:

Stabilizes the pelvis at the hip joint

Origin, proximal attachment, arises from:

Anterior pubis between the crest and symphysis

Insertion, distal attachment, attaches to:

Middle one third of the medial lip of the linea aspera of the femur

Innervation:

Obturator nerve (L2 to L4)

Major synergists:

The adductor group of the thigh is synergistic, as is the iliopsoas.

Major antagonists:

Gluteus medius and gluteus minimus, tensor fasciae latae, and hamstrings

Trigger points:

Within the belly of each muscle and near the ischial tuberosity attachment

Referred pain pattern:

Deep in the groin, into the medial thigh and downward to the knee and leg; may mimic hamstring tension

Concentric action:

Adduction and extension of the thigh at the hip joint and posterior tilt of the pelvis at the hip joint

Eccentric action:

Restrains abduction and flexion of the thigh and anterior tilt of the pelvis

Isometric action:

Stabilizes the pelvis at the hip joint

Origin, proximal attachment, arises from:

Inferior ramus of the pubis and the ramus of the ischium (anterior fibers); posterior fibers attach to the ischial tuberosity

Insertion, distal attachment, attaches to:

Gluteal tuberosity, linea aspera, medial supracondylar line, and adductor tubercle of the femur

Innervation:

Obturator and tibial division of sciatic nerves (L2 to L4)

Major synergists:

The adductor group of the thigh is synergistic, as are the hamstrings.

Major antagonists:

Gluteus medius and gluteus minimus, tensor fasciae latae, and iliopsoas

Trigger points:

Within the belly of each muscle and near the ischial tuberosity attachment

Referred pain pattern:

Deep in the groin, into the medial thigh and downward to the knee and leg; may mimic hamstring tension

Gracilis (gra-SIL-iss)

Gracilis means "slender."

Anterior

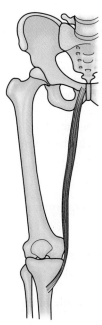

Concentric action:

Adduction and flexion of the thigh at the hip joint, anterior tilt of the pelvis at the hip joint, and flexion and medial rotation of the leg at the knee joint (The knee joint must be semiflexed for medial rotation to occur.)

Eccentric action:

Restrains abduction and extension of the thigh and allows posterior tilt of the pelvis and extension and lateral rotation of the leg

Isometric action:

Stabilizes the pelvis at the hip joint and assists in controlling and stabilizing the valgus angulation of the knee joint

Origin, proximal attachment, arises from:

Inferior half of the symphysis pubis and inferior ramus of the pubic bone

Insertion, distal attachment, attaches to:

Proximal anteromedial tibia at the pes anserinus tendon

Innervation:

Obturator nerve (L2 to L3)

Major synergists:

The adductor group of the thigh is synergistic, as are the iliopsoas and sartorius.

Major antagonists:

Gluteus medius and gluteus minimus, tensor fasciae latae, and hamstrings

Trigger points:

Within the belly of each muscle and near the ischial tuberosity attachment

Referred pain pattern:

Deep in the groin, into the medial thigh and downward to the knee and leg; may mimic hamstring tension

ACTIVITY 9-24

Draw and color the **muscles of the medial thigh** in the spaces provided. For each muscle, do the following:

1. Label the origin and insertion attachment points: *O* for origin; *I* for insertion.
2. Place an X on the trigger points.
3. Palpate this muscle; identify the attachment points and the bellies of the muscles.
4. Move these muscles on yourself.

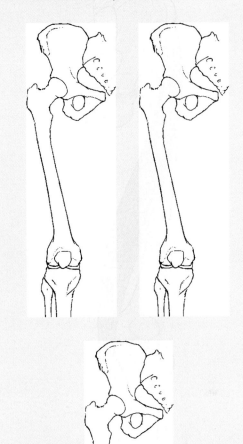

Muscles of the Anterior Thigh

▌ Sartorius (sar-TOR-ee-us)

Sartorius means "tailor."

Anterior

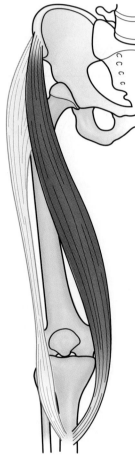

Concentric action:

Flexion, lateral rotation, and abduction of the thigh at the hip joint; flexion and medial rotation of the leg at the knee joint (the knee joint must be semiflexed for medial rotation to occur); and anterior tilt of the pelvis at the hip joint

Eccentric action:

Restrains extension, medial rotation, and adduction of the thigh and allows extension and lateral rotation of the leg and posterior tilt of the pelvis

Isometric action:

Stabilizes the knee and hip joints

Origin, proximal attachment, arises from:

Anterior superior iliac spine

Insertion, distal attachment, attaches to:

Proximal anteromedial tibia at the pes anserinus tendon

Innervation:

Femoral nerve (L2 to L3)

Major synergists:

Iliopsoas, rectus femoris, lateral rotator group of the thigh, and gluteus medius

Major antagonists:

Hamstrings, tensor fasciae latae, adductor group of the thigh, and quadriceps femoris group

Trigger points:

Three or four areas along the belly of the muscle

Referred pain pattern:

Entire anterior thigh, with concentration at the knee

Rectus femoris (REK-tus FEM-or-iss)

The first muscle of the quadriceps femoris group, *rectus* means "straight" or "upright"; *femoris* means "related to the thigh." *Quadriceps* means "four headed."

Anterior

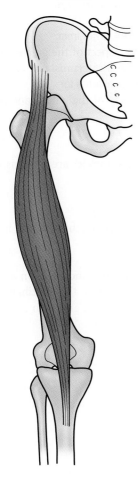

Concentric action:

Extension of the leg at the knee joint, flexion of the thigh at the hip joint, and anterior tilt of the pelvis at the hip joint

Eccentric action:

Restrains flexion of the leg and allows extension of the thigh and posterior tilt of the pelvis

Isometric action:

Stabilizes the knee and hip joints

Origin, proximal attachment, arises from:

Anterior inferior iliac spine; groove above the rim of the acetabulum

Insertion, distal attachment, attaches to:

Tibial tuberosity, by way of the patella and patellar ligament

Innervation:

Femoral nerve (L2 to L4)

Major synergists:

All quadriceps femoris muscles are synergistic, as are the iliopsoas and sartorius.

Major antagonists:

Hamstrings and gluteus maximus

Trigger points:

Near the attachment at the pelvis

Referred pain pattern:

Entire anterior thigh, with concentration at the knee

Vastus lateralis (VAS-tus LAT-ter-al-us)

The second muscle of the quadriceps femoris group, *vastus* means "vast" or "large"; *lateralis* means "related to the side." *Quadriceps* means "four headed."

Anterior

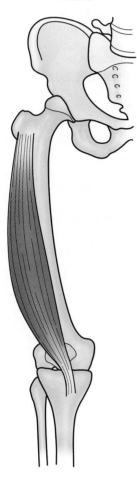

Concentric action:

Extension of the leg at the knee joint (The vastus lateralis also exerts a lateral pull on the patella.)

Eccentric action:

Restrains flexion of the leg at the knee joint (The vastus lateralis also restrains the medial pull on the patella by the vastus medialis.)

Isometric action:

Stabilizes the patella and the knee joint (and the iliotibial band)

Origin, proximal attachment, arises from:

Linea aspera, anterior aspect of the greater trochanter, gluteal tuberosity, and lateral intermuscular septum

Insertion, distal attachment, attaches to:

Tibial tuberosity, by way of the patella and patellar ligament

Innervation:

Femoral nerve (L2 to L4)

Major synergists:

All quadriceps femoris muscles are synergistic.

Major antagonists:

Hamstrings

Trigger points:

Several locations at each attachment and in the belly of the muscle

Referred pain pattern:

Entire anterior thigh, with concentration at the knee

A tight vastus lateralis, not the iliotibial band, is usually responsible for shortening and pain in the lateral thigh.

Vastus medialis (VAS-tus MEE-dee-al-us)

The third muscle of the quadriceps femoris group, *vastus* means "vast" or "large"; *medialis* means "related to the middle." *Quadriceps* means "four headed."

Anterior

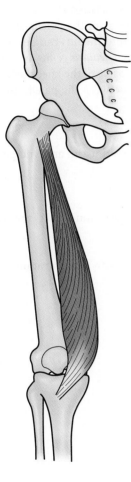

Concentric action:

Extension of the leg at the knee joint (The vastus medialis also exerts a medial pull on the patella.)

Eccentric action:

Restrains flexion of the leg at the knee joint (The vastus medialis also restrains the lateral pull on the patella by the vastus lateralis.)

Isometric action:

Stabilizes the patella and the knee joint

Origin, proximal attachment, arises from:

Linea aspera, intertrochanteric line, medial supracondylar line, and medial intermuscular septum

Insertion, distal attachment, attaches to:

Tibial tuberosity, by way of the patella and patellar ligament

The lower fibers of the vastus medialis often are called the *VMO (vastus medialis oblique)*; the upper fibers often are called the *VML (vastus medialis longus)*.

Innervation:

Femoral nerve (L2 to L4)

Major synergists:

All quadriceps femoris muscles are synergistic.

Major antagonists:

Hamstrings

Trigger points:

In the belly of the muscle, near the attachment just above the knee, and in the oblique portion (vastus medialis oblique)

Referred pain pattern:

Entire anterior thigh, with concentration at the knee

Vastus intermedius (VAS-tus in-ter-MEE-dee-us)

The fourth muscle of the quadriceps femoris group, *vastus* means "vast" or "large"; *intermedius* means "among the middle." *Quadriceps* means "four headed."

Anterior

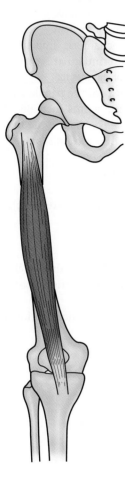

Concentric action:

Extension of the leg at the knee joint

Eccentric action:

Restrains flexion of the leg

Isometric action:

Stabilizes the patella and the knee joint

Origin, proximal attachment, arises from:

Linea aspera, anterior and lateral surfaces of the proximal two thirds of the shaft of the femur, and intermuscular septum

Insertion, distal attachment, attaches to:

Tibial tuberosity, by way of the patella and patellar ligament

A portion of vastus intermedius can be considered a separate muscle called the *articularis genus,* which is responsible for lifting the joint capsule of the knee during extension so that it is not pinched between the patella and femur.

Innervation:

Femoral nerve (L2 to L4)

Major synergists:

All quadriceps femoris muscles are synergistic.

Major antagonists:

Hamstrings

Trigger points:

Near the proximal attachment at the musculotendinous junction

Referred pain pattern:

Entire anterior thigh, with concentration at the knee

✎ ACTIVITY 9-25

Draw and color the **muscles of the medial and anterior thigh** in the spaces provided. For each muscle, do the following:
1. Label the origin and insertion attachment points: *O* for origin; *I* for insertion.

2. Place an X on the trigger points.
3. Palpate this muscle; identify the attachment points and the bellies of the muscles.
4. Move these muscles on yourself.

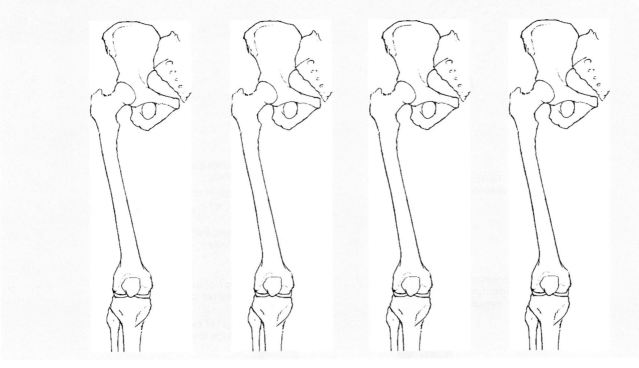

Muscles of the Anterior and Lateral Leg

The muscles of the leg are primarily important for their actions at the foot (Figure 9-23). These muscles produce dorsiflexion and plantar flexion movements of the foot at the ankle joint and inversion and eversion movements of the foot at the tarsal (subtalar) joints. Many of these muscles also flex and extend the toes at the metatarsophalangeal and interphalangeal joints. The muscles of the anterior leg primarily provide dorsiflexion of the foot at the ankle joint and extension of the toes at the metatarsophalangeal and interphalangeal joints. The muscles of the posterior leg primarily provide plantar flexion of the foot at the ankle joint and flexion of the toes at the metatarsophalangeal and interphalangeal joints. Dorsiflexion of the foot is important in preventing the toes from dragging during walking; plantar flexion of the foot is important for pushing off during walking. The lateral leg muscles evert the foot at the tarsal (subtalar) joints and provide plantar flexion of the foot at the ankle joint.

The deep fascia of the leg is continuous with the iliotibial band, which expands and ensheathes the thigh and binds the leg muscles together. This construction helps prevent excessive swelling of the muscles during exercise. This same fascial sheath supports a pumping action that aids the circulation of blood and lymph, particularly venous return flow. The fascia divides the leg muscles into the anterior, lateral, and posterior compartments, each with its own nerve and blood supply. The leg fascia thickens at the ankles to form the retinacula, which secure the muscle tendons in place as they cross the ankles into the feet. Because of this extensive fascial structure, massage is effective when applied in a slow, sustained manner with a drag that addresses the viscous quality of the tissue. Although most of these muscles primarily produce movements of the foot, any muscle that crosses the knee joint is involved in the function and dysfunction of the knee joint. Because the hip, knee, and ankle joints function as a complex unit and closed kinematic chain when standing, all muscles affecting these joints interact with one another.

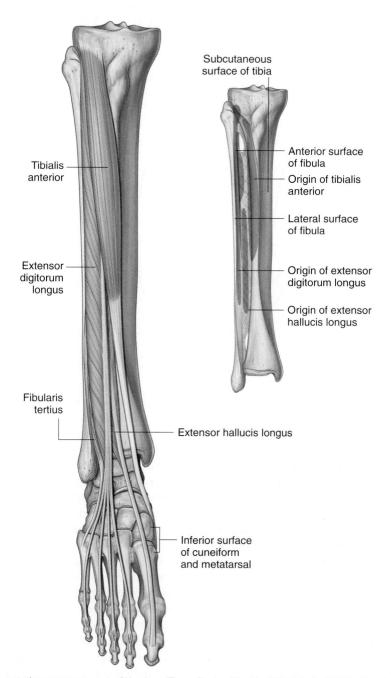

FIGURE 9-23 Muscles of the anterior compartment of the leg. (From Drake RL, Vogl W, Mitchell WM: *Gray's anatomy for students,* ed 2, Edinburgh, 2010, Churchill Livingstone.)

Anterior Muscles

Tibialis anterior (TIB-ee-AL-iss)

Tibialis means "related to the shin bone"; *anterior* means "before" or "in front."

Lateral

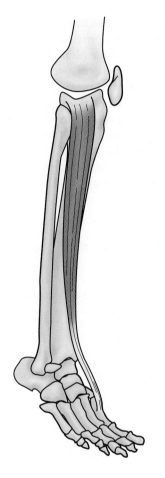

Concentric action:
Dorsiflexion of the foot at the ankle joint and inversion of the foot at the tarsal joints

Eccentric action:
Restrains plantar flexion and eversion of the foot

Isometric action:
Stabilizes the ankle joint

Origin, proximal attachment, arises from:
Lateral condyle and proximal two thirds of the anterior surface of the tibia, interosseous membrane, deep fascia, and lateral intermuscular septum

Insertion, distal attachment, attaches to:
At the foot on the medial plantar surface of the medial cuneiform bone and base of the first metatarsal bone

Innervation:
Deep fibular nerve (L4 to L5)

Major synergists:
Extensor digitorum longus, extensor hallucis longus, and tibialis posterior

Major antagonists:
Gastrocnemius, soleus, and fibularis muscles

Trigger points:
In the belly of the muscle

Referred pain pattern:
Down the leg to the ankle and into the toes

Extensor digitorum longus
(ex-STEN-sur DIH-jih-TOR-um LONG-us)

Extensor means "one that stretches," *digitorum* means "of the fingers and toes," and *longus* means "long."

Lateral

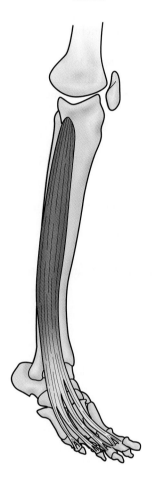

Concentric action:

Extension of toes 2 to 5 at the metatarsophalangeal and interphalangeal joints, dorsiflexion of the foot at the ankle joint, and eversion of the foot at the tarsal joints

Eccentric action:

Restrains flexion of the toes and allows plantar flexion and inversion of the foot

Isometric action:

Stabilizes joints of the ankle and foot

Origin, proximal attachment, arises from:

Lateral condyle of the tibia, proximal two thirds of the anterior surface of the shaft of the fibula, interosseous membrane, deep fascia, and intermuscular septa

Insertion, distal attachment, attaches to:

By four tendons to the second through fifth digits; each tendon divides into an intermediate slip, which attaches to the base of the middle phalanx, and two lateral slips, which attach to the base of the distal phalanx.

The distal tendons of the extensor digitorum longus create the dorsal digital expansion of toes 2 to 5.

Innervation:

Deep fibular nerve (L5 to S1)

Major synergists:

Extensor digitorum brevis, tibialis anterior, and fibularis muscles

Major antagonists:

Flexor digitorum longus, flexor digitorum brevis, tibialis anterior, and tibialis posterior

Trigger points:

In the belly of the muscle

Referred pain pattern:

Down the leg to the ankle and into the toes

Extensor hallucis longus
(ex-STEN-sur HAL-uh-siss LONG-us)

Extensor means "one that stretches," *hallucis* means "related to the big toe," and *longus* means "long."

Lateral

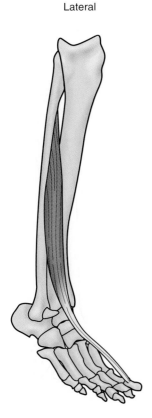

Concentric action:
Extension of the big toe at the metatarsophalangeal and interphalangeal joints, dorsiflexion of the foot at the ankle joint, and inversion of the foot at the tarsal joints
Eccentric action:
Restrains flexion of the great toe and allows plantar flexion and eversion of the foot
Isometric action:
Stabilizes the great toe and assists in stabilizing the ankle
Origin, proximal attachment, arises from:
Middle third of the anterior surface of the fibula and adjacent interosseous membrane
Insertion, distal attachment, attaches to:
Base of the distal phalanx of the great toe
Innervation:
Deep fibular nerve (L5 to S1)
Major synergists:
The tibialis anterior, digitorum longus, peroneus tertius, and extensor hallucis longus are synergistic for dorsiflexion.
Major antagonists:
Eversion and inversion—tibialis anterior, digitorum longus
Dorsiflexion—gastrocnemius, soleus, peroneus longus and peroneus brevis, flexors of the toes, tibialis posterior
Trigger points:
In the belly of each muscle
Referred pain pattern:
Down the leg to the ankle and into the toes

Fibularis (peroneus) tertius (fib-you-LAR-iss TER-she-us)

Fibularis means "related to the pin or fibula"; *tertius* means "the third."

Lateral

Concentric action:
Dorsiflexion of the foot at the ankle joint and eversion of the foot at the tarsal joints
Eccentric action:
Restrains plantar flexion and inversion of the foot
Isometric action:
Assists in stabilizing the ankle joint
Origin, proximal attachment, arises from:
Distal one third of the anterior surface of the fibula, interosseous membrane, and intermuscular septum
Insertion, distal attachment, attaches to:
Dorsal surface of the base of the fifth metatarsal bone
Innervation:
Deep fibular nerve (L5 to S1)
Major synergists:
Extensor hallucis brevis and tibialis anterior
Major antagonists:
Flexor hallucis longus, flexor hallucis brevis, and fibularis muscles
Trigger points:
In the belly of the muscle
Referred pain pattern:
Down the leg to the ankle and into the toes

✎ ACTIVITY **9-26**

Draw and color the **anterior leg muscles** in the spaces provided. For each muscle, do the following:

1. Label the origin and insertion attachment points: *O* for origin; *I* for insertion.

2. Place an X on the trigger points.
3. Palpate this muscle; identify the attachment points and the bellies of the muscles.
4. Move these muscles on yourself.

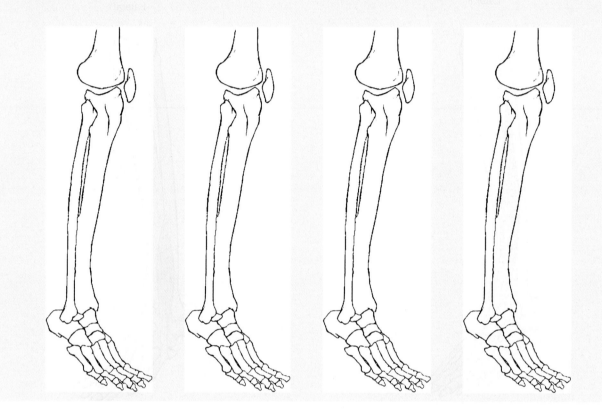

Lateral Muscles

▌ *Fibularis (peroneus) longus* (fib-you-LAR-iss LONG-us)

Fibularis means "related to the pin or fibula"; *longus* means "long."

Lateral

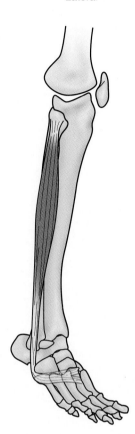

▌ *Fibularis (peroneus) brevis* (fib-you-LAR-iss BREV-us)

Fibularis means "related to the pin or fibula"; *brevis* means "smaller."

Lateral

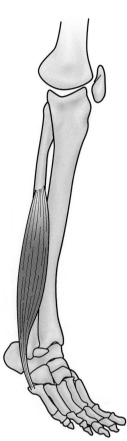

Concentric action:
Eversion of the foot at the tarsal joints and plantar flexion of the foot at the ankle joint
Eccentric action:
Restrains inversion and dorsiflexion of the foot
Isometric action:
Stabilizes the ankle joint
Origin, proximal attachment, arises from:
Lateral condyle of the tibia, head and proximal half of the lateral surface of the fibula, intermuscular septa, and adjacent deep fascia
Insertion, distal attachment, attaches to:
Lateral side of the base of the first metatarsal bone and the medial cuneiform bone
Innervation:
Superficial fibular nerve (L5 to S1)
Major synergist:
Fibularis brevis
Major antagonist:
Tibialis anterior
Trigger points:
Located at the origin and insertion near the musculotendinous junction
Referred pain pattern:
To the lateral malleolus and the heel

Concentric action:
Eversion of the foot at the tarsal joints and plantar flexion of the foot at the ankle joint
Eccentric action:
Restrains inversion and dorsiflexion of the foot
Isometric action:
Stabilizes the ankle joint
Origin, proximal attachment, arises from:
Distal half of the lateral surface of the fibula and adjacent intermuscular septum
Insertion, distal attachment, attaches to:
Tuberosity at the base of the fifth metatarsal bone on the lateral side
Innervation:
Superficial fibular nerve (L5 to S1)
Major synergist:
Fibularis longus
Major antagonist:
Tibialis anterior
Trigger points:
Located at the origin and insertion near the musculotendinous junction
Referred pain pattern:
To the lateral malleolus and the heel

✎ ACTIVITY 9-27

Draw and color the **lateral leg muscles** in the spaces provided. For each muscle, do the following:
1. Label the origin and insertion attachment points: *O* for origin; *I* for insertion.

2. Place an X on the trigger points.
3. Palpate this muscle; identify the attachment points and the bellies of the muscles.
4. Move these muscles on yourself.

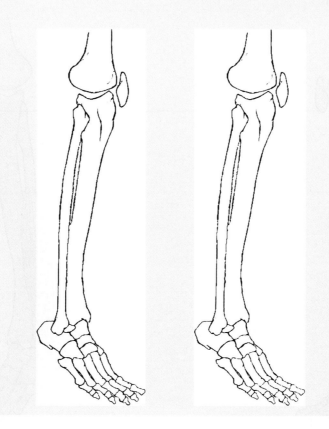

Muscles of the Posterior Leg

The majority of the posterior leg muscles provide plantar flexion of the foot at the ankle joint and invert the foot at the tarsal joints; many of them also flex the toes at the metatarsophalangeal and interphalangeal joints (Figure 9-24). Plantar flexion lifts the entire weight of the body to allow a person to stand on tiptoe and provides the necessary forward thrust for walking and running. Plantar flexion is a powerful movement.

The popliteus muscle, which crosses the knee, is important in unlocking the extended knee (by medial rotation of the leg at the knee joint) in preparation for flexion of the leg at the knee joint. Because they cross the knee joint posteriorly, the gastrocnemius and plantaris muscles assist with flexion of the leg at the knee joint. The gastrocnemius and soleus can become adhered together, which interferes with the function of the gastrocnemius, often causing knee pain, stiffness, and ankle restriction.

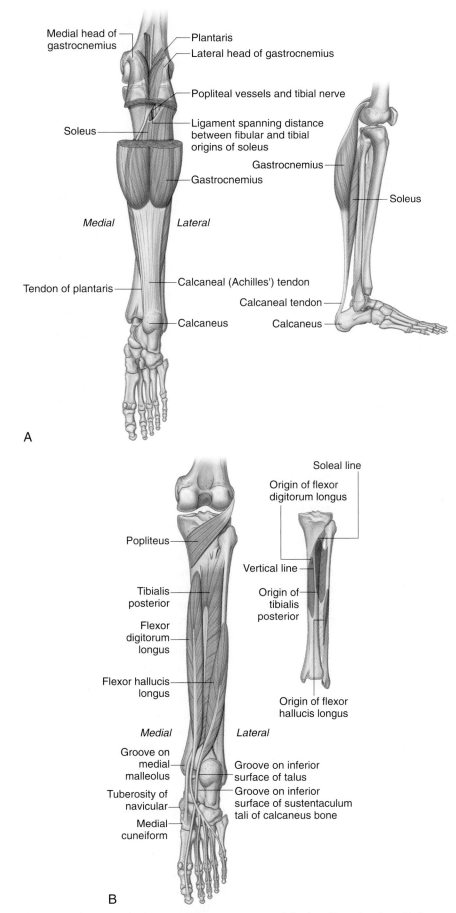

Medial head of gastrocnemius

Plantaris

Lateral head of gastrocnemius

Popliteal vessels and tibial nerve

Ligament spanning distance between fibular and tibial origins of soleus

Soleus

Gastrocnemius

Soleus

Medial

Lateral

Gastrocnemius

Tendon of plantaris

Calcaneal (Achilles') tendon

Calcaneal tendon

Calcaneus

Calcaneus

A

Soleal line

Origin of flexor digitorum longus

Popliteus

Vertical line

Tibialis posterior

Origin of tibialis posterior

Flexor digitorum longus

Flexor hallucis longus

Medial

Lateral

Origin of flexor hallucis longus

Groove on medial malleolus

Groove on inferior surface of talus

Groove on inferior surface of sustentaculum tali of calcaneus bone

Tuberosity of navicular

Medial cuneiform

B

FIGURE 9-24 A, Superficial group of muscles in the posterior compartment of the leg. Posterior view. **B,** Deep group of muscles in the posterior compartment of the leg. (From Drake RL, Vogl W, Mitchell WM: *Gray's anatomy for students,* ed 2, Edinburgh, 2010, Churchill Livingstone.)

▌*Popliteus* (pop-LIT-ee-us)

Popliteus means "hollow of the knee."

Posterior

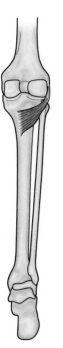

Concentric action:

With the proximal attachment (origin) fixed, medial rotation and flexion of the leg at the knee joint. The medial rotation of the knee joint is considered to be important for flexing the fully extended knee. The reverse action of lateral rotation of the thigh at the knee joint is also important for beginning flexion of the thigh at the knee joint in a weight-bearing lower extremity. The popliteus also moves the lateral meniscus posteriorly during knee flexion.

Eccentric action:

Restrains lateral rotation and extension of the leg

Isometric action:

Stabilizes the knee joint

Origin, proximal attachment, arises from:

Lateral surface of the lateral condyle of the femur, oblique popliteal ligament, and lateral meniscus of the knee

Insertion, distal attachment, attaches to:

Triangular area above the soleal line on the posterior and medial surfaces of the tibia, as well as the fascia covering its surface

Innervation:

Tibial nerve (L4 to S1)

Major synergists:

Semitendinosus, semimembranosus, sartorius, and gracilis

Major antagonists:

Biceps femoris and the quadriceps femoris group

Trigger points:

Belly of the muscle

Referred pain pattern:

To the back of the knee

▌*Tibialis posterior* (TIB-ee-AL-iss)

Tibialis means "related to the shin bone"; *posterior* means "coming after" or "behind."

Posterior/Inferior

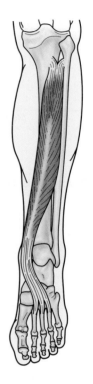

Concentric action:

Plantar flexion of the foot at the ankle joint and inversion of the foot at the tarsal joints

Eccentric action:

Restrains dorsiflexion and eversion of the foot

Isometric action:

Stabilizes the ankle joint

Origin, proximal attachment, arises from:

Proximal two thirds of the posterior surface of the tibia, fibula, and the interosseous membrane and intermuscular septa

Insertion, distal attachment, attaches to:

Tuberosity of the navicular bone, calcaneus, three cuneiform bones and the cuboid bone, and bases of the second through fourth metatarsal bones (sole of foot)

Innervation:

Tibial nerve (L4 to L5)

Major synergists:

Tibialis anterior, flexor digitorum longus, and flexor hallucis longus

Major antagonists:

Fibularis longus, fibularis brevis, and tibialis anterior

Trigger points:

Belly of the muscle near the knee joint

Referred pain pattern:

Down the posterior leg to the heel and the sole of the foot into the plantar surface of the toes; can be a factor in knee pain and restricted mobility of the knee and ankle

Flexor digitorum longus (FLEKS-or DIH-jih-TOR-um LONG-us)

Flexor means "to bend," *digitorum* means "related to the fingers or toes," and *longus* means "long."

Posterior/Inferior

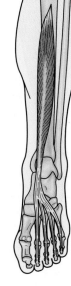

Concentric action:
Flexion of toes 2 to 5 at the metatarsophalangeal and inter-phalangeal joints, plantar flexion of the foot at the ankle joint, and inversion of the foot at the tarsal joints

Eccentric action:
Allows extension of the toes and allows dorsiflexion and ever-sion of the foot

Isometric action:
Stabilizes the ankle joint and the toes

Origin, proximal attachment, arises from:
Middle one third of the posterior surface of the shaft of the tibia and the fascia covering the tibialis posterior

Insertion, distal attachment, attaches to:
Bases of the distal phalanges of the second through fifth digits (sole of foot)

Innervation:
Tibial nerve (L5 to S2)

Major synergist:
Flexor digitorum brevis

Major antagonists:
Extensor digitorum longus and extensor digitorum brevis

Trigger points:
In the belly of the muscle

Referred pain pattern:
Down the posterior leg to the heel and the sole of the foot into the plantar surface of the toes; can be a factor in knee pain and restricted mobility of the knee and ankle

Flexor hallucis longus (FLEKS-or HAL-uh-siss LONG-us)

Flexor means "to bend," *hallucis* means "related to the big toe," and *longus* means "long."

Posterior/Inferior

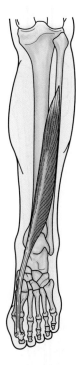

Concentric action:
Flexion of the big toe at the metatarsophalangeal and inter-phalangeal joints, plantar flexion of the foot at the ankle joint, inversion of the foot at the tarsal joints

Eccentric action:
Restrains extension of the big toe and dorsiflexion and ever-sion of the foot

Isometric action:
Stabilizes the big toe, ankle, and foot

Origin, proximal attachment, arises from:
Distal two thirds of the posterior surface of the fibula, interos-seous membrane, and adjacent intermuscular septum and fascia

Insertion, distal attachment, attaches to:
Plantar aspect of the base of the distal phalanx of the big toe (sole of foot)

Innervation:
Tibial nerve (L5 to S2)

Major synergist:
Flexor hallucis brevis

Major antagonists:
Extensor hallucis longus and extensor hallucis brevis

Trigger points:
In the belly of the muscle

Referred pain pattern:
Down the posterior leg to the heel and the sole of the foot into the plantar surface of the toes; can be a factor in knee pain and restricted mobility of the knee and ankle

Plantaris (plan-TAR-iss)

Plantaris means "the sole of the foot."

Posterior

Soleus (SOL-ee-us)

Soleus means "sandal" or "sole of the foot."

Posterior

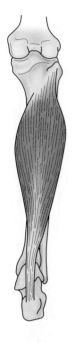

Concentric action:
Plantar flexion of the foot at the ankle joint and flexion of the leg at the knee joint
Eccentric action:
Restrains dorsiflexion of the foot and extension of the leg
Isometric action:
Stabilizes the ankle and knee joints
Origin, proximal attachment, arises from:
Distal part of the lateral supracondylar line of the femur and oblique popliteal ligament
Insertion, distal attachment, attaches to:
Posterior medial part of the calcaneus with the calcaneal tendon
Innervation:
Tibial nerve (S1 to S2)
Major synergists:
Gastrocnemius and soleus
Major antagonists:
Tibialis anterior and quadriceps femoris group
Trigger points:
In the belly of the muscle at the back of the knee joint
Referred pain pattern:
Down the posterior leg to the heel and the sole of the foot into the plantar surface of the toes; can be a factor in knee pain and restricted mobility of the knee and ankle

Concentric action:
Plantar flexion of the foot at the ankle joint and inversion of the foot at the tarsal joints
Eccentric action:
Restrains dorsiflexion and eversion of the foot
Isometric action:
Stabilizes the ankle joint
Because of its thick, large venous sinuses, tough fascial covering, and vein structure, the soleus is an effective musculovenous pump that functions as a "second heart," especially during strenuous running and jumping activities.
Origin, proximal attachment, arises from:
Posterior surface of the head and proximal one third of the posterior surface of the fibula, soleal line of the tibia, and fibrous band between the tibia and the fibula
Insertion, distal attachment, attaches to:
Calcaneus (with the gastrocnemius) via the calcaneal (Achilles) tendon
Innervation:
Tibial nerve (S1 to S2)
Major synergist:
Gastrocnemius
Major antagonists:
Tibialis anterior, extensor digitorum longus, and extensor hallucis longus
Trigger points:
Near the proximal and distal attachments
Referred pain pattern:
Down the posterior leg to the heel and the sole of the foot into the plantar surface of the toes; can be a factor in knee pain and restricted mobility of the knee and ankle

Gastrocnemius (GAS-trok-NEEM-ee-us)

Gastrocnemius means "belly" and "leg."

Posterior

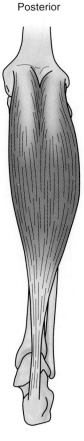

Concentric action:

Plantar flexion of the foot at the ankle joint, inversion of the foot at the tarsal joints, and flexion of the leg at the knee joint

Eccentric action:

Allows dorsiflexion and eversion of the foot and allows extension of the leg

Isometric action:

Stabilizes the knee and ankle joints and is involved in maintaining balance in static standing

Origin, proximal attachment, arises from:

Medial head—proximal posterior part of the medial condyle of the femur and capsule of the knee joint

Lateral head—distal part of the lateral supracondylar line and lateral condyle of the femur and capsule of the knee joint

Insertion, distal attachment, attaches to:

Calcaneus (with the soleus) by way of the calcaneal (Achilles) tendon

Innervation:

Tibial nerve (S1 to S2)

Major synergists:

Soleus and hamstring muscles

Major antagonists:

Tibialis anterior, extensor digitorum longus, extensor hallucis longus, and quadriceps femoris muscles

Trigger points:

In the belly of the muscle and at the attachment near the knee in each head of this muscle

Referred pain pattern:

Down the posterior leg to the heel and the sole of the foot into the plantar surface of the toes; can be a factor in knee pain and restricted mobility of the knee and ankle

ACTIVITY 9-28

Draw and color the **posterior leg muscles** in the spaces provided. For each muscle, do the following:

1. Label the origin and insertion attachment points: *O* for origin; *I* for insertion.

2. Place an X on the trigger points.
3. Palpate this muscle; identify the attachment points and the bellies of the muscles.
4. Move these muscles on yourself.

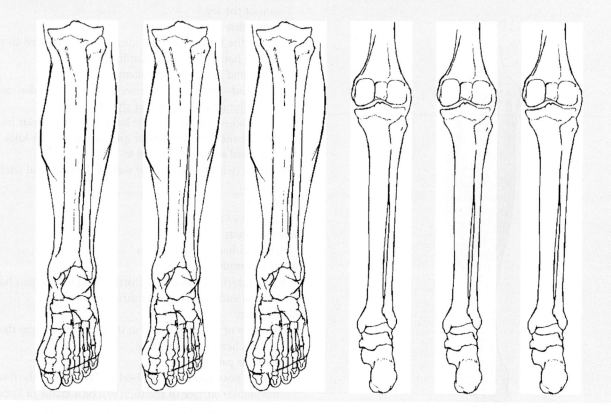

Intrinsic Muscles of the Foot

Intrinsic muscles of the foot are small muscles located entirely within the foot (i.e., they originate and insert within the foot). The muscles of the sole of the foot work concentrically and eccentrically to help flex, extend, abduct, and adduct the toes; they also work isometrically with the tendons of the leg muscles to support the arches of the foot. These muscles are numerous, their arrangement is complex, and their actions are interdependent. Although only the classic concentric mover functions of these muscles are listed, note that the primary function of these muscles is stabilization and proprioceptive feedback on foot position (Figure 9-25).

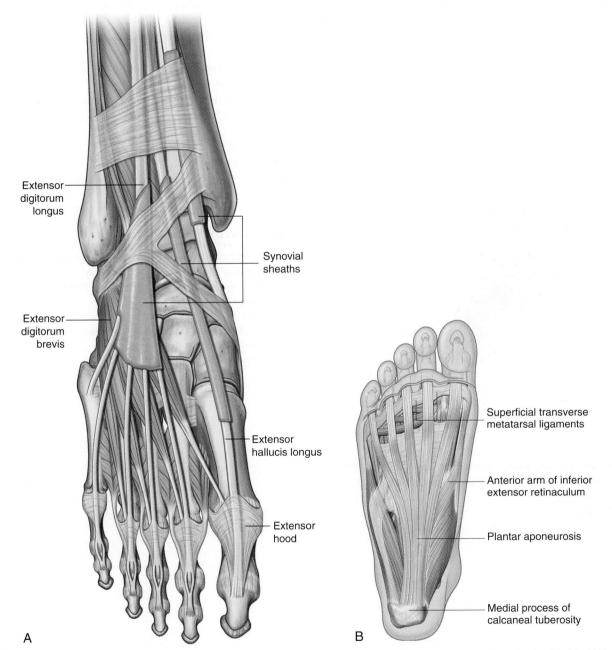

Extensor
digitorum
longus

Synovial
sheaths

Extensor
digitorum
brevis

Extensor
hallucis longus

Extensor
hood

Superficial transverse
metatarsal ligaments

Anterior arm of inferior
extensor retinaculum

Plantar aponeurosis

Medial process of
calcaneal tuberosity

A   B

FIGURE 9-25 A, Extensor digitorum brevis and dorsal interossei pedis muscles. **B,** Plantar aponeurosis. (From Drake RL, Vogl W, Mitchell WM: *Gray's anatomy for students,* ed 2, Edinburgh, 2010, Churchill Livingstone.)

Dorsal Aspect

Extensor digitorum brevis
(ex-STEN-sur DIH-jih-TOR-um BREV-us)

Extensor means "to stretch," *digitorum* means "related to the fingers or toes," and *brevis* means "short."

The most medial portion of the extensor digitorum brevis inserts into the dorsal surface of the base of the proximal phalanx of the big toe and sometimes is called the *extensor hallucis brevis muscle.*

Lateral

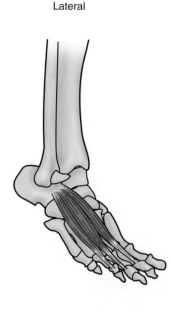

Concentric action:

Extension of the big toe at the metatarsophalangeal joint and extension of toes 2 to 4 at the metatarsophalangeal and interphalangeal joints

Eccentric action:

Restrains flexion of the big toe and flexion of toes 2 to 4

Origin, proximal attachment, arises from:

Dorsal surface of the calcaneus, lateral talocalcaneal ligament, and inferior extensor retinaculum

Insertion, distal attachment, attaches to:

First tendon into the dorsal surface of the base of the proximal phalanx of the great toe and lateral sides of the tendons of the extensor digitorum longus (dorsal digital expansion) to the second, third, and fourth toes

Innervation:

Deep fibular nerve (L5 to S1)

Major synergists:

Extensor digitorum longus and extensor hallucis longus

Major antagonists:

Flexor digitorum longus, flexor hallucis longus, and flexor digitorum brevis

Trigger points:

The belly of the muscle

Referred pain pattern:

The entire foot, with areas concentrated at the large toe, the ball of the foot, and the heel

ACTIVITY 9-29

Draw and color the **muscle of the dorsal aspect of the foot** in the space provided. Do the following:

1. Label the origin and insertion attachment points: *O* for origin; *I* for insertion.
2. Place an X on the trigger points.
3. Palpate this muscle; identify the attachment points and the bellies of the muscles.
4. Move muscle on yourself.

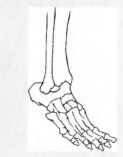

Plantar Aspect: Superficial Layer

Abductor hallucis (ab-DUCK-tur HAL-uh-siss)

Abductor means "to lead away from"; *hallucis* means "big toe."

Inferior

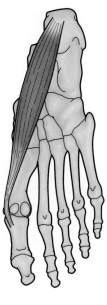

Flexor digitorum brevis (FLEKS-or DIH-jih-TOR-um BREV-us)

Flexor means "to bend," *digitorum* means "related to fingers or toes," and *brevis* means "short."

Inferior

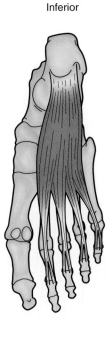

Concentric action:

Abduction and flexion of the big toe at the metatarsophalangeal joint

Eccentric action:

Restrains adduction and extension of the big toe

Origin, proximal attachment, arises from:

Medial process of the calcaneal tuberosity, flexor retinaculum, plantar aponeurosis, and adjacent intermuscular septum

Insertion, distal attachment, attaches to:

Medial side of the base of the proximal phalanx of the great toe

Innervation:

Medial plantar nerve (S1 to S2)

Major synergist:

Flexor hallucis brevis

Major antagonist:

Adductor hallucis

Trigger points:

The belly of the muscle

Referred pain pattern:

The entire foot, with areas concentrated at the large toe, the ball of the foot, and the heel

Concentric action:

Flexion of toes 2 to 5 at the metatarsophalangeal and proximal interphalangeal joints

Eccentric action:

Restrains extension of toes 2 to 5

Origin, proximal attachment, arises from:

Medial process of the calcaneal tuberosity, plantar aponeurosis, and adjacent intermuscular septa

Insertion, distal attachment, attaches to:

Medial and lateral sides of the middle phalanges of the second through fifth toes

Innervation:

Medial plantar nerve (S1 and S2)

Major synergists:

Flexor digitorum longus and quadratus plantae

Major antagonists:

Extensor digitorum longus and extensor digitorum brevis

Trigger points:

The belly of the muscle

Referred pain pattern:

The entire foot, with areas concentrated at the large toe, the ball of the foot, and the heel

Abductor digiti minimi pedis
(ab-DUCK-tur DIH-jih-tee MIN-ih-mee PEE-dis)

Abductor means "to lead away from," *digiti* means "related to the fingers or toes," *minimi* means "smallest," and *pedis* means "of the foot."

Inferior

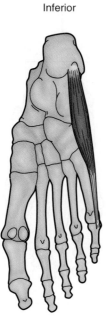

Concentric action:
Abduction and flexion of the little toe at the metatarsophalangeal joint

Eccentric action:
Restrains adduction and extension of the little toe

Origin, proximal attachment, arises from:
Lateral process of the calcaneal tuberosity, plantar aponeurosis, and intermuscular septum

Insertion, distal attachment, attaches to:
Lateral side of the base of the proximal phalanx of the fifth toe

Innervation:
Lateral plantar nerve (S2 to S3)

Major synergists:
Flexor digitorum brevis

Major antagonist:
Plantar interosseous (No. 3)

Trigger points:
The belly of the muscle

Referred pain pattern:
The entire foot, with areas concentrated at the large toe, the ball of the foot, and the heel

---

✏ **ACTIVITY 9-30**

Draw and color the **muscles of the plantar aspect (superficial layer) of the foot** in the spaces provided. For each muscle, do the following:
1. Label the origin and insertion attachment points: *O* for origin; *I* for insertion.
2. Place an X on the trigger points.
3. Palpate this muscle; identify the attachment points and the bellies of the muscles.
4. Move these muscles on yourself.

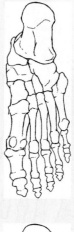

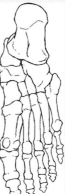

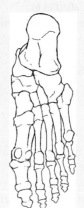

Plantar Aspect: Second Layer

Quadratus plantae (kwad-RATE-us PLAN-tie)

Quadratus means "square shaped"; *plantae* means "for the sole of the foot."

Inferior/Plantar surface

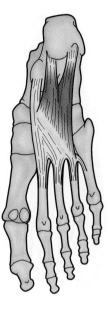

Lumbricals pedis (LUM-brih-kals PEE-dis)

Lumbricals means "earthworms"; *pedis* means "of the foot."

Inferior/Plantar surface

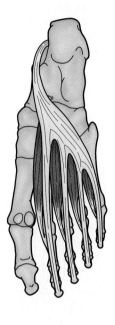

Concentric action:

Flexion of toes 2 to 5 at the metatarsophalangeal and interphalangeal joints (The quadratus plantae acts to modify the line of pull of the flexor digitorum longus.)

Eccentric action:

Restrains extension of toes 2 to 5

Origin, proximal attachment, arises from:

Medial head—medial surface of the calcaneus and medial border of the long plantar ligament

Lateral head—lateral inferior surface of the calcaneus, lateral border of the plantar surface of the calcaneus, and lateral border of the long plantar ligament

Insertion, distal attachment, attaches to:

Lateral margin of the flexor digitorum longus tendon

Innervation:

Lateral plantar nerve (S2 to S3)

Major synergists:

Flexor digitorum longus and flexor digitorum brevis

Major antagonists:

Extensor digitorum longus and extensor digitorum brevis

Trigger points:

The belly of the muscle

Referred pain pattern:

The entire foot, with areas concentrated at the large toe, the ball of the foot, and the heel

Concentric action:

Flexion of toes 2 to 5 at the metatarsophalangeal joints and extension of toes 2 to 5 at the proximal and distal interphalangeal joints

Eccentric action:

Restrains extension and flexion of toes 2 to 5

Origin, proximal attachment, arises from:

First—From the medial side of the first flexor digitorum longus tendon

Second—From adjacent sides of the first and second flexor digitorum longus tendons

Third—From adjacent sides of the second and third flexor digitorum longus tendons

Fourth—From adjacent sides of the third and fourth flexor digitorum longus tendons

Insertion, distal attachment, attaches to:

Distal tendons of the extensor digitorum longus (dorsal digital expansion) into the base of the middle and distal phalanges of the second through fifth toes

Innervation:

Medial and lateral plantar nerves (S1 to S3)

Major synergists:

Flexor digitorum longus and extensor digitorum longus

Major antagonists:

Flexor digitorum longus and extensor digitorum longus

Trigger points:

The belly of the muscle

Referred pain pattern:

The entire foot, with areas concentrated at the large toe, the ball of the foot, and the heel

ACTIVITY 9-31

Draw and color the **muscles of the plantar aspect (second layer) of the foot** in the spaces provided. For each muscle, do the following:

1. Label the origin and insertion attachment points: *O* for origin; *I* for insertion.
2. Place an X on the trigger points.
3. Palpate this muscle; identify the attachment points and the bellies of the muscles.
4. Move these muscles on yourself.

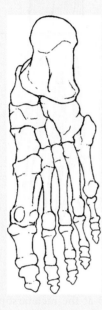

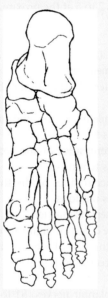

Plantar Aspect: Third Layer

Flexor hallucis brevis (FLEKS-or HAL-uh-siss BREV-us)

Flexor means "to bend," *hallucis* means "big toe," and *brevis* means "short."

Inferior

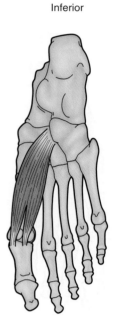

Concentric action:
Flexion of the big toe at the metatarsophalangeal joint
Eccentric action:
Restrains extension of the big toe
Origin, proximal attachment, arises from:
Medial aspect of the plantar surface of the cuboid bone, lateral cuneiform bone, and from the tendon of the tibialis posterior
Insertion, distal attachment, attaches to:
Medial and lateral sides of the base of the proximal phalanx of the great toe
Innervation:
Medial plantar nerve (S1 to S2)
Major synergist:
Flexor hallucis longus
Major antagonists:
Extensor hallucis longus and extensor digitorum brevis (medial part)
Trigger points:
The belly of the muscle
Referred pain pattern:
The entire foot, with areas concentrated at the large toe, the ball of the foot, and the heel

Adductor hallucis (ad-DUCK-tur HAL-uh-siss)

Adductor means "to lead toward"; *hallucis* means "big toe."

Inferior/Plantar surface

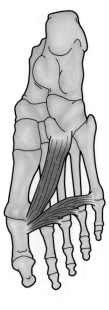

Concentric action:

Adduction and flexion of the big toe at the metatarsophalangeal joint

Eccentric action:

Restrains abduction and extension of the big toe

Origin, proximal attachment, arises from:

Oblique head—bases of the second, third, and fourth metatarsal bones and sheath of the tendon of the fibularis longus

Transverse head—plantar metatarsophalangeal ligaments of the third, fourth, and fifth digits and deep transverse metatarsal ligament of the sole

Insertion, distal attachment, attaches to:

Lateral side of the base of the proximal phalanx of the big toe

Innervation:

Lateral plantar nerve (S2 to S3)

Major synergists:

Flexor hallucis longus and flexor hallucis brevis

Major antagonist:

Abductor hallucis

Trigger points:

The belly of the muscle

Referred pain pattern:

The entire foot with areas concentrated at the large toe, the ball of the foot, and the heel

Flexor digiti minimi pedis
(FLEKS-or DIH-jih-tee MIN-ih-mee PEE-dis)

Flexor means "to bend," *digiti* means "related to the fingers and toes," *minimi* means "smallest," and *pedis* means "of the foot."

Occasionally, some of the deeper fibers of the flexor digiti minimi pedis reach the lateral part of the distal half of the fifth metatarsal bone; this sometimes is described as a distinct muscle, the opponens digiti minimi pedis.

Inferior

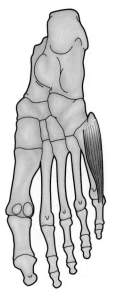

Concentric action:

Flexion of the little toe at the metatarsophalangeal joint

Eccentric action:

Restrains extension of the little toe

Origin, proximal attachment, arises from:

Medial part of the plantar surface of the base of the fifth metatarsal bone and sheath of the fibularis longus

Insertion, distal attachment, attaches to:

Plantar surface of the base of the proximal phalanx of the little toe

Innervation:

Lateral plantar nerve (S2 to S3)

Major synergists:

Flexor digitorum longus and flexor digitorum brevis

Major antagonist:

Extensor digitorum longus

Trigger points:

The belly of the muscle

Referred pain pattern:

The entire foot, with areas concentrated at the large toe, the ball of the foot, and the heel

✏ ACTIVITY 9-32

Draw and color the **muscles of the plantar aspect (third layer) of the foot** in the spaces provided. For each muscle, do the following:

1. Label the origin and insertion attachment points: *O* for origin; *I* for insertion.
2. Place an X on the trigger points.
3. Palpate this muscle; identify the attachment points and the bellies of the muscles.
4. Move these muscles on yourself.

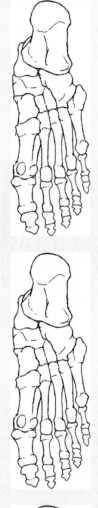

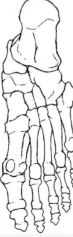

Plantar Aspect: Fourth Layer

▌ *Plantar interossei* (plan-TAR INT-er-OSS-ee-eye)

Plantar means "sole of the foot"; *interossei* means "between the bones."

Inferior

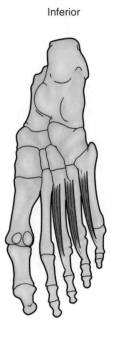

Concentric action:

Adduction of toes 3 to 5 at the metatarsophalangeal joints (adduction of a toe is a movement toward an imaginary line drawn through the middle of the second toe), flexion of toes 3 to 5 at the metatarsophalangeal joints, and extension of toes 3 to 5 at the proximal and distal interphalangeal joints

Eccentric action:

Restrains abduction, extension, and flexion of toes 3 to 5

Origin, proximal attachment, arises from:

Three plantar interossei arise from the base and medial sides of the shafts of the third, fourth, and fifth metatarsals.

Insertion, distal attachment, attaches to:

Medial sides of the bases of the proximal phalanges of the same toes and the dorsal digital expansion

Innervation:

Lateral plantar nerve (S2 to S3)

Major synergists:

Lumbricals pedis

Major antagonists:

Dorsal interossei pedis

Trigger points:

The belly of the muscle

Referred pain pattern:

The entire foot, with areas concentrated at the large toe, the ball of the foot, and the heel

Dorsal interossei pedis
(DOOR-sul INT-er-OSS-ee-eye PEE-dis)

Doral means "on or near the back," *interossei* means "between the bones," and *pedis* means "of the foot."

Inferior

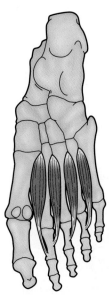

Concentric action:

Abduction of toes 2 to 4 at the metatarsophalangeal joints (abduction of a toe is a movement away from an imaginary line drawn through the middle of the second toe), flexion of toes 2 to 4 at the metatarsophalangeal joints, and extension of toes 2 to 4 at the proximal and distal interphalangeal joints

Eccentric action:

Restrains adduction, extension, and flexion of toes 2 to 4.

Origin, proximal attachment, arises from:

Each arises by way of two heads from adjacent sides of the metatarsal bones between which they are placed.

Insertion, distal attachment, attaches to:

Bases of the proximal phalanges of toes 2 to 4 and distal tendons of the extensor digitorum longus (dorsal digital expansion)

Innervation:

Lateral plantar nerve (S2 to S3)

Major synergists:

Lumbricals pedis

Major antagonists:

Plantar interossei

Trigger points:

The belly of the muscle

Referred pain pattern:

The entire foot, with areas concentrated at the large toe, the ball of the foot, and the heel

---

ACTIVITY 9-33

Draw and color the **muscles of the plantar aspect (fourth layer) of the foot** in the spaces provided. For each muscle, do the following:
1. Label the origin and insertion attachment points: *O* for origin; *I* for insertion.
2. Place an X on the trigger points.
3. Palpate this muscle; identify the attachment points and the bellies of the muscles.
4. Move these muscles on yourself.

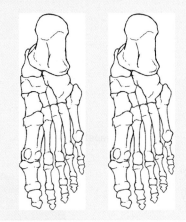

Muscles of Scapular Stabilization

The muscles of scapular stabilization hold the scapula to the rib cage (wall of the thorax) when acting isometrically and move the scapula during concentric and eccentric function (Figure 9-26). The arrangement of the muscle attachments to the scapula requires cooperative concentric, eccentric, and isometric interaction to produce movement. Several muscles must act together to elevate or depress the scapula or to create other scapular movements at the scapulocostal joint.

The prime movers of scapular elevation at the scapulocostal joint (shrugging the shoulder) are the upper trapezius and the levator scapulae. The opposite rotational effects of the trapezius and levator scapulae on the scapula counterbalance each other.

Scapular depression at the scapulocostal joint results largely from gravitational pull, but when the scapula is depressed against resistance, the lower trapezius and serratus anterior are active. Serratus anterior activity creates the forward (pushing) movements of protraction (abduction) of the scapula at the scapulocostal joint on the chest wall. The trapezius and the rhomboid muscles provide retraction (adduction) of the scapula at the scapulocostal joint.

Although the serratus anterior and trapezius muscles are antagonists in the anterior/posterior movements of the scapula, they act together to create upward rotation of the scapula at the scapulocostal joint.

Clavicular movements accompany scapular movements. The clavicles rotate around their own axes as they move with scapular movements, giving stability and precision to these movements. Therapeutic massage methods easily address these more superficial muscles.

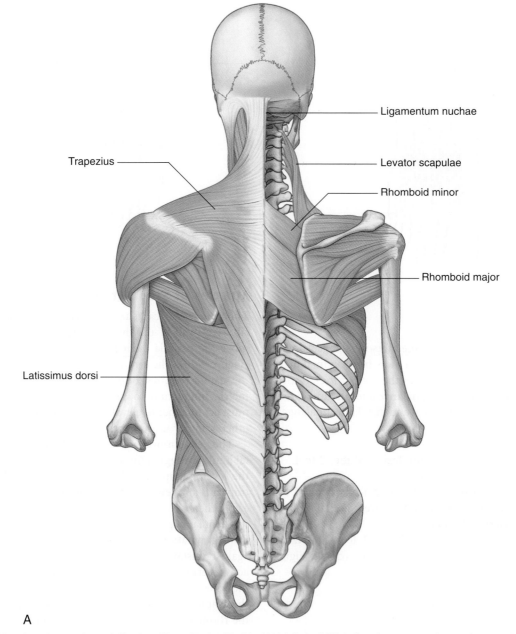

A

FIGURE 9-26 Muscles of scapular stabilization. (From Drake RL, Vogl W, Mitchell WM: *Gray's anatomy for students,* ed 2, Edinburgh, 2010, Churchill Livingstone.)

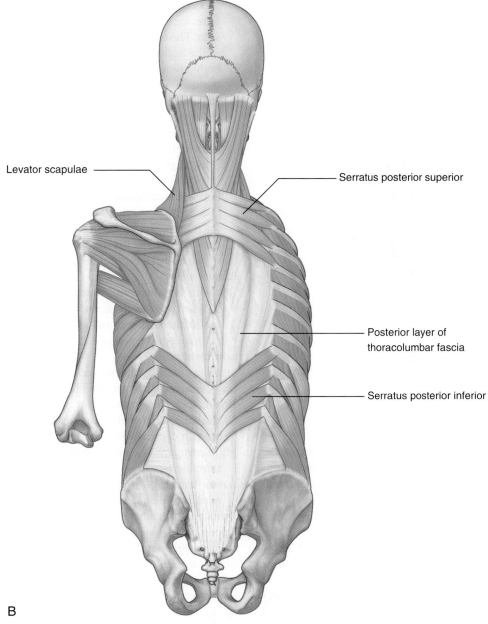

Levator scapulae

Serratus posterior superior

Posterior layer of
thoracolumbar fascia

Serratus posterior inferior

B

FIGURE 9-26, cont'd.

Trapezius (tra-PEE-zee-us)

Trapezius means "a figure with four unequal sides" (a trapezoid).

The trapezius usually is considered to consist of three functional parts: the upper trapezius, middle trapezius, and lower trapezius. Concentric, eccentric, and isometric contraction can occur simultaneously in different aspects of the muscle.

Posterior

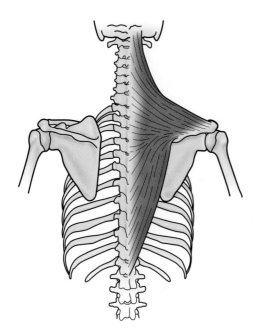

Concentric action:

Extension, lateral flexion, and contralateral rotation of the neck and head at the spinal joints (upper trapezius); elevation of the scapula at the scapulocostal joint (upper trapezius); retraction of the scapula at the scapulocostal joint (entire trapezius); depression of the scapula at the scapulocostal joint (lower trapezius); upward rotation of the scapula at the scapulocostal joint (upper and lower trapezius); and extension of the trunk at the spinal joints (middle and lower trapezius)

Many books divide the actions of the trapezius (and other muscles of the neck and trunk) into the actions created when the muscle contracts on one side (unilaterally) and when the right and left muscles contract (bilaterally). In this division they often describe these actions in a manner that may be misleading. For example, they might state that the unilateral contraction of the upper trapezius causes lateral flexion and contralateral rotation of the neck at the spinal joints and that bilateral contraction of the upper trapezius muscles causes extension of the neck at the spinal joints. Although the bilateral trapezius contraction causes extension of the neck (and is pure extension because the

opposite lateral flexions and opposite rotations cancel each other out), unilateral trapezius contraction also causes extension of the neck. This may not be immediately understood when actions are worded this way. No muscle can cause extension bilaterally if it cannot cause extension unilaterally.

What is valuable to take from this type of description is that when any muscle of the neck and trunk contracts bilaterally, its lateral flexion and rotation components always cancel each other out, and the resulting joint action is a pure sagittal plane movement—that is, flexion or extension. The other important thing to realize with all muscles of the neck and trunk is that the muscle on one side of the body always can be an antagonist to the same muscle on the other side of the body. For example, the right upper trapezius causes right lateral flexion of the neck, and the left upper trapezius causes left lateral flexion of the neck; hence they are antagonistic. Also, the right upper trapezius causes left rotation of the neck, and the left upper trapezius causes right rotation of the neck; hence they are antagonistic. Of course, regarding extension of the neck, because both sides can cause extension of the neck, they are synergistic. These principles are true and should be kept in mind for all muscles of the neck and trunk. As a rule, this text does not usually list the same muscle on the opposite side of the body in the synergist and antagonist sections.

Eccentric action:

Restrains flexion, contralateral lateral flexion, and ipsilateral rotation of the neck and head; depression, protraction (abduction), elevation, and downward rotation of the scapula; and flexion of the trunk

Isometric action:

Stabilizes the scapula and cervical spine

Origin, proximal attachment, arises from:

Upper trapezius—external occipital protuberance; superior nuchal line, nuchal ligament; and spinous process of the seventh cervical vertebrae

Middle trapezius—spinous processes of the first through fifth thoracic vertebrae

Lower trapezius—spinous processes of the sixth through twelfth thoracic vertebrae

Insertion, distal attachment, attaches to:

Upper trapezius—lateral one third of the clavicle and acromion process of the scapula

Middle trapezius—acromion process and spine of the scapula

Lower trapezius—root of the spine of the scapula

Innervation:

Spinal accessory nerve (cervical nerve XI) and ventral rami of third and fourth cervical spinal nerves

Major synergists:

Upper trapezius—semispinalis capitis, levator scapulae, serratus anterior, and sternocleidomastoid

Middle trapezius—rhomboid muscles and spinal extensors

Lower trapezius—serratus anterior, pectoralis minor, and spinal extensors

Major antagonists:

Upper trapezius—lower trapezius, rhomboid muscles, and flexors of the neck

Middle trapezius—pectoralis minor and serratus anterior
Lower trapezius—upper trapezius and levator scapulae
Trigger points:
Upper trapezius near the acromion and clavicular attachments, middle trapezius near the spine of the scapula, and lower trapezius in the belly of the muscle
Referred pain patterns:
Neck posterior to the ear and to the temple, subscapular area, and acromial pain

Rhomboid major (ROM-boyd) (rhomboideus major)

Rhomboideus means "shaped like a rhombus" (a diamond shape); *major* means "larger."

Posterior

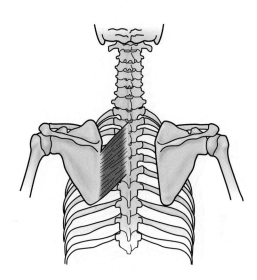

Concentric action:
Retraction (adduction), elevation, and downward rotation of the scapula at the scapulocostal joint
Eccentric action:
Restrains protraction (abduction), depression, and upward rotation of the scapula
Isometric action:
Stabilizes the scapula
Origin, proximal attachment, arises from:
Spinous processes of the second through fifth thoracic vertebrae
Insertion, distal attachment, attaches to:
Medial border of the scapula, between the spine and the inferior angle
Innervation:
Dorsal scapular nerve (C4 to C5)
Major synergists:
Rhomboideus minor, trapezius, levator scapulae, and pectoralis minor
Major antagonists:
Serratus anterior, pectoralis minor, and trapezius
Trigger points:
At the attachment point near the scapular border
Referred pain pattern:
Scapular region

▌*Rhomboid minor (ROM-boyd) (rhomboideus minor)*

Rhomboideus means "shaped like a rhombus" (a diamond shape); *minor* means "smaller."

Posterior

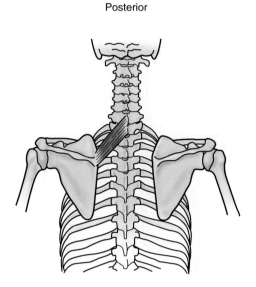

Concentric action:

Retraction (adduction), elevation, and downward rotation of the scapula at the scapulocostal joint

Eccentric action:

Restrains protraction, depression, and upward rotation of the scapula

Isometric action:

Stabilizes the scapula

Origin, proximal attachment, arises from:

Ligamentum nuchae and spinous processes of the seventh cervical and first thoracic vertebrae

Insertion, distal attachment, attaches to:

Medial border of the scapula at the root of the spine of the scapula

Innervation:

Dorsal scapular nerve (C4 to C5)

Major synergists:

Rhomboideus major, trapezius, levator scapulae, and pectoralis minor

Major antagonists:

Serratus anterior, pectoralis minor, and trapezius

Trigger points:

At the attachment point near the scapular border

Referred pain pattern:

Scapular region

▌*Levator scapulae* (le-VAY-tor SKAP-you-lee)

Levator scapulae means "to elevate the scapula."

Posterior

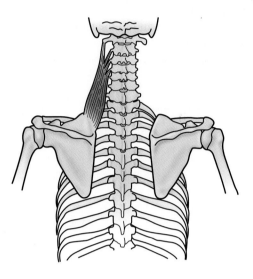

Concentric action:

Elevation and retraction (adduction) of the scapula at the scapulocostal joint and extension, lateral flexion, and ipsilateral rotation of the neck at the spinal joints

Eccentric action:

Allows depression and protraction (abduction) of the scapula and restrains flexion, contralateral lateral flexion, and contralateral rotation of the neck

Isometric action:

Stabilizes cervical/scapular function

Origin, proximal attachment, arises from:

Transverse processes of the atlas and axis and the third and fourth cervical vertebrae

Insertion, distal attachment, attaches to:

Medial border of the scapula between the superior angle and the root of the spine

The levator scapulae is a large muscle and has a rotation, or twist, that occurs in its design such that the attachments at the atlas and axis are from muscle fibers that attach to the inferior portion of the medial border of the scapula and the attachments at C4 are from fibers at the superior portion of the medial border.

Innervation:

Dorsal scapular nerve (C3 to C5)

Major synergists:

Splenius cervicis and the upper trapezius

Major antagonists:

Serratus anterior and the sternocleidomastoid

Trigger points:

Belly of the muscle just as it begins the twist in its fibers and at the attachment near the scapula

Referred pain patterns:

Angle of the neck at the trigger point and along the vertebral border of the scapula and stiff neck in rotation

Pectoralis minor (PEK-tor-al-iss)

Pectoralis means "related to the chest"; *minor* means "smaller."

Anterior

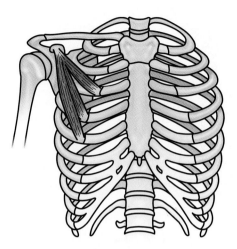

Concentric action:

Protraction (abduction), depression, and downward rotation of the scapula at the scapulocostal joint and elevation of ribs 3 to 5 at the sternocostal and costovertebral joints (This action assists in forced inspiration; therefore, the pectoralis minor is an accessory respiratory muscle.)

Eccentric action:

Allows retraction (adduction), elevation, and upward rotation of the scapula and allows depression of ribs 3 to 5

Isometric action:

Stabilizes the scapula

Origin, proximal attachment, arises from:

Third, fourth, and fifth ribs near the cartilage and the aponeurosis covering the intercostal muscles

Insertion, distal attachment, attaches to:

Coracoid process of the scapula

Innervation:

Medial and lateral pectoral nerves (C5 to T1)

Major synergists:

Serratus anterior, rhomboid muscles, and lower trapezius

Major antagonists:

Rhomboid muscles and upper trapezius

Trigger points:

Near the attachment at the coracoid process and at the belly of the muscle

Referred pain pattern:

May mimic angina; front of the chest from the shoulder and down the ulnar side of the arm into the fingers

Serratus anterior (suhr-RATE-us)

Serratus means "sawlike"; *anterior* means "toward the front."

Lateral

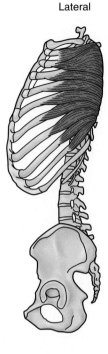

Concentric action:

Protraction (abduction) and upward rotation of the scapula at the scapulocostal joint and elevation of ribs 7 to 9 (assisting forced inspiration; therefore the serratus anterior is an accessory muscle of respiration)

Eccentric action:

Restrains retraction and downward rotation of the scapula

Isometric action:

Holds the medial border of the scapula firmly against the thorax, thereby preventing winging of the scapula

Origin, proximal attachment, arises from:

External surfaces and superior borders of the upper eight or nine ribs

Insertion, distal attachment, attaches to:

Costal surface of the medial border of the scapula

This muscle lies along the rib cage and is deep to the scapula.

Innervation:

Long thoracic nerve (C5 to C7)

Major synergists:

Pectoralis minor and upper trapezius

Major antagonists:

Rhomboid muscles and middle trapezius

Trigger points:

Along the midaxillary line near the ribs

Referred pain patterns:

Side and back of the chest and down the ulnar aspect of the arm into the hand

Injury may result in shortness of breath and pain during inhalation.

✎ ACTIVITY **9-34**

Draw and color the **muscles of scapular stabilization** in the spaces provided. For each muscle, do the following:

1. Label the origin and insertion attachment points: *O* for origin; *I* for insertion.

2. Place an X on the trigger points.
3. Palpate this muscle; identify the attachment points and the bellies of the muscles.
4. Move these muscles on yourself.

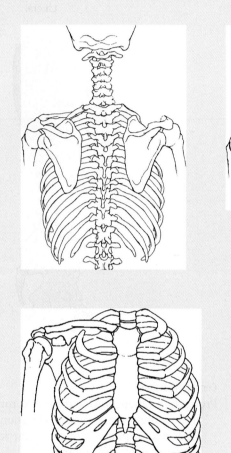

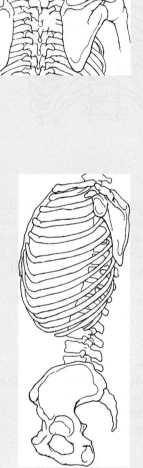

Muscles of the Musculotendinous (Rotator) Cuff

Nine muscles cross over the ball-and-socket joint of the shoulder to stabilize and move this joint (Figure 9-27). Of these nine, the four "SITS" muscles are known as the rotator cuff muscles: the *s*upraspinatus, *i*nfraspinatus, *t*eres minor, and *s*ubscapularis. These muscles originate on the scapula, and their distal tendons blend into each other (and with the fibrous capsule of the shoulder joint). The main functions of these muscles are to hold the head of the humerus in the glenoid cavity and to reinforce the joint capsule; therefore they often sustain isometric contraction. The massage therapist can access all these muscles (except for the subscapularis) easily during massage. Because the subscapularis is located deep to the scapula, the best access position is supine with pressure applied through the axilla and toward the scapula. Caution must be taken not to press on the nerves and vessels in the area.

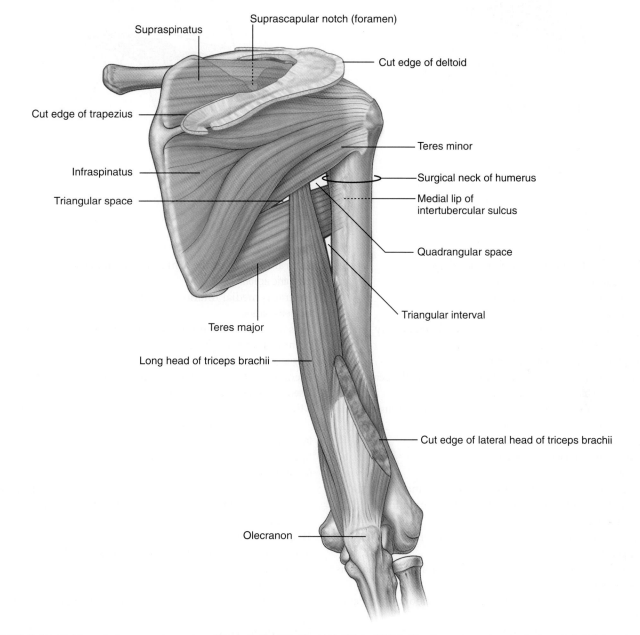

FIGURE 9-27 Right posterior scapular region. (From Drake RL, Vogl W, Mitchell WM: *Gray's anatomy for students,* ed 2, Edinburgh, 2010, Churchill Livingstone.)

Supraspinatus (SOO-prah-spy-NAH-tus)

Supraspinatus means "above the spine" (of the scapula).

Posterior

Infraspinatus (in-fra-spy-NAH-tus)

Infraspinatus means "below the spine" (of the scapula).

Posterior

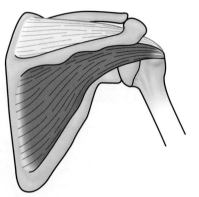

Concentric action:
Abduction of the arm at the shoulder joint
Eccentric action:
Restrains adduction of the arm
Isometric action:
Acts to stabilize the humeral head in the glenoid cavity during movements of the arm
Origin, proximal attachment, arises from:
Medial two thirds of the supraspinous fossa of the scapula
Insertion, distal attachment, attaches to:
Superior facet of the greater tubercle of the humerus and the capsule of the shoulder joint
Innervation:
Suprascapular nerve (C5 to C6)
Major synergist:
Deltoid (The rotator cuff muscles assist one another in stabilizing the head of the humerus in the glenoid fossa.)
Major antagonists:
Latissimus dorsi, teres major, and pectoralis major
Trigger points:
In the belly of the muscle and near the tendon at the humerus
Referred pain pattern:
Shoulder, deltoid, and down the arm to the elbow, often experienced as a dull ache

Concentric action:
Lateral rotation of the arm at the shoulder joint
Eccentric action:
Restrains medial rotation of the arm
Isometric action:
Acts to stabilize the humeral head in the glenoid cavity during movements of the arm
Origin, proximal attachment, arises from:
Medial two thirds of the infraspinous fossa
Insertion, distal attachment, attaches to:
Middle facet of the greater tubercle of the humerus and the capsule of the shoulder joint
Innervation:
Suprascapular nerve (C5 to C6)
Major synergists:
Teres minor and posterior deltoid (The rotator cuff muscles assist one another in stabilizing the head of the humerus in the glenoid fossa.)
Major antagonists:
Subscapularis, pectoralis major, anterior deltoid, latissimus dorsi, and teres major
Trigger points:
Belly of the muscle below the spine of the scapula and near the medial border of the scapula
Referred pain patterns:
Deep into the shoulder and deltoid area, down the arm, suboccipital area, and medial border of the scapula, which limits the ability to reach behind the back

▌*Teres minor* (TER-eez)

Teres means "smooth and round"; *minor* means "smaller."

Posterior

▌*Subscapularis* (sub-SKAP-you-LAR-iss)

Subscapularis means "under (deep to) the shoulder blade." This muscle often is implicated in "frozen shoulder" syndromes.

Anterior

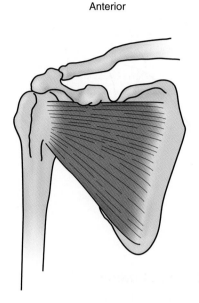

Concentric action:
Lateral rotation and adduction of the arm at the shoulder joint
Eccentric action:
Restrains medial rotation and abduction of the arm
Isometric action:
Acts to stabilize the humeral head in the glenoid cavity during movements of the arm
Origin, proximal attachment, arises from:
Superior two thirds, dorsal surface of the lateral border of the scapula
Insertion, distal attachment, attaches to:
Inferior facet of the greater tubercle of the humerus and the capsule of the shoulder joint
Innervation:
Axillary nerve (C5 to C6)
Major synergists:
Infraspinatus, posterior deltoid, and latissimus dorsi (The rotator cuff muscles assist one another in stabilizing the head of the humerus in the glenoid fossa.)
Major antagonists:
Subscapularis, pectoralis major, anterior deltoid, and supraspinatus
Trigger points:
Belly of the muscle closer to the attachment on the humerus
Referred pain pattern:
Posterior deltoid region often has limited range of motion for reaching behind the back, such as putting hands in the back pocket of pants.

Concentric action:
Medial rotation of the arm at the shoulder joint
Eccentric action:
Restrains lateral rotation of the arm
Isometric action:
Acts to stabilize the humeral head in the glenoid cavity during movements of the arm
Origin, proximal attachment, arises from:
Subscapular fossa of the scapula
Insertion, distal attachment, attaches to:
Lesser tubercle of the humerus and the capsule of the shoulder joint
Innervation:
Upper and lower subscapular nerves (C5 to C6)
Major synergists:
Pectoralis major, anterior deltoid, latissimus dorsi, and teres major (The rotator cuff muscles assist one another in stabilizing the head of the humerus in the glenoid fossa.)
Major antagonists:
Infraspinatus, teres minor, and posterior deltoid
Trigger points:
Access through the axilla near the attachment at the humerus and in the belly of the muscle
Referred pain pattern:
Posterior deltoid, scapular region, triceps area and into the wrist; often mistaken for bursitis because the pain often refers to insertion at the shoulder

✎ ACTIVITY **9-35**

Draw and color the **muscles of the rotator cuff** in the spaces provided. For each muscle, do the following:

1. Label the origin and insertion attachment points: *O* for origin; *I* for insertion.

2. Place an X on the trigger points.

3. Palpate this muscle; identify the attachment points and the bellies of the muscles.

4. Move these muscles on yourself.

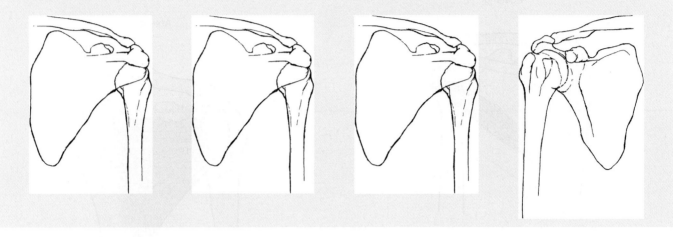

Muscles of the Shoulder Joint

In general, any muscle that crosses the shoulder joint anteriorly can flex the arm at the shoulder joint, and any muscle that crosses the shoulder joint posteriorly can extend the arm at the shoulder joint (Figure 9-28). The deltoid is the prime mover of arm abduction at the shoulder joint but also is involved in flexion and extension of the arm at the shoulder joint. The main antagonists to abduction of the arm at the shoulder joint are the pectoralis major anteriorly and the latissimus dorsi posteriorly. Depending on the location and insertion points, the various muscles acting on the arm also provide lateral (external) and medial (internal) rotation of the arm at the shoulder joint. The interaction of these muscles is complex, and each muscle contributes to more than one movement.

Because these muscles are active during walking, all gait reflexes are involved with the shoulder muscles to promote the appropriate counterbalancing arm swing to the thigh swing. Facilitation occurs between muscles of the arms that flex and extend in conjunction with thigh muscles during contralateral gait patterns. The massage therapist often needs to consider the muscles of the shoulder joint with muscles of the hip joint and provide massage in a correlated pattern to be most effective. Although not listed with synergists, the shoulder joint flexors on one side work with hip joint flexors on the opposite side. Adductors and medial rotators of the arm at the shoulder joint on one side work with adductors and medial rotators of the thigh at the hip joint on the opposite side. The same pattern applies to lateral rotation. These muscles inhibit muscles on the same side of the body—that is, medial rotation of the arm at the shoulder joint and thigh at the hip joint on the right inhibit each other, as do the lateral rotators. Obviously, the same patterns occur on the left. Also, during normal gait, flexors and extensors of the arm at the shoulder joints interact. The flexors on the right work with extensors on the left and inhibit flexors on the left, and vice versa. The extensors on the right work with flexors on the left and inhibit the extensors on the left, and vice versa. Although this seems confusing, the patterns become apparent when observing gait. To understand this, the student should take a step—freeze—and then notice which muscles are interacting.

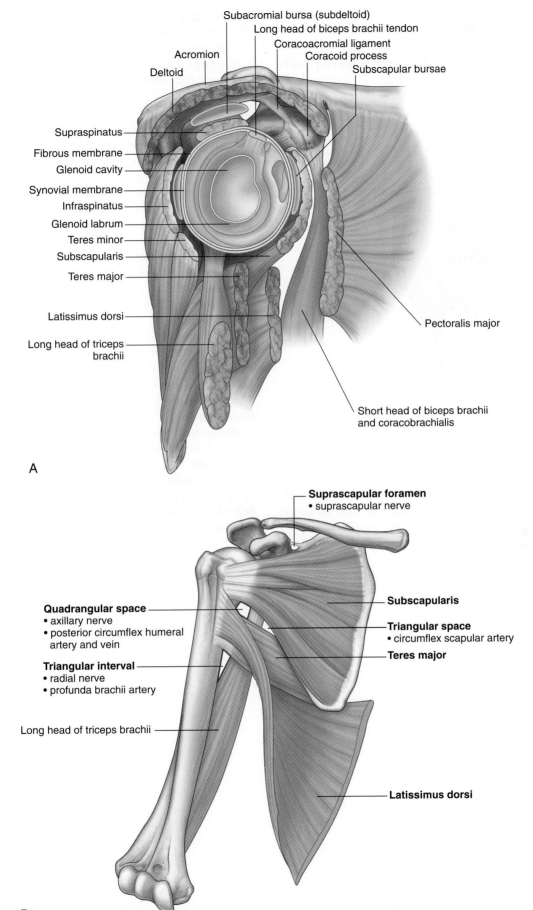

Subacromial bursa (subdeltoid)
Long head of biceps brachii tendon
Coracoacromial ligament
Coracoid process
Acromion
Subscapular bursae

Deltoid

Supraspinatus

Fibrous membrane

Glenoid cavity

Synovial membrane

Infraspinatus

Glenoid labrum

Teres minor

Subscapularis

Teres major

Latissimus dorsi

Long head of triceps
brachii

Pectoralis major

Short head of biceps brachii
and coracobrachialis

A

Suprascapular foramen
• suprascapular nerve

Quadrangular space
• axillary nerve
• posterior circumflex humeral
artery and vein

Triangular interval
• radial nerve
• profunda brachii artery

Long head of triceps brachii

Subscapularis

Triangular space
• circumflex scapular artery

Teres major

Latissimus dorsi

B

FIGURE 9-28 A, Lateral view of right glenohumeral joint and surrounding muscles with proximal end of humerus removed. **B,** Posterior wall of the axilla. (From Drake RL, Vogl W, Mitchell WM: *Gray's anatomy for students,* ed 2, Edinburgh, 2010, Churchill Livingstone.)

Deltoid (DEL-toyd) (deltoideus)

Deltoid means "triangular."

This muscle functions in three distinct patterns and can be thought of as three different muscles.

Lateral

Concentric action:

Anterior deltoid—flexion, medial rotation, and abduction of the arm at the shoulder joint

Middle deltoid—abduction of the arm at the shoulder joint

Posterior deltoid—extension, lateral rotation, and abduction of the arm at the shoulder joint

Eccentric action:

The anterior deltoid muscle restrains extension, lateral rotation, and adduction of the arm. The middle deltoid muscle restrains adduction of the arm. The posterior deltoid muscle restrains flexion, medial rotation, and adduction of the arm.

Isometric action:

Stabilizes glenohumeral joint during arm movement

Origin, proximal attachment, arises from:

Anterior deltoid—superior surface, lateral third of the clavicle

Middle deltoid—lateral margin of the spine of the scapula and superior surface of the acromion

Posterior deltoid—posterior border of the spine of the scapula

Insertion, distal attachment, attaches to:

Deltoid tuberosity of the humerus

Innervation:

Axillary nerve (C5 to C6)

Major synergists:

Anterior deltoid—coracobrachialis, clavicular head of the pectoralis major, and biceps brachii

Middle deltoid—supraspinatus

Posterior deltoid—latissimus dorsi, teres major, and infraspinatus

Major antagonists:

Pectoralis major and latissimus dorsi; the anterior and posterior deltoid muscles are antagonistic to each other.

Trigger points:

Anterior deltoid—near the clavicular attachment

Posterior and middle deltoid—in the belly of the muscles

Referred pain pattern:

Deltoid region and down the lateral side of the arm

Pectoralis major (PEK-tor-al-iss)

Pectoralis means "of the chest"; *major* means "larger."

Anterior

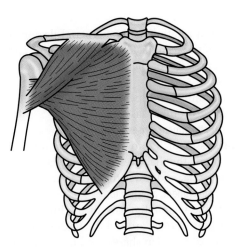

Concentric action:
Entire muscle—adduction and medial rotation of the arm at the shoulder joint
Clavicular head—flexion of the arm at the shoulder joint
Sternocostal head—extension of the arm at the shoulder joint
Eccentric action:
Restrains abduction and lateral rotation of the arm and also can restrain extension and flexion of the arm
Isometric action:
Stabilizes the shoulder during overhead activity
Origin, proximal attachment, arises from:
Ventral surface of the sternum down to the seventh rib, medial half of the clavicle, cartilage of ribs 1 to 7, and aponeurosis of the external abdominal oblique muscle
Insertion, distal attachment, attaches to:
Lateral lip of the bicipital groove of the humerus
The attachment pattern for this muscle is complex and consists of several overlapping sheets of muscles in a fan arrangement with a spiraling distal attachment. The muscle is divided into clavicular, sternal, costal, and abdominal sections, each able to function independently.
Innervation:
Medial and lateral pectoral nerves (C5 to T1)
Major synergists:
Clavicular head—anterior deltoid and coracobrachialis
Sternocostal head—latissimus dorsi and teres major
Major antagonists:
Clavicular head—latissimus dorsi and teres major
Sternocostal head—anterior deltoid, supraspinatus, infraspinatus, and teres minor
Trigger points:
Belly of the muscle
Referred pain pattern:
Chest and breast and down the ulnar aspect of the arm and forearm to the fourth and fifth fingers

Subclavius (sub-KLAVE-ee-us)

Subclavius means "below" and "little key" (referring to the clavicle).
This muscle often is considered with the clavicular portion of the pectoralis major.

Anterior

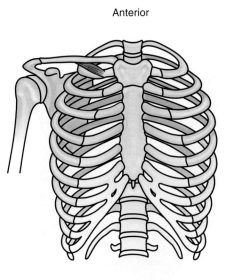

Concentric action:
Protraction and depression of the clavicle at the sternoclavicular joint
Eccentric action:
Restrains retraction and elevation of the clavicle at the sternoclavicular joint
Isometric action:
Stabilizes the clavicle
Origin, proximal attachment, arises from:
Junction of the first rib and its costal cartilage
Insertion, distal attachment, attaches to:
Inferior surface of the clavicle
Innervation:
Fifth and sixth cervical nerves (C5 to C6)
Major synergists:
Deltoid muscle and pectoralis major
Major antagonists:
Sternocleidomastoid and upper trapezius
Trigger points:
Belly of the muscle
Referred pain pattern:
Chest and breast region

Latissimus dorsi (la-TISS-ih-mus DOR-see)

Latissimus means "widest"; *dorsi* means "belonging to the back."

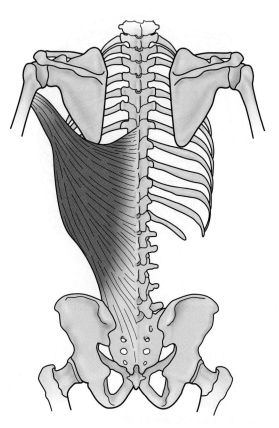

Posterior

Concentric action:

Medial rotation, adduction, and extension of the arm at the shoulder joint; depression of the scapula at the scapulocostal joint; extension of the trunk at the spinal joints; and anterior tilt and elevation of the pelvis at the lumbosacral joint

Eccentric action:

Restrains lateral rotation, abduction, and flexion of the arm, elevation of the scapula, flexion of the trunk, and posterior tilt and depression of the pelvis

Isometric action:

Stabilizes the lumbar and pelvic area by maintaining tension on the thoracolumbar fascia

Origin, proximal attachment, arises from:

Spinous processes of T7 to L5, posterior one third of the external lip of the iliac crest, posterior layer of the thoracolumbar fascia, and lower three or four ribs

Insertion, distal attachment, attaches to:

Medial lip of the bicipital groove of the humerus just as the muscle begins to twist around the teres major

The latissimus dorsi is fan shaped and has a twist in its fibers such that the superior fibers attach more distally on the humerus and the inferior fibers attach more proximally on the humerus. Shortening in this muscle limits arm movement over the head and can cause the back of the lumbar area to feel tight.

Innervation:

Thoracodorsal nerve (C6 to C8)

Major synergists:

Teres major, the long head of the triceps brachii, sternocostal head of the pectoralis major, subscapularis, and anterior deltoid muscle

Major antagonists:

Clavicular head of the pectoralis major, teres minor, infraspinatus, deltoid muscle, supraspinatus, levator scapulae, and rectus abdominis

Trigger points:

Posterior axillary area and belly of the muscle near the rib attachments

Referred pain pattern:

Just below the scapula and into the ulnar side of the arm and anterior deltoid region and abdominal oblique area

Teres major (TER-eez)

Teres means "smooth and round"; *major* means "larger." This muscle may be fused with the latissimus dorsi.

Posterior

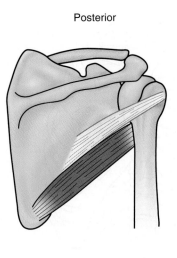

Concentric action:
Medial rotation, adduction, and extension of the arm at the shoulder joint and upward rotation of the scapula at the scapulocostal joint

Eccentric action:
Restrains lateral rotation, abduction, and flexion of the arm and restrains downward rotation of the scapula

Isometric action:
Stabilizes the glenohumeral joint

Origin, proximal attachment, arises from:
Dorsal surfaces of inferior angle and lower third of lateral border of scapula

Insertion, distal attachment, attaches to:
Medial lip of bicipital groove of the humerus

Innervation:
Lower subscapular nerve (C5 to C7)

Major synergists:
Latissimus dorsi, subscapularis, and trapezius

Major antagonists:
Teres minor, infraspinatus, supraspinatus, anterior deltoid muscle, and pectoralis minor

Trigger points:
Near the musculotendinous junction at both attachments and points at the attachments at the humerus; can be best reached through the axilla

Referred pain pattern:
Posterior deltoid region and down the dorsal portion of the arm

Coracobrachialis (KORE-a-koe-BRAY-kee-AL-iss)

Coracobrachialis means "crow's beak" and "of the arm."

Anterior

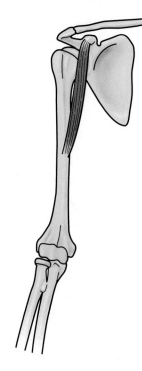

Concentric action:
Flexion and adduction of the arm at the shoulder joint

Eccentric action:
Restrains extension and abduction of the arm

Isometric action:
Stabilizes the shoulder and scapula

Origin, proximal attachment, arises from:
Tip of the coracoid process of the scapula

Insertion, distal attachment, attaches to:
Anteromedial surface of the middle of the shaft of the humerus, opposite the deltoid tuberosity

Innervation:
Musculocutaneous nerve (C5 to C7)

Major synergists:
Pectoralis major and short head of biceps brachii

Major antagonist:
Posterior deltoid muscle

Trigger points:
Near the musculotendinous junction and the coracoid attachment

Referred pain pattern:
Front of shoulder and posterior aspect of the arm down the triceps and posterior forearm into the posterior hand

ACTIVITY 9-36

Draw and color the **muscles of the shoulder joint** in the spaces provided. For each muscle, do the following:

1. Label the origin and insertion attachment points: *O* for origin; *I* for insertion.

2. Place an X on the trigger points.

3. Palpate this muscle; identify the attachment points and the bellies of the muscles.

4. Move these muscles on yourself.

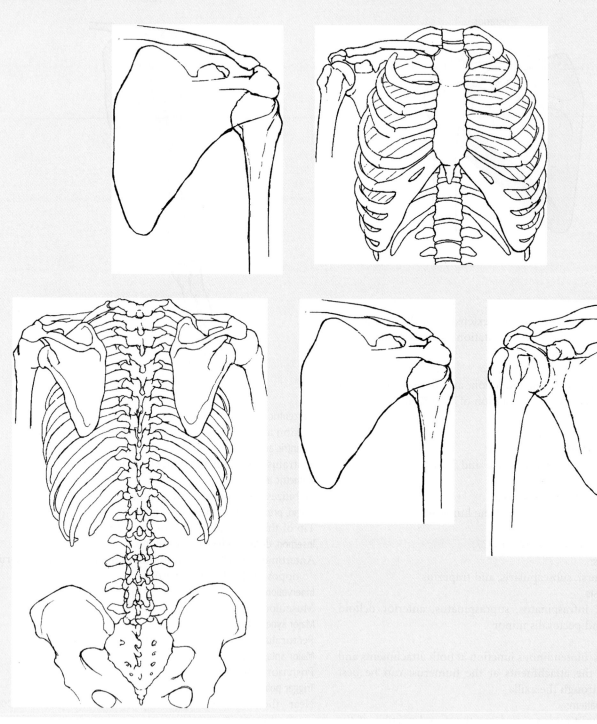

Muscles of the Elbow and Radioulnar Joints

The elbow is a hinge joint, and movements produced by the muscles at the elbow joint are limited entirely to flexion and extension of the forearm. Posterior arm muscles produce extension of the forearm at the elbow joint; anterior arm muscles produce flexion of the forearm at the elbow joint. The strongest elbow flexor is the brachialis. **Reverse actions** of flexion and extension of the arm at the elbow joint are also common. Pronation and supination take place at the radioulnar joints. Because of contralateral joint reflexes involved with gait, flexors of the forearm at the elbow joint work with flexors of the leg at the knee joint on the opposite side of the body, and extensors of the forearm at the elbow joint work with extensors of the leg at the knee joint on the opposite side of the body. Massage application is more effective when the massage therapist observes these interactions and considers the bodywide patterns. Dysfunction is common with static posture. Static position requires these muscles to hold contraction for prolonged periods. Examples are driving a car, holding a phone, computer work, and using hand tools. Repetitive-use activities such as using a hammer or wrench also strain this group of muscles (Figure 9-29).

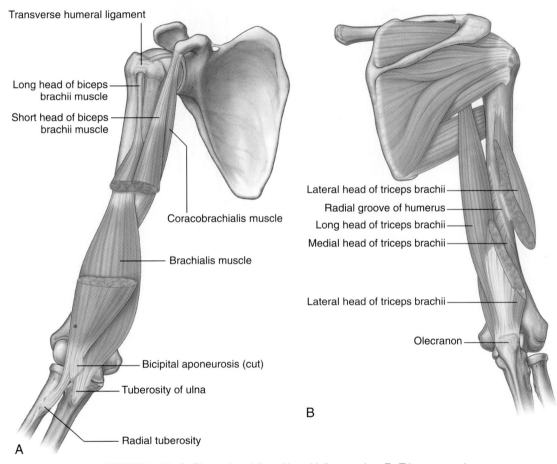

FIGURE 9-29 A, Biceps brachii and brachialis muscles. **B,** Triceps muscle.

Continued

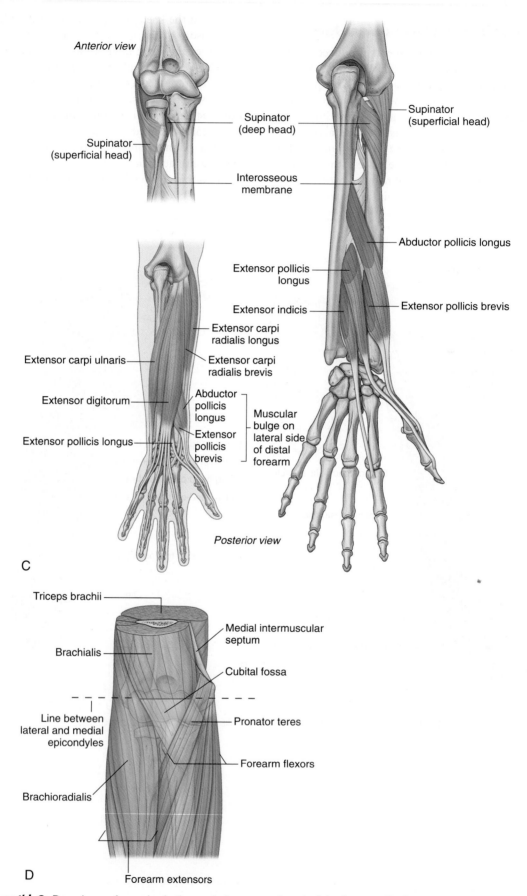

Anterior view

Supinator (deep head)

Supinator (superficial head)

Supinator (superficial head)

Interosseous membrane

Abductor pollicis longus

Extensor pollicis longus

Extensor indicis

Extensor pollicis brevis

Extensor carpi radialis longus

Extensor carpi ulnaris

Extensor carpi radialis brevis

Extensor digitorum

Abductor pollicis longus

Muscular bulge on lateral side of distal forearm

Extensor pollicis longus

Extensor pollicis brevis

Posterior view

C

Triceps brachii

Medial intermuscular septum

Brachialis

Cubital fossa

Line between lateral and medial epicondyles

Pronator teres

Forearm flexors

Brachioradialis

D

Forearm extensors

FIGURE 9-29, cont'd C, Deep layer of muscles in the posterior compartment of the forearm. **D,** Cross section of arm. (From Drake RL, Vogl W, Mitchell WM: *Gray's anatomy for students,* ed 2, Edinburgh, 2010, Churchill Livingstone.)

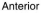

Biceps brachii (BI-seps BRAY-kee-eye)

Biceps means "two heads"; *brachii* means "of the arm."

Anterior

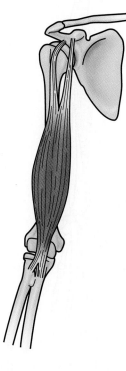

Concentric action:

Flexion of the forearm at the elbow joint, supination of the forearm at the radioulnar joints, and flexion of the arm at the shoulder joint (A common reverse action is flexion of the arm at the elbow joint such as when doing a pull-up or chin-up.)

Eccentric action:

Restrains extension and pronation of the forearm and extension of the arm

Isometric action:

Stabilizes the humerus at the shoulder and elbow joints during full extension and stabilizes the elbow joint when flexed and holding a weight

Origin, proximal attachment, arises from:

Long head—supraglenoid tubercle of the scapula

Short head—tip of the coracoid process of the scapula

Insertion, distal attachment, attaches to:

Tuberosity of the radius and aponeurosis of the proximal attachment (origin) of the wrist flexor muscles in the forearm

Innervation:

Musculocutaneous nerve (C5 to C6)

Major synergists:

Brachialis, brachioradialis, supinator, and anterior deltoid muscle

Major antagonists:

Triceps brachii, pronator teres, pronator quadratus, and posterior deltoid muscle

Trigger points:

In the belly of the long and short heads, closer to the elbow

Referred pain pattern:

Front of the shoulder at the anterior deltoid region and into the scapular region and also into the antecubital space (front of the elbow)

Brachialis (BRAY-kee-AL-iss)

Brachialis means "of the arm."

Anterior

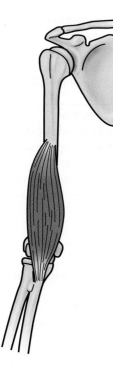

Concentric action:

Flexion of the forearm at the elbow joint

Eccentric action:

Restrains extension of the forearm

Isometric action:

Stabilizes the elbow joint

Origin, proximal attachment, arises from:

Distal one half of the anterior surface of the humerus and the medial and lateral intermuscular septae

Insertion, distal attachment, attaches to:

Coronoid process and tuberosity of the ulna

Innervation:

Musculocutaneous nerve (C5 to C7)

Major synergists:

Biceps brachii and brachioradialis

Major antagonist:

Triceps brachii

Trigger points:

Several locations in the belly of the muscle

Referred pain pattern:

Primarily to the thumb, with some pain in the anterior deltoid area and at the elbow

Brachioradialis (BRAY-kee-oh-RAY-dee-AL-iss)

Brachioradialis means "related to the arm" and "radius."

Anterior

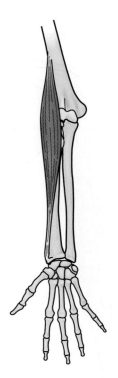

Concentric action:

Flexion of the forearm at the elbow joint; the brachioradialis also can assist in pronation and supination of the forearm at the radioulnar joints to midposition (halfway between full pronation and full supination)

Eccentric action:

Restrains extension of the forearm and can restrain pronation and supination of the forearm (beyond midposition)

Isometric action:

Stabilizes the elbow joint

Origin, proximal attachment, arises from:

Proximal two thirds of the lateral supracondylar ridge of the humerus and lateral intermuscular septum

Insertion, distal attachment, attaches to:

Lateral side of the base of the styloid process of the radius

Innervation:

Radial nerve (C5 to C6)

Major synergists:

Biceps brachii, brachialis, supinator, pronator teres, and pronator quadratus

Major antagonists:

Triceps brachii, supinator, pronator teres, and pronator quadratus

Trigger points:

Belly of the muscle

Referred pain pattern:

Wrist and base of the thumb in the web space between the thumb and index finger and to the lateral epicondyle at the elbow

▌*Pronator teres* (PRO-nay-tor TER-eez)

Pronator means "one that causes pronation"; *teres* means "round and smooth."

Anterior

Concentric action:
Pronation of the forearm at the radioulnar joints and flexion of the forearm at the elbow joint
Eccentric action:
Restrains supination and extension of the forearm
Isometric action:
Stabilizes the elbow joint and the radioulnar joints
Origin, proximal attachment, arises from:
Humeral head—medial epicondyle of the humerus, common flexor tendon, and deep antebrachial fascia
Ulnar head—medial side of the coronoid process of the ulna
Insertion, distal attachment, attaches to:
Middle of lateral surface of radius
Innervation:
Median nerve (C6 to C7)
Major synergists:
Pronator quadratus and all forearm flexors
Major antagonists:
Supinator, biceps brachii, and triceps brachii
Trigger points:
Belly of the muscle near the elbow attachment
Referred pain pattern:
Radial side of the forearm into the wrist and thumb; may mimic carpal tunnel syndrome

▌*Supinator* (SOOP-in-ATE-or)

Supinator means "one that causes supination."

Posterior

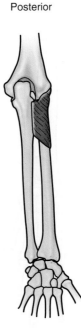

Concentric action:
Supination of the forearm at the radioulnar joints
Eccentric action:
Restrains pronation of the forearm
Isometric action:
Stabilizes the elbow and radioulnar joints
Origin, proximal attachment, arises from:
Lateral epicondyle of the humerus, radial collateral ligament of the elbow joint, annular ligament of the radius, and supinator crest of the ulna
Insertion, distal attachment, attaches to:
Lateral surface of the proximal one third of the shaft of the radius, covering part of the anterior, medial, and posterior surfaces
The supinator is a large muscle that wraps around the bones of the forearm.
Innervation:
Deep branch of the radial nerve (C6 to C7)
Major synergist:
Biceps brachii
Major antagonists:
Pronator teres and pronator quadratus
Trigger points:
Near the radius in the antecubital space
Referred pain pattern:
Local area

▌*Pronator quadratus* (PRO-nay-tor kwad-RATE-us)

Pronator means "one that causes pronation"; *quadratus* means "square shaped."

Anterior

▌*Triceps brachii* (TRY-seps BRAY-kee-eye)

Triceps means "three heads"; *brachii* means "of the arm."

Posterior

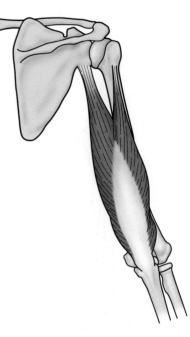

Concentric action:
Extension of the forearm at the elbow joint; in addition, the long head adducts and extends the arm at the shoulder joint
Eccentric action:
Restrains flexion of the forearm and abduction and flexion of the arm
Isometric action:
Stabilizes the elbow and shoulder joints
Origin, proximal attachment, arises from:
Long head—infraglenoid tubercle of the scapula
Lateral head—lateral and posterior surfaces of the proximal one half of the shaft of the humerus and the lateral intermuscular septum
Medial (deep) head—distal half of the medial and posterior surfaces of the shaft of the humerus distal to the radial groove and the medial intermuscular septum
Insertion, distal attachment, attaches to:
Posterior surface of the olecranon process of the ulna and antebrachial fascia
Innervation:
Radial nerve (C6 to C8)
Major synergist:
Anconeus
Major antagonists:
Brachialis and biceps brachii
Trigger points:
Belly of each head
Referred pain pattern:
Length of the posterior arm

Concentric action:
Pronation of the forearm at the radioulnar joints
Eccentric action:
Restrains supination of the forearm
The pronator quadratus is the prime mover of pronation of the forearm.
Origin, proximal attachment, arises from:
Medial side and anterior surface of the distal one fourth of the ulna
Insertion, distal attachment, attaches to:
Lateral side and anterior surface of the distal one fourth of the radius
Innervation:
Anterior interosseous branch of the median nerve (C7 to C8)
Major synergist:
Pronator teres
Major antagonists:
Supinator and biceps brachii
Trigger points:
Belly of muscle
Referred pain pattern:
Local area

Anconeus (an-KO-nee-us)

Anconeus means "elbow."

Posterior

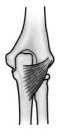

Concentric action:

Extension of the forearm at the elbow joint

Eccentric action:

Restrains flexion of the forearm

Isometric action:

Stabilizes the elbow joint

Origin, proximal attachment, arises from:

Posterior surface of the lateral epicondyle of the humerus

Insertion, distal attachment, attaches to:

Lateral side of the olecranon process and proximal one fourth
   of the posterior surface of the shaft of the ulna

Innervation:

Radial nerve (C6 to C8)

Major synergist:

Triceps brachii

Major antagonists:

Biceps brachii and brachialis

Trigger points:

In the belly

Referred pain pattern:

Elbow at the lateral epicondyle

Muscles of the Wrist and Hand Joints

If all the muscles that move the hand actually were located in the hand, the hand would be too bulky to be functional. Instead, the bellies of these muscles are located closer to the elbow, tapering to long insertion tendons in the wrist and hand. Strong ligaments, called the *flexor* and *extensor reti-nacula*, secure the long, tendinous insertions much like a bracelet at the wrist. Synovial tendon sheaths surround the tendons to assist their movements and reduce friction. Many of the forearm muscles attach on the humerus and cross the elbow and the wrist joints; however, their action on the elbow is usually insignificant. The forearm muscles are subdivided by fascial sheets into the anterior and posterior compartments,

ACTIVITY 9-37

Draw and color the **muscles of the elbow and radioulnar joints** in the spaces provided. For each muscle, do the following:

1. Label the origin and insertion attachment points: *O* for origin; *I* for insertion.
2. Place an X on the trigger points.
3. Palpate this muscle; identify the attachment points and the bellies of the muscles.
4. Move these muscles on yourself.

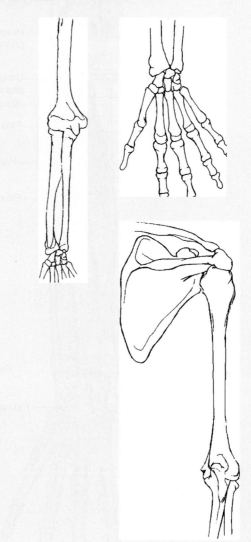

each having a superficial and a deep layer of muscles. Most muscles of the anterior compartment are wrist and finger flexors; the muscles of the posterior compartment are mainly wrist and finger extensors. These muscles have distinct layers, and massage application requires careful and gradual access to the deeper layers by penetrating through the superficial layers using a broad-base compressive force. A narrow-pointed contact with the tissue usually results in tensing and guarding by the superficial muscles (Figure 9-30).

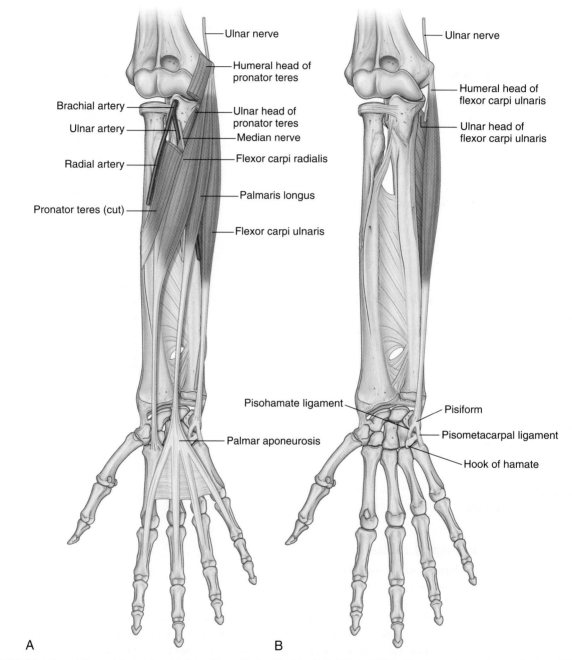

A   B

FIGURE 9-30 Muscles of the wrist and hand joints. (From Drake RL, Vogl W, Mitchell WM: *Gray's anatomy for students,* ed 2, Edinburgh, 2010, Churchill Livingstone.)

Anterior Flexor Group: Superficial Layer

Flexor carpi radialis (FLEKS-or KAR-pee RAY-dee-AL-iss)

Flexor means "to bend," *carpi* means "of the wrist," and *radialis* means "related to the radius."

Anterior

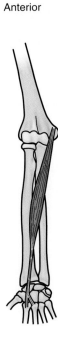

Concentric action:

Flexion and radial deviation (abduction) of the hand at the wrist joint, flexion of the forearm at the elbow joint, and pronation of the forearm at the radioulnar joints

Eccentric action:

Restrains extension and ulnar deviation (adduction) of the hand and extension and supination of the forearm

Isometric action:

Stabilizes the wrist

Origin, proximal attachment, arises from:

Common flexor tendon from the medial epicondyle of the humerus and deep antebrachial fascia

Insertion, distal attachment, attaches to:

Base of the second and third metacarpal bones

Innervation:

Median nerve (C6 to C7)

Major synergists:

All flexors of the hand and the extensor carpi radialis longus and extensor carpi radialis brevis

Major antagonists:

All extensors of the hand and the flexor carpi ulnaris

Palmaris longus (pal-MAR-iss LONG-us)

Palmaris means "related to the palm"; *longus* means "long."

Anterior

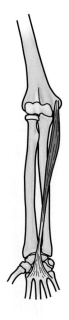

Concentric action:

Flexion of the hand at the wrist joint, flexion of the forearm at the elbow joint, and pronation of the forearm at the radioulnar joints

Eccentric action:

Restrains extension of the hand and extension and supination of the forearm

Isometric action:

Tenses the palmar fascia

Origin, proximal attachment, arises from:

Common flexor tendon from the medial epicondyle of the humerus and deep antebrachial fascia

Insertion, distal attachment, attaches to:

Flexor retinaculum and palmar aponeurosis

Innervation:

Median nerve (C7 to C8)

Major synergists:

All flexors of the hand and the palmaris brevis

Major antagonists:

All extensors of the hand

The tendon of the palmaris longus is superficial to the antebrachial fascia of the wrist and is visible if one cups the hand and slightly flexes the wrist. This muscle is absent in about one fourth of the population.

Flexor carpi ulnaris (FLEKS-or KAR-pee ul-NAR-iss)

Flexor means "to bend," *carpi* means "of the wrist," and *ulnaris* means "related to the ulna."

Anterior

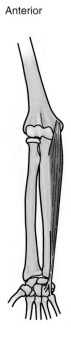

Concentric action:

Flexion and ulnar deviation (adduction) of the hand at the wrist joint and flexion of the forearm at the elbow joint

Eccentric action:

Restrains extension and radial deviation (abduction) of the hand and extension of the forearm

Isometric action:

Stabilizes the wrist

Origin, proximal attachment, arises from:

Humeral head—common flexor tendon from the medial epicondyle of the humerus

Ulnar head—olecranon, proximal two thirds of the posterior border of the ulna, and deep antebrachial fascia

Insertion, distal attachment, attaches to:

Pisiform bone and, indirectly, by ligaments to the hamate and fifth metacarpal bones

Innervation:

Ulnar nerve (C7 to C8)

Major synergists:

All flexors of the hand and the extensor carpi ulnaris

Major antagonists:

All extensors of the hand and the flexor carpi radialis

ACTIVITY 9-38

Draw and color the **muscles of the anterior flexor group: superficial layer** in the spaces provided. For each muscle, do the following:

1. Label the origin and insertion attachment points: *O* for origin; *I* for insertion.
2. Place an X on the trigger points.
3. Palpate this muscle; identify the attachment points and the bellies of the muscles.
4. Move these muscles on yourself.

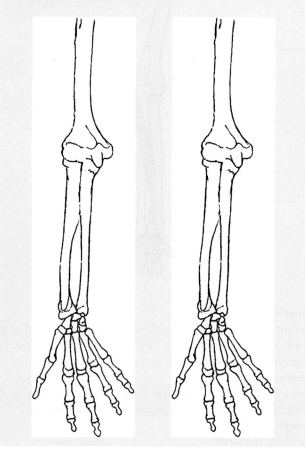

Anterior Flexor Group: Intermediate Layer

Flexor digitorum superficialis
(FLEKS-or DIH-jih-TOR-um SOO-per-fish-ee-AL-us)

Flexor means "to bend," *digitorum* means "of the fingers or toes," and *superficialis* means "related to the top or surface."

Anterior

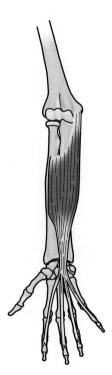

Concentric action:

Flexion of fingers 2 to 5 at the metacarpophalangeal and proximal interphalangeal joints and flexion of the hand at the wrist joint

Eccentric action:

Restrains finger extension and hand extension

Isometric action:

Stabilizes wrist and finger joints

Origin, proximal attachment, arises from:

Humeral head—common flexor tendon from the medial epicondyle of the humerus, ulnar collateral ligament of the elbow joint, and deep antebrachial fascia

Ulnar head—medial side of the coronoid process of the ulna

Radial head—oblique line of the radius

Insertion, distal attachment, attaches to:

Sides of the palmar surface of the middle phalanges of the second through fifth fingers

Innervation:

Median nerve (C7 to T1)

Major synergist:

Flexor digitorum profundus

Major antagonist:

Extensor digitorum

✎ ACTIVITY 9-39

Draw and color the **muscle of the anterior flexor group: intermediate layer** in the space provided. Do the following:

1. Label the origin and insertion attachment points: *O* for origin; *I* for insertion.
2. Place an X on the trigger points.
3. Palpate this muscle; identify the attachment points and the belly of the muscle.
4. Move this muscle on yourself.

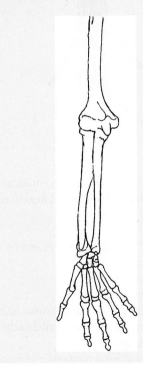

Anterior Flexor Group: Deep Layer

Flexor digitorum profundus
(FLEKS-or DIH-jih-TOR-um pro-FUND-us)

Flexor means "to bend," *digitorum* means "related to the fingers or toes," and *profundus* means "deep."

Flexor pollicis longus (FLEKS-or POLL-is-iss LONG-us)

Flexor means "to bend," *pollicis* means "of the thumb," and *longus* means "long."

Anterior

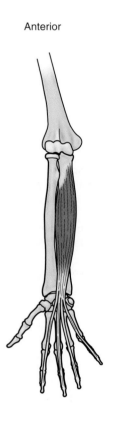

Anterior

Concentric action:
Flexion of fingers 2 to 5 at the metacarpophalangeal, proximal, and distal interphalangeal joints and flexion of the hand at the wrist joint

Eccentric action:
Restrains extension of the fingers and extension of the hand

Isometric action:
Stabilizes wrist and finger joints

Origin, proximal attachment, arises from:
Medial and anterior surfaces of the proximal half of the ulna, interosseous membrane, and deep antebrachial fascia

Insertion, distal attachment, attaches to:
By four tendons into the distal phalanges of fingers 2 to 5 on the anterior surface

Innervation:
Ulnar nerve and interosseous branch of the median nerve (C7 to T1)

Major synergist:
Flexor digitorum superficialis

Major antagonist:
Extensor digitorum

Concentric action:
Flexion of the thumb at the carpometacarpal, metacarpophalangeal, and interphalangeal joints

Eccentric action:
Restrains extension of the thumb

Isometric action:
Stabilizes the thumb

Origin, proximal attachment, arises from:
Anterior surface of the radius medial epicondyle of the humerus, the coronoid process of the ulna, and interosseous membrane

Insertion, distal attachment, attaches to:
Palmar surface of the base of the distal phalanx of the thumb

Innervation:
Anterior interosseous branch of the median nerve (C7 to C8)

Major synergist:
Flexor pollicis brevis

Major antagonists:
Extensor pollicis longus and extensor pollicis brevis
Elements common to the anterior flexion group:

Trigger points:
In the belly

Referred pain pattern:
Into the wrist, associated fingers, or thumb and occasionally into the elbow

ACTIVITY 9-40

Draw and color the **muscles of the anterior flexor group: deep layer** in the spaces provided. For each muscle, do the following:

1. Label the origin and insertion attachment points: *O* for origin; *I* for insertion.
2. Place an X on the trigger points.
3. Palpate this muscle; identify the attachment points and the bellies of the muscles.
4. Move these muscles on yourself.

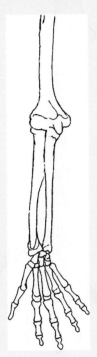

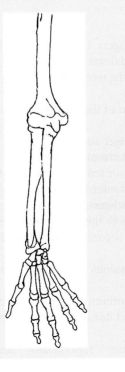

Posterior Extensor Group: Superficial Layer

Extensor carpi radialis longus
(ex-STEN-sur KAR-pee RAY-dee-AL-iss LONG-us)

Extensor means "one that stretches," *carpi* means "related to the wrist," *radialis* means "related to the radius," and *longus* means "long."

Posterior

Concentric action:
Extension and radial deviation (abduction) of the hand at the wrist joint, flexion of the forearm at the elbow joint
Eccentric action:
Restrains flexion and ulnar deviation (adduction) of the hand, extension of the forearm, and pronation of the forearm at the radioulnar joint
Isometric action:
Stabilizes wrist and elbow joints
Origin, proximal attachment, arises from:
Distal one third of the lateral supracondylar ridge of the humerus and lateral intermuscular septum
Insertion, distal attachment, attaches to:
Dorsal surface of the base of the second metacarpal bone on the radial side
Innervation:
Radial nerve (C5 to C6)
Major synergists:
All extensors of the hand and the flexor carpi radialis
Major antagonists:
All flexors of the hand and the extensor carpi ulnaris

Extensor carpi radialis brevis
(ex-STEN-sur KAR-pee RAY-dee-AL-iss BREV-us)

Extensor means "one that stretches," *carpi* means "of the wrist," *radialis* means "related to the radius," and *brevis* means "short."

Posterior

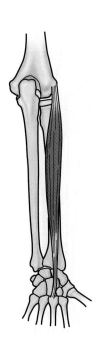

Extensor digitorum (ex-STEN-sur DIH-jih-TOR-um)

Extensor means "one that stretches"; *digitorum* means "of the fingers or toes."

Posterior

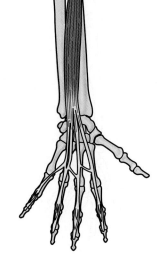

Concentric action:

Extension and radial deviation (abduction) of the hand at the wrist joint and flexion of the forearm at the elbow joint

Eccentric action:

Restrains flexion and ulnar deviation (adduction) of the hand and extension of the forearm

Isometric action:

Stabilizes the wrist joint

Origin, proximal attachment, arises from:

Common extensor tendon from the lateral epicondyle of the humerus, radial collateral ligament of the elbow joint, and deep antebrachial fascia

Insertion, distal attachment, attaches to:

Dorsal surface of the base of the third metacarpal bone

Innervation:

Posterior interosseous branch of the radial nerve (C7 to C8)

Major synergists:

All extensors of the hand and the flexor carpi radialis

Major antagonists:

All flexors of the hand and the extensor carpi ulnaris

Concentric action:

Extension of fingers 2 to 5 at the metacarpophalangeal and proximal and distal interphalangeal joints and extension of the hand at the wrist joint

Eccentric action:

Restrains flexion of the fingers and flexion of the hand

Isometric action:

Stabilizes the finger and wrist joints

Origin, proximal attachment, arises from:

Common extensor tendon from the lateral epicondyle of the humerus and intermuscular septa

Insertion, distal attachment, attaches to:

By four tendons to the lateral and dorsal surface of the phalanges of the second through fifth digits

Innervation:

Posterior interosseous branch of the radial nerve (C7 to C8)

Major synergists:

Extensor digiti minimi, extensor indicis, lumbricals, palmar interossei, and dorsal interossei manus

Major antagonists:

Flexor digitorum superficialis and flexor digitorum profundus

The distal tendon of this muscle forms the dorsal digital expansion of fingers 2 to 5.

Extensor digiti minimi (ex-STEN-sur DIH-jih-tee MIN-ih-mee)

Extensor means "one that stretches," *digiti* means "of the fingers or toes," and *minimi* means "smallest."

Posterior

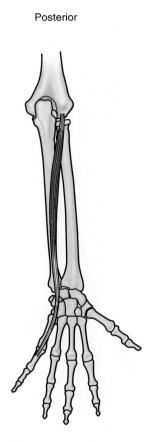

Concentric action:

Extension of the little finger at the metacarpophalangeal, proximal, and distal interphalangeal joints

Eccentric action:

Restrains flexion of the little finger

Isometric action:

Stabilizes the little finger

Origin, proximal attachment, arises from:

Common extensor tendon from the lateral epicondyle of the humerus and intermuscular septa

Insertion, distal attachment, attaches to:

Into the dorsal digital expansion of the little finger with the extensor digitorum tendon

Innervation:

Posterior interosseous branch of the radial nerve (C7 to C8)

Major synergist:

Extensor digitorum

Major antagonists:

Flexor digitorum superficialis and flexor digitorum profundus

Extensor carpi ulnaris (ex-STEN-sur KAR-pee ul-NAR-iss)

Extensor means "one that stretches," *carpi* means "of the wrist," and *ulnaris* means "related to the ulna."

Posterior

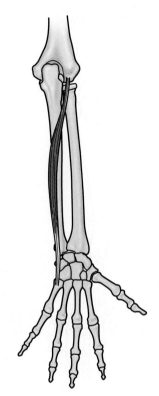

Concentric action:

Extension and ulnar deviation (adduction) of the hand at the wrist joint

Eccentric action:

Restrains flexion and radial deviation (abduction) of the hand

Isometric action:

Stabilizes the wrist joint

Origin, proximal attachment, arises from:

Common extensor tendon from the lateral epicondyle of the humerus and the aponeurosis from the posterior border of the ulna

Insertion, distal attachment, attaches to:

Posterior side of the base of the fifth metacarpal bone

Innervation:

Posterior interosseous branch of the radial nerve (C7 to C8)

Major synergists:

All extensors of the hand and the flexor carpi ulnaris

Major antagonists:

All flexors of the hand and the extensor carpi radialis longus and extensor carpi radialis brevis

✎ ACTIVITY 9-41

Draw and color the **muscles of the posterior extensor group: superficial layer** in the spaces provided. For each muscle, do the following:

1. Label the origin and insertion attachment points: *O* for origin; *I* for insertion.
2. Place an X on the trigger points.
3. Palpate this muscle; identify the attachment points and the bellies of the muscles.
4. Move these muscles on yourself.

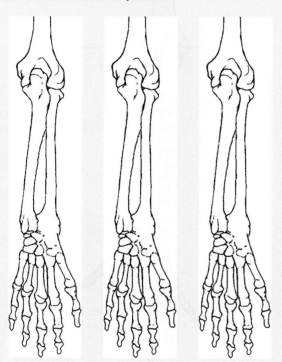

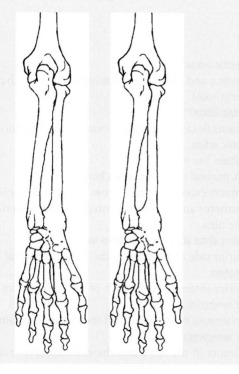

Posterior Extensor Group: Deep Layer

Extensor pollicis brevis
(ex-STEN-sur POLL-is-iss BREV-us)

Extensor means "one that stretches," *pollicis* means "of the thumb," and *brevis* means "short."

Posterior

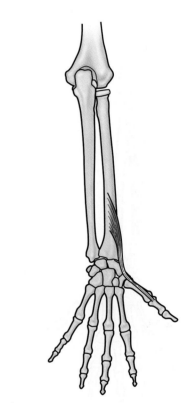

Concentric action:

Extension of the thumb at the carpometacarpal and metacarpophalangeal joints, abduction of the thumb at the carpometacarpal joint, radial deviation (abduction) of the hand at the wrist joint, and supination of the forearm at the radioulnar joints

Eccentric action:

Restrains flexion and adduction of the thumb, ulnar deviation (adduction) of the hand, and pronation of the forearm

Isometric action:

Stabilizes the thumb

Origin, proximal attachment, arises from:

Posterior surface of the shaft of the radius distal to the origin of the abductor pollicis longus and the interosseous membrane

Insertion, distal attachment, attaches to:

Base of the proximal phalanx of the thumb on the dorsal surface

Innervation:

Posterior interosseous branch of the radial nerve (C7 to C8)

Major synergists:

Extensor pollicis longus, abductor pollicis longus, and abductor pollicis brevis

Major antagonists:

Flexor pollicis longus, flexor pollicis brevis, and adductor pollicis

Abductor pollicis longus
(ab-DUCK-tur POLL-is-iss LONG-us)

Abductor means "one that leads away," *pollicis* means "of the thumb," and *longus* means "long."

Posterior

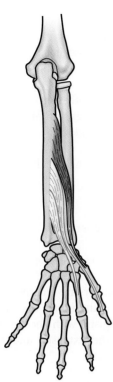

Concentric action:

Abduction and extension of the thumb at the carpometacarpal joint, radial deviation (abduction) and flexion of the hand at the wrist joint, and supination of the forearm at the radioulnar joints

Eccentric action:

Restrains adduction and flexion of the thumb, ulnar deviation (adduction) and extension of the hand, and pronation of the forearm

Isometric action:

Stabilizes the thumb and the wrist joint

Origin, proximal attachment, arises from:

Posterior surface of the shaft of the ulna distal to the origin of the supinator, interosseous membrane, and posterior surface of the middle one third of the shaft of the radius

Insertion, distal attachment, attaches to:

Base of the first metacarpal bone of the thumb on the lateral side

Innervation:

Posterior interosseous branch of the radial nerve (C7 to C8)

Major synergists:

Abductor pollicis brevis, extensor pollicis longus, and extensor pollicis brevis

Major antagonists:

Adductor pollicis, flexor pollicis longus, and flexor pollicis brevis

Extensor pollicis longus
(ex-STEN-sur POLL-is-iss LONG-us)

Extensor means "one that stretches," *pollicis* means "of the thumb," and *longus* means "long."

Posterior

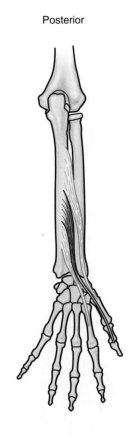

Concentric action:

Extension of the thumb at the carpometacarpal, metacarpophalangeal, and interphalangeal joints; radial deviation (abduction) of the hand at the wrist joint; and supination of the forearm at the radioulnar joints

Eccentric action:

Restrains flexion of the thumb, ulnar deviation (adduction) of the hand, and pronation of the forearm

Isometric action:

Stabilizes the thumb and the wrist joint

Origin, proximal attachment, arises from:

Middle one third of the posterior surface of the ulna distal to the origin of the abductor pollicis longus and the interosseous membrane

Insertion, distal attachment, attaches to:

Dorsal surface of the base of the distal phalanx of the thumb

Innervation:

Posterior interosseous branch of the radial nerve (C7 to C8)

Major synergist:

Extensor pollicis brevis

Major antagonists:

Flexor pollicis longus and flexor pollicis brevis

Extensor indicis (ex-STEN-sur IN-dih-siss)

Extensor means "one that stretches"; *indicis* means "of the index finger."

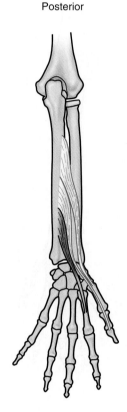

Posterior

Concentric action:

Extension of the index finger at the metacarpophalangeal, proximal, and distal interphalangeal joints; adduction of the index finger at the metacarpophalangeal joint; and supination of the forearm at the radioulnar joints

Eccentric action:

Restrains flexion and abduction of the index finger and pronation of the forearm

Isometric action:

Stabilizes the index finger

Origin, proximal attachment, arises from:

Posterior surface of the ulna and the interosseous membrane

Insertion, distal attachment, attaches to:

Into the dorsal digital expansion of the index finger with the extensor digitorum tendon

Innervation:

Posterior interosseous branch of the radial nerve (C7 to C8)

Major synergist:

Extensor digitorum

Major antagonists:

Flexor digitorum superficialis and flexor digitorum profundus

Elements common to the posterior extensor group muscles

Major synergists:

For extension, all extensors are synergistic with each other; for radial deviation of the hand, the extensor carpi radialis muscles are synergistic with the flexor carpi radialis; for ulnar deviation, the extensor and flexor carpi ulnaris muscles are synergistic.

Major antagonists:

The flexor group; the ulnar deviation and radial deviation groups are antagonistic to each other

Trigger points:

Belly of each muscle, located nearer the elbow

Referred pain pattern:

From the lateral epicondyle at the elbow down the dorsum of the forearm to various parts of the hand, especially to the web of the thumb

Draw and color the **muscles of the posterior extensor group: deep layer** in the spaces provided. For each muscle, do the following:

1. Label the origin and insertion attachment points: *O* for origin; *I* for insertion.
2. Place an X on the trigger points.
3. Palpate this muscle; identify the attachment points and the bellies of the muscles.
4. Move these muscles on yourself.

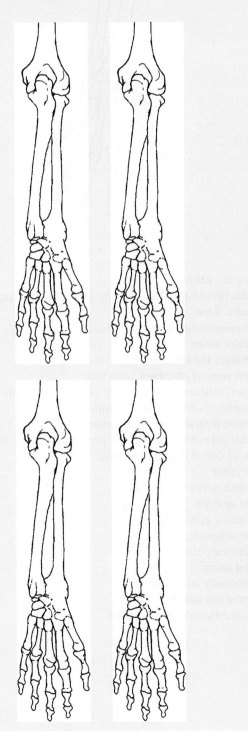

Intrinsic Muscles of the Hand

Intrinsic muscles of the hand are small muscles that are located wholly within the hand (i.e., they originate and insert within the hand). The complex and intricate nature of these muscles allows for an almost limitless variety of fine hand movements. The delicacy of the muscles and the interactive pattern of their layout are unique to the human hand (Figure 9-31).

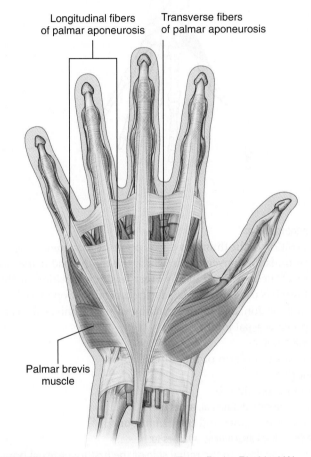

FIGURE 9-31 Palmar aponeurosis. (From Drake RL, Vogl W, Mitchell WM: *Gray's anatomy for students,* ed 2, Edinburgh, 2010, Churchill Livingstone.)

Thenar Eminence Muscles

Opponens pollicis (oh-PONE-ens POLL-is-iss)

Opponens means "opposing"; *pollicis* means "of the thumb."

Anterior

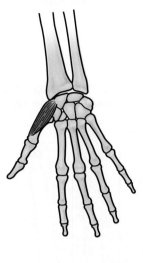

Concentric action:
Opposition of the thumb at the carpometacarpal joint (Opposition is the movement in which the thumb pad comes to meet the finger pad of any other finger; opposition of the thumb is usually considered to be a combination of abduction, flexion, and medial rotation of the thumb at the carpometacarpal joint.)

Eccentric action:
Restrains reposition of the thumb

Isometric action:
Stabilizes the thumb

Origin, proximal attachment, arises from:
Flexor retinaculum and trapezium bone

Insertion, distal attachment, attaches to:
Anterior surface on the radial side of the first metacarpal bone

Innervation:
Median and ulnar nerves (C8 to T1)

Major synergists:
Flexor pollicis brevis and abductor pollicis brevis

Major antagonists:
Extensor pollicis longus, extensor pollicis brevis, and adductor pollicis

Trigger points:
In the belly of the muscle

Referred pain pattern:
Into the thumb and the wrist

Abductor pollicis brevis (ab-DUCK-tur POLL-is-iss BREV-us)

Abductor means "one that leads away," *pollicis* means "of the thumb," and *brevis* means "short."

Anterior

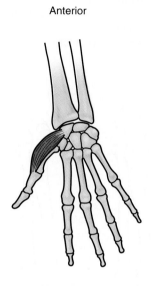

Concentric action:
Abduction of the thumb at the metacarpophalangeal joint

Eccentric action:
Restrains adduction of the thumb

Isometric action:
Stabilizes the thumb

Origin, proximal attachment, arises from:
Flexor retinaculum, tubercle of the trapezium bone, and tubercle of the scaphoid bone

Insertion, distal attachment, attaches to:
Radial side of the base of the proximal phalanx of the thumb and dorsal digital expansion

Innervation:
Median nerve (C8 to T1)

Major synergist:
Abductor pollicis longus

Major antagonist:
Adductor pollicis

Trigger points:
In the belly of the muscle

Referred pain pattern:
Into the thumb and the wrist

Flexor pollicis brevis (FLEKS-or POLL-is-iss BREV-us)

Flexor means "one that bends," *pollicis* means "of the thumb," and *brevis* means "short."

Anterior

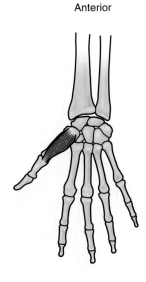

Concentric action:
Flexion of the thumb at the carpometacarpal and metacarpophalangeal joints
Eccentric action:
Restrains extension of the thumb
Isometric action:
Stabilizes the thumb
Origin, proximal attachment, arises from:
Superficial head—flexor retinaculum and trapezium bone
Deep head—trapezoid and capitate bones
Insertion, distal attachment, attaches to:
Radial side of the base of the proximal phalanx of the thumb and dorsal digital expansion
Innervation:
Median and ulnar nerves (C8 to T1)
Major synergist:
Flexor pollicis longus
Major antagonists:
Extensor pollicis longus and extensor pollicis brevis
Trigger points:
In the belly of the muscle
Referred pain pattern:
Into the thumb and the wrist

ACTIVITY 9-43

Draw and color the **thenar eminence muscles** in the spaces provided. For each muscle, do the following:
1. Label the origin and insertion attachment points: *O* for origin; *I* for insertion.
2. Place an X on the trigger points.
3. Palpate this muscle; identify the attachment points and the bellies of the muscles.
4. Move these muscles on yourself.

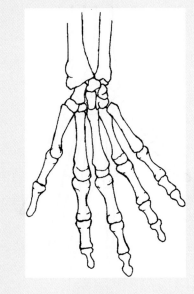

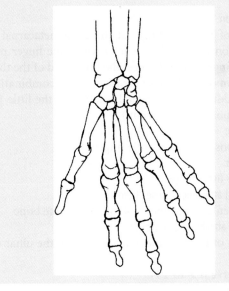

Hypothenar Muscles

Opponens digiti minimi
(oh-PONE-ens DIH-jih-tee MIN-ih-mee)

Opponens means "opposing," *digiti* means "of the fingers or toes," and *minimi* means "smallest."

Anterior

Abductor digiti minimi manus
(ab-DUCK-tur DIH-jih-tee MIN-ih-mee MAN-us)

Abductor means "one that leads away," *digiti* means "of the fingers or toes," *minimi* means "smallest," and *manus* means "of the hand."

Anterior

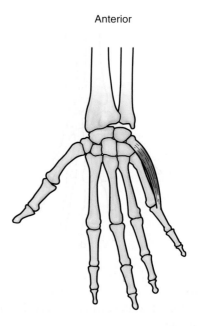

Concentric action:

Opposition of the little finger at the carpometacarpal joint (Opposition is the movement in which the finger pad of the little finger comes to meet the finger pad of the thumb. Opposition of the little finger is actually a combination of flexion, adduction, and lateral rotation of the little finger at the carpometacarpal joint.)

Eccentric action:

Restrains reposition of the little finger

Isometric action:

Stabilizes the little finger

Origin, proximal attachment, arises from:

Flexor retinaculum and the hook of the hamate bone

Insertion, distal attachment, attaches to:

Entire length of the fifth metacarpal bone on the ulnar side

Innervation:

The ulnar nerve (C8 to T1)

Major synergists:

Flexor digitorum superficialis, flexor digitorum profundus, and palmar interossei (No. 3)

Major antagonists:

Extensor digitorum, extensor digiti minimi, and abductor digiti minimi manus

Trigger points:

In the belly of the muscle

Referred pain pattern:

Into the little finger and wrist

Concentric action:

Abduction of the little finger at the metacarpophalangeal joint

Eccentric action:

Restrains adduction of the little finger

Isometric action:

Stabilizes the little finger

Origin, proximal attachment, arises from:

Tendon of the flexor carpi ulnaris and the pisiform bone

Insertion, distal attachment, attaches to:

Base of the proximal phalanx of the little finger on the ulnar side and dorsal digital expansion

Innervation:

Ulnar nerve (C8 to T1)

Major synergists:

No major synergists

Major antagonists:

Palmar interossei (No. 3)

Trigger points:

In the belly of the muscle

Referred pain pattern:

Into the little finger and wrist

Flexor digiti minimi manus
(FLEKS-or DIH-jih-tee MIN-ih-mee MAN-us)

Flexor means "one that bends," *digiti* means "of the fingers or toes," *minimi* means "smallest," and *manus* means "of the hand."

Anterior

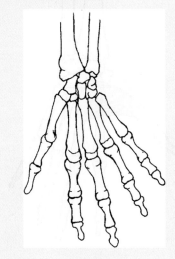

Concentric action:
Flexion of the little finger at the metacarpophalangeal joint
Eccentric action:
Restrains extension of the little finger
Isometric action:
Stabilizes the little finger
Origin, proximal attachment, arises from:
Hook of the hamate bone and flexor retinaculum
Insertion, distal attachment, attaches to:
Base of the proximal phalanx of the little finger on the ulnar side
Innervation:
Ulnar nerve (C8 to T1)
Major synergists:
Flexor digitorum superficialis and flexor digitorum profundus
Major antagonists:
Extensor digitorum and extensor digiti minimi
Trigger points:
In the belly of the muscle
Referred pain pattern:
Into the little finger and wrist

ACTIVITY 9-44

Draw and color the **hypothenar muscles** in the spaces provided. For each muscle, do the following:
1. Label the origin and insertion attachment points: *O* for origin; *I* for insertion.
2. Place an X on the trigger points.
3. Palpate this muscle; identify the attachment points and the bellies of the muscles.
4. Move these muscles on yourself.

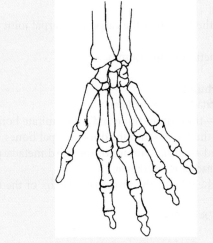

Central Compartment Muscles

Adductor pollicis (ad-DUCK-tur POLL-is-iss)

Adductor means "one that leads toward"; *pollicis* means "of the thumb."

Anterior

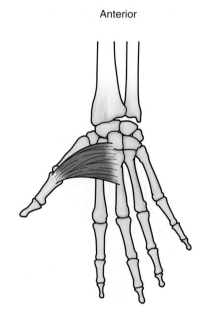

Concentric action:
Adduction of the thumb at the carpometacarpal joint
Eccentric action:
Restrains abduction of the thumb
Isometric action:
Stabilizes the thumb
Origin, proximal attachment, arises from:
Oblique head—trapezium, trapezoid, and capitate bones and the base of the second and third metacarpal bones
Transverse head—palmar surface of the third metacarpal
Insertion, distal attachment, attaches to:
Ulnar side of the base of the proximal phalanx of the thumb
Innervation:
Ulnar nerve (C8 to T1)
Major synergists:
There are no major synergists.
Major antagonists:
Abductor pollicis longus and abductor pollicis brevis
Trigger points:
In the belly of the muscle
Referred pain pattern:
Into the associated finger; commonly associated with Heberden's nodes, which develop on the dorsolateral or dorsomedial aspect of the terminal phalanx at its joint

Palmar interossei (PAL-mar INT-er-OSS-ee-eye)

Interossei means "between the bones"; *palmar* means "of the palm."

Anterior

Concentric action:
Adduction of the index, ring, and little fingers (2, 4, and 5) at the metacarpophalangeal joints (adduction of a finger is a movement toward an imaginary line drawn through the middle of the middle finger); flexion of fingers 2, 4, and 5 at the metacarpophalangeal joints; and extension of fingers 2, 4, and 5 at the proximal and distal interphalangeal joints
Eccentric action:
Restrains abduction, extension, and flexion of fingers 2, 4, and 5
Isometric action:
Stabilizes fingers 2, 4, and 5
Origin, proximal attachment, arises from:
First—ulnar side of the base of the second metacarpal bone
Second—radial side of the base of the fourth metacarpal bone
Third—radial side of the base of the fifth metacarpal bone
Insertion, distal attachment, attaches to:
First—ulnar side of the proximal phalanx of the index finger
Second—radial side of the proximal phalanx of the ring finger
Third—radial side of the proximal phalanx of the little finger
Innervation:
Ulnar nerve (C8 to T1)
Major synergists:
Lumbricals manus
Major antagonists:
Dorsal interossei
Trigger points:
In the belly of the muscle
Referred pain pattern:
Into the associated finger; commonly associated with Heberden's nodes, which develop on the dorsolateral or dorsomedial aspect of the terminal phalanx at its joint

Dorsal interossei dorsales manus
(DOR-sal INT-er-OSS-ee-eye MAN-us)

Interossei means "between the bones," *dorsales* means "related to the back," and *manus* means "of the hand."

Posterior

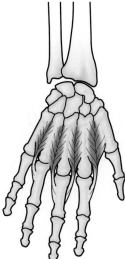

Concentric action:

Abduction of the index, middle, and ring fingers (fingers 2 to 4) at the metacarpophalangeal joints (abduction of a finger is a movement away from an imaginary line drawn through the middle of the middle finger); flexion of fingers 2 to 4 at the metacarpophalangeal joints; and extension of fingers 2 to 4 at the proximal and distal interphalangeal joints

Eccentric action:

Restrains adduction, extension, and flexion of fingers 2 to 4

Isometric action:

Stabilizes fingers 2 to 4

Origin, proximal attachment, arises from:

First—adjacent sides of the first and second metacarpal bones

Second—adjacent sides of the second and third metacarpal bones

Third—adjacent sides of the third and fourth metacarpal bones

Fourth—adjacent sides of the fourth and fifth metacarpal bones

Insertion, distal attachment, attaches to:

First—radial side of the proximal phalanx of the index finger

Second—radial side of the proximal phalanx of the middle finger

Third—ulnar side of the proximal phalanx of the middle finger

Fourth—ulnar side of the proximal phalanx of the ring finger

Innervation:

Ulnar nerve (C8 to T1)

Major synergists:

Lumbricals manus

Major antagonists:

Palmar interossei

Trigger points:

In the belly of the muscle

Referred pain pattern:

Into the associated finger; commonly associated with Heberden's nodes, which develop on the dorsolateral or dorsomedial aspect of the terminal phalanx at its joint

Lumbricals manus (LUM-brih-kals MAN-us)

Lumbricals means "earthworms"; *manus* means "of the hand."

Anterior

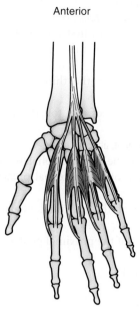

Concentric action:

Extension of the index, middle, ring, and little fingers at the interphalangeal joints and flexion of the index, middle, ring, and little fingers at the metacarpophalangeal joints

Origin, proximal attachment, arises from:

First and second—radial surface of the flexor digitorum profundus tendons of the index and middle fingers, respectively

Third—adjacent sides of the flexor digitorum profundus tendons of the middle and ring fingers

Fourth—adjacent sides of the flexor digitorum profundus tendons of the ring and little fingers

Insertion, distal attachment, attaches to:

Into the radial border of the dorsal digital expansion on the dorsal aspect of the digits

Innervation:

Median and ulnar nerves (C8 to T1)

Major synergists:

Palmar interossei and dorsal interossei manus, flexor digitorum superficialis, flexor digitorum profundus, and extensor digitorum

Major antagonists:

Flexor digitorum superficialis, flexor digitorum profundus, extensor digitorum

Trigger points:

In the belly of the muscle

Referred pain pattern:

Into the associated finger; commonly associated with Heberden's nodes, which develop on the dorsolateral or dorsomedial aspect of the terminal phalanx at its joint

✐ ACTIVITY 9-45

Draw and color the **central compartment muscles** in the spaces provided. For each muscle, do the following:

1. Label the origin and insertion attachment points: *O* for origin; *I* for insertion.
2. Place an X on the trigger points.
3. Palpate this muscle; identify the attachment points and the bellies of the muscles.
4. Move these muscles on yourself.

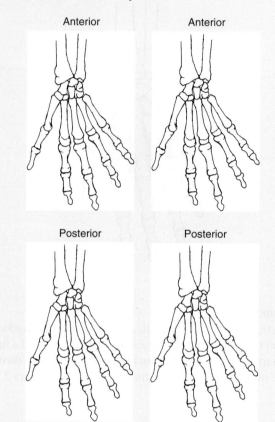

Anterior   Anterior

Posterior   Posterior

PATHOLOGIC CONDITIONS

SECTION OBJECTIVES

Chapter objective covered in this section:

13. Identify common pathology related to muscles and explain indications and contraindications for massage

After completing this section, the student will be able to perform the following:

- Identify common pathology related to muscles and explain indications and contraindications for massage

Mechanisms of Disease

Whenever the myofascial system is stressed, a fairly predictable sequence of events occurs[1]:

1. Causal factors and reflex factors can lead to increased muscle tension and retention of metabolic wastes. Causal factors include congenital factors or predisposition, overuse, misuse, abuse and disuse of the body, postural stress, chronic stressful emotional states, and so forth.

Reflex factors include trigger points, dysfunctional firing patterns, and so forth.

2. Increased tension leads to localized ischemia and edema.
3. Pain results.
4. Pain increases tension or spasm, which increases pain.
5. Inflammation or chronic irritation may result.
6. Neurologic reporting stations in tense tissue bombard the central nervous system with information, which leads to hyperactivity.
7. Macrophages and fibroblasts are activated.
8. Connective tissue production increases, with increasing shortening of fascia.
9. Because fascia is continuous throughout the body, any distortions in one area could create distortions elsewhere, affecting structures supported by or attached to the fascia, including the nerves, muscles, lymph, and blood vessels.
10. Changes occur in the muscular tissues, leading to chronic tension and ultimately to fibrotic changes. Increased tension in a muscle causes inhibition of the antagonist muscles and facilitation in the synergists.
11. Chain reactions in myotatic units occur. Typically, muscles used for posture become shortened, and muscles used for motion tend to weaken. This effect alters gait reflexes, and synergists can become dominant, causing muscle firing patterns to be altered.
12. Sustained increases in muscle tension cause ischemia in tendinous areas, and areas of periosteal pain develop.
13. Abnormal biomechanics and bodywide compensatory patterns develop. Torsion patterns at the shoulder and pelvic girdle are common. Gait patterns are compromised.
14. Joint restriction or imbalance or both develop, and fascial shortening and immobility increase.
15. Trigger points develop or worsen.
16. Generalized fatigue develops as a result of wasted energy used to maintain unproductive patterns and of an interrupted sleep pattern.
17. Sympathetic arousal is heightened, generalizing the pattern.
18. Immune response is altered, increasing susceptibility to disease.

Massage Intervention

Muscle dysfunction in the concentric action often results in short, tense muscles that do not relax and lengthen when necessary. Trigger points often set up in the muscle belly. Concentric contraction dysfunction is an important place to begin treatment, and the muscle needs to be relaxed and lengthened. Ideally, the shortened muscles will respond to strengthening procedures, and trigger points normalize.

Muscle dysfunction in the eccentric action phase often results in tense but elongated and strained muscles that are not shortening, so they attempt recruitment of synergists to function. Trigger points often set up in the attachments. The massage therapist should not treat any eccentric tight patterns with any methods that would relax and elongate the muscle further.

Isometric muscle dysfunction usually results in agonist and antagonist patterns interacting simultaneously to stabilize a joint dysfunction. This dysfunction is usually joint laxity, guarding an injury, or overuse. If this continues for a time, fibrosis is common, as is a reduced ability in concentric and eccentric functions. Mobility and coordination decrease because stabilizing function supersedes mobility.

Intervention focuses on reversing nonproductive patterns and supporting resourceful compensation patterns that develop in response to chronic problems. The goal is to support circulation and connective tissue pliability and calm the nervous system. Compression and stroking techniques support circulation. Connective tissue responds to methods that affect the viscoelastic, plastic, and colloid properties. Muscle shortening patterns respond to compression and drag that stimulates proprioceptors. Muscle energy methods systematically use contraction and relaxation of muscles combined with lengthening to restore normal length of the muscles. Trigger points respond to methods that reduce hyperactivity such as muscle energy methods and compression. Calming the sympathetic arousal is also necessary.

Medications

Pathologic conditions of the muscles are treated with antibiotics. Steroidal and nonsteroidal antiinflammatory medications ease inflammation. Muscle relaxants soothe spasm and hypertonic muscles, and analgesics treat pain. Low doses of antidepressants sometimes assist the client with sleep restoration and support of other restorative processes.

These drugs may be prescription or over-the-counter medications or herbal or homeopathic substances. Any form of medication or herbal remedy may have effects on the client that need to be taken into consideration when developing a treatment plan. Consideration must also be given to the interaction between massage and the effects of medication. Many medications used to treat muscle dysfunction determine the intensity of pressure and the duration and amount of stretch one can apply to the tissues.

Any time infection is present and is being treated with antibiotics, the system already is stressed. Therapeutic methods support the healing process by promoting general relaxation but are to be performed gently so as not to place additional demand on the system to respond. When clients use antiinflammatory drugs, the practitioner should avoid methods that produce therapeutic inflammation. Muscle relaxants interfere with the normal feedback systems of the stretch and tension receptors; because these medications interrupt this protective mechanism, the massage therapist must take care with any type of lengthening or stretching methods. Because analgesics interfere with the normal pain response, feedback from the client may be inaccurate. It is necessary to adjust intensity and duration.

Massage can support the use of these medications, helping make them more effective. In some instances the dosage of medication can be reduced or the medication can be replaced by massage therapy. Ice applications can support and sometimes reduce the use of analgesics and antiinflammatory drugs. Because all medications have side effects, the ability to take smaller doses of medication for short durations is beneficial. Any change in medication use must be set in place and carefully monitored by the prescribing health care provider.

Specific Disorders
Conditions
Stress-Induced Muscle Tension and Headache

Stress-induced muscle tension can result in myalgia, or muscle pain. The contracted muscles exert pressure on the nerves and blood vessels in the area, causing the pain. The stress-induced headache is a dull, persistent ache with feelings of tightness around the head, temples, forehead, and occipital area. It is often accompanied by stiffness in the neck and back. The headache may be less intense in the morning and worsen as the day goes on.

INDICATIONS/CONTRAINDICATIONS for *Therapeutic Massage*

Various strategies are used to treat stress-induced muscle tension headaches, including massage and other forms of soft-tissue work, biofeedback, relaxation training, exercise, and stretching methods. Chronic patterns often indicate connective tissue shortening, which can be alleviated with myofascial techniques. Headaches respond best to whole-body therapy, which not only addresses the immediate areas but also relaxes the entire body.

Cramps/Spasms

Cramps are painful muscle spasms or involuntary twitches. Cramps involve the whole muscle; spasms involve individual motor units within a muscle. Cramps often result from mild myositis or fibromyositis, but they can be a symptom of any irritation or of an electrolyte imbalance. Clonic spasms alternate contraction and relaxation in the muscle. Tonic spasms, or tetany, are sustained muscle contractions usually caused by disorders of the central nervous system.

Cramps and spasms may seem benign, but they can be symptomatic of more severe underlying conditions. If there does not seem to be a logical reason for the cramps or spasms or if the cramps or spasms occur frequently, the practitioner should refer the client for a diagnosis.

INDICATIONS/CONTRAINDICATIONS for *Therapeutic Massage*

Simple cramps or spasms can be managed by firmly pushing the belly of the muscle together or by initiating reciprocal inhibition, which involves positioning the muscle so that the proximal and distal attachment of the cramping muscle closer together and then contracting the antagonist. The practitioner lengthens the muscle gently after the cramp or spasm has subsided.

Fibromyalgia

Fibromyalgia is a syndrome with symptoms of widespread pain or aching, persistent fatigue, generalized morning stiffness, nonrestorative sleep, and multiple tender points. The

symptoms often are found with headaches, irritable bladder, dysmenorrhea, cold sensitivity, Raynaud's phenomenon, restless legs, atypical patterns of numbness and tingling, and complaints of weakness. The onset usually is gradual, often following prolonged exposure to damp cold, a bacterial or viral infection, or prolonged physical or emotional stress. Chronic fatigue syndrome also may be present.

A neurochemical imbalance, central nervous system hypersensitivity, and a disrupted sleep pattern, coupled with the dysfunction of myofascial repair mechanisms, seem to be contributing factors. Treatment protocols aim at sleep restoration and a gradual rebuilding of the myofascial system. Diet and lifestyle changes, moderate exercise, and various forms of complementary therapies and mind/body approaches are beneficial. If necessary, low doses of antidepressants often can help restore sleep patterns.

INDICATIONS/CONTRAINDICATIONS for *Therapeutic Massage*

General constitutional approaches seem to work best to aid in symptomatic pain reduction and restoration of the sleep pattern. The practitioner should avoid any form of therapy that causes therapeutic inflammation, including intense exercise and stretching programs, until healing mechanisms in the body are functioning. Exercise programs should be gentle and slow. If tender points have been injected with antiinflammatory medications, anesthetics, or other substances, the massage therapist should not massage over the area.

Contracture

Contracture is the chronic shortening of a muscle, especially the connective tissue component. Volkmann's ischemic contracture occurs in the upper or lower extremity when the blood supply is cut off and can be caused by tight casts, tourniquets, fractures, dislocations, or vascular spasms. The ischemia can lead to fibrosis and can result in the contracture of the muscles, tendons, and fascia.

INDICATIONS/CONTRAINDICATIONS for *Therapeutic Massage*

Gentle, slow intervention using connective tissue methods and stretching may improve contractures. Applying soft tissue and movement methods may prevent or slow the development of a contracture. The reason for the contracture must be taken into consideration when developing a treatment plan for managing this condition.

Dupuytren's Contracture

The first sign of Dupuytren's contracture is a thickened plaque overlying the tendon of the ring finger and occasionally the little finger at the level of the distal palmar crease. The skin in this area puckers, and a thickened, fibrotic cord develops between the palm and the finger. Flexion contracture of the fingers may increase gradually.

INDICATIONS/CONTRAINDICATIONS for *Therapeutic Massage*

Treatment is contraindicated regionally if methods increase symptoms.

Torticollis

Torticollis, or wry neck, involves a spasm or shortening of one of the sternocleidomastoid muscles. The condition may be congenital, acute, or chronic. Congenital torticollis can be caused by the fetal position or by a birth injury; acute torticollis is associated with cold or flu symptoms; chronic torticollis results from emotional stress, trauma, or infection.

INDICATIONS/CONTRAINDICATIONS for Therapeutic Massage

> Management of torticollis with massage therapy involves relaxing the neck, releasing trigger points, stretching the contracted muscles, and improving range of motion. Avoiding pressure on the vessels under the sternocleidomastoid muscle is important.

Anterior Compartment Syndrome

The anterior compartment of the leg is surrounded by a tough fascial sheath containing the tibialis anterior, the extensor digitorum longus, the extensor hallucis longus, and the peroneus (fibularis) tertius, as well as nerves and blood vessels. Any condition that increases pressure in this compartment interferes with blood flow and compresses the nerves. The affected person usually has a tight feeling in the calf and pain, numbness, and tingling. Overuse, repetitive stress, and accelerated growth of the muscles are common causal factors.

INDICATIONS/CONTRAINDICATIONS for Therapeutic Massage

> Treatment is contraindicated regionally unless supervised by the diagnosing or treating health care provider. Massage methods may soften the connective tissue sheath, relieving some of the pressure, but they also could aggravate the inflammatory process. Massage methods also can relieve fluid congestion, but by enhancing circulation, they also could increase blood flow to the area, thereby increasing the pressure. Elevation and ice may help.

Flaccidity and Spasticity

A muscle with decreased tone is flaccid; a muscle with excessive tone is spastic. Flaccid or spastic muscles often are associated with motor neuron disorders. The reason for the change in tone determines the appropriateness of massage or movement therapy. These conditions differ from general muscle tension or weakness in that the dysfunction has a physical cause rather than a functional one.

INDICATIONS/CONTRAINDICATIONS for Therapeutic Massage

> Massage therapy is indicated for both conditions for general relaxation and pain management. However, if these conditions result from a nervous system dysfunction, it is unlikely that massage will alter the specific condition. Caution is necessary because normal feedback mechanisms are altered and the client is unable to provide accurate feedback. Increased spacity can be a result of massage; therefore it is necessary to carefully monitor the result of massage. Flaccid muscles offer little resistance to compressive force, and the tissues may be injured if pressure is excessive.

Injuries

Muscle Strain

Injury to skeletal muscles caused by overexertion or trauma can result in muscle strain. Muscle strains involve overstretching or tearing of muscle fibers and associated connective tissue. Although the inflammation may subside in a few hours or days, repair of damaged muscle fibers usually takes weeks, and some damaged muscle cells may be replaced by fibrous tissue, forming scars.

INDICATIONS/CONTRAINDICATIONS for Therapeutic Massage

> Direct work over the area of injury is contraindicated regionally until all signs of inflammation have dissipated. The use of ice and gentle range of motion exercises can support healing. Methods to manage distortion in posture resulting from compensation in the rest of the body are helpful.

Contusion

Minor trauma to the muscles may cause a muscle bruise, or contusion, that involves local internal bleeding and inflammation. Severe trauma to a skeletal muscle may cause a crush injury that damages the affected muscle tissue and releases the muscle fiber contents into the bloodstream. This situation can be life-threatening because the reddish muscle pigment myoglobin can accumulate in the blood and cause kidney failure.

INDICATIONS/CONTRAINDICATIONS for Therapeutic Massage

> Direct work over the area of injury is contraindicated regionally until all signs of inflammation have dissipated.

Whiplash

Whiplash is an injury to the soft tissues of the neck caused by sudden hyperextension or flexion (or both) of the neck. The most common cause is an automobile accident resulting in pain, swelling, stiffness, and spasm in the shoulders and neck. In extension injuries the muscles most likely to be injured are the sternocleidomastoid, scalenes, infrahyoid muscles, suprahyoid muscles, levator scapulae, longus colli, suboccipital muscles, and rhomboid muscles. In flexion injuries the muscles most likely to be injured are the trapezius, splenius capitis, and semispinalis capitis. A side injury affects the sternocleidomastoid, suboccipital muscles, levator scapulae, splenius capitis, and splenius cervicis. Vestibular system damage to the inner ear may result in dizziness, nausea, vomiting, headache, and gait problems.

INDICATIONS/CONTRAINDICATIONS for Therapeutic Massage

> Direct intervention during the acute phase is contraindicated unless closely supervised by a physician or other qualified health care professional. Massage is a valuable part of rehabilitation in the subacute phase and can help restore function if the condition is chronic. Extension injury is more severe and requires careful intervention.

Rotator Cuff Tear

Repeated impingement, overuse, or other conditions may weaken the rotator cuff and eventually cause partial or complete tears. The condition is more common after age 40. Prior injury may increase the likelihood of a tear. Symptoms include weakness, atrophy of the supraspinatus and infraspinatus muscles, pain, and tenderness. A complete tear of the supraspinatus tendon severely impairs active abduction at the glenohumeral joint. An attempt to abduct the arm instead produces a characteristic shoulder shrug.

INDICATIONS/CONTRAINDICATIONS for Therapeutic Massage

> Work on acute myofascial tears is contraindicated. However, massage therapy may be indicated in the rehabilitative process and as part of a supervised treatment protocol. Compensatory patterns can be managed or improved with massage.

Myopathies

Muscular Dystrophy

The term *muscular dystrophy* encompasses a group of disorders characterized by atrophy of skeletal muscles with no malfunction of the nervous system. The muscle protein dystrophin declines or is lacking. Some forms of muscular dystrophy can be fatal.

The most common form of muscular dystrophy is Duchenne's muscular dystrophy (DMD), also called *pseudohypertrophy* (meaning "false muscle growth") because the atrophy of muscle is masked by excessive replacement of muscle by fat and fibrous tissue. DMD usually begins with mild leg muscle weakness that progresses rapidly to include the shoulder muscles.

The first signs of DMD become apparent at about 3 years of age, and the child usually is affected severely within 5 to 10 years. Death from respiratory or cardiac muscle weakness often occurs by 21 years of age.

Many pathophysiologists believe that DMD is caused by a missing fragment in the X chromosome, although other factors may be involved. Because girls have two X chromosomes and boys only one, genetic diseases involving X chromosome abnormalities are more likely to occur in boys. This is true because girls with one affected X chromosome may not exhibit an X-linked disease if the other X chromosome is normal.

Some less devastating forms of muscular dystrophy are fascioscapulohumeral dystrophy, which affects the fascia and shoulder girdle muscles, and limb-girdle dystrophy, which affects the pelvic and shoulder girdle muscles.

INDICATIONS/CONTRAINDICATIONS for Therapeutic Massage

> Careful intervention may slow the atrophy. Passive and active range of motion methods not only directly affect the muscles and joints but also aid in the circulation and elimination processes. Abdominal massage may help with constipation. Methods that cause any inflammation should not be used.

Myositis Ossificans

Myositis ossificans involves an inflammatory process that stimulates the formation of osseous tissue in the fascial components of muscles. The disease may occur with no apparent cause or may occur after a fracture or contusion. The onset of muscle pain is gradual.

INDICATIONS/CONTRAINDICATIONS for Therapeutic Massage

> Treatment is contraindicated regionally in myositis ossificans.

Muscle Infections

Several bacteria, viruses, and parasites may infect muscle tissue, often producing local or widespread myositis (muscle inflammation). Trichinosis, which is caused by a parasite, is an example of such an infection. The muscle pain and stiffness that sometimes accompany influenza is another example of myositis. Poliomyelitis is a viral infection of the nerves that control skeletal muscle movement. Polio is usually asymptomatic in populations where there is poor sanitation. It enters the body by way of a fecal-oral route and usually passes through the body without causing disease, but in a small number of cases it enters the central nervous system and causes the "polio" symptoms we recognize. Poliomyelitis often causes paralysis that may progress to death. Virtually eliminated in the United States through an effective vaccine, polio nonetheless still affects millions around the world who have not been vaccinated.

More common is the occurrence of postpolio syndrome in persons who had polio years ago. The symptoms are weakness, fatigue, intolerance to cold, and general aching pain.

INDICATIONS/CONTRAINDICATIONS for Therapeutic Massage

> For postpolio syndrome general constitutional approaches seem to work best to aid in overall pain reduction and restoration of the sleep pattern. Any form of therapy that causes therapeutic inflammation, including intense exercise and stretching programs, should not be used.

Acquired Metabolic and Toxic Myopathies

Acquired metabolic myopathies often result from disorders of the endocrine system. Nutritional and vitamin deficiency, especially protein deficiency and lack of vitamins C, D, and E, may lead to myopathy.

INDICATIONS/CONTRAINDICATIONS for Therapeutic Massage

> Treatment for these types of myopathy usually is not contraindicated, as long as the therapeutic approaches are general and focus on supporting body restoration and the healing processes. Regional avoidance of steroid injection sites is indicated. Massage can support detoxification efforts because these methods enhance circulation. The massage therapist must take care in toxic conditions not to tax an already overloaded system. A general therapeutic approach over a longer period is indicated.

Toxic myopathies are related to certain drugs and chemicals. Corticosteroid therapy may cause steroid-induced muscle weakness. An excessive alcohol intake can result in breakdown of striated muscles, which can affect the skeletal and other muscles.

SUMMARY

Just as muscles are able to function concentrically, eccentrically, and isometrically, massage professionals play various roles. You, the massage professional, are the one who provides the massage application, educates the client in wellness strategies, supports other professions in multidisciplinary teams, and maintains stability in scope of practice and ethical boundaries in the professional relationship. Much like muscles, your job requires a specific action depending on the demands and usually is an ever-changing dynamic process. Competency is measured by how you are able to take information and use it in a multidimensional way and in functional units. This chapter presented functional patterns of interaction of the muscles. This information is used functionally in the massage practice in multiple ways as well. Understanding the location and various actions of muscles and their relationship to the rest of the body influences skilled assessment, clinical reasoning, decision making regarding appropriate methods to achieve outcomes for the session, charting and other forms of written documentation, and interaction with other health and training professionals.

This chapter has taken an in-depth look at the muscular system. We have explored individual muscles and mapped the interdependent nature of muscular action in the synergist and antagonist pattern of each muscle. We have identified common trigger points and their referred pain patterns. We have discussed the progression of pathologic conditions in muscle dysfunction along with the indications and contraindications for massage for specific muscle-related dysfunctions.

We explore the larger picture of dynamic movement in the next chapter, where we see all the parts—bones, joints, and muscles—as a functioning unit that is more than the sum of its parts.

The author would like to thank Joseph E. Muscolino, Sandra K. Anderson, and Christopher Jones for their diligent reviews of this chapter. Their expertise is much appreciated.

⊝volve

http://evolve.elsevier.com/Fritz/essential

Activity 9-1 Play a hangman game to familiarize yourself with key terms from this chapter.

Activity 9-2 Complete a crossword that reviews the anatomy and physiology of muscle fibers.

Activity 9-3 A matching exercise helps you review muscle shapes.

Activity 9-4 Drag and drop muscle names onto anterior and posterior views of the human body.

Activity 9-5 Reinforce your knowledge of muscle identification by studying the individual muscles on flashcards.

Additional Resources:

Scientific animations and cadaver dissection video

Weblinks: Access weblinks that lead to research articles and an anatomy lesson from a Georgetown University instructor.

Remember to study for your certification and licensure exams! Review questions for this chapter are located on Evolve.

REFERENCES

1. Chaitow L: The amazing fascial web, part I, *Massage Today*, May, 2005.
2. Chaitow L: *Muscle energy techniques*, ed 3, London, 2006, Churchill Livingstone.
3. Drake R, Vogl W, Mitchell AWM: *Gray's anatomy for students*, ed 2, Edinburgh, 2010, Churchill Livingstone.
4. Greenman PE: *Principles of manual medicine*, ed 3, Philadelphia, 2003, Lippincott Williams & Wilkins.
5. Muscolino JE: *The muscular system manual: the skeletal muscles of the human body*, ed 3, St Louis, 2007, Mosby.
6. Myers T: *Anatomy trains: myofascial meridians for manual and movement therapists*, ed 2, New York, 2009, Churchill Livingstone.
7. Pollack GH, Cameron I, Wheatley D: *Water and the cell*, New York, 2006, Springer.
8. Stecco A et al: Anatomical study of myofascial continuity in the anterior region of the upper limb, *J Bodyw Mov Ther* 13(1):53–62, 2009.

RECOMMENDED READINGS

Muscolino JE: *The muscular system manual: the skeletal muscles of the human body*, ed 3, St Louis, 2010, Mosby.

Muscolino JE: *Kinesiology: the skeletal system and muscle function*, ed 2, St Louis, 2011, Mosby.

Salvo SG: *Mosby's pathology for massage therapists*, ed 2, St Louis, 2009, Mosby.

Workbook Section

Short Answer

1. List and describe the functions of muscles.

_____
_____
_____
_____
_____
_____
_____
_____
_____
_____
_____
_____
_____

2. List and describe the three types of muscles.

_____
_____
_____
_____
_____
_____
_____
_____
_____
_____
_____
_____
_____

3. List and describe the three types of skeletal muscle fibers.

_____
_____
_____
_____
_____
_____
_____
_____
_____
_____

4. List and describe the four components of myotatic units.

_____
_____
_____
_____
_____
_____
_____
_____
_____
_____
_____
_____

Fill in the Blank

An agonist is a muscle that causes or controls joint motion through a specified plane of motion and also is known as a primary or (1) _____ mover.

The (2) _____ occurs when a muscle contraction is initiated and all the muscle fibers contract to their full ability, or they do not contract at all.

A/An (3) _____ is a muscle that usually is located on the opposite side of the joint from the agonist and that has the opposite action.

(4) _____ and antagonist muscles can contract together at the same time in what is called a (5) _____.

Contractility is the ability of a muscle to (6) _____ forcibly with adequate stimulation.

(7) _____ forms a coarse sheet of fibrous connective tissue that binds muscles into functional groups and forms partitions, called *intermuscular septa,* between muscle groups.

Dynamic force produces (8) _____ in or of an object.

Elasticity is the ability of a muscle to recoil and resume its original resting length after being (9) _____. Applying force is called (10) _____, and releasing force is called *unloading.*

(11) _____ is the ability of a muscle to receive and respond to a stimulus.

(12) _____ is the ability of a muscle to be stretched or extended.

A/An (13) _____ is a stabilizing muscle located at a joint that contracts to fixate, or stabilize, an area, enabling another limb or body segment to exert force and move.

The insertion is the most movable part of a muscle, or the part that attaches (14) _____ from the midline or center of the body.

Maximal stimulus is the point at which all the motor units of a muscle have been recruited and the muscle is unable to (15) _____ in strength.

A (16) _____ consists of the muscle fibers innervated by a single motor neuron.

The (17) _____ is the part of a muscle considered the least movable, or the part that attaches closest to the midline or center of the body.

Oxygen debt is the extra amount of oxygen that must be taken in to convert (18) _____ to glucose or glycogen.

(19) _____ force applied to an object does not produce movement.

Synergist muscles aid or assist the action of the agonists but are not primarily responsible for the action; synergists are also known as (20) _____ muscles.

The (21) _____ is the stimulus at which the first observable muscle contraction occurs.

Tone is a state of slight (22) _____ in all skeletal muscle that enables the muscle to respond to stimulation.

A trigger point, as described by Janet Travell, is a (23) _____ locus within a taut band of skeletal muscle, located in the muscular tissue or its associated fascia or both. The spot is painful on compression and can evoke characteristic (24) _____ pain and autonomic phenomena. (25) _____ involves neurochemical responses of the muscle fiber. Stretching involves a (26) _____ force directed to altering connective tissue structure.

According to Myers, (27) _____ refers to structures that maintain their integrity primarily because of a balance of continuous tensile forces through the structure.

Problem Solving

Read the problem presented. There is no correct answer; rather the exercise is intended to assist the student in developing the analytical and decision-making skills necessary in a professional practice. After reading the problem, follow the next six steps:
1. Identify the facts presented in the information.
2. Identify the possibilities ("what if" statements), or develop your own possibilities that relate to the facts.
3. Evaluate each possibility in terms of the logical cause and effect and pros and cons.
4. Consider the effect on the persons involved.
5. Write each answer in the space provided.
6. Develop your solution by answering the question posed.

Problem

Massage professionals focus on the muscular system as they work with clients. Therefore thinking in terms of individual muscles certainly seems logical when working with

assessment—or is it? This chapter described the way muscles work in functional units. The nervous system controls muscles. Connective tissue is a huge component of muscles. Muscle tension increases with sympathetic arousal, as in the fight-or-flight response. Is it possible that therapeutic massage really has little to do with muscle tissue?

Many testing processes focus extensively on the functional aspect of individual muscles and little on the more systemic effects of massage. This situation may influence the curriculum at schools that teach massage therapies. One wonders if such an education may overemphasize the study of individual muscles and underemphasize the nervous system, endocrine system, and systemic homeostatic processes. The study of muscles is important. The truth is that the massage practitioner really understands functional patterns of movement only when he or she has a solid comprehension of the components of movement—the bones, the joints, the connective tissue, and the muscles. Also true is that the major benefits of massage are based on the systems of control and support of connective tissue structures.

Question

In this age of "too much to know," what learning is necessary to function as a competent health professional?

Facts

1. Massage professionals focus on the muscular system.
2. _____
3. _____

Possibilities

1. Curricula at schools that teach massage therapies may be influenced by examination requirements.
2. _____
3. _____

Logical Cause and Effect

1. Important areas of study are not covered effectively because of lack of time.
2. _____
3. _____

Effect

1. Students may be frustrated with studying information that seems less important.
2. _____
3. _____

On the basis of your analysis, how will you respond to the following question: In this age of "too much to know," what learning is necessary to function as a health professional?

Professional Application

What additional knowledge base would the practitioner need to work with stress-induced muscle tension and headache for therapeutic massage? Where might a massage practitioner find this information and get additional training?

_____

_____

_____

_____

_____

_____

_____

_____

Assess Your Competencies

1. Explain the various terminologies used to describe muscles.
   - Identify areas of terminology confusion.
   - Explain the importance of the Terminologia Anatomica.
   - Use muscle attachment terminology based on both anatomy and physiology.

Muscle Structure and Function

2. Describe the relationship between structure and function of muscles.
3. Describe the anatomy and physiology of skeletal muscle fibers.
4. List the components of myotatic units.
5. Identify the different muscle shapes and fiber arrangements.
6. Describe the response of proprioceptors to stimuli and the most common reflexes.
7. Describe the process of muscle firing patterns/muscle activation sequences.
   - Explain the function of muscles.
   - List the three types of muscles.
   - List and describe four functional characteristics of muscle.
   - Define and demonstrate two types of muscle actions and the variations of each.
   - Describe a muscle as an organ and the structural and functional components.
   - Explain the length-tension relationship.
   - Define *resting muscle tone*.
   - Identify the energy source for muscle contraction.
   - Explain the difference between red slow-twitch and white fast-twitch muscle fibers.
   - Describe the connective tissue component of muscle.
   - Explain how muscles attach to bone or related tissue.
   - List the components of myotatic units.
   - List and draw four distinct muscle shapes.
   - Describe the nervous system functions of proprioception and reflexes related to muscle function.
   - Define *muscle activation sequences*.

8. Describe the integrated connective tissue structure of muscle.
   - Describe the biochemical activities of connective tissue.
   - Define fascia.
   - Define biomechanical terms relating to fascia.
   - Describe the concept of myofascial continuity.
   - Explain pathologic connective tissue changes.
9. Explain and demonstrate the three types of muscle actions.
10. Describe how muscles are named.
11. Learn how to palpate individual muscles.
12. Identify the attachments, action, synergist, antagonist, and common trigger points of individual muscles.
    - Draw muscles, identifying location, fiber direction, attachments, and common trigger point location.
    - Apply knowledge of the muscular system to therapeutic massage application.
13. Identify common pathology related to muscles and explain indications and contraindications for massage.
    - Identify common pathology related to muscles and explain indications and contraindications.

Next, on a separate piece of paper or using an audio or video recorder, prepare a short narrative that reflects how you would explain this content to a client and how the information relates to how you would provide massage. See the example in Chapter 1 on p. 22. When read or listened to, the narrative should not take more than 5 to 10 minutes to complete. Simpler is better. Use examples, tell stories, and use metaphors. It is important to understand that there is no precisely correct way to complete this exercise. The intent is to help you identify how effectively you understand the content and how relevant your application is to massage therapy. An excellent learning activity is to work together with other students and share your narratives. Also share these narratives with a friend or family member who is not familiar with the content. If that person can understand what you have written or recorded, that indicates that you understand it. There are many different ways to complete this learning activity. Yes, it may be confusing to do this, but that's all right. Out of confusion comes clarity. By the time you do this 12 times, once for each chapter in this book, you will be much more competent.

Further Study

Using additional resource material (see the Works Consulted list at the back of this book), find the content that pertains to the information presented in this chapter. As a study guide, elaborate by writing a paragraph of additional information on each of the following:
Force

_____

_____

_____

_____

Motor points

_____
_____
_____
_____

Repair of muscle

_____
_____
_____
_____

Cardiac muscle

_____
_____
_____
_____

Smooth muscle

_____
_____
_____
_____

CHAPTER OBJECTIVES

After completing this chapter, the student will be able to perform the following:

1. Explain the basic principles of biomechanics
2. Explain and assess function of the kinetic chain
3. List principles of a massage intervention plan based on efficient biomechanical movement.
4. Assess biomechanical function using individual joint assessment.
5. Assess biomechanical functions for regions of the body.
6. Identify and describe the three main biomechanical dysfunctional patterns and the associated indications and contraindications for massage.

CHAPTER OUTLINE

BIOMECHANICS, 469
Force, 469
Levers and Fulcrums, 470
Balance, Equilibrium, and Stability, 473
Posture, 473
KINETIC CHAIN, 476
Inner Unit, 477
Outer Unit, 478
Postural Stabilization, 478
Sitting, Standing, and Bending, 478
Walking/Gait, 478
Muscle Firing Patterns/Activation Sequences, 494
ASSESSMENT BASED ON BIOMECHANICS, 494
Individual Joint Assessment, 494
Biomechanics by Region, 498
PATHOLOGIC CONDITIONS, 537
Common Postural Deviations, 542
Nonoptimal Motor Function, 543
Neuromuscular-related Dysfunction, 543
Myofascial-related Dysfunction, 543
Joint-related Dysfunction, 544
Degrees and Stages of Dysfunction, 545
SUMMARY, 546

KEY TERMS

Acceleration The rate of change in speed.
Balance The ability to control equilibrium.
Biomechanics The science concerned with the internal and external forces acting on the human body and the effects produced by these forces.

Center of gravity An imaginary midpoint or center of the weight of a body or object, where the body or object could balance on a point.
Effort The force applied to overcome resistance.
Equilibrium All forces acting on an object are equal.
Force Push or pull on an object in an attempt to affect motion or shape.
Gait The rhythmic and alternating motions of the legs, trunk, and arms resulting in the propulsion of the body.
Gait cycle Subdivided into the stance phase and swing phase, this cycle begins when the heel of one foot strikes the floor and continues until the same heel strikes the floor again.
Inertia (in-NUR-shuh) The property of matter in which it remains at rest or in uniform motion in the same straight line unless acted upon by some external force.
Kinesiology (ki-NE-SE-ol-O-JE) The study of movement that combines the fields of anatomy, physiology, physics, and geometry and relates them to human movement.
Kinetic chain An integrated functional unit. The kinetic chain is made up of the myofascial system (muscle, ligament, tendon, and fascia), articular (joint) system, and nervous system. Each of these systems works interdependently to allow structural and functional efficiency in all three planes of motion: sagittal, frontal, and transverse.
Lever (LEV-er) A solid mass such as a crowbar or a person's arm that rotates around a fixed point called the *fulcrum*. The rotation is produced by a force applied to a lever at some distance from the fulcrum.
Resistance Resistance opposes force.
Stability The resistance to change in the acceleration of the body or the resistance to the disturbance of the equilibrium of the body.
Vector The direction of the force.

Chapter 10 is the final chapter in the kinesiology and biomechanics section of this textbook. Chapters 7, 8, and 9 targeted kinesiology. In Chapters 7, 8, and 9, the information about bones, joints, and muscles provided the foundation for learning about biomechanics. Chapter 10 (this chapter) is biomechanics. These four chapters combine to create an understanding of why, how, and what happens when we move. As you begin the study of biomechanics you will find that it is necessary to understand the kinesiology before you can comprehend the effects of movement on the body.

There is a difference between learning the names of parts and what parts can do and learning about how various parts work together to create a combined outcome. Think of a bike. It has a multiple parts. One of the parts is a wheel. The wheel is part of the bike, but the wheel is not the bike. Okay: a little weird, but consider a movement such as walking. Walking requires bones, joints, muscles, and at least the nervous system and circulatory system, if not the rest. So muscles are part of walking, but walking is a lot more than muscles.

This chapter is not specifically about parts. You learned the parts in previous chapters. This chapter is about understanding the relationships of those parts. If you do not remember the names of the parts (e.g., bones, joints, and muscles), you will be confused. If you do not remember the meaning of a word, you will have to look it up. The best way to study this chapter is to make up examples. There are lots of examples in the chapter, but the examples you make up are even better.

The information in this chapter is also about doing. For example: Pressure is the amount of force on a specific area. During massage application the method called *compression* generates a compressive force. The amount of pressure used during the massage depends on variations of the compressive force applied to the body.

Now do something: get a balloon, blow it up, and then watch and feel what happens when you press on it.

Have fun.

Recall that kinesiology is:

1. The science dealing with the interrelationship of anatomy and the physiology of the body with respect to movement.
2. The study of movement that blends anatomy, physiology, physics, and geometry and relates them to human movement.

Kinesiology is the study of body movement. It involves a lot of anatomy and physiology. Where we apply massage requires understanding kinesiology. Biomechanics is the study of the effects of movement on the body. It involves a lot of math and measurement. What occurs because of the mechanical forces applied to the body during massage requires understanding biomechanics. You need to understand biomechanics before you are able to perform physical assessment and develop care/treatment plans for clients with goals related to posture and movement.

BIOMECHANICS

SECTION OBJECTIVES

Chapter objective covered in this section:

1. Explain the basic principles of biomechanics.

After completing this section, the student will be able to perform the following:

- Define biomechanics.
- Identify the center of gravity of the body
- Describe force
- Describe and demonstrate the effects of force.
- Explain lever and fulcrum and the application of force
- Demonstrate mechanical advantage and disadvantage.
- Describe and demonstrate balance, equilibrium and stability.
- Describe and demonstrate good posture.
- Perform a postural assessment
- Identify common postural deviations
- Explain gait
- Demonstrate the adult walking cycle

Biomechanics is the science concerned with the internal and external forces acting on the human body and the effects produced by these forces. Movement is a fundamental characteristic of human behavior and is accomplished by contraction of skeletal muscles acting within a system of levers and pulleys formed by bones, tendons, and ligaments that network into the unified tensegric system of the body.

Biomechanics involves investigating in detail the body, its alignment, and how it functions. Because a variety of forces may act on the human body and lead to movement, rest, or stress, the massage therapist must have a basic understanding of biomechanical principles. Understanding these principles helps us in assessing and observing the body and in clinical reasoning methods used to develop treatment plans.

The study of biomechanics involves looking at the static (nonmoving) or dynamic (moving) aspects of various activities. An understanding of biomechanics includes:

- Application of the mechanical principles in the study of living organisms.
- The science of movement of a living body including how muscles, bones, tendons, and ligaments work together to produce movement.
- The study of mechanical principles and actions applied to living bodies. This may involve looking at the static (nonmoving) or dynamic (moving) systems associated with various activities.
- The application of mechanical principles such as engineering to human movement.

Physical therapists, occupational therapists, exercise physiologists, and athletic trainers deal with the performance-specific and rehabilitative analysis of human movement. They undertake extended studies to address problems with biomechanics or to develop specific training and exercise protocols. Therapeutic massage can be a valuable adjunct modality to the rehabilitation programs developed by these health care specialists. However, clients should first be referred to these professionals if movement problems are found during assessment.

Force

Because biomechanics is the science concerned with the internal and external forces acting on the human body and the effects produced by these forces, we need to understand the properties of force. Throughout the textbook mechanical forces have been described and discussed. Recall that the types of mechanical forces are compression, tension, bend, shear, and torsion.

Force causes change. Forces push or pull on an object in an attempt to affect motion or shape. The human body moves because of internal forces, such as muscle contraction, and external forces, such as being pulled by a dog on leash. Therapeutic massage applies external forces to create change in the homeostatic mechanisms of the body. Forces generated by massage include tension, torsion, bend, shear, and compression. Chapters 8 and 9 define these forces in detail.

Technically, force is the product of mass multiplied by acceleration. A **vector** is the direction of the force. The magnitude of a vector is the result of the horizontal and vertical components of an applied force. For example, an 80-pound force being applied downward at 60 degrees is the result of a horizontal force of 40 pounds and a vertical force of 69.3 pounds. Mass is the amount of matter or material substance that forms or comprises a body. For our purposes, weight and mass are the same. The weight times the speed or acceleration determines the amount of force. A feather floating softly down to touch our arm exerts less force than a bowling ball thrown down an alley.

The following elements influence or are related to force and massage application:

Pressure: Pressure is the amount of force on a specific area. During massage application the method called *compression* generates a compressive force. The amount of pressure used during the massage depends on variations of the compressive force applied to the body.

Inertia: Inertia is the property of matter in which it remains at rest or in uniform motion in the same straight line unless acted upon by some external force. Because force is required to change inertia, any activity that is carried out at a steady pace, in a consistent direction, conserves energy. Any irregularly paced or multidirectional activity costs energy. A movement example is handball, which is more fatiguing than dancing. To support the body mechanics of the massage therapist, massage methods should be applied using a steady pace in a consistent direction. For example, massage strokes are typically slow, even, and rhythmic.

Acceleration: Acceleration is the rate of change in speed. To begin to move the body and attain speed generally requires a strong muscular force. Weight (mass) coupled with the influence of gravity affects speed and acceleration during physical movements. Accelerating a 200-lb adult takes more muscle force than accelerating a 50-lb child. Acceleration occurs in the same direction as the force that caused it. The change in acceleration is directly proportional to the force causing it and inversely proportional to the mass of the body. This means that a large force provides a greater degree of acceleration than a small force. Given the same amount of force, more acceleration occurs on a light body than on a heavy one.

Speed: Speed is a variable of massage application. Typically, the speed of a massage method is slow; however, some, such as percussion (tapotement) methods, are fast. The concept of acceleration would suggest that each time a new massage stroke begins, more muscle effort is required by the massage therapist, and massage methods that are applied at a fast speed require the most effort.

Resistance: Resistance opposes force. Newton's law of reaction says that for every action, there is an opposite and equal reaction. As we place force on the floor by walking on it, the floor provides an equal resistance back in the opposite direction to the soles of our feet. Walking on a wood floor is easier than walking on a sandy beach because of the difference in the reaction of the two surfaces. The wood floor resists the weight and pushes back, making walking easier, whereas the sand dissipates the force and requires more effort with each step.

The massage client's body tissues provide resistance to the force created by the massage stroke. The surface of the body—especially with the application of a lubricant—offers little resistance to the massage application. However, more resistance is experienced when the pressure increases and the deeper tissues are accessed. Also, some individuals have much denser tissue and therefore offer more resistance to the mechanical forces created by massage.

Effort: Effort is the force applied to overcome resistance. It takes more effort by the massage therapist to work on deep tissues that are dense and thick. It also takes effort to hold surface tissue at their binding end points, such as when performing certain myofascial release methods. It takes less effort to work on surface tissues of the body, especially when using a lubricant that increases the slipperiness of the skin.

Practical Application

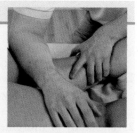

Because massage therapy is the application of mechanical forces, it is helpful to relate the elements that influence force to massage.

When applying pressure to a client, especially during a gliding stroke, it is always more efficient to go uphill than downhill. Whenever a force vector is applied at an angle, the force can be broken down into its horizontal and vertical component. When applying a force into a client going uphill, both the horizontal and vertical components of the force go into the client's tissue. However, when applying a force downhill, only the vertical component of the force goes into the client's tissue; the horizontal component goes out into space away from the body like pushing into the air and is wasted (Figure 10-1).

Levers and Fulcrums

Force is more easily achieved using a lever. Levers help a given effort move a heavier load or move a load farther than could otherwise be done. A **lever** is a rigid bar or mass that rotates around a fixed point called the *axis of rotation*, or *fulcrum*. Rotation is produced by applying force to a lever at some distance from the fulcrum. A force applied to a lever reduces the effort needed to overcome resistance.

In the body joints are the fulcrums and bones are the levers. Muscle contraction provides the effort and applies it at the muscle attachment points on a bone. The load that is

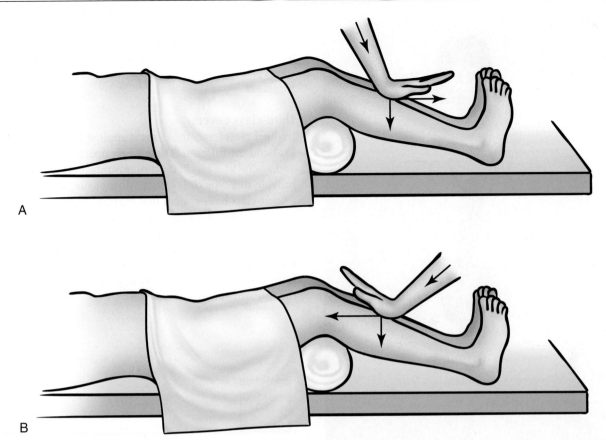

FIGURE 10-1 A, When applying a force downhill, only the vertical component of the force goes into the client's tissue; the horizontal component goes out into space like pushing into air and is wasted. **B,** When applying a force into a client going uphill, both the horizontal and vertical components of the force go into the client's tissue.

moved includes the bone, the overlying tissues, and anything else one tries to move with that particular lever, such as a book bag. Forces, when working on a joint that is a fulcrum in the body, cause a rotational effect. This is known as a moment (or torque). The body may be considered a series of interconnected levers. For example, in the forearm the radius and ulna act as a lever, with the elbow joint as the fulcrum (Figure 10-2).

Mechanical Advantage and Disadvantage

Mechanical advantage means that less effort is required to move an object, and mechanical disadvantage requires more effort to move the same object (Figure 10-3).

Regardless of the type, all levers follow the same basic principles:

- Lever systems that operate at a mechanical advantage are slower, more stable, and used where strength is a priority.
- In lever systems that operate at a mechanical disadvantage, force is lost but speed is gained.

There are three types of levers: first class, second class, and third class.

First-class Levers

In first-class levers the effort is applied at one end of the lever and the load at the other, with the fulcrum somewhere between them. Seesaws, scissors, and crowbars are familiar examples of first-class levers. Use of a first-class lever occurs when you lift your head off your chest. Some first-class levers in the body operate at a mechanical advantage when the effort is farther from the joint than the load and is less than the load to be moved. Other muscles operate at a mechanical disadvantage when the effort is closer to the joint and greater than the load to be moved (Figure 10-4).

Second-class Levers

In second-class levers the effort is applied at the end of the lever and the fulcrum is located at the other end, with the load at some intermediate point between them. A wheelbarrow is an example of this type of lever. Second-class levers are uncommon in the body, and the best example of their use is standing on your toes. Joints forming the ball of the foot act together as the fulcrum. The load is the entire body weight. The calf muscles inserted into the calcaneus exert the effort, pulling the heel upward. All second-class levers in the body

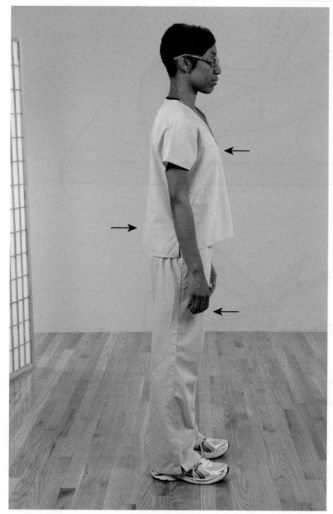

FIGURE 10-2 The lumbar area acts as the fulcrum, and the postural muscles working together act as a first-class lever where effort and resistance balance to maintain upright posture. Soft-tissue structures that surround the fulcrum are called the core and consist of all lumbar and abdominal structures.

work at a mechanical advantage because the muscle distal attachment is always farther from the fulcrum than is the load to be moved. Second-class levers are levers of strength, with speed and range of motion sacrificed (Figure 10-5).

Third-class Levers

In third-class levers the effort is applied at a point between the load and the fulcrum. These levers operate with greater speed and always at a mechanical disadvantage. Tweezers or forceps provide this type of leverage. Most of the body operates with a third-class lever system that permits a muscle to be inserted close to a joint, allowing rapid extensive movement with little shortening of the muscle. As an example, the biceps muscle of the arm provides the effort, the fulcrum is the elbow, and the force is exerted on the proximal radius. The load to be lifted is the distal forearm and anything carried in the hand or over the forearm (Figure 10-6).

Evolve Activity 10-1

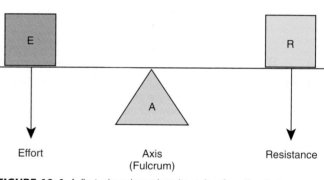

Effort   Axis   Resistance
                        (Fulcrum)

FIGURE 10-4 A first-class lever has its axis of motion between the force of effort and the force of resistance. (Modified from Roberts SL, Falkenburg SA: *Biomechanics: problem solving for functional activity,* St Louis, 1992, Mosby.)

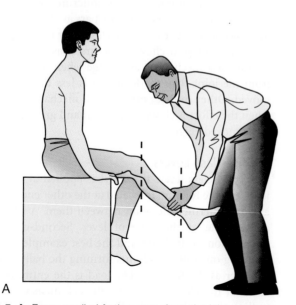

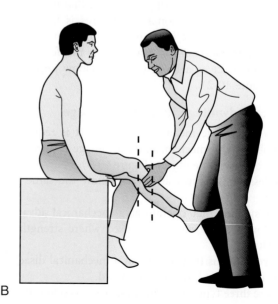

FIGURE 10-3 A, Force applied farther away from the joint results in mechanical advantage. **B,** Force applied near the joint results in mechanical disadvantage.

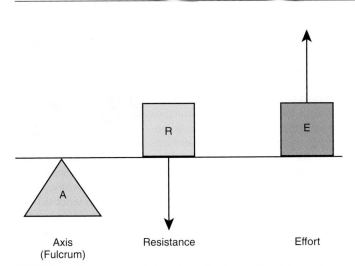

FIGURE 10-5 In a second-class lever the force of resistance lies between the axis of movement and the force of effort. (Modified from Roberts SL, Falkenburg SA: *Biomechanics: problem solving for functional activity,* St Louis, 1992, Mosby.)

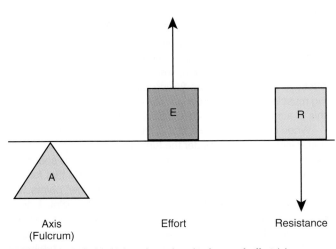

FIGURE 10-6 A third-class lever has its force of effort lying between the axis and the force of resistance. (Modified from Roberts SL, Falkenburg SA: *Biomechanics: problem solving for functional activity,* St Louis, 1992, Mosby.)

Balance, Equilibrium, and Stability

Balance is the ability to control equilibrium. The two types of balance are static or still balance and dynamic or moving balance.

Equilibrium means that all forces acting on an object are equal. Equilibrium may be static or dynamic. A body at rest or completely motionless is in static equilibrium. Dynamic equilibrium occurs when all of the applied and internal forces acting on the moving body are in balance, resulting in movement with no change in speed or direction. For us to control equilibrium to achieve balance, we need to maximize stability.

Stability is the resistance to change in the acceleration of the body or the resistance to the disturbance of the equilibrium of the body. Determining the center of gravity of the body and changing it appropriately may enhance stability.

In biomechanical terms the concept of center refers to the **center of gravity,** the midpoint or center, of the weight of a body or object. The center of gravity is the point at which all the mass, or weight, of the body is balanced equally or distributed equally in all directions. The anatomic center of gravity can be calculated if the body is at rest; however, the anatomic center of gravity changes constantly as the body moves. The position of the center of gravity depends on the arrangement of the body segments and changes with every movement. Any loss of biomechanical stability, such as occurs with a missing limb or altered posture, alters not only the total body weight distribution but also the center of gravity.

Physiologic functions of the nervous system contribute to balance. The tonic neck reflex is a reflex pattern stimulated by head movement that stimulates flexion and extension of the limbs, arms, and neck. The semicircular canals of the inner ear, vision, touch, pressure, and proprioceptive sense provide balance information. The body is in a constant dynamic state of adjustment to maintain balance, reflecting dynamic homeostasis.

Balance Principles

- A person is balanced when his or her center of gravity falls within the base of support.
- A person is balanced in direct proportion to the size of the base of support. The larger the base of support, the more balance.
- A person is balanced depending on his or her weight, or mass. The greater the weight, the more balance.
- A person's balance depends on the height of the center of gravity. The lower the center of gravity, the more balance.
- A person's balance depends on where his or her center of gravity is in relation to the base of support. If the center of gravity is near the edge of the base, less balance is present. However, in anticipation of an oncoming force, a person may improve stability by placing the center of gravity closer to the side of the base of support expected to receive the force.
- In anticipation of an oncoming force, a person may increase stability by enlarging the size of the base of support in the direction of the anticipated force.
- A person may enhance equilibrium by increasing the friction between the body and the surface it contacts.
- Rotation around an axis is easier to balance. A bike that is moving is easier to balance than a bike that is stationary (Activity 10-1) (Thompson and Floyd, 2000).

Posture

The postural muscles help us to maintain our upright position in gravity. This is quite a task because the center of gravity

✏ ACTIVITY 10-1

Kinetic chain protocol for posture stabilization
Assessment and Intervention: Practical Application (Posture)

The possible combination of these neurologic patterns is almost endless, yet one can assess for and treat these by applying the following principles:

Kinetic Chain Protocol: Posture-Movement Segments
The trunk moves and is balanced in the following areas:
Top of head and atlas/axis
Atlas/axis and C6/C7 vertebrae
C6/C7 and T12 (thoracolumbar junction)
T12 and S1 (sacrolumbar junction)
S1 and hips (acetabula)
Hips and knees
Knees and ankles
Ankles and tips of toes
Each of these areas can be considered a fulcrum

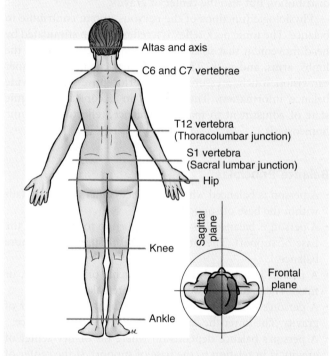

1. Identify the most prominent symptom, from pain or positional distortion. Usually these areas are in the soft tissue between the movement points (fulcrums).
2. Methodically assess the tissues diagonally from right to left and front to back in each soft-tissue segment, using the figure above. Search above and below the segment that contains the targeted area for related tension and pain. For example, if a symptom is on the back left between T12 and S1, begin assessment in segments above and below the segment with the symptom, on the opposite side (in this example, *right*), and in the front. Continue to the next segments above and below the area just checked using diagonal patterns until all areas are covered.
3. Provide intervention. Use any massage method to reduce tension and pain in each segment before addressing the main symptom, and then reassess the proximal attachmental symptom pattern, which should be reduced.

Practical Application

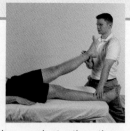

Muscles have properties and are able to function in multiple ways to meet various tasks, such as maintaining balance. Most daily activities require the coordination of complex neuromuscular interactions. Sometimes muscles are required to function for long periods without fatiguing, and at other times muscles must provide maximal effort for only a few seconds. Muscles have three major actions: isometric, concentric, and eccentric. Muscles must be able to shorten and lengthen to provide range of motion at joints, yet they must generate enough power to move a load at each end of the range. Muscles must be able to hold a static position to provide stability. The nervous system accomplishes the fine control of muscle contraction over a wide range of lengths, tensions, speeds, and loads.

When giving a massage, we have to assess for these functions. Massage application depends on accurate functional assessment. We can observe as a muscle contracts through its range of motion. When muscles move a joint, its ability to stabilize is decreased, and vice versa. Muscles that span a long distance, such as the biceps brachii of the arm, are most efficient supplying movement through a longer range of motion. Other muscles are more effective at stabilizing the joint than moving it. The coracobrachialis of the shoulder joint is a good example; its line of pull is mostly vertical and close to the axis of the shoulder joint. Therefore the coracobrachialis has a short range of motion, which makes this muscle more effective at stabilizing than flexing the shoulder joint. Opposing muscle groups generate parallel forces to provide stability; this is achieved through co-contraction (Figure 10-7).

When considering the effect of the massage, the massage therapist must also consider the function. For example, it may be important to lengthen and stretch a muscle that spans a distance and is primarily a mover muscle. A muscle that functions primarily as a stabilizer may develop trigger points to help keep the muscle short and support the stabilizing function necessary for balance. Because the trigger point is assisting stabilization of a joint, it is important during the massage to address the trigger point but not interfere with the stabilization function of the muscles.

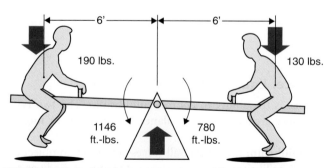

FIGURE 10-7 Parallel forces demonstrated by the seesaw with counterforce in the middle. To balance, the person at the left must move closer to the center. In order for the 190-lb person to generate 780 ft.-lbs., the person needs to be 4.1 feet (780/190) from the fulcrum.

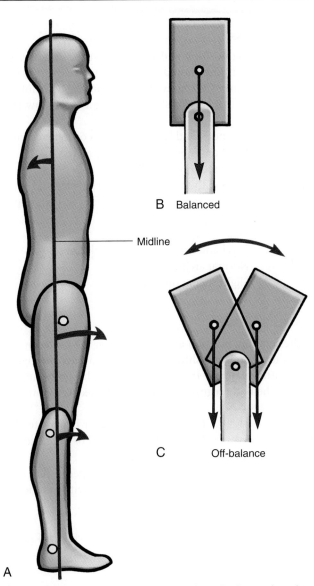

FIGURE 10-8 A, In normal, relaxed standing, the leg and trunk tend to rotate slightly off the midline of the body but maintain a counterbalance force. Balance is achieved in **B** and not in **C.** Whenever the trunk moves off this midline balance point, the body must compensate. (From Fritz S: *Mosby's fundamentals of therapeutic massage,* ed 4, St Louis, 2009, Mosby.)

thoracic and sacral curves are concave anteriorly and convex posteriorly. Conversely, the lumbar and cervical curves are convex anteriorly and concave posteriorly. Any change of these vertebral curves, such as an increase or decrease, results in poor posture. For example, a sway back is an increased lumbar curve, or *lordosis,* whereas a flat back is a decreased thoracic curve. Any lateral curvature of the spine is a pathologic condition called *scoliosis.*

The pelvis should be in a neutral position, defined as follows:

1. When the anterior superior iliac spine and posterior superior iliac spine are level with each other in a transverse plane
2. When the anterior superior interior spine is in the same vertical plane as the symphysis pubis

When the pelvis is in a neutral position, the lumbar curve has the optimal amount of curvature. When the pelvis is tilted anteriorly, the amount of lumbar curvature increases, causing lordosis. When the pelvis is tilted posteriorly, the amount of curve decreases, causing flat back.

When weight is distributed evenly on both legs, the pelvis should remain level from side to side, with the anterior superior iliac spine and anterior superior interior spine being at the same level. During the normal walking gait, the pelvis dips from side to side as weight shifts from stance to swing phase. This lateral pelvic tilt is controlled by the hip abductors, mainly the gluteus medius and gluteus minimus, and the trunk lateral flexors, primarily the erector spinae and quadratus lumborum.

In the upright position, posture depends primarily on muscle contractions and fascial support to remain upright in gravity. The muscles most involved are called *antigravity muscles.* The antigravity muscles are primarily the hip and knee extensors and the trunk and neck extensors. Other muscles maintaining the upright position are the trunk and neck flexors and lateral flexors, hip abductors and adductors, and the ankle pronators (everters) and supinators (inverters). If all of these muscles were to relax, the body would collapse.

The ankle plantar flexors and dorsiflexors are also antigravity muscles and are important in controlling postural sway. Postural sway is anterior-posterior motion of the upright body caused by motion occurring primarily at the ankles. This sway results from the constant displacement and correction of the center of gravity within the base of support.

A person's posture can be assessed most accurately using a plumb line suspended from the ceiling or a posture grid placed behind the person as a point of reference (Figure 10-9). A plumb line is a string or cord with a weight attached to the lower end. Because the string is weighted, it makes a perfectly straight vertical line in gravity. It is important to remember we are all slightly asymmetrical. When comparing an individual's body against a postural grid, it is unrealistic to expect that someone's posture will line up perfectly, nor is it a realistic massage outcome goal to expect to shift posture to perfect symmetry. The grid helps identify exaggerated areas of postural asymmetry that may be problematic.

constantly changes with each movement. When we lie down, we relieve the postural muscles of this task.

Good posture is important because it decreases the amount of stress placed on ligaments, muscles, and tendons and improves function and decreases the amount of muscle energy needed to keep the body upright (Figure 10-8).

Recall from Chapter 7 that the vertebral column is a column of block-shaped bones stacked in counterbalancing anterior-posterior curves. At birth the entire vertebral column is concave anteriorly and called the *primary curve.* As the child grows, anteriorly convex curves of the cervical and lumbar regions develop. These curves are maintained during rest and activity and function as shock absorbers. The thoracic and sacral curves counter the cervical and lumbar curves. The

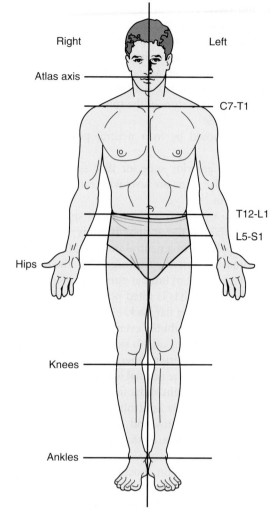

Right   Left

Atlas axis

C7-T1

T12-L1

L5-S1

Hips

Knees

Ankles

FIGURE 10-9 Posture grid. Gridlines help identify symmetry or deviations in symmetry. Just as seen in the figure, no one is perfectly symmetrical. It is the degree of variation and the limitation in function that determines degree of dysfunction.

Lateral View

In the standing position and viewed from the lateral position, the plumb line should be aligned so that it passes slightly in front of the lateral malleolus. For ideal posture the body segments should be aligned so that the plumb line passes through the listed landmarks as follows:

Head	Through the ear lobe
Shoulder	Through the tip of the acromion process
Thoracic spine	Anterior to the vertebral bodies
Lumbar spine	Through the vertebral bodies
Pelvis	Level
Hip	Through the greater trochanter (slightly posterior to the hip joint axis)
Knee	Slightly posterior to the patella (slightly anterior to the knee joint axis) with the knees in extension
Ankle	Slightly anterior to the lateral malleolus with the ankle joint in a neutral position between dorsiflexion and plantar flexion

Anterior View

In the standing position and viewed from the anterior position, the plumb line should be aligned to pass through the midsagittal plane of the body, thus dividing the body into two halves. The body segments should be aligned as follows:

Head	Extended and level, not flexed or hyperextended
Shoulders	Level and not elevated or depressed
Sternum	Centered in the midline
Hips	Level with the anterior superior iliac and anterior superior interior spines in the same plane
Legs	Slightly apart
Knees	Level and not bowed or knock-kneed
Ankles	Normal arch in feet
Feet	Slight toeing outward

Posterior View

In the standing position and viewed from the posterior position, the plumb line should be aligned to pass through the midsagittal plane of the body, dividing the body into two halves. The body segments should be aligned as follows:

Head	Extended, not flexed or hyperextended
Shoulders	Level and not elevated or depressed
Spinous processes	Centered in the midline
Hips	Level with posterior superior iliac spine and in the same plane with anterior superior iliac spine
Legs	Slightly apart
Knees	Level and not bowed or knock-kneed
Ankles	Calcaneus should be straight

KINETIC CHAIN

SECTION OBJECTIVES

Chapter objective covered in this section:
2. Explain and assess function of the kinetic chain.
After completing this section, the student will be able to perform the following:
- Define *the kinetic chain.*
- List the muscles and function of the inner and outer units.
- Explain postural stabilization.
- Assess posture.
- Demonstrate correct sitting, standing, and bending positions.
- Describe and analyze gait.
- Demonstrate and analyze the adult walking cycle.
- Assess gait.
- Describe and assess muscle firing patterns/activation sequences.

The **kinetic chain** is an integrated functional unit (Figure 10-10). The kinetic chain is different than previously described open and closed kinematic chains, which refer to single or multiple linked joint function. The kinetic chain networked systems of the body involved human movement. Kinetic means force(s), and chain means connected or linked together.

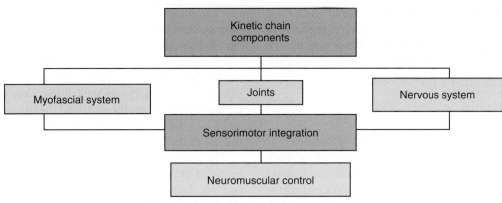

FIGURE 10-10 Kinetic chain components.

Specifically, the kinetic chain is made up of the myofascial system (muscle, ligament, tendon, and fascia), articular (joint) system, and nervous system. Each of these systems works interdependently to allow structural and functional efficiency in all three planes of motion: sagittal, frontal, and transverse. If one or more of the systems do not work efficiently, compensations and adaptations occur in the remaining systems, leading to stress in the body and eventually resulting in the development of dysfunctional patterns.

For example: If you change the position of one joint either by faulty movement patterns or posture it will effect the position and forces on all other joints and the associated soft tissue. Recall the three main functions of the nervous system:

Sensory function: Sense changes in either external or internal environmental.

Integrative function: Combines and interprets the information gathered from all the senses to plan a response to restore homeostasis.

Motor function: Directs the neuromuscular system to produce the response based on the integrative plan.

The result of the integration of the kinetic chain is effective and efficient functional movement.

All functional movement patterns involve acceleration provided by concentric muscle action, stabilization provided by isometric muscle action, and deceleration provided by eccentric action. All three actions occur at every joint in the kinetic chain and in all three planes of motion with each movement pattern. Muscles also must react proprioceptively to gravity, momentum, external forces, and forces created by other functioning muscles.

This kinetic chain model considers the body as a linked system of interdependent segments involving the entire neuromuscular connective tissue articular system linking each segment to the next. The parts of the body act as a system of chain links so that the energy or force generated by one part of the body can be transferred successively to the next link. The optimum coordination (timing) of these body segments and their movements will allow for the efficient transfer of energy and power up through the body, moving from one body segment to the next. Each movement in the sequence builds upon the previous motion.

Biomechanical principles are used to analyze the movement of the body. Dysfunction in the kinetic chain is often caused by muscle imbalances that allow for faulty movement patterns at a joint or joints somewhere along the chain. Length-tension relationships are very important because if muscle lengths are altered as a result of postural distortion or joint dysfunction, they will not be able to produce an efficient movement pattern. Faulty length-tension relationships are also responsible for most common postural problems. Connective tissue binding, joint injury, or degeneration or neurological and balance problems are also causes of dysfunction. Regardless of where the problem begins, eventually the entire chain is affected. Massage therapy techniques can be used to facilitate joint and soft tissue mobility and neuromuscular function.

Muscles function cooperatively in integrated groups to provide neuromuscular control during movements and can be divided into two main groups (each with multiple names, depending on the resource): the inner unit (stabilizers/postural muscles) and the outer unit (movers/phasic muscles).

Inner Unit

The inner unit primarily consists of intrinsic muscles that function at only one joint and are involved predominantly in joint support or stabilization. Joint support systems consist of muscles that are not movement specific but that provide stability to allow movement of a joint. Joint support systems also have a broad spectrum of attachments to the joint capsule that make them ideal for increasing joint stability. This group provides stability to the core and peripheral joints.

The postural/core/stabilization portion of the inner unit of the kinetic chain consists of the lumbo-pelvic-hip complex, thoracic spine, and cervical spine and operates as an integrated functional unit to stabilize the kinetic chain dynamically during functional movements of the limbs and head.

The joint support system of the core consists of muscles that have their proximal attachment into the spine. The major muscles include the deep erector spinae, deep cervical muscles, transverse abdominis, abdominal obliques, diaphragm, lumbar multifidus, and the muscles of the pelvic floor.

The peripheral joints in the shoulders, pelvic girdle, and the limbs also contain inner units of muscles. An example of a peripheral joint support system is the rotator cuff for the glenohumeral joint that provides dynamic stabilization for the humeral head in the glenoid fossa during movement.

Outer Unit

The outer unit muscles are predominantly responsible for movement and typically consist of more superficial extrinsic muscles that attach from the limbs and shoulder and pelvic girdles to the trunk (core). Examples of these muscles include the rectus abdominis, external obliques, erector spinae, latissimus dorsi, hamstrings, gluteus maximus, adductors, and quadriceps. The outer unit muscles are usually larger than the inner unit and are associated with movement of the trunk and limbs.

There are other ways to classify functional movement groups, including the following:
- The erector spinae, thoracolumbar fascia, sacrotuberous ligament, and biceps femoris assist in stabilizing the sacroiliac joint. Dysfunction in these structures can lead to sacroiliac joint pain.
- The superficial erector spinae, psoas, deep erector spinae, transverse abdominis, abdominal obliques, diaphragm, lumbar multifidus, and muscles of the pelvic floor provide intersegmental stabilization of the trunk during functional movement. Dysfunction in any of these structures can lead to sacroiliac joint instability and low back pain.
- The internal oblique, external oblique, adductor group, external rotator hip group, contralateral gluteus maximus and latissimus dorsi, anterior and posterior tibialis, soleus and gastrocnemius, and fibularis group create a stabilizing force for the sacroiliac joint function, aid in the stability and rotation of the pelvis, and contribute to leg swing. Dysfunction in this group often leads to sacroiliac joint dysfunction and rotational strain in the lumbar spine, pelvic area, and knee and also can affect the ankle. The weakening of the gluteus maximus or latissimus dorsi (or both) also may lead to increased tension in the hamstrings and therefore cause recurring hamstring strains.
- The gluteus medius, tensor fasciae latae, adductor group, and quadratus lumborum are responsible for pelvofemoral stability. During single-leg functional movements such as in walking, lunges, or stair climbing, the ipsilateral gluteus medius, tensor fasciae latae, and adductors combine with the contralateral quadratus lumborum to control the pelvis and femur. Dysfunction can create instability and strain during walking, running, and jumping activities.

Postural Stabilization

Stabilization of the body during normal movement occurs in soft tissues between movement segments. For example, the muscles located between the base of the skull and the top of the shoulders or the muscles located between the last thoracic vertebrae and the top of the hips are considered segments. These patterns balance each other to provide postural stability

in a diagonal counterbalancing function. Compensation and dysfunction can occur as well. For example, if the right hip is elevated because of muscles tensing in the back, typically there is a compensation tension pattern in the anterior muscles on the left between vertebrae C7 and T12. Another example is pain in the quadriceps on the left that shows a compensation pattern in the calf on the right and the tissue between the hips and S1 on the right posterior. Tension also may develop in the tissues on the top of the left foot.

The body must be balanced in three dimensions against the forces of gravity to provide stability in the upright position and for locomotion. Balanced daily against the forces of gravity, the body reacts to pain, injury, and other stimuli through complex compensations involving many polysynaptic reflex arcs. Some compensation patterns are resourceful, such as when the body is required to adapt to a trauma or repetitive use pattern. Massage application should support these changes. Some compensation patterns become pathologic or maladaptive and increase strain in the system. Therapeutic massage can assist in reversing some of these nonproductive patterns. Any form of compensation can yield a confusing combination of signs and symptoms. Symptoms may range from complaints of left scapular pain after a right quadriceps injury to complaints of pain on the front left side of the neck after injury to the right calf. Signs such as decreased movement of extremities, splinting, and lack of bilateral symmetry also may be observable.

Massage therapists can use a systematic application of assessment and intervention to help understand and address this array of signs, symptoms, and compensations. Such a system is developed in this text as the kinetic chain protocol for posture stabilization, which gives recommendations for assessing and treating postural patterns (see Activity 10-1 on p. 474). The kinetic chain also involves movement, particularly walking and running or gait. Assessment and treatment of gait patterns are described in Activity 10-2.

Sitting, Standing, and Bending

Squatting down to pick up an object is more efficient than bending over at the hip joint and then lifting up. Bending over puts an enormous strain on the back. Half the body weight is being moved in addition to the weight of the object being lifted. When squatting down and then moving from a squat to a standing position, keep weight distributed over the entire bottom of the foot, particularly the heels. The tendency is to bear weight on the ball of the foot and toes. This position causes instability in the ankle and knee.

When in the seated position, moving to a standing position begins by leaning forward at the hips and leading with the head. The momentum carries the body forward into a semisquat. The leg muscles then lift the body into a standing position (Figure 10-11).

Walking/Gait

Locomotion, or walking, is the act of moving from one place to another. Gait is the means of achieving this action. Despite

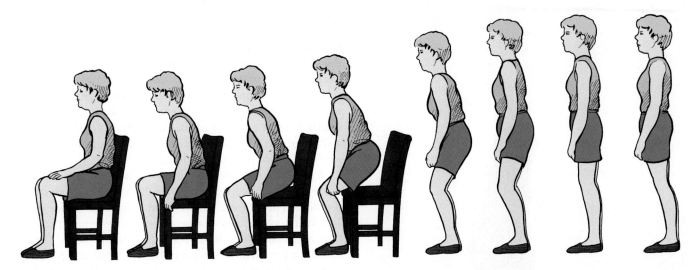

FIGURE 10-11 Sit-to-stand viewed laterally. (Modified from Gillen G, Burkhardt A: *Stroke rehabilitation: a function-based approach,* ed 3, St Louis, 2011, Mosby.)

years of scientific study, we still do not know exactly why we stand upright and walk. The question remains as to how much of locomotion is innate and how much is learned. Human beings certainly are driven to walk. Most authorities agree that the urge and the "hardwiring" for bipedal (two-legged) loco-motion are with us from birth, and the coordination of all the components necessary to accomplish the task is learned.

Controlling bipedal locomotion is not an easy task. Reflex-ive coordination by the central nervous system is an essential part of the walking pattern. The central nervous system coor-dinates muscles to generate the locomotion pattern through the following actions:

- Producing the effort necessary to move the body
- Adapting changes in the center of gravity
- Coordinating the movements and projected movements of the limbs
- Adapting to changing conditions and joint positions
- Coordinating visual, auditory, vestibular, and peripheral afferent information

Understanding reflex patterns is an important part of understanding how we walk. Because most reflex actions involve a great many reflex arcs, local stimulation of a small number of receptors leads to a large number of outgoing impulses to muscles and glands. The result is a widespread and generalized reflex response. Most reflexes are polysynaptic, using many sensory neurons, interneurons, and motor neurons. Breaking down these complex functional patterns is often confusing (Whittle, 2007; Sahrmann, 2002). We can sim-plify this process for understanding gait.

Walking is an activity in which a person moves his or her body into and out of balance with each step. When standing and while walking, our center of gravity is located in our pelvis at the upper sacral region anterior to the second sacral verte-bra. Our head is balanced on top of the spine, and the center of gravity for the head is in front of the ear by the cheek.

The pivot point for movement of the head is behind the center of gravity, which means that posterior occipital and cervical muscles must exert force to hold up the head. The benefit is that to begin forward movement, all a person has to do is relax the muscles at the back of the head. The head moves forward and, because of its weight, this movement takes the whole body with it. Beginning an action requires effort. Once started, movement takes on a momentum of its own. The same principle can be applied to a moving car. A car needs the most power when it starts off from a stationary position and little energy to keep it going at a constant speed. Therefore the body moves not by requiring increased force but by using the head to initiate the movement. "Lead all movement with your head" is a biomechanically sound principle.

Watching toddlers as they start to walk clearly reveals that from the beginning, walking is counterbalanced by activity of the arms, hands, head, and pelvis. This counterbalancing action becomes important in understanding the complex system of reflex control of gait patterns.

Normal Adult Walking Cycle

Simply stated, we walk around on two legs composed of three segments each: the thigh, lower leg, and foot. On top of our legs are the trunk, head, and arms. The whole arm unit is used as a counterbalance and for momentum and moves opposite the leg movement. This pattern is linked by the contralateral reflex arc mechanism (Figure 10-12).

When we walk, peripheral receptors in our joints and muscles detect changes in muscle length and force, joint posi-tion, and weight-bearing status of the limbs. Righting reflexes involving the eyes and ears, together with tonic neck reflexes, maintain an upward, level, and forward head position, whereas ocular/pelvic reflexes balance the head and pelvis position. Pressure receptors (baroreceptors) on the soles of the feet relay postural information about weight distribution. The relation-ship between the movement of the legs when walking and the independent use of the arm/hand complex depends on the task and environment.

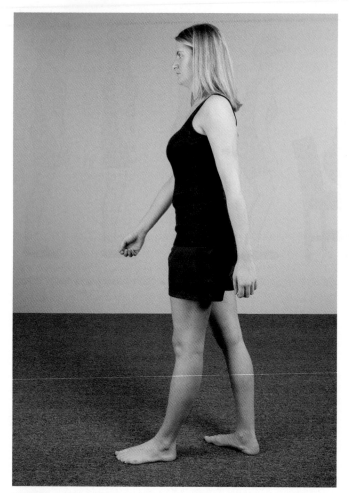

FIGURE 10-12 Counterbalance is shown as the arm moves opposite the leg. (From Fuhr A: *The activator method*, ed 2, St Louis, 2008, Mosby.)

Flexion and extension of the hip joints cause some rotation in the lumbar spine, and to keep the head facing forward and the eyes level, the thorax and cervical spine rotate in the opposite direction. Reciprocal movements of the upper and lower limbs occur with the right upper limb flexing at the shoulder joint simultaneously with flexion at the left hip joint. Normally, the shoulder joint starts to flex or extend slightly before the same movement occurs in the elbow joint. These movements again serve to keep the head and trunk oriented and to counterbalance the body weight in gravity.

Gait Cycle

Gait is defined as the rhythmic and alternating movement of the legs along with the trunk and the arms, which results in the propulsion of the body mass. Gait is an automatic function coordinated by innate and learned reflexes. Muscles certainly work together to produce movement, but an interesting note is that in large portions of the gait cycle, little or no muscle activity occurs in most of the muscle groups, pointing to the energy-efficient nature of walking.

A **gait cycle** is the period during which a complete sequence of events takes place; it begins when the heel of one foot strikes the floor. The gait cycle is subdivided into the stance phase and swing phase. The stance phase occurs when the limb under consideration is in contact with the floor. During walking a period always occurs when both feet are in contact with the floor; this is called *double stance.* The swing phase occurs when the foot is not in contact with the floor.

In the average walking pattern, the stance phase takes about 60% of the gait cycle and the swing phase about 40%. As the speed of walking, or cadence, increases, the length of time in the stance phase decreases. Double-stance time increases with slow walking.

The components of the stance phase are heel strike, foot flat, midstance, heel-off, and toe-off (Figure 10-13). The components of the swing phase are acceleration, midswing, deceleration, and arm swing (Figure 10-14 and Activity 10-2).

Practical Application

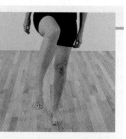

The massage practitioner often can trace dysfunctional patterns through these basic reflex principles. For example, a client complains of a stiff left shoulder and cannot remember how the pain began but can remember walking around an amusement park with a blister on the right heel. This dysfunctional pattern may result from a change in gait, developed from an alteration in the reciprocal counterbalancing pattern, which eventually led to the shoulder pain. The shoulder difficulty may be relieved by addressing neuromuscular tension patterns in the right leg and hip. Many such patterns could develop in different clients. By paying attention to the reflex pattern operating in the body and understanding the gait cycle and the kinetic chain, the massage therapist can manage this type of soft-tissue dysfunction more effectively.

Text continued on page 494.

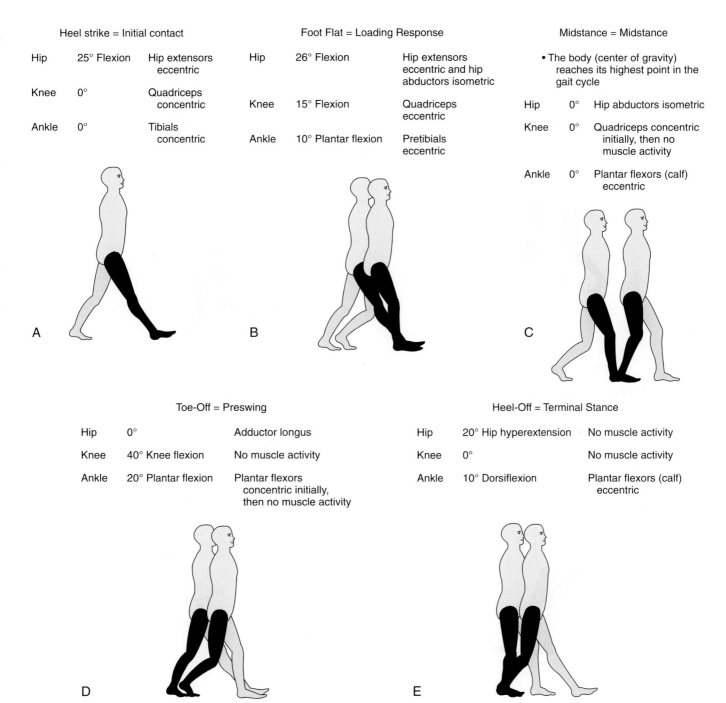

Heel strike = Initial contact

Hip	25° Flexion	Hip extensors eccentric
Knee	0°	Quadriceps concentric
Ankle	0°	Tibials concentric

Foot Flat = Loading Response

Hip	26° Flexion	Hip extensors eccentric and hip abductors isometric
Knee	15° Flexion	Quadriceps eccentric
Ankle	10° Plantar flexion	Pretibials eccentric

Midstance = Midstance

• The body (center of gravity) reaches its highest point in the gait cycle

Hip	0°	Hip abductors isometric
Knee	0°	Quadriceps concentric initially, then no muscle activity
Ankle	0°	Plantar flexors (calf) eccentric

A   B   C

Toe-Off = Preswing

Hip	0°	Adductor longus
Knee	40° Knee flexion	No muscle activity
Ankle	20° Plantar flexion	Plantar flexors concentric initially, then no muscle activity

Heel-Off = Terminal Stance

Hip	20° Hip hyperextension	No muscle activity
Knee	0°	No muscle activity
Ankle	10° Dorsiflexion	Plantar flexors (calf) eccentric

D   E

FIGURE 10-13 Gait cycle. Components of the stance phase.

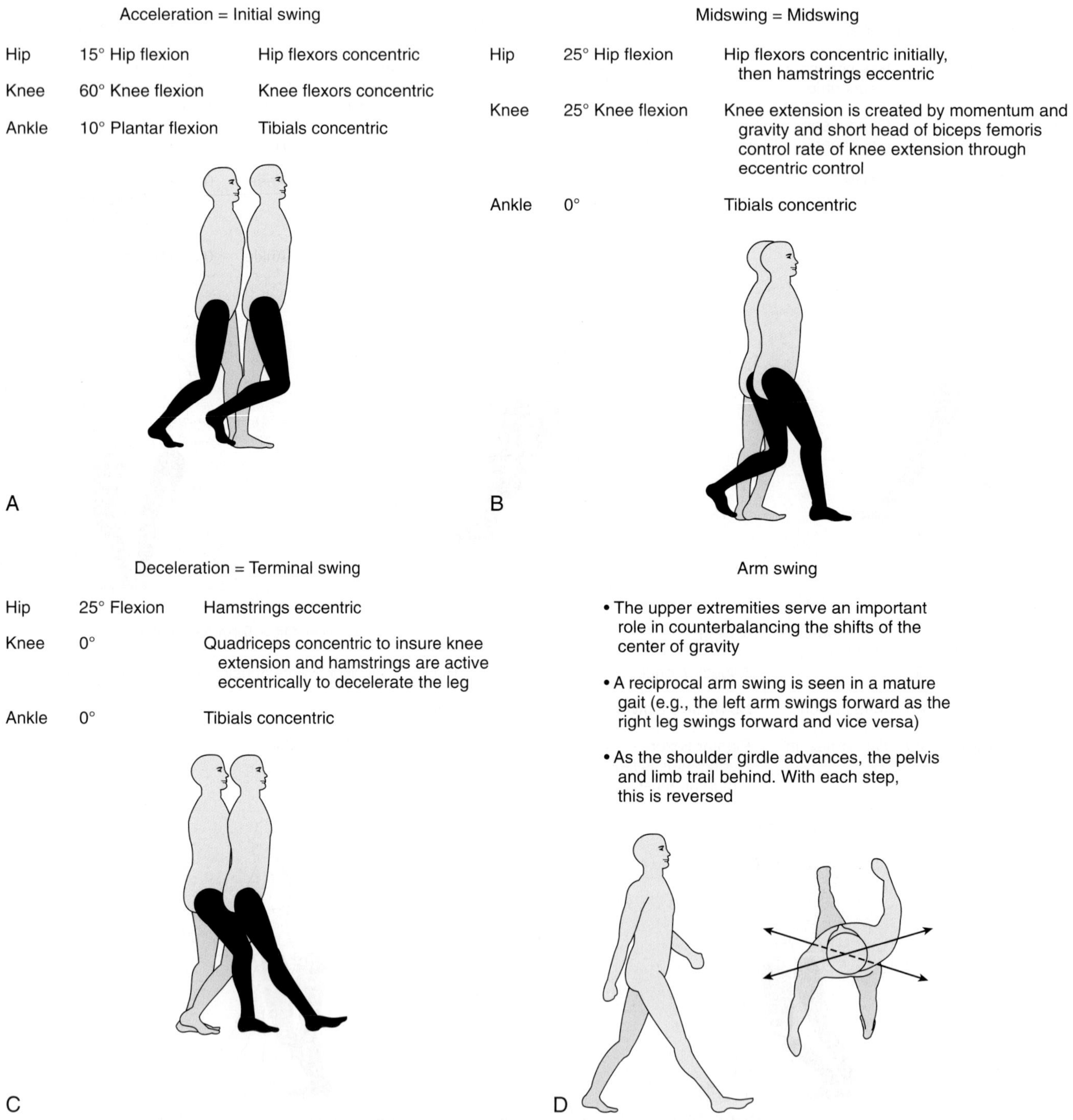

Acceleration = Initial swing

Hip	15° Hip flexion	Hip flexors concentric
Knee	60° Knee flexion	Knee flexors concentric
Ankle	10° Plantar flexion	Tibials concentric

A

Midswing = Midswing

Hip	25° Hip flexion	Hip flexors concentric initially, then hamstrings eccentric
Knee	25° Knee flexion	Knee extension is created by momentum and gravity and short head of biceps femoris control rate of knee extension through eccentric control
Ankle	0°	Tibials concentric

B

Deceleration = Terminal swing

Hip	25° Flexion	Hamstrings eccentric
Knee	0°	Quadriceps concentric to insure knee extension and hamstrings are active eccentrically to decelerate the leg
Ankle	0°	Tibials concentric

C

Arm swing

- The upper extremities serve an important role in counterbalancing the shifts of the center of gravity

- A reciprocal arm swing is seen in a mature gait (e.g., the left arm swings forward as the right leg swings forward and vice versa)

- As the shoulder girdle advances, the pelvis and limb trail behind. With each step, this is reversed

D

FIGURE 10-14 Gait cycle. Components of the swing phase.

✎ ACTIVITY **10-2**   KINETIC CHAIN PROTOCOL: GAIT

Think of the two main actions involved with gait:

1. On opposite sides: Right arm flexors concentrically contract with left leg flexors.
2. On the same side: Right arm flexors concentrically contract with right leg extensors.

   The reciprocal is then also true:

1. On opposite sides: Left arm extensors concentrically contract with right leg extensors.
2. On the same side: Left arm extensors concentrically contract with left leg flexors.

Muscle Contraction

Muscles that concentrically contract together in these patterns should maintain a strong, steady contraction simultaneously during muscle testing. Weakness in the muscle being tested would indicate dysfunction.

The massage therapist should test muscles (antagonists) that are inhibited in these patterns. The antagonist patterns should not hold easily against a force of resistance. This response should not be confused with a dysfunctional, weak muscle. Instead, reciprocal inhibition from the prime mover produces an appropriate "letting go" sensation. If a muscle that should be inhibited remains locked in concentric contraction as indicated by "testing strong," a dysfunction in the reflex arc is present.

How To Assess

1. Isolate muscle groups. Ask client to apply force (10% to 20%) or to hold against your opposing pressure with the muscles of the control group.
2. Test the desired muscle group for strong, steady contraction in the concentric pattern or inhibition in the eccentric pattern.

Kinetic Chain Protocol: Gait Assessment

Control group: The group that serves as standard or reference for comparison with a test group and is the group of muscles that initiates the reflex response

Test group: The muscle group that responds to the stimulus from the control group

There are many gait-related kinetic chain patterns. We will concentrate on the main patterns involved in flexion, extension, abduction, and adduction at the shoulder and pelvic girdle. For testing the arm flexors/extensors, stabilize the humerus superior to the elbow joint and the femur above the knee.

The control group is activated first, the test group is next, and then both contractions are held simultaneously. Both groups should hold strong and steady during the test. Chart the data to show any inhibitions.

The antagonist pattern should be inhibited during the test. The antagonists should let go. If they do not, the contraction maintained is concentric instead of eccentric. Chart the data.

See page 493 for suggested corrective interventions.

I. CONTRALATERAL FLEXORS

A. Left Arm Flexor Test (Pictured below and next page)

1. Isolate and stabilize left arm and right leg in supine flexion.
2. Control group: Use right leg as control, and have client hold right leg position against therapist's inferior/caudal pressure.
3. Test group: Test left arm flexors by having client hold left arm position against practitioner's inferior/caudal pressure.
4. Both groups should hold equally strong and steady. If test group is inhibited, chart the data.

Antagonist test: Test left arm extensors by having client hold against practitioner's superior/cranial pressure. These muscles should inhibit (let go). If test group remains concentrically contracted and holds, chart data.

B. Right Arm Flexor Test

1. Isolate and stabilize left leg and right arm in supine flexion.
2. Control group: Use left leg as control, and have client hold left leg position against practitioner's inferior/caudal pressure.
3. Test group: Test right arm flexors by having client hold right arm position against practitioner's inferior/caudal pressure.
4. Both groups should hold equally strong and steady. If test group is inhibited, chart data.

Antagonist test: Test right arm extensors by having client hold right arm position against practitioner's superior/cranial pressure. These muscles should inhibit (let go). If test group remains concentrically contracted and holds, chart data.

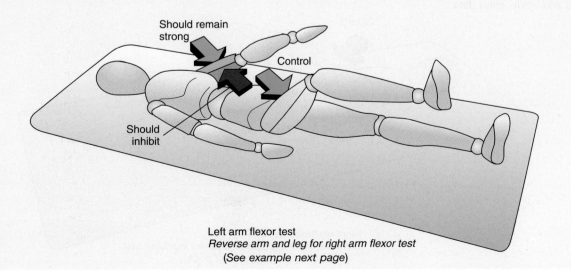

Should remain strong

Control

Should inhibit

Left arm flexor test
Reverse arm and leg for right arm flexor test
(*See example next page*)

Continued

✎ ACTIVITY **10-2**   KINETIC CHAIN PROTOCOL: GAIT—cont'd

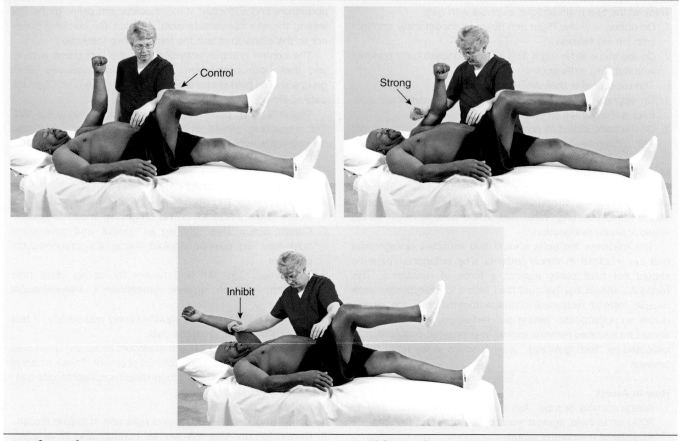

C. Left Leg Flexor Test

1. Isolate and support/stabilize left leg and right arm in supine flexion.
2. Control group: Use right arm as control, and have client hold right arm position against therapist's inferior/caudal pressure.
3. Test group: Test left leg flexors by having client hold left leg position against practitioner's inferior/caudal pressure.
4. Both groups should hold equally strong and steady. If the test group is inhibited, chart data.

   Antagonist test: Test left leg extensors by having client hold against practitioner's superior/cranial pressure. These muscles should inhibit (let go). If test group remains concentrically contracted and holds, chart data.

D. Right Leg Flexor Test (Pictured below and on next page)

1. Isolate and stabilize left arm and right leg in supine flexion.
2. Control group: Use left arm as control, and have client hold left arm position against practitioner's inferior/caudal pressure.
3. Test group: Test right leg flexors by having client hold right leg position against practitioner's inferior/caudal pressure.
4. Both groups should hold equally strong and steady. If test group is inhibited (let go), chart data.

   Antagonist test: Test right leg extensors by having client hold right leg position against practitioner's superior/cranial pressure. These muscles should inhibit (let go). If test group remains concentrically contracted and holds, chart data.

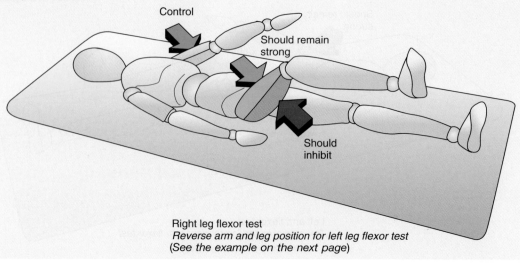

Right leg flexor test
Reverse arm and leg position for left leg flexor test
(See the example on the next page)

✎ ACTIVITY 10-2 KINETIC CHAIN PROTOCOL: GAIT—cont'd

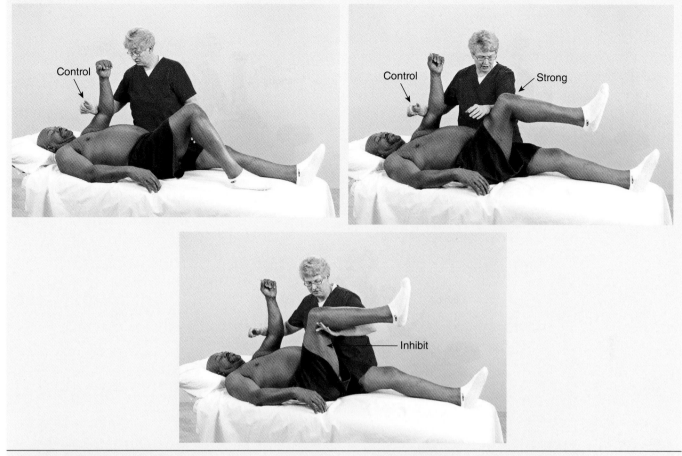

II. CONTRALATERAL EXTENSORS

A. Left Arm Extensor Test (Pictured below and on next page)

1. Isolate and stabilize left arm and right leg in supine flexion.
2. Control group: Right leg is control. Have client hold leg position against practitioner's superior/cephalad pressure.
3. Test group: Test left arm extensors by having client hold arm position against practitioner's superior/cephalad pressure.
4. Both groups should stay equally strong and steady. If test group is inhibited, chart data.

Antagonist test: Test left arm flexors by having client hold left arm position against practitioner's inferior/caudal pressure. These muscles should inhibit (let go). If test group remains concentrically contracted and holds, chart data.

B. Right Arm Extensor Test

1. Isolate and stabilize left leg and right arm in supine flexion.
2. Control group: Left leg is control. Have client hold leg position against practitioner's superior/cephalad pressure.
3. Test group: Test right arm extensors by having client hold arm position against practitioner's superior/cephalad pressure.
4. Both groups should stay equally strong and steady. If test group is inhibited, chart data.

Antagonist test: Test right arm flexors by having client hold right arm position against practitioner's inferior/caudal pressure. These muscles should inhibit (let go). If test group remains concentrically contracted and holds, chart data.

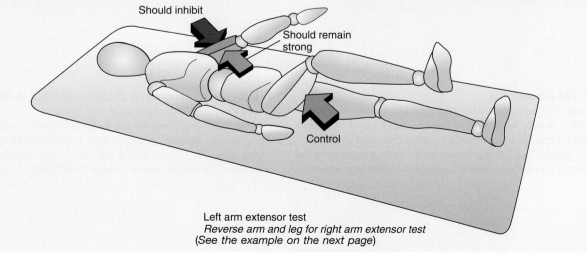

Left arm extensor test
Reverse arm and leg for right arm extensor test
(See the example on the next page)

Continued

✎ ACTIVITY **10-2**   KINETIC CHAIN PROTOCOL: GAIT—cont'd

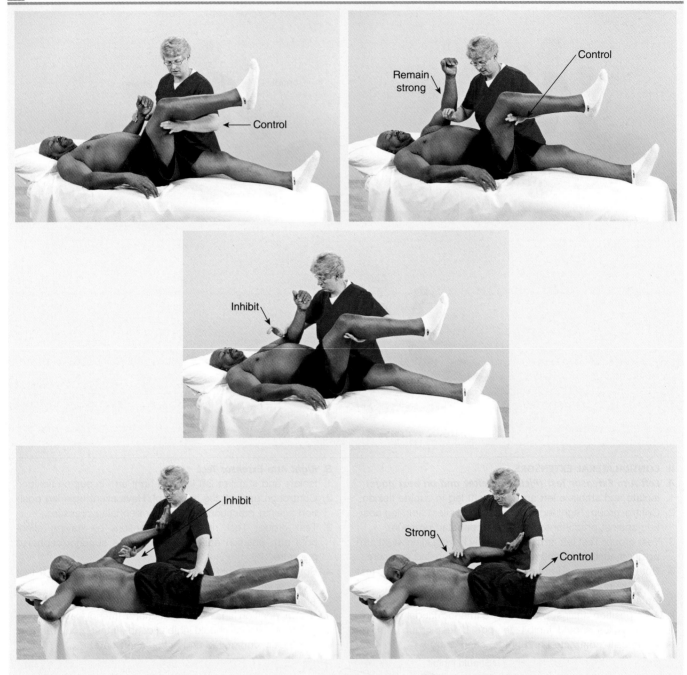

C. *Left Leg Extensor Test*

1. Isolate and stabilize left leg and right arm in supine flexion.
2. Control group: Right arm is control. Have client hold arm position against practitioner's superior/cephalad pressure.
3. Test group: Test left leg extensors by having client hold leg position against practitioner's superior/cephalad pressure.

4. Both groups should stay equally strong and steady. If test group is inhibited, chart data.

   Antagonist test: Test left leg flexor by having client hold left leg position against practitioner's inferior/caudal pressure. These muscles should inhibit (let go). If test group remains concentrically contracted and holds, chart data.

✎ ACTIVITY **10-2** KINETIC CHAIN PROTOCOL: GAIT—cont'd

D. Right Leg Extensor Test (Pictured below)
1. Isolate and stabilize left arm and right leg in supine flexion.
2. Control group: Left arm is control. Have client hold arm position against practitioner's superior/cephalad pressure.

3. Test group: Test right leg extensors by having client hold leg position against practitioner's superior/cephalad pressure.
4. Both groups should stay equally strong and steady. If the test group is inhibited, chart data.

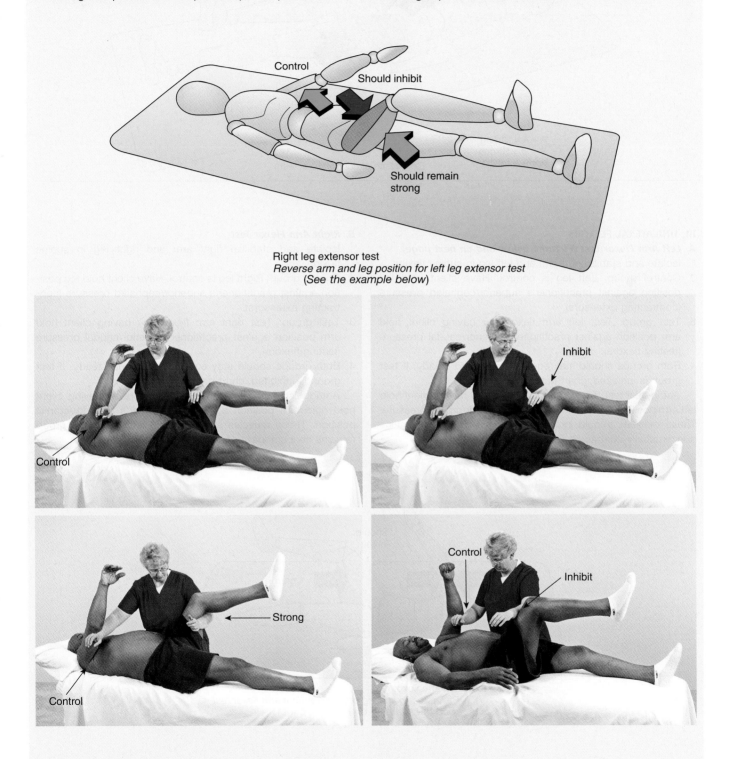

Right leg extensor test
Reverse arm and leg position for left leg extensor test
(See the example below)

Antagonist test: Test right leg flexors by having client hold right leg position against practitioner's inferior/caudal pressure.

These muscles should inhibit (let go). If test group remains in concentrically contracted and holds, chart data (pictured).

Continued

✎ ACTIVITY **10-2**   KINETIC CHAIN PROTOCOL: GAIT—cont'd

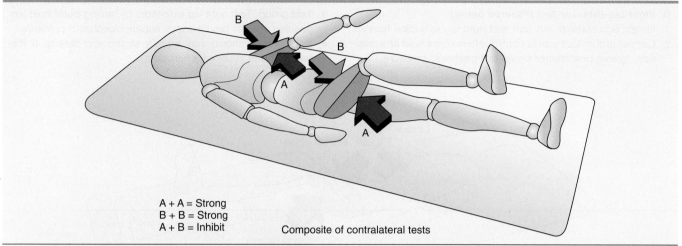

A + A = Strong
B + B = Strong
A + B = Inhibit   Composite of contralateral tests

III. UNILATERAL FLEXORS

A. *Left Arm Flexor Test (Pictured below and on next page)*

1. Isolate and stabilize left arm and left leg in supine flexion.
2. Control group: Left leg is control. Have client hold leg position against practitioner's superior/cephalad pressure (contracting extensors).
3. Test group: Test left arm flexors by having client hold arm position against practitioner's inferior/caudal pressure (testing flexors).
4. Both groups should stay equally strong and steady. If test group is inhibited, chart data.

Antagonist test: Test left arm extensors by having client hold left arm position against practitioner's superior/cranial pressure. These muscles should inhibit (let go). If test group remains concentrically contracted and holds, chart data.

B. *Right Arm Flexor Test*

1. Isolate and stabilize right arm and right leg in supine flexion.
2. Control group: Right leg is control. Have client hold leg position against practitioner's superior/cephalad pressure (contracting extensors).
3. Test group: Test right arm flexors by having client hold arm position against practitioner's inferior/caudal pressure (testing flexors).
4. Both groups should stay equally strong and steady. If test group is inhibited, chart data.

Antagonist test: Test right arm extensors by having client hold right arm position against practitioner's superior/cranial position. These muscles should inhibit (let go). If test group remains concentrically contracted and holds, chart data.

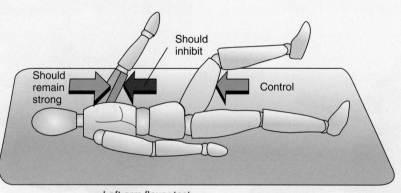

Should inhibit

Should remain strong

Control

Left arm flexor test
Reverse arm and leg position for right arm flexor test
(See the example on the next page)

✎ ACTIVITY **10-2** KINETIC CHAIN PROTOCOL: GAIT—cont'd

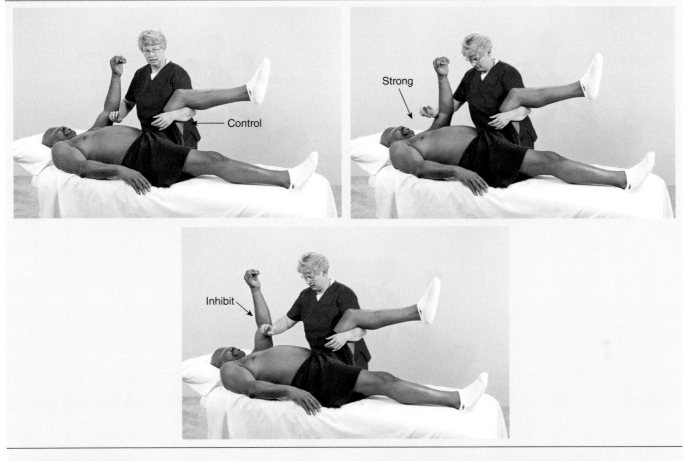

C. Left Leg Flexor Test

1. Isolate and stabilize left arm and left leg in supine flexion.
2. Control group: Left arm is control. Have client hold arm position against practitioner's superior/cephalad pressure (contracting extensors).
3. Test group: Test left leg flexors by having client hold leg position against practitioner's inferior/caudal pressure (testing flexors).
4. Both groups should stay equally strong and steady. If test group is inhibited, chart data.

Antagonist test: Test left leg flexors by having client hold left leg position against practitioner's inferior/caudal pressure. These muscles should inhibit (let go). If test group remains concentrically contracted and holds, chart data.

D. Right Leg Flexor Test (Pictured on next page)

1. Isolate and stabilize right arm and right leg in supine flexion.
2. Control group: Right arm is control. Have client hold arm position against practitioner's superior/cephalad pressure (contracting extensors).
3. Test group: Test right leg flexors by having client hold leg position against practitioner's inferior/caudal pressure (testing flexors).
4. Both groups should stay equally strong and steady. If test group is inhibited, chart data.

Antagonist test: Test right leg extensors by having client hold leg position against practitioner's superior/cranial position. These muscles should inhibit (let go). If test group remains concentrically contracted and holds, chart data.

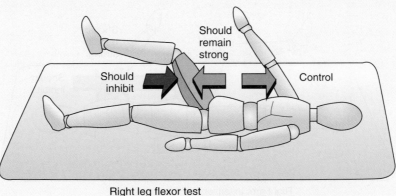

Right leg flexor test
Reverse arm and leg position for left leg flexor test
(See the example on the next page)

Continued

✎ ACTIVITY **10-2**   KINETIC CHAIN PROTOCOL: GAIT—cont'd

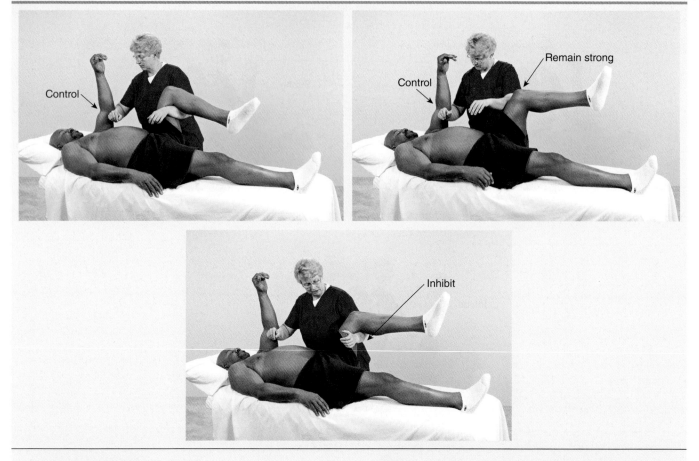

IV. UNILATERAL EXTENSORS

A. Left Arm Extensor Test

1. Isolate and stabilize left arm and left leg in supine flexion.
2. Control group: Left leg is control. Have client hold leg position against practitioner's inferior/caudal pressure (contracting flexors).
3. Test group: Test left arm extensors by having client hold arm position against practitioner's superior/cephalad pressure (testing extensors).
4. Both groups should stay equally strong and steady. If test group is inhibited, chart data.

Antagonist test: Test left arm flexors by applying inferior/caudal pressure. These muscles should inhibit (let go). If test group remains concentrically contracted and holds, chart data.

B. Right Arm Extensor Test (Pictured on next page)

1. Isolate and stabilize right arm and right leg in supine flexion.
2. Control group: Right leg is control. Have client hold leg position against practitioner's inferior/caudal pressure (contracting flexors).
3. Test group: Test right arm extensors by having client hold arm position against practitioner's superior/cephalad pressure (testing extensors).
4. Both groups should stay equally strong and steady. If test group is inhibited, chart data.

Antagonist test: Test right arm flexors by applying inferior/caudal pressure. These muscles should inhibit (let go). If test group remains concentrically contracted and holds, chart data.

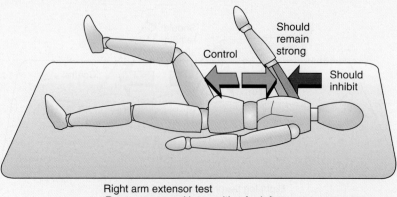

Right arm extensor test
Reverse arm and leg position for left arm extensor test
(See the example on the next page)

✎ ACTIVITY **10-2** KINETIC CHAIN PROTOCOL: GAIT—cont'd

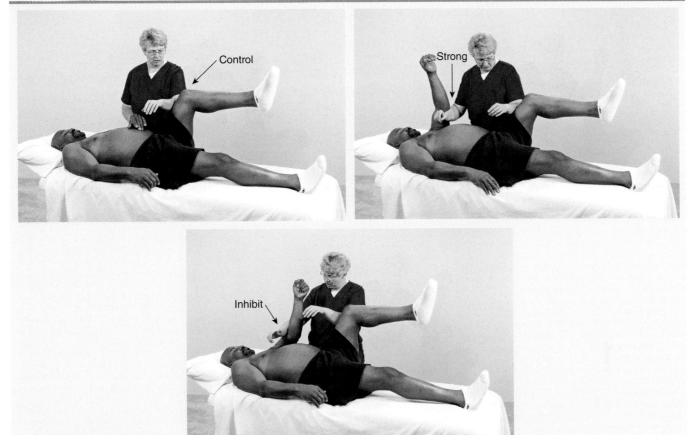

C. Left Leg Extensor Test

1. Isolate and stabilize left arm and left leg in supine flexion.
2. Control group: Left arm is control. Have client hold arm position against practitioner's inferior/caudal pressure (contracting flexors).
3. Test group: Test left leg extensors by having client hold leg position against practitioner's superior/cephalad pressure (testing extensors).
4. Both groups should stay equally strong and steady. If test group is inhibited, chart data.

   Antagonist test: Test left leg flexors by applying inferior/caudal pressure. These muscles should inhibit (let go). If test group remains in concentric contraction and holds, chart data.

D. Right Leg Extensor Test (Pictured below and on next page)

1. Isolate and stabilize right arm and right leg in supine flexion.
2. Control group: Right arm is control. Have client hold arm position against practitioner's inferior/caudal pressure (contracting flexors).
3. Test group: Test right leg extensors by having client hold leg position against practitioner's superior/cephalad pressure (testing extensors).
4. Both groups should stay equally strong and steady. If test group is inhibited, chart data (pictured).

   Antagonist test: Test right leg flexors by applying inferior/caudal pressure. These muscles should inhibit (let go). If test group remains concentrically contracted, chart data.

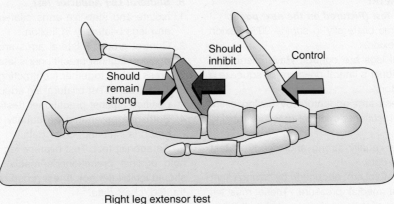

Right leg extensor test
Reverse arm and leg position for left leg extensor test
(See the example on the next page)

Continued

✎ ACTIVITY 10-2 KINETIC CHAIN PROTOCOL: GAIT—cont'd

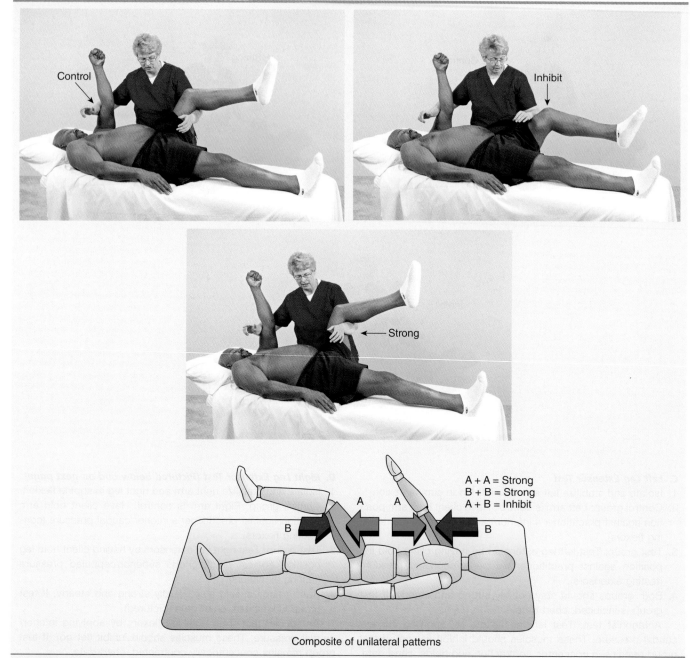

Composite of unilateral patterns

A + A = Strong
B + B = Strong
A + B = Inhibit

V. MEDIAL/LATERAL SYMMETRY

A. Bilateral Arm Adductor Test (Pictured on the next page)

1. Isolate and stabilize arms bilaterally in supine 90% flexion and legs bilaterally in flexion.
2. Control group: Bilateral legs are control. Have client hold position against practitioner's lateral pressure or squeeze a ball (contracting adductors).
3. Test group: Test bilateral arm adductors by having client hold position against practitioner's lateral pressure (testing adductors).
4. Both groups should be equally strong and steady. If test group is inhibited, chart data.

   Antagonist test: Test bilateral arm abduction by having client hold arm position against medial pressure. These muscles should inhibit (let go). If test group remains concentrically contracted, chart data.

B. Bilateral Leg Adductor Test

1. Isolate and stabilize arms bilaterally in supine 90% flexion and legs bilaterally in flexion.
2. Control group: Bilateral arms are control. Have client hold position against practitioner's lateral pressure or have client press palms together (contracting adductors).
3. Test group: Test bilateral leg adductors by having client hold position against practitioner (testing adductors).
4. Both groups should be equally strong and steady. If test group is inhibited, chart data.

   Antagonist test: Test bilateral leg abductors by having client hold against practitioner's medial pressure. These muscles should inhibit (let go). If test group remains concentrically contracted, chart data.

✎ ACTIVITY 10-2   KINETIC CHAIN PROTOCOL: GAIT—cont'd

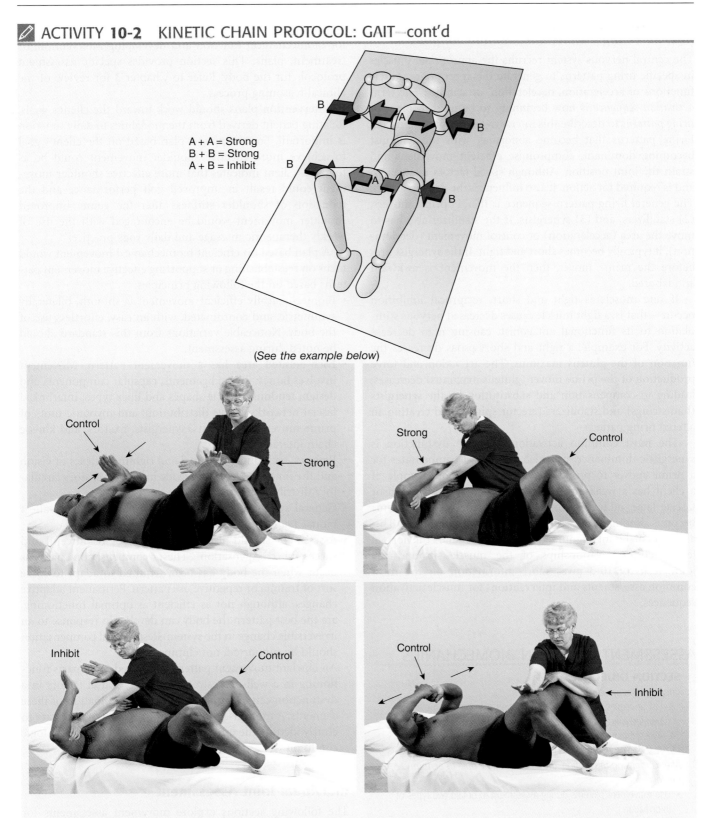

A + A = Strong
B + B = Strong
A + B = Inhibit

(See the example below)

Intervention: Use any massage method to inhibit muscles that test too strong by remaining in concentric contraction patterns when they should inhibit (let go). Appropriate methods are slow compression, kneading, gliding, and shaking. Strengthen muscles that inhibit when they should hold strong. Appropriate methods are tapotement and rhythmic tensing of inhibited muscles. Then retest pattern; it should be normal.

Muscle Firing Patterns/Activation Sequences

The central nervous system recruits the appropriate muscles in specific firing patterns to generate the appropriate muscle functions of acceleration, deceleration, or stability. The term *activation sequence* is now beginning to be used in place of *firing patterns* to describe this interactive function of muscles. Firing patterns that become abnormal, with the synergist becoming dominant, compromise efficient movement and strain the joint position. Although speed factors in strength and is required for action, it also influences the firing patterns. The general firing pattern sequence is the (1) prime movers, (2) stabilizers, and (3) synergists. If the stabilizer also has to move the area (acceleration) or control movement (deceleration), it typically becomes short and tight. If the synergist fires before the prime mover, then the movement is awkward and labored.

If one muscle is tight and short, reciprocal inhibition occurs—that is, a tight muscle causes decreased nervous stimulation to its functional antagonist, causing it to decrease activity. For example, a tight and short psoas decreases the function of the gluteus maximus. The activation and force production of the prime mover (gluteus maximus) decreases, leading to compensation and substitution by the synergists (hamstrings) and stabilizers (erector spinae) and creating an altered firing pattern.

The most common activation sequence dysfunction is synergistic dominance, in which a synergist compensates for a prime mover to produce the movement. For example, if a client has a weak gluteus medius, then synergists (tensor fasciae latae, adductor complex, and quadratus lumborum) become dominant to compensate for the weakness. This alters normal joint alignment, which further alters the normal length-tension relationships of the muscles around the joint. Activity 10-3 gives more information on the most common assessments and interventions for muscle activation sequences.

ASSESSMENT BASED ON BIOMECHANICS

SECTION OBJECTIVES

Chapter objective covered in this section:
  3. List principles of a massage intervention plan based on efficient biomechanical movement.
  4. Assess biomechanical function using individual joint assessment.
  5. Assess biomechanical functions for regions of the body.
After completing this section, the student will be able to perform the following:
  • Use movement patterns during assessment to obtain two types of information
  • Demonstrate applications of resistance and stabilization during assessment
  • Apply clinical reasoning to individual joint assessment
  • Develop a massage care/treatment plan based on efficient biomechanical movement
  • Assess individual joint function.
  • Assess the body by region
  • Use a clinical reasoning process to interpret assessment information

The clinical reasoning process is essential when assessing for biomechanical function and developing intervention, or treatment, plans. This section provides specific assessment protocols for the body. Refer to Chapter 3 for review of the clinical reasoning process.

Intervention plans should work toward the client's goals. Relating benefit derived from the modalities to daily function is important. For example, a plan based on the client's goal to achieve more effective shoulder movement could be as follows: "Client indicates that more effective shoulder movement could result in improved golf performance and the reduction of shoulder stiffness after the game. Improved shoulder movement would be encouraged with the use of weekly therapeutic massage and daily yoga practice."

A plan based on efficient biomechanical movement would focus on reestablishing or supporting effective movement patterns based on the following principles:

• Biomechanically efficient movement is smooth, bilaterally symmetric, and coordinated, with an easy, effortless use of the body. Noticeable variations from this standard should be noted during assessment.
• Each jointed area has a movement pattern. Movement involves bones; joints; ligaments; capsular components and design; tendons; muscle shapes and fiber types; interlinked fascial networks; nerve distribution; and myotatic units of prime movers, antagonists, synergists, fixators, and kinetic chain interactions.
• Reflexes, including positional and righting reflexes of vision and the inner ear, have bodywide influence, as does circulatory distribution.
• General systemic balance and nutritional influences affect biomechanical movement.
• Assessment should also identify areas of resourceful and successful compensation. These compensation patterns occur when the body has been required to adapt to some sort of trauma or repetitive use pattern. Permanent adaptive changes, although not as efficient as optimal functioning, are the best pattern the body can develop in response to an irreversible change in the system. Resourceful compensation should be supported, not eliminated.
• An efficient movement pattern is assessed as all parts functioning in a well-orchestrated manner. Causal factors in a dysfunction can be from any one or a combination of these elements. A multidisciplinary diagnosis is often necessary to clearly identify the interconnected pattern of the pathologic condition.

Individual Joint Assessment

The following sections explore movement assessments for individual jointed areas by applying a force to load the muscles to determine a response in the jointed area.

Remember that each joint movement pattern is part of an interconnected aspect of the kinetic chain and the tensegric nature of the design of the body. Posture and movement dysfunction should be identified in an individual joint pattern and then addressed in broader terms of kinetic chain

Text continued on p. 498.

ACTIVITY **10-3** COMMON MUSCLE FIRING PATTERNS

Trunk Flexion (Pictured below)
Palpate either side of the rectus abdominis to assess contraction of the obliques and transverse abdomen.

1. Normal firing pattern
   a. Transverse abdominis
   b. Abdominal obliques
   c. Rectus abdominis
2. Assessment
   a. Client is supine with knees and hips at approximately 90 degrees of flexion.
   b. Client is instructed to perform a normal curl-up.
   c. Massage practitioner assesses the ability of the abdominal muscles functionally to stabilize the lumbar-pelvic-hip complex by having the client draw the abdominal muscle

in (as when bringing the umbilicus toward the back) and then do a curl, just lifting the scapula off the table while keeping both feet flat. Inability to maintain the drawing-in position and/or to activate the rectus abdominis during the assessment demonstrates an altered firing pattern of the abdominal stabilization mechanism.

3. Altered firing pattern
   a. Weak agonist: abdominal complex
   b. Overactive antagonist: erector spinae
   c. Overactive synergist: psoas, rectus abdominis
4. Symptoms
   a. Low back pain
   b. Buttock pain
   c. Hamstring shortening

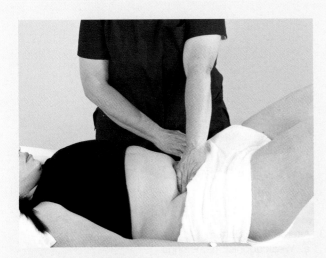

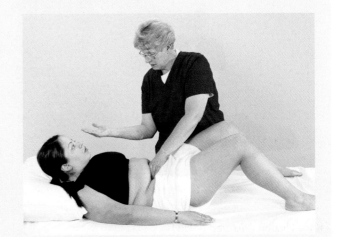

Hip Extension (Pictured below)

1. Normal firing pattern
   a. Gluteus maximus
   b. Opposite erector spinae
   c. Same-side erector spinae and hamstring
   or
   a. Gluteus maximus
   b. Hamstring
   c. Opposite erector spinae
   d. Same-side erector spinae
2. Assessment
   a. Client is prone.
   b. Massage practitioner palpates the erector spinae with the fingers of one hand while palpating the muscle belly of

the opposite gluteus maximus and hamstring with the little finger and thumb of the other hand.
   c. Client is instructed to raise the hip more than 15 degrees off the table.
3. Altered firing pattern
   a. Weak agonist: gluteus maximus
   b. Overactive antagonist: psoas
   c. Overactive stabilizer: erector spinae
   d. Overactive synergist: hamstring
4. Symptoms
   a. Low back pain
   b. Buttock pain
   c. Recurrent hamstring strains

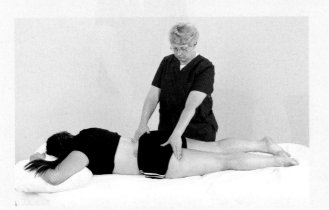

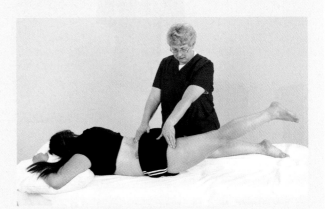

Continued

✎ ACTIVITY 10-3   COMMON MUSCLE FIRING PATTERNS—cont'd

Hip Abduction *(Pictured below)*
1. Normal firing pattern
   a. Gluteus medius
   b. Tensor fasciae latae
   c. Quadratus lumborum
2. Assessment
   a. Client is in side-lying position.
   b. Massage practitioner stands next to the client and palpates the quadratus lumborum with one hand and the tensor fasciae latae and gluteus medius with the finger of the other hand.
   c. Client is instructed to abduct the leg from the table.

3. Altered firing pattern
   a. Weak agonist: gluteus medius
   b. Overactive antagonist: adductors
   c. Overactive synergist: tensor fasciae latae
   d. Overactive stabilizer: quadratus lumborum
4. Symptoms
   a. Low back pain
   b. Sacroiliac joint pain
   c. Buttock pain
   d. Lateral knee pain
   e. Anterior knee pain

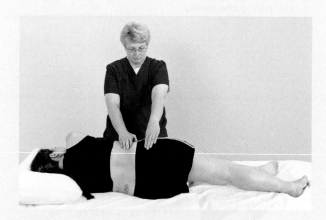

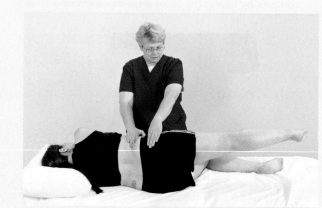

Knee Flexion *(Pictured below)*
1. Normal firing pattern
   a. Hamstrings
   b. Gastrocnemius
2. Assessment
   a. Client is prone.
   b. Massage practitioner places fingers on the hamstring and gastrocnemius.
   c. Client flexes the knee.

3. Altered firing pattern
   a. Weak agonist: hamstrings
   b. Overactive synergist: gastrocnemius
4. Symptoms
   a. Pain behind the knee
   b. Achilles tendinitis

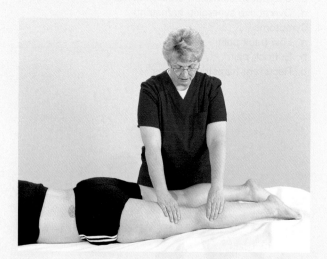

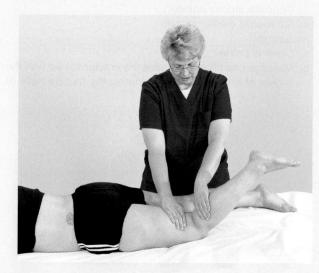

✎ ACTIVITY **10-3** COMMON MUSCLE FIRING PATTERNS—cont'd

Knee Extension *(Pictured below)*
1. Normal firing pattern
   a. Vastus medialis
   b. Vastus intermedius and vastus lateralis
   c. Rectus femoris
2. Assessment
   a. Client is supine with the leg flat.
   b. Client is asked to pull the patella cranially (toward the head).

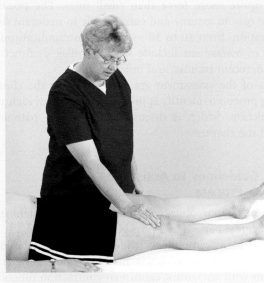

Shoulder Flexion *(Pictured below)*
1. Normal firing pattern
   a. Supraspinatus
   b. Deltoideus
   c. Infraspinatus
   d. Middle and lower trapezius
   e. Contralateral quadratus lumborum
2. Assessment
   a. Massage practitioner stands behind seated client with one hand on the client's shoulder and the other on the contralateral quadratus area.

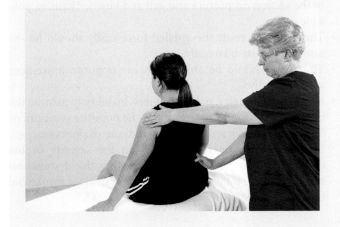

   c. Massage practitioner places the finger on the vastus medialis oblique portion, vastus lateralis, and rectus femoris.
3. Altered firing pattern
   a. Weak agonist: vastus medius, primarily oblique portion
   b. Overactive synergist: vastus lateralis
4. Symptoms
   a. Knee pain under patella
   b. Patellar tendinitis

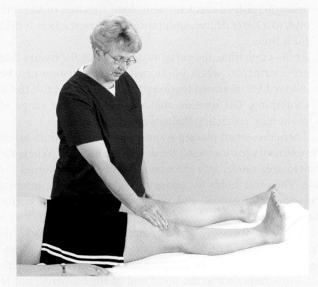

   b. Client is asked to abduct the shoulder to 90 degrees.
3. Altered firing pattern
   a. Weak agonist: levator scapula
   b. Overactive agonist: upper trapezius
   c. Overactive stabilizer: ipsilateral quadratus lumborum
4. Symptoms
   a. Shoulder tension
   b. Headache at the base of the skull
   c. Upper chest breathing
   d. Low back pain

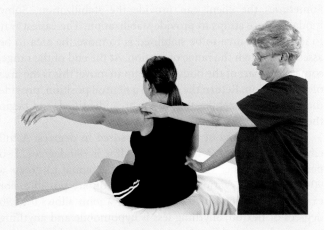

Intervention for Altered Firing Patterns
Use appropriate massage application to inhibit the dominant muscle. Then strengthen the weak muscles.

interactions, muscle tension-length relationships, and the effects of stress and strain on the entire system.

Assessing a movement pattern gives two types of information:

1. When a jointed area moves into flexion and the joint angle decreases, the prime mover and synergists concentrically shorten, antagonists eccentrically lengthen, and the fixators isometrically stabilize. Bodywide stabilization patterns also come into play to assist in allowing the motion. During assessment apply resistance to load the prime mover groups and synergists to check for neurologic function of strength and, to a lesser degree, endurance as the contraction is held for a time.

2. At the same time, the antagonist pattern of the tissues that are lengthened when positioned as in step one can be assessed for increased tension patterns or connective tissue shortening. Dysfunction shows itself in limited range of motion by restricting the movement pattern.

Therefore, when placing a jointed area into flexion, assess the extensors for increased tension or shortening. When the jointed area moves into extension, the opposite becomes the case. The same holds for adduction and abduction, internal and external rotation, and plantar and dorsal flexion, for example.

Resistance (pressure against) applied to the muscles is focused at the end of the lever system for mechanical advantage. For example, when assessing the function of the shoulder, focus resistance at the distal end of the humerus, not at the wrist. When assessing extension of the hip, place resistance at the end of the femur. When assessing flexion of the knee, place resistance at the distal end of the tibia. The practitioner applies resistance slowly, smoothly, and firmly at an appropriate intensity determined by the size of the muscle mass.

Stabilization is essential to assess movement patterns accurately. Allow only the area being assessed to move. Movement in any other part of the body needs to be stabilized. The massage therapist usually applies a stabilizing force. As one hand applies resistance, the other provides the stabilization. Sometimes the client can provide the stabilization. Some modalities use straps to provide stabilization. The easiest way to identify the area to be stabilized is to move the area to be assessed through the range of motion. At the end of the range, some other part of the body will begin to move; this is the area of stabilization. Return the body to a neutral position, provide the appropriate stabilization to the area identified, and begin the assessment procedure.

Range of motion of a joint is measured in degrees. A full circle is 360 degrees. A flat horizontal line is 180 degrees. Two perpendicular lines (as in the shape of a capital L) create a 90-degree angle. Various ranges of motion are possible. For example, when the range of motion of a joint allows 0 to 90 degrees of flexion, anything less is hypomobile and anything more is hypermobile. A great degree of variability exists among individuals as to the actual normal range of motion; the degrees provided are general guidelines (Figure 10-15). Range of motion is measured from the anatomic position. Regardless of whether the client is standing, supine, or sidelying, anatomic position is considered 0 degree of motion.

In actual professional practice, the practitioner picks and chooses which assessments to perform according to the client's goals and intervention processes. The activities are arranged to represent (agonist/antagonist) myotonic units (e.g., trunk extension/flexion and hip adduction/abduction).

During assessments muscles should be able to hold against appropriate resistance without strain or pain from the pressure and without recruiting or using other muscles. Apply appropriate resistance slowly and steadily and with just enough force for the muscles to respond to the stimulus. Large muscle groups require more force than small ones. The position should be easy to assume and comfortable to maintain for a short duration, from 10 to 30 seconds. Contraindications to this type of assessment include joint and disk dysfunction, acute pain, recent trauma, and inflammation.

Results of the assessment are analyzed using the clinical reasoning process to identify appropriate function of each area or dysfunction, which is discussed later in the pathology section of the chapter.

General Guidelines To Assist the Clinical Reasoning Process

- If an area is hypomobile, consider tension or shortening in the antagonist pattern as a possible cause.
- If an area is hypermobile, consider instability of the joint structure or muscle weakness in the fixation pattern or problems with antagonist/agonist co-contraction function.
- If an area cannot hold against resistance, consider weakness from reciprocal inhibition of the muscles of the prime mover and synergist pattern and tension in the antagonist pattern as possible causes.
- If pain occurs on passive movement, consider joint capsular dysfunction and nerve entrapment syndromes as possible causes.
- If pain occurs on active movement, consider muscle and fascial involvement as a possible cause.
- Always consider bodywide reflexive patterns, as discussed in the section on posture and gait and kinetic chain, as possible causes.
- The ability to resist the applied force easily should be the same or similar bilaterally.
- The client should be able to assume opposite movement patterns easily.
- Bilateral asymmetry, pain, weakness, inability to assume the isolation position or to move into the opposite position, or fatigue or a heavy sensation may indicate dysfunction.
- Intervention or referral depends on the severity of the condition (stage 1, 2, or 3) and whether the dysfunction is related to the joints, neuromuscular system, or myofascial tissues.

Biomechanics by Region

This part of Chapter 10 describes the kinesiology and biomechanics of the body in a regional format. Each region will be discussed, and then activities will help you integrate the information. Assessment activities will teach you how to muscle

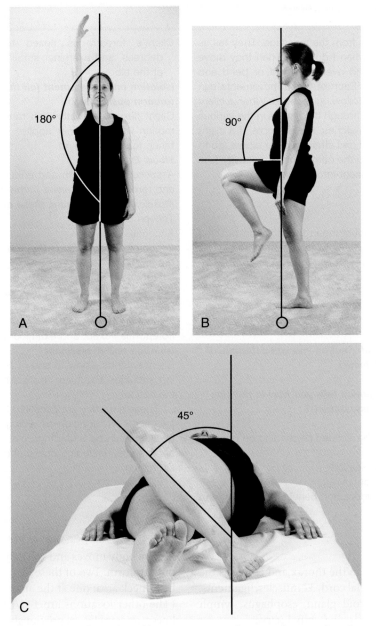

FIGURE 10-15 Examples of how to measure degrees of range of motion.

test and assess for range of motion. For each jointed region the following information will be provided:

Name of the movement
Muscles Involved
Range of Motion
Position of Client
Isolation and Assessment

The activities are organized so those movements within the same plane are adjacent. For example: Trunk flexion/trunk extension, shoulder adduction/abduction. This means that the muscles involve for the movements would be agonist/antagonist pairs.

- For example: the muscles that produce truck flexion would have the trunk exterior muscles as the antagonist. The shoulder adductors would be antagonist for the shoulder abductors.

This is important since a decrease in range of motion of a joint is often due to shortening in the antagonist muscles.

- For example: If the shoulder cannot abduct to the indicated range of motion, it may be that the shoulder adductors are short.

If you are not sure about a specific muscle listed, return to Chapter 9 and review. If you are not clear of how the specific joint is designed, return to Chapters 7 and 8 for review.

The information in this section consolidates content you learned in Chapters 7, 8, and 9. In these chapters you learned about individual parts of the anatomy and physiology. However, none of the individual structures can operate individually. Bones, joints, and muscles all work together under the direction of the nervous system. In this section you will learn how all the bones, joints, muscles, and associated connective tissue function together.

Practical Application

Massage clients expect results from the massage. They tell us during assessment, "It hurts when I do this." Then they move their head or arm or then bend over and twist or bend and straighten their knee or ankle. Each of those movements can be found in the activities in the following sections. When a client makes a joint movement, look through the figures in the various activities to find the one that matches. For example, if a client shows you that it hurts to bend and straighten her elbow, go to the section on the elbow and to the corresponding activity (see Activity 10-10) to find the pertinent information.

Examples:

Elbow Flexion

Assesses for strength and endurance in the isolation position and tension or shortening in the elbow extension pattern

Muscles Involved (from this list you can look up in Chapter 9 specific information on the muscles involved)

Biceps brachii (short head)

Brachialis

Brachioradialis

Pronator teres

Range of Motion (from this information you can determine if the joint movement is problematic)

0 to 150 degrees

Position of Client (this information tells you how to position the joint area to do various assessments)

Seated, with arms at sides

Three separate muscles can be isolated depending on position of forearm:

Biceps brachii: forearm in supination

Brachialis: forearm in pronation

Brachioradialis: forearm in midposition between pronation and supination

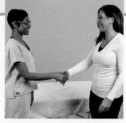

Client's forearm is flexed to 90 degrees, and examiner stabilizes it at the elbow.

Isolation and Assessment (all three forearm positions)

Client flexes elbow through range of motion while examiner applies resistance to distal forearm.

Elbow Extension

Assesses for strength and endurance in the isolation position and tension or shortening in the elbow flexion pattern

Muscles Involved (again, these are the muscles involved)

Triceps brachii

Anconeus

Range of Motion (this is the normal functional range of the joint)

No range of motion

Position of Client (here is how you position the client)

Standing or seated with arm to be tested able to extend without touching table

Forearm is flexed, and examiner stabilizes it at the elbow.

Isolation and Assessment

Client extends elbow to end of available range without extending shoulder. Examiner applies resistance at wrist to prevent the action.

These activities are excellent for helping you provide results for clients. In addition to aiding in assessment, each of the positions can be a starting point for various types of massage applications, including active and passive joint movement and stretching.

Head/Neck Region

The neck connects to the head in the thorax and contains the C1 to C7 cervical vertebrae, spinal cord, 32 muscles, ligaments, pharynx, larynx, trachea, thyroid gland, esophagus, lymph glands, hyoid bone, blood vessels, and spinal nerves.

The cervical vertebrae allow the head and neck to be moved into flexion, extension, lateral flexion, and rotation. Combinations of these movements are also possible. The small bodies and thick disks of the cervical vertebrae tend to increase mobility. Side bending is somewhat restricted by the rectangular shape of the vertebral bodies. The atlas and axis (C1 and C2) form a pivot joint that allows the head and C1 to rotate almost 90 degrees, such as in a "no" motion. The short spinous processes of C3 to C6 allow for good extension of the head and neck.

Intervertebral disks make up approximately 25% of the height of the cervical spine. The ligaments connecting the occiput to the atlas are dense and broad. These ligaments protect the entrance of the spinal cord through the foramen magnum into the skull. The atlantoaxial (C1 and C2) joint almost totally depends on ligamentous structure. The cervical spine from C2 to C7 is reinforced by anterior and posterior longitudinal ligaments. These ligaments limit the amount of flexion and extension.

The body moves and is balanced at certain points throughout our form. Two of these movement segments fall within the head/neck area: one at the atlas and skull and one at C6 to C7. (The other locations are T12/L1, L4/L5/S1, acetabulum/hips, knees, and ankles, as previously described in Activity 10-1.)

All muscles that act on the head attach on the skull. Those that are anterior to the coronal midline are termed *capital flexors*. Those muscles that lie behind the coronal midline are termed *capital extensors*. Their center of motion is in the atlantooccipital or atlantoaxial joints.

Muscles that act on the cervical spine are attached to the skull and the cervical and thoracic vertebrae, sternum, clavicle, ribs, and scapula. Most movement occurs at C6 to C7.

The muscles of the erector spinae group are considered stabilizers of the spinal column. The deep muscles extend, rotate, laterally flex, and stabilize the cervical region. All the muscles serve to maintain the correct position of the head and spine while we are moving (e.g., walking, sitting). These muscles are adapted physiologically to work in a relay manner so that they do not fatigue under normal conditions.

The sternocleidomastoid is primarily responsible for flexion and rotation of the head and neck. Extension, particularly extension and rotation, involves the splenius muscles together with the erector spinae and the upper trapezius muscles. The neck extensors, trapezius, scalenes, sternocleido-mastoid, and levator scapulae are considered major postural muscles in the body. The responsibility of these muscles is taxing even when the body has good posture and no pathologic condition is present. Many muscles of the neck are called on to assist in breathing if incorrect breathing patterns exist.

Trunk and Thorax Region

Biomechanics of the trunk and thorax are unique because the vertebral column is composed of 24 intricate and complex articulating vertebrae and 31 pairs of spinal nerves. Vertebral motion is greatest where the articulating surfaces and disks are large.

Spinal or Vertebral Movements

Movement depends on a finely integrated system of muscles that are deep—composed of numerous small bundles that attach from vertebra to vertebra—or superficial—arranged in large, broad sheets.

The name given to the region of movement often precedes the descriptions of spinal or vertebral movements. For example, flexion of the trunk at the lumbar spine is known as *lumbar flexion,* and extension of the neck often is referred to as *cervical extension.* Movement of the head between the cranium and the first cervical vertebra is called *capital movement.* Movements occurring among the other cervical vertebrae are called *cervical movements.* These motions usually occur together.

The five spinal movements are as follows (Activity 10-4):

- *Spinal flexion:* Spinal flexion is anterior movement of the spine in the sagittal plane. In the cervical region, the head moves toward the chest. In the thoracic and lumbar regions, the thorax moves toward the pelvis.
- *Spinal extension:* Spinal extension is posterior movement of the spine in the sagittal plane to return from flexion. In the cervical region the head moves away from the chest. The thorax moves away from the pelvis.
- *Lateral flexion (side bending):* Lateral flexion in the frontal plane occurs in the cervical region when the head moves laterally toward the shoulder. In the thoracic and lumbar regions, the thorax moves laterally toward the pelvis. Movement can be to the left or right.
- *Reduction:* Reduction is the return movement from lateral flexion to neutral.

- *Spinal rotation (left or right):* Spinal rotation in the transverse plane is the rotary or twisting movement of the spine. In the cervical region the chin rotates from neutral toward the shoulder. In the thoracic and lumbar regions, the thorax rotates to one side.

As explained previously, each pair of vertebrae constitutes a vertebral motion segment, the basic movable unit of the back. Except for the atlantoaxial joint formed by the first two cervical vertebrae, little movement is possible between any two vertebrae. The amount of movement varies depending on the shape of the vertebrae, the thickness of the intervertebral disk—with thicker disks providing greater mobility—and any rib articulations. However, the cumulative effect of the movements from several adjacent vertebrae allows for substantial movements within a given area. Most of the spinal column movement occurs in the cervical and lumbar regions. Of course, some thoracic movement occurs, but it is slight compared with that of the neck and low back.

Rotation screws the superior vertebra down into the adjacent vertebra, compressing the disk. Prime mover muscles contract while the contralateral muscles lengthen. Ligament structures are twisted.

In flexion the anterior muscles contract, the posterior muscles lengthen, the superior vertebra tilts toward the front, and the disks are compressed anteriorly and expand posteriorly while the nucleus moves slightly to the back. The superior articular facets slide forward on the inferior ones. The posterior ligaments are stretched, and the anterior ligaments slacken.

In extension, just the opposite occurs. The posterior muscles contract and the anterior muscles lengthen. The superior vertebra tilts toward the back. The disk is compressed posteriorly and expands anteriorly, and the nucleus moves slightly to the front. The articular facets are pressed together. The anterior ligaments are stretched, and the posterior ligaments slacken. Lateral flexion follows the same pattern (Figure 10-16; Activity 10-5).

Thoracic Vertebral Column Region

The thoracic vertebrae are structured to articulate with the ribs, with stability as the main function of this outer unit region. This area does not move extensively, but small

---

✎ ACTIVITY 10-4

From a standing position, slowly move your head into flexion. Then follow with your cervical region, thoracic region, and lumbar region, each moving into flexion. Pay attention to the limitation of each region, and notice the increased range of motion as each area is brought into play. Now move into extension following the same pattern. Repeat this activity for lateral flexion and rotation on both sides. Describe the experience.

Example

I noticed that it was difficult to isolate head flexion by itself.

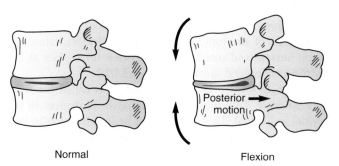

Normal   Flexion

FIGURE 10-16 Movement of the spine from a position of extension into flexion causes the nucleus to move in a posterior direction. (Adapted from Shankman GA: *Fundamental orthopedic management for the physical therapist assistant,* ed 3, St Louis, 2011, Mosby.)

✎ ACTIVITY 10-5

In the space provided, write the sequence for lateral flexion with side bending to the right.

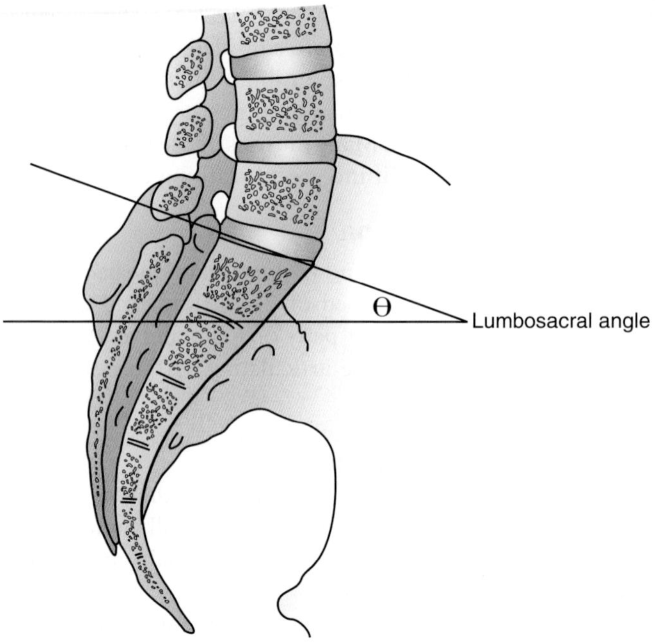

FIGURE 10-17 The lumbosacral angle. (Modified from Malone TR, McPoil T, Nitz AJ: *Orthopedic and sports physical therapy,* ed 3, St Louis, 1997, Mosby.)

movements at the facet joints are ongoing with the breathing process.

A few large extrinsic muscles and numerous small intrinsic muscles are found in this area. Extrinsic muscles are defined as muscles that link a limb to the trunk of the body. Intrinsic muscles are muscles that are entirely within the body part or segment (inner unit). The largest muscle is the erector spinae (sacrospinalis), which extends on each side of the spinal column from the pelvic region to the cranium.

The erector spinae muscles function best when the pelvis is held up in front, thus pulling them down slightly in back.

As the spine is held straight and the ribs are raised, the chest raises and consequently makes the abdominal muscles more effective in holding the pelvis up in front and flattening the abdominal wall.

Lumbar Vertebral Column Region

The five lumbar vertebrae are the most massive of the spinal column. These vertebrae carry a large share of the upper body weight, balancing the torso on the sacrum. The combined unit of the vertebrae and disks in the upright position forms the lumbar spinal curve. The lumbar vertebral disks are strong, short, and thick. The ligaments provide stability in all directions. This is the most frequently injured area of the back.

The lumbar vertebral group has less mobility than the cervical region but more than the thoracic region. Because of the absence of ribs and the shape of the spinous processes, the lumbar spine is freer in flexion and extension. Rotation, however, is limited by the amount of tension created in the surrounding ligaments and annulus fibrosis of the disks.

Motions of the lumbar spine include flexion, extension, lateral flexion, and rotation. More motion takes place at L5/S1 (the lumbosacral junction) than at L1/L2.

The angle formed between L5 and S1 is called the *lumbosacral angle.* This angle is approximately 41 degrees in the normal individual. This is typically a neutral position in that no erector spinae force needs to be exerted as a counterbalance. When special conditions exist such as obesity, pregnancy, abdominal muscle weakness, wearing of high heels, foot pronation, and poor posture, this angle increases undesirably, which can lead to lumbar pain and dysfunction (Figure 10-17).

Abdominal muscles initiate flexion, whereas the erector spinae resist flexion. Intrinsic muscles of the back provide extension, whereas the abdominal muscles (mainly the rectus abdominis) resist. Lateral bending occurs with spinal rotation. Ipsilateral structures tend to relax, whereas contralateral structures resist. Lumbosacral rotation takes place with a variety of complex tension and relaxation patterns. Rotation is limited by the straight, posteriorly oriented spinous processes.

Abdomen Region

Abdominal muscles do not extend from bone to bone but attach into tendinous bands and an aponeurosis (fascia) around the rectus abdominis area. The abdominal muscles are the rectus abdominis, external oblique, internal oblique, and transversus abdominis.

The rectus abdominis muscle controls the tilt of the pelvis and the consequent curvature of the lower spine. Holding the pelvis up in front makes the erector spinae muscle more effective as an extensor of the spine and makes the hip flexors such as the iliopsoas more effective.

The internal oblique muscles run diagonally in the direction opposite to that of the external oblique muscles. The left internal oblique muscle causes rotation to the left, and the right internal oblique muscle causes rotation to the right. In rotary movements the internal oblique muscle and the opposite-side external oblique muscle always work together.

The transversus abdominis is the chief muscle of forced expiration. The transversus abdominis and the external oblique and internal oblique muscles are effective in helping to hold the abdomen flat.

Thorax Region

As discussed in Chapter 7, the skeletal foundation of the thorax is formed by 12 pairs of ribs, the manubrium, the body of the sternum, and the xiphoid process. Breathing is a major function of the thorax. Breathing involves inspiration, or inhaling, and expiration, or exhaling. The primary muscles of inspiration are the diaphragm and the external intercostal muscles.

During quiet respiration the diaphragm may act alone, or a slight rhythmic activity may occur in the scalenus anterior and scalenus medius and in the intercostal muscles. In deep inspiration the action of the primary muscles increases, and the sternocleidomastoid and scalenes assist in raising the ribs. Forced inspiration involves any muscles that stabilize or elevate the shoulder girdle to elevate the ribs directly or indirectly.

Expiration is primarily passive as relaxation of the prime movers and the weight of gravity pulls the rib cage down. The primary muscles of expiration are the internal intercostal muscles. Forced expiration involves muscles that force the rib cage down (quadratus lumborum) or compress the abdominal cavity (oblique and transverse abdominal muscles), forcing the diaphragm upward.

There are two different types of breathing patterns: diaphragmatic and thoracic. Diaphragmatic, or abdominal, breathing is the natural way to breathe and occurs in infants and sleeping adults. Inhalation deep into the lungs occurs by the contraction of the diaphragm, flattening its dome shape and resulting in negative pressure in the lungs, which fill with air to equalize the pressure. The diaphragm then relaxes, expelling the air by its upward movement. Diaphragmatic breathing is even and relaxed.

Thoracic, or chest, breathing is common in persons with anxiety or other emotional distress. Anxious persons may experience breath holding, hyperventilation syndrome, constricted breathing, shortness of breath, or fear of fainting. Thoracic breathing occurs in persons who wear restrictive clothing, actively hold in their abdominal muscles, or lead sedentary or stressful lives. Chest breathing is often shallow, irregular, and rapid. On inhalation the chest expands and the shoulders rise to take in air. Dysfunctional patterns can develop if the accessory muscles of respiration (scalenes, sternocleidomastoid, serratus posterior superior, levator scapulae, rhomboid muscles, abdominal muscles, and quadratus lumborum) are used constantly for regular breathing when forced inhalation and expiration are not required (Activity 10-6).

✎ ACTIVITY **10-6**

In this activity, you will be working with a partner to assess individual movement patterns, normal function, and possible dysfunction in each other. One of you is first to isolate the specified movement patterns on each side of your partner, one side at a time, and assess for normal function by applying a gentle pressure opposite to the action of the isolation position. The body should be stabilized so that only the isolated area is moving. In some instances the ability to assume the position and maintain it indicates normal function. Muscles should be able to hold against gravity or the applied pressure without strain or pain. The position itself should be easy to assume and comfortable to maintain for a short duration, from 10 to 30 seconds. The bilateral movement patterns should be the same. The opposite movement pattern also should be able to be easily performed.

Dysfunction may be indicated by bilateral asymmetry, pain, weakness, fatigue, a heavy sensation (binding), and inability to assume the isolation position or move into the opposite position. Intervention or referral depends on the severity of the condition and whether the dysfunction is neuromuscular, myofascial, or joint related.

Note: Do not perform these assessments if contraindications exist. Contraindications to this type of assessment include joint and disk dysfunction, acute pain, recent trauma, and inflammation.

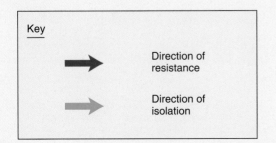

Key	
→	Direction of resistance
→	Direction of isolation

Trunk Extension

Assesses for strength and endurance in the isolation position and tension or shortening in the flexion pattern

Muscles Involved

Erector spinae (sacrospinalis) group: iliocostalis, longissimus, and spinalis

Splenius cervicis and splenius capitis

Semispinalis

Multifidus

Range of Motion

Thoracic spine: No range of motion

Lumbar spine: 0 to 25 degrees

Position of Client

Prone, with hands clasped behind head; client may hold hands behind back.

Isolation and Assessment

Client extends the lumbar spine until the head and chest are raised from the table. Ability to perform test indicates normal function. No resistance is required.

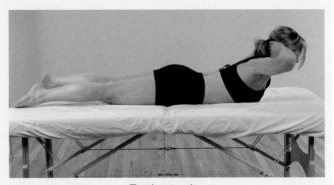

Trunk extension

Continued

✎ ACTIVITY **10-6**—cont'd

Trunk Flexion

Assesses for strength and endurance in the isolation position and tension or shortening in the extension pattern

Muscles Involved

Rectus abdominis

Internal and external obliques

Psoas major and psoas minor

Range of Motion

0 to 50 degrees (beyond 50 degrees, any additional flexion comes from pelvic rotation)

Position of the Client

Supine, with hands clasped behind head or crossed in front and placed on shoulders, knees bent, feet flat

Note: Client is not to lift head with hands.

Isolation and Assessment

Client tucks chin to chest and brings shoulders toward thighs. Ability to clear scapulae from the table indicates good function. No resistance is required.

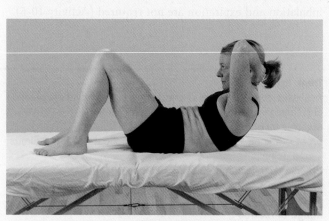

Trunk flexion

Trunk Rotation

Assesses for strength and endurance in the isolation position and tension or shortening in the contralateral pattern

Muscles Involved

External obliques

Internal obliques

Latissimus dorsi

Rectus abdominis

Deep back muscles (unilateral test)

Range of Motion

0 to 45 degrees

Position of Client

Supine, with knees bent and feet flat, hands clasped across chest or held beside ears

Note: Client is not to lift head with hands.

Isolation and Assessment

Client slowly flexes and rotates trunk to one side. After returning to supine position, movement is repeated on opposite side. Ability to clear scapulae from the table indicates good function.

Right shoulder to left knee tests the right external obliques and left internal obliques. Left shoulder to right knee tests the left external obliques and right internal obliques.

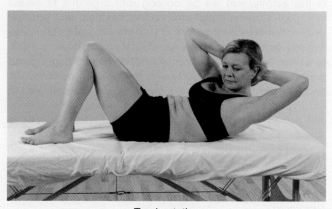

Trunk rotation

✐ ACTIVITY **10-6**—cont'd

Elevation of the Pelvis (More Correctly Known as *Lateral Tilt*)
Assesses for strength and endurance in the isolation position and tension or shortening in the contralateral pattern

Muscles Involved
Quadratus lumborum
Latissimus dorsi
Internal abdominal obliques
Iliocostalis lumborum

Range of Motion
Not applicable

Position of Client
Prone with hip and lumbar spine in extension, hip slightly abducted, feet off end of table; the client grasps the edges of the table to provide stabilization during resistance.

Isolation and Assessment
Client brings iliac crest toward ribs on one side while examiner applies resistance to lower leg to pull hip down.

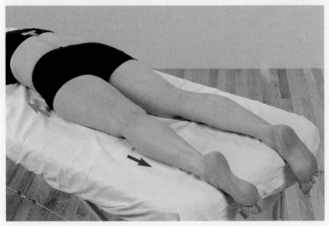

Elevation of the pelvis, lateral tilt

Capital Extension
Assesses for strength and endurance in the isolation position and tension or shortening in the flexion pattern

Muscles Involved
Rectus capitis posterior major
Rectus capitis posterior minor
Longissimus capitis
Obliquus capitis superior
Obliquus capitis inferior
Splenius capitis
Semispinalis capitis

Range of Motion
0 to 25 degrees

Position of Client
Prone with head off end of table, arms at sides
Note: Do not do this test if client has cervical disk problems.

Isolation and Assessment
Client lifts chin up away from chest, as if beginning to nod "yes"; cervical spine is not extended. Examiner applies resistance to the back of the head.

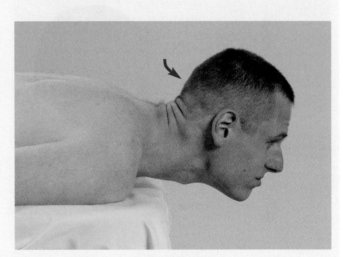

Capital Extension

Continued

ACTIVITY **10-6**—cont'd

Cervical Extension

Assesses for strength and endurance in the isolation position and tension or shortening in the flexion pattern

Muscles Involved

Longissimus cervicis

Semispinalis cervicis

Iliocostalis cervicis

Splenius capitis and splenius cervicis

Range of Motion

0 to 25 degrees

Position of Client

Prone, with head off end of table, arms along sides

Note: Do not do this test if client has cervical disk problems.

Isolation and Assessment

Client extends neck by lifting head toward ceiling. No resistance is required. Ability to hold head up against gravity indicates normal function.

Capital Flexion

Assesses for strength and endurance in the isolation position and tension or shortening in the extension pattern

Muscles Involved

Rectus longus

Capitis anterior

Range of Motion

0 to 10 or 15 degrees

Position of Client

Supine

Note: Do not do this test if client has cervical disk problems.

Isolation and Assessment

Client tucks chin into neck as in nodding "yes." Head remains on table. No motion should occur at the cervical spine. No resistance is required.

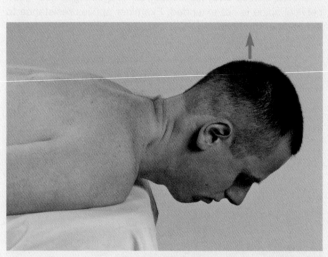

Cervical Extension

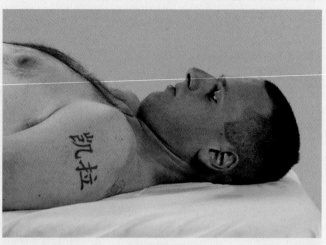

Capital Flexion

✎ ACTIVITY **10-6**—cont'd

Cervical Flexion

Assesses for strength and endurance in the isolation position and tension or shortening in the extension pattern

Muscles Involved

Scalenus anterior, scalenus medius, and scalenus posterior
Sternocleidomastoid
Longus colli

Range of Motion

0 to 35 or 45 degrees
Note: Women usually have greater cervical lordosis than men, so they likely could have a greater arc of motion.

Position of Client

Supine, with arms at sides and head supported on table
Note: Do not do this test if client has cervical disk problems.

Isolation and Assessment

Client lifts head off table and tucks chin. This is a weak muscle group, so no resistance is required.

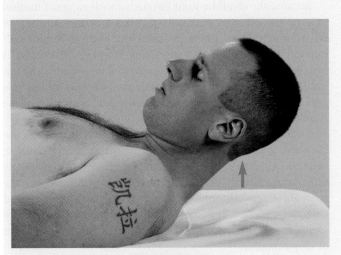

Cervical Flexion

Cervical Rotation

Assesses for strength and endurance in the isolation position and tension or shortening in the contralateral pattern

Muscles Involved

Sternocleidomastoid
Rectus capitis posterior major
Obliquus capitis inferior
Longissimus capitis

Range of Motion

0 to 45 or 55 degrees
Two separate actions will be tested.

Position of Client

Supine
Begin with head supported on table and turned to one side.

Isolation and Assessment

Client lifts head off table without any additional rotation, returns to start position, and repeats on other side. No resistance is required.

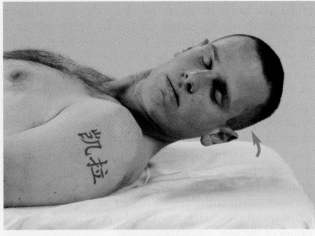

Cervical Rotation 1

Position of Client

Supine, with cervical spine in neutral flexion and extension
Begin with head supported on table and turned to one side.

Isolation and Assessment

Client rotates head to neutral (nose facing ceiling) against resistance. Make sure client does not lift head off table. Repeat on opposite side.

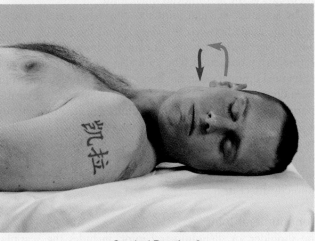

Cervical Rotation 2

Shoulder Region

The complicated framework of the shoulder not only is extremely mobile but also provides a secure and stable immovable point for specific actions such as lifting, thrusting, shoving, and pushing heavy objects. This region consists of the shoulder girdle and the shoulder, or glenohumeral joint.

Shoulder Girdle Region

The shoulder girdle is made up of the scapula and clavicle (which generally move as a unit) and associated soft tissues. The clavicle has two synovial gliding joints. The sternoclavicular joint is medial, and the acromioclavicular joint is lateral. When analyzing scapulothoracic movements, realize that the scapula moves on the rib cage because the joint motion actually occurs at the sternoclavicular joint and, to a lesser extent, at the acromioclavicular joint.

The movements of the sternoclavicular joint include elevation, depression, rotation, protraction, and retraction. For full abduction to occur, the clavicle must rotate 50 degrees posteriorly. Movement at the joint occurs indirectly as a result of scapular movement. The characteristics of the joint are influenced indirectly by the movement of the glenohumeral joint. Although no direct muscular attachments cross this joint, several muscles have indirect influence on the movement, especially the pectoralis major, subclavius, sternocleidomastoid, sternothyroid and sternohyoid, scalenus medius and scalenus posterior, and upper trapezius.

The acromioclavicular joint contributes little to scapular movement because its joint surfaces do not allow much angular movement. A rotary and hingelike motion takes place at this joint, chiefly with elevation of the arm above 90 degrees. The S shape of the clavicle provides the extra motion during elevation of the arm.

The scapulae rotate at the acromioclavicular joint at the beginning of scapular movement. Of the approximately 60 degrees that scapular movement contributes to the elevation of the arm, about 30 degrees occurs at the sternoclavicular joint and the remaining 30 degrees occurs from the combined effects of clavicular rotation, which causes the clavicular joint surfaces to face upward, and the acromioclavicular movement that occurs at the acromioclavicular joint.

The acromioclavicular joint allows widening and narrowing of the angle between the clavicle and the scapula (from above). Narrowing occurs during protraction; widening occurs during retraction. The joint also allows for rotation of the scapula upward when the inferior angle moves away from the midline, and rotation of the scapula downward when the inferior angle moves toward the midline. The acromioclavicular joint also allows rotation of the scapula in such a way that the inferior angle swings anteriorly and posteriorly. Although no muscles directly cause movements of the acromioclavicular joint, the deltoid, upper trapezius, and subclavius muscles indirectly affect it.

Glenohumeral Joint

The shoulder, or glenohumeral joint, includes the scapula, humerus, and associated soft tissues. The only attachment of the shoulder joint to the axial skeleton is the clavicle at the sternoclavicular joint.

The glenohumeral joint is a ball-and-socket joint and is the articulation between the glenoid fossa of the scapula and the head of the humerus. Movements of the shoulder joint are many and varied. This mobile joint allows adduction, abduction, flexion, extension, hyperextension, horizontal adduction and abduction, and lateral and medial rotation of the humerus in all planes: sagittal, frontal, and transverse.

Movement of the humerus without scapular movement is unusual. Much of the movement of the scapula is related to movement at the glenohumeral joint. Flexion and abduction of the humerus elevates and abducts the scapula with upward rotation. Adduction and extension of the humerus results in depression, rotation downward, and adduction of the scapula. The scapula is abducted with humeral internal rotation and horizontal adduction. Scapular adduction accompanies external rotation and horizontal abduction of the humerus.

Because the shoulder joint has such a wide range of motion in so many different planes, it also has a certain amount of laxity, which often results in instability such as rotator cuff impingement and dislocations. Often the price of mobility is instability. The concept that the more mobile a joint is, the less stable it is, and that the more stable it is, the less mobile it is applies generally throughout the body but especially in the shoulder joint.

An important, protective fibroosseous arch over the glenohumeral arch is formed by the coracoacromial ligament, together with the acromion (or the lateral end of the clavicle articulating directly with the acromion and indirectly with the coracoid process through the coracoclavicular ligaments) and coracoid process. This arch forms a secondary restraining socket for the humeral head, preventing superior dislocation or displacement.

At the brim of the glenoid fossa is a fibrocartilaginous ring called the *glenoid labrum* that adds stability and substance to this shallow and mobile articulation.

The glenoid labrum merges with several ligaments and tendons to form the joint capsule of the glenohumeral joint. Tendons that connect at this joint are from the muscles of the subscapularis, infraspinatus, teres minor, and the supraspinatus, also known as SITS, or rotator cuff muscles, because they contribute to the rotation of the humerus. In reality, numerous muscles and tendons intersect the glenohumeral joint, and because of their attachment points, they contribute to the stability of the joint through their tension lines of pull. The deltoid forms a hood over the small muscles that closely surround the joint and acts as a shock absorber to protect the joint from impact.

The deep fascia covering the deltoid, known as the *deltoid aponeurosis,* is a fibrous layer that covers the outer surface of the muscle. The deep fascia is thick and strong behind, where it is continuous with the infraspinatus fascia, and thinner over the rest of the muscle. In front, the deltoid aponeurosis is continuous with the fascia covering the pectoralis major. Above, the deltoid aponeurosis is attached to the clavicle, the acromion, and spine of the scapula; below, it is continuous with the deep fascia of the arm. This extensive fascial network provides dynamic stability.

Scapulothoracic Junction

The scapulothoracic junction meets the criteria of a joint in that it allows the scapula to glide over the ribs and is separated by muscle, fascia, and bursae. The junction is not a true synovial joint because it does not have regular synovial features and its movement depends totally on the sternoclavicular and acromioclavicular joints. Even though scapular movement occurs as a result of motion at the sternoclavicular and acromioclavicular joints, the scapula can be described as having a total range of 25 degrees of abduction-adduction, 60 degrees of upward-downward rotation, and 55 degrees of elevation-depression. A large subscapular bursal sheet and fat pad enhance the gliding of this junction.

In analyzing shoulder girdle movements, focusing on a specific bony landmark such as the inferior angle (posteriorly), glenoid fossa (laterally), and acromion process (anteriorly) often is helpful. All the following movements have their pivotal point where the clavicle joins the sternum at the sternoclavicular joint. Movements of the shoulder girdle can be described as movements of the scapula.

Movements of the Scapula

The following movements involve the scapula:

Abduction (protraction): Movement of the scapula laterally away from the spinal column

Adduction (retraction): Movement of the scapula medially toward the spinal column

Upward rotation: Turning the glenoid fossa upward and moving the inferior angle superiorly and laterally away from the spinal column

Downward rotation: Returning the inferior angle medially and inferiorly toward the spinal column and the glenoid fossa to its normal position

Elevation: Upward or superior movement, as in shrugging the shoulders

Depression: Downward or inferior movement, as in returning to normal position

Movements of the Glenohumeral Joint

The glenohumeral joint allows the following movements:

Abduction: Lateral movement of the humerus out to the side and away from the body

Adduction: Movement of the humerus medially toward the body from abduction

Flexion: Movement of the humerus anteriorly

Extension: Movement of the humerus posteriorly

Horizontal adduction (flexion): Movement of the humerus in a horizontal or transverse plane toward and across the chest

Horizontal abduction (extension): Movement of the humerus in a horizontal or transverse plane away from the chest

External rotation: Movement of the humerus laterally around its long axis away from the midline

Internal rotation: Movement of the humerus medially around its long axis toward the midline

Table 10-1 Shoulder Joint

Shoulder Joint	Shoulder Girdle
Abduction	Upward rotation
Adduction	Downward rotation
Flexion	Elevation, upward rotation, protraction
Extension	Depression, downward rotation, retraction
Internal rotation	Abduction (protraction)
External rotation	Adduction (retraction)
Horizontal abduction	Adduction (retraction)
Horizontal adduction	Abduction (protraction)

✎ ACTIVITY 10-7

Slowly and deliberately move your scapula and glenohumeral joint through each of the movement patterns just described. Identify the interplay between the shoulder girdle movements and the shoulder joint movements. Pay attention to the limitation of each region, and notice the increase in range of motion as each area is brought into play. Describe the experience.

Example

I noticed that it was confusing to attempt to isolate scapular movements by themselves.

The shoulder joint and shoulder girdle work together in carrying out upper extremity activities. Table 10-1 shows a pairing of shoulder girdle and shoulder joint movements (Activity 10-7).

Shoulder Girdle Muscles

Five muscles are involved primarily in shoulder girdle movements: trapezius, levator scapulae, rhomboid muscles, serratus anterior, and pectoralis minor. Grouping the muscles of the shoulder girdle separately from the shoulder joint is helpful to avoid confusion. All five shoulder girdle muscles have their proximal attachment on the axial skeleton, with their distal attachment located on the scapula or clavicle. Shoulder girdle muscles do not attach to the humerus, nor do they cause actions of the shoulder joint. The shoulder girdle muscles are essential in providing dynamic stability of the scapula so that it can serve as a base of support for shoulder joint activities. A force couple occurs when muscles work in conjunction, pulling in different directions, to accomplish a specific movement (Figure 10-18).

The trapezius muscle fixates the scapula for deltoid action by preventing the glenoid fossa from being pulled down when the arms lift objects. The muscle is used strenuously when lifting with the hands, as in picking up a heavy wheelbarrow. The trapezius must prevent the scapula from being pulled downward, such as when an object is held overhead or a person is carrying an object that is resting on the tip of his or her shoulder.

Shrugging the shoulder calls the levator scapulae muscle into play, along with the upper trapezius muscle.

The rhomboids fix the scapula in adduction/retraction when the muscles of the shoulder joint adduct or extend the

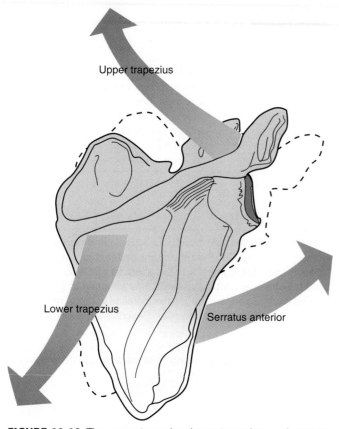

Upper trapezius

Lower trapezius

Serratus anterior

FIGURE 10-18 The upper trapezius, lower trapezius, and serratus anterior pull in three different directions to achieve one type of motion-upward rotation of the scapula. This is called a *force couple.*

arm. The trapezius and rhomboid muscles work together to produce adduction, with slight elevation of the scapula. To prevent this elevation, the latissimus dorsi muscle is called into play. The serratus anterior muscle acts in movements drawing the scapula forward with slight upward rotation and works along with the pectoralis major muscle in actions such as throwing a baseball. A winged scapula condition indicates a definite weakness of the serratus anterior.

The pectoralis minor muscle is used, along with the serratus anterior muscle, in true abduction (protraction) without rotation. When true abduction of the scapula is necessary, the serratus anterior draws the scapula forward with a slight upward rotation and the pectoralis minor pulls forward with slight downward rotation. The two pulling together give true abduction. These muscles work together in most movements of pushing with the hands.

Glenohumeral Joint Muscles

Muscles of the glenohumeral joint contribute to more than one action when the humerus is in a sequence of movement. The muscles involved in flexion of the shoulder and glenohumeral joint cross the joint anteriorly. The primary flexors are the pectoralis major, anterior deltoid, and coracobrachialis. Synergists to flexion are the biceps brachii and the subscapularis.

In extension of the glenohumeral joint, when movement meets no resistance, gravity is the prime mover, with the flexor muscles eccentrically contracting to control the action of extension. When resistance occurs, the posterior muscles of the glenohumeral joint go to work, specifically the teres major, latissimus dorsi, and sternocostal pectoralis. Synergists for extension are the posterior deltoid, particularly when the humerus is rotated externally, and the triceps brachii (long head) when the elbow is flexed.

Two primary movers are involved in abduction of the glenohumeral joint: the middle deltoid and supraspinatus. Both muscles intersect the shoulder superior to the glenohumeral joint. The supraspinatus begins the movement of abduction for approximately the first 110 degrees. The middle deltoid is active from approximately 90 degrees to 180 degrees. To counteract superior dislocation, the infraspinatus, subscapularis, and teres major shorten to control the action of the middle deltoid.

Adduction of the glenohumeral joint is another movement in which, if no resistance occurs, gravity is the prime mover, with the abductors as the antagonist controlling the speed of the motion. With resistance, the principal adductors are the latissimus dorsi, teres major, and pectoralis major sternal, all positioned inferior to the glenohumeral joint. The synergists are the biceps (short head) and triceps (long head).

Medial rotation of the humerus results from the subscapularis and teres major as the prime movers. Both attach to the anterior aspect of the humerus. Synergists to medial rotation are the pectoralis major, anterior deltoid, latissimus dorsi, and biceps brachii (short head).

Muscles attaching into the posterior aspect of the humerus generate the lateral rotation, specifically the infraspinatus and teres minor.

Horizontal adduction results from the actions of anterior muscles, which include the anterior deltoid, pectoralis major, and coracobrachialis. The synergist to horizontal adduction is the biceps brachii (short head).

Horizontal abduction is affected by the middle and posterior deltoid, infraspinatus, and teres minor, muscles located on the posterior aspect of the joint. The synergists to horizontal abduction are the teres major and latissimus dorsi (Activity 10-8).

Text continued on p. 517.

ACTIVITY **10-8**

In this activity you will be working with a partner to assess individual movement patterns, normal function, and possible dysfunction in each other. One of you is first to isolate the specified movement patterns on each side of your partner, one side at a time, and assess for normal function by applying a gentle pressure opposite the action of the isolation position. The body should be stabilized so that only the isolated area is moving. In some instances the ability to assume the position and maintain it indicates normal function. Muscles should be able to hold against gravity or the applied pressure without strain or pain. The position itself should be easy to assume and comfortable to maintain for a short duration, from 10 to 30 seconds. The bilateral movement patterns should be the same. The opposite movement pattern also should be able to be done easily.

Dysfunction may be indicated by bilateral asymmetry, pain, weakness, fatigue, a heavy sensation (binding), and the inability to assume the isolation position or move into the opposite position. Intervention or referral depends on the severity of the condition and whether the dysfunction is neuromuscular, myofascial, or joint related.

Note: Do not perform these assessments if contraindications exist. Contraindications to this type of assessment include joint and disk dysfunction, acute pain, recent trauma, and inflammation.

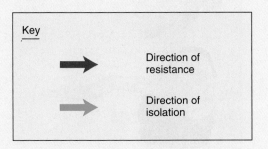

Key

→ Direction of resistance

→ Direction of isolation

Before starting scapular motion assessments, do a visual assessment of your partner to check for variations in position and symmetry. Asymmetry often shows as one shoulder or scapula that is higher, especially in those who carry briefcases, purses, or babies on one side.

Working with your partner, determine the position of the scapulae at rest and whether the two sides are symmetric. The normal scapula lies close to the rib cage with the vertebral border nearly parallel and from 1 to 3 inches lateral to the spinous processes. The inferior angle is tucked in. If the inferior angle of the scapula is tilted away from the rib cage, check for tightness of the pectoralis minor and weakness of the trapezius.

The most prominent abnormal posture of the scapula is "winging," in which the vertebral border tilts away from the rib cage, a sign of serratus weakness.

Within the total arc of 180 degrees of shoulder forward flexion, 120 degrees is glenohumeral motion and 60 degrees is scapular motion. Because these movements are not isolated, saying that the glenohumeral and scapular motions coexist after 60 degrees and up to 150 degrees is more correct.

Passively raise your partner's test arm in forward flexion completely above his or her head to determine scapular mobility. The scapula should start to rotate at about 60 degrees, although considerable individual variation exists.

Check that the scapula basically remains in its rest position at ranges of shoulder flexion less than 60 degrees, with some variation among individuals. If the scapula moves as the glenohumeral joint moves below 60 degrees (i.e., within this range they move as a unit), limited glenohumeral motion is evident, but the scapula may move through a complete or even excessive range.

From greater than 60 degrees and to about 150 or 160 degrees in active and passive motion, the scapula moves in concert with the humerus.

Continued

✎ ACTIVITY **10-8**—cont'd

Scapular Abduction (Protraction)

Assesses for strength and endurance in the isolation position and tension or shortening in the scapular adduction pattern

Muscles Involved

Serratus anterior

Pectoralis minor

Range of Motion

Reliable values are not available.

Position of Client

Seated, with legs over end or side of table, and hands at sides on top of table

Isolation and Assessment

Client flexes the straight arm to approximately 130 degrees and reaches forward to protract the scapula. The examiner palpates the medial border of the scapula and applies resistance to the arm.

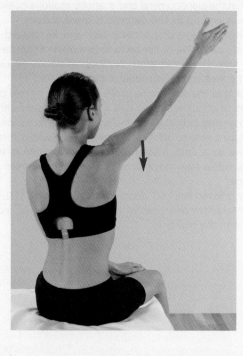

Scapular Adduction (Retraction)

Assesses for strength and endurance in the isolation position and tension or shortening in the scapular abduction pattern

Muscles Involved

Trapezius (middle fibers)

Rhomboideus major and rhomboideus minor

Latissimus dorsi

Range of Motion

Reliable values are not available.

Position of Client

Seated with legs over edge of table

Shoulder is abducted to 90 degrees and externally rotated.

Elbow is flexed to a right angle and held at shoulder level.

Isolation and Assessment

Client horizontally abducts arm to adduct the scapula while examiner applies resistance to the posterior arm above the elbow to push the arm into horizontal adduction.

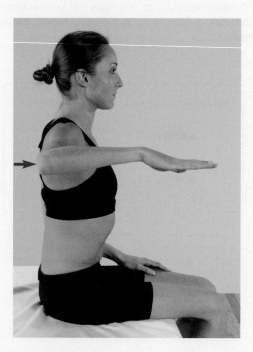

✎ ACTIVITY 10-8—cont'd

Scapular Elevation

Assesses for strength and endurance in the isolation position and tension or shortening in the scapular depression pattern

Muscles Involved
Trapezius (upper fibers)
Levator scapulae
Rhomboideus major and rhomboideus minor

Range of Motion
Reliable values are not available.

Position of Client
Seated, with legs over side of table and arms relaxed

Isolation and Assessment
Client lifts shoulders toward ears, as in shrugging, while examiner applies resistance to push the shoulders down.

Scapular Upward Rotation with Abduction

Assesses for strength and endurance in the isolation position and tension or shortening in the scapular downward rotation pattern

Muscles Involved
Upper and lower trapezius
Anterior serratus
Pectoralis minor

Range of Motion
Reliable values are not available.

Position of Client
Seated, with legs over side of table, arms resting at sides

Isolation and Assessment
Client flexes shoulder forward to 120 degrees with no rotation or horizontal movement while examiner applies resistance to arm just above elbow to push it down.

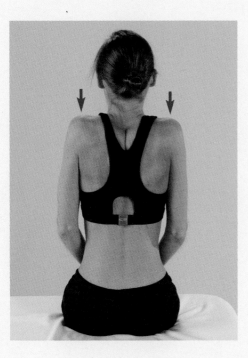

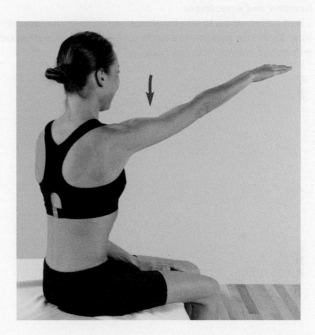

Continued

✎ ACTIVITY **10-8**—cont'd

Scapular Depression with Adduction and Downward Rotation

Assesses for strength and endurance in the isolation position and tension or shortening in the scapular elevation and upward rotation pattern

Muscles Involved

Lower trapezius

Lower anterior serratus

Levator scapula

Rhomboideus major and rhomboideus minor

Latissimus dorsi

Range of Motion

Reliable values are not available.

Position of Client

Prone

Head may be turned to either side for comfort.

Internally rotate shoulder, flex elbow, and adduct arm across back.

Hand rests on low back near waist.

Isolation and Assessment

Client further adducts arm by attempting to touch the opposite side. Examiner applies resistance to the medial side of upper arm to pull it away from the body.

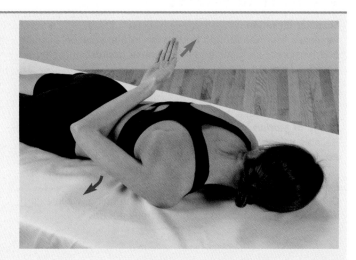

✎ ACTIVITY **10-8**—cont'd

Shoulder Flexion

Assesses for strength and endurance in the isolation position and tension or shortening in the shoulder extension and adduction pattern

Muscles Involved

Deltoid (anterior and middle)

Supraspinatus

Pectoralis major (upper)

Coracobrachialis

Biceps brachii

Subscapularis

Range of Motion

0 to 180 degrees

Position of Client

Seated with knees bent off table, arms at sides, elbows slightly flexed, and forearm pronated

Isolation and Assessment

Client flexes shoulder to 90 degrees without rotation or horizontal movement while examiner applies resistance to upper arm above elbow to push arm down.

Shoulder Extension

Assesses for strength and endurance in the isolation position and tension or shortening in the shoulder flexion pattern

Muscles Involved

Latissimus dorsi

Deltoid (posterior)

Teres major

Triceps brachii (long head)

Range of Motion

0 to 45 degrees

Position of Client

Prone, with arms at sides and shoulder internally rotated (palm up)

Elbow remains extended throughout isolation.

Isolation and Assessment

Client lifts arm off table and holds while examiner applies resistance to posterior arm above elbow to push it down.

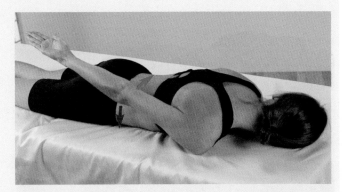

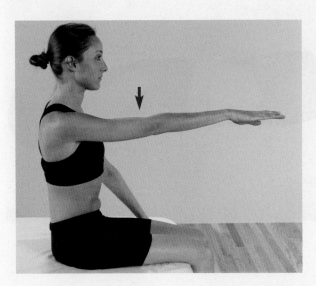

Continued

✎ ACTIVITY 10-8—cont'd

Shoulder Horizontal Abduction

Assesses for strength and endurance in the isolation position and tension or shortening in the shoulder horizontal adduction pattern

Muscles Involved

Deltoid (posterior fibers)

Infraspinatus

Teres minor

Range of Motion

0 to 90 degrees (beginning at 90 degrees flexion)

Position of Client

Prone with shoulder abducted to 90 degrees, elbow flexed, upper arm supported on table, and forearm off edge of table

Isolation and Assessment

Client horizontally (posteriorly) abducts shoulder (lifts elbow toward ceiling) while examiner applies resistance to the posterior arm above elbow to push arm down.

Shoulder Horizontal Adduction

Assesses for strength and endurance in the isolation position and tension or shortening in the shoulder horizontal abduction pattern

Muscles Involved

Pectoralis major

Deltoid (anterior fibers)

Range of Motion

0 to 40 degrees when starting from a position of 90 degrees of forward flexion

Position of Client

Supine

Shoulder abducted to 90 degrees, upper arm supported on table, and elbow flexed to 90 degrees

Isolation and Assessment

Client horizontally adducts arm to move it across the chest while examiner applies resistance to medial side of upper arm above elbow to push it down.

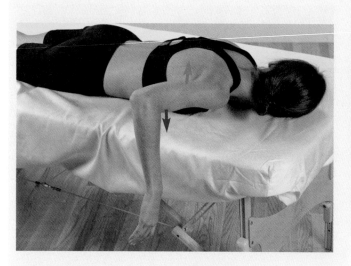

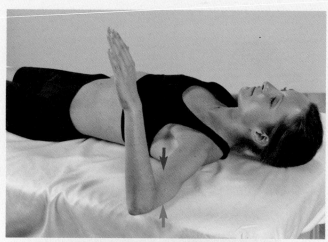

✎ ACTIVITY **10-8**—cont'd

Shoulder External or Lateral Rotation

Assesses for strength and endurance in the isolation position and tension or shortening in the shoulder internal or medial rotation pattern

Muscles Involved

Infraspinatus

Teres minor

Deltoid (posterior)

Range of Motion

0 to 90 degrees

Position of Client

Prone, with head turned toward test side

Shoulder is abducted to 90 degrees with upper arm fully supported on table, elbow flexed, and forearm hanging over edge of table.

Isolation and Assessment

Client moves forearm upward toward the level of the table, keeping upper arm on table, while examiner applies resistance to distal forearm above wrist to push it down.

Shoulder Internal or Medial Rotation

Assesses for strength and endurance in the isolation position and tension or shortening in the shoulder external or lateral rotation pattern

Muscles Involved

Subscapularis

Pectoralis major

Latissimus dorsi

Teres major

Deltoid (anterior)

Range of Motion

0 to 80 degrees

Position of Client

Prone with shoulder abducted to 90 degrees, upper arm supported on table, elbow flexed, and forearm hanging over edge of table

Examiner stabilizes upper arm.

Isolation and Assessment

Client moves forearm through internal rotation (backward and upward) while examiner applies resistance to forearm above wrist to push it down.

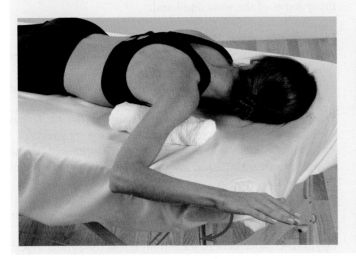

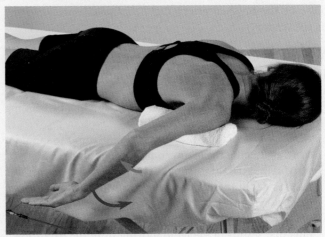

Elbow Region

The elbow is considered a stable joint with firm osseous support and is composed of three articulations: the humeroulnar joint, humeroradial joint, and radioulnar joint. The elbow is a uniaxial hinge joint that moves in only one plane along a single axis. The action of the elbow is flexion/extension. The elbow is capable of moving from 0 degree of extension to approximately 145 to 150 degrees of flexion.

After the elbow flexes beyond 20 degrees, its bony stability is somewhat unlocked, allowing for more side-to-side laxity. In flexion the stability of the elbow depends on the lateral or radial collateral ligament, with most of the work by the medial or ulnar collateral ligament.

The radioulnar joint is classified as a trochoid or pivot-type joint. The radial head rotates around its location at the proximal ulna. This rotary movement is accompanied by the distal radius rotating around the distal ulna. The radial head is maintained in its joint by the annular ligament. The radioulnar joint can supinate approximately 80 to 90 degrees from the neutral position. Pronation varies from 70 to 90 degrees.

Practically any movement of the upper extremity involves the elbow and radioulnar joints. Often these joints are grouped together because of their close anatomic relationship. Radioulnar joint motion may be attributed incorrectly to the wrist joint because it appears to occur there. However, with close inspection the elbow joint and its movements may be distinguished clearly from those of the radioulnar joints, just as the radioulnar movements may be distinguished from those of the wrist.

When the arm is in an anatomic extended position, the longitudinal axes of the upper arm and forearm form a

ACTIVITY 10-9

Slowly and deliberately move your humeroulnar joint, humero-radial joint, and radioulnar joint through each of the movement patterns described. Describe your own experience.

Example

I noticed that it took less effort to pronate than to supinate.

valgus angle at the elbow joint known as the *carrying angle;* this angle approximates 5 degrees in men and between 10 and 15 degrees in women. Anatomically, the carrying angle is designed to fit closely into the waist depressions immediately superior to the iliac crest. The carrying angles should be bilaterally symmetric.

The olecranon fossa of the humerus, which receives the olecranon of the ulna during extension, is filled with fat and covered by a portion of the triceps muscle and aponeurosis.

The cubital fossa is defined by the brachioradialis laterally and the pronator teres medially, with the biceps tendon, brachial artery, and median and musculocutaneous nerves passing through this area. The biceps tendon is a taut, long structure that is medial to the brachioradialis muscle, and the pulse of the brachial artery can be palpated medial to the biceps tendon.

Movements of the Elbow

The elbow allows the following movements (Activities 10-9 and 10-10):

Flexion: Movement of the forearm to the shoulder by bending the elbow to decrease its angle

Extension: Movement of the forearm away from the shoulder by straightening the elbow to increase its angle

Pronation: Internal rotary movement of the radius on the ulna that results in the hand moving from the palm-up to the palm-down position

Supination: External rotary movement of the radius on the ulna that results in the hand moving from the palm-down to the palm-up position

Elbow Muscles

The elbow flexors are the biceps brachii, brachialis, and brachioradialis. The triceps brachii is the primary elbow extensor, assisted by the anconeus. The pronator group consists of the pronator teres, pronator quadratus, and brachioradialis. The brachioradialis also assists with supination, which is controlled mainly by the supinator muscle and the biceps brachii.

Wrist and Hand Region

The joints of the wrist, hand, and fingers often are taken for granted, even though the fine motor characteristics of this area are essential in skilled activities requiring precise functioning of the wrist and hand. Anatomically and structurally, the human wrist and hand have highly developed, complex mechanisms capable of a variety of movements. The amazing diversity of motion results from the arrangement of the 29 bones, more than 25 joints, and more than 30 muscles (of which 15

are intrinsic muscles with proximal attachment and distal attachment found inside the hand). This complexity may be simplified by relating the functional anatomy to the major actions of the joints: flexion, extension, abduction, and adduction of the wrist and hand.

Wrist motion occurs primarily between the distal radius and the proximal carpal row, consisting of the scaphoid, lunate, and triquetrum. The joint allows 70 to 90 degrees of flexion and 65 to 85 degrees of extension. The wrist can abduct 15 to 25 degrees and adduct 25 to 40 degrees.

Each finger has three joints. In these joints 0 to 40 degrees of extension and 85 to 100 degrees of flexion are possible. The proximal interphalangeal joint, classified as a hinge joint, can move from full extension to 90 to 120 degrees of flexion. The distal interphalangeal joints, also classified as hinge joints, can flex 80 to 90 degrees from full extension.

The thumb has only two joints. The metacarpophalangeal joint moves from full extension into 40 to 90 degrees of flexion. The interphalangeal joint can flex 80 to 90 degrees. The carpometacarpal joint of the thumb is a unique saddle-type joint having 50 to 70 degrees of abduction and can flex approximately 15 to 45 degrees and extend 0 to 20 degrees. Numerous ligaments support and provide static stability to many joints of the wrist and hand.

Movements of the Wrist and Hand

The following are movements of the wrist and hand (see Activity 10-10):

Flexion: Moving the palm of the hand or the phalanges toward the anterior or volar aspect of the forearm

Extension: Moving the back of the hand or the phalanges toward the posterior or dorsal aspect of the forearm

Abduction (radial flexion or deviation): Movement of the thumb side of the hand toward the lateral aspect or radial side of the forearm

Adduction (ulnar flexion or deviation): Movement of the little-finger side of the hand toward the medial aspect or ulnar side of the forearm

Opposition: Movement of the thumb across the palmar aspect to oppose any or all of the phalanges

Muscles of the Wrist and Hand

The extrinsic muscles of the wrist and hand may be grouped according to function and location. The wrist flexor-pronator muscle group includes the pronator teres, flexor carpi radialis, flexor carpi ulnaris, and palmaris longus.

All the wrist flexors generally have their proximal attachments on the anteromedial aspect of the proximal forearm and medial epicondyle of the humerus, whereas their distal attachments are on the anterior aspect of the wrist and hand.

The wrist extensors include the extensor carpi radialis longus, extensor carpi radialis brevis, and extensor carpi ulnaris muscles. The wrist extensors generally have their proximal attachments on the posterolateral aspect of the proximal forearm and lateral humeral epicondyle, and their distal attachments are located on the posterior aspect of the hand and wrist.

Text continued on page 525.

✎ ACTIVITY **10-10**

In this activity you will be working with a partner to assess individual movement patterns, normal function, and possible dysfunction in each other. One of you is first to isolate the specified movement patterns on each side of your partner, one side at a time, and assess for normal function by applying gentle pressure opposite to the action of the isolation position. The body should be stabilized so that only the isolated area is moving. In some instances the ability to assume the position and maintain it indicates normal function. Muscles should be able to hold against gravity or the applied pressure without strain or pain. The position itself should be easy to assume and comfortable to maintain for a short duration, from 10 to 30 seconds. The bilateral movement patterns should be the same. The opposite movement pattern also should be able to be done easily.

Dysfunction may be indicated by bilateral asymmetry, pain, weakness, fatigue, a heavy sensation, binding, and inability to assume the isolation position or move into the opposite position. Intervention or referral depends on the severity of the condition and whether the dysfunction is neuromuscular, myofascial, or joint related.

Note: Do not perform these assessments if contraindications exist. Contraindications to this type of assessment include joint and disk dysfunction, acute pain, recent trauma, and inflammation.

Elbow Flexion

Assesses for strength and endurance in the isolation position and tension or shortening in the elbow extension pattern

Muscles Involved

Biceps brachii (short head)
Brachialis
Brachioradialis
Pronator teres

Range of Motion

0 to 150 degrees

Position of Client

Seated, with arms at sides
Three separate muscles can be isolated depending on position of forearm:
    Biceps brachii: forearm in supination
    Brachialis: forearm in pronation
    Brachioradialis: forearm in midposition between pronation and supination
Client's forearm is flexed to 90 degrees, and examiner stabilizes it at the elbow.

Isolation and Assessment (All Three Forearm Positions)

Client flexes elbow through range of motion while examiner applies resistance to distal forearm.

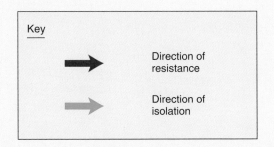

Key

→   Direction of resistance

→   Direction of isolation

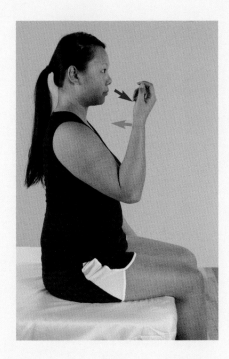

Continued

✎ ACTIVITY **10-10**—cont'd

Elbow Extension

Assesses for strength and endurance in the isolation position and tension or shortening in the elbow flexion pattern

Muscles Involved

Triceps brachii

Anconeus

Range of Motion

No range of motion

Position of Client

Standing or seated with arm to be tested able to extend without touching table

Forearm is flexed, and examiner stabilizes it at the elbow.

Isolation and Assessment

Client extends elbow to end of available range without extending shoulder. Examiner applies resistance at wrist to prevent the action.

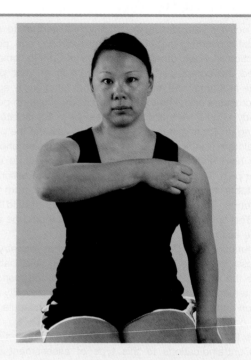

✎ ACTIVITY **10-10**—cont'd

Forearm Supination

Assesses for strength and endurance in the isolation position and tension or shortening in the pronation pattern

Muscles Involved

Supinator

Biceps brachii

Range of Motion

0 to 90 degrees

Position of Client

Seated, arm at side and elbow flexed to 90 degrees, and forearm in neutral or midposition

Examiner stabilizes at elbow with one hand and grasps forearm above wrist with other hand.

Isolation and Assessment

Client supinates the forearm until the palm faces the ceiling while examiner resists the motion.

Forearm Pronation

Assesses for strength and endurance in the isolation position and tension or shortening in the supination pattern

Muscles Involved

Pronator teres

Pronator quadratus

Flexor carpi radialis

Range of Motion

0 to 80 degrees

Position of Client

Seated, with arm at side and elbow flexed to 90 degrees, and forearm in neutral position

Examiner stabilizes at elbow with one hand and grasps forearm at wrist with other hand.

Isolation and Assessment

Client pronates the forearm until the palm faces downward while examiner resists the motion.

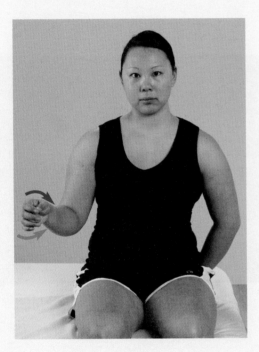

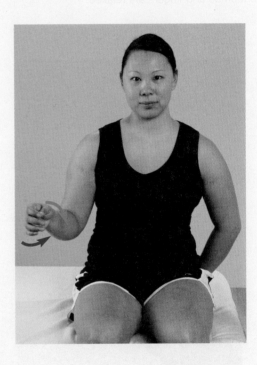

Continued

✎ ACTIVITY 10-10—cont'd

Wrist Flexion

Assesses for strength and endurance in the isolation position and tension or shortening in the extension pattern

Muscles Involved

Flexor carpi radialis
Flexor carpi ulnaris
Palmaris longus
Abductor pollicis longus
Flexor digitorum superficialis
Flexor pollicis longus
Flexor digitorum profundus

Range of Motion

0 to 80 degrees

Position of Client

Seated with elbow flexed if needed and the forearm supinated while supported on its dorsal surface on a table
Wrist position is neutral.

Isolation and Assessment

Client flexes the wrist while examiner resists action. Make sure client's thumbs and fingers are relaxed.

Wrist Extension

Assesses for strength and endurance in the isolation position and tension or shortening in the flexion pattern

Muscles Involved

Extensor carpi radialis longus
Extensor carpi radialis brevis
Extensor carpi ulnaris
Extensor digitorum
Extensor digiti minimi
Extensor indicis
Extensor pollicis longus

Range of Motion

0 to 85 degrees

Position of Client

Seated, with elbow flexed as needed, and forearm pronated while arm is supported on table

Isolation and Assessment

Client hyperextends wrist while examiner resists action. Client's thumb and fingers stay relaxed.

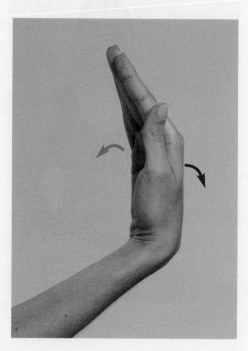

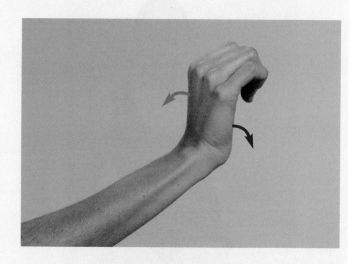

✎ ACTIVITY **10-10**—cont'd

Finger Flexion

Assesses for strength and endurance in the isolation position and tension or shortening in the finger extension pattern

Muscles Involved

Lumbricales

Dorsal interossei

Palmar interossei

Flexor digitorum superficialis

Flexor digitorum profundus

Range of Motion

0 to 100 degrees

Position of Client

Seated, with elbow flexed and forearm supinated and supported on a table

Wrist is maintained in neutral position.

Begin with metacarpophalangeal joints fully extended and interphalangeal joints flexed.

Each finger is to be isolated separately.

Isolation and Assessment

Client flexes the metacarpophalangeal joint (bends knuckles) and extends the interphalangeal (finger) joints while examiner resists metacarpophalangeal flexion. Make sure client does not flex interphalangeal joint.

Finger Extension

Assesses for strength and endurance in the isolation position and tension or shortening in the finger flexion pattern

Muscles Involved

Extensor digitorum

Extensor indicis

Extensor digiti minimi

Range of Motion

0 to 15 degrees

Position of Client

Seated, with forearm in pronation and supported on a table and wrist in neutral

Isolation and Assessment

No resistance is required. Ability to perform isolation indicates normal function.

Extensor digitorum: Client extends metacarpophalangeal joints (all fingers simultaneously), allowing the interphalangeal joints to be in slight flexion.

Extensor indicis: Client extends the metacarpophalangeal joint of the index finger.

Extensor digiti minimi: Client extends the joint of the fifth digit.

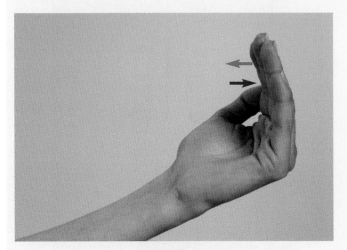

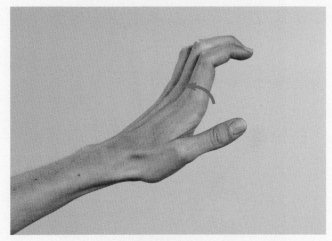

Continued

✎ ACTIVITY **10-10**—cont'd

Finger Abduction

Assesses for strength and endurance in the isolation position and tension or shortening in the finger adduction pattern

Muscles Involved

Dorsal interossei

Abductor digiti minimi

Range of Motion

0 to 20 degrees

Position of Client

Seated, with forearm pronated and supported and wrist in neutral position

Fingers are abducted (separated), and metacarpophalangeal joints remain neutral.

Isolation and Assessment

Each finger is isolated separately against resistance given near distal end of finger to push it together with other fingers.

Dorsal interossei:

Abduction of ring finger toward little finger (includes abductor digiti minimi)

Abduction of middle finger toward ring finger

Abduction of middle finger toward index finger

Abduction of index finger toward thumb

Finger Adduction

Assesses for strength and endurance in the isolation position and tension or shortening in the finger abduction pattern

Muscles Involved

Palmar interossei

Range of Motion

0 to 20 degrees

Position of Client

Seated, with elbow flexed, forearm pronated and supported, wrist in neutral, and fingers extended and adducted (together)

Metacarpophalangeal joints are neutral.

Isolation and Assessment

Fingers are tested separately; middle finger is not tested because it has no palmar interossei muscle. Examiner applies resistance near distal end of finger to pull it away from other fingers. Adduction of little finger is toward ring finger. Adduction of ring finger is toward middle finger. Adduction of index finger is toward middle finger. Adduction of thumb is toward index finger.

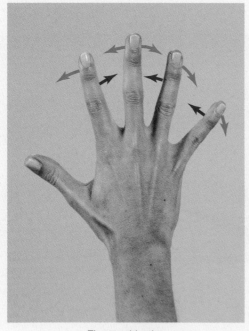

Finger adduction

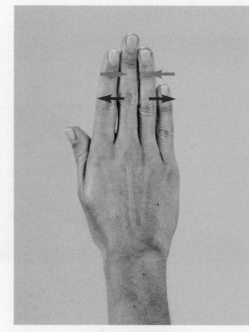

Finger adduction

✏ ACTIVITY **10-10**—cont'd

Thumb Adduction, Flexion, and Medial Rotation
Assesses for strength and endurance in the isolation position and tension or shortening in the thumb extension pattern
> Thumb extensors are extrinsic muscles.
> The thumb has 0 to 20 degrees of extension.

Muscles Involved
Flexor pollicis brevis
Flexor pollicis longus
Adductor pollicis

Range of Motion
Metacarpophalangeal flexion: 0 to 50 degrees
Interphalangeal flexion: 0 to 80 degrees
Adduction: 0 to 70 degrees

Position of Client
Seated, with forearm supinated and supported and wrist in neutral position
Carpometacarpal joint and interphalangeal joints are neutral.
Thumb is in adduction.

Isolation and Assessment
Client flexes the metacarpophalangeal joint of the thumb to slide thumb across palm while examiner applies resistance to pull thumb back between carpometacarpal and interphalangeal joints. Interphalangeal joint does not flex.

Thumb Opposition
Assesses for strength and endurance in the isolation position and tension or shortening in the thumb opposition pattern

Muscles Involved
Opponens pollicis
Opponens digiti minimi

Range of Motion
0 to 70 degrees

Position of Client
Seated, with forearm supinated and supported, wrist in neutral position, and thumb in palmar abduction
Opponens pollicis: Apply resistance for the opponens pollicis at the head of the first metacarpal in the direction of lateral rotation, extension, and adduction.

Isolation and Assessment
Client medially rotates and flexes thumb toward little finger while little finger flexes and rotates toward thumb such that pads of digits touch (not tips of digits).
> The examiner applies resistance on palmar surface of thumb and fifth metacarpal to bring them apart.

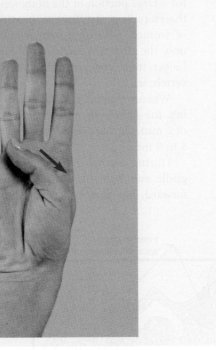

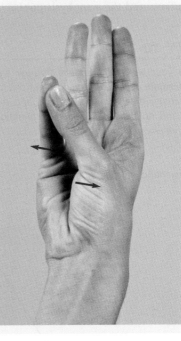

The wrist abductors include the flexor carpi radialis, extensor carpi radialis longus, extensor carpi radialis brevis, abductor pollicis longus, extensor pollicis longus, and extensor pollicis brevis. These muscles generally cross the wrist joint anterolaterally and posterolaterally to insert on the radial side of the hand. The flexor carpi ulnaris and extensor carpi ulnaris adduct the wrist and cross the wrist joint anteromedially and posteromedially to insert on the ulnar side of the hand.

Nine other muscles function primarily to move the phalanges but also are involved in wrist joint actions because they originate on the forearm and cross the wrist. These muscles are generally weaker in their actions on the wrist. The flexor digitorum superficialis and flexor digitorum profundus are finger flexors, and they also assist in wrist flexion along with the flexor pollicis longus, which is a thumb flexor. The extensor digitorum, extensor indicis, and extensor digiti minimi are finger extensors and also assist in wrist extension, along with the extensor pollicis longus and extensor pollicis brevis, which extend the thumb. The abductor pollicis longus abducts the thumb and assists in wrist abduction.

Intrinsic hand muscles have their proximal attachment and distal attachment within the hand. They are primarily responsible for fine and precise movements of the fingers and thumb. Those acting on the thumb, located in the thenar eminence, include the opponens pollicis, abductor pollicis brevis, and flexor pollicis brevis. Those acting on the little finger are the opponens digiti minimi, abductor digiti minimi, and flexor digiti minimi brevis. These muscles are located in the hypothenar eminence. Acting with the thenar muscles, they function in opposition, allowing effective grasping movements.

The lumbricales flex the metacarpophalangeal joint and extend the interphalangeal joints. The dorsal and palmar interossei muscles are involved with adduction and abduction of the fingers. The adductor pollicis and abductor pollicis muscles adduct and abduct the thumb. With these actions the hand is able to hold and manipulate small objects such as a pencil (Activity 10-11).

Pelvic Girdle and Hip Joint Region

The pelvis consists of three bones and three joints. The bones are the two fused coxal bones (made up of the ilium, ischium, and pubis) and the sacrum. The three joints are the two sacroiliac articulations and the symphysis pubis.

ACTIVITY 10-11

Slowly move your wrist and fingers through the movement patterns described. Isolate wrist action from finger action. Combine as many different wrist, finger, and thumb actions as possible, and notice the endless combinations. Describe your own experience.

Example
I can make my hand dance.

Motion in the Pelvic Girdle

The pelvic girdle functions as one unit, with all three bones moving at all three joints. The lower extremities, the vertebral column, and the trunk influence the pelvic girdle. The unit moves around a vertical axis. In a movement to the left, the symphysis turns left of the midline, the right coxal turns forward, the left coxal turns backward, and the sacrum turns a little to the left. The reverse happens when rotating to the right.

The pelvic girdle moves back and forth within three planes for a total of six different movements. Analyzing the pelvic girdle activity to determine the exact location of the movement is important to prevent confusion.

All pelvic girdle rotation results from motion at the right hip, left hip, or lumbar spine. Although it is not essential for movement to occur in all three of these areas, it must occur in at least one area for the pelvis to rotate in any direction. Even though the sacroiliac joints are synovial joints, they permit little movement and even fuse in many persons later in life. This general reduction of motion is related to degenerative changes such as osteoarthritis (Figure 10-19).

Four groups of ligaments form the main bond that keeps the ilium and sacrum in approximation. Stability of the sacroiliac joints is crucial because they maintain support for a large portion of the body weight. More movement (and therefore less stability) is present in the sacroiliac joints of women, who have smaller and flatter surfaces involving only the first two sacral vertebrae, than in men, who have longer, more concave surfaces involving the first three sacral vertebrae.

When weight shifts from one leg to the other while standing, the symphysis may show an upward/downward motion of 2 mm. During pregnancy the symphysis may separate from 5 to 9 mm.

During normal walking, motions involve the entire pelvic girdle and both hip joints. When the pelvic girdle rotates forward, hip flexion occurs; when it rotates backward, hip

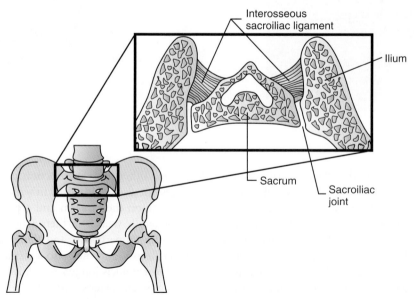

FIGURE 10-19 Cross section of the sacroiliac joints.

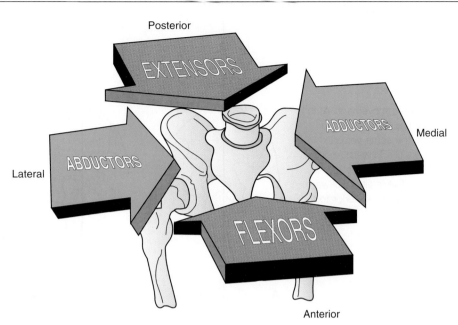

FIGURE 10-20 Position and function of hip to support multiaxial joint function.

extension occurs. The symphysis pubis serves as the axis for the rotation. Jogging and running result in faster and greater range of these movements.

Muscular attachments to the pelvic girdle are extensive, but no muscles directly influence the sacroiliac joint. Indirect actions come from the abdominal muscles, which insert on the superior aspect of the pelvic girdle and are joined by the quadratus lumborum.

Six groups of hip and thigh muscles are attached to the pelvic girdle and lower extremities. These hip muscles highly influence the movement of the two coxal bones within the pelvic girdle. Anterior to the sacroiliac joint are two important muscles, the psoas and piriformis.

The psoas crosses over the anterior aspect of the sacroiliac joint and goes from the lumbar region to insert into the lesser trochanter of the femur. The right and left piriformis muscles originate from the anterior surface of the sacrum, pass through the sciatic notch, and insert into the greater trochanter of the femur. Muscle imbalance of any of these groups can affect pelvic function adversely.

The pelvic girdle is thought to be of importance within the craniosacral system. Theory indicates that the sacrum has a mobility between the two coxals as part of the craniosacral rhythm. Any changes or alteration in biomechanical function of the pelvic girdle can influence the craniosacral mechanism negatively; the reverse is also true.

Because the pelvis is the supporting base of the spine, dysfunctions in its joints have a great effect on the lumbar spine. Sacroiliac pain is usually a dull ache in the bones above the buttock on one side. Because the nerves in that region are not specific, pain caused by the sacroiliac joint can be felt in the groin, back of the thigh, and lower abdomen.

One of the most common dysfunctions occurs when leaning forward to lift some heavy object instead of going into the bent-knee position. If the abdominal muscles are strong and support the anterior pelvis, stabilizing the trunk to maintain a more or less constant balance between the trunk and the pelvis, no dysfunction happens. But if the abdominal muscles and the sacrotuberous ligaments are weak, dysfunction and pain could occur.

Hip Joint

Except for the glenohumeral joint, the hip joint is one of the most mobile joints of the body, largely because of its multiaxial arrangement. Unlike the glenohumeral, the bony architecture of the hip joint provides a great deal of stability, resulting in few hip joint dislocations. An extremely strong and dense ligamentous capsule reinforces the joint, especially the anterior portion (Figure 10-20).

Because of individual differences, some disagreement exists regarding the exact range of each movement in the hip joint, but the ranges are generally 0 to 130 degrees of flexion, 0 to 30 degrees of extension, 0 to 35 degrees of abduction, 0 to 30 degrees of adduction, 0 to 45 degrees of internal rotation, and 0 to 50 degrees of external rotation.

Movements of the Pelvis and Hip Joints

Anterior and posterior pelvic rotations occur in the sagittal plane, whereas right and left lateral rotation occurs in the frontal plane. Right transverse (clockwise) rotation and left transverse (counterclockwise) rotation occur in the horizontal or transverse plane of motion. The movements are as follows:

Anterior pelvic rotation: Anterior movement of the upper pelvis; the iliac crest tilts forward in a sagittal plane.

Posterior pelvic rotation: Posterior movement of the upper pelvis; the iliac crest tilts backward in a sagittal plane (Figure 10-21).

Left lateral pelvic rotation (tilt): In the frontal plane the left pelvis moves superiorly in relation to the right pelvis; the left pelvis rotates upward or the right pelvis rotates downward.

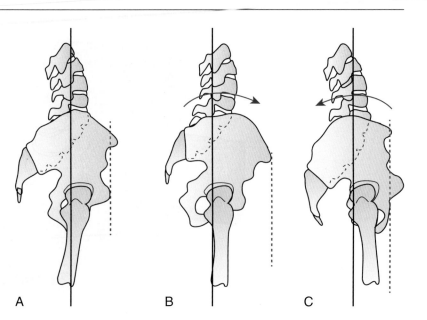

FIGURE 10-21 Sagittal plane pelvic movement. **A,** In the neutral position the anterior superior iliac spine and the pubic symphysis are in the same vertical plane. **B,** Anterior rotation. Pelvis tilts forward, moving the anterior superior iliac spine anterior to the pubic symphysis. **C,** Posterior rotation. Pelvis tilts backward, moving the anterior superior iliac spine posterior to the pubic symphysis.

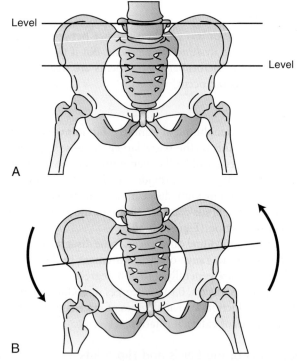

FIGURE 10-22 Frontal plane pelvic movement tilt. When standing upright, the iliac crests should be level in the frontal plane, and the anterior superior iliac spines on the left and right should be level.

Right lateral pelvic rotation (tilt): In the frontal plane the right pelvis moves superiorly in relation to the left pelvis; the right pelvis rotates upward, or the left pelvis rotates downward (Figure 10-22).

Left transverse pelvic rotation: In a transverse (horizontal) plane of motion, the pelvis rotates to the left of the body; the right iliac crest moves anteriorly in relation to the left iliac crest, which moves posteriorly.

Right transverse pelvic rotation: In a transverse (horizontal) plane of motion, the pelvis rotates to the right of the body;

Table 10-2	Pelvic Girdle, Lumbar Spine, and Hip Joint Movements		
Pelvic Rotations	**Lumbar Spine Motion**	**Right Hip Motion**	**Left Hip Motion**
Anterior rotation	Extension	Flexion	Flexion
Posterior rotation	Flexion	Extension	Extension
Right lateral rotation	Right lateral flexion	Adduction	Abduction
Left lateral rotation	Left lateral flexion	Abduction	Adduction
Right transverse rotation	Left lateral rotation	Internal rotation	External rotation
Left transverse rotation	Right lateral rotation	External rotation	Internal rotation

the left iliac crest moves anteriorly in relation to the right iliac crest, which moves posteriorly (Figures 10-23).

Hip flexion: Movement of the femur straight anteriorly toward the pelvis

Hip extension: Movement of the femur straight posteriorly away from the pelvis

Hip abduction: Movement of the femur laterally to the side away from the midline

Hip adduction: Movement of the femur medially toward the midline

Hip external rotation: Rotary movement of the femur laterally around its longitudinal axis away from the midline

Hip internal rotation: Rotary movement of the femur medially around its longitudinal axis toward the midline

The lumbar spine, hip joint, and pelvic girdle work together in carrying out lower extremity activities.

Table 10-2 shows a comparison of pelvic girdle, lumbar spine, and hip joint movements (Activity 10-12).

Muscles of the Hip Joint

At the hip joint are six two-joint muscles that have one action at the hip and another at the knee. The muscles usually

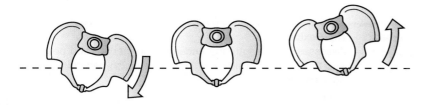

A   Left forward rotation   B   Normal   C   Left backward rotation

FIGURE 10-23 A superior view of transverse rotation of the pelvis in the transverse plane. **A,** Forward rotation. **B,** Neutral position of the pelvis. **C,** Backward rotation of the pelvis.

✎ ACTIVITY **10-12**

Slowly and deliberately move your joints through each of the movement patterns described. Identify the interplay between the hip movements and the pelvic girdle movements, paying close attention to the secondary movement of the pelvic girdle during hip movement. Describe your own experience.

Example
I could feel the rotation at the symphysis pubis when I walked if I placed my fingers on the joint.

---

involved in hip and pelvic girdle motions depend largely on the direction of the movement and the position of the body in relation to the earth and its gravitational forces. In addition, note that the body part that moves the most is the part least stabilized. For example, when a person is standing on both feet and contracting the hip flexors, the trunk and pelvis flex anteriorly; however, when the person is lying supine and contracting the hip flexors, the thighs move forward into flexion on the stable pelvis. In another example, the hip flexor muscles are used in moving the legs toward the trunk, but the extensor muscles are used eccentrically when the pelvis and trunk move downward slowly on the femur and concentrically when the trunk is raised on the femur, such as when rising to the standing position.

In the downward phase of the knee-bend exercise, the movement at the hips and knees is flexion. The muscles involved primarily are the hip and knee extensors in eccentric contraction to control the trunk.

The iliopsoas muscle provides stabilization and powerful actions such as raising the legs from a supine position on the floor. The proximal attachment in the lower back tends to move the lower back anteriorly or, in the supine position, pulls the lower back up as it raises the legs. For this reason lower back problems are common with this activity because leg raising is primarily hip flexion, not abdominal action. Strong abdominal muscles prevent lower back strain by pulling up on the front of the pelvis and thus flattening the back.

The sartorius, a two-joint muscle, is effective as a hip or knee flexor and is weak when both actions occur at the same time. When the knees are extended, the sartorius becomes a more effective hip flexor.

The rectus femoris muscle pulls from the anterior inferior iliac spine of the ilium to rotate the pelvis anteriorly. Only the abdominal muscles, particularly the rectus abdominis, can prevent this from occurring. In older adults the pelvis may be tilted forward permanently. The relaxed abdominal wall does not hold the pelvis up, and therefore an increased lumbar curve results. The rectus femoris muscle is a powerful extensor of the knee when the hip is extended but is weak when the hip is flexed.

The pectineus muscles tend to rotate the pelvis anteriorly. The abdominal muscles pulling up on the pelvis in front counteract this tilting.

The tensor fasciae latae muscle is used when flexion and internal rotation take place. This muscle also aids in preventing external rotation of the femur as it is flexed by other flexor muscles.

Typical action of the gluteus medius and gluteus minimus muscles occurs in walking. As the weight of the body shifts to one leg, these muscles prevent the opposite hip from sagging. Weakness in the gluteus medius and gluteus minimus can result in what is known as the *Trendelenburg gait*. With this weakness, the individual's opposite hip sags on weight bearing because the hip abductors cannot maintain proper alignment. As the body ages, the gluteus medius and gluteus minimus muscles tend to lose their effectiveness. Walking loses its easy spring and becomes more labored.

The gluteus maximus muscle comes into action when movement between the pelvis and the femur approaches and goes beyond 15 degrees of extension. As a result, the gluteus maximus is not used extensively in ordinary walking but is important in extension of the thigh with external rotation and stabilization between the lumbar dorsal fascia and iliotibial band.

The six deep lateral rotator muscles—piriformis, gemellus superior, gemellus inferior, obturator externus, obturator internus, quadratus femoris—provide powerful movements of external rotation of the femur. Standing on one leg and forcefully turning the body away from that leg is accomplished by contraction of these muscles.

The hamstrings (semitendinosus, semimembranosus, and biceps femoris), together with the gluteus maximus muscle, act in extension of the thigh when the knees are straight. These muscles are used in ordinary walking as extensors of the hip and allow the gluteus maximus to stabilize the movement. When the trunk is bent forward with the knees straight, the hamstring muscles have a powerful pull on the rear pelvis and tilt it down in back. If the knees are flexed when this movement takes place, the gluteus maximus chiefly does the work.

The adductor brevis, adductor longus, adductor magnus, and gracilis provide powerful movement of the thighs toward each other and are important postural muscles (Activity 10-13).

✏️ ACTIVITY 10-13

In this activity, you will be working with a partner to assess individual movement patterns, normal function, and possible dysfunction in each other. One of you is first to isolate the specified movement patterns on each side of your partner, one side at a time, and assess for normal function by applying gentle pressure opposite to the action of the isolation position. The body should be stabilized so that only the isolated area is moving. In some instances the ability to assume the position and maintain it indicates normal function. Muscles should be able to hold against gravity or the applied pressure without strain or pain. The position itself should be easy to assume and comfortable to maintain for a short duration, from 10 to 30 seconds. The bilateral movement patterns should be the same. The opposite movement pattern also should be able to be done easily. Dysfunction may be indicated by bilateral asymmetry, pain, weakness, fatigue, a heavy sensation (binding), and the inability to assume the isolation position or move into the opposite position.

Intervention or referral depends on the severity of the condition and whether the dysfunction is neuromuscular, myofascial, or joint related.

Note: Do not perform these assessments if contraindications exist. Contraindications to this type of assessment include joint and disk dysfunction, acute pain, recent trauma, and inflammation.

Hip Flexion
Assesses for strength and endurance in the isolation position and tension or shortening in the hip extension pattern

Muscles Involved
Psoas major
Iliacus
Rectus femoris
Sartorius
Tensor fasciae latae
Pectineus
Adductor brevis
Adductor longus
Adductor magnus

Range of Motion
0 to 130 degrees

Position of Client
Seated, knees bent with thighs fully supported on table and feet
   hanging over the edge
Client may use arms for stability.

Isolation and Assessment
Client flexes hip through full range while examiner applies resistance on anterior thigh above knee to push leg down.

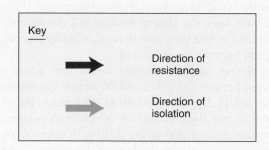

Key

→ Direction of resistance

→ Direction of isolation

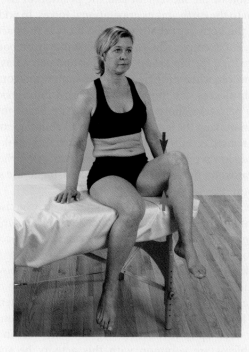

✎ ACTIVITY **10-13**—cont'd

Hip Extension

Assesses for strength and endurance in the isolation position and tension or shortening in the hip flexion pattern

Muscles Involved

Gluteus maximus
Semitendinosus
Semimembranosus
Biceps femoris (long head)

Range of Motion

0 to 30 degrees

Position of Client

Prone, with arms overhead or abducted to hold sides of table
Place pillows under hips to help flex hips for start position.

Isolation and Assessment

Client extends hip through entire available range of motion while knee is extended. The entire leg should clear the table. Examiner applies resistance to posterior thigh above knee to push leg down.

Hip Abduction

Assesses for strength and endurance in the isolation position and tension or shortening in the hip adduction pattern

Muscles Involved

Gluteus medius
Gluteus minimus
Tensor fasciae latae
Gluteus maximus (upper fibers)

Range of Motion

0 to 35 degrees

Position of Client

Side-lying on nontest side, hip and knee flexed for stability
Hip is slightly extended on leg to be tested.

Isolation and Assessment

Client abducts hip through range of motion leading with heel to prevent flexing or rotating the hip. Examiner applies resistance to lateral aspect of thigh above knee to push leg down.

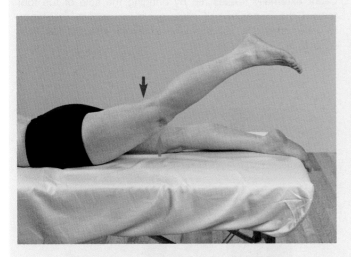

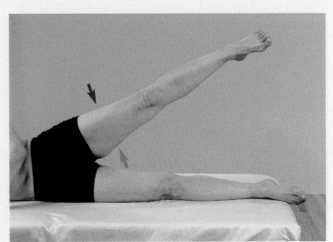

Continued

✏ ACTIVITY **10-13**—cont'd

Hip Adduction

Assesses for strength and endurance in the isolation position and tension or shortening in the hip abduction pattern

Muscles Involved

Adductor magnus
Adductor brevis
Adductor longus
Pectineus
Gracilis

Range of Motion

0 to 15 to 30 degrees

Position of Client

Side-lying on test side with uppermost limb in 25 degrees of abduction, supported by the examiner
The therapist cradles the leg with the forearm; the hand supports the limb on the medial surface of the leg.

Isolation and Assessment

Client adducts hip until the lower limb contacts the upper one. No resistance is required.

Hip External or Lateral Rotation

Assesses for strength and endurance in the isolation position and tension or shortening in the hip internal or medial rotation pattern

Muscles Involved

Obturator externus
Obturator internus
Quadratus femoris
Piriformis
Gemellus superior
Gemellus inferior
Gluteus maximus
Sartorius

Range of Motion

0 to 45 degrees

Position of Client

Seated, with hips flexed but not rotated
Patella in line with anterior superior interior spine
Examiner stabilizes outer thigh above knee.
Trunk is supported by placing hands at sides.

Isolation and Assessment

Client externally rotates hip by bringing the sole of the foot toward the opposite calf while examiner applies resistance to inner ankle. It is important to avoid knee stress with resistance.

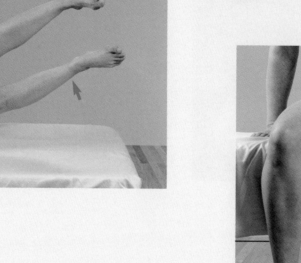

✐ ACTIVITY **10-13**—cont'd

Hip Internal or Medial Rotation

Assesses for strength and endurance in the isolation position and tension or shortening in the lateral or external hip rotation pattern

Muscles Involved

Gluteus minimus

Gluteus medius

Tensor fasciae latae

Range of Motion

0 to 50 degrees

Position of Client

Seated, with hips flexed, patella in line with anterior superior iliac spine

Arms at sides to support the trunk

Examiner stabilizes medial thigh just above knee.

Isolation and Assessment

Client internally rotates hip, turning sole of foot to the side and bringing the knee toward the opposite leg while examiner applies resistance to outer ankle, avoiding knee strain.

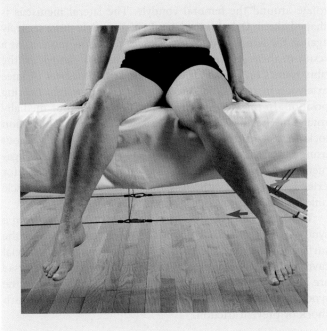

Knee Region

The knee joint is the largest and most complex joint in the body and is primarily a hinge joint. The combined functions of weight bearing and locomotion place considerable stress and strain on the knee joint. The ligaments provide static stability to the knee joint, and contractions of the quadriceps and hamstrings produce dynamic stability.

The knee includes the articulation of the femur and tibia and the patella, which covers it anteriorly. The knee acts as part of a closed kinematic chain with the lumbar spine, hip, and ankle. Weight-bearing forces normally bisect the knee even though it has a slight valgus angulation. A slight hyperextension of both knees when standing is normal (more in females). The extension ends when the capsule and ligaments twist and draw tight, locking the joint in its close-packed position. The range of motion of the knee is 5 to 10 degrees of hyperextension, 135 to 150 degrees of flexion with soft tissue of the calf and thigh limiting flexion, and 10 degrees of internal or external tibial rotation. With the knee flexed 30 degrees or more, approximately 30 degrees of internal rotation and 45 degrees of external rotation can occur. The external rotation of the tibia toward the end of extension and internal rotation during the beginning of flexion are automatic because of the shape of the articulating bones.

The quadriceps pull the patella in line with the femur. The patellar tendon pulls the patella in line with the tibia. The quadriceps (Q) angle is the angle formed by these two pulls. The tension from the quadriceps and patellar tendon plus the anterior projection of the lateral femoral condyle and the deep patellar groove in the femur hold the patella in place during flexion. As the muscle contracts, the patella moves out of the groove and lateral, and the Q angle decreases. The lateral femoral condyle and the contraction of the vastus medialis muscle (oblique pattern) help prevent lateral dislocation of the patella. This is particularly important for a woman because her broader pelvis causes a greater Q angle and a stronger lateral pull (Figure 10-24).

The superior tibiofemoral joint aids the knee in supporting one sixth of the body weight. The joint glides anteriorly during knee flexion and rotates with ankle dorsiflexion. Joint dysfunctions such as hypomobility can lead to lateral knee, leg, or ankle pain.

Other Major Knee Components

Two cartilaginous menisci partially fill the space between the articulating surfaces of the tibia and femur. Both menisci are thicker on the periphery than in the center margin. They move with the tibia during flexion or extension and with the femur in rotation. Menisci improve weight distribution by increasing the contact area between the two long bones. They act as shock absorbers by spreading the stress over the articulating surfaces, decreasing friction and cartilage wear. They are part of the locking mechanism of the knee, which prevents hyperextension by directing the movement of the articulating condyles.

The medial (tibial) collateral ligament is a strong, broad, triangular strap that attaches to the medial epicondyle of the

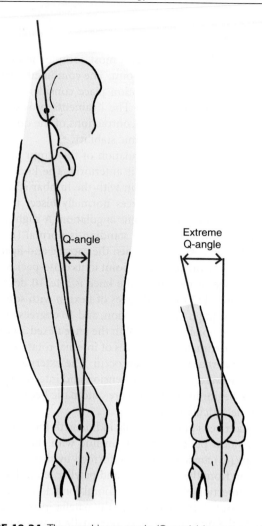

FIGURE 10-24 The quadriceps angle (Q angle) is measured from the anterior superior iliac spine through the axis of the patella and distally to the distal attachment of the patellar tendon on the tibial tuberosity. (Modified from Shankman GA: *Fundamental orthopedic management for the physical therapist assistant,* ed 3, St Louis, 2011, Mosby.)

femur. The ligament helps prevent anterior tibial displacement on the femur. The lateral collateral ligament is shorter and more rounded than the medial collateral ligament and is located between the biceps femoris tendon externally and the popliteus tendon internally. The lateral collateral ligament does not attach to the lateral meniscus. Its fibers are tight, especially during knee extension, tibial adduction, and lateral rotation. The lateral collateral ligament helps protect the lateral aspect of the knee from varus stress. Excessive varus (bow legs) and valgus (knock-knees) are two of the more common deformities of the knee joint (Figure 10-25).

The medial collateral ligament and lateral collateral ligament twist in relationship with each other to protect the knee externally from excessive tibial rotation and extension. The cruciate ligaments are the main rotary stabilizers and cross each other within the knee capsule. These ligaments are vital in maintaining the anterior, posterior, and rotary stability of the knee joint. They aid the rolling and gliding movements of

ACTIVITY 10-14

Slowly and deliberately move your joints through each of the movement patterns described. Describe your own experience.

Example

I could feel the rotation of my knee during the last phase of extension and noticed how solid it felt when the screw-home mechanism kicked in.

---

the tibia on the femur and are rotary guides for the screw-home, or locking, mechanism of the knee.

The screw-home mechanism occurs with rotary movement of the knee (Figure 10-26). This rotary motion results not from muscle action but instead from joint and menisci structure. The articular surface of the medial femoral condyle is longer than that of the lateral condyle. In addition, the C shape of the medial meniscus allows the medial tibial condyle to rotate around the femoral condyle. The lateral meniscus is shaped like an O, holds the lateral tibial condyle more securely against the femoral condyle, and does not allow motion. As a result of these structural features, the medial condyle of the tibia rotates on the femur during the last 15 degrees of knee extension in an external direction in the non–weight-bearing position. In the weight-bearing position, the femur medially rotates on the tibia when the knee is extended fully. This action locks the knee into extension, which allows us to stand without using muscle action but instead being supported on the ligaments at the hip. This saves energy and allows us to stand for extended periods without fatigue. The popliteus muscle unlocks the knee to begin flexion.

The knee joint is well supplied with synovial fluid from a synovial cavity that lies under the patella and between the surfaces of the tibia and the femur. Commonly, this synovial cavity is called the *capsule* of the knee. More than 10 bursae are located in the knee, some of which are connected to the synovial cavity. Bursae are located where they can absorb shock or prevent friction.

Movements of the Knee

Flexion and extension of the knee occurs in the sagittal plane, whereas internal and external rotation occurs in the horizontal plane (Activity 10-14):

Flexion: Bending or decreasing the angle of the knee, characterized by the heel moving toward the buttocks

Extension: Straightening or increasing the angle of the knee

External rotation: Rotary motion of the lower leg laterally away from the midline

Internal rotation: Rotary motion of the lower leg medially toward the midline

Muscles of the Knee

The muscles that flex and medially rotate the knee are the hamstrings, sartorius, gracilis, gastrocnemius, and popliteus. The popliteus muscle is the only flexor of the leg found only at the knee. All other flexors are two-joint muscles. Two-joint muscles are most effective when the proximal attachment or distal attachment is fixed by the contraction of the muscles that prevent movement in the direction of the pull.

The popliteus provides posterolateral stability to the knee and assists the medial hamstrings in internal rotation of the lower leg at the knee. The plantaris and gastrocnemius assist with flexion.

The quadriceps extend the knee. All quadriceps muscles attach to the patella and by the patellar tendon to the tibial tuberosity. All these muscles are superficial and palpable except the vastus intermedius, which is under the rectus femoris. The quadriceps muscles generally are desired to be 25% to 33% stronger than the hamstring muscle group (knee flexors). Proper tracking of the patella is provided by the relationship between the vastus medialis (primarily oblique portion) and vastus lateralis.

The tensor fasciae latae assists with flexion and extension. The semimembranosus and semitendinosus (medial hamstrings) muscles are assisted by the popliteus to rotate the knee internally, whereas the biceps femoris (lateral hamstrings) is responsible for external knee rotation. The pes anserinus is the tendinous expansions of the sartorius, gracilis, and semitendinosus muscles at the medial border of the tibial tuberosity (Activity 10-15).

Ankle and Foot Region

The ankle joint is made up of the talus, distal tibia, and distal fibula. The ankle joint allows approximately 50 degrees of plantar flexion and 15 to 20 degrees of dorsiflexion. Greater range of dorsiflexion is possible when the knee is flexed, which reduces the tension of the biarticular gastrocnemius muscle.

Inversion and eversion, although commonly thought to be ankle joint movements, technically occur in the subtalar and transverse tarsal joints. These joints combine to allow approximately 20 to 30 degrees of inversion and 5 to 25 degrees of eversion. Minimal movement occurs within the remainder of the intertarsal and tarsometatarsal arthrodial joints.

The structural complexity of the foot is demonstrated by its 26 bones, 19 large muscles, many small (intrinsic) muscles, and more than 100 ligaments. The bones of the foot connect with the upper bony structure of the upper body through the fibula and tibia. Body weight is transferred from the tibia to the talus and calcaneus.

Support and propulsion are the two functions of the foot. Proper functioning and adequate development of the muscles of the foot and the practice of proper foot mechanics are essential for everyone. In our modern society, foot trouble is one of the most common ailments. Poor foot mechanics begun in early life invariably lead to foot discomfort in later years.

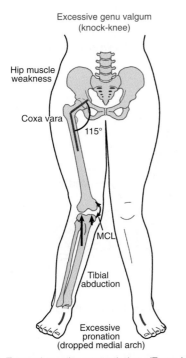

FIGURE 10-25 Excessive valgus angulation. (From Neumann DA: *Kinesiology of the musculoskeletal system: foundations for rehabilitation*, ed. 2. St Louis, 2010, Mosby.)

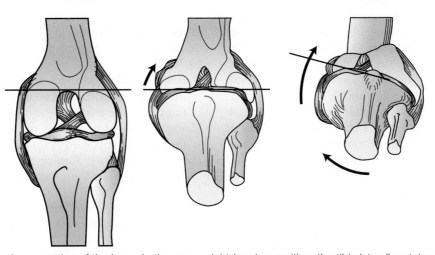

FIGURE 10-26 The screw-home motion of the knee. In the non–weight-bearing position, the tibia laterally rotates on the femur as the knee moves into the last few degrees of extension.

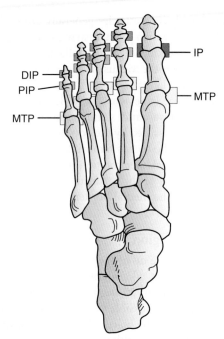

FIGURE 10-27 Joints of the phalanges of the foot. *DIP,* Distal interphalangeal; *PIP,* proximal interphalangeal; *MTP,* metatarsophalangeal; *IP,* interphalangeal.

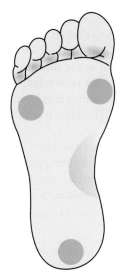

FIGURE 10-28 The main weight-bearing surfaces of the foot.

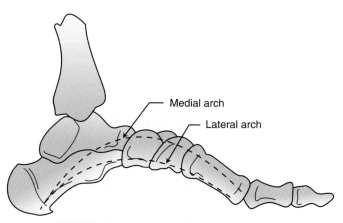

FIGURE 10-29 Longitudinal arches of the foot.

ACTIVITY 10-15

Slowly and deliberately move your ankle and then your toes through the movement patterns. Then move the ankle and toes together, and differentiate between extrinsic and intrinsic muscle activity.

On a separate piece of paper, describe the experience.

Example
It was hard to isolate the intrinsic muscles.

The metatarsophalangeal joint of the great toe flexes 45 degrees and extends 70 degrees, whereas the interphalangeal joint can flex from 0 degree of full extension to 90 degrees of flexion. The metatarsophalangeal joints of the four lesser toes allow approximately 40 degrees of flexion and 40 degrees of extension. The metatarsophalangeal joints also adduct minimally. The proximal interphalangeal joints in the lesser toes flex from 0 degree of extension to 35 degrees of flexion. The distal interphalangeal joints flex 60 degrees and extend 30 degrees. Much variation exists from joint to joint and person to person in all of these joints (Figure 10-27).

Ligaments in the foot and the ankle have the difficult task of maintaining the position of the arches in the foot. The foot has three longitudinal arches: the medial, lateral, and transverse. Individual long arches vary from high, medium, and low, but a low arch is not necessarily a weak arch.

The medial longitudinal arch is located on the medial side of the foot and extends from the calcaneus to the talus, the navicular, the three cuneiform bones, and the proximal ends of the three medial metatarsals. The lateral longitudinal arch is located on the lateral side of the foot and extends from the calcaneus to the cuboid bone and proximal ends of the fourth

and fifth metatarsals. The transverse arch extends across the foot from one metatarsal bone to the other. A vast network of fascia in the sole of the foot supports the arches. Plantar fascia with the muscles provides the spring to the arch structure (Figures 10-28 and 10-29).

Movements of the Ankle and Foot

The following are movements of the ankle and foot (Figure 10-30):

Dorsiflexion: Movement of the top of the ankle and foot toward the anterior tibial bone, accomplished by the flexor muscles of the ankle

Plantar flexion: Movement of the ankle and foot away from the tibia, accomplished by the extensor muscles of the ankle

Eversion (pronation): Turning the ankle and foot outward, away from the midline, with weight on the medial edge of the foot

Inversion (supination): Turning the ankle and foot inward, toward the midline, with weight on the lateral edge of the foot

Toe flexion: Movement of the toes toward the plantar surface of the foot

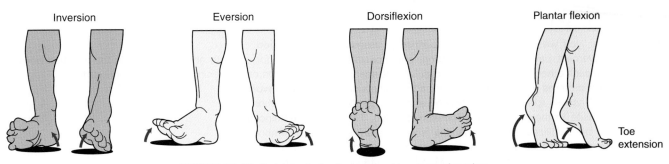

FIGURE 10-30 Quick tests for foot and ankle range of motion.

Toe extension: Movement of the toes away from the plantar surface of the foot

Muscles of the Ankle and Foot

The large number of muscles in the ankle and foot may be grouped according to location and function. In general, the muscles located on the anterior of the ankle and foot are the dorsal flexors. Those to the posterior are plantar flexors. Muscles that are everters are located more to the lateral side, and the invertors are located medially. The muscular strength patterns are not balanced. Plantar flexion is dominant over dorsiflexion, and inversion dominates eversion.

The gastrocnemius muscle is more effective as a knee flexor if the foot is elevated and more effective as a plantar flexor of the foot if the knee is held in extension. You can observe this when someone sits too close to the wheel when driving a car. When the knees are bent, the muscle becomes an ineffective plantar flexor, and the person finds it difficult to depress the brakes.

The soleus muscle is one of the most important plantar flexors of the ankle. This is especially true when the knee is flexed. When the knee is slightly flexed, the effect of the gastrocnemius is reduced, thereby placing more work on the soleus.

The tibialis posterior muscle pulls down from the underside and contracts to invert and plantar flex the foot. Use of the tibialis posterior in plantar flexion and inversion gives support to the longitudinal arch of the foot.

Passing down the back of the lower leg under the medial malleolus and then forward, the flexor digitorum longus muscle draws the four lesser toes down into flexion toward the heel as it plantar flexes the ankle. This muscle is important in helping other foot muscles maintain the longitudinal arch.

Pulling from the underside of the great toe, the flexor hallucis muscle may work independently of the flexor digitorum longus muscle or with it.

The fibularis longus muscle passes behind and beneath the lateral malleolus and under the foot from the outside to the inner surface. Because of its line of pull, the peroneus longus is a strong everter and assists in plantar flexion.

When the fibularis longus muscle is used effectively with the other ankle flexors, it helps support the transverse arch as it flexes.

The fibularis brevis muscle passes down behind and under the lateral malleolus to pull on the base of the fifth metatarsal. The fibularis brevis is a primary everter of the foot and assists in plantar flexion. In addition, the fibularis brevis aids in maintaining the longitudinal arch as it depresses the foot.

The tibialis anterior muscle holds up the inner margin of the foot. However, as it contracts, the tibialis anterior muscle dorsiflexes the ankle and is an antagonist to the plantar flexors of the ankle. The tibialis anterior is forced to contract strongly when a person ice skates or walks on the outside of the foot, and the muscle strongly supports the long arch in inversion.

Strength is necessary in the extensor digitorum longus muscle to maintain balance between the plantar and the dorsal flexors. The strength of the ankle is evident when the gastrocnemius, soleus, tibialis posterior, fibularis longus, fibularis brevis, digitorum longus, flexor digitorum brevis, and flexor hallucis longus muscles are all used effectively in walking.

Intrinsic Muscles of the Foot

The intrinsic muscles of the foot have their proximal attachment and distal attachment on the bones within the foot. Four layers of these muscles are found on the plantar surface of the foot. These muscles are involved with dorsiflexion and plantar flexion of the toes:

First layer (most superficial): Adductor hallucis, flexor digitorum brevis, and abductor digiti quinti pedis

Second layer: Quadratus plantae and lumbricales (four)

Third layer: Flexor hallucis brevis, flexor digiti quinti brevis pedis, and adductor hallucis

Fourth layer (deepest): Interossei (seven) (Activity 10-16)

PATHOLOGIC CONDITIONS

SECTION OBJECTIVES

Chapter objective covered in this section:

6. Identify and describe the three main biomechanical dysfunctional patterns and the associated indications and contraindications for massage.

After completing this section, the student will be able to perform the following:

- Categorize biomechanical dysfunction into postural deviation, nonoptimal motor function, neuromuscular-related dysfunction, myofascial-related dysfunction, and joint-related dysfunction.
- Describe three degrees of postural imbalance.
- Describe three degrees of distorted motor function.
- Classify biomechanical dysfunction into three stages.
- Define three stages of pathobiomechanical disturbances

Evolve Activity 10-2

✎ ACTIVITY 10-16

In this activity, you will be working with a partner to assess individual movement patterns, normal function, and possible dysfunction in each other. One of you is first to isolate the specified movement patterns on each side of your partner, one side at a time, and assess for normal function by applying gentle pressure opposite to the action of the isolation position. The body should be stabilized so that only the isolated area is moving. In some instances the ability to assume the position and maintain it indicates normal function. Muscles should be able to hold against gravity or the applied pressure without strain or pain. The position itself should be easy to assume and comfortable to maintain for a short duration, from 10 to 30 seconds. The bilateral movement patterns should be the same. The opposite movement pattern also should be able to be done easily.

Dysfunction may be indicated by bilateral asymmetry, pain, weakness, fatigue, a heavy sensation (binding), and the inability to assume the isolation position or move into the opposite position. Intervention or referral depends on the severity of the condition and whether the dysfunction is neuromuscular, myofascial, or joint related.

Note: Do not perform these assessments if contraindications exist. Contraindications to this type of assessment include joint and disk dysfunction, acute pain, recent trauma, and inflammation.

Key

➡ (black arrow)   Direction of resistance

➡ (gray arrow)   Direction of isolation

Knee Flexion

Assesses for strength and endurance in the isolation position and tension or shortening in the extension pattern.

Muscles Involved

Biceps femoris
Semitendinosus
Semimembranosus
Popliteus
Gastrocnemius

Range of Motion

0 to 150 degrees

Position of Client

Prone, with limbs straight and toes hanging over the edge of the table.

Examiner applies light to moderate counterpressure to hamstrings.

Isolation and Assessment

Client flexes knee through full range, keeping thigh in contact with table. Examiner applies resistance gradually to posterior leg proximal to ankle joint after knee reaches 45 degrees to straighten leg.

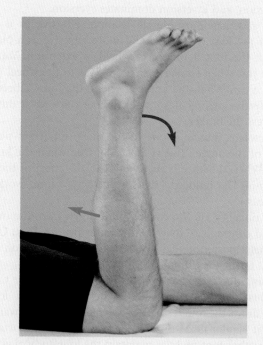

✐ ACTIVITY **10-16**—cont'd

Knee Extension

Assesses for strength and endurance in the isolation position and tension or shortening in the flexion pattern.

Muscles Involved

Rectus femoris
Vastus intermedius
Vastus lateralis
Vastus medialis

Range of Motion

0 to 135 degrees

May extend 10 degrees beyond 0 in those with hyperextension.

Position of Client

Seated, with hips flexed and small pillow under thigh to maintain 90 degrees of hip flexion

Client grasps table edge for stabilization while examiner places one hand on distal anterior thigh.

Isolation and Assessment

Client extends knee through available range of motion as examiner applies resistance to distal end of anterior leg to bend it at the knee. Do not allow the client to hyperextend the knee or lift thigh off table.

Plantar Flexion

Assesses for strength and endurance in the isolation position and tension or shortening in the dorsiflexion pattern

Muscles Involved

Gastrocnemius
Soleus
Flexor digitorum longus
Flexor hallucis longus
Plantaris
Tibialis posterior

Range of Motion

0 to 50 degrees

Position of Client

Gastrocnemius: Prone, with ankle dorsiflexed off end of table and knee extended

Soleus: Prone, with knee flexed and ankle dorsiflexed

Isolation and Assessment (Both Positions)

Client initiates plantar flexion of the ankle through the available range of motion while examiner applies resistance to posterior calcaneus or sole of foot to push foot into dorsiflexion.

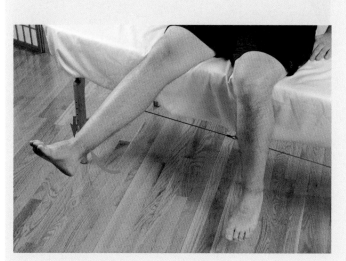

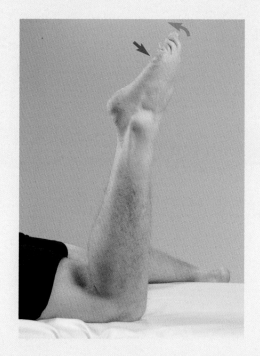

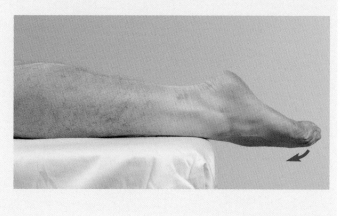

Continued

✎ ACTIVITY **10-16**—cont'd

Foot Dorsiflexion
Assesses for strength and endurance in the isolation position and tension or shortening in the plantar flexion pattern

Muscles Involved
Tibialis anterior
Fibularis tertius
Extensor digitorum longus (extensor of lesser toes)
Extensor hallucis longus (greater toe extensor)

Range of Motion
0 to 20 degrees

Position of Client
Supine with leg straight

Isolation and Assessment
Client initiates dorsiflexion of the ankle, keeping toes relaxed, and examiner applies resistance to pull foot into plantar flexion.

Foot Inversion
Assesses for strength and endurance in the isolation position and tension or shortening in the eversion pattern

Muscles Involved
Tibialis anterior
Tibialis posterior
Flexor digitorum longus (flexor of lesser toes)
Flexor hallucis longus (great toe flexor)
Gastrocnemius (medial head)

Range of Motion
0 to 30 degrees

Position of Client
Supine or side-lying on test side with ankle in neutral position

Isolation and Assessment
Client inverts foot through available range of motion as examiner applies resistance to medial edge of forefoot to pull it into eversion. Client keeps toes relaxed.

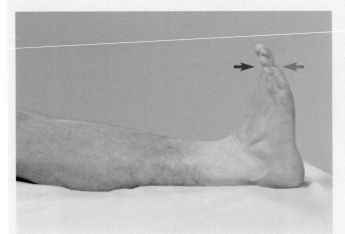

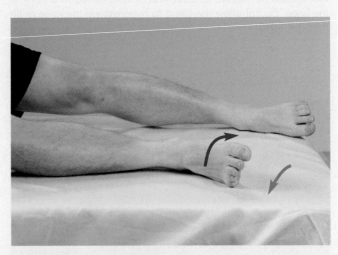

✏ ACTIVITY **10-16**—cont'd

Foot Eversion

Assesses for strength and endurance in the isolation position and tension or shortening in the inversion pattern

Muscles Involved

Fibularis longus
Fibularis brevis
Fibularis tertius
Extensor digitorum longus

Range of Motion

0 to 15 degrees

Position of Client

Supine or side-lying on nontest side with ankle in neutral position

Isolation and Assessment

Client everts foot through full range while examiner applies resistance to lateral edge of foot to pull it into inversion.

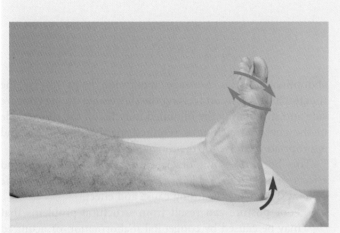

Toe Flexion

Assesses for strength and endurance in the isolation position and tension or shortening in the extension pattern

Muscles Involved

Flexor digitorum longus
Flexor digitorum brevis
Flexor hallucis longus
Flexor hallucis brevis
Flexor digiti minimi brevis
Lumbricales
Interossei (dorsal and plantar)

Range of Motion

Great toe: 0 to 45 degrees
Lateral four toes: 0 to 40 degrees

Position of Client

Supine with foot and ankle in neutral position
Examiner stabilizes metatarsals.

Isolation and Assessment

Great toe is tested separately from lateral four toes. Client flexes great toe while examiner applies light resistance to plantar surface of proximal phalange to push it into extension. Client flexes four toes while examiner applies light resistance to plantar surface of proximal phalanges to push each toe into extension.

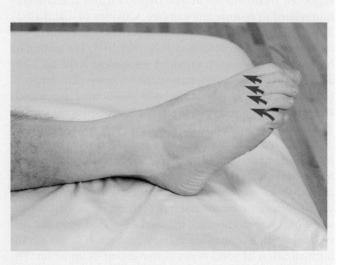

Continued

✎ ACTIVITY **10-16**—cont'd

Toe Extension
Assesses for strength and endurance in the isolation position and tension or shortening in the flexion pattern
Muscles Involved
Extensor digitorum longus
Extensor digitorum brevis
Extensor hallucis longus
Range of Motion
Great toe: 0 to 70 degrees
Lateral four toes: 0 to 40 degrees
Position of Client
Supine with foot and ankle in neutral position
Examiner stabilizes metatarsals.
Isolation and Assessment
Great toe is tested separately from lateral four toes. Client extends great toe while examiner applies light resistance to dorsal surface of proximal phalange to pull it into flexion. Client extends four toes while examiner applies light resistance to dorsal surface of proximal phalanges to pull each toe into flexion.

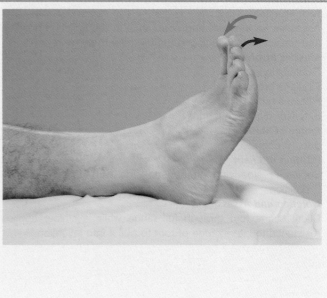

The activities in this chapter have provided assessment and suggested treatment for kinetic chain function and dysfunction related to posture and gait (see Activities 10-1 and 10-2). Muscle activation sequences (firing patterns) assessment and treatment were also described in Activity 10-3. The section on biomechanics by region provided assessment activities using active and passive joint movement to assess for range of motion as well as providing body positioning for muscle strength testing. Together these assessment provide data to determine biomechanical dysfunction.

Biomechanical dysfunctions include local functional block, local hypermobility or hypomobility, altered firing patterns, and postural imbalance, which lead to changes in motor function. Differential diagnosis to determine the causal factors of biomechanical dysfunction is beyond the scope of this text. However, the modalities studied in the specific application of massage therapy have much to offer in the normalization of some types of movement dysfunction. The four areas most effectively addressed by these methods are postural, neuromuscular-, myofascial-, and joint-related dysfunction.

Common Postural Deviations

Because standing is a closed kinetic chain activity (see Chapter 8) and because of the tensegric nature of body form, the position or motion of one joint affects the positions or motions of other joints.

Generally, if a person tends to maintain a posture in which a curve is increased, the muscles on the concave side tend to shorten and tighten, whereas the muscles on the convex side tend to become long and weak but still feel tight (Jacobs, 2007). For example, a client with a lumbar lordosis will likely have tight and short back extensors and weak and long

abdominal muscles. Massage application helps reverse the functional strain by addressing the shortening on the concave side and stimulating the inhibited muscles on the convex side of the curve. Stretching is required for the short areas and appropriate exercise for the long areas (Figure 10-31).

This book does not describe the individual causes and effects of postural problems. However, we can make some general statements regarding cause and effect.

- Poor posture can result from structural problems that may be caused by congenital malformation or acquired by trauma such as a compression fracture.
- Postural deviations also may result from neurologic conditions causing paralysis or spasticity.
- However, most postural problems are functional, or nonstructural. For example, a person who sits or stands for long periods tends to slouch, resulting in a muscle imbalance, which causes positional strain.
- Many postural problems are due to problems with core stability and distortion in normal vertebral curves.
- Postural problems can occur if the arches of the feet are abnormal or if the ankles are unstable.

Efficient posture can be achieved as follows:
- Lift head up and draw chin back.
- Eyes should be forward and level with the horizontal plane.
- Shoulders roll back and down. Medial border of scapula move toward each other.
- The thorax at the sternum moves out and down.
- The core muscles engage as the abdomen is drawn in and the lumbar area moves back and flattens a bit reducing lordosis.
- The pelvis tips slightly posteriorly as the low back flatten and the symphysis pubis moves up.
- The sacrum moves down vertically.

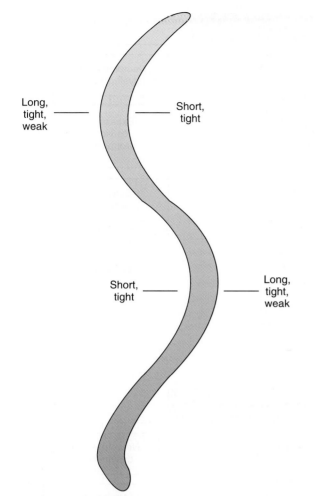

Long,
tight,
weak

Short,
tight

Short,
tight

Long,
tight,
weak

FIGURE 10-31 First, massage application with stretching lengthens the short, tight areas. Coupled with therapeutic exercise, massage then stimulates the long, tight, and weak areas.

- The thighs shift back, the leg (below the knee) shifts forward.
- The weight is distributed to the feet.
- The feet are flat with the weight distributed somewhat evenly but with a slight increase to the heel of the foot, which will act to lift the body up vertically.

This pattern should be taught to clients with postural problems. When in this posture the person will feel taller.

Regional Postural Muscular Imbalance

Muscles and muscle groups have constant muscular tone that is regulated by the central nervous system. Some muscles have higher tone, such as those that support the vertical position of the body, and others are necessary for functions such as eating and breathing. Postural stress, pattern overload, repetitive movement, lack of core stability, and lack of neuromuscular efficiency cause biomechanical neuromuscular imbalances. Most often, the tone of postural muscles, which have greater tone to begin with, increases and thus the imbalance appears. The muscles tense and shorten, inhibiting muscles that function for movement and causing sensations of fatigue and heaviness in the limbs.

Predictable neuromuscular chain reactions can occur. As described by Vladimir Janda, these chain reactions can be divided into two patterns: the upper and lower crossed syndromes (Figures 10-32 and 10-33) (Chaitow and Delany, 2008).

Nonoptimal Motor Function

All human beings create optimal carriage —how they uniquely hold and move their bodies—and optimal motor function. Optimal motor function defines the degree of mobility that the body needs to operate in the most economical way. When all goes well, movement usually proceeds efficiently. With pathologic changes, however, motor function changes as well. Carriage is disturbed, joint mobility becomes limited, tissues and joints are altered, and the tone-strength balance in the tissues is altered. The person spends more energy performing normal movements, which causes fatigue more quickly. The change of the optimal motor function influences the work of the viscera, which in turn influences the condition of the muscles and joints and in turn alters motor function and carriage even more. Thus a vicious circle starts in which the worsening of different processes negatively contributes to each process.

Neuromuscular-related Dysfunction

Neuromuscular-related dysfunction manifests as a breakdown or confusion in the nervous system interaction with muscle activity. Neuromuscular dysfunction can develop in many forms, including the following:
- Neurotransmitter fluctuations
- Hypermuscular or hypomuscular activity and altered muscle activation sequences (firing patterns)
- Increased tension in individual motor units or the entire muscle
- Hypersensitivity or hyposensitivity in the proprioceptive feedback loop and reflex arcs
- Central nervous system processing difficulties
- Gait reflex and kinetic chain disturbance

The myotonic unit becomes disrupted with patterns of overly tense muscles and corresponding weakened or reciprocally inhibited muscles. All these patterns can be reduced to two: regional postural muscular imbalance and nonoptimal motor function.

Myofascial-related Dysfunction

Connective tissue changes occur as function is altered or as the result of trauma, including microtrauma caused by accumulated overuse. We have described and discussed connective tissue in previous chapters of this textbook; reviewing these sections, primarily in Chapters 8 and 9, would be prudent.

Practically speaking, most often connective tissue loses hydration, which affects the viscous and plastic qualities and results in shortening and reduced pliability. Connective tissues also can become overstretched and lax, reducing their ability to stabilize the body.

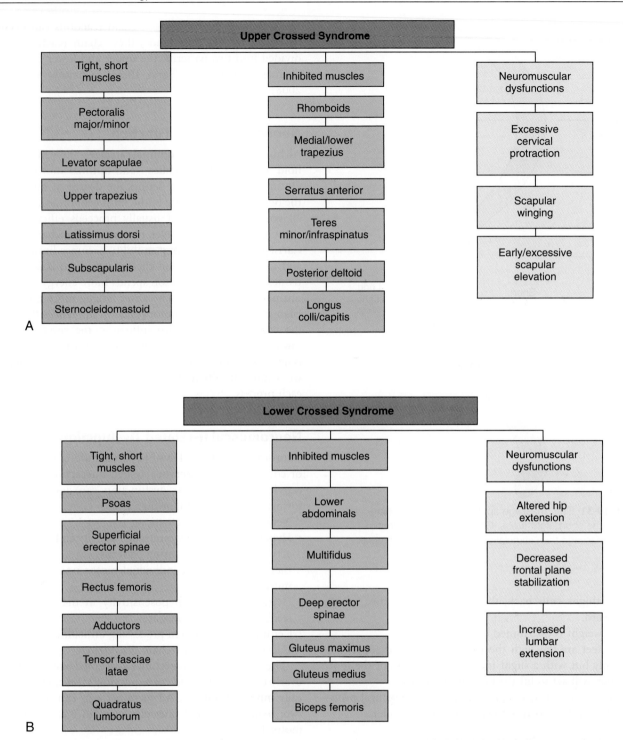

FIGURE 10-32 A, Upper crossed syndrome flow chart. **B,** Lower crossed syndrome flow chart. (Modified from Chaitow L, DeLany J: *Clinical applications of neuromuscular techniques*, vol 1, *The upper body*, Edinburgh, 2001, Churchill Livingstone.)

Joint-related Dysfunction

Joint-related dysfunction can be within the capsule itself or noncapsular. The most common noncapsular pattern is the *functional block*, which is the reversible limitation of range of movement that occurs because of change in connective tissue after long-term muscle spasms. The muscle spasm first appears as a reflex defense mechanism against painful movement in an affected jointed area. Immobility of the joint increases stagnation of tissues, which leads to more pain, resulting in the development of the pain-spasm-pain cycle.

Contributing factors to functional block development include the following:

• Holding a weight that is too heavy for too long
• Constant loading on the spine, such as occurs during work situations that demand long-term sitting

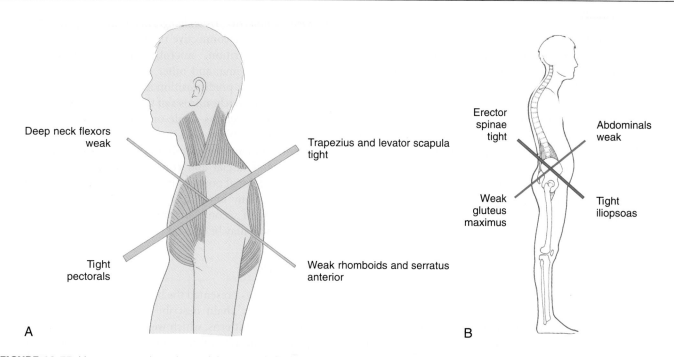

FIGURE 10-33 Upper crossed syndrome (after Janda). **B,** Lower crossed syndrome (after Janda). (Modified from Chaitow L, DeLany J: *Clinical applications of neuromuscular techniques,* vol 1, *The upper body,* ed 2, Edinburgh, 2008, Churchill Livingstone.)

- Powerful effort, such as that used in lifting during sport or work
- Passive overstretching, such as holding a heavy weight in the hand, which can cause development of functional block in the shoulder joint
- Reflex influences on muscles near joints
- Long-term immobility, such as when wearing a cast or when bedridden

The appropriate medical professional needs to assess, diagnose, and treat specific joint dysfunction. Massage application can complement the intervention of professionals such as orthopedic physicians, osteopathic physicians, chiropractors, physical therapists, and athletic trainers.

> **INDICATIONS/CONTRAINDICATIONS** for Therapeutic Massage
>
> In postural imbalance some postural muscles are shortened and their antagonists are weakened. Motor function is altered as a result. Postural imbalance often manifests as lumbar and cervical hyperlordosis but also could lead to other changes in the spine and joints of the limbs. These changes often play a pathogenic role in movement. Functional block may be treated successfully by massage techniques for relaxation and pain management, mobilization techniques such as repeated passive movement and traction, muscle energy techniques such as various forms of active muscle contraction followed by muscle lengthening, and stretching programs.

Degrees and Stages of Dysfunction

It is common to categorize dysfunction as an aid for the development of treatment plans. There are generally three degrees of postural imbalance and distorted motor function.

Depending on the combined dysfunctions, the client's condition can be categorized in three stages of severity.

Postural Imbalance

Three degrees of postural imbalance of muscles may occur:
- *First degree:* Shortening or weakening of some muscles or the formation of local changes in tension or connective tissue in these muscles
- *Second degree:* Moderately expressed shortening of postural muscles and weakening of antagonist muscles
- *Third degree:* Clearly expressed shortening of postural muscles and weakening of antagonist muscles with the appearance of specific, nonoptimal movement

Assessment defines mobility through active and passive movements of the affected parts and observation of a distortion in these movements. In addition, muscle testing can show the functional relationships of the muscles. To determine appropriate therapeutic intervention, defining which muscles are shortened and which are inhibited is important for chronic joint, muscular, and nervous system disorders.

Distorted Motor Function

There are three degrees of distorted motor function:
- *First degree:* For usual and simple movements, a person has to use additional muscles from different parts of the body. As a result, movement becomes uneconomical and labored.
- *Second degree:* Moderately peculiar postures and movements of some parts of the body are present. Postural and movement distortion, such as altered firing patterns, begin to occur.
- *Third degree:* Significantly expressed peculiarity in postures and movement occurs. Increased postural and movement distortions result.

Biomechanical Dysfunction

Pathobiomechanical disturbances may occur in all age groups. Based on the three degrees of distorted motor function, there are three stages in the development of postural and movement pathologic conditions:

• *Stage 1, functional tension:* At this stage a person tires more quickly than normal. This fatigue is accompanied by some functional block in the first- or second-degree limitation of mobility, painless local myodystonia (changes in the muscle tension/length relationship), postural imbalance in the first or second degree, and nonoptimal motor function of the first degree.

• *Stage 2, functional stress:* This stage is characterized by a feeling of fatigue after moderate activity; discomfort, slight pain, and the appearance of singular or multiple functional blocks; and any degree of limited mobility. Functional block may be painless or result in first-degree pain; it may be accompanied by local hypermobility. Functional stress also is characterized by fascial/connective tissue changes, regional postural imbalance, and distortion of motor function in the first or second degree.

INDICATIONS/CONTRAINDICATIONS for Therapeutic Massage

Working with stages 2 and 3 functional stress and connective tissue changes usually requires more training and proper supervision using a multidisciplinary approach.

Stage 1 functional tension can often be managed effectively by massage modalities and with training equivalent to 500 to 1000 hours that includes an understanding of the information presented in this text and technical training in the practitioner's chosen modality.

Any massage modality influences the systems, tissues, and viscera of the body mechanically and reflexively. Massage modalities improve blood circulation, decrease chronic muscle tension, normalize range of motion of the joint, and rebuild proper proprioception.

The body perceives any technique first as a tactile sensation because the surface of the skin is altered by various degrees, depending on the methods used. Second, massage modalities alter the degree of muscle tension. Proprioceptors of the deep tissues report to the central nervous system regarding the condition of muscle tension, capillary pressure, and blood pressure of muscles and vessels.

The tissues produce warmth. This heat acts as a thermal stimulant that signals the sympathetic and parasympathetic systems to cause vasodilation or vasoconstriction.

Chemical substances such as histamine and acetylcholine are formed in the tissues. Histamine stimulates the discharge of adrenaline. These substances are carried with the blood throughout the body, altering circulation, influencing the functions of inner organs (viscera), speeding up nerve impulses, mobilizing the immune system, normalizing blood pressure, and stimulating muscle activity.

All these signals create the reaction of the central nervous system. The goal is to generate, through massage methods, the stimulation required to generate self-regulating mechanisms, allowing the body to self-correct and restore dynamic balance, or homeostasis.

• *Stage 3, connective tissue changes in the musculoskeletal system:* The reasons for connective tissue changes are overloading, tissue malnutrition, microtraumas, microhemorrhages, unresolved edema, and other endogenous and exogenous factors. Genetic predisposition is also a consideration. In the third stage, osteochondrosis of the spine and weight-bearing joints may appear as single or multiple functional blocks, local hypermobility and instability of several vertebral motion segments, hypomobility, widespread painful muscle tension and fascial and connective tissue changes in the muscles, regional postural imbalance in the second or third degree in many joints, and temporary nonoptimal motor function with second- or third-degree distortion. Visceral disturbances may be present (Gurevich, 1992).

SUMMARY

This chapter has presented the basic principles of biomechanics. The kinetic chain describes three main biomechanical dysfunctional patterns, which we discussed with intervention suggestions and referral recommendations. A practice assessment protocol for biomechanical function was provided.

The concepts in this chapter may seem complex and at times difficult to understand. Comprehending the ways in which all the aspects of movement work together requires knowledge and an understanding of the relationship of the pieces and how they function. Sometimes the information may be overwhelming, and being able to use reference texts effectively is helpful.

Many students find themselves lost in the terminology of all the pieces: the bones, ligaments, names of the joints, actions of movement, names of the muscles, and directions for isolation. When this happens, the student should slow down and actually perform the movement while saying the words. The entire unit has been about movement. Movement is best understood by moving. The student should continue to look up the definitions of the words that are confusing. Persist in understanding biomechanical concepts. Competency in therapeutic massage is based on the integrated applications described in this chapter.

Balance and center may be the most important concepts of all. The student should remember that the importance of being centered often is expressed as being present in the moment and responding resourcefully to each unfolding second of life.

⊖volve

http://evolve.elsevier.com/Fritz/essential
Activity 10-1 Review information about levers by completing a tic tac toe game.
Activity 10-2 Video clips of muscle testing, posture, and gait assessment are located on the Evolve site.
Additional Resources:
Scientific animations
Weblinks
Remember to study for your certification and licensure exams! Review questions for this chapter are located on Evolve.

REFERENCES

Chaitow L, DeLany J: *Clinical applications of neuromuscular techniques. Vol 1: The upper body*, Edinburgh, 2001, Churchill Livingstone.

Cummings NH, Stanley-Green S, Higgs P: *Perspectives in athletic training*, St. Louis, 2009, Mosby.

Donatelli R: *Sport-specific rehabilitation*, St. Louis, 2007, Churchill Livingstone.

Goodman CC, Snyder TEK: *Differential diagnosis for physical therapists: screening for referral*, ed. 4, St. Louis, 2007, Saunders.

Greene DP, Roberts SL: *Kinesiology: movement in the context of activity*, ed 2, St. Louis, 2005, Mosby.

Gurevich D: *Russian medical massage*, Flint, Mich., 1992.

Hislop HJ, Montgomery J: *Daniels & Worthingham's muscle testing: techniques of manual examination*, ed 8, St. Louis, 2007, Saunders.

Huber FE, Wells CL: *Therapeutic exercise treatment planning for progression*, St. Louis, 2006, Saunders.

Jacobs K: *Ergonomics for therapists*, ed 3, St. Louis, 2007, Mosby.

Magee DJ: *Orthopedic physical assessment*, ed 5, St. Louis, 2008, Saunders.

Olson KA: *Manual physical therapy of the spine*, St. Louis, 2009, Saunders.

Reese NB, Bandy WD: *Joint range of motion and muscle length testing*, Philadelphia, 2009, Saunders.

Reese NB et al: *Muscle and sensory testing*, ed 2, St. Louis, 2005, Saunders.

Sahrmann S: *Diagnosis and treatment of movement impairment syndromes*, St. Louis, 2002, Mosby.

Seidel HM et al: *Mosby's physical examination handbook*, ed 6, St. Louis, 2006, Mosby.

Thompson GW, Floyd RT: *Manual of structural kinesiology with dynamic movement*, ed 14, St Louis, 2000, Mosby.

Whittle MW, Gait Analysis: an Introduction, ed 4, 2007, Butterworth Heinemann.

Workbook Section

Short Answer

1. Explain the basic principles of balance.

_____
_____
_____
_____
_____
_____
_____
_____
_____

2. Describe the steps in the normal adult walking cycle.

_____
_____
_____
_____
_____
_____
_____
_____
_____
_____

3. Identify the three main biomechanical dysfunctional patterns.

_____
_____
_____

Fill in the Blank

(1) _____ is the study of mechanical actions as applied to living bodies.

(2) _____ is the study of movement that emerges and blends the knowledge of anatomy, physiology, physics, and geometry and relates them to human movement. Dynamic systems can be divided into kinetics and kinematics. A (3) _____ is the direction of the force.

(4) _____ is a fundamental characteristic of human behavior accomplished by the contraction of skeletal muscles acting within a system of levers and pulleys.

In biomechanical terms the concept of *center* refers to the (5) _____, the midpoint or center of weight of a body or object. Any loss of biomechanical (6) _____, such as what occurs with a missing limb or altered posture, alters not only the total body weight distribution but also the center of gravity.

External forces acting on the body include (7) _____ and those forces generated by the

interaction with (8) _____, such as lifting a box or managing an umbrella in the wind. Therapeutic massage attempts to alter body function by exerting (9) _____ forces to generate (10) _____ forces, which then cause change in the homeostatic mechanisms of the body. Forces generated by massage include tension, torsion, bend, shear, and compression.

(11) _____ is the reluctance of matter to change its state of motion. Any irregularly paced or multidirectional activity is costly to energy reserves.

(12) _____ may be defined as the rate of change in velocity and occurs in the same direction as the force that caused it.

(13) _____ is the ability to control equilibrium. *Equilibrium* refers to a state of zero acceleration in which no change occurs in the speed or direction of the body.

(14) _____ equilibrium occurs when the body is at rest or completely motionless.

(15) _____ equilibrium occurs when all of the applied or internal forces acting on the moving body are in balance, resulting in movement with unchanging speed or direction.

(16) _____ is the resistance to change in the acceleration of a body or the resistance to the disturbance of the equilibrium of a body.

The (17) _____ is made up of the myofascial system (muscle, ligament, tendon, and fascia), articular (joint) system, and nervous system. If one or more of the systems do not work efficiently, compensations and adaptations occur in the remaining systems, leading to stress in the body and eventually resulting in the development of dysfunctional patterns. All functional movement patterns involve acceleration provided by (18) _____, stabilization provided by (19) _____, and deceleration provided by (20) _____. All three actions occur at every joint in the kinetic chain and in all three planes of motion with each movement pattern.

Problem Solving and Professional Application

Design an assessment form. On this form, list each of the activity assessments in this chapter and provide room for your responses. As you develop this form, consider how you would use it to organize the information in this chapter as you take a physical assessment. Possibilities for design of the form include a checklist or a silhouette drawing that provides areas that can be marked to indicate function and dysfunction during the assessment process. You may come up with a different idea. Be creative. However, be sure to develop a comprehensive form to use as a tool that will remind you of the information in this chapter as you work professionally with a client. (The activity assessments begin with the section on Biomechanics by Region, starting with the head and neck and trunk and thorax.)

Assess Your Competencies

1. Explain the basic principles of biomechanics
   - Define *biomechanics*.
   - Identify the center of gravity of the body
   - Describe force
   - Describe and demonstrate the effects of force.
   - Explain lever and fulcrum and the application of force
   - Demonstrate mechanical advantage and disadvantage.
   - Describe and demonstrate balance, equilibrium and stability.
   - Describe and demonstrate good posture.
   - Perform a postural assessment
   - Identify common postural deviations
   - Explain gait
   - Demonstrate the adult walking cycle
2. Explain and assess function of the kinetic chain
   - Define *the kinetic chain*.
   - List the muscles and function of the inner and outer units.
   - Explain postural stabilization.
   - Assess posture.
   - Demonstrate correct sitting, standing, and bending positions.
   - Describe and analyze gait.
   - Demonstrate and analyze the adult walking cycle.
   - Assess gait.
   - Describe and assess muscle firing patterns/activation sequences.
3. List principles of a massage intervention plan based on efficient biomechanical movement.
4. Assess biomechanical function using individual joint assessment.
5. Assess biomechanical function for regions of the body.
   - Use movement patterns during assessment to obtain two types of information
   - Demonstrate applications of resistance and stabilization during assessment
   - Apply clinical reasoning to individual joint assessment
6. Identify and describe the three main biomechanical dysfunctional patterns and the associated indications and contraindications for massage.
   - Categorize biomechanical dysfunction into postural deviation, nonoptimal motor function, neuromuscular-related dysfunction, myofascial-related dysfunction, and joint-related dysfunction.
   - Describe three degrees of postural imbalance.
   - Describe three degrees of distorted motor function.
   - Classify biomechanical dysfunction into three stages.

Next, on a separate piece of paper or using an audio or video recorder, prepare a short narrative that reflects how you would explain this content to a client and how the information relates to how you would provide massage. See the example in Chapter 1 on p. 22. When read or listened to, the narrative should not take more than 5 to 10 minutes to complete. Simpler is better. Use examples, tell stories, and use metaphors. It is important to understand that there is no precisely correct way to complete this exercise. The intent is to help you identify how effectively you understand the content and how relevant your application is to massage therapy. An excellent learning activity is to work together with other students and share your narratives. Also share these narratives with a friend or family member who is not familiar with the content. If that person can understand what you have written or recorded, that indicates that you understand it. There are many different ways to complete this learning activity. Yes, it may be confusing to do this, but that's all right. Out of confusion comes clarity. By the time you do this 12 times, once for each chapter in this book, you will be much more competent.

Further Study

Using additional resource material (see the Works Consulted list at the back of this text), identify chapters pertaining to the information presented in this chapter. As a study guide, locate the information presented in this text and then elaborate by writing a paragraph of additional information on each of the following:

Center of gravity
_____
_____
_____
_____
_____
_____
_____
_____
_____

Levers
_____
_____
_____
_____
_____
_____
_____
_____
_____

Gait
_____
_____
_____
_____
_____
_____
_____
_____
_____

CHAPTER
11

Integumentary, Cardiovascular, Lymphatic, and Immune Systems

e http://evolve.elsevier.com/Fritz/essential

CHAPTER OBJECTIVES

After completing this chapter, the student will be able to perform the following:

1. Explain the physiology of touch.
2. List and describe the components and functions of the integumentary system.
3. Identify pathologies of the integumentary system and describe indications and contraindications for massage.
4. List and describe the components and functions of the cardiovascular system.
5. Identify pathologies of the cardiovascular system and describe indications and contraindications for massage.
6. List and describe the components and functions of the lymphatic system.
7. Identify pathologies of the lymphatic system and describe indications and contraindications for massage.
8. Define immunity.
9. List and describe nonspecific and specific immune responses of the body.
10. Explain how the mind/body connection affects immunity.
11. Identify pathologies of the immune system and describe indications and contraindications for massage.

CHAPTER OUTLINE

INTEGUMENTARY SYSTEM, 552
  Physiology of Touch, 552
  Structure of the Integument, 552
  Pathologic Conditions of the Integumentary System, 556
CARDIOVASCULAR SYSTEM, 562
  Heart, 562
  Vascular System, 565
  Blood, 575
  Pathologic Conditions of the Cardiovascular System, 576
LYMPHATIC SYSTEM, 583
  Lymph, 584
  Lymph Vessels, Nodes, and Organs, 584
  Pathologic Conditions of the Lymphatic System, 586
IMMUNE SYSTEM, 589
  Nonspecific Defenses, 591
  Specific Immunity, 593
  Mind/Body Connection, 594
  Pathologic Conditions of the Immune System, 595
SUMMARY, 597

KEY TERMS

Antibodies (AN-ti-bod-eez) Serum proteins of the immunoglobulin class that are secreted by plasma cells.

Arterioles Small blood vessels that connect arteries to capillaries.

Arteriosclerosis (ar-tee-ree-o-skle-RO-sis) A term meaning "hardening of the arteries"; refers to arteries that have lost their elasticity.

Artery (AR-ter-ee) A blood vessel that transports oxygenated blood from the heart to the body or deoxygenated blood from the heart to the lungs.

Atherosclerosis (ath-er-o-skle-RO-sis) A condition in which fatty plaque is deposited in medium-sized and large arteries.

Atrium (AY-tree-um) One of the two small, thin-walled upper chambers of the heart.

Blood A thick, red fluid that provides oxygen, nourishment, and protection to the cells and carries away waste products.

Blood pressure The measurement of pressure exerted by the blood on the walls of the blood vessels. The highest pressure exerted is called *systolic pressure,* which results when the ventricles contract. Diastolic pressure, the lowest pressure, results when the ventricles relax.

Capillary (KAP-i-lair-ee) The smallest blood vessel; found between arteries and veins. Capillaries allow the exchange of gases, nutrients, and waste products.

Coronary arteries (KOR-o-nair-ee) The arteries that supply oxygenated blood to the heart muscle itself; they are located in grooves between the atria and ventricles and between the two ventricles.

Dermatitis (der-mah-TIE-tis) A general term for acute or chronic skin inflammation characterized by redness, eruptions, edema, scaling, and itching.

Dermis (DER-mis) The deep layer of skin that contains collagen and elastin fibers, which provide much of the structure and strength of the skin.

Epidermis (ep-i-DER-mis) The superficial layer of skin; composed of epithelial tissue in sublayers called *strata.*

Heart A hollow, cone-shaped, muscular organ responsible for pumping blood. It is about the size of a fist and is located in the mediastinum of the thoracic cavity.

Heart valves Four sets of valves that keep the blood flowing in the correct direction through the heart.

Hemorrhage (HEM-or-ej) The passage of blood outside of the cardiovascular system.

Immunity Resistance to disease; the immune system is a functional system rather than an organ system in the anatomic sense.

Integument (in-TEG-yoo-ment) The skin and its appendages: hair, sebaceous and sweat glands, nails, and breasts.

Lymph (limf) Fluid derived from interstitial fluid; contains lymphocytes, returns plasma proteins that have leaked out through capillary walls, and transports fats from the gastrointestinal system to the bloodstream.

Lymph nodes Small, round structures distributed along the network of lymph vessels; they filter wastes and pathogens out of lymph.

Pericardium (pair-i-KAR-dee-um) A double-membrane, serous sac that surrounds and protects the heart.

Plasma (PLAZ-mah) A thick, straw-colored fluid that makes up about 55% of the blood.

Standard Precautions Safety measures established by the Centers for Disease Control and Prevention. The precautions were instituted to prevent the spread of bacterial and viral infections by setting up specific methods of dealing with human fluids and waste products.

Superficial fascia The subcutaneous tissue that comprises the third layer of skin; consists of loose connective tissue and contains fat or adipose tissue.

Tumor Also referred to as a *neoplasm,* a tumor is a growth of new tissues that may be benign or malignant.

Veins Blood vessels that collect blood from the capillaries and transport it back to the heart.

Ventricles (VEN-tri-kulz) The two large lower chambers of the heart; they are thick-walled and are separated by a thick interventricular septum.

Venules (VEN-yoolz) Small blood vessels that connect capillaries to veins.

LEARNING HOW TO LEARN

As we begin this study of these final two chapters, eight body systems will be covered. Visualizing is a valuable learning tool. When you are learning about each system, also think about the applications for massage. Ask yourself the following questions: How would I apply massage to this area? What would be the outcomes of massage for this system? Actually visualize yourself massaging the area and learn massage application and the structure and function of each body system. Incorporate all you have learned about learning, and remember to take brain breaks.

Previous chapters have provided an overview of anatomy and physiology, mechanisms of health and disease, and scientific language. This information set the stage for the complex study of the body systems that monitor and control the physiology: namely, the nervous and endocrine systems. The information on kinesiology and biomechanics presented core content for the practice of massage.

This unit has only two chapters. Chapter 11 covers four body systems, and Chapter 12 covers four body systems. The reason is that although massage therapy benefits occur for these body systems, typically it is because these benefits are secondary effects of the nervous system, primarily the autonomic portion, and the endocrine system. Additionally, the organs of these systems are primarily found in the thoracic, abdominal, and pelvic cavities of the torso. To some extent massage can work mechanically to affect the connective tissue and membrane secretions and support normal sliding for the organs within the cavities, but specific direct massage application is unlikely.

For a massage therapy student in entry-level education, the basic study of the body systems presented in Chapters 11 and 12 supports learning the most pertinent information relative to massage. It is not necessary to memorize all the content. Instead, the information can be used as a basis for asking questions and seeking appropriate answers. If, in the future, you decide to specialize in an area related to one of the eight body systems presented, then more in-depth study of the system would be essential.

For example, if you want to work with clients who have respiratory disorders such as asthma, you will need to know more about the respiratory system.

If you want to work with clients with various types of cancer, such as breast and gastrointestinal cancer, you will need to know more about the integumentary and digestive systems.

If you want to work with a cosmetic surgeon, you will need to know more about the integumentary system.

If you want to work with cardiac rehabilitation specialists, you will need to learn more about the cardiovascular system.

If you want to work with clients who have autoimmune diseases, such as lupus and multiple sclerosis, you will need to know more about the immune system.

If you want to work with clients who have diabetes, in addition to the endocrine system, you will need to know more about the digestive system, nutrition, and the urinary system (because diabetes affects the kidneys).

If you want to perform prenatal and postnatal massage, you will need to know about the reproductive system.

If you want to work with clients who have postinjury swelling, such as occurs with various athletic injuries, you will need to learn more about the lymphatic system.

The Evolve site for this chapter provides links to some sites that can reinforce the information provided in the chapters. As has been stated before, learning requires repetition.

Much of the outdated information and myths about massage therapy are related to the eight body systems described in Chapters 11 and 12. It is important to learn to examine the evidence of any massage claim. Even when textbooks are revised on a regular basis, some of the content can become outdated. Your critical thinking skills will help you keep current on the latest information regarding massage therapy.

Massage therapy is moving to a practice based on research and consensus of groups of experts. In the past, massage therapy benefits, mechanisms of action, and the underlying physiology of the effects of massage methods were often mistakenly based on opinion, perpetuating myths and outdated information. With an increase in scholarly research and greater scrutiny of massage claims, this situation is changing. The Massage Therapy Foundation is committed to supporting the development of best practices for massage therapy. Best practices are methods and techniques that have consistently shown results superior to those achieved by other means.

Best practices are based on evidence. An evidence-based practice uses the best available information. Because of the need for a way to classify evidence, in 1996 the U.S. Preventive Services Task Force offered a methodology to assess the strength of evidence and the levels of recommendation to be made on the basis of that evidence. The quality of evidence can be scored as follows:

I. Evidence obtained from at least one properly designed randomized controlled trial.

II-1. Evidence obtained from well-designed controlled trials without randomization.

II-2. Evidence obtained from well-designed cohort or case-controlled analytic studies, preferably from more than one center or research group.

II-3. Evidence obtained from multiple time series with or without the intervention.

III. Opinions of respected authorities, based on clinical experience, descriptive studies, or reports of expert committees.

INTEGUMENTARY SYSTEM

SECTION OBJECTIVES

Chapter objective covered in this section:

1. Explain the physiology of touch.
2. List and describe the components and functions of the integumentary system.
3. Identify pathologies of the integumentary system and describe indications and contraindications for massage.

After completing this chapter, the student will be able to perform the following:

- Explain the importance of touch.
- Describe the function of the integumentary system.
- Describe two main concerns with integumentary pathologic conditions.

Physiology of Touch

The skin is the most sensitive of our organs. It is the home of the touch receptors of the nervous system. Touch is one of the five basic senses, along with taste, vision, smell, and hearing; it expands the ways in which we experience the world. Touch is the first sense to develop in the embryo, and the need for touch remains throughout our lives. As massage professionals, we touch our clients, obviously, and the skin is our contact point; therefore we must understand the effects of skin stimulation.

We can survive without sight, hearing, taste, and smell, but without the ability to feel, we are in constant danger. In fact, a complete loss of the sense of touch can cause a psychotic breakdown. Not being touched can be life-threatening and can contribute to a condition called *marasmus* (wasting away), especially in infants, the elderly, and those with weakened immune systems. Sensory stimulation is essential to well-being at all stages of life, and touch is a necessary component. Deprivation of this sense leads to reduced production of the neuroendocrine chemicals necessary for well-being. It is common for touch-deprived individuals to develop inappropriate forms of sensory stimulation or abusive or addictive behavior (often food or drugs) in an attempt to stimulate the production of chemicals the body needs.

✎ ACTIVITY 11-1

This exercise is done with a partner. Your partner sits quietly with his or her eyes closed through the entire exercise while you think of a time when you were nurturing, angry, parental, fearful, happy, comforting, playful, and so on. Hold the thought in your mind while you touch your partner on the forearm with your hand. See whether your partner can guess what emotion is being expressed.

Repeat the exercise, but this time deliberately attempt to communicate each of the emotions listed (nurturing, angry, parental, fearful, happy, comforting, playful, and so forth), using the touch of your hand on your partner's forearm. See whether your partner can identify the emotion being expressed.

Then change roles. Finally, describe the experience in the space provided.

Note: Remember that the touch is limited to using your hand on your partner's forearm.

Example

Distinguishing between a nurturing touch and a comforting touch was difficult. When touching my partner, I found it easy to communicate playfulness but difficult to communicate parental feelings. I did not like keeping my eyes closed while I was touched but found it easier to touch someone else if he or she could not see me.

As a survival mechanism, touch alerts us to danger through variations in temperature, vibration, and pressure received by millions of sensory receptors in the skin. Touch informs us of differences in texture, shape, resistance, and tension. About one third of the 5 million or so sensory receptors are in the skin of our hands. The fingertips alone have more than 1000 nerve endings per square inch, and the lips and tongue have even more.

Different types of touch are identified by different receptors in the skin. The degree of pressure in light touch as opposed to deep touch is sensed by specific sensory receptor mechanisms and can evoke entirely different responses. A slow, light touch can relay compassion or intimacy. A deeper slow touch can evoke relaxation or security, whereas an abrupt touch startles and alerts. Touch can evoke pleasure, which we seek, and pain or discomfort, which we avoid. Each of these sensations triggers the manufacture and release of specific neurochemicals (see Chapters 4 through 6).

What form of communication is more intimate than touch? Its importance is reflected even in the language: That was a touching experience; what you said touched me; you hurt my feelings; let's stay in touch. The various kinds of touch—nurturing, angry, parental, fearful, sexual, happy, comforting, and playful—are, in some amazing way, understood by the neuropathways of the skin (Activity 11-1).

Structure of the Integument

The word **integument** means "covering." The integumentary system, which covers our bodies, is made up of the skin and its appendages: hair, sebaceous glands, sweat glands, nails, and breasts (Figure 11-1).

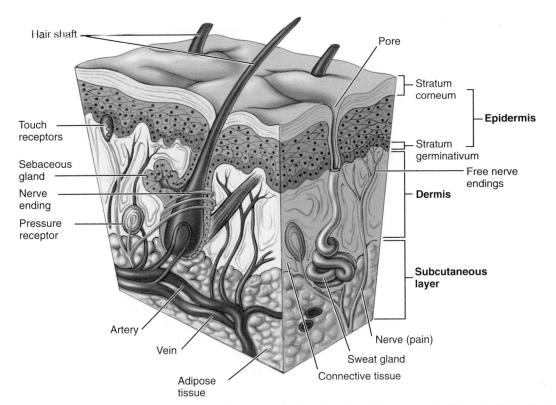

FIGURE 11-1 Skin structure. (From Herlihy H: *The human body in health and disease,* ed 4, St Louis, 2011, Mosby.)

The following are some of the major functions of the integumentary system:

- Protecting the internal organs and structures from trauma, sun exposure, chemicals, and water loss
- Assisting in **immunity** by preventing the entry of bacteria and viruses
- Synthesizing vitamin D when exposed to ultraviolet rays of the sun
- Detecting the stimuli sensed through touch, temperature, pain, and pressure
- Regulating body temperature
- Excreting sweat and salts and secreting sebum

Skin

The skin is the largest and heaviest organ of the body and is composed of two major layers: the **epidermis** and the **dermis.**

The epidermis is the outer layer of the skin. It contains no nerves or blood vessels and consists of sublayers called *strata.* Most areas have four layers, but areas subject to pressure or friction, such as the palms and the soles, have five layers. In all areas the outermost layer is the stratum corneum. This layer is made up of 20 to 30 layers of flat, keratin-filled dead cells that are continuously shed and are replaced from the layer deep to it. The innermost layer is the stratum basale, which produces a continuous supply of new cells. As the new cells develop and mature, they move up through the other layers until they reach the top and are shed, a process that takes about 2 to 3 weeks. This lowest layer also contains melanocytes, which produce melanin, a pigment that colors the skin.

The melanin pigment protects the skin from the harmful effects of ultraviolet radiation. The cumulative effects of exposure to ultraviolet radiation can damage fibroblasts located in the dermis, leading to faulty manufacture of connective tissue and wrinkling of the skin. Also, damage to the chromosomes of multiplying cells in the stratum germinativum (basale) can cause skin cancer.

Keratin is produced in the epidermis by keratinocytes. Keratin is the fibrous protein that protects the skin and makes it waterproof.

The dermis, the layer of skin deep to the epidermis, is much thicker than the epidermis. The dermis is composed of dense connective tissue that contains collagen and elastin fibers, which provide much of the structure and strength of the skin. The fibers are arranged so that the skin can be moved in many directions. Stretch marks result when these fibers are overstretched. The top layer of the dermis forms into ridges and presses up into the epidermis to create our fingerprints. Hair, sebaceous and sweat glands, and nails originate in the dermis and also push upward through the epidermis. Blood vessels and nerves are found in the dermis as well.

Figure 11-2 shows lines of the cleavage of the skin. This pattern of collagen and elastin fiber bundles in the dermis follows the lines of tension in the skin. Injuries to the skin that are at right angles to the lines tend to gap because the cut elastin fibers recoil and pull the wound apart. Healing is slower, and more scarring occurs in these kinds of injuries than in injuries that are parallel to the lines. Surgeons attempt to make their incisions parallel to lines of cleavage so as to promote healing and reduce scarring.

The subcutaneous layer, consisting of loose connective tissue and adipose tissue, is found below the dermis. This layer, also known as the **superficial fascia,** attaches to muscle and

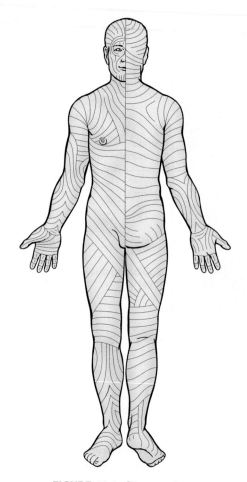

FIGURE 11-2 Cleavage lines.

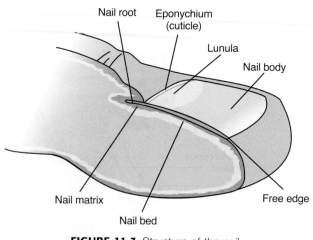

FIGURE 11-3 Structure of the nail.

bone. The subcutaneous layer is not actually a part of the integument, but because it contains loose connective tissue that attaches to the dermis, it usually is described along with the integumentary system. The adipose tissue insulates and provides padding; its distribution varies in men and women and is affected by genetic factors.

The skin has an extensive blood supply. The volume of blood flowing in the vessels of the skin varies according to the need to replace heat lost from the body. A simple assessment of circulation is to apply pressure to the nail body for 2 to 3 seconds and then release. Watch the color change as the blood refills the area. If this refilling process is longer than 2 to 3 seconds, circulation is sluggish.

The appendages of the skin are special structures that perform a variety of functions.

Hair

Hair protects the skin and orifices of the body, keeps us warm, and assists our sense of touch. It is found all over the body except on the palms of the hands, the soles of the feet, the palmar and plantar surfaces of the digits, the lips, the nipples, and portions of the external genitalia. Even though some parts of the body appear to be hairless, they actually have fine hair. Hair is composed of dead cells that have become keratinized, or hardened. Follicles, including the hair root and connective tissues, hold the hair in place. A root hair plexus is a nerve that is stimulated each time the hair is moved. Tiny muscles called

erector pili attach to hair follicles and cause the hair to stand on end at times. When this happens, the body is more sensitive to changes in air pressure and more alert to movements that may be possible signs of danger. One reason forms of energy bodywork are thought to be effective is that the touch and gentle movements stimulate the root hair plexuses, providing sensory stimulation.

Nails

Toenails and fingernails are hard, keratinized cells that protect the ends of the digits and assist us in grasping. The lunula is the crescent-shaped white area at the base of the nail. It is white because the blood vessels are covered with connective tissue and do not show. The nail actually grows from the lunula; the clear, visible portion of the nail is the nail body (Figure 11-3).

Sebaceous (Oil) Glands

Most oil glands are connected to hair follicles by small ducts. They can be found over most of the body except on the palms and soles. By secreting an oily substance known as *sebum*, the oil glands prevent dehydration, soften the skin and hair, and slow the growth of bacteria. Hormones, primarily androgens, stimulate the secretion of sebum. If the sebum builds up and blocks the oil gland, a whitehead can form. If the sebum dries and makes contact with oxygen, a blackhead can form. Acne is a bacterial inflammation of the sebaceous glands.

Sweat Glands

Also known as *sudoriferous glands,* sweat glands are found in most areas of the body, primarily on the forehead, palms, and soles. They are classified according to their structures and locations; the two main types are the eccrine glands and the apocrine glands.

The eccrine glands, which are the most common, are responsible for the moisture that appears on the surface of the body when body temperature rises, particularly during physical activity. Eccrine glands cool the body and provide minor elimination of metabolic waste. Sweat is 99% water and 1% solutes in the water. The sympathetic division of the autonomic nervous system regulates sweating. Heat-induced sweating tends to begin on the forehead and then spreads to the rest of the body, whereas emotion-induced sweating, stimulated by fright, embarrassment, or anxiety, begins on the palms and in the axillae and then spreads to the rest of the body.

The apocrine glands, which are located in areas of body hair—primarily in the axillary and anogenital areas—begin to function during puberty. When a person is under stress, these glands produce secretions that are thicker and have a stronger odor than those of the eccrine glands. The exact function of these glands has yet to be determined, but because they are stimulated during sexual arousal and phases of the menstrual cycle, they may be similar to the sexual scent glands in other animals.

Ceruminous glands are modified apocrine glands found in the external ear canal. They secrete a sticky substance called *cerumen,* or earwax, that prevents foreign material from entering the ear and repels insects.

Mammary Glands

Mammary glands develop in the pectoral region of the chest, specifically the *breasts.* They are accessory reproductive structures in the female but are flat, nonfunctional organs in the male. Developmentally, the mammary glands are modified apocrine sweat glands. Each mammary gland is contained within a rounded, skin-covered breast anterior to the pectoral muscles of the thorax. A ring of pigmented skin called the *areola* surrounds the nipple. Internally, each mammary gland consists of 15 to 25 lobes located around the nipple. The lobes are padded and separated from each other by fibrous connective tissue and fat. Ligaments attach the breast to the underlying muscle fascia and to the overlying skin, providing support. During lactation glandular alveoli produce milk, which collects in lobules within the lobes and passes through lactiferous ducts to the nipple.

Skin Color

Skin color is created by combinations of pigments in the skin and in the blood flowing through the skin. These pigments are melanin, carotene, and hemoglobin.

Melanin, which is found in the epidermis, ranges in color from yellow to black. Melanin makes up most of our skin color. All of us have the same number of melanocytes, or melanin-producing cells, but the amount of melanin produced depends on genetic factors and exposure to ultraviolet light. Melanin is a natural sunscreen that protects us from ultraviolet rays by darkening our skin; this is an adaptive homeostatic function. Freckles, moles, age spots, and actinic keratoses result from increases in the melanin concentration or from changes in melanocytes.

Carotene is a yellow pigment found in the dermis that naturally gives the skin of some individuals a yellow tint. If plant foods containing carotene make up a large part of a person's diet, carotene can accumulate in the skin and adipose tissue and give the skin a temporary yellow or orange color, especially on the face and the palms.

Hemoglobin is the oxygen-carrying red pigment molecule in the blood. In persons with light skin, the color of the hemoglobin shows through as pink.

The color of the skin can indicate health or a pathologic condition. For example, a blue tint to the skin is called *cyanosis,* a condition caused by defective or deficient oxygenation of the blood. A yellow-gold color of the skin may result from jaundice or liver disorders. A bronze or metallic hue often is a sign of Addison's disease, a hypofunction of the adrenal cortex. Black-and-blue marks on the skin, or bruises, result when blood leaves the blood vessels and clots in the surrounding tissues. Most commonly caused by trauma or injury, constant bruising may indicate a vitamin C deficiency or a blood-clotting disorder.

Pallor, or whiteness of the skin, may be caused by emotional factors. The skin can contain as much as 5% of the blood in our bodies. During sympathetic autonomic activation, when the muscles need blood, the vessels of the skin contract to move the blood out. Sudden pallor may be caused by stressful situations, such as those provoking anger or fear. Anemia is a decrease in functioning red blood cells or hemoglobin; people with anemia appear pale. Some people, however, are naturally pale as a result of the opaqueness of the epidermis. Excessive redness may be caused by embarrassment resulting in blushing, an increase in body temperature or fever, hypertension, inflammation, allergy, rosacea, or hormonal fluctuations.

Practical Application

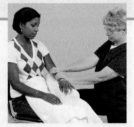

Observation of a person's skin color and changes in the appearance, texture, and suppleness of the skin and the appendages can provide information about changes in a person's health status. Because massage practitioners are likely to touch the skin more than any other professional, they should be especially observant of the skin and its appendages, which can be indicators of dysfunction or of improved health.

Stem Cells, Wound Healing, and Scar Tissue

Stem cells are cells that can become, or differentiate into, any of several types of cells. There are stem cells located within the skin. Stem cells are a major focus of medical research. One of the major obstacles to stem cell research is obtaining stem cells. Recently, researchers at Rockefeller University have identified two proteins that enable skin stem cells to renew themselves. Scientists have created liver cells in a laboratory using these reprogrammed cells from human skin, paving the way for the potential development of new treatments for liver diseases that kill thousands each year.

Delayed healing of skin wounds is a major health care concern. The research on massage benefits for wound healing is scant, but there is some indication that massage is helpful. The majority of the research involves burn healing. Massage may reduce itching and pain related to wound healing, and although not directly related to skin, massage also reduced anxiety and improved mood. Massage may also support productive scar tissue development. A recent research study found

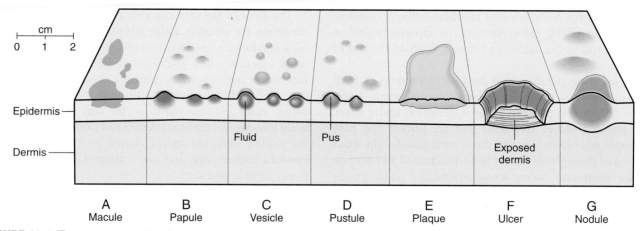

FIGURE 11-4 The appearance of various skin lesions. (From Damjanov I: *Pathology for the health-related professions,* ed 4, Philadelphia, 2012, Saunders.)

that connective tissue growth factor (CTGF) was reduced after 24 hours of cell stretching. These findings suggest that cyclic stretching of fibroblasts contributes to antifibrotic processes by reducing CTGF production. Massage is a method of producing cell stretching. Whether massage produces a significant effects on scar development has not been substantiated, but it may be possible.

Pathologic Conditions of the Integumentary System

Pathologic conditions of the integument give rise to two main concerns related to impairment of the structural integrity of the skin. The first concern is loss of the protection of internal structures. The second concern is loss of the ability of the skin to prevent the pathogens of contagious disease from entering the body. Observing the **Standard Precautions** guidelines established by the Centers for Disease Control and Prevention and proper sanitation methods maintains the security of the skin and its protective barriers. Pathologic conditions of the skin, especially sores, rashes, and changes in color and texture (Figures 11-4 and 11-5), can indicate more serious systemic disease, and the practitioner should refer the client to a physician for diagnosis.

Bacterial Infections

Acne

Acne vulgaris, the common form of acne, is a chronic inflammation of the sebaceous glands and hair follicles caused by the interaction of bacteria, sebum, and sex hormones. Acne vulgaris is most common at puberty and may recur in women during menopause. The condition can produce blackheads, whiteheads, cysts, pustules, and inflamed nodules.

Boils

Boils are local staphylococcus infections similar to acne, but they are not caused by an interaction with sex hormones. Boils look like acne except that the lesions are bigger and more painful, and they usually occur singly rather than being spread over a large area. Sometimes they occur in a cluster called a *carbuncle*. The bacteria that cause boils are virulent

and communicable. Local massage is contraindicated, and the therapist should take care to make sure that the infection is not systemic.

Impetigo

Impetigo is an acute, highly contagious bacterial skin infection usually found on the face. Impetigo is characterized by small red spots that develop into vesicles, which become filled with pus; burst; and develop a thick, yellow crust.

Cellulitis

Cellulitis is a rapidly spreading, acute bacterial infection of the skin usually found in the lower extremities. Bacteria enter through damaged skin or as a result of complications of diabetes or poor circulation. Symptoms include redness, heat, swelling, and pain.

Erysipelas

Erysipelas is a streptococcus infection that kills skin cells, leading to painful inflammation of the skin. Erysipelas usually occurs on the face or lower legs. The bacterial infection can invade the **lymph** and circulatory systems. Massage is systemically contraindicated until the infection has passed completely.

Ecthyma

Ecthyma is a skin infection that is similar to impetigo but more deeply invasive. Usually caused by a streptococcus infection, ecthyma goes through the epidermis to the dermis of skin, possibly causing scars.

Viral Skin Infections

Chicken Pox

Chicken pox is a viral infection that causes a blisterlike rash on the surface of the skin and mucous membranes. Chicken pox blisters usually appear first on the trunk and face and then spread to almost every other area of the body, including the scalp and penis and inside the mouth, nose, ears, and vagina. Chicken pox blisters are about 0.2 to 0.4 inch (5 to 10 mm) wide, have a reddish base, and appear in crops over 2 to 4 days. Some persons get only a few blisters, and others have several

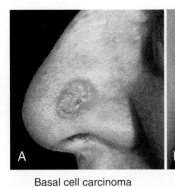
A
Basal cell carcinoma

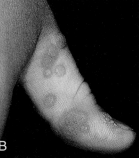
B
Common warts

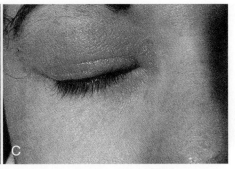
C
Contact dermatitis caused by shampoo

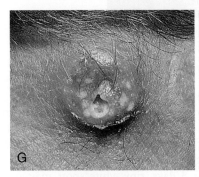
D
Contact dermatitis
caused by shoes

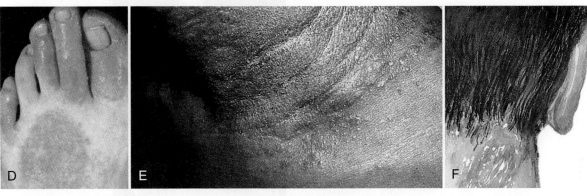
E
Contact dermatitis caused by
application of Lanacane

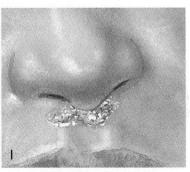
F
Dermatitis

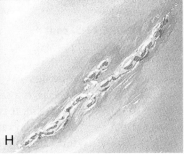
G
Furuncle (boil)

H
Herpes zoster (shingles)

I
Impetigo contagiosa

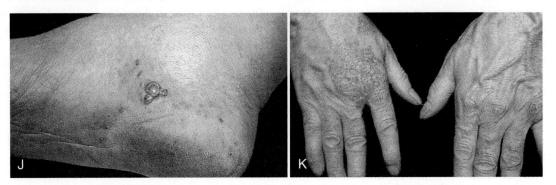
J
Kaposi's sarcoma

K
Nummular eczema

FIGURE 11-5 Common skin disorders. Skin problems may result from various causes, such as parasitic infestations; fungal, bacterial, or viral infections; reactions to substances encountered externally or taken internally; and new growths. Many of the skin manifestations have no known cause; others are hereditary. (**A** and **M** from Habif TP: *Clinical dermatology: a color guide to diagnosis and therapy,* ed 4, St Louis, 2004, Mosby; **B** from Habif TP, *Clinical dermatology,* ed 2, Mosby; **G,** from Jaime A Tschen, MD, Department of Dermatology, Baylor College of Medicine, Houston; **C, D, K, L,** and **P** reprinted with permission from the American Academy of Dermatology. Copyright © 2012 All rights reserved; **F, H, I, N,** and **O** from Bork K, Brauninger W: *Skin diseases in clinical practice,* ed 2, Philadelphia, 1998, WB Saunders; **J** from Habif TP: *Clinical dermatology: a color guide to diagnosis and therapy,* ed 3, 1996, Mosby; **E,** from Zitelli BJ, Davis HW: *Atlas of pediatric physical diagnosis,* ed 5, Philadelphia, 2007, Mosby.) *Continued*

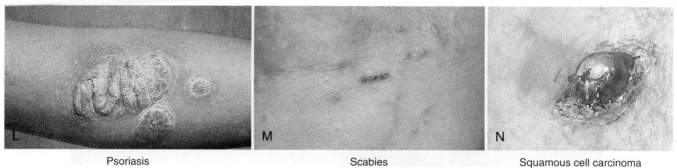

Psoriasis   Scabies   Squamous cell carcinoma

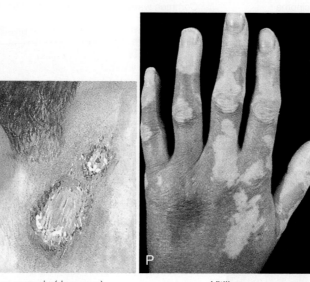

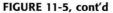

Tinea corporis (ringworm)   Vitiligo

FIGURE 11-5, cont'd

hundred. As blisters itch and break, scabs form and the blisters may become infected by bacteria, which is considered a secondary bacterial infection.

Some individuals may experience fever, abdominal pain, or a vague sick feeling along with their skin blisters. These symptoms usually last for 3 to 5 days, and temperature stays in the range of 101° to 103° F (38.3° to 39.4° C). Younger children often have milder symptoms and fewer blisters than older children or adults. Generally, chicken pox is a mild illness, but it can be deadly in persons who have leukemia or other diseases that weaken the immune system.

Usually a person has only one attack of chicken pox in his or her lifetime. But the virus that causes chicken pox can stay dormant in the body and can cause a different type of skin eruption, called *shingles*, later in life.

Herpes Simplex

Herpes simplex is a viral infection resulting in cold sores or fever blisters on the face or in the mouth (type 1) or around the genitals, thighs, or buttocks (type 2). All the herpes viruses are contagious. As with all herpes viruses, herpes simplex remains dormant in the nerves of the body until resistance is low, at which time it travels down the nerve to cause the eruption. Herpes outbreaks often are preceded by 2 to 3 days of tingling, itching, or pain. Blisters then appear, gradually crust, and disappear, usually within 2 weeks.

Measles

Measles is a serious infection that spreads easily from person to person. It is caused by the measles virus. Symptoms begin 10 to 12 days after contact with an infected person and include fever (often high), fatigue, runny nose, cough, and watery red eyes. After 2 or 3 days, tiny white spots may appear in the mouth, and after 2 more days, a raised, red rash starts on the face and spreads down the body and out to the arms and legs. The rash usually lasts 4 to 7 days. Symptoms usually last from 1 to 2 weeks, and measles is contagious for about 1 week before to 1 week after the rash begins. Serious complications of measles can occur. Those with measles should stay away from others until at least 4 full days have passed since the time the rash first appeared.

Measles is spread from person to person by the droplets issuing from the mouth, nose, and throat of an infected person. The infected droplets spread through the air or directly onto other person's hands and face through coughing and sneezing.

German measles, or rubella, is a mild viral illness caused by the rubella virus. It involves fever and a rash, along with aches in the joints when it affects adults. The major reason to eradicate this virus is the serious effects it has on an unborn baby when a pregnant woman contracts it in early pregnancy.

Children usually are not affected seriously. Commonly, the first manifestation is a fine, pink rash spreading from the forehead and face downward. The rash may last 1 to 5 days. Glands (lymph nodes) are enlarged, especially those behind the ears and on the back of the head. Adults often feel more unwell before the rash appears and may have arthritis-type pain in the joints.

Molluscum Contagiosum

Molluscum contagiosum is a superficial skin infection. The virus invades the skin, causing the appearance of firm, flesh-colored, doughnut-shaped bumps 2 to 5 mm in diameter. Their sunken centers contain a white, curdlike material. The bumps can occur almost anywhere on the body, including the buttocks, thighs, and external genitalia. They often remain unchanged for many months, then disappear.

Molluscum contagiosum is caused by a virus belonging to the poxvirus family. Close physical contact is usually necessary for transmission; indirect transmission through shared towels, swimming pools, and so forth also may be responsible for infection. The incubation period varies from several weeks to several months. Shaving or scratching may cause the infection to spread.

Warts

A wart is a benign growth of the keratin-producing cells of the epidermis and mucous membranes that is caused by the human papillomavirus. Warts are transmitted through direct contact. The common wart (*Verruca vulgaris*) has a rough, elevated surface and is found mainly on the hands and fingers of children and young adults. Filiform warts are longer, slender growths on the face, neck, and axillae. Periungual warts are found around the nails of the fingers and toes. Flat warts are flesh colored and form when several warts spread, through scratching or shaving. Plantar warts have rough surfaces and are located in the thickened skin of the sole of the foot. They may be mistaken for calluses but often have small, dark spots that calluses do not have. Normal skin lines stop at the edge of the wart.

Fungal Skin Infections

Candidiasis

Candidiasis is an infection of the skin or mucous membranes, most often caused by the organism *Candida albicans*. Red, scaly patches may appear in the creases of the axillae and groin and under the breasts, as well as between the fingers and toes. Associated candidal infections can occur in the ear, vagina, and mouth. When it develops in the mouth, it is called *thrush. C. albicans* is a common cause of diaper rash in infants.

Dermatophytosis

More commonly known as *ringworm*, tinea is a group of common fungal infections contracted by touching contaminated items or an infected person's skin. The types of tinea are named by their location on the body. Tinea corporis appears on the nonhairy portions of the skin as fast-growing, reddish, elevated lesions surrounded by a dry and scaly or moist and crusty, raised, ringlike border, which gives it the ringworm appearance. Tinea pedis, or athlete's foot, is marked by blisters

and cracking of the skin between the toes and on the ball of the foot. Tinea cruris, or jock itch, is ringworm of the pubic area.

Parasitic Skin Infections

Lice

Lice are parasites, and three types affect human beings. Head lice (*Pediculosis capitis*) are the most common type. They are found mainly on the scalp and sometimes in the eyebrows and eyelashes, and they cause intense itching. Outbreaks generally occur among schoolchildren. The bite of the body louse (*Pediculosis corporis*) leaves visible, itchy red spots primarily on the shoulders, buttocks, and abdomen. Genital lice (*Pediculosis pubis*; crab lice) usually are found in the pubic area and are transmitted during sexual activity or contact with contaminated bedding.

Scabies

Scabies is a contagious skin disease characterized by intense itching caused by a microscopic, parasitic mite that burrows under the epidermis. Scabies can attack any area of the body, but the parts most susceptible are the finger webs, anterior wrists, elbows, axillary regions, areolae of the breasts, genitals, and lower buttocks. The parasite is transmitted by skin-to-skin contact with human beings or pets or by direct contact with contaminated items.

(Note: Although bed bugs are not technically a skin infection, it might be useful to be familiar with the appearance of their bites.)

Ulcers

An ulcer is a round open sore of the skin or mucous membrane that results from the tissue damage that accompanies inflammation, infection, or malignancy.

Decubitus Ulcer

A decubitus ulcer is an open sore that develops primarily over the bony areas of the heels and hips of those who are immobile, bedridden, or in wheelchairs. Continuous pressure on the skin diminishes or stops circulation, and the tissue dies.

Neurotrophic Ulcer

Neurotrophic ulcers develop at pressure-point areas on the feet when pain sensation is diminished or absent, as in diabetic neuropathy. Although often deep and infected, these ulcers are painless. Callus formation around the ulcer, like the ulcer itself, results from chronic pressure.

Benign Tumors and Growths

A neoplasm or **tumor** is a growth of new tissues that may be benign or malignant. The following are considered benign.

Mole

A mole, or nevus, is a benign pigmented skin growth formed of melanocytes.

Callus

A callus is an area of thickened, hardened skin, like a corn, that develops in an area of friction or a region of recurrent pressure. A callus involves skin that normally is thick, such as the sole of the foot or the palm of the hand, and usually is painless. If a callus is painful, an underlying plantar wart may be present.

Corn

A corn is a painful, conical thickening of skin over bony prominences of the feet caused by continual pressure and friction on normally thin skin. Corns located in moist areas, such as between the toes, are called *soft corns*.

Lipoma

A lipoma is a benign tumor formed of mature fat cells. The tumor appears as a soft, movable subcutaneous nodule that is typically found on the trunk, forearms, or neck.

Sebaceous Cyst

A sebaceous cyst is a slow-growing, benign tumor caused by the blockage of a sebaceous gland. The cyst contains keratin, sebum, and hair follicle cells.

Seborrheic Keratosis

A seborrheic keratosis is a slightly raised skin lesion most commonly seen on the chest, back, neck, and face. These benign growths usually appear in middle-aged and elderly individuals as light brown or black flat areas. They may grow quickly and can be mistaken for moles or warts.

Skin Tag

A skin tag is a small, soft, flesh-colored or pigmented benign growth found on the neck or in the axillary or groin region.

Angioma

An angioma is a benign tumor composed of blood or lymphatic vessels. Angiomas, or angiomata, are common in newborns and usually disappear during childhood.

Malignant Skin Tumors

Skin cancer is the most common of all malignancies. Most skin cancers appear on the head, neck, and other areas frequently exposed to the sun. Too much sun exposure damages the skin by causing the elastin fibers to clump, leading to leathery skin and wrinkling. Immune function may be depressed temporarily, and DNA is altered, leading to skin cancer. Three types of malignancy can occur.

Basal Cell Carcinoma

The most common form of skin cancer, basal cell carcinoma is associated with exposure to ultraviolet light. It grows slowly and is the easiest type to treat successfully when recognized early.

Squamous Cell Carcinoma

Also related to exposure to ultraviolet light, squamous cell carcinoma is responsible for one third of all skin cancers. Like basal cell carcinoma, squamous cell carcinoma is best treated in the earlier stages, before it metastasizes. Persons with fair skin, blond or red hair, and chronic skin inflammation who are exposed to the sun or who suffered sun damage when young are at greater risk for basal cell and squamous cell carcinomas.

Malignant Melanoma

Malignant melanoma is the least common and the most dangerous of the skin cancers. It is not connected directly to sun exposure. Because melanoma spreads rapidly, it must be identified and treated quickly.

The memory device that helps in identifying a melanoma is "ABCD": asymmetry, border irregularity, color change, and increase in diameter. Most melanomas are not evenly round but have irregular borders with white, blue, or red edges turning to brown or black. Moles are especially susceptible to transformation into melanomas.

Breast Disorders

Fibrocystic Disease

Fibrocystic disease is the most common disorder of the breast. The condition involves the growth of small, lumpy cysts that develop because of changes in the milk-producing glands. The disease affects about 50% of women. No treatment is necessary, but because the incidence of breast cancer is higher in these women, health care providers must address recommendations for breast self-examination and the frequency of mammograms for each person.

Breast Cancer

Breast cancer is the second leading cause of cancer death in women (the first is lung cancer). One in eight women in the United States faces the possibility of developing breast cancer. The peak incidence occurs in the early menopausal age group, when some women develop a painless, firm lump, often in the upper outer quadrant. In one form of breast cancer, no lump develops. The diagnosis is made by using low-voltage soft-tissue radiographs called *mammograms* and by performing fine-needle biopsy. The standard medical treatment is based on many factors, including the size of the lump, the patient's age and physical condition, and the involvement of lymph nodes and other tissues. Muscle tissue and lymph nodes are removed when metastasis has occurred.

Surgical intervention consists of one of the following procedures: a lumpectomy (removal of the tumor), a simple mastectomy (removal of the affected breast only), a radical mastectomy (removal of the breast, pectoralis major and pectoralis minor muscles, and the axillary lymph nodes), an extended radical mastectomy (in addition to the aforementioned, removal of the internal mammary lymph nodes near the sternum), or a modified radical mastectomy (removal of the breast and axillary lymph nodes, preserving the pectoralis major muscle). Radiation therapy, chemical therapy (chemotherapy), and hormone therapy are other methods of intervention, which may be used alone or with surgery.

Although the number of men who develop breast cancer is small, lumps and changes in the tissues of a man's breast cannot be ignored, and such clients should be referred to a physician for examination.

Anatomic and Physiologic Problems after a Mastectomy

With removal of the pectoralis major muscle, some flexion and adduction of the arm is lost. The client may develop the anterior part of the deltoid, as well as the coracobrachialis and the long head of the biceps, to help with flexion.

Loss of lymphatic channels in the axillae causes obstruction of lymph flow from the arm, and localized edema develops. Elevation of the arm and use of a special sleeve to provide compression are helpful. Massage may help in mild cases.

Burns

The term *burn* refers to cells that have been destroyed or inflamed because of heat, chemicals, radiation, or electricity. Fluid loss and secondary bacterial infection can occur as a consequence of the tissue damage. Burns are classified by the depth of damage and are identified by degree.

In a first-degree burn, only the epidermis sustains injury. Signs and symptoms include redness, mild stinging or pain, and mild swelling. These burns usually heal within a matter of days or weeks. A mild sunburn is a first-degree burn.

In a second-degree burn, the epidermis and the dermis are damaged. Along with redness and moderate to intense pain and swelling, blisters usually develop. In deeper burns the tissues may be white because of damage to the vascular supply. Second-degree burns can take 6 weeks to a few months to heal and commonly leave scars.

In a third-degree burn, the epidermis and entire dermis are damaged severely or destroyed. Damage to nerves can interrupt pain signals in the actual area of the burn. The skin may appear white, black, or charred, and no blisters form. Dehydration and infection may occur because of the loss of the protective skin barrier. A third-degree burn develops scars and may require a skin graft and a long healing period.

Other Skin Disorders

Dermatitis and Eczema

Dermatitis is a general term for an acute or chronic skin inflammation characterized by redness, eruptions, edema, scaling, and itching. The term *eczema* is used interchangeably with the term *dermatitis*, but many medical references limit the designation *dermatitis* to conditions caused by internal factors. Three major types of dermatitis have been recognized:

1. *Atopic dermatitis:* Caused by an allergy or hypersensitivity, most commonly pollens, cosmetics, or foods. The condition is commonly associated with other hypersensitivity disorders. Symptoms include inflammation, oozing and crusting, and intense itching.
2. *Seborrheic dermatitis:* A chronic condition that manifests in inflammation, scales, and crusting. The skin may be dry or greasy. The adult form of seborrheic dermatitis is a mild form of dandruff, most commonly seen at the eyebrows and on the scalp as a dry or greasy scaling. Cradle cap is the associated childhood form. Genetic predisposition, weather, stress, and some neurologic diseases may be risk factors.
3. *Contact dermatitis:* Caused by sensitivity to a substance that damages or irritates the skin, such as poison ivy, a medication, cosmetics, or rubber. The condition may be marked by blisters or itchy, flaky skin.

Pseudofolliculitis barbae (razor bumps) is a common condition of the beard area that occurs in African-American men and other persons with curly hair. The problem results when highly curved hairs grow back into the skin, causing inflammation and a foreign-body reaction. Over time, this can cause keloidal scarring, which looks like hard bumps on the beard area and neck.

Psoriasis

Psoriasis is a common, noncontagious chronic skin disease characterized by reddened skin covered by dry, silvery scales. It is found most commonly on the scalp, elbows, knees, back, or buttocks.

Rosacea

Rosacea is a noncontagious chronic skin problem in which the small blood vessels of the forehead, cheeks, and nose become dilated. Rosacea may affect a small area or the entire face. Eye inflammation (conjunctivitis) may develop. Rosacea may lie dormant for a time and then be activated by stress, infection, hot or spicy food, sunlight, or physical activity.

Urticaria (Hives)

Urticaria, or hives, is a condition of localized skin eruptions, called *wheals,* in the dermis. Hives are caused by allergy, exposure to heat or cold, or an emotional reaction. Urticaria may be accompanied by local pruritus (itching).

Alopecia

Alopecia is hair loss or baldness on parts or all of the body. Alopecia can be caused by aging, genetic predisposition, local diseases, chemotherapy, stress, or nutritional imbalances. Androgens seem to play a part in hair loss. Male-pattern baldness features hair loss on the forehead and top of the head, whereas female-pattern baldness involves thinning of the hair in the frontal and parietal regions.

Scleroderma

Scleroderma (systemic sclerosis) is an autoimmune disorder of the connective tissue that is characterized by the inflammation and overproduction of collagen. The resulting scarring causes the tissues to stiffen and compress the capillaries, thus diminishing or halting blood flow. The disease usually appears in persons between 30 and 50 years of age and affects women more often than men. Characteristics include increased joint stiffness, muscle weakness, swelling of the fingers, and skin-thickening collagen deposits. Collagen deposits can invade not only the integument but also many of the body systems, such as the gastrointestinal tract, reducing the absorption of nutrients, and the lungs, diminishing respiratory effectiveness. Hypersensitivity to cold in the fingers, toes, ears, and nose, as occurs in Raynaud's syndrome, may be present. In the most serious cases, heart and lung failure may occur.

Vitiligo

Vitiligo is a disease marked by loss of skin pigmentation in irregular patches. Vitiligo usually affects exposed areas of the

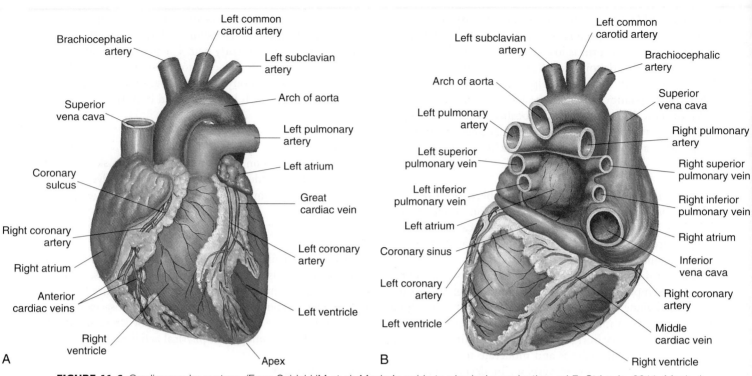

FIGURE 11-6 Cardiovascular system. (From Seidel HM et al: *Mosby's guide to physical examination,* ed 7, St Louis, 2011, Mosby.)

skin in persons under 30 years of age who have a family history of the disease.

INDICATIONS/CONTRAINDICATIONS for Therapeutic Massage

Integumentary System

Therapeutic massage usually is not contraindicated in localized skin conditions, but local (regional) avoidance of the affected area is necessary. Localized touch can irritate most skin disorders. Massage is contraindicated if the skin is inflamed or if the condition is contagious or transmissible through touch.

A wound is any injury to the skin that has not healed and that is vulnerable to infection if exposed to bacteria or other microorganisms. Skin injuries are vulnerable as long as a visible crust or scab remains. Massage is contraindicated locally for any unhealed skin injury in which bleeding has occurred. When the underlying epidermis has been replaced completely, the scab falls off and the wound no longer is at risk for infection. Massage may be contraindicated systemically if the skin injury is connected to a contraindicated underlying condition, such as diabetes.

Standard Precautions are indicated for all skin pathologies. Malignancy is a contraindication unless the appropriate medical personnel supervise the therapy.

CARDIOVASCULAR SYSTEM

SECTION OBJECTIVES

Chapter objective covered in this section:

4. List and describe the components and functions of the cardiovascular system.
5. Identify pathologies of the cardiovascular system and describe indications and contraindications for massage.

After completing this chapter, the student will be able to perform the following:

- List and describe the components of blood.
- Describe the functions of the cardiovascular system.
- Determine massage indications and contraindications for pathologic conditions of the cardiovascular system.

The cardiovascular system is a transport system composed of the heart, blood vessels, and blood (Figure 11-6). The **heart** is the pump that sends the oxygen and nutrient-rich blood out to the body by way of the arteries and **arterioles.** The oxygen and nutrients in the blood leave the capillaries and enter the tissues. Carbon dioxide and metabolic wastes leave the tissues, reenter the capillaries, and pass through the **venules** and **veins** on their way back to the heart. The heart then pumps the blood to the lungs, where carbon dioxide diffuses out of the blood so it can be eliminated from the body. The blood also picks up oxygen and travels back to the heart, where the cycle starts all over again.

Heart

The heart is the major organ of the cardiovascular system (Figure 11-6). The heart is a hollow, muscular pump about the size of a clenched fist located in the mediastinum (the space between the lungs). The heart rests on the diaphragm. The **pericardium** is a sac that surrounds the heart and secretes a lubricating fluid that prevents friction resulting from the movement of the heart. The pericardium also secures the heart within the thoracic cavity.

The myocardium is the heart muscle that makes up the thickest part of the heart. Contractions of the myocardium perform the pumping action of the heart. The outer

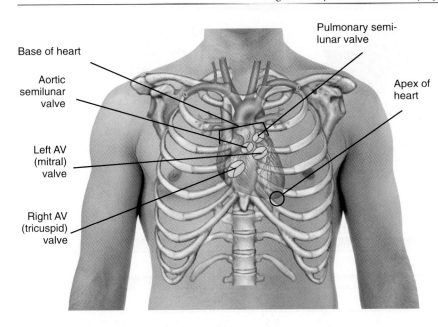

Base of heart

Aortic
semilunar
valve

Left AV
(mitral)
valve

Right AV
(tricuspid)
valve

Pulmonary semi-
lunar valve

Apex of
heart

FIGURE 11-7 Relation of the heart to the anterior wall of the thorax. Valves of the heart are projected on the anterior thoracic wall. *AV,* Atrioventricular. (From Seidel HM et al: *Mosby's guide to physical examination,* ed 7, St Louis, 2011, Mosby.)

membrane of the heart is called the *epicardium* and is continuous with the pericardium. The endocardium is the smooth, thin inner lining of the heart. The blood actually slides along the endocardium as it flows through the heart.

The heart is divided into four chambers. The two small, thin-walled superior chambers are the atria, known separately as the left **atrium** and the right atrium; they are separated by the interatrial septum. The two larger, inferior chambers are the left and right **ventricles;** their thick walls are separated by the interventricular septum. The atria and ventricles are separated by a fibrous structure called the *skeleton* of the heart.

Heart Valves

Created from the folds of the endocardium and maintained within the skeleton of the heart are the **heart valves.** This set of four valves regulates the flow of blood through the heart. Atrioventricular valves allow blood to flow from the atria into the ventricles and keep it from returning back into the atria when the ventricles contract. The ventricles contract quite forcefully, shooting blood upward. Strings of connective tissue known as *chordae tendineae cordis* connect between the ventricle wall and the valves. They keep the cusps, or flaps, of the valve closed when the ventricle contracts to keep the force of the blood from pushing open the valve. This ensures that the blood moves forward into the aorta and pulmonary arteries, not back into the atria. The bicuspid, or mitral (left atrioventricular), valve is located between the left atrium and the left ventricle; the tricuspid (right atrioventricular) valve is located between the right atrium and the right ventricle.

Semilunar valves control the blood flow out of the ventricles into the aorta and pulmonary arteries. They prevent backflow of blood into the ventricles. The aortic valve is between the left ventricle and the aorta, and the pulmonary valve is between the pulmonary **artery** and the right ventricle. These valves open in response to pressure generated when the blood leaves the ventricle. They close when blood pools in small

pockets of the cusps of the valves and pushes the valves closed (Figure 11-7).

Blood Vessels

Arteries carry oxygenated blood away from the heart. The only exceptions are the pulmonary arteries. They carry blood away from the heart to the lungs, but it is deoxygenated blood. Veins carry deoxygenated blood from the body to the heart. The only exceptions are the pulmonary veins. They carry blood to the heart from the lungs, but it is oxygenated blood.

Arteries branch into small vessels called *arterioles.* These enter the tissues and branch into capillaries. Capillaries are the smallest blood vessels. They allow the exchange of gases, nutrients, and waste products between the blood and tissue cells. Capillaries join into venules, which in turn join into veins. Arteries, arterioles, capillaries, venules, and veins are discussed in more detail in the section on the vascular system.

The term *great vessels* refers to the large blood vessels entering or leaving the heart that transport blood to the lungs and the rest of the body. The three great vessels are as follows:

1. *Aorta:* The artery that carries oxygen and nutrients away from the heart to the body
2. *Pulmonary trunk:* The artery that carries blood to the lungs to release carbon dioxide and take in oxygen
3. *Superior vena cava:* The vein that returns deoxygenated blood to the right atrium from the upper venous circulation

Other major blood vessels include the following:

- Inferior vena cava: The vein that returns deoxygenated blood from the lower venous circulation to the right atrium
- Pulmonary veins: The four veins, two from each lung, that take oxygenated blood to the left atrium

Blood Supply to and from the Heart

The two **coronary arteries,** which originate from the base of the aorta, supply oxygenated blood to the heart muscle.

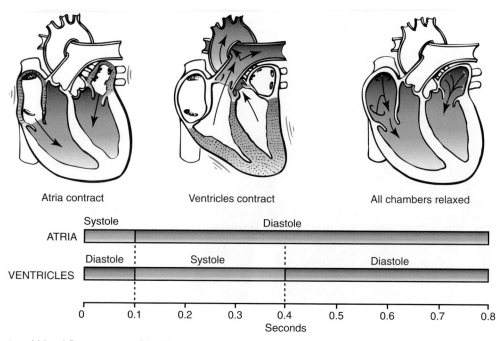

FIGURE 11-8 Heart and blood flow patterns. (Modified from Applegate E: *The anatomy and physiology learning system*, ed 4, St Louis, 2011, Saunders.)

Coronary veins follow parallel to the arteries and return the blood to the right atrium by way of the coronary sinus. Both types of coronary vessels run in grooves between the atria and ventricles and between the two ventricles. All the veins of the heart drain into the coronary sinus, which drains the deoxygenated blood from the heart tissues into the right atrium.

Blood Flow through the Heart

Blood moves into and out of the heart in a well-coordinated and precisely timed rhythm. The rhythm can be divided into the following stages (see Figure 11-8):

Stage 1: Deoxygenated blood from the body enters the superior and inferior venae cavae. Deoxygenated blood from the heart drains into the coronary sinus. All three empty into the right atrium. When the blood reaches a certain volume, it pushes open the tricuspid valve and blood empties into the right ventricle. The right atrium then contracts to squeeze a little more blood into the right ventricle.

Stage 2: The right ventricle contracts and pushes blood through the pulmonary valve into the pulmonary artery. This artery divides into the left and right pulmonary arteries and takes the blood to each lung.

Stage 3: This process takes place at the same time as the process described in stage 1. Four pulmonary veins leave the lungs, carrying oxygenated blood back to the left atrium. When the blood reaches a certain volume, it pushes open the bicuspid (mitral) valve and blood empties into the left ventricle. The left atrium then contracts to squeeze a little more blood into the left ventricle.

Stage 4: This process takes place at the same time as the process described in stage 2. The left ventricle contracts and pushes blood through the aortic valve into the aorta. Arteries branch off the aorta and the descending aorta to carry oxygenated blood to all parts of the body. The myocardium of the left ventricle is much thicker than the myocardium of the right ventricle to provide the extra strength needed to pump blood out into the entire body.

The heart has its own built-in rhythm. Not only can each cardiac cell contract without nerve stimulus, but the heart can contract (for a short time) even if removed from the body. However, the autonomic nervous system does affect the rate of the rhythm and the force of contraction through sympathetic and parasympathetic activation.

As seen in the previous section, both atria contract while both ventricles are relaxed, and when the atria relax, the ventricles contract. This synchronization leads to the sequence of events known as the *cardiac cycle*, which consists of one heartbeat. *Diastole* is the term for relaxation, and *systole* is the term for contraction. Therefore the ventricles are in diastole when the atria are in systole, and the atria are in diastole when the ventricles are in systole. Because the myocardium of the ventricles is much thicker than the myocardium of the atria, the heartbeat felt is ventricular systole.

The heart rate is identified by the number of cardiac cycles that occur in 1 minute. The average healthy person has 60 to 70 cycles, or beats, per minute.

Conduction System of the Heart

The coordinated rhythm of the heart is initiated by a built-in electrical system called the *conduction system of the heart*. The sinoatrial node, located in the right atrium, sets the pace of the heart rate. A nerve impulse originates in the sinoatrial node and travels to the left atrium, causing the atria to contract. At the precise moment the atria have completed their contraction, the signal travels through the atrioventricular bundle, located in the interventricular septum, to the right ventricle and into the left ventricle, causing the ventricles to contract. The rhythm can be checked by an electrocardiogram (ECG), which monitors the electrical changes in the heart. A portable ECG machine, known as a *Holter monitor*, can measure the heart signals over 24 hours. If difficulty with the electrical system develops in the sinoatrial node, physicians can implant a device known as a *pacemaker* to assist or take over the initiation of the signal.

Heart Sounds

Heart sounds can be heard through a stethoscope. These heart sounds are caused by closure of the heart valves. Valves usually are quiet as they open. Closure of the valves produces two main sounds. The first is a low-pitched "lubb" generated by blood turbulence as the mitral and tricuspid valves close. The second is a higher-pitched "dubb" caused by blood turbulence as the aortic and pulmonary valves close. Extra sounds, such as those resulting from faulty valves, are referred to as *murmurs*.

Blood Volume and Flow

Cardiac output is the amount of blood pumped by the left ventricle in 1 minute. The average output under normal conditions is 5 to 6 liters of blood. To pump more oxygen and nutrients to the cells during exercise and in times of stress, output may rise to 20 liters or more. The output increases because the heart beats faster and stronger. The speed of the blood flow is fastest in arteries and moderate in veins. The slowest blood movement is in the capillaries to allow for the exchange of nutrients and waste products between tissues and blood.

Entrainment

Entrainment is the coordination or synchronization with a rhythm (see Chapter 2). Research at the Institute of Heart-Math and other facilities indicates that the heart rhythm tends to be the guide that the other body rhythms follow. The heart rate, respiratory rate, and thalamus synchronization combine to support the entrainment process, and the other, more subtle body rhythms follow. Most meditation processes and relaxation methods create an environment in which this entrainment can occur.

The heart is considered the seat of love and the home of emotions relating to relationships. The heart is the symbol of love on Valentine's Day cards. We speak of how a person's heart can be broken by loss and grief. We have lost heart when we give up hope. We have a big heart when we are compassionate and nurturing. Is it possible that the strong rhythm of the heart, of which we can easily become conscious, also brings us awareness of how experience affects us? The heart's rate and strength of contraction can change in a moment in response to the demands of life. Living with awareness of our hearts is a way to live with awareness of our responses to experience.

Vascular System

The vascular system is the other part of the cardiovascular system. It consists of blood vessels that carry blood from the heart to the lungs and body tissues and back to the heart in a continuous cycle. As discussed previously in the section on blood vessels, a blood vessel that transports blood from the heart is called an *artery*. Arteries eventually branch off into smaller and smaller arteries, the smallest of which are called *arterioles*. A **capillary** is one of the tiny blood vessels located between the arterioles and the venules, the smallest of the veins. The veins get larger and larger as they get closer to the heart. The largest veins return blood to the right atrium of the heart (Figure 11-9).

Arteries

The body has three types of arteries:

1. Elastic arteries are the large arteries capable of undergoing passive stretching. They have thick walls that contain a great deal of elastic tissue. They recoil when the ventricles relax, which maintains the pressure necessary to move the blood. The aorta and pulmonary artery are elastic arteries.

2. Muscular arteries constitute most of the arteries in the body. These are small to medium-sized arteries that distribute blood to all tissues by contracting or dilating to control blood flow. Located between the elastic layers are many smooth muscle cells and some collagen. Although the walls of muscular arteries are distensible to a certain extent, as they become smaller and smaller with each successive branching, the amount of elastic tissue decreases and the amount of smooth muscle increases. Muscular arteries vary in size from about 1 cm in diameter close to their origin at the elastic arteries to about 0.5 mm in diameter. Muscular arteries are composed almost entirely of smooth muscle. The larger arteries may have 30 or more layers of smooth muscle cells, whereas the smallest peripheral arteries have only 2 or 3 layers. These arteries are highly contractile; the degree of their contraction and relaxation is controlled by the autonomic nervous system and by endothelium-derived vasoactive substances. A few fine elastic fibers are scattered among the smooth muscle cells but are not organized into sheets. These are most numerous in the large muscular arteries, which are a direct continuation of the distal end of the elastic arteries.

3. Arterioles are the smallest branches of the arterial tree. Arterioles vary in diameter ranging from 30 μm (0.03 mm) to 400 μm (0.4 mm). Any artery smaller than 0.5 mm in diameter is considered to be an arteriole. The arterioles offer considerable resistance to blood flow because of their small radius. This resistance has several functions. First, together with the elastic arteries, the resistance converts the pulsing ejection of blood from the heart into a steady flow through the capillaries; the arterioles constrict and dilate to control the amount of blood entering the capillaries. Second, if no resistance was present and a high pressure persisted into the capillaries, a considerable loss of blood volume into the tissue would occur through the movement of the fluid across the capillary wall and around the cells. The arterioles are also important in determining the blood supply to various tissues and regions.

Capillaries (Microvasculature)

Capillaries are small-diameter blood vessels with thin, partially permeable walls that permit the diffusion of substances through them. This is how nutrients, oxygen, ions, and other

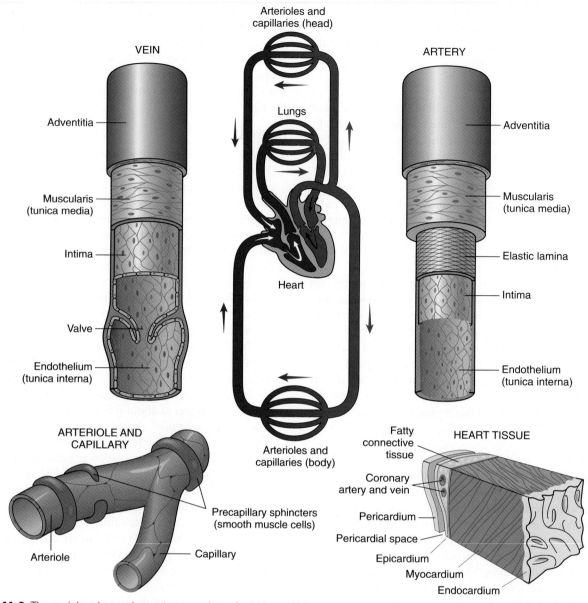

FIGURE 11-9 The peripheral vascular system consists of arteries, which carry oxygenated blood (red), and capillaries and veins, which carry deoxygenated blood (blue). The thick wall of the arteries is composed of distinct layers of smooth muscle cells and elastic laminae that separate these layers. In comparison, the veins have much thinner walls. The walls of the capillaries consist of a single layer of endothelium. The cross-section of the heart tissue is included for comparison. (From Damjanov I: *Pathology for the health-related professions*, ed 4, Philadelphia, 2012, Saunders.)

Practical Application

The massage therapist may be able to increase arterial blood flow in two ways. First, stimulating sympathetic autonomic functions increases the heart rate, providing more push to the blood in the arteries. The action is a reflexive, indirect method that involves the use of homeostatic mechanisms to maintain balance. Massage can be structured so that it is stimulating to the sympathetic autonomic nervous system. In general, the methods used are brisk and involve active contraction of the muscles, which increases the client's respiratory rate.

Second, the massage therapist may be able to increase arterial blood flow mechanically through the pump-and-tube mechanism of the cardiovascular system, which functions in the same way as the fluid dynamics of hydraulics. Arteries are pliable muscular tubes that carry blood (a fluid) under pressure from the heart pump. Crimping or closing causes pressure to build up between the pump (the heart) and the barrier, like water

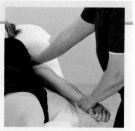

behind a dam. With removal of the barrier, the buildup of pressure provides an initial extra push to the fluid. Compression over more superficial arteries to close off the flow of blood temporarily results in the same phenomenon. Back pressure builds, and on release of the compression the blood pushes forward with more force than would have been available from the heart action alone. The massage therapist applies compression against the arteries in the legs and arms to assist peripheral circulation. The rhythm of compression and release is a rate of approximately 60 beats per minute, to coincide with the heart rhythm. The increase in blood flow is temporary, and in healthy individuals with adequate blood flow, the effect may be negligible (Figures 11-10 and 11-11).

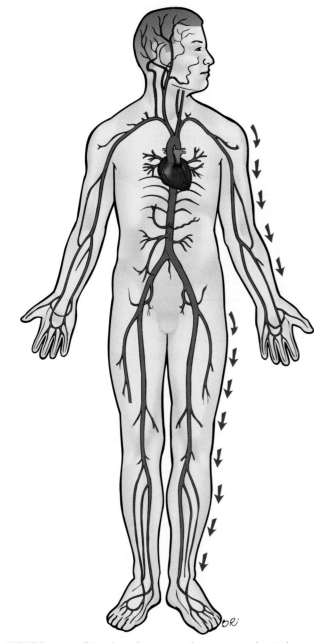

FIGURE 11-10 Direction of compression over arteries to increase arterial flow. (From Fritz S: *Mosby's fundamentals of therapeutic massage,* ed 5, St Louis, 2013, Mosby.)

molecules move from the blood into tissue cells, and how wastes, carbon dioxide, cell products such as hormones, and other molecules move from the cells into the blood.

The smallest vessels of the circulatory system, capillaries form a complex interlinking network. Specialized regions near the junctions between the terminal (smallest) arterioles and the capillaries, known as *precapillary sphincters,* consist of a few smooth muscle cells arranged circularly. Relaxed sphincters allow the capillary beds distal to the sphincters to be open and full of blood, partially constricted sphincters reduce blood flow to the capillaries, and fully contracted sphincters allow no blood flow.

The efficient exchange between capillary blood and the surrounding tissue fluid occurs because the capillaries are so

numerous and so small that the blood within them flows at its slowest rate, which ensures the maximum contact time between blood and tissue. This flow of blood through the capillary bed is referred to as the *microcirculation.*

Some tissues have a much more abundant network of capillaries than others. For example, dense connective tissue has a poor capillary network compared with cardiac tissue or that of the kidneys and liver.

Capillary networks drain into a series of venules and veins that have increasingly larger diameters.

Arteriovenous shunts, or arteriovenous anastomoses are direct connections between the arterial and venous systems that bypass the capillary beds. These short connecting vessels have strongly developed muscular control and are directed by the sympathetic nervous system. They are found in many tissues and organs; for example, in the skin these connections enable cutaneous blood flow to increase so as to allow the dissipation of heat from the body surfaces.

Practical Application

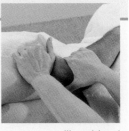

The massage practitioner can use compression and kneading to encourage the movement of blood through the capillaries. Research evidence does support the effect of massage on local capillary circulation. The mechanical forces created by massage support the exchange between capillary blood and the surrounding tissue fluid, somewhat like what happens when a sponge is squeezed.

Veins

The venous system acts as a collecting system, returning blood from the capillary networks to the heart passively, as blood flows down a pressure gradient (Figure 11-12). The capillaries merge to form venules, which in turn unite to form larger but fewer veins, which eventually converge into the venae cavae. Some of the superficial veins in the hands and arms are visible, but they all empty into the deeper veins that usually are found near arteries.

The walls of veins consist of the same three layers found in the arteries, but with less smooth muscle. In general, the walls of veins are thinner and more expandable than those of arteries. Veins have a relatively large diameter (the venae cavae are 2 to 3 cm in diameter) and thus offer low resistance to blood flow. Some veins, especially in the arms and legs, have internal folds in the endothelial lining that form valves. These valves prevent backflow of blood, allowing it to flow only *toward* the heart. The veins of the legs contain more valves than the veins of the arms because they must fight the effects of gravity and prevent blood from pooling in the feet. Long periods of high venous pressures can damage these valves by overstretching them; this occurs during pregnancy and in persons who stand for extended periods. The valves become weak and lose their ability to function; varicose veins develop and may lead to edema and varicose ulcers.

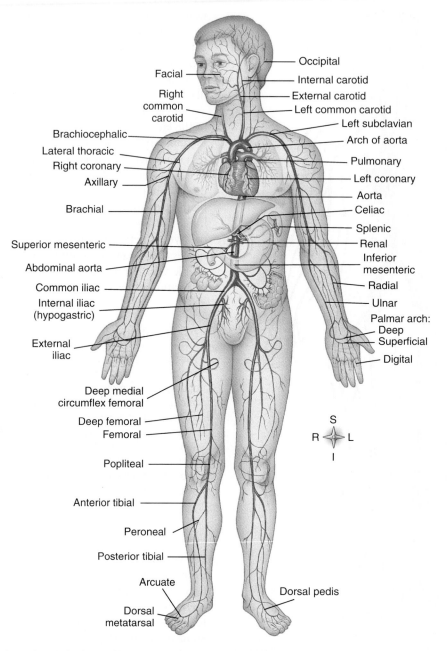

FIGURE 11-11 Principal arteries of the body. (From Thibodeau GA, Patton KT: *Anatomy and physiology,* ed 6, St Louis, 2006, Mosby.)

As much as 75% of the body's total blood volume is contained in the venous system, so veins sometimes are referred to as "capacity vessels." The capacity of the venous system can be modified by altering the lumen size of the venules and veins, which is accomplished by changing the venomotor tone (the degree of smooth muscle contraction in the vein). Venomotor tone is controlled predominantly by the sympathetic nervous system, and changes in the venomotor tone increase or decrease the capacity of the venous circulation. Therefore they can compensate partially for variations in the effective circulating blood volume.

Venous Return

Venous blood flow occurs along pressure gradients, and even small variations in resistance and vessel size affect the flow.

The effect of gravity slows venous return. When a person is upright, blood tends to collect in the feet and legs because the veins are more distended and because of the hydrostatic pressure of blood in the veins below the level of the heart. The leg veins take on a more circular diameter that provides greater capacity. When a person is horizontal, the veins take on a more elliptical diameter that provides less capacity. Increasing the venomotor tone, which reduces the diameter and hence the capacity of the veins, helps reduce venous pooling. This pooling is not blood stagnation; rather, it indicates that the veins are accommodating a greater volume of blood.

Maintaining adequate venous return to the heart at all times is vital because cardiac output is determined by venous return, which is considered cardiac input. In most instances the cardiac output equals the venous return. Thus if the

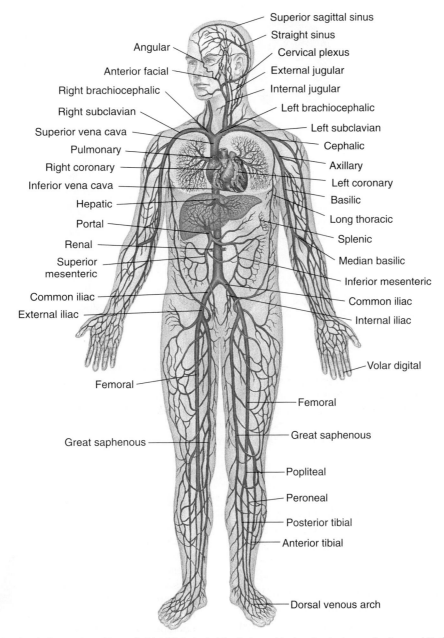

FIGURE 11-12 Systemic circulation: veins. (From Seidel HM et al: *Mosby's guide to physical examination,* ed 7, St Louis, 2011, Mosby.)

venous return falls, cardiac output and blood pressure also may drop. There are several mechanisms that help maintain the venous return at all times. Increasing the venomotor tone is an important mechanism because it decreases the capacity of the venous system and so aids in increasing venous return. After a long period of bed rest when the veins have not had to compensate, venomotor tone is reduced, and this method of reducing the effects of gravity is temporarily less efficient. The practitioner should remember this when helping someone up from a massage session. Move the client slowly and steadily and support the person in case he or she becomes dizzy or feels faint.

Two additional systems, sometimes referred to as the "skeletal muscle pump" and the "respiratory pump," also assist venous return. Skeletal muscle contraction, especially in the limbs, squeezes the veins and pushes blood in the extremities toward the heart; the numerous valves prevent backflow. Many communicating channels also allow the emptying of blood from the superficial veins of the limbs into the deep veins when rhythmic muscular contractions occur. Consequently, every time a person moves the legs or tenses the muscles, these actions push a certain amount of blood toward the heart. The more frequent and powerful such rhythmic contractions are, the more efficient their action. Sustained continuous muscle contractions, unlike rhythmic contractions, impede blood flow because of continuous blocking of the veins. When an individual stands still for long periods of time, muscle pumping decreases and venous return decreases. The result is fainting as the result of inadequate cerebral blood flow. When standing still for long periods, it is advisable to contract the muscles of the legs and buttocks periodically to encourage venous return.

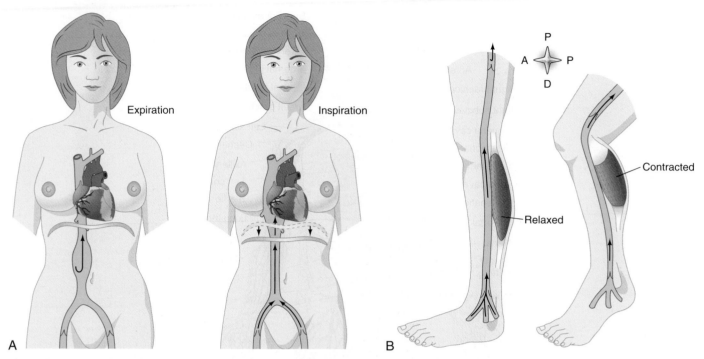

FIGURE 11-13 Venous pumping mechanisms. **A,** The respiratory pump operates by alternately decreasing thoracic pressure during inspiration (thus pulling venous blood into the central veins) and increasing pressure in the thorax during expiration (thus pushing central venous blood into the heart). **B,** The skeletal muscle pump operates by the alternate increase and decrease in peripheral venous pressure that normally occurs when the skeletal muscles are used for the activities of daily living. Both pumping mechanisms rely on the presence of semilunar valves in the veins to prevent backflow during the low-pressure points in the pumping cycle. (From Thibodeau GA, Patton KT: *Anatomy and physiology,* ed 6, St Louis, 2007, Mosby.)

Respiration produces variations in intrapleural and intrathoracic pressure. Each inspiration lowers the pressure in the thorax and the right atrium of the heart. It also increases the pressure gradient, helping blood to flow back to the heart. At the same time, the movement of the diaphragm into the abdomen raises the intraabdominal pressure and increases the gradient to the thorax, again promoting venous return. With expiration the pressure gradients reverse, and blood tends to flow in the opposite direction; the valves in the medium-sized veins prevent this.

Maintaining adequate circulating blood volume also is necessary. If the blood volume is depleted for some reason, such as with dehydration or hemorrhage, the body increases the effective circulating volume in the short term by means of venoconstriction and vasoconstriction in the blood reservoirs of the body, such as the skin, liver, lungs, and spleen. More blood is then available to flow to the other organs. However, fluid replacement is eventually necessary to restore the blood volume. The pressures in the central regions of the venous system directly reflect the blood volume. Thus central venous pressure, or right atrial pressure, is a good indicator of blood volume, unlike arterial pressures, which are regulated and controlled reflexively (Figure 11-13).

Pulse and Blood Pressure

Blood forced into the aorta during systole sets up a pressure wave that travels along the arteries and expands the arterial wall. This expansion can be palpated by pressing the artery

Practical Application

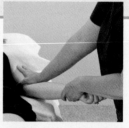

The practitioner can incorporate the principles affecting venous return into massage by using approaches that encourage venous return flow:

- Muscular pump: Rhythmic contraction and relaxation of the muscles during movement encourages venous return flow. Restoring normal muscle function and reducing muscle tension supports venous return flow.
- Gravity: Positioning the limbs higher than the heart passively assists venous return flow.
- Respiratory pump: Slow, deep diaphragmatic breathing enhances venous return flow.
- Massage application: Stroking over the veins toward the heart passively moves the blood in the veins. This method is particularly effective in the limbs. The practitioner can encourage rhythmic contraction of the muscles by having the person move his or her limbs through a complete range of motion against movement resistance in a contract-and-relax rhythm of approximately 60 cycles per minute. The therapist then applies short strokes (1 or 2 inches long) over the veins, stroking toward the heart with sufficient pressure to move the blood in the superficial veins. At the same time, the therapist places the client's limbs in a supported position above the heart so that gravity can help the return flow. The client should be encouraged to relax and breathe deeply (Figure 11-14).

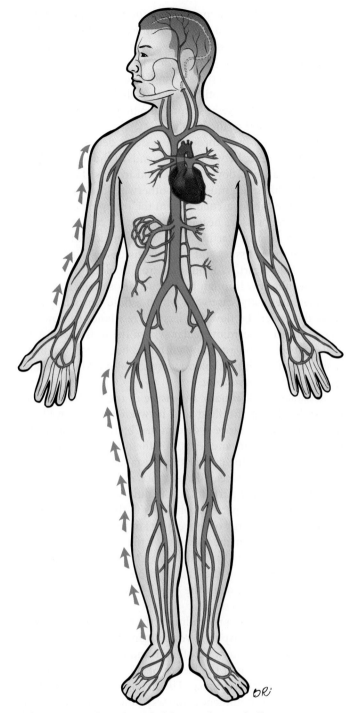

FIGURE 11-14 Direction of gliding strokes to facilitate venous flow. (From Fritz S: *Mosby's fundamentals of therapeutic massage,* ed 5, St Louis, 2013, Mosby.)

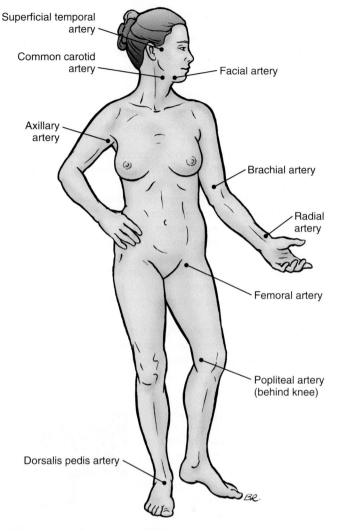

FIGURE 11-15 Pulse points. Each pulse point is named after the artery with which it is associated.

against tissue. The number of waves is known as the *pulse,* which is a direct reflection of the heart rate. The pulse rate, measured when a person is at rest, may be regular or irregular, strong or weak. An irregular pulse occurs commonly with atrial fibrillation and premature contractions. A strong pulse occurs with hyperthyroidism; a weak one with shock and myocardial infarction. A resting heart rate greater than 100 beats per minute is known as *tachycardia;* a heart rate less than 50 or 60 beats per minute is known as *bradycardia* (Figure 11-15).

The amount of pressure exerted by the blood on the walls of the blood vessels is called **blood pressure.** The higher pressure, called *systolic pressure,* occurs when the ventricles contract. The lower pressure, called *diastolic pressure,* occurs when the ventricles relax. Blood pressure is measured with a sphygmomanometer, a cloth-covered rubber bag that is wrapped around the arm over the brachial artery.

Sympathetic nerves in the arterioles regulate blood pressure. Normally, arterioles are in a state of partial constriction called *arteriole tone.* Stimulation of the sympathetic system causes further arteriolar constriction and an increase in blood pressure. Nonstimulation results in a decrease in blood pressure. With hypertension the sympathetic system is in a state of continuous stimulation, resulting in constant high blood pressure.

As the vessels become more and more remote from the heart, the systolic and diastolic pressures equalize. As the vessels change from arteries to arterioles to capillaries to venules to veins, the pressure decreases until, in the large veins, the pressure may be zero or negative. For this reason it is necessary to pull back on the syringe when drawing venous blood.

Blood pressure depends on the person's size.

The average newborn has a blood pressure of 90/60.

At 15 years of age, the average blood pressure is approximately 120/60.

An average, healthy young adult has a blood pressure less than 120/80.

A blood pressure with a systolic reading of less than 90 is considered hypotension.

A pressure of 120/80 or higher is considered prehypertension.

A pressure of 140/90 or higher is considered stage I, or mild, hypertension.

A pressure of 160/100 or higher is considered stage II, or moderate to severe, hypertension.

The blood pressure changes under various conditions, and a single reading should never be used as a final determinant.

A systolic increase occurs under temporary conditions such as anxiety and exercise.

Hypertension involves an increase in the systolic and diastolic pressures.

Hypotension is a decrease in the systolic and diastolic pressures and is an important manifestation of shock, which results from an inadequate blood supply to vital organs.

Practical Application

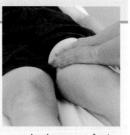

The practitioner can monitor the pulses during assessment of the client. In general, the pulses should feel bilaterally equal. Should the practitioner note differences, he or she should refer the client for diagnosis. The pulse rate ranges from 50 to 70 beats per minute at rest. A rate much slower or faster indicates the need for referral. If the general intent of the therapy session is stress management focused on relaxation and parasympathetic predominance, the pulse rate should slow somewhat over the duration of the session. The opposite is true if the goal is increased arousal of the sympathetic system to energize the client. Many Asian medical practices use the pulse in assessing the meridian system, a form of diagnosis that takes years to perfect.

A blood pressure reading is the number of millimeters of mercury (mm Hg) displaced by the changes in pressure. The first number is the systolic pressure, and the second number is the diastolic pressure. When recording the pressure, only the numbers are written; "mm Hg" usually is dropped (Box 11-1).

Hydrostatic Pressure

All fluids in a confined space exert pressure. The term *hydrostatic pressure* refers to the force a liquid exerts against the walls of its container, as in the pressure blood exerts in the vascular system (the blood pressure). Pascal's principle states that if pressure is exerted on a confined fluid, the pressure is transmitted equally in all directions. The flexibility of the container, as with veins, influences the hydrostatic pressure. If the

container is flexible, the pressure in the fluid is lower than it is in a rigid container. If a weak point exists in the wall of the container and the pressure exerted is great enough, the container wall may break. This is what happens when an aneurysm bursts. In a hypertensive individual the blood vessels harden (undergo sclerotic changes called **arteriosclerosis**), which prevents the vessels from bursting as a result of the increased pressure of the blood.

The flow of a fluid through a vessel is determined by the pressure difference between the two ends of the vessel and also by the resistance to flow. For any fluid to flow along a vessel, a pressure difference must exist; otherwise, the fluid will not move. In the cardiovascular system the pumping of the heart generates the pressure head, or force, and a continuous drop in pressure occurs, starting in the left ventricle of the heart and going to the tissues and from the tissues back to the right atrium of the heart. Without this drop in blood pressure, no blood would flow through the circulatory system. Resistance is a measure of the ease with which a fluid flows through a tube: the easier the flow, the less the resistance to flow, and vice versa. In the cardiovascular system the resistance usually is described as the *vascular resistance,* because it originates mainly in the peripheral blood vessels; it also is known simply as the *peripheral resistance.*

Resistance is essentially a measure of the friction between the molecules of the fluid and between the tube wall and the fluid. The resistance is determined by the viscosity of the fluid and the radius and length of the tube. The smaller the radius of a vessel, the greater the resistance to the movement of particles. This increased resistance results from a greater probability that the particles of the fluid will collide with the vessel wall. When a particle collides with the wall, some of the kinetic energy (energy of movement) of the particle is lost on impact, resulting in the slowing of the particle. Thus, in a vessel that has a smaller diameter, a greater number of collisions occur, reducing the energy content and speed of the particles moving through the vessel. The result is a decrease in the hydrostatic pressure.

Small alterations in the radius of the blood vessels, particularly of the more peripheral vessels, can influence the flow of blood. Changes in the walls of large and medium-sized arteries cause narrowing of the lumen of the vessels and result in increased vascular resistance. The nature of the lining of the tube or vessel also influences the way fluids flow. If the lining of the blood vessel is smooth, the fluid flows evenly because there is less friction; this is known as *streamlined,* or *laminar, flow.* However, if the lining is rough or uneven, friction increases. The fluid itself can flow irregularly. In both cases the fluid flows turbulently. Laminar flow is characteristic of most parts of the vascular system and is silent, whereas turbulent flow is audible, such as during blood pressure measurements with a sphygmomanometer.

Viscosity of the Fluid

Viscosity is a measure of the tendency of a liquid to resist flow. The greater the viscosity (thickness) of a fluid, the greater the force required to move that liquid. For example, water has less viscosity than a milkshake.

Normally, the viscosity of blood remains constant, but in polycythemia, in which the red cell content is high, the viscosity of the blood can be considerably greater, reducing the blood flow. Severe dehydration, in which loss of plasma occurs, and cooling of the blood also can lead to increased viscosity.

Medulla and Baroreceptors

In the medulla of the brain, the cells of the reticular formation regulate three vital signs: heart rate, blood pressure, and respiration. They work with signals from the various nerve centers in the body. One type of nerve center in the cardiovascular system is the baroreceptor.

Baroreceptors are stretch receptors in the carotid arteries, the aorta, and nearly every large artery of the neck and thorax. When blood pressure increases, arteries stretch. The baroreceptors transmit signals about sudden, brief changes in blood pressure, such as when we change position. When blood pressure is elevated for a long period, the baroreceptor reflex resets to the new blood pressure level.

When blood pressure suddenly drops, the frequency of signals from the baroreceptors declines. This change sets off a response in the cardioregulatory center of the medulla that increases sympathetic stimulation and decreases parasympathetic stimulation, resulting in an increase in the heart rate and blood pressure. Conversely, when blood pressure increases, the signal increases, and the medulla changes its output to slow the heart rate and blood pressure by increasing parasympathetic signals. This is another example of how a negative feedback system works in the body.

Practical Application

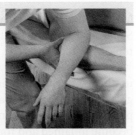

Stress management programs include methods of movement and moderate aerobic exercise, stretching programs, massage, and other forms of soft-tissue methods. Although these approaches initially elevate blood pressure, when continued, they activate parasympathetic quieting responses, such as slow, deep breathing and progressive relaxation. Therefore they tend to have a normalizing effect on the blood pressure. These methods are classified as nonspecific constitutional approaches; they allow the homeostatic mechanisms to reset to a more effective pattern after disruption.

Names of Specific Arteries and Veins

The names of most arteries and veins are derived from the anatomic structures they serve. The femoral artery and the femoral vein, for example, are found close to the femur, where these blood vessels serve the tissues of the upper and lower legs. The renal artery is so named because it exits the abdominal aorta and enters the kidney. The renal vein exits the kidney and enters the inferior vena cava. Arteries and veins are found on both sides of the body and are identified as right or left (e.g., the right common carotid artery, the left common carotid artery).

Practical Application

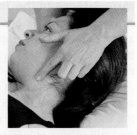

Stimulation of baroreceptors during therapeutic massage could affect blood pressure. The blood pressure could drop, and the client may be lightheaded and show other signs of low blood pressure. It is important to monitor the client for signs of being lightheaded, dizzy, or faint. You may be able to reduce the potential of dizziness and lightheadedness that occur with low blood pressure by instructing the client to move slowly as he or she changes position. After a massage, instruct the client to breathe deeply for a few minutes and then slowly sit up before standing. Should a client become dizzy while standing, have him or her cross the thighs in a scissors fashion and squeeze them together or put one foot on a ledge or chair and lean as far forward as possible. These maneuvers encourage blood to flow from the legs to the heart.

The following is a list of the main arteries and veins. Many of them change names as they enter into and pass through certain areas of the body. Use the illustrations to trace the locations of these vessels (see Figures 11-11 and 11-12).

Arteries

Main Arteries of the Head and Neck
The arch of the aorta gives rise to three arteries; from right to left, they are the brachiocephalic (or innominate) artery, the left common carotid artery, and the left subclavian artery. The subclavian artery supplies the upper extremities.

The brachiocephalic artery, a short artery, becomes the right common carotid artery and the right subclavian artery.

The common carotid arteries branch at the level of the upper part of the thyroid cartilage to become the external and internal carotid arteries. The common carotid artery is an important pulse-taking artery; damage to this artery may result in a transient ischemic attack. The internal carotid artery supplies the brain; the external carotid artery supplies the face, head, and neck.

The superficial temporal artery is the cranial termination of the external carotid artery. The superficial temporal artery is a pulse-taking artery located superior and anterior to the ear.

The two vertebral arteries become the basilar artery, which helps supply the brain.

Main Arteries of the Upper Extremities
The subclavian artery becomes the axillary artery at the clavicle.

Near the head of the humerus, the axillary artery becomes the brachial artery. The brachial artery is the main artery for measuring blood pressure and is also a pulse-taking artery.

The brachial artery divides at the elbow region into the ulnar and radial arteries.

The ulnar artery lies deep and medial. The radial artery lies more superficial and lateral. Both arteries communicate in the hand by way of two deep interconnected vessels called *anastomoses* and a superficial and a deep palmar arch.

Main Arteries of the Trunk

After supplying the head, neck, and upper extremities, the aorta descends posteriorly as the thoracic aorta, sending branches to the intercostal muscles as the right and left intercostal arteries.

The intercostal arteries anastomose anteriorly with the left and right internal thoracic arteries. If the aorta is damaged, the intercostal muscles, which are important for breathing, may still receive a blood supply by way of the internal thoracic arteries.

Main Arteries of the Abdomen

When the thoracic aorta penetrates the diaphragm, it is known as the *abdominal aorta,* which supplies the abdominal organs. The following structures, listed in a cranial to caudal direction, are the main branches of the abdominal aorta.

- Celiac trunk: Supplies the stomach, spleen, and liver by way of the gastric, splenic, and hepatic arteries
- Superior mesenteric artery: Supplies the small intestine, part of the pancreas, and half of the colon
- Renal arteries: Supply the kidneys
- Testicular or ovarian arteries: Supply the gonads
- Inferior mesenteric artery: Supplies the remaining half of the colon to the rectum

The abdominal aorta then divides into the left and right common iliac arteries. The common iliac divides into the internal iliac artery, which supplies the pelvic organs, and the external iliac artery.

Main Arteries of the Lower Extremities

After passing under the inguinal ligament, the external iliac artery becomes the femoral artery. The femoral artery lies superficially at the femoral triangle and then descends posteriorly through the adductor muscles. The femoral artery is an important pulse-taking artery. When the femoral artery emerges behind the knee in the popliteal region, it becomes the popliteal artery. The popliteal artery then divides to become the anterior and posterior tibial arteries.

The anterior tibial artery becomes the dorsalis pedis artery on the dorsal aspect of the foot. The dorsalis pedis is an important pulse-taking artery.

The posterior tibial artery descends behind the medial malleolus and is also a pulse-taking artery but usually is more difficult to find than the dorsalis pedis.

Veins

Main Veins of the Head and Neck

The following are veins of the head and neck:

- Superficial: The right and left external jugular veins drain blood from the face, head, and neck. Each external jugular vein empties into a subclavian vein.
- Deep: Venous drainage from the brain is accomplished by the internal jugular veins. Each internal jugular vein joins a subclavian vein to form a brachiocephalic vein.

Main Veins of the Upper Extremities

Superficial veins originate on the dorsum of the hand as the dorsal venous plexus. They curve around the wrist to the ventral side as the cephalic vein, which runs along the lateral aspect of the forearm and arm, goes deep at the deltoid muscle; the basilic vein, which runs along the medial aspect of the forearm and arm, goes deep at the biceps muscle. The medial cubital vein is an anastomosis between the basilic and cephalic veins.

The deep veins form from branches in the hand and forearm. Although sometimes an individual has a short brachial vein, most often the first main deep vein is the axillary vein. The axillary vein becomes the subclavian vein when it passes under the clavicle.

Main Veins of the Trunk

The subclavian vein joins the internal jugular vein to become the brachiocephalic vein. The subclavian vein is an important central vein for intravenous infusion.

Two brachiocephalic veins join to become the superior vena cava, which empties into the right atrium.

The azygos system, which lies on the posterior body wall, drains the intercostal veins. The azygos vein empties into the superior vena cava.

The inferior vena cava drains blood from the abdominal viscera into the right atrium. The digestive organs and spleen first drain into the portal vein, which empties into the liver. The following veins, listed from cranial to caudal, are branches of the inferior vena cava:

- Hepatic veins from the liver
- Right and left renal veins from the kidneys
- Right and left testicular or ovarian veins from the gonads
- Two common iliac veins (the continuation of the femoral veins)

Main Veins of the Lower Extremities

Superficial veins of the leg begin as a dorsal venous arch on top of the foot.

The great saphenous vein ascends medially from the foot up the leg to the thigh and drains into the femoral vein. The great saphenous veins may become chronically dilated in some persons and develop into varicose veins. They then may become inflamed and form blood clots, a condition known as *thrombophlebitis.*

The small saphenous vein runs laterally from the foot along the gastrocnemius muscle and drains into the popliteal vein.

The anterior tibial vein and posterior tibial vein drain into the popliteal vein.

The popliteal vein becomes the femoral vein after it passes the knee. The deep veins of the leg may become inflamed, a condition referred to as *deep vein thrombosis,* which is a more serious condition than superficial thrombophlebitis. The clot may break off and travel to the heart and then lodge in the lung as a pulmonary embolism (see Figure 11-12).

Hepatic Portal System

A portal system is one in which blood drains from one venous system into another without arteries in between. This occurs between the hypothalamus and pituitary gland, which is how hormones from the hypothalamus travel to the pituitary gland. Another portal system is in the abdomen between the digestive tract and the liver.

The hepatic portal system begins in the capillaries of organs of the digestive tract and ends in the portal vein. The splenic vein and the superior mesenteric vein anastomose to form the portal vein. The inferior mesenteric vein typically joins with the splenic vein at some point along its course deep to the pancreas. The portal vein is deep to the proper hepatic artery and common bile duct and runs within the free right edge of the lesser omentum. This set of three structures—the hepatic artery, bile duct, and portal vein—is called the *hepatic triad.* The portal veins enter the liver and become smaller and smaller until reaching the second venous capillary bed, called the *sinusoids* of the liver. Portal blood contains substances absorbed by the stomach and intestines. As this blood passes through the liver, the liver cells absorb, excrete, or convert nutrients and toxins.

Once filtered, the blood passes into the central vein, which is the beginning of the second venous system. This venous system is filled with progressively larger veins known as *hepatic veins.* The hepatic veins eventually drain the filtered blood through the three large hepatic veins. Restriction of outflow through the hepatic portal system can lead to portal hypertension. Portal hypertension most often is associated with cirrhosis.

The liver receives approximately 30% of resting cardiac output and is therefore a vascular organ. The hepatic vascular system has a considerable ability to store and release blood, and it functions as a reservoir within the general circulation. Normally, 10% to 15% of the total blood volume is in the liver, with roughly 60% of that in the sinusoids. With loss of blood, the liver dynamically adjusts its blood volume and can eject enough blood to compensate for a moderate amount of hemorrhage. Conversely, when vascular volume increases acutely, as with rapid infusion of fluids, the hepatic blood volume expands, providing a buffer against acute increases in systemic blood volume.

Blood

Blood is a thick red liquid form of connective tissue. Blood transports nutrients to the individual cells and removes waste products. Whole blood consists of solid, formed elements and the liquid matrix, or plasma.

Red blood cells, white blood cells, and platelets are the formed elements of blood that float in the plasma, a thick straw-colored fluid. Amino acids, carbohydrates, electrolytes, hormones, lipids, proteins, vitamins, and waste materials are the other constituents of blood. A person who weighs 140 to 150 lb has about 5 quarts of blood.

In an adult, blood cells form mainly in the red marrow of the bones of the chest, vertebrae, and pelvis. Yellow marrow can convert to red marrow if the body requires increased production of blood cells. *Hematopoiesis* is the term for the stages of blood cell development in red marrow. All blood cells, whether they are red, white, or platelets, originate from a common precursor cell called the *stem cell.* Immature blood cells are blast cells. When the cells are mature, they move into the bloodstream. In certain types of leukemia, blast cells may be seen in peripheral blood because the body sends them out before they are mature.

Red Blood Cells

Red blood cells, also known as *erythrocytes* or *red blood corpuscles,* make up more than 90% of the formed elements. They are round with raised edges and a flattened middle. Their function is to transport oxygen to the cells and carbon dioxide away from the cells. Inside red blood cells oxygen and carbon dioxide bind to an iron and protein molecule called *hemoglobin,* but not at the same time. A red blood cell loses its nucleus and most of its organelles during development so that a great deal of hemoglobin can fit inside it. Because it does not have organelles necessary for cell division, red blood cells cannot divide.

Men have slightly more red blood cells than women, and the cells live slightly longer in men (about 120 days) than in women (110 days). The body recycles dead red blood cells, using their hemoglobin in new red blood cells and their proteins either in new red blood cells or other body cells. Because red blood cells cannot divide, they must be produced frequently to replace dead cells. Red bone marrow produces enough red blood cells daily to replace dead blood cells. The body needs a proper intake and assimilation of iron, vitamin B_{12}, and folic acid to produce new red blood cells. An abnormal increase in red blood cells is known as *polycythemia;* an abnormal decrease is called *anemia.*

A variety of chemical markers, or antigens, are present in red blood cells. Some of these chemical markers commonly are called *factors* and are used to identify the type of blood. The best-known grouping method is the ABO system. This system has four blood groups: A, B, AB, and O. These are commonly called the "blood types." The Rh system, the most complex of all the blood grouping methods, has 42 different groups. The most commonly known fact about the Rh system is whether the red blood cells have it or not. If a person's red blood cells have it, his or her blood type is positive. If a person's blood cells do not have it, his or her blood type is negative.

White Blood Cells

White blood cells also are called *leukocytes* or *white blood corpuscles.* Their white color results from their lack of hemoglobin. The usual ratio of white to red blood cells is 1 to 500. The main function of the white blood cells is to protect the body from pathogens and remove dead cells and substances. White blood cells are divided into the following five groups:

1. Neutrophils: Neutrophils are granular leukocytes; more than half of all white blood cells are neutrophils. These cells fight disease phagocytizing pathogens. A buildup of neutrophils and the debris they collect is called *pus.*
2. Lymphocytes: Lymphocytes account for about 30% of the total number of white blood cells in the body. They produce **antibodies** and chemicals that are active in regulating disease and allergic reactions and controlling tumors.
3. Monocytes: Monocytes are the largest of the white blood cells, yet they account for only about 6% of the total

number. They also protect the body through phagocytosis. Monocytes are unique because when they leave the blood and enter the tissues, they can develop into large phagocytic cells called *macrophages*.

4. Eosinophils: About 3% of the total white blood cell count is made up of eosinophils. However, the number increases greatly with parasitic infections or allergic reactions (e.g., hay fever). Eosinophils are capable of phagocytic activity, and they release chemicals during the inflammatory process.

5. Basophils: Basophils are also granular white blood cells, and they make up about 1% of the total white blood cell count. Their exact function is not yet understood clearly.

Platelets

Thrombocytes, also called *platelets*, are the smallest cellular elements of the blood. They are involved in blood clotting, which prevents blood loss when blood vessels are damaged.

Damage to a blood vessel causes the release of chemicals. Special proteins, called *clotting factors,* are activated and then form additional clotting factors. A special protein called *fibrin* forms and seals the damaged blood vessels by trapping red blood cells, platelets, and fluid to form a clot, or thrombus. Fibrin then anchors the clot. The clotting process starts the instant the blood vessel is damaged and takes only a few minutes to complete. Calcium and vitamin K are important to the success and speed of the clotting process.

Plasma

Plasma is the straw-colored liquid found in blood and lymph and is about 90% water; the rest comprises nutrients, gases, and waste products. Plasma constitutes about 55% of blood and plays a major role in the movement of water between the tissues and the blood.

Pathologic Conditions of the Cardiovascular System

Cardiovascular disease is a major cause of death. Many risk factors are associated with cardiovascular disease. The aging process and hereditary predisposition are risk factors that cannot be altered. Many people with cardiovascular disease have elevated or high cholesterol levels. Low levels of high-density lipoprotein (HDL) cholesterol (known as the "good" cholesterol) and high levels of low-density lipoprotein (LDL) cholesterol (known as the "bad" cholesterol) are more specifically linked to cardiovascular disease than is total cholesterol. A blood test, administered by most health care professionals, is used to determine cholesterol levels. Hypertension is a major risk factor for cardiovascular disease Abdominal fat, as opposed to fat that accumulates on the hips, is associated with increased risk of cardiovascular disease and heart attack. Overweight individuals are more likely to have additional risk factors related to heart disease, specifically hypertension, high blood sugar levels, high cholesterol, high triglycerides, and diabetes. People with cardiovascular disease may not have any distinct symptoms but may experience difficulty in breathing during exertion or when lying down, fatigue, lightheadedness, dizziness, fainting, depression, memory problems, confusion,

frequent waking during sleep, chest pain, an awareness of the heartbeat, sensations of fluttering or pounding in the chest, swelling around the ankles, or a large abdomen. All of these symptoms can be attributed to other conditions, especially generalized stress, which is why many with cardiovascular disease go undiagnosed.

Cardiac Disorders

Bradycardia

In bradycardia the resting heart rate is less than 60 beats per minute. However, healthy athletes often have heart rates between 50 and 60 beats per minute, which in these individuals is not necessarily a pathologic condition. Primary treatment, when necessary, involves administration of atropine, a parasympathetic blocking agent.

Tachycardia

In most healthy persons the heart rate increases in response to extra demands on it, such as those imposed by exercise. In tachycardia the heartbeat increases suddenly without any increase in physical or emotional stress. Treatment ranges from no intervention to administration of sympathetic blocking agents. Interventions for persons with paroxysmal supraventricular tachycardia include interrupting the sympathetic signals by methods such as holding the breath or rinsing the face with cool water. Because stimulation of the vagus nerve slows the heart rate, the Valsalva maneuver (forced expiration against a closed airway) may help. A physician may massage the carotid baroreceptor or inject medication to reduce the heart rate.

Arrhythmia

In arrhythmias the rhythm of the heart may be partly or completely irregular, or it may be regular but with a frequency that is too slow or too fast. Treatment may include medication, installation of a pacemaker to initiate the heartbeat, or use of a defibrillator to restore normal heart rhythm.

Mitral Valve Dysfunction

Although all valves may undergo some changes in structure or function, the mitral valve is the one most commonly affected. This is because the left ventricle contracts so forcefully that pressure of the blood against the mitral valve may damage it. Mitral valve prolapse is a deformity that may be congenital or may result from rheumatic fever or some other heart disease. The valve does not close completely, and blood leaks back into the left atrium. Although many persons do not notice any symptoms, others may experience chest pain, palpitation, fatigue, or shortness of breath. This condition may be a factor in anxiety-related disorders.

Mitral valve stenosis is scarring that causes the parts of the valve to stick together and gradually narrow. Blood backs up in the left atrium and pressure increases, which causes blood to back up into the pulmonary veins.

Angina Pectoris

Angina pectoris is chest pain or discomfort that results when the amount of oxygen supplied to the heart declines. However, there is no lasting tissue damage to the heart. Angina pectoris is caused mainly by coronary artery disease but also can be a sign of heart disease, anemia, or hyperthyroidism. Symptoms most often occur during exertion, emotional upset, or cold weather. The pain begins in the center of the chest and often spreads to the arms, neck, or jaw. In severe cases pain may occur when the person is at rest. Rest or the use of nitroglycerin usually relieves the symptoms.

Myocardial Infarction (Heart Attack)

An infarct is an area of dead tissue that results when the blood supply to that area is cut off. Most heart attacks occur because of blockage of a coronary artery by a blood clot, especially in arteries narrowed by coronary artery disease. The blocking of blood flow damages or destroys the heart muscle. The first symptom is usually a crushing pain in the center of the chest over the sternum (Figure 11-16). Pain also may occur in the arms, neck, jaw, and upper abdomen and occasionally in the back. The person also may perspire heavily and complain of dizziness, chills, or nausea. Immediate treatment is essential.

Congestive Heart Failure

Heart failure occurs when the heart muscle weakens and cannot pump sufficient blood; when the heart valves are damaged; or when hypertension exists or excessive demands are made on the heart. Blood pools in the veins, and not enough of it reaches the heart. The heart compensates by pumping out more blood, causing even more pooling in the veins and organs. This buildup of fluid is called *congestion*; thus the condition is called

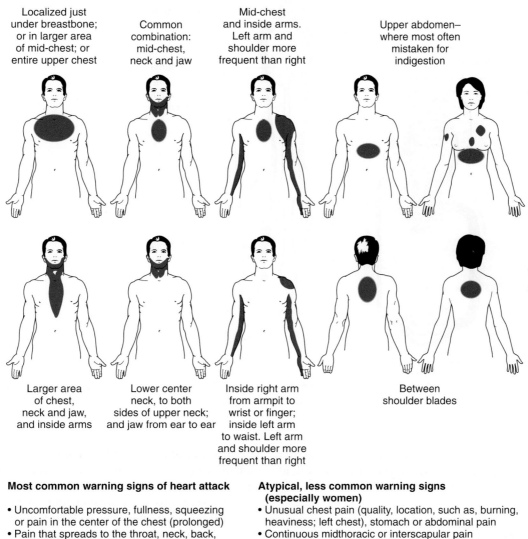

FIGURE 11-16 Early warning signs of heart attack. (From Goodman CG: *Differential diagnosis for physical therapists: screening for referral,* ed 5, St Louis, 2013, Saunders.)

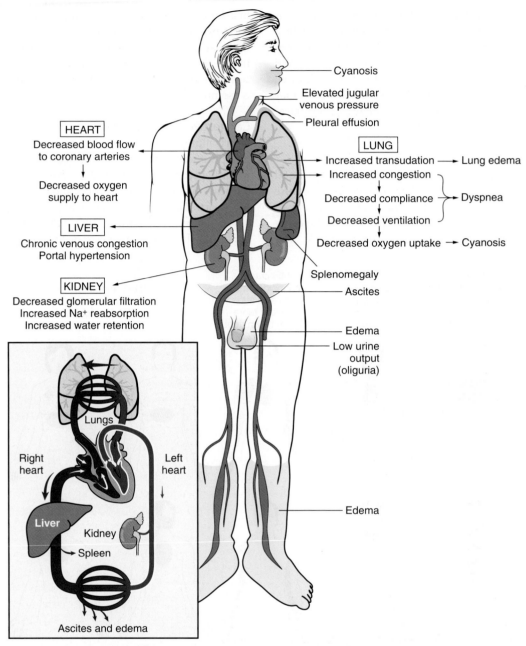

FIGURE 11-17 Congestive heart failure. Left heart failure leads to pulmonary edema. Right ventricular failure causes peripheral edema that is most prominent in the lower extremities. (From Damjanov I: *Pathology for the health-related professions,* ed 4, Philadelphia, 2012, Saunders.)

congestive heart failure. Treatment usually includes use of a diuretic such as furosemide (Lasix) to eliminate excess fluid and reduce blood pressure (Figure 11-17).

Rheumatic Heart Disease

Rheumatic fever may occur in young children after an untreated streptococcal throat infection; it is an immunologic response to bacterial substances remaining in the body. Besides its signature rash, other signs and symptoms include joint pain, swelling, fever, and endocarditis. If left untreated, the endocarditis may cause rheumatic heart disease, in which the inflamed heart valves, particularly the mitral valve, become deformed.

Heart and Pericardial Inflammation

Inflammation that affects the heart and pericardial sac is uncommon. Pericarditis is an inflammation of the pericardium; myocarditis is an inflammation of the heart muscle. Endocarditis may affect the endocardium, heart valves, or both. Inflammation usually follows acute or chronic viral or bacterial infections or accompanies alcohol abuse or radiation therapy. The symptoms usually are mild but can lead to heart failure or arterial blockage if the condition is not treated early.

Vascular Disorders

Ischemia

Ischemia is a temporary deficiency or a diminished supply of blood to a tissue.

Arteriosclerosis and Atherosclerosis

Often the two terms are used interchangeably, but that is incorrect. *Arteriosclerosis* is a general term that means "hardening of the arteries" and refers to arteries that have lost their elasticity. In **atherosclerosis,** the most common type of arteriosclerosis, small fat deposits from cholesterol in the blood build up at stress points in the arteries. These stress points occur where the arteries branch out or incur damage. The fat combines with connective tissue sent to repair the damage and forms plaque. As this process continues, the arterial walls harden and blood flow diminishes. Symptoms do not usually appear until a major blockage occurs. The body compensates by enlarging the artery, if possible. Sometimes the artery enlarges, forms an aneurysm, and ruptures. Problems also occur when the plaque breaks off and travels elsewhere in the body. It can lodge in a vessel smaller in diameter than it is and completely block the vessel. In the brain it can cause a stroke.

People in countries where it is common to consume high-fat diets, particularly diets high in saturated fatty acids and cholesterol, have higher incidences of atherosclerosis. Nonsurgical interventions, such as modifying the diet and taking part in aerobic exercise, may be able to enlarge an artery, increasing the blood flow. Also, collateral circulation may develop around the blockage as new vessels develop. Surgical interventions may include creating a bypass out of blood vessels transferred from other parts of the body, excising the blockage, or enlarging the vessel (Figure 11-18).

Coronary Artery Disease

Coronary artery disease is commonly caused by arteriosclerosis, atherosclerosis, and thrombus formation in one or more of the coronary arteries. Occlusion, or blockage, of the artery diminishes the amount of oxygen and nutrients reaching the heart tissues. Partial occlusion causes the transient chest and arm pain of angina pectoris. Total occlusion causes the crushing or squeezing pain of myocardial infarction and heart tissue death. Some of the many risk factors that contribute to coronary artery disease can be controlled, such as diet, weight, and avoidance of smoking. Treatment commonly includes the use of beta blockers and calcium channel blockers to slow the heart rate and reduce the strength of the contraction. In addition to lowering the blood pressure, calcium channel blockers dilate the coronary arteries.

Hypertension

Most authorities consider hypertension to be a sustained blood pressure greater than 140/90 mm or higher Hg. Hypertension is graded as mild, moderate, borderline high, or severe, depending on the diastolic reading. In most cases the cause is unknown (called *essential hypertension*), although kidney disease and arteriosclerosis may play roles. With hypertension, continuous sympathetic stimulation constricts arterioles. Chronic untreated hypertension leads to hypertensive heart disease. The heart becomes enlarged because of the increased work of the left ventricle against arteriolar resistance, and heart failure or infarction may result. Other important complications of untreated hypertension are stroke and kidney disease.

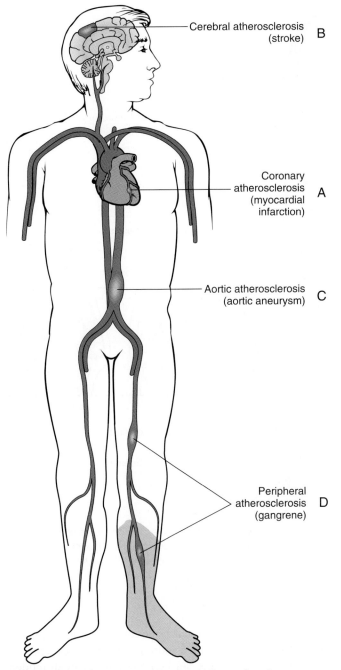

FIGURE 11-18 The four major forms of atherosclerosis are classified as coronary **(A)**, cerebral **(B)**, aortic **(C)**, and peripheral vascular **(D)**. (From Damjanov I: *Pathology for the health-related professions,* ed 4, Philadelphia, 2012, Saunders.)

Nondrug therapy consists of restricting salt (which reduces fluid retention), losing weight (which reduces the resistance against which the heart must pump), reducing the consumption of alcohol, avoiding smoking, and participating in stress management and aerobic exercise programs.

Medical treatment may include a diuretic, a beta blocker, a calcium channel blocker, an angiotensin-converting enzyme inhibitor, or a combination of these medications as needed.

Varicose Veins

Varicose veins result when veins stretch so much that the valves cannot close sufficiently. More women than men are

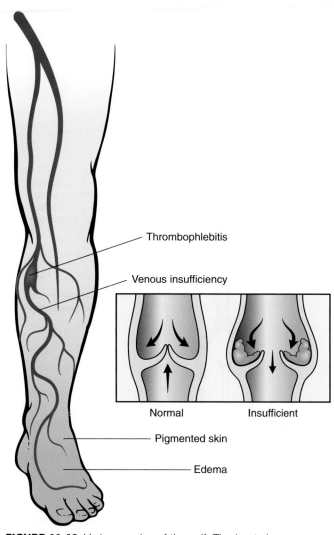

FIGURE 11-19 Varicose veins of the calf. The *inset* shows venous valvular insufficiency, which accounts for the reflux of blood. (From Damjanov I: *Pathology for the health-related professions,* ed 4, Philadelphia, 2012, Saunders.)

affected because estrogen makes the connective tissue, including that in veins, in women more pliable than in men. This means that venous walls can become more easily distended. The condition may be congenital and may result from remaining in one position, especially standing, too long or may be caused by obesity, pregnancy, or menopause. The great and small saphenous veins are affected most commonly. Hemorrhoids are another common type of varicose vein.

Treatment includes rest, elevating the legs, wearing compression stockings, surgical removal of the vein, or sclerotherapy (injection of a saline solution into the vein) (Figure 11-19).

Aneurysm

An aneurysm is a permanent bulge in the wall of a vessel because of weakness or damage to its structure. Although the usual result of arteriosclerosis is an aneurysm, the condition also may be congenital or may result from inflammation. The most common sites are the aorta and the arteries of the brain.

Aneurysms are dangerous because they may rupture and hemorrhage.

Shock

Shock is a condition that results when the blood supply to vital organs becomes inadequate, causing diminished function by these organs. The blood vessels dilate rapidly, and blood pressure drops. The brain receives insufficient oxygen and can be damaged. Treatment usually consists of administering intravenous fluids until the person's condition stabilizes and the cause can be determined.

The four main types of shock are hypovolemic shock, which results from a loss of blood or other bodily fluids; cardiogenic shock, which occurs when the heart does not pump sufficient blood; septic shock, which is caused by a bacterial infection (e.g., toxic shock syndrome); and anaphylactic shock, which results from an allergy or overreaction by the immune system.

Arterial Inflammation

Endarteritis obliterans is a defect in which the artery walls become inflamed, blocking the opening of the vessel and blocking the smaller vessels.

Raynaud's Disease and Phenomenon

Raynaud's disease, a primary condition, and Raynaud's phenomenon, a secondary condition, are primarily disorders that affect the blood supply to the fingers and toes and occasionally to the nose. Temporary spasms in the small arteries reduce or stop blood flow to the area, and the skin turns pale and then blue. Tissue damage, ulceration, or both may follow. The Raynaud's disorders are aggravated by cold and emotional disturbances and often occur in individuals with connective tissue disorders or other systemic disorders.

Temporal Arteritis

Temporal arteritis is an inflammation of the temporal arteries, which causes pain, swelling, and tenderness. The condition also can cause a decrease in or a loss of vision and, in severe cases, stroke.

Blood Disorders

Anemia

Anemia is a decrease in the normal number of red blood cells or in the amount of hemoglobin or iron in the blood. The various anemias are classified according to whether the cause is a loss in the number or a change in the usability of red cells or whether it involves a decline in the production of red cells.

Nutritional Anemias

Iron deficiency anemia may result from the inability to absorb sufficient iron in the small intestine or maintain iron levels in the blood. Pernicious anemia usually results from the lack of intrinsic factor in the stomach, which leads to the inability to absorb vitamin B_{12}. Other nutritional anemias may result from deficiencies in nutrients such as folic acid. Folic acid is necessary for the production of red blood cells.

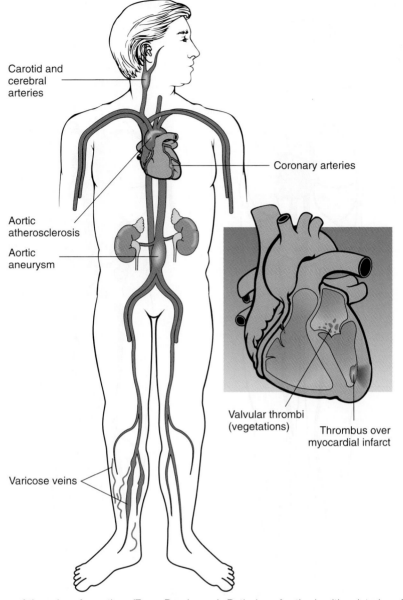

Carotid and
cerebral
arteries

Coronary arteries

Aortic
atherosclerosis

Aortic
aneurysm

Valvular thrombi
(vegetations)

Thrombus over
myocardial infarct

Varicose veins

FIGURE 11-20 Common sites of thrombus formation. (From Damjanov I: *Pathology for the health-related professions,* ed 4, Philadelphia, 2012, Saunders.)

Intrinsic factor is needed to absorb vitamin B_{12} from the digestive tract.

Bone Marrow Suppression Anemia
Various types of anemia result from bone marrow suppression. Marrow suppression may occur in individuals undergoing chemotherapy or taking certain antibiotics, as a complication of radiation therapy, or in persons with chronic diseases. The red blood cells may be damaged or destroyed, and the body often tries to compensate by producing new ones and sending them out before they mature. Severe cases require blood transfusions, along with bone marrow transplantation.

Thrombosis
A thrombosis is clotting in an unbroken blood vessel. If it breaks loose, it becomes an embolus (Figures 11-20 and 11-21).

Phlebitis, Thrombophlebitis, and Deep Vein Thrombosis
The term *phlebitis* refers to the inflammation of a vein caused by injury, infection, or swelling. These insults diminish blood flow, which may cause thromboses to develop. If the thrombosis becomes inflamed, a condition known as *thrombophlebitis* develops. The superficial leg veins are the most common sites, primarily the saphenous veins. Clots also may form in the deep veins, especially in the legs and abdomen, a condition known as *deep vein thrombosis* (DVT). The clot can break off and travel in the bloodstream as an embolus.

Embolus
An embolus is a blood clot (thrombus), plaque, air or gas, fat, tumor cells, tissue, or clumps of bacteria in the bloodstream. If the embolus lodges in a blood vessel smaller in diameter than it is, it can block blood flow.

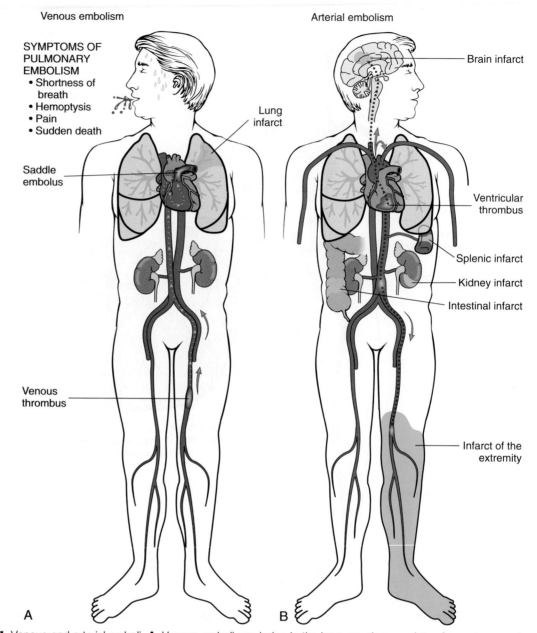

Venous embolism

Arterial embolism

SYMPTOMS OF
PULMONARY
EMBOLISM
• Shortness of
  breath
• Hemoptysis
• Pain
• Sudden death

Lung
infarct

Saddle
embolus

Venous
thrombus

Brain infarct

Ventricular
thrombus

Splenic infarct

Kidney infarct

Intestinal infarct

Infarct of the
extremity

A   B

FIGURE 11-21 Venous and arterial emboli. **A,** Venous emboli can lodge in the lung, causing a variety of symptoms and conditions. **B,** Arterial emboli may occlude arteries in many organs. (From Damjanov I: *Pathology for the health-related professions,* ed 4, Philadelphia, 2012, Saunders.)

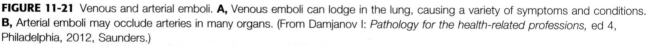

In pulmonary embolism a clot detaches from a deep vein in the leg or pelvis and travels to the right atrium, then to the right ventricle, and on to the pulmonary artery. Predisposing factors for clot formation are obesity, heart failure, surgery and immobilization, and a history of thrombophlebitis. A clot that lodges at the junction of the pulmonary trunk and the pulmonary arteries may cause death. A clot that moves into a pulmonary artery and lodges there destroys lung tissue and is called a *pulmonary infarction.* The person suddenly becomes short of breath. Other signs and symptoms are chest pain, fever, and wheezing. Diagnosis is made by means of a lung scan and pulmonary angiogram. Treatment consists of intravenous anticoagulant (heparin) therapy to prevent

further clotting and the use of a clot-dissolving medication. Subsequent therapy often involves orally administered warfarin (Coumadin).

Hemorrhage

Hemorrhage refers to passage of blood outside of the cardiovascular system. Depending on the source, hemorrhage may be classified as cardiac, aortic, arterial, capillary, or venous. Clinically, hemorrhage may be of sudden onset, such as from an acute puncture wound; may be chronic, such as from an ulcer; or may be recurrent and marked by repeated episodes of blood loss. The following are clinical terms that describe various forms of hemorrhage:

Hemoptysis: Respiratory tract bleeding with expectoration, which means expelling from the lungs or throat by coughing and spitting

Hematemesis: Vomiting of blood

Melena: Passage of black, discolored blood in the stool. This represents upper gastrointestinal tract bleeding in which the blood is exposed to hydrochloric acid, which produces the color change.

Hematuria: Blood in the urine

Metrorrhagia: Uterovaginal bleeding. Heavy menstrual bleeding is called *menorrhagia.*

Sickle Cell Disease

Sickle cell disease causes premature destruction of red blood cells. These blood cells contain hemoglobin S because of an amino acid substitution in the hemoglobin molecules. These cells collapse and form a sickle or crescent shape. Because of their abnormal shape, they do not flow smoothly through the vessels and can block them. When the sickle cells block small blood vessels, multiple infarctions can result throughout the body. Common signs and symptoms are jaundice, diminished growth and development, and pain in the arms, legs, and abdomen resulting from the lack of oxygen. Infection or a cerebrovascular accident causes death. The primary treatment is symptomatic and includes administration of oxygen, blood transfusions, and use of analgesics.

Sickle cell disease is a genetic disease that affects mainly those who live, or are descendants of those who lived, in the malaria belt around the world. The malaria belt includes parts of the Mediterranean region, sub-Saharan Africa, and tropical Asia. People with two sickle cell genes have severe anemia; those with only one defective gene have minor problems. The gene that causes the red blood cells to sickle also changes the permeability of the cell membranes of sickled cells, causing potassium ions to leak out. Low levels of potassium kill the malaria parasites that may infect sickled cells. Because of this, a person with one normal gene and one sickled gene has a higher than average resistance to malaria. Thus the single sickle cell gene gives a survival advantage.

Hemophilia

Hemophilia is a genetic disorder in which factor VIII, a vital clotting factor in the blood, is greatly diminished or absent, resulting in the blood's inability to clot. It is recessively sex-linked. This means that it is carried on the X chromosome. Therefore a female can carry the gene but not develop severe symptoms because a corresponding nondefective gene on her other X chromosome prevents the gene from becoming fully active. A male with the hemophilia gene on his X chromosome, however, does not have a corresponding, nondefective gene on his Y chromosome so the gene becomes fully active. Although hemophilia is passed on by females, they usually have only minor bleeding problems or no symptoms. Men with hemophilia may experience extended episodes of bleeding and may be susceptible to internal bleeding caused by minor trauma.

Polycythemia

Polycythemia is an abnormally high amount of red blood cells. This raises the viscosity of blood and makes blood more difficult for the heart to pump. Increased viscosity also contributes to high blood pressure and increased risk of stroke. Causes of polycythemia include abnormal increases in red blood cell production, low amounts of oxygen in the tissues, dehydration, and blood doping or the use of EPO in athletes. EPO is erythropoietin, and it increases red blood cell production. Blood doping involves boosting the number of red blood cells in the bloodstream through the use of transfusions in order to enhance athletic importance. The increased red blood cells means more oxygen can be carried to tissues.

Thrombocytopenia

Thrombocytopenia is a decrease in platelets, which diminishes the ability of the blood to clot. Common causes include blood loss, infection, cancer (especially Hodgkin's disease and leukemia), and lupus. The condition also may result from radiation therapy or chemotherapy. Idiopathic thrombocytopenic purpura is an autoimmune disease in which antiplatelet antibodies are present. Common signs include easy bruising, nosebleeds, bleeding gums, and blood in the urine. Complications include cerebral hemorrhage and bleeding into nerve tissue, which can cause paralysis.

INDICATIONS/CONTRAINDICATIONS for Therapeutic Massage

Cardiovascular System

In general, cardiovascular disease presents contraindications for therapeutic massage. If the contraindication does not arise from the disease itself, the medication taken to control the disease may pose problems. Blood thinners, for example, increase the possibility of bruising and hemorrhage. Nonetheless, therapeutic massage often is indicated as part of a supervised treatment program. The key is supervision by a qualified health care provider, because cardiovascular diseases can be complex in the presenting pathologic conditions and in the treatment protocols. The general stress management and homeostatic normalization effects of therapeutic massage treatments are desirable for most cardiovascular difficulties as long as the treatments are supervised as part of a total therapeutic program.

Take care to refrain from performing any type of therapeutic massage over sites of thrombophlebitis or DVT. Systemic contraindications also may be present. The practitioner should refer for diagnosis any client with unexplained leg pain, a cardinal sign of thrombophlebitis or DVT.

LYMPHATIC SYSTEM

SECTION OBJECTIVES

Chapter objective covered in this section:

6. List and describe the components and functions of the lymphatic system.
7. Identify pathologies of the lymphatic system and describe indications and contraindications for massage.

After completing this chapter, the student will be able to perform the following:

- List and describe the components of the lymphatic system.
- List and describe the components of lymph.

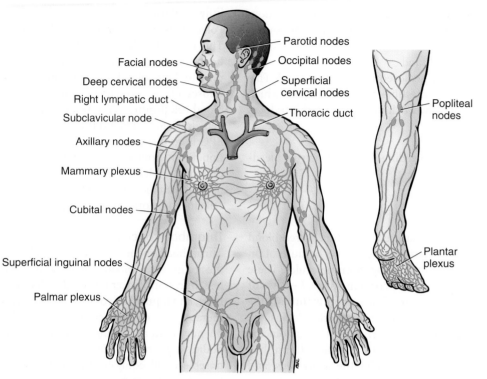

FIGURE 11-22 The lymphatic system: principal lymph vessels and nodes.

- Describe the functions of the lymphatic system.
- Explain the role of the lymph nodes, spleen, thymus, and lymph nodules.
- Describe how lymph moves through the body.
- Determine massage indications and contraindications for pathologic conditions of the lymphatic system.

The lymphatic system comprises the spleen; thymus; lymph nodes and lymph nodules; the lymph capillaries, vessels, trunks, and ducts; and lymph and lymphocytes. It is a one-way system that begins in the tissues and ends when it reaches the blood vessels. The system helps the body maintain homeostasis by collecting accumulated tissue fluid around the cells and returning it to the blood circulation. The lymph nodes play an active part in the immune defenses of the body by filtering out and destroying foreign substances and microorganisms. Special lymph capillaries called *lacteals* absorb lipids from the small intestine so the lymph can transport them to the bloodstream (Figure 11-22).

Lymph

Interstitial fluid comes from blood plasma that seeps through capillaries. Interstitial fluid becomes lymph when it moves into the lymph capillaries. Lymph contains proteins and other cells products as well as pathogens and cell debris. As lymph travels through lymph vessels, it is filtered by lymph nodes that remove pathogens and cell debris. Lymph then travels to the bloodstream and once again becomes plasma.

Lymph Vessels, Nodes, and Organs

Lymph Vessels

The lymph capillaries are tiny open-ended channels located in tissue spaces throughout the entire body except for the brain, spinal cord, and cornea (Figure 11-23). A lymphatic capillary network of vessels slightly larger than blood capillaries drains tissue fluid from nearly all tissues and organs that have blood vascularization. The cardiovascular system is a closed system, whereas the lymphatic system is an open-ended system, beginning in the interstitial spaces.

The moment interstitial fluid enters a lymph capillary, a flap valve prevents it from returning to the interstitial space. Lymph capillaries join to form larger lymph vessels that resemble veins but have thinner, more transparent walls. Like veins, they have valves to prevent backflow. The large vessels continue to merge and eventually become two main ducts called the *right lymphatic duct* and the *thoracic duct* (left lymphatic duct). The right lymphatic duct drains the upper right half of the body and empties into the right subclavian vein. The thoracic duct drains the rest of the body and empties into the left subclavian vein.

Lymph Nodes

Lymph nodes are small, round structures located along the lymph vessels. For the most part, they are clustered at the joints; movement of the joints helps pump lymph through the nodes. The superficial lymph nodes are most numerous in the groin, axillae, and neck, whereas most of the deep lymph nodes are found alongside blood vessels in the pelvic,

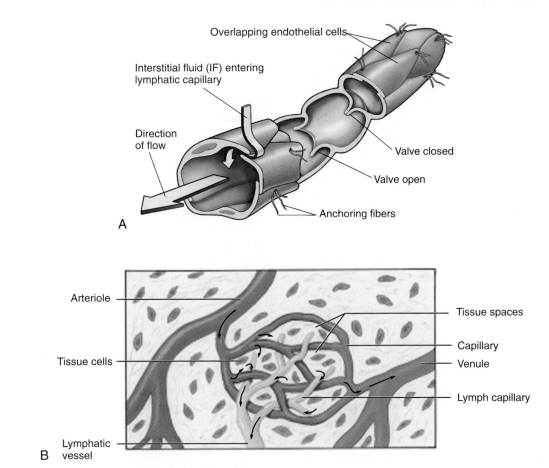

FIGURE 11-23 A, Structure of a typical lymphatic capillary. The interstitial fluid enters through clefts between overlapping endothelial cells that form the wall of the vessel. Semilunar valves ensure one-way flow of lymph out of the tissue. **B,** Distribution on lymphatic capillaries in the tissue. (**A,** from Patton KT, Thibodeau GA: *Anatomy and physiology,* ed 7, St Louis, 2010, Mosby. **B,** from Applegate E: *The anatomy and physiology learning system,* ed 4, Philadelphia, 2011, Saunders.)

abdominal, and thoracic cavities. All lymph passes through one or more nodes before it enters the bloodstream. Lymph nodes contain mature lymphocytes, white blood cells that destroy bacteria, virus-infected cells, pathogens, foreign matter, and waste materials. During periods of infection an immune response is occurring (discussed in more detail in the section on immunity) in which the number of lymphocytes increases. The additional activity in the nodes and the buildup of the lymphocytes can make the nodes swollen and painful. The nodes also provide a filtering system that removes waste products and transfers them for detoxification in the other systems of the body.

The locations of the lymph nodes are as follows:

- Preauricular lymph nodes are located just in front of the ear and drain the superficial tissues and skin on the lateral side of the head and face.
- Submental and submaxillary nodes are located in the floor of the mouth and drain lymph from the nose, lips, and teeth.
- Cervical lymph nodes are located at the neck.
- Superficial cubital or supratrochlear nodes are located just above the bend of the elbow and drain lymph from the forearm.
- Axillary lymph nodes located deep in the underarm and upper chest drain lymph from the arm and upper part of the thoracic wall, including the breast.

- Inguinal lymph nodes located in the groin drain lymph from the leg and external genitals.
- Popliteal lymph nodes are located behind the knee.

Spleen

The spleen, the largest of the lymphatic organs, is located near the stomach under the diaphragm. Macrophages in the spleen filter out worn-out red blood cells and destroy microorganisms in the blood. The spleen serves as a blood reservoir and can release small amounts of blood into the circulation during times of emergency or blood loss. The spleen functions with the lymphatic system by storing lymphocytes and releasing them as part of the immune response.

Thymus

The thymus is a triangular gland composed of lymphatic tissue. It is located in the upper chest, superior to the superior vena cava and inferior to the thyroid gland. This gland is most prominent in the newborn and begins to atrophy after puberty, becoming only a small remnant in the adult. The thymus is important in the development and maturation of certain lymphocytes and in programming them to become T cells in the immune system.

Lymph Nodules

Lymph nodules are small masses of lymph tissue (up to approximately 1 mm in diameter) that contain lymphocytes enmeshed within reticular fibers. Collectively, this tissue is referred to as *mucosa-associated lymph tissue,* and along with the spleen and thymus, it is involved in the development of immunity. This tissue does not filter lymph but is positioned strategically to protect the respiratory and gastrointestinal tracts from microbes and other foreign material. Lymph nodules are scattered throughout loose connective tissue, especially in the mucous membrane lining the upper respiratory tract, digestive tract, reproductive tract, and urinary tract. Lymph nodules appear to be distributed strategically to defend the body against disease-causing organisms that could penetrate the linings of passageways that open outside the body.

Most lymphatic nodules are small and solitary. However, some are found in large clusters. For example, large aggregates of lymph nodules occur in the wall of the lower portion (ileum) of the small intestine. These masses of lymph nodules are known as *Peyer's patches.* Tonsils, strategically located under the epithelial lining of the oral cavity and pharynx so that they can defend against invading bacteria, are also aggregates of lymph nodules. The lingual tonsils are located at the base of the tongue. The single pharyngeal tonsil is located in the posterior wall of the nasal portion of the pharynx above the soft palate and often is referred to as the *adenoid.*

Lymph nodules include the following:
- Palatine and lingual tonsils located between the mouth and the oral part of the pharynx
- Pharyngeal tonsil located on the wall of the nasal part of the pharynx
- Solitary lymphatic follicles dispersed throughout the body
- Aggregated lymphatic follicles (Peyer's patches) located in the wall of the small intestine
- Vermiform appendix, an outgrowth from the cecum (the first part of the large intestine)

Lymphatic Pump and Drainage

Although the lymph system has no muscular pumping organ such as the heart, the movement of joints provides some pumping action, and lymph moves along slowly and steadily. It flows through the thoracic duct and reenters the general circulation at the rate of about 3 liters per day, despite the fact that most of the flow is against gravity. Lymph moves through the system in the correct direction because of the large number of valves that permit fluid to flow only toward the center of the body.

The movement of lymph is known as *lymphatic drainage.* It begins when lymph moves out of the interstitial spaces and into the lymph capillaries, movement that is assisted by the pressure exerted by the compression of skeletal muscles against the vessels during movement; by changes in internal pressure during respiration; and by the opening of lymph vessels resulting from the pull of the skin and fascia during movement. Major lymph plexuses are found on the soles and the palms, possibly because the rhythmic pumping of walking and grasping facilitates lymphatic flow. Current research suggests that the lymph vessels themselves may have an intrinsic pumping

action. Every 6 to 20 mm, there is a valve that lies directly between two or three layers of spiral smooth muscle. The unit is called a *lymphangion.* The rhythmic smooth muscle contraction causes the lymph vessels to undulate, almost in the manner of intestinal tract peristalsis. Some researchers think that this contraction is the sensation felt by those who sense a rhythmic pulsation in the human body.

Specialized application of massage may be effective in increasing lymph removal from stagnant or edematous tissue. Massage that uses light pressure to drag the skin has the potential to increase superficial lymph movement. Crosswise and lengthwise stretching of the lymph vessels' anchoring filaments opens the lymph capillaries, thus allowing the interstitial fluid to enter the lymphatic system. The practitioner applies the massage strokes in the direction of normal lymphatic drainage, thus speeding up lymph movement.

The lymph in the left arm flows from the fingers toward the axilla and from there to the neck, where it joins the thoracic duct. Lymph from the right arm does the same, except that it drains into the smaller right lymphatic duct. Both ducts empty at the junction of the subclavian and internal jugular veins. The lymph from the right side of the chest, face, and scalp also flows toward the right axilla and into the right lymphatic duct. The lymph from the left side of the face and scalp flows into the thoracic duct.

The lymph from the feet and legs drains upward toward the groin and into the abdomen and empties into the lower end of the thoracic duct, called the *cisterna chyli.*

Of the lymph flow from the chest, 85% drains into the respective axillary nodes. The remaining lymph drains into nodes located behind the sternum and into lymph vessels located in the pectoralis muscle. In general, lymph moves toward the groin and the axillae.

The alteration of valves and smooth muscles gives a characteristic moniliform shape to these vessels, like pearls on a string. Lymphatic circulation is separated into two layers:
1. The superficial circulation, which constitutes 60% to 70% of lymph circulation, is located just under the skin in the junction between the **superficial fascia** and the dermoepidermis. The superficial circulation is not stimulated directly by exercise but is influenced by the stretching and pulling of the skin and superficial fascia during movement.
2. The deep muscular and visceral circulation, below the fascia, is activated by muscular contraction.

Pathologic Conditions of the Lymphatic System

The lymphatic system clears away infection and keeps body fluids in balance. When it is not working properly, fluid builds in the tissues and causes swelling, called *lymphedema.* Other lymphatic system problems can include blockage infections, cancer, and lymphatic malformation.

Edema

Edema is the accumulation of abnormal amounts of fluid in tissue spaces and often accompanies congestion, which is an

Practical Application

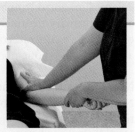

Simple muscle tension and binding by connective tissues puts pressure on the lymph vessels and may block them, interfering with efficient drainage. Therapeutic massage can relax muscle tension and connective tissue pliability. As the muscles relax and the connective tissue has more space, the lymph vessels open. Lymphatic massage mechanically stimulates the flow of lymph by tracing the lymphatic routes with light pressure. This pull on the skin and superficial connective tissues affects the anchoring filaments of the lymph capillaries, ultimately opening the capillaries. The focus of the pressure is on the dermis. Little pressure is required to reach the area; too much pressure squeezes the capillaries closed and nullifies any effect. Rhythmic, gentle, passive and active joint movement and rhythmic muscle contraction reproduce the way the body normally pumps lymph, especially in the deep lymphatic circulation. During massage the practitioner can stimulate this process by using rhythmic compression with enough depth to compress the muscles. The client helps the process by breathing slowly and deeply, which stimulates lymph flow. When possible, position the area being massaged above the heart so that gravity can assist the lymph flow. Because lymph capillary plexuses are present on the bottoms of the feet, rhythmic compression on the soles also enhances lymph flow. When applying lymph drainage techniques, the practitioner must take care not to promote excessive increases in the volume of lymph flow in persons who have heart and kidney conditions because the venous system must accommodate the load once the fluid has been delivered to the subclavian veins. Significantly increasing the load could place excessive strain on the heart and kidneys (Figure 11-24).

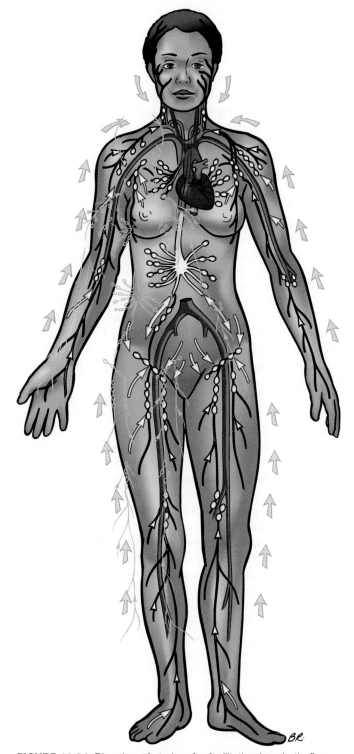

FIGURE 11-24 Direction of strokes for facilitating lymphatic flow. (From Fritz S: *Mosby's fundamentals of therapeutic massage,* ed 5, St Louis, 2013, Mosby.)

increase in the volume of blood in dilated vessels. Common causes of edema are heart failure, kidney disease, and liver disease. Localized edema occurs with inflammation and lymphatic obstruction.

Lymphedema

Lymphedema is an increase in tissue fluid caused by inflammation or obstruction by scar tissue, parasites, or trauma. For example, after a radical mastectomy in which axillary lymph channels are removed, arm drainage may be partially blocked, causing the arm to swell. The primary treatment for generalized edema is cautious use of diuretics to remove the fluid. Some forms of massage are effective for managing moderate lymphedema. External pumping sleeves that rhythmically compress the area are beneficial in chronic cases. The practitioner should refer a client with any form of edema for diagnosis because edema is symptomatic of many disease processes, particularly cardiovascular disease.

Lymphatic Filariasis

Lymphatic filariasis is a tropical parasitic disease caused by microscopic threadlike worms. The adult worms live only in the human lymph system. Lymphatic filariasis is spread from person to person by mosquitoes. People with the disease can suffer from lymphedema and elephantiasis, which is a condition caused by long-term obstruction of lymphatic vessels that leads to engorgement and thickened skin. It causes disfigurement, often of the leg. Lymphatic filariasis is a leading cause of permanent disability worldwide. The condition is treated with antiparasitic medication.

Infectious Mononucleosis

Infectious mononucleosis is a contagious viral infection that occurs most commonly in teenagers and young adults. Mononucleosis affects the lymphocytes, causing an increase in the number and a change in the structure of some of these cells. The infection is transmitted primarily by kissing, hence its nickname, the "kissing disease." Common signs and symptoms are fever, sore throat, enlarged cervical lymph nodes, a rash and, in some, anemia. Complications include ruptured spleen, hepatitis, encephalitis, meningitis, and depression. The primary treatment is bed rest for several weeks or months.

Leukemia

Leukemia is the term for any of a number of cancers of the white blood cells in which the body produces abnormal cells at a faster rate than normal or the cells live longer than normal (or both). Because the cancerous cells do not have the same structure as healthy white blood cells, they do not function properly. They build up and invade the organs of the body, interfering with organ function. The increased abnormal white blood cells crowd out functioning red blood cells and platelets. Leukemia may also affect red blood cell and platelet production, resulting in anemia or diminished clotting ability. Brain hemorrhage and infection may follow.

Acute leukemia progresses rapidly; chronic leukemia progresses slowly. Usually, the acute forms show mostly immature blast cells, and the chronic forms show mostly mature cells. Two categories of leukemia are described by the white blood cell they affect. Lymphocytic leukemia affects the cells that become lymphocytes; myelocytic leukemia affects the cells that develop into granulocytes or monocytes. The myelocytic leukemias also may be identified by the terms *granulocytic* or *monocytic leukemia.*

The following are common leukemias:

Acute myelogenous leukemia: Develops rapidly and demonstrates such symptoms as an increase in infections, sores in the mouth, and a greater tendency to bruise or bleed

Chronic myelogenous leukemia: Found in young adults and most often associated with a chromosome abnormality

Acute lymphoblastic (acute lymphocytic) leukemia: Affects children; incidence peaks at 5 years of age; commonly can be cured by chemotherapy, and complete remission often occurs.

Chronic lymphocytic leukemia: Affects older persons; the increase in abnormal white cells reduces the number and effectiveness of the normal white blood cells, sometimes resulting in anemia and an increase in infections. Often, no therapy is required unless symptoms are evident.

Lymphomas

A lymphoma is a tumor of the lymphatic system that is almost always malignant. Most lymphomas, or lymphomata, are first felt as enlarged, painless lymph nodes or lymphoid tissues. Lymphomata generally are divided into two categories: Hodgkin's disease and non-Hodgkin's lymphoma.

Hodgkin's Disease

Hodgkin's disease is a cancer that involves painless swelling of the lymph nodes, primarily in the neck and groin, caused by enlarged, mutated lymphocytes. Radiation and chemotherapy are the primary treatment methods, and this disease has one of the highest cure rates of any form of cancer. Some individuals may require bone marrow transplantation.

Non-Hodgkin's Lymphoma

Non-Hodgkin's lymphoma is any cancer of lymphatic tissue that is not classified as Hodgkin's disease. Most non-Hodgkin's lymphomas involve mutation of lymphocytes, correlation with retroviruses, or T-cell leukemia. As with Hodgkin's disease, the first symptom is swollen lymph nodes, most often in the neck, axilla, or groin. But unlike Hodgkin's disease, non-Hodgkin's lymphoma is a group of diverse lymphomas that may manifest different primary and secondary symptoms, such as enlarged lymph nodes, swollen abdomen (belly), feeling full after eating small amounts of food, chest pain or pressure, shortness of breath or cough, fever, weight loss, night sweats, and fatigue. Non-Hodgkin's lymphoma often is subcategorized by grade and area of tumor involvement.

Some forms of leukemia may be classified as lymphomas because they involve lymphocytes. However, not all types of leukemia are disorders of lymphatic tissue; instead, some could be classified as blood disorders.

Lymphatic Malformation

Lymphatic malformation (LM) is a spongelike collection of abnormal channels and cystic spaces that contain clear fluid. They occur as localized swelling and sometimes more extensive enlargement of soft tissues and bones. LM in the superficial skin presents as tiny clear bubbles (vesicles) that often become dark red as a result of bleeding. LM is a common basis for enlargement of any structure (e.g., lip, cheek, ear, tongue, limb, finger, toe). Generalized swelling caused by trapped tissue fluid, called *lymphedema,* can also be caused by a type of LM. Old terms for LM are "cystic hygroma" and "lymphangioma." Lymphatic channels sprout from veins in early embryonic life. Although the precise cause is unknown, LMs are believed to be caused by an error in the formation of these tiny thin-walled sacs and tubes in the embryonic period. Two ways to manage LMs are sclerotherapy (direct injection of an irritating solution) and surgical removal.

INDICATIONS/CONTRAINDICATIONS for Therapeutic Massage

Lymphatic System

Massage is contraindicated in the presence of malignant and infectious conditions until the client's health care professional gives approval. Do not specifically massage a lymphatic malformation. Modification of massage application is necessary according to the type of treatment the client is receiving and his or her stress and fatigue levels. Massage that relaxes the client supports well-being and is helpful.

The massage practitioner can manage simple edema by using a massage application focused on supporting the lymphatic system. The appropriate health professional must supervise massage in clients with more complicated lymphedema.

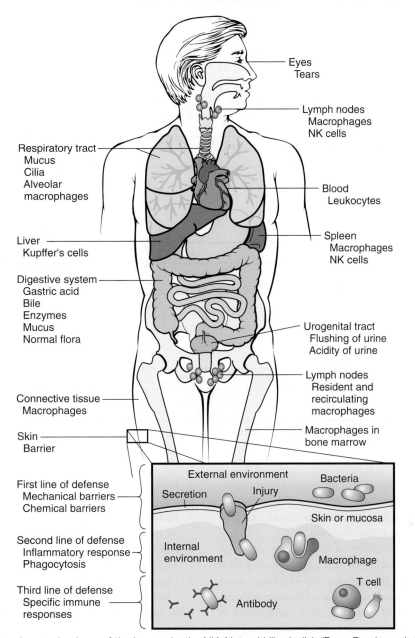

Eyes
Tears

Lymph nodes
Macrophages
NK cells

Respiratory tract
Mucus
Cilia
Alveolar
macrophages

Blood
Leukocytes

Liver
Kupffer's cells

Spleen
Macrophages
NK cells

Digestive system
Gastric acid
Bile
Enzymes
Mucus
Normal flora

Urogenital tract
Flushing of urine
Acidity of urine

Lymph nodes
Resident and
recirculating
macrophages

Connective tissue
Macrophages

Macrophages in
bone marrow

Skin
Barrier

First line of defense
Mechanical barriers
Chemical barriers

External environment

Bacteria

Secretion

Injury

Skin or mucosa

Second line of defense
Inflammatory response
Phagocytosis

Internal
environment

Macrophage

Third line of defense
Specific immune
responses

T cell

Antibody

FIGURE 11-25 Natural protective mechanisms of the human body. *NK,* Natural killer (cells). (From Damjanov I: *Pathology for the health-related professions,* ed 4, Philadelphia, 2012, Saunders.)

IMMUNE SYSTEM

SECTION OBJECTIVES

Chapter objective covered in this section:

8. Define immunity.
9. List and describe nonspecific and specific immune responses of the body.
10. Explain how the mind/body connection affects immunity.
11. Identify pathologies of the immune system and describe indications and contraindications for massage.

After completing this chapter, the student will be able to perform the following:

- Explain the difference between nonspecific and specific immunity.
- Determine massage indications and contraindications for pathologic conditions of the immune system.

Immunity is a complex response that involves all the systems of the body as they join together to eliminate any pathogen, foreign substance, or toxic material that could damage the body. The immune system is not a specific structural organ system but rather a functional system (Figures 11-25 and 11-26) that draws on the structures and processes of each organ, tissue, and cell and the chemicals produced in them. The immune system responds in one of two ways. In a nonspecific (innate) immune response, the body responds exactly the same way to all substances that are not identified as part of the body. People are born with nonspecific immunity. Specific immunity involves particular responses to each foreign substance identified. Special memory cells are called upon to identify a pathogen if it reappears. Specific immunity

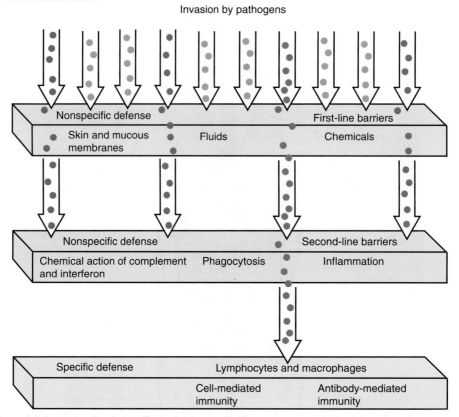

FIGURE 11-26 Overview of defense mechanisms. (From Applegate E: *The anatomy and physiology learning system,* ed 4, St Louis, 2011, Saunders.)

can be acquired in two ways: through natural immunity, which is the result of exposure; and through artificial immunity, in which a substance, such as a vaccine, is introduced into the body to stimulate the immune response.

The key to immunity is the ability of the body to recognize self and nonself. The recognition of self begins during fetal development and continues throughout life. The body must be able to identify the substances capable of causing a threat before it initiates any kind of response; such recognition is immunologic. An antigen—any substance that causes the body to produce antibodies—is usually something that has been identified as harmful or potentially dangerous to the body. A foreign antigen comes from outside the body; a self-antigen comes from within. An antibody is a specific protein produced to destroy or suppress antigens.

Microorganisms are minute life forms that may be damaging to the body or may interfere with its function. All microorganisms are microscopic. Many microorganisms do not normally cause disease in human beings but exist either in a state of commensalism, in which they give little or no benefit or harm to human beings, or in a state of mutualism, in which both gain some benefit. This nonharmful balance exists when the immune system works well, but these same organisms can cause infection if the immune system does not function properly. Many other microorganisms can cause infectious disease and are called *pathogens.* Pathogens, as explained in Chapter 2, fall into five main groups:

1. Viruses
2. Bacteria
3. Fungi
4. Protozoa
5. Pathogenic animals

In addition, two other classes of small agents can cause disease:

1. Ticks and mites
2. Mesozoa and leeches

These organisms live in and on the body, causing infestations rather than the infectious disease caused by bacteria or virus.

Infectious disease is by far the greatest cause of disease and death worldwide. Respiratory infections and gastrointestinal infections cause more deaths worldwide than all other diseases added together. General symptoms of infectious diseases are as follows:

• Fever
• Increased catabolism
• Malaise

Opportunistic infections occur when the normal human defenses are so weak that they allow infection by organisms that generally would not cause infection in a healthy human being. Nosocomial infections are transmitted in hospitals; some of these may be opportunistic infections, or they may occur because of the special nature of the hospital environment.

The time between exposure to a pathogen and the first appearance of symptoms is called the *incubation period,* and although no symptoms are apparent, the organism may be causing substantial damage during this time. There may follow a period known as the *prodrome,* in which nonspecific signs and symptoms, such as headache, fever, and lethargy, appear before the development of the acute phase and specific symptoms. Once the acute stage has passed, there is a period of resolution, in which the severity of the symptoms gradually decreases. Finally, during convalescence the symptoms have largely disappeared, but the body is still recovering.

The time, course, and severity of the disease are determined by the balance between the virulence (strength) of the infecting agent and the success with which the immune system combats the organism. Infections that are not sufficiently severe to produce clinical symptoms are called *asymptomatic* or *subclinical infections.* Clinical infections have a number of outcomes, ranging from death to complete recovery. The term *latency* refers to a situation in which a pathogen persists in a dormant, inactive form without causing damage but could reactivate to cause problems at a later date. An example is the herpes simplex virus, which lies dormant within dorsal root ganglia after the primary infection but may reactivate periodically to cause cold sores.

Microorganisms are everywhere. They are in the air we breathe and in or on the food we eat. Thus our epithelial surfaces (skin, respiratory tract, gastrointestinal tract, and genitourinary tract) are exposed to microorganisms continuously. Disease occurs when microorganisms invade epithelial surfaces. However, given our constant exposure to microorganisms, it is surprising that we enjoy such long infection-free periods and that infections are the exception rather than the rule.

When the immune system is operating effectively, it protects the body from infectious microorganisms and any of the cells of the body that have turned against it (i.e., cells that have overreacted in their response or that have begun to develop and grow at an unhealthy rate or have mutated into cancer). The immune system performs this protection directly by attacking the cells and indirectly by releasing mobilizing chemicals and protective antibodies.

Nonspecific Defenses

Nonspecific (innate or natural) immunity involves mechanical barriers, such as intact skin and mucous membranes, and chemical barriers, such as stomach acid. No matter what the invading substance is, the body responds in the same manner, with the same chemicals and cells mediating the actions. This general response is a preventive measure and the first reaction to pathogenic invasion.

Sanitary practices such as hand washing, disinfecting, and sterilizing support immunity by preventing exposure to pathogens.

Each body area has mechanical and chemical aspects of innate immunity.

Skin

Just as the husk of a fruit or berry protects it from drying up in drought or swelling in rain, so the skin protects the body from undue entry or loss of water. When intact the skin is virtually impermeable to microorganisms and also protects

from chemicals (e.g., weak acids, alkalis) and most gases (although some gases developed for use in chemical warfare can be absorbed through the skin). The integument provides some protection from physical trauma. Sebum from sebaceous glands is composed of triglycerides, waxes, and cholesterol. The main function of the sebum is to waterproof the skin, but sebum is also antibacterial.

Each square centimeter of skin may contain as many as 3 million microorganisms, most of which are harmless. The skin does not provide a hospitable environment for bacteria unless they have adapted through evolution to living there. The application of deodorants and the use of strong soaps that change the skin pH from acid to alkaline upset the fine balance that exists between our parasites and us. These agents tend to kill or inhibit the normal flora, leaving the area open to potential colonization by pathogens.

Arms and legs have the fewest microorganisms (only 1000 to 10,000 per square centimeter), whereas the forehead may contain as many as 1 million per square centimeter and the area between the toes may have as many as 1 billion per square centimeter.

Microorganisms thrive in moist conditions, so the axillae (armpits) and groin provide favorable areas for their growth. The skin can never be sterilized completely. The topical application of alcohol and iodine-based lotions may cause the death of a large percentage of resident organisms, but such applications do not remove those bacteria that inhabit the hair follicles and make up at least 20% of the resident bacteria.

Eye

Tears produced by the lacrimal glands constantly irrigate the surface of the eyeball. Tears contain high levels of lysozyme— in fact, the highest levels of any of the body secretions—so they form an effective barrier against infection. If the diet is lacking in vitamin A, the production of lysozyme in the tears decreases and can predispose a person to eye infection. Blinking is a defense reflex that eliminates irritants and ensures even distribution of the tears.

In some conditions, such as facial paralysis and stroke, this reflex is lost, and preventing the eye from drying up by keeping it closed or covered and performing regular irrigation becomes necessary.

Ear

Ceruminous glands located in the outer ear canal are modified sweat glands that produce cerumen, or ear wax. Cerumen provides a sticky barrier to foreign agents entering the ear canal.

Mouth

The mouth is lined with mucous membrane that is constantly irrigated by saliva. This flow is directed toward the throat and has the dual purpose of preventing microorganisms from infecting the salivary glands and of trapping the organisms so that they can be swallowed and disposed of in the digestive tract.

Saliva contains an enzyme called *lysozyme* that is antibacterial and mucus that contains immunoglobulin A. Dehydrated persons have a reduced flow of saliva and are at a higher risk for mouth infections.

The resident bacteria of the mouth are generally harmless. Indeed some, such as alpha-hemolytic streptococcus, are of benefit because they produce hydrogen peroxide, which helps keep the mouth clean.

Persons who are on prolonged courses of oral antibiotics run the risk of having their normal flora (bacteria) wiped out, which can result in the opportunistic infection of the mouth by other microorganisms. A common organism that can become problematic is the unicellular fungus *Candida albicans,* which causes thrush.

The tonsils also assist in protecting the oral cavity.

Stomach

The hydrochloric acid present in the gastric juices produced by the stomach lining is of a sufficiently low pH to kill most organisms entering the body with food or drink or by being swallowed. Some organisms, however, can resist this strong acid. Examples include the tubercule bacillus, enteroviruses, salmonella, and the eggs of parasitic worms.

Milk and proteins are effective buffers against stomach acid, and organisms that enter the stomach accompanied by this type of food stand more chance of escaping the damaging effects of hydrochloric acid. Thus contaminated meat and dairy products tend to be more dangerous in terms of an infection.

Vomiting may be considered a defense mechanism because it rids the body of irritants and toxins such as alcohol, drugs, and bacterial toxins in some instances, although this protection is by no means fully effective.

Intestines

The small and large intestines rely to a great extent on the bactericidal action of the stomach. In addition, the normal beneficial flora of the area, such as *Escherichia coli,* nonhemolytic streptococci, and anaerobic bacteroides, contribute to the normal functioning of the intestines. Their importance becomes more evident when the administration of broad-spectrum antibiotics or indiscriminate use of laxatives removes them. The intestines then are open to colonization by pathogenic bacteria, such as *Staphylococcus pyogenes,* that may be resistant to antibiotics.

In addition, the small and large intestines are supplied liberally with lymphatic tissue throughout their length. The lymph participates in the nonspecific and acquired immune defense systems of the body.

Like vomiting, diarrhea can also be considered a defense mechanism, although in most instances it occurs far too late in the course of an infection to be of much benefit.

Respiratory Tract

Upper Respiratory Tract

Hairs in the nose prevent insects and large particles from entering the upper respiratory tract. The ciliated nasal mucosa secretes a backward-flowing stream of mucus that is sticky and traps smaller particles. It also has bactericidal and virucidal properties. Lysozyme is also present in nasal secretions.

The epithelium of the upper respiratory tract is thin and unfortunately is prone to infections by rhinoviruses and adenoviruses, which are not affected by the nasal secretions. Sneezing is a protective reflex that expels irritants.

Trachea and Lungs

The trachea and bronchi are lined with a ciliated mucous membrane that traps any organisms in debris that may have escaped from the upper tract. The cilia beat upward and shift a stream of mucus away from the lungs and toward the pharynx to be swallowed. Should any organisms reach the alveoli, alveolar macrophages phagocytize them. The lung is well supplied with lymph nodes that act as another filter.

Coughing is a defensive reflex that removes particulate matter or excessive mucus in the lower tract.

Genitourinary Tract

The constant downward flow of urine through the ureter and bladder tends to protect against ascending infections. Urination irrigates the urethra. Urination is an effective response in the long male urethra but is less so in the female. The adult female urethra is only 2 to 3 cm long and forms a short and readily available entry point for organisms to invade the bladder.

Sexual activity in the female may predispose to the occurrence of urethritis (an inflammation of the urethra) and cystitis (a bladder infection). The most common offending organism is a coliform bacillus from the perineal area.

The beneficial resident florae of the vagina, especially lactobacillus, help maintain an acidic environment, creating an inhospitable habitat for invading pathogens. Some vaginal deodorants disturb the pH balance of the vaginal area and can result in infection, often by the opportunistic *C. albicans.*

Inflammatory Response

Complements are proteins found in blood that combine to create substances that phagocytize bacteria. Interferon, a protein produced by cells infected by viruses, forms antiviral proteins to help protect uninfected cells.

Cellular response is the action of the blood cells, primarily white blood cells, that deal with pathogens. Natural killer cells are a subset of lymphocytes that can eliminate virus-infected cells. Cells such as macrophages and neutrophils begin to phagocytize, or to surround and destroy, pathogens. Basophils and mast cells (from connective tissue) release chemicals that initiate inflammation. Eosinophils release chemicals that slow or stop the inflammatory response.

Inflammatory response is a sequence of events involving chemical and cellular activation that destroys pathogens and aids in the repair of tissues (see Chapter 2). For example, when damage occurs to tissue, basophils and mast cells release chemicals that increase the blood flow, which brings neutrophils and macrophages to the area. The phagocytic white cells, mainly macrophages, enter the tissues to destroy any bacteria. At the same time, the chemical response changes the permeability of the blood vessel wall so that fibrin can enter the tissues to repair the damage. This process continues until the

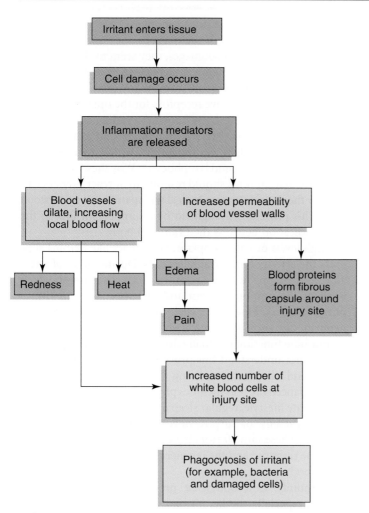

FIGURE 11-27 Inflammatory response. Tissue damage caused by bacteria triggers a series of events that produces the inflammatory response and promotes phagocytosis at the site of injury. These responses tend to inhibit or destroy the bacteria.

Table 11-1	Types of Adaptive Immunity
Type	**Description or Example**
Natural immunity	Exposure to the causative agent is not deliberate.
Active (exposure)	A child develops measles and acquires an immunity to a subsequent infection.
Passive (exposure)	A fetus receives protection from the mother through the placenta, or an infant receives protection through the mother's milk.
Artificial immunity	Exposure to the causative agent is deliberate.
Active (exposure)	Injection of the causative agent, such as a vaccination against polio, confers immunity.
Passive (exposure)	Injection of protective material (antibodies) that was developed by another individual's immune system.

From Patton KT, Thibodeau GA: *Anatomy and physiology,* ed 7, St Louis, 2010, Mosby.

damage has been repaired and all bacteria have been removed (Figure 11-27).

Specific Immunity

Specific immunity is the ability to recognize certain antigens and destroy them (Table 11-1).

Lymphocytes are the cells of specific immunity because they can recognize and destroy specific molecules. When a person has a disease such as measles, memory cells set up a lymphocyte pattern at the time of the first infection that can respond to a second exposure and prevent reinfection. Lymphocytes develop in the following three ways:

1. All lymphocytes form in the red bone marrow. T cells are matured in the thymus, then travel to lymphatic tissue such as is found in the spleen, lymph nodules, and lymph nodes. They are able to recognize antigens and respond by releasing inflammatory and toxic substances. Specialized T cells also regulate immune responses. These cells release molecules that amplify the response, whereas other T cells suppress the response of the body when the infection has been

contained. Some T cells develop into memory cells and handle secondary responses on reexposure to antigens that have already produced a primary response.

2. B cells stay in the bone marrow to mature and then travel to lymphatic tissue. They differentiate into plasma cells, which produce antibodies. Antibodies are in the immunoglobulin class of proteins. They circulate in body fluids and destroy specific antigens. Some B cells modify and become antigen nonspecific, which provides them with a greater ability to respond to bacterial and viral pathogens. Some B cells, like T cells, become memory cells and handle reexposure to antigens.

3. A few lymphocytes do not develop the same structural or functional characteristics as the T cells and B cells. These cells are known as natural killer cells. They too develop in the bone marrow and, when mature, can attack and kill tumor cells and virus-infected cells during their initial developmental stage, before the immune system is activated.

Specific defense responses can develop quickly. Because lymph capillaries pick up proteins and pathogens from nearly all body tissues, immune cells in lymph nodes are in a strategic position to encounter a large variety of antigens. Lymphocytes and macrophages in the tonsils act primarily against microorganisms that invade the oral and nasal cavities, and the spleen acts as a filter to trap blood antigens.

Lymphocytes fight infection in three ways:

1. Elimination of extracellular microorganisms

In response to infection, B cells mature into plasma cells that secrete antibodies. B cells recognize microbes because they have a protein in their cell membrane that acts as an antigen receptor. An antibody recognizes structures on the surfaces of microorganisms as well as proteins, carbohydrates, and lipids. Thus each person's plasma contains many different types of antibodies, each of which recognizes different microorganisms. As discussed previously, antibodies circulate in body fluids to target extracellular microorganisms. When the antibody binds to a microorganism, it activates mechanisms that eliminate the microorganism.

In the primary response, at the time of first infection, no antibody exists in blood, and the level of antibody does not begin to increase until 7 to 10 days later. The level of antibody rises slowly to a low peak and then gradually declines toward baseline.

In the secondary response, on subsequent exposure to the same microorganisms, the level of antibody begins to increase within 24 hours and reaches and sustains a high level.

2. Production of local hormones to stimulate T cells

Helper T cells, also known as *CD4 T cells*, secrete local hormones called *cytokines*. Cytokines stimulate another type of T cell, called *killer T cells, CD8 T,* or *cytotoxic T cells,* to multiply and lymphatic tissue to search for microorganisms inside body cells.

3. Elimination of microorganisms that have infected body cells

The most common type of microorganism that infects body cells is viruses. During intracellular replication, virus proteins appear on the surface of the infected cell. CD8 T cells recognize these viral antigens as foreign and secrete cytotoxic molecules that kill the infected cells.

Practical Application

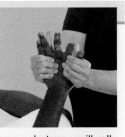

Homeopathy is a form of health care that introduces minute energetic forms of various plants and other substances into the body. The premise is that if large doses of a substance cause a particular physiologic response (e.g., vomiting), minuscule energetic tracings of the same substance will rally the defenses of the body to restore balance to whatever is causing the disruption.

The concept of vaccination is similar to, and may have been based on, the concept of homeopathy. The difference is the strength of the product. Vaccines are weakened or killed forms of the actual pathogen, whereas homeopathic substances are energetic forms of the actual substance. Live vaccines can cause disease, as is shown by the symptoms babies sometimes develop when they receive their immunizations. However, both systems seek to activate the body's immunity so it can protect and heal itself.

Mind/Body Connection

The sheer power of the mind to affect the body as a whole and the general state of health is amazing. Scientists have confirmed that a witch doctor can cause death simply by telling those who believe in his powers that they are going to die. Moreover, scientists have confirmed that we can think ourselves to health.

Studies of neuroimmunomodulation have discovered that left-handed persons are more likely to suffer immune system disorders than are right-handed persons. These studies indicate that the left hemisphere most directly controls the immune cells through the T cell response but that the right hemisphere

enhances and modulates the response. Other investigations have shown that although the nervous and immune systems have different chemical languages, they seem to share a few of the more important chemical signals, such as those of the opiate neuropeptides. Like neurons, many cells involved with the immune response have receptors for the opiate neuropeptides, which have long been known to influence mood and behavior. Many scientists are convinced that macrophages have receptors for these neuropeptides, which are released by pain-sensing neurons and lymphocytes. Why these cells, which are active in immunity, should respond to or react to chemicals used by the nervous system to deal with pain is not understood fully. This process is thought to be an important link in the communication between the brain and body.

High levels of natural opiates (which act like heroin) suppress the activity of natural killer cells. During times of stress and severe depression, the number of T cells is lower, which weakens the immune system and increases susceptibility to physical illness. Hormones such as corticosteroids and epinephrine also provide chemical links between the two systems.

Immune function gradually declines as humans age. Scientists do not understand this process, but studies of longevity have found a link between living vitally in the advanced years and a balanced life that includes physical activity, a simple diet, a moderate lifestyle, regular sleep and wake cycles, loving relationships, a sense of purpose or reason for being, and spiritual strength. These same factors have been shown to support the immune response and the regeneration and healing capacities of the body.

Immunity is a bodywide process. The integumentary system, especially the keratinized epithelial cells, provides a mechanical barrier, and these same cells act as an alarm system, triggering responses when the integument is breached. The skeletal system provides the bone marrow as the developmental home for the lymphocytes and macrophages. Heat from the muscle system actively initiates fever-like effects. The nervous and endocrine systems interact directly, linking the mind/body effects of the immune response through a shared chemical language. The cardiovascular system provides the travel network, lymphatic system, and filtering system. The respiratory system provides oxygen needed by immune cells, and the digestive system nourishes the immune cells and secretes acids hostile to pathogens. The urinary system eliminates waste and maintains the protective acid balance. The reproductive system works with the endocrine system to influence the process through hormone function.

The immune system is the best example of teamwork, or of a multidisciplinary approach, in the body, and a lesson can be learned here. When any one of us does not do our job, others are overtasked; in the body this is immune deficiency. When we overreact, our hypersensitivities are unproductive and we feel miserable, wasting energy that could be better used in other ways. When we are unaware of ourselves (autoimmunity), we not only attack ourselves but also fail to combine efforts to support others. Energy for the common good is wasted, and the lack of self-recognition destroys us, little by little. The amazing multidimensional links of the immune system support the idea that we truly are what we think, eat, do, hate, love, breathe, support, and become. Living well in our own bodies and sharing space with all forms of life on this planet reflect the ancient spiritual wisdom of living in a balanced way with cooperation and respect.

Pathologic Conditions of the Immune System

The organizational structures and responses of the immune system can break down (Box 11-2). The imbalances that occur in that circumstance are immune deficiencies, hypersensitivities, and autoimmune diseases.

Immune deficiency is a condition in which the body is unable to mount the proper immune response to a pathogen. An analogy is an office that has too much work and not enough workers to get the job done. The work piles up, the

---

| Box 11-2 | Four Classes of Immune Hypersensitivity Malfunction |

Type I: Immediate Anaphylactic Hypersensitivity
Type 1 hypersensitivity is best exemplified by allergic asthma, atopic dermatitis (eczema), allergic rhinitis (hay fever), and acute urticaria (hives).
- Type I hypersensitivity is considered to be one of the most powerful effector mechanisms of the immune system. This reaction begins rapidly. The most serious and extreme systemic form is anaphylaxis.
- Allergies now are recognized as common, affecting 20% of all persons in the United States. Allergies are considered the most common immune disorder in the world.

Type II: Antibody-Dependent Cytotoxic Hypersensitivity
Type II hypersensitivity, which involves antibody responses against antigens on cells, is also an immediate reaction, such as that which occurs when incompatible blood is given during a transfusion.
- Exposure to certain medications can cause a similar process; the drug molecules probably combine with a protein in the blood before being misidentified as an antigen.
- Penicillin and its derivatives are responsible for most of the recorded allergic reactions to drugs and 97% of the deaths caused each year by drug allergies.
- Symptoms are typically mild: hives, some fever, chills, swelling of lymph nodes, and sometimes arthritis-like discomfort.

Type III: Immune Complex-Mediated Hypersensitivity
In type III hypersensitivity the immune system misidentifies a protein in antiserum as potentially harmful and develops a response against the antiserum.
- Type III response is similar to type I response in that some of the same effects occur: blood vessel dilation, sneezing, coughing, and itching.

Type IV: Cell-Mediated (Delayed Type) Hypersensitivity
Type IV hypersensitivity involves T cells and macrophages, not antibodies.
- This type of reaction is an important part of the process of immune reactions to many intracellular infectious agents, and this response also is involved in graft rejection and tumor immunity.

---

workers get further and further behind, and eventually the office system breaks down. Some immune deficiencies are present at birth. These congenital problems affect the development of lymphocytes and result in a severe inability to respond to disease. Other immune deficiencies can arise later in life, such as acquired immunodeficiency syndrome (AIDS). Chronic stress also suppresses the immune system. Stress can be caused by physical mechanisms (e.g., chronic pain), other forms of chronic disease, and unresolved emotional or spiritual disturbances. When immunosuppressed, the body is more likely to be susceptible to a variety of bacterial, viral, and toxic pathogenic activities.

Hypersensitivity

The immune system also can become overactive, a condition called *hypersensitivity* or *allergy*. Few persons die of allergies, but the symptoms can make life miserable. Allergies are an overblown immune response to an allergen, something that causes the allergic reaction. Anaphylactic shock is the exception, and although rare, it is life-threatening. Anaphylactic shock is a severe, usually immediate reaction to a substance that causes respiratory distress, anxiety, and weakness. In extreme cases, anaphylactic shock also can involve arrhythmia and can result in death if not treated immediately (see Box 11-2).

AIDS and HIV Infection

AIDS is caused by a dysfunction in the immune system of the body. The diseases of AIDS are caused by pathogens encountered in everyday life. In fact, some of these pathogens live permanently in small numbers inside the human body. When the immune system weakens, these pathogens have the opportunity to multiply freely; thus the diseases these pathogens cause are called *opportunistic diseases.*

The human immunodeficiency virus (HIV) is a ribonucleic acid (RNA) virus. In most RNA viruses the viral RNA directly hijacks the host cell. However, HIV is different. After the virus enters the host cell, the RNA strand "writes" dual strands of viral DNA. This backward writing is called *reverse transcription.* The newly written DNA strands then go on to hijack the cell and oversee the production of new RNA replicas. Reverse-writing viruses such as HIV are called *retroviruses.*

As a group, retroviruses can live in their hosts for a long time without causing any sign of illness. In most animals such infections last for life. Retroviruses are not tough; they die when exposed to heat, are killed by many common disinfectants, and usually do not survive if the tissue or blood they are in dries. However, they have a high rate of mutation, and as a result, they tend to evolve quickly into new strains or varieties. HIV seems to share this trait and others with other known retroviruses.

HIV replicates in T cells and macrophages. The favorite target of the virus is the CD4 T cell. HIV infection of the CD4 T cells creates a defect in the immune system that eventually may cause AIDS. After HIV hijacks a T cell, the lymphocyte stops functioning normally, although this change is not immediately apparent. Little or no viral replication takes place for an indefinite period. The HIV takeover is a quiet event. When the CD4 T cell does become active, rather than functioning normally, it manufactures viral RNA strands. An infected CD4 T cell no longer detects invaders and triggers alarms. Eventually, the infected CD4 T cells begin to die, gradually reducing the CD4 T cell alarm network and allowing opportunistic diseases to enter and grow within the body.

HIV must travel from the inside of one person to the inside of another person, arriving with its RNA strands intact. Then the virus, or its intact RNA strands, must get into the bloodstream of the new host and find and enter a T cell. Once inside a host cell, HIV can prepare for replication. After replication replica viruses infect other host cells, probably attaching to new host cells when the infected host cell collides with other cells in the bloodstream.

Viruses generally are not able to enter the body through intact skin. Therefore viruses must enter the body through an open wound or one of a number of possible body openings. Most of these openings contain mucous membranes that protect the body. These membranes secrete mucus, which contains germicidal chemicals and keeps the surrounding tissues moist. Mucous membranes are found in the mouth, inside the eyelids, in the nose and air passages leading to the lungs, in the stomach, along the digestive tract, in the vagina, in the anus, and inside the opening of the penis. Many viruses, if placed on the surface of a mucous membrane, can travel through the membrane and enter the tiny blood vessels inside.

The danger with HIV is different; the major infection sites are the bloodstream and the central nervous system. Although HIV-carrying macrophages (roving white blood cells that engulf invaders but are susceptible to HIV infection) are found in the connective tissues of the lungs and in oral and mucous membranes, the number of viral organisms present does not appear to be great. This means that HIV is present in low concentrations, if at all, in saliva and sputum, so coughing should not expel a large quantity of HIV, if any. Apparently, HIV cannot easily cross the mucous membrane, and large concentrations of HIV probably are necessary for it to do so.

HIV can be found in any bodily fluid or substance that contains lymphocytes—blood, semen, vaginal and cervical secretions, breast milk, saliva, tears, urine, and feces—but the presence of HIV in a substance does not necessarily mean that it is capable of transmitting infection. All of these substances are, in theory, able to transmit disease, but in reality the most dangerous substances seem to be blood, semen, cervical and vaginal secretions, and perhaps feces. Despite an extensive search, no one has been able to find a clear-cut case in which saliva caused transmission, although kissing theoretically could.

The concentration of HIV in these substances is important when it comes to infection. The higher the concentration of viral organisms in a substance, the more likely it is to transmit HIV. Below a certain concentration, the substance cannot effectively transmit infection.

Hepatitis

Hepatitis is an inflammatory process and an infection of the liver caused by a virus. Hepatitis A, the least serious form, usually is transmitted by fecal contamination of food and water and does not become chronic. Once infected, a person becomes immune to future hepatitis A infections.

Hepatitis B, transmitted by routes similar to those of HIV, may be acute or chronic. The acute symptoms are similar to those of hepatitis A, but hepatitis B is much more severe in the chronic and acute stages. As liver cells die, liver function is impaired and death can result. Two types of vaccines are available for preventing hepatitis B, but more than 1 million persons in the United States are estimated to be carriers of the hepatitis B virus, which is 100 times more contagious than HIV.

Hepatitis C accounts for 85% of the new cases of hepatitis each year. This form is transmitted mostly by blood transfusions or when intravenous drug users share needles, and it usually becomes chronic.

Hepatitis D infects only those who have hepatitis B, and the symptoms are more severe than other forms of hepatitis. Vaccines do not appear to be effective for hepatitis D.

Hepatitis E is transmitted by food and water contaminated with feces and is usually a self-limited type of hepatitis that may occur after a natural disaster if sanitation is not maintained.

The treatment for all forms of hepatitis is rest and a high-protein diet. Observance of the Standard Precautions can prevent the spread of hepatitis. Obviously, people must avoid all behaviors that could transmit HIV and hepatitis B.

Autoimmune Disease

Autoimmune diseases occur when the body cannot distinguish self from nonself; self-antigens are treated as foreign antigens. When the recognition of self breaks down, the immune cells begin to attack the self. Some of the autoimmune diseases are multiple sclerosis, Graves' disease, rheumatoid arthritis, and juvenile diabetes.

The inflammatory response triggered by the immune complex is the pathogenic mechanism of tissue injury in a number of autoimmune diseases, including arthritis,

---

INDICATIONS/CONTRAINDICATIONS for Therapeutic Massage

Immune System

Therapeutic massage approaches help immune function by supporting balanced homeostatic functions. No specific methods are used for the immune system, yet any behavior that supports wellness, including regular massage, supports immunity. Any modality that normalizes autonomic nervous system functions supports immunity.

Any activity, including therapeutic massage, that causes the body to adapt puts stress on the system. If the client is basically healthy, he or she will be able to adapt without overstressing the body. However, if a client's immunity is suppressed, the reserves needed for adaptation are already at the breakdown point. The practitioner must gauge the intensity and duration of bodywork methods against the ability of the body to adapt so that the stress introduced supports a return to balance and is not "the straw that breaks the camel's back." The premise of "less is more" is a wise approach for individuals with immune dysfunction. Massage professionals should follow Standard Precautions to prevent spreading contagious diseases.

Table 11-2	**Examples of Autoimmune Diseases**	
Disease	Possible Self-Antigen	Description
Addison disease	Surface antigens on adrenal cells	Hyposecretion of adrenal hormones, resulting in weakness, reduced blood sugar, nausea, loss of appetite, and weight loss
Cardiomyopathy	Cardiac muscle	Disease of cardiac muscle (i.e., the myocardium), resulting in loss of pumping efficiency (heart failure)
Diabetes mellitus (type I)	Pancreatic islet cells, insulin, insulin receptors	Hyposecretion of insulin by the pancreas, resulting in extremely elevated blood glucose levels (in turn causing host of metabolic problems, even death if untreated)
Glomerulonephritis	Blood antigens that form immune complexes that deposited in kidney	Disease of the filtration apparatus of the kidney (renal corpuscle), resulting in fluid and electrolyte imbalance and possibly total kidney failure and death
Graves disease (type of hyperthyroidism)	TSH receptors on thyroid cells	Hypersecretion of thyroid hormone and resulting increase in metabolic rate
Hemolytic anemia	Surface antigens on RBCs	Condition of low RBC count in the blood resulting from excessive destruction of mature RBCs (hemolysis)
Hypothyroidism	Antigens in thyroid cells	Hyposecretion of thyroid hormone in adulthood, causing decreased metabolic rate and characterized by reduced mental and physical vigor, weight gain, hair loss, and edema
Multiple sclerosis (MS)	Antigens in myelin sheaths of nervous tissue	Progressive degeneration of myelin sheaths, resulting in widespread impairment of nerve function (especially muscle control)
Myasthenia gravis	Antigens at neuromuscular junction	Muscle disorder characterized by progressive weakness and chronic fatigue
Pernicious anemia	Antigens on parietal cells; intrinsic factor	Abnormally low RBC count resulting from the inability to absorb vitamin B_{12}, a substance critical to RBC production
Reproductive infertility	Antigens on sperm or tissue surrounding ovum (egg)	Inability to produce offspring (in this case, resulting from the destruction of gametes)
Rheumatic fever	Cardiac cell membranes (cross reaction with group A streptococcal antigen)	Rheumatic heart disease; inflammatory cardiac damage (especially to the endocardium valves)
Rheumatoid arthritis (RA)	Collagen	Inflammatory joint disease characterized by synovial inflammation that spreads to other fibrous tissues
Systemic lupus erythematosus (SLE)	Numerous	Chronic inflammatory disease with widespread effects and characterized by arthritis, a red rash on the face, and other signs
Ulcerative colitis	Mucous cells of colon	Chronic inflammatory disease of the colon characterized by watery diarrhea containing blood, mucus, and pus

From Patton KT, Thibodeau GA: *Anatomy and physiology,* ed 7, St Louis, 2010, Mosby.

vasculitis, and glomerulonephritis (Table 11-2). Immune complex injury may result from the activation of resident inflammatory cells and the recruitment of circulating monocytes or neutrophils at various sites. A growing consensus among scientists is that common disorders such as atherosclerosis, colon cancer, and Alzheimer's disease are caused in part by a chronic inflammatory syndrome.

SUMMARY

The justification activity at the end of this chapter and provided again at the end of Chapter 12 represents the outcomes of a competency-based education. In fact, all the problem-solving activities support competency. Being a competent massage therapist requires much more than recall of factual data, and competence is based on how you use those data in professional application of massage. Clinical reasoning is necessary if you are to use information in professional practice. How do you plan and organize an effective massage session? How

do you provide assessment to determine indications for and contraindications to massage? How do you choose a massage application based on physiologic effects? How do you collect and analyze data to develop appropriate treatment plans and then obtain informed consent? How do you know whether you are functioning within your scope of practice? How do you identify the most logical approach to massage application, including time management, body mechanics and ergonomic practice, and type of equipment needed? How do you evaluate the behaviors, feelings, and outcomes of the professional relationship as measured against the outcomes of the massage? All these issues are relevant to ethical, professional practice, as are the principles of respect and the provision of benefits that outweigh the burden of treatment and do no harm.

This chapter began with a discussion of touch, an important topic that certainly could be explored in greater depth, because massage therapy depends on touch not only for therapeutic benefit but also for the compassionate, nurturing connection that is established between practitioner and client.

Evolve Activity 11-4

✎ ACTIVITY 11-2

Note: This activity may seem difficult, but it is very important to be able to justify the work we do. The only way to become proficient is to practice.

We must be able to explain and justify the therapeutic value of the work we do. The following activity will assist you in developing the skills necessary to explain the effectiveness of therapeutic massage to clients and other health care professionals. Use the clinical reasoning model that follows to accomplish this task. The focus should be the primary massage method applied to one of the systems discussed in this chapter: the integumentary, cardiovascular, lymphatic, or immune system. You can either pick one of the common pathologies of the system or justify how massage supports effective function of that system. (See example in Appendix C.)

Methods/Applications

1. What are the facts?
   a. Which system is involved, and which structures of that system can be reached directly or indirectly?
   b. What is considered normal or balanced function?
   c. How are the functions of this system related to the homeostasis of the body?
   d. Which of these structures are most affected by this massage?
   e. Which physiologic functions are affected by the massage?
   f. When the treatment is applied, what changes in function will occur in:
      (1) this system?
      (2) the whole body?
   g. What has worked or has not worked?
   h. Where could you find information that would support the use of massage as a therapeutic intervention?
   i. What research is available to support the use of therapeutic massage?
   j. How does the intervention support a healthy state?
   k. Under which pathologic, or dysfunctional, condition is the therapeutic massage most likely to be beneficial?

2. What are the possibilities?
   a. What do the facts suggest?
   b. List at least three applications of massage that would affect the structure and function of the system involved.
   c. What are other ways to look at the situation?
   d. What other methods could provide similar benefits?

3. What is the logical outcome of therapeutic intervention?
   a. What would be the logical progression of the symptom pattern, contributing factors, and current behaviors?
   b. What are the benefits and drawbacks of each intervention suggested?
      Benefits:
      Drawbacks:
   c. What are the costs in terms of time, resources, and finances?
   d. What is likely to happen if massage is not used?
   e. What is likely to happen if massage is used?

4. What would be the effects on the persons involved, specifically the client, practitioner, and other professionals working with the client?
   a. How does each person involved (including, in addition to the aforementioned, the client's family and support system) feel about the possible massage interventions?
   b. Does the practitioner feel qualified to work with the situation and apply massage to the particular person?
   c. Does a feeling of cooperation and agreement exist among all those involved, and how would the practitioner recognize this feeling?

Justification

Using the information developed in the clinical reasoning model, present a clear, concise statement of how massage would be beneficial in supporting the particular body system in a healthy condition or as part of a treatment plan for a pathologic or dysfunctional condition.

We presented basic anatomy, physiology, and pathologic conditions of the integumentary, cardiovascular, lymphatic, and immune systems.

The justification exercises began the process of explaining and validating therapeutic massage. Being able to justify the effectiveness of therapeutic massage in supporting health maintenance or as part of a multidisciplinary approach for pathologic conditions will become increasingly important as more persons use these methods. The ability to explain the benefits of therapeutic massage and the skills each professional has to offer, based on a solid foundation of anatomy and physiology, adds to professional development and supports the use of these important treatments.

It is common for the student to find the justification activities difficult. Rising above the discomfort to achieve an integrated practice is necessary. The student should go back and do the activities again and again, using different scenarios and conditions. The student should remember that in professional practice, clinical reasoning, problem solving, and the integration of knowledge with application is the measure of a competent massage therapist (Activity 11-2).

℮volve

http://evolve.elsevier.com/Fritz/essential

Activity 11-1 Complete a word search with terms relating to the heart.

Activity 11-2 Review blood cells by completing a word chart exercise.

Activity 11-3 Read a case study on a heart attack client with questions at the end for review.

Activity 11-4 Drag-and-drop labelling exercises on the Evolve site help you review the structures of the systems of the body discussed in this chapter.

Additional Resources:

Scientific animations and Electronic Coloring Book

Weblinks

Remember to study for your certification and licensure exams! Review questions for this chapter are located on Evolve.

Workbook Section

Short Answer

1. What are some of the major functions of the integumentary system?

_____

_____

_____

_____

2. List the appendages of the skin.

_____

_____

3. What are the two main concerns involving integumentary pathologic conditions?

_____

_____

_____

4. List and describe the three types of arteries, and give an example of each type.

_____

_____

_____

_____

_____

_____

_____

_____

5. List the four sets of heart valves, and explain what each set does.

_____

_____

_____

_____

_____

_____

_____

_____

6. Why is venous blood return important? List factors that can affect it.

_____

_____

_____

_____

_____

_____

_____

7. What are the five groups of white blood cells?

_____

_____

_____

8. How is blood supplied to the heart? What happens if this supply is interrupted?

_____

_____

_____

_____

_____

9. What are the normal and abnormal heart sounds, and how are they produced?

_____

_____

_____

_____

_____

_____

_____

_____

10. What are the normal ranges of blood pressure, based on size, and what are the terms used for high blood pressure and low blood pressure?

_____

_____

_____

_____

11. What are the two main lymphatic ducts? How are they formed, and into what do they empty?

_____

_____

_____

_____

_____

12. What are lymph nodes, and where are they found?

_____

13. What is the name of the defense system of the body, and in what way does it respond to threats?

_____

_____

_____

_____

_____

_____

_____

14. How is nonspecific immunity provided?

_____

_____

_____

_____

_____

Fill in the Blank

The (1) _____ is made up of the skin and its appendages: hair, sebaceous glands, sweat glands, nails, and breasts.

The (2) _____ is the outer layer of skin; it consists of sublayers called *strata*. Four or five layers of strata make up the outer layer of skin, depending on the location on the body.

The (3) _____, the inner layer of skin, is much thicker than the epidermis and is composed of dense connective tissue that contains collagen and elastin fibers. The various appendages of the skin originate in the dermis and push upward through the epidermis. Blood vessels and nerves are present in the dermis but not in the epidermis. Subcutaneous tissue, which is located below the dermis, is also called (4) _____. It consists of loose connective tissue and contains fat (adipose) tissue.

The (5) _____ is a transport system composed of the heart, blood vessels, and blood. It functions to bring nutrients to the tissues and remove waste products from them.

One part of the cardiovascular system, the (6) _____, is a hollow, muscular pump about the size of a closed fist. It is located in the (7) _____, the space between the lungs. The (8) _____ is a sac that surrounds the heart. It secretes a lubricating fluid that prevents friction caused by the movement of the heart.

The two small, thin-walled upper chambers of the heart are the (9) _____, known separately as the right atrium and left atrium. They are separated by the thin interatrial septum. The two large lower chambers are the left and right (10) _____. Their thick walls are separated by the interventricular septum.

(11) _____ is the amount of blood pumped by the left ventricle in 1 minute. The average output is 5 to 6 liters of blood under normal conditions.

The (12) _____ is the sequence of events in one heartbeat. It consists of diastole and systole. The average person has 60 to 70 cardiac cycles per minute. The number of cardiac cycles in 1 minute is known as the (13) _____.

The vascular system is the other part of the cardiovascular system. The vascular system consists of blood vessels that carry blood from the heart to the lungs and body tissues and back to the heart in a continuous cycle. Blood vessels that transport blood from the heart are called (14) _____; these branch off into smaller and smaller arteries. The smallest of the arteries are called the (15) _____.

(16) _____ are the tiny blood vessels located between the arterioles and the veins. The function of the (17) _____ is to collect blood from the capillaries and transport the blood back to the heart. The smallest of the veins are the (18) _____. The veins get larger as they get closer to the heart. The largest veins return blood to the right atrium of the heart.

The amount of pressure exerted by the blood on the walls of the blood vessels is called (19) _____. The maximal pressure is called (20) _____; this occurs when the ventricles contract. (21) _____ occurs when the ventricles relax. Blood pressure is measured with a (22) _____, a cloth-covered rubber bag that is wrapped around the arm over the brachial artery. Blood pressure is highest during contraction of the heart (systole), which produces the systolic blood pressure. Blood pressure is lowest when the heart is relaxing (diastole), which gives the diastolic pressure.

The hepatic portal system begins in the capillaries of the digestive organs and ends in the (23) _____. Portal blood contains substances absorbed by the stomach and intestines. Portal blood is passed through the (24) _____, which absorbs, excretes, or converts nutrients and toxins. Restriction of outflow through the hepatic portal system can lead to (25) _____.

(26) _____, the thick, red fluid in our bodies, is a form of connective tissue. It transports nutrients to the individual cells and removes waste products.

The cellular substances in blood are red blood cells, white blood cells, and platelets. Blood cells float in a thick, straw-colored fluid called (27) _____. Red blood cells, also called (28) _____, or red blood corpuscles, constitute more than 90% of the formed elements in blood. Their function is to transport oxygen to the cells and carbon dioxide away from the cells.

White blood cells also are called (29) _____, or white blood corpuscles. Their white color is due to the lack of hemoglobin.

Thrombocytes, also called (30) _____, are the smallest cellular elements of the blood. They are important in the blood-clotting process and are manufactured in the bone marrow. A special protein, called (31) _____, is formed to seal damaged blood vessels by trapping red blood cells, platelets, and fluid to form a clot. This protein also anchors the clot in place.

The term (32) _____ means "hardening of the arteries" and refers to arteries that have become brittle and have lost their elasticity. Although the condition has several causes, the most common and important cause is (33) _____, the deposit of fatty plaques in medium and large arteries.

The (34) _____ collects accumulated tissue fluids from the entire body and returns them to the blood circulation. The system is one way, beginning in the tissues and ending in the blood vessels. The lymphatics work as an active part of our immunity by filtering and destroying foreign substances and microorganisms. Foreign particulate matter and pathogenic bacteria are screened out by the (35) _____ that are spaced along the course of the vessels. They also play an active role in digestion by absorbing fats from the small intestine.

(36) _____ is a clear interstitial tissue fluid that bathes the cells. The tiny (37) _____ are open-ended channels found in the tissue spaces of the entire body except for the brain, spinal cord, and cornea. They join to form larger lymph vessels that look like veins but have thinner, more transparent walls. Like veins, they have valves to prevent backflow.

(38) _____ is a complex response that networks all of the systems in the body to eliminate any pathogen, foreign substance, or toxic material that can be damaging to the body. The immune system is not a specific structural organ system but rather a functional system. The immune system protects the body directly by cell attack and indirectly by releasing mobilizing chemicals and protective (39) _____.

(40) _____ are the cells of specific immunity because they recognize and destroy specific molecules and have the ability to remember that particular pathogen.

Assess Your Competencies

Review the following objectives for this chapter:

1. Explain the physiology of touch.
2. List and describe the components and functions of the integumentary system.
   - Explain the importance of touch.
   - Describe the function of the integumentary system.
   - Describe two main concerns with integumentary pathologic conditions.
3. Identify pathologies of the integumentary system and describe indications and contraindications for massage.
4. List and describe the components and functions of the cardiovascular system.
   - List and describe the components of blood.
   - Describe the functions of the cardiovascular system.
   - Determine massage indications and contraindications for pathologic conditions of the cardiovascular system
5. Identify pathologies of the cardiovascular system, and describe indications and contraindications for massage.
6. List and describe the components of the lymphatic system.
7. Identify pathologies of the lymphatic system, and describe indications and contraindications for massage.
   - List and describe the components of the lymphatic system. List and describe the components of lymph.
   - Describe the functions of the lymphatic system.
   - Explain the role of the lymph nodes, spleen, thymus, and lymph nodules.
   - Describe how lymph moves through the body.
   - Determine massage indications and contraindications for pathologic conditions of the lymphatic system.
8. Define *immunity*.
9. List and describe nonspecific and specific immune responses of the body.
10. Explain how the mind/body connection affects immunity.
11. Identify pathologies of the immune system, and describe indications and contraindication for massage.
    - Explain the difference between nonspecific and specific immunity.
    - Determine massage indications and contraindications for pathologic conditions of the immune system.
    - Justify the effectiveness of therapeutic massage in supporting health maintenance for the integumentary, cardiovascular, lymphatic, and immune systems.

Next, on a separate piece of paper or using an audio or video recorder, prepare a short narrative that reflects how you would explain this content to a client and how the information relates to how you would provide massage. See the example in Chapter 1 on p. 22. When read or listened to, the narrative should not take more than 5 to 10 minutes to complete. Simpler is better. Use examples, tell stories, and use metaphors. It is important to understand that there is no precisely correct way to complete this exercise. The intent is to help you identify how effectively you understand the content and how relevant your application is to massage therapy. An excellent learning activity is to work together with other students and share your narratives. Also share these narratives with a friend or family member who is not familiar with the content. If the person can understand what has been written or recorded by you, that indicates that you understand it. There are many different ways to complete this learning activity. Yes, it may be confusing to do this, but that's all right. Out of confusion comes clarity. By the time you have done this 12 times, once for each chapter in this book, you will be much more competent.

Exercise: Skin Structure

In the cross-section of the skin structure pictured on the next page, write the name of each component next to the corresponding letter. Color each part after you label it.

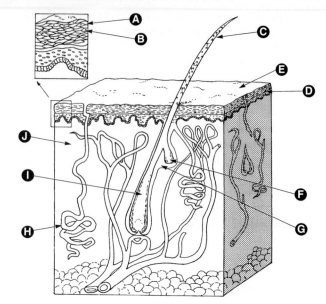

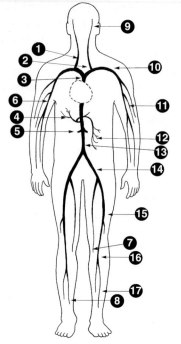

Dermis
Epidermis
Hair
Hair follicle
Horny tissue
Melanin
Sebaceous gland
Sebum
Skin
Sweat gland

A. _____
B. _____
C. _____
D. _____
E. _____
F. _____
G. _____
H. _____
I. _____
J. _____

Radial
Renal
Right common carotid

Label the figure by writing the names of the veins listed
     below next to the matching number in the illustration.

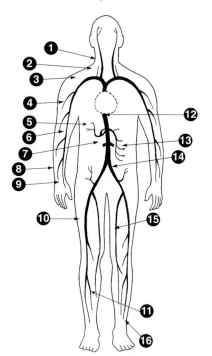

Labeling

Label the figure by writing the names of the arteries listed
below next to the matching number in the illustration.

Abdominal aorta
Anterior tibial
Aorta
Brachial
Brachiocephalic
Celiac
Deep femoral
External iliac
Femoral
Left external carotid
Left subclavian
Mesenteric
Peroneal
Popliteal

Anterior tibial
Basilic
Brachial
Common iliac
Femoral
Great saphenous
Hepatic
Inferior vena cava

Mesenteric
Posterior tibial
Radial
Renal
External jugular
Internal jugular
Right subclavian
Ulnar

Respiratory, Digestive, Urinary, and Reproductive Systems

CHAPTER OBJECTIVES

After completing this chapter, the student will be able to perform the following:

1. List and describe the components and function of the respiratory system.
2. Explain the mechanics of breathing.
3. Describe pathologic conditions of the respiratory system and the associated indications and contraindications for massage.
4. Describe how the decisions about what and when to eat influence health.
5. List and describe the components of the digestive system.
6. Describe the process of digestion.
7. Explain the importance of nutrition.
8. List and describe the main food groups.
9. Explain metabolic rate, energy balance, and body weight.
10. Describe pathologic conditions of the digestive system and the associated indications and contraindications for massage.
11. List the functions of the urinary system.
12. List and describe the components of the urinary system.
13. Describe urinary function and the processes of fluid electrolyte balances.
14. Describe pathologic conditions of the urinary system and the associated indications and contraindications for massage.
15. List and describe the components and functions of the male reproductive system.
16. List and describe the components and functions of the female reproductive system.
17. Explain the three stages of pregnancy and the process of lactation.
18. Describe pathologic conditions of the reproductive system and the associated indications and contraindications for massage.

CHAPTER OUTLINE

RESPIRATORY SYSTEM, 604
  Organs of the Respiratory System, 604
  Nerves and Vessels of the Lungs and Respiratory Muscles, 607
  Mechanics of Breathing, 607
  Pathologic Conditions of the Respiratory System, 610
DIGESTIVE SYSTEM, 613
  Organs and Structures of the Digestive System, 615
  Digestion, 617
  Nutrition, 618
  Pathologic Conditions of the Digestive System, 623
URINARY SYSTEM AND FLUID ELECTROLYTE BALANCES, 626
  Functions of the Urinary System, 626
  Organs of the Urinary System, 627
  Urinary Function, 628
  Water Balance, 629
  Pathologic Conditions of the Urinary System, 631
REPRODUCTIVE SYSTEM, 634
  Male Reproductive System, 635
  Female Reproductive System, 636
  Pathologic Conditions of the Reproductive System, 641
SUMMARY, 645

KEY TERMS

Absorption The movement of food molecules from the digestive tract to the cardiovascular and lymphatic systems so they can be transported to the cells of the body.

Basal metabolic rate (BA-sal) The rate of energy expenditure of the body in a quiet, resting, fasting state.

Breathing pattern disorder A complex set of behaviors that leads to overbreathing without the presence of a pathologic condition.

Diaphragm A dome-shaped sheet of muscle attached to the thoracic wall that separates the lungs and thoracic cavity from the abdominal cavity. As the chest cavity enlarges, the diaphragm moves downward and flattens to create a vacuum that allows air to flow into the lungs. As the chest contracts and the diaphragm relaxes, the diaphragm arches upward, helping air to flow out of the lungs.

Digestion The mechanical and chemical breakdown of food from its complex form into simple molecules.

Elimination (egestion) The removal and release of undigested and unabsorbed food as solid waste products.

External respiration The exchange of oxygen and carbon dioxide between the lungs and the bloodstream.

Gestation (jes-TAY-shun) The period of fetal growth from conception until birth.

Hyperventilation (hye-per-ven-ti-LAY-shun) Abnormally deep or rapid breathing in excess of physical demands.

Ingestion (in-JEST-chun) Taking food into the mouth.

Internal respiration The exchange of gases between the tissues and blood.

Lower respiratory tract The larynx, trachea, bronchi, and alveoli.

Lungs The primary organs of respiration. The lungs are soft, spongy, highly vascular structures that are separated into the left and right lungs by the mediastinum. Each lung is separated into lobes. The right lung has three lobes: upper, middle, and lower; the left lung has two lobes: upper and lower.

Peristalsis (pair-ih-STAL-sis) The rhythmic contraction of smooth muscles that propels products of digestion along the tract from the esophagus to the anus.

Respiration The movement of air in and out of the lungs, the exchange of oxygen and carbon dioxide between the lungs and the blood, and the exchange between the blood and the body tissues.

Sinuses (SYE-nus-ez) Four groups of air-filled spaces that open into the internal nose. They are located in the frontal, ethmoid, sphenoid, and maxillary bones of the skull. They lighten the weight of the skull and play a role in sound production.

Thorax (THOR-aks) Also known as the *chest cavity*. The thorax is the upper region of the torso. It is enclosed by the sternum, ribs, and thoracic vertebrae and contains the lungs, heart, and great blood vessels.

Upper respiratory tract The nasal cavity and all its structures and the pharynx.

LEARNING HOW TO LEARN

All the body systems discussed in this chapter are indirectly affected by massage through the nervous system and endocrine system. Massage therapy can have a more direct effect on the respiratory and digestive systems because techniques can mechanically address anatomy related to these systems. Massage supports the mechanics of breathing, which include muscle and connective tissue function and mobility of the ribs and entire thorax. The large intestine of the digestive system in particular can be addressed by massage to support waste movement in the body. One of the functions of the urinary system is to control blood pressure massage can support this by affecting the autonomic nervous systems and the cardiovascular system. Study of the reproductive system supports a massage population specialty of prenatal and postnatal massage.

RESPIRATORY SYSTEM

SECTION OBJECTIVES

Chapter objectives covered in this section:

1. List and describe the components and function of the respiratory system.
2. Explain the mechanics of breathing.
3. Describe pathologic conditions of the respiratory system and the associated indications and contraindications for massage.

After completing this section, the student will be able to perform the following:

- Define respiration.
- Explain external and internal respiration.
- Locate and describe the organs of the respiratory system.
- List the nerves and vessels of the respiratory system.
- Locate the muscles involved in respiration.
- Explain the mechanisms of breathing.
- Define lung volume.
- Explain the transport of oxygen and carbon dioxide.
- Describe the central nervous system control of breathing.
- List the reflexes of the respiratory system.
- Determine indications and contraindications of massage to respiratory system pathology.

Of all the basic life support systems in the body, the respiratory system is the only one under voluntary and automatic control. The respiratory system obtains the oxygen necessary to create energy for body functions and eliminate the carbon dioxide produced during cellular metabolism. Respiratory movements are under voluntary control, most often in connection with speech. This voluntary control of breathing helps regulate the autonomic nervous system. Therefore control of breathing becomes important in many relaxation and meditation practices. Respiration and breath are intimately connected to the expression of emotion, such as in laughing, crying, exploding in anger, holding one's breath in fear, and sighing with relief.

The respiratory system may have one of the most vital functions because the heart and brain require a continuous supply of oxygen to function. Apnea, the lack of spontaneous breathing, can cause irreversible brain damage if it continues for more than 3 or 4 minutes.

Respiration is the movement of air in and out of the lungs. Breathing is a mechanical action of inhalation and exhalation that draws oxygen into the lungs and releases carbon dioxide into the atmosphere.

Respiration is also the exchange of oxygen and carbon dioxide between the lungs and the blood and between the blood and the body tissues. **External respiration** is the exchange of oxygen and carbon dioxide between the lungs and the bloodstream. The exchange of gases between the body cells and the blood is called **internal respiration.**

On average, we breathe 12 to 16 times per minute. Each breath contains approximately 500 mL of air (about 2 cups), so in 1 hour we breathe about 360 liters, or 82 gallons, of air.

The organs of the respiratory system are divided into upper and lower regions. The **upper respiratory tract** consists of the nasal cavity, all its structures, and the pharynx; the **lower respiratory tract** consists of the larynx, trachea, and bronchi and alveoli in the lungs (Figure 12-1).

Organs of the Respiratory System

Nose and Nasal Cavity

The nose is divided into two parts, the external and internal portions. The lower two thirds of the external nose are composed mostly of cartilage. The upper third, or bridge of the nose, is formed by two small, hard nasal bones. The tip of the nose is the apex, and the nostrils are the nares. Air enters the external nares and passes across internal nasal hairs that trap particles of dirt and other foreign material; the air then flows into the nasal cavity.

The internal nose is the continuation of the nose inside the skull and above the mouth and includes the sinuses. The roof is formed by a small portion of the frontal bone and the ethmoid and sphenoid bones, and the floor is formed by the hard palate, consisting of the maxillae and palatine bones. The internal nares are the portion of the internal nose that communicates with the throat. The nasal cavity is the actual space inside the external and internal nose structures and is separated into left and right sides by the septum, a partition

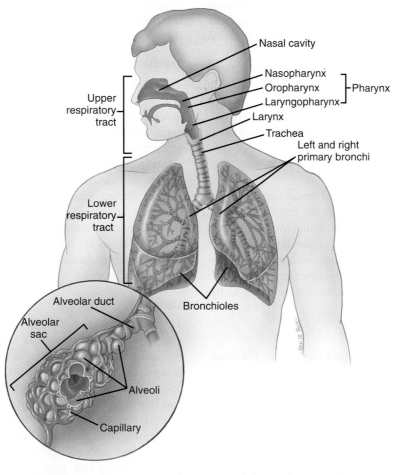

FIGURE 12-1 The organs and structures of the respiratory system.

composed of cartilage and bone. At the upper portion of the nasal cavity, three thin, curled bones, the turbinates, or conchae, project inward from the two outer walls. These turbinates separate into small, grooved passageways, each called a *meatus,* that continue to move the air.

Mucous membranes line the entire respiratory tract, starting in the nasal cavity. Deep to the mucous membrane are small blood vessels. Air that passes through the upper respiratory tract is warmed by blood in the blood vessels and moistened by the mucous membranes. Sticky mucus traps smaller inhaled particles, which helps prevent infection. Small hairs that line the nasal cavity and cilia that line the throat and air passageways in the lungs transport these foreign particles upward, where they are either swallowed (and destroyed in the digestive tract) or expelled from the body through coughing or sneezing.

The ends of the olfactory nerve lie in the upper third of both sides of the nasal septum, the olfactory region, and are stimulated by odor particles. Olfactory nerve fibers pass through small holes in the ethmoid bone to the olfactory bulb and then to the cortex, which interprets the impulses as smell.

Venous areas called *swell bodies* are located on the turbinates. About every half hour, the swell bodies on one side of

the nasal cavity engorge with blood, resulting in decreased air flow on that side, with good flow on the other side. Then the process reverses. These periodic changes permit the inside of the nose to recover from drying. This same mechanism becomes important during sleep. When a person lies with his or her head to one side, the swell bodies of the lower nostril become congested. The chamber narrows, and the lumen closes. Therefore a person breathes through only one nostril at a time while sleeping. The closure of the nostril then initiates movement of the head from one side to the other, which in turn causes a major movement and turning of the body. This head-body moving cycle, initiated by the nose, ensures maximal rest during sleep. A poorly functioning nose may allow the body and head to remain in one position and can cause symptoms such as backaches, numbness, cramps, and circulatory dysfunction.

The nasal septum is supplied with sensory nerves and blood vessels. Nasal reflex responses and referred phenomena are well established among the nose, ears, throat, larynx, heart, lungs, diaphragm, nervous system, and body temperature. Contained in the coordination of these various reflex patterns is the mechanism of entrainment among heart rate, breathing rate, and synchronization of other body rhythms. Most relaxation methods and the methods of ritual, meditation, and many healing practices incorporate a form of structured breathing. This practical application of coordinating body rhythms seems to be accomplished through the coordination of air flow through the nose.

A deviated septum is a condition in which the cartilage is bent, usually as the result of a blow to the nose. It results in difficulty in breathing through one side of the nose. As simple as this seems, because of reflex patterns, any disruption of air flow through the nose can lead to bodywide effects, such as disturbed sleep patterns.

Sinuses

The **sinuses** are four groups of air-filled spaces that open into the internal nose. They are located in the frontal, ethmoid, sphenoid, and maxillary bones of the skull. Sinuses are lined with mucosa and lighten the weight of the skull, making it easier to hold up the head. They also help with the production of sound, also known as *phonation*. Because the sinus mucosa communicates with the nasal cavity, sinuses are prone to the same infections as the nasal cavity.

Pharynx

The pharynx, or throat, is divided into three areas. The nasopharynx is the continuation of the nasal cavity into the throat; it transports air. The auditory or eustachian tubes from the inner ear open into the nasopharynx; they help equalize pressure in the head, nose, and pharynx. The oropharynx is the portion of the throat that you can see; it contains the tonsils and functions as a passageway for food between the mouth and the esophagus and as a passageway for air between the nose, mouth, and trachea. The laryngopharynx begins at the hyoid bone and separates into the esophagus and larynx; it is a pathway for both air and food. At the entrance to the larynx is a small cartilaginous flap, the epiglottis. As food is swallowed, the epiglottis closes over the glottis, preventing food and fluids from entering the lungs.

Larynx

The larynx, or voice box, connects the pharynx to the trachea and consists of cartilage, ligaments, connective tissue, muscles, and the vocal cords. The cartilage provides a rigid structural framework for the larynx and trachea below, ensuring that the airway is open at all times. The thyroid cartilage, known as the *Adam's apple*, is located on the anterior portion of the larynx and is larger in men than in women. The vocal cords and the spaces between the cords are located inside the glottis.

The function of the larynx, in addition to permitting air passage to and from the lungs, is to produce sound. As we exhale, the vocal cords vibrate to produce high or low sounds, or pitch. In high-pitched sounds, the glottis is narrower and the vocal cords are more tense, whereas in low-pitched sounds, the glottis is more open and the vocal cords are more relaxed. The lips and the tongue create speech.

Laryngitis is an inflammation of the vocal cords caused by overuse, infection, or irritation by cigarette smoke or a tumor. Laryngitis can cause hoarseness or loss of the voice.

Obstruction of the glottis (e.g., by food) can be fatal. Bacterial infection of the epiglottis (epiglottitis) in children is a life-threatening but rare cause of obstruction.

Trachea

The trachea, or windpipe, is the main airway to the lungs and is a 4- to 5-inch tube that begins at the glottis and ends at the junction of the two main bronchi near the level of the sternal angle. The trachea consists of 16 to 20 horseshoe-shaped rings of cartilage that have connective tissue between them. When a foreign particle enters the trachea, mucus and cilia trap it and initiate the cough reflex.

The trachea branches off into two bronchi, which have the same structural framework as the trachea except that they have more smooth muscle. The first branches of the bronchial tubes are the right and left primary bronchi. Each main bronchus divides into two (left lung) or three (right lung) lobar bronchi.

Lungs

The two **lungs** are the primary organs of respiration. These soft, spongy, highly vascular structures are separated into the left and right lungs by the mediastinum. Each lung is separated into lobes. The right lung has three lobes: upper, middle, and lower; the left has two lobes: upper and lower.

Each of the lobar bronchi, which extend from the trachea, divide into 10 segmental bronchi, which then divide further. The amount of cartilage in each tube gradually decreases until the tubes lack cartilage. At that point the tubes are about 1 mm in diameter and are known as the *bronchioles*, which terminate in the air sacs, or alveoli. The alveoli are surrounded by capillaries, and this is where external respiration takes place.

The lungs are enclosed in a pleural cavity lined by two pleural membranes. One connects directly to the surface of the lung, and the other attaches to the mediastinum and inside chest wall. This cavity created by the membranes contains approximately a half teaspoon of lubricating fluid that reduces friction between the two layers as we breathe. Increases in the amount of fluid often occur with diseases such as lung cancer and pulmonary edema and can make breathing difficult. Pneumothorax is a condition in which air enters the pleural cavity as a result of trauma or rupture of part of the lung. This can be caused by a penetrating injury, such as from a bullet or knife, or in a disease process, such as emphysema. A chest tube, called a *thoracotomy tube*, inserted between the ribs and connected to a pump removes the air. In hemothorax, blood is in the pleural cavity; physicians can drain blood from the pleural space in a manner similar to how air is drained.

Diaphragm

The **diaphragm** is a dome-shaped sheet of muscle attached to the thoracic wall that separates the lungs and thoracic cavity from the abdominal cavity. As the chest cavity enlarges, the diaphragm moves downward and creates a vacuum that allows air to flow into the lungs. As the chest contracts and the diaphragm relaxes, the diaphragm arches upward, which helps push air out of the lungs.

Thorax

The **thorax**, or chest cavity, is the upper region of the torso. It is enclosed by the sternum, ribs, and thoracic vertebrae and contains the lungs, heart, and great vessels.

Nerves and Vessels of the Lungs and Respiratory Muscles

The autonomic nervous system supplies the bronchi and bronchioles. Stimulation of the vagus nerve, a major parasympathetic nerve, causes contraction of the smooth muscles and narrows the diameter of the tubes; this is called *bronchoconstriction.* Stimulation of sympathetic nerves initiates smooth muscle relaxation, resulting in widening of the tubes; this is called *bronchodilation.*

The nerve supply to the intercostal muscles extends from spinal nerves T1 to T11. The phrenic nerve originates at C3 to C5 and innervates the diaphragm. The reason the nerve supply originates in such a distant location is that during fetal development, the diaphragm actually begins its growth in the neck and then descends from the neck to the abdomen. A broken neck that injures the spinal cord below C5 allows the person to continue breathing because the diaphragm does most of the breathing. Injury to both phrenic nerves or a spinal cord injury above C3 to C5 severely compromises breathing. A person with such an injury needs to be on a ventilator, which essentially does their breathing for them.

The pulmonary arteries and veins participate in the exchange of oxygen and carbon dioxide between the capillaries and alveoli. Branches of the aorta and upper intercostal arteries supply blood to most of the lung tissue. Venous drainage takes place from the azygos vein on the right side of the thorax and from the first intercostal vein on the left.

Mechanics of Breathing

During the moments before we take a breath, the pressure inside the lungs and outside the body is equal, whereas the pressure inside the pleural space is slightly lower. When we begin to inhale, the external intercostal muscles between the ribs contract, lifting the lower ribs up and out. This creates a vacuum that expands the lungs, causing the pressure inside the lungs to decrease. The diaphragm moves down, increasing the volume of the pleural cavities and decreasing lung pressure even more. Elastic fibers in the alveolar walls stretch, permitting expansion of the air sacs. The lungs draw in air until the pressure is equal again.

Exhalation mainly results from elastic recoil of the alveoli. Additionally, as we exhale, the pressure inside the pleural cavity increases; the external intercostals, diaphragm, and alveolar walls relax; the volume inside the lungs decreases; and the pressure in the lungs increases until it again equals the atmospheric pressure.

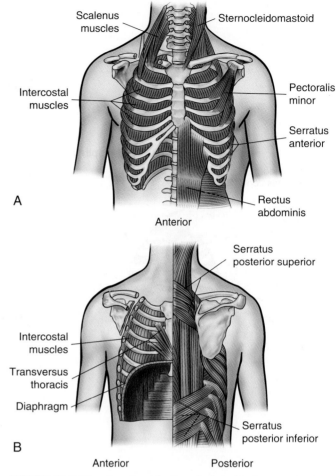

FIGURE 12-2 Muscles of respiration. **A,** Anterior view. **B,** Posterior view. (Modified from Seidel HM et al: *Mosby's guide to physical examination,* ed 5, St Louis, 2003, Mosby.)

In diseases such as asthma, bronchitis, and emphysema, the accessory muscles of respiration are often used. Contraction of the sternocleidomastoid and other muscles of the neck aid inspiration, whereas use of the internal intercostals and abdominal muscles aids expiration (Figures 12-2, 12-3, and 12-4).

Practical Application

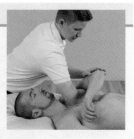

Massage therapy that targets the trunk, including the back chest and abdomen, can be applied to support normal breathing. The main goal is for the soft tissues to be sufficiently pliable that the ribs can move efficiently during inspiration and expiration.

A hiccup (singultus) is a sudden involuntary contraction of the inspiratory muscles, producing the sound of inspiration with the glottis closed. Most cases involve food or alcohol, are short-lived, and resolve without therapy. The reflex is primitive, similar to yawning, coughing, sneezing, and vomiting. Often, sedatives and home remedies work. In prolonged cases a tranquilizer may be necessary.

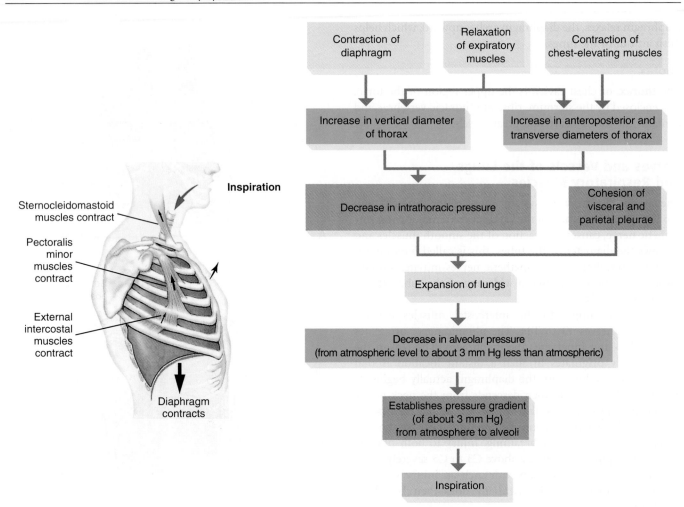

FIGURE 12-3 Mechanism of inspiration. (From Patton KT, Thibodeau GA: *Anatomy and physiology,* ed 5, St Louis, 2003, Mosby.)

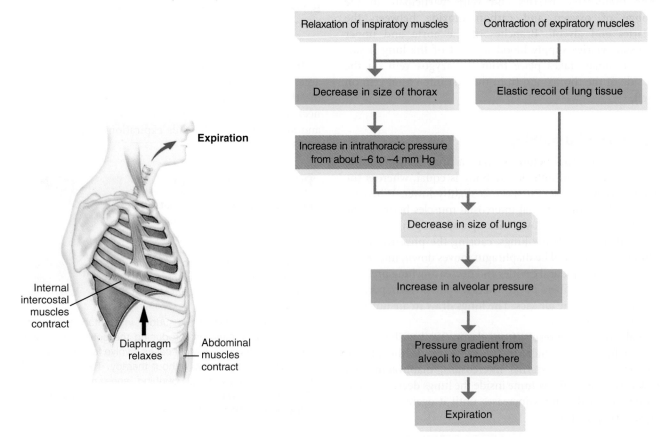

FIGURE 12-4 Mechanism of expiration. (From Patton KT, Thibodeau GA: *Anatomy and physiology,* ed 5, St Louis, 2003, Mosby.)

Lung Volumes

There are various volumes of air that can be breathed in and out. It is possible to measure four different pulmonary volumes that may be used as guidelines in health assessments. The tidal volume is the amount of air taken in or exhaled in a single breath during normal breathing, usually while the person is resting. It is about half a liter. Inspiratory reserve volume is the amount of air that can be inhaled forcefully after normal tidal volume inspiration; it is about 3 liters in the average male and almost 2 liters in the average female (the difference is because males usually have larger body sizes so they have larger lungs).

Expiratory reserve volume is the amount of air that can be exhaled forcefully after a normal exhalation; it is a little more than a liter in males and a little less than a liter in females. Reserve volume is the amount of air that remains in the lungs and passageways after a maximal expiration. Vital capacity is the total of the tidal volume, inspiratory reserve volume, and expiratory reserve volume. In the normal, healthy adult lung, vital capacity usually is about 5.5 liters of air for men and 3.5 liters of air for women.

In diseased lungs, such as those affected by asthma or emphysema, the vital capacity and expiratory reserve volumes are abnormal. A person with asthma, for example, may have a normal tidal volume and vital capacity but decreased expiratory reserve volume, whereas a person with emphysema may have a normal (but often decreased) tidal volume and decreased vital capacity and expiratory reserve volume. Ultimately, because of the pathologic condition of the lung tissues, the person cannot exhale effectively.

Transport of Oxygen and Carbon Dioxide

The pulmonary arteries bring oxygen-deficient blood from the right ventricle of the heart to the lungs. Carbon dioxide diffuses from the bloodstream through the capillary and alveolar membranes into the alveoli. Oxygen diffuses in the opposite direction, from the alveoli through both membranes and into the bloodstream. The carbon dioxide is then exhaled from the lungs while the pulmonary veins return oxygen-rich blood to the left atrium of the heart.

The amount of oxygen in the blood depends on the amount of oxygen available in the atmosphere. The air in the average room is composed of the following:

- Nitrogen (N_2): 79%
- Oxygen (O_2): 20.96%
- Carbon dioxide (CO_2): 0.04%.

Red blood cells transport oxygen in the blood as oxyhemoglobin. Red blood cells move into the capillaries. At the arteriole end of the capillary, oxygen leaves the red blood cell and then diffuses through the capillary membrane into the tissue fluid. Oxygen then diffuses into cell membranes to be used for cellular metabolism.

Carbon dioxide moves out of the tissue cell in the reverse direction, through the same membranes, into the red blood cells, where most of it is converted into a bicarbonate ion (HCO_3). The plasma transports bicarbonate to the lungs, where bicarbonate ion is converted back into carbon dioxide in the alveolar membrane so that it can be exhaled.

Control of Breathing

The respiratory center is a group of nerve cells in the medulla and pons of the brain. A variety of stimuli affect the center. Impulses from the cerebral cortex under voluntary control modify respiration, as do changes in the carbon dioxide content and acidity of blood and cerebrospinal fluid. Chemoreceptors, nerve cells found near the baroreceptors, are sensitive to the oxygen level and to a lesser extent to carbon dioxide and pH (acid/base balance) levels in the bloodstream. Two chemoreceptors, called *aortic bodies,* are located near the arch of the aorta. There is also one in each carotid artery; these are called *carotid bodies.* The aortic bodies transmit impulses to the respiratory center in the medulla through the vagus nerve; the carotid bodies transmit by way of the glossopharyngeal nerve. A low concentration of oxygen in the body stimulates these chemoreceptors, and the respiratory rate increases as a result.

Respiratory Rate

The respiratory rate in an adult is about 12 to 16 breaths per minute and in a newborn about 35, which gradually decreases to adult values at about age 20. Emotions are powerful stimuli for respiratory changes. Fear, grief, and shock slow the rate, whereas excitement, anger, and sexual arousal increase the respiratory rate.

Besides the effects of emotions, changes in breathing rates can occur as a result of increased oxygen requirements induced by exercise; in obesity as a result of increased vessel resistance; during infections and fever because of increased energy requirements; in heart failure as a result of decreased oxygen flow; during pain because of increased nervous stimulation; with anemia because of decreased oxygen transport; in hyperthyroidism because of an increase in metabolic rate; and during emphysema because of blockage of oxygen. Hyperpnea is fast breathing, and tachypnea is rapid, shallow breathing. These types of breathing can lead to acute **hyperventilation** or chronic overbreathing, called **breathing pattern disorder,** which causes a variety of signs and symptoms, as discussed later in this section. Bradypnea, or slow breathing, occurs in intoxication by alcohol and other depressant drugs because of the depressive action of these substances in the brain. Bradypnea also occurs in cases of increased intracranial pressure on account of pressure on the respiratory center and in diabetic coma. Periods of hyperpnea alternating with periods of apnea (no breathing) sometimes occur in the sleep of infants, particularly premature ones. These patterns also appear in those with brain injury and in the terminally ill.

Reflexes That Affect Breathing

Foreign matter or other irritants in the trachea or bronchi stimulate the cough reflex. The epiglottis and glottis reflexively close, and contraction of the expiratory muscles causes air pressure in the lungs to increase. The epiglottis and glottis open suddenly, resulting in an upward force of air in a cough that removes the irritant from the throat.

The sneeze reflex is similar to the cough reflex, except that contaminants or irritants in the nasal cavity provide the stimulus. A burst of air moves through the nose and mouth, forcing the contaminant out of the respiratory tract.

A hiccup is an involuntary, spasmodic contraction of the diaphragm that causes the glottis to close suddenly, producing the characteristic sound. A yawn is slow, deep inspiration through the open mouth. Scientists still have not found the actual physiologic mechanism of yawning.

Pathologic Conditions of the Respiratory System

Respiratory diseases can arise from a number of causes. Infections, genetic predisposition, inhalation of toxic substances, accidents, and lifestyle choices such as smoking can cause respiratory pathology. People with lung disease have difficulty breathing. The term *lung disease* refers to many disorders affecting the lungs, such as asthma, chronic obstructive pulmonary disease, and cancer.

Common Cold

More than 200 viruses can cause the common cold; these viruses are easily spread. Usually affecting the nasal mucosa, the viruses may spread to the sinuses and pharynx and down the respiratory tract. The person's temperature rises to eliminate the virus. Irritation in the nose and pharynx causes coughing and sneezing. Fluids and bed rest are recommended.

Influenza

Influenza is commonly called *flu.* It is a common viral infection of the entire body, resulting in fever, muscle aches and weakness, backache, and cough. Primary treatment, as with most viral infections, is bed rest and fluids.

Sinusitis

Sinusitis is inflammation of the sinuses; most commonly, it accompanies a nasal infection. Congestion, edema, and pain are present because of irritation of the sensory nerve endings in the periosteum. Pain takes the form of a headache, particularly if the frontal sinus is involved. Congestion blocks drainage into the nasal cavity. The maxillary sinus lies over the upper teeth, and sometimes a person has difficulty telling whether the problem is a sinus attack or a toothache because of the similarity of the pain pattern. Treatment often consists of an antibiotic and a decongestant.

Sore Throat

Sore throat, or pharyngitis, is an inflammation of the pharynx. If the tonsils are involved, the condition is tonsillitis. The cause is usually viral, but a throat culture may show a *Streptococcus* species, the organism that causes rheumatic fever, rheumatic heart disease, or glomerulonephritis as complications in certain individuals. Common signs and symptoms are a red, tender throat; enlarged cervical lymph nodes; and fever. Treatment consists of rest, an analgesic, saline gargles, and an antibiotic if the culture is positive for *Streptococcus* species.

Croup

Croup is a viral infection in children that most commonly affects boys between 3 months and 5 years of age. The larynx, trachea, and bronchi are red and swollen and may block the glottis. A "seal bark" cough is usually present. A high-pitched whistling inhalation is sometimes present, and affected children must use their neck and abdominal muscles to breathe. Humidified air often eases the symptoms; if not, oxygen therapy may help.

Pneumonia

Pneumonia is an acute infection of the lungs caused by bacteria or viruses, fungi, exposure to certain chemicals, or inhaled substances. Symptoms include fever, chills, chest pain, difficulty breathing, headache, loss of appetite, muscle and joint pain, a cough usually accompanied by yellow or green sputum, and rales (the sound of movement of air and fluid in the bronchial tree). The diagnosis is usually made by reviewing the patient's history and test results, most often a chest radiograph showing an abnormal white area. Evaluation of sputum and blood tests commonly show an elevated white count. Primary treatment for bacterial pneumonia is an antibiotic, bed rest, and fluids. In serious cases the person must be hospitalized and given oxygen and antibiotics.

Asthma

Asthma is the reversible narrowing of the small airways for reasons other than cardiovascular disease. Asthma manifests as acute attacks that constrict and obstruct these airways. Asthma attacks may be triggered by allergic reactions, air pollutants, exercise, hypersensitivity to substances such as wood and flour, chemicals, viral infections, and emotional upsets. During an episode the smooth muscle layer of the bronchi and bronchioles goes into bronchoconstricting spasms, and the glands of the bronchi hypersecrete mucus. The airways fill with thick mucus, and air cannot leave the lungs. Breathlessness, coughing, chest tightness, and wheezing occur as the person tries to force air out of the lungs. Arterial blood gases may initially show a low amount of carbon dioxide, leading to a condition called *respiratory alkalosis.* Long-term therapy may include the use of a bronchodilator, a mast cell stabilizer, or corticosteroids. Antibiotics may benefit the person if the trigger is a respiratory infection.

Chronic Obstructive Pulmonary Disease

Although the processes involved in the evolution of emphysema and bronchitis are different, the result is irreversible respiratory insufficiency, sometimes called *chronic obstructive pulmonary disease* (COPD). In emphysema the obstruction is in the alveoli; in bronchitis the obstruction is in the bronchi. A component of each appears in heavy smokers. The lung tissue changes, and the person becomes less able to tolerate exercise and activity.

Acute bronchitis often occurs along with an upper respiratory infection, measles, or the flu. A virus usually causes infection, but the cause also may be bacterial. Symptoms include a mild fever, an increase in secreted mucus, and coughing in an attempt to loosen and remove the phlegm, which may be yellow or green. Prolonged irritation by cigarette smoke is the usual cause of chronic bronchitis. Sputum production increases in response to the constant irritation of the tissues. The smoke damages the cilia such that excessive mucus cannot be moved out of the airway, and the person usually has a chronic cough. The person may also make wheezing noises. The evidence suggests that the condition does not reverse, but further deterioration can be halted after quitting smoking. Treatment involves the use of bronchodilators and oxygen therapy.

Pleurisy

Pleurisy (pleuritis) is an inflammation of the pleural membrane, usually the result of a lung infection such as pneumonia. The inflamed membranes rub against each other, causing stabbing pain that is worse during inhalation.

Lung Cancer

About 90% of all cases of lung cancer are caused by smoking tobacco. Primary tumors usually develop in the bronchi and block air passages. Cancer in the lung can spread to other parts of the body. Symptoms commonly begin with cough, blood in the phlegm, wheezing, chest pain, and fever. A large tumor may cause problems in swallowing. Diagnosis is by physical examination, radiographs, and computed tomography (CT) scans.

Pulmonary Edema

Pulmonary edema is the accumulation of fluid in the lungs. The most common cause is heart failure, although kidney disease, pneumonia, and other disorders may also cause pulmonary edema. Treatment usually involves diuretics and oxygen therapy.

Tuberculosis

Tuberculosis is an infection that develops as chronic inflammatory lesions caused by the bacillus *Mycobacterium tuberculosis*. It is contagious and is contracted by inhaling or ingesting infected droplets dispersed by infected persons by way of coughing and nasal discharge. Once thought to occur rarely, tuberculosis is on the rise again in adults who are immunosuppressed. Although any site of the body may be affected, pulmonary tuberculosis is by far the most common. In rare cases tuberculosis may also affect the bones and kidneys. Early symptoms include listlessness and fatigue, chest pain, fever, and weight loss. The disease progresses to impair respiratory function severely and spreads to involve other body sites. Treatment includes rest, nutritional support, and a medication regimen that may last more than 1 year. The disease is no longer infectious once sputum tests are free of bacteria, although the bacteria may lie dormant.

Cystic Fibrosis

Cystic fibrosis is a genetic disorder that causes abnormally thick and sticky mucus to be produced throughout the body. In the lungs the mucus cannot be moved out by the cilia, so bacteria and viruses are held in instead of released by the body. Infections develop, causing obstruction of the smaller airways.

(See the section on pathologic conditions of the digestive system for more information.)

Choking

Choking commonly occurs when a person is talking while eating and inhales at the same time as swallowing. The piece of food, usually meat, obstructs the larynx. The person coughs, which often dislodges the object. If not, the airway can become completely blocked. The person usually appears distressed, grasps his or her neck, and cannot inhale or exhale. The term *café coronary* has been used because it is common for choking to occur in a restaurant, and it superficially resembles a heart attack. Other objects, such as chewing gum or balloons, are frequently the cause of obstructions in children.

First aid for choking is the Heimlich maneuver (Box 12-1).

Box 12-1 Heimlich Maneuver/Abdominal Thrust

The Heimlich maneuver, also called *abdominal thrust,* is an effective and often lifesaving technique used to open a suddenly obstructed windpipe. The maneuver uses air already present in the lungs to expel the object obstructing the trachea. Individuals trained in emergency procedures must be able to tell the difference between airway obstruction and other conditions such as heart attacks that produce similar symptoms. The key question to ask the person who appears to be choking is, "Can you talk?" A person with an obstructed airway will not be able to speak, even while conscious. The rescuer makes a fist with one hand, grasps it with the other, and then delivers an upward thrust against the victim's diaphragm just below the xiphoid process of the sternum. The thrust compresses air trapped in the lungs, forcing the object that is choking the victim out of the airway.

Technique If Victim Can Be Lifted
1. Rescuer stands behind the victim and wraps both arms around the victim's waist.
2. Rescuer makes a fist with one hand, places the thumb side of the fist against the victim's upper abdomen, below the ribcage and above navel.
3. The rescuer grabs his or her first with the other hand and presses into the victim's upper abdomen with a quick, upward thrust. The rescuer should not squeeze the ribcage; the force of the thrust should be confined to the hands.
4. The maneuver should be repeated until the object is expelled.

When Victim is Unconscious or Rescuer Cannot Reach Around Victim
1. Rescuer places victim on back.
2. Facing victim, rescuer straddles the victim's hips.
3. Rescuer places one hand on top of the other, the heel of the bottom hand on the upper abdomen below the ribcage and above the navel.
4. Using body weight, rescuer presses into the victim's upper abdomen with a quick, upward thrust.
5. The maneuver should be repeated until the object is expelled.

www.heimlichinstitute.com

Sleep Apnea

In sleep apnea the person stops breathing for a period of 10 seconds or more while sleeping, at least a few times per hour. Each time breathing stops, oxygen levels fall and cause the person to wake, which results in resumption of breathing. Sleep apnea commonly occurs because of obstructed breathing, which is identified as obstructive sleep apnea (OSA). OSA results in drowsy episodes accompanied by snoring and apneic spells. It is more common in men, especially those who are overweight and are heavy drinkers. OSA also occurs in persons with enlarged tonsils, small jaws, large tongues and soft palates, and other subtle anatomic abnormalities. Persons taking medications such as sleeping pills can suffer from OSA because the upper airway muscles can relax too much. The tongue appears to fall back and block the airway during sleep periods that are without rapid eye movement.

Infant apnea is associated with infections that obstruct the airway; sometimes the cause is not identifiable. Sudden infant death syndrome (SIDS) may be a variation. Central nervous system and obstructive problems may cause SIDS, but OSA seems to be an important component. Additional risk factors for SIDS include male sex, low birth weight, decreased carotid body substance, and upper respiratory infection.

Carbon Monoxide Poisoning

Carbon monoxide poisoning is the leading cause of gas-related deaths in this country. Carbon monoxide is odorless and binds to hemoglobin 210 times more readily than oxygen, forming the molecule carboxyhemoglobin.

Red blood cells are able to carry very little oxygen. Most deaths occur as the result of smoke inhalation during fires. Some deaths are caused by automobile exhaust fumes and poorly ventilated or defective gasoline heaters and charcoal stoves. Poisonings also occur in machine shops in which ventilation is poor. The symptoms are headache, dizziness, weakness, and nausea; they occur when the blood has approximately 6% to 7% carboxyhemoglobin.

Emphysema can result from long-term irritation of the bronchi and bronchioles. Mucus and pus accumulate, and the air in the alveoli becomes trapped. When the pressure exceeds the elastic limit, the alveoli become permanently ballooned, making exhalation difficult. The person typically develops a barrel-chest from using the internal intercostals as well as the abdominal and neck muscles to breathe. Inflammation brings in more white blood cells, which break down the walls of the alveoli, which merge to form larger sacs. Alveolar destruction results in less surface area for the internal exchange of gases, so oxygen in the blood decreases. As emphysema progresses, the person becomes breathless with minor exertion. Emphysema is the most common cause of respiratory failure. Bronchodilators and oxygen therapy may help.

Drowning

In drowning the victim inhales and swallows water. In 10% of cases the larynx goes into spasm on inhalation of the first small amount of fluid, and asphyxia, or suffocation caused by lack of oxygen, takes place, even with no fluid in the lungs.

Survival depends mostly on the continued presence of a pulse, not necessarily on the length of time of immersion. Treatment in near-drowning consists of cardiopulmonary resuscitation and hospitalization; oxygen and bicarbonate are administered for the acidosis caused by high carbon dioxide levels.

Breathing Pattern Disorder

Physiologists define *hyperventilation* as abnormally deep or rapid breathing in excess of physical demands. Now called breathing pattern disorder, it is a complex set of behaviors that leads to overbreathing in the absence of a pathologic condition. Hyperventilation is a functional condition in which all the parts are working effectively, so a pathologic condition does not exist, but the breathing pattern is inappropriate for the situation, resulting in confused signals to the central nervous system, setting up a whole chain of events. Persons experiencing this difficulty often are told that nothing is wrong, which may add to their anxiety, or they are told to take a few deep breaths, which increases their symptoms. One review indicates that as many as 28% of patients in various medical populations may experience functional breathing pattern disorder.

Increased ventilation is a common component of fight-or-flight responses, but when breathing increases while actions and movements are restricted, a person is breathing in excess of metabolic need. Blood levels of carbon dioxide fall, and symptoms may occur. As a person exhales too much carbon dioxide too quickly, the blood becomes more alkaline. These biochemical changes can cause many of the following signs and symptoms:

Respiratory: Symptoms include shortness of breath, typically after exertion; irritable cough; tightness or oppression in chest; difficulty breathing; asthma; air hunger; inability to take a satisfying breath; excessive sighing, yawning, and sniffing.

Cardiovascular: Symptoms include palpitations; missed beats; tachycardia; sharp or dull atypical chest pain; angina; vasomotor instability; cold extremities; Raynaud's phenomenon; blotchy flushing of blush area; and capillary vasoconstriction in the face, arms, and hands.

Neurologic: Cerebrovascular blood vessel constriction, a primary response to breathing pattern disorder, can reduce the oxygen available to the brain by about one half. Symptoms include dizziness, unsteadiness, or instability; feelings of fainting but rarely actual fainting; visual disturbance such as blurred or tunnel vision; headache (often migraine); paresthesia (i.e., numbness, heaviness, "pins and needles,") burning, limbs feeling out of proportion or "not belonging," commonly of hands, feet, or face, sometimes scalp or whole body; intolerance of light or noise; enlarged pupils; and sensation of giddiness.

Psychologic: Symptoms include tension; anxiety; tearfulness; emotional instability; feelings of unreality; depersonalization; feeling "out of one's body"; hallucinations; impaired concentration, memory, and performance; disturbed sleep, including nightmares; emotional sweating in the axillae, palms, and sometimes the whole body; fear of insanity; panic; phobias; and agoraphobia. A fear of not

INDICATIONS/CONTRAINDICATIONS for Therapeutic Massage

Respiratory System

In any of the disorders of the respiratory system that are of viral or bacterial origin, massage is usually contraindicated until the disease has run its course. Whenever the body is under stress, as with respiratory infection, further stress on the system can worsen the condition. Simple palliative measures to provide comfort and encourage sleep are appropriate. The practitioner should follow all sanitary procedures and Standard Precautions.

In chronic conditions such as asthma and emphysema, general stress management and maintenance of normal function of the muscles of respiration are beneficial as long as the appropriate added stress levels caused by the stimulation of massage are considered. In cystic fibrosis, percussion helps loosen the phlegm but should not be attempted without medical supervision and training.

Therapeutic massage approaches and moderate application of movement therapies, such as tai chi, yoga, or aerobic exercise, often help breathing pattern disorder. Almost every meditation and relaxation system uses breathing patterns because they are a direct link to altering autonomic nervous system patterns, which in turn alter mood, feelings, and behavior. Other ways to modulate breathing are through singing and chanting.

Constant activation of the accessory muscles of respiration when these muscles are not needed during normal activity results in dysfunctional muscle patterns. The accessory breathing muscles such as the scalenes, sternocleidomastoid, serratus posterior superior, levator scapulae, rhomboids, abdominals, and quadratus lumborum, should only be activated for forced inhalation and expiration during heavy exertion such as running. Therapeutic massage can bring balance into these areas to encourage a more effective breathing pattern. General stress management reduces anxiety and helps normalize the breathing pattern.

Although a detailed discussion of the many forms of meditation, breathing modulation, and retraining measures is beyond the scope of this text, two basic types of systems exist: One leads to physiologic hyperarousal, and one to hypoarousal. Both processes facilitate the reestablishment of homeostasis, just as a muscle can be encouraged to relax by tensing it first and then releasing it or by using the antagonist pattern to initiate reciprocal inhibition, thus allowing the muscle to relax. Hyperarousal systems increase sympathetic activity and elicit a secondary parasympathetic balance. Aerobic exercise is an example. Hypoarousal systems directly activate parasympathetic responses. Examples are quiet reflection or meditative prayer combined with a chant to promote exhalation. Many resources use retraining programs to improve breathing patterns, and the recommendation is to find one that is comfortable and use it regularly.

Herbs such as eucalyptus give off a vapor that is soothing to the respiratory system. Aromatherapy uses different scents that are taken into the body through the respiratory system. Some scents have a stimulating effect, and others have a calming effect.

getting enough air is a core factor in the cause of panic attacks.

Gastrointestinal: Symptoms include difficulty in swallowing, dry mouth and throat, acid regurgitation, heartburn, hiatal hernia, nausea, flatulence, belching, air swallowing, abdominal discomfort, and bloating.

Muscular: Symptoms include cramps; muscle pains, particularly in the occipital region, neck, shoulders, and between scapulae and less commonly in the lower back and limbs; tremors, twitching, weakness, stiffness, or tetany (seizing up) in muscles involved in the attack posture—affected persons hunch their shoulders, thrust their heads and necks forward, scowl, and clench their teeth. There can also be generalized body tension, feeling of weakness, and a chronic inability to relax.

All the aforementioned symptoms can lead to exhaustion.

DIGESTIVE SYSTEM

SECTION OBJECTIVES

Chapter objectives covered in this section:

4. Describe how the decisions about what and when to eat influence health.
5. List and describe the components of the digestive system.
6. Describe the process of digestion.
7. Explain the importance of nutrition.
8. List and describe the main food groups.
9. Explain metabolic rate, energy balance, and body weight.
10. Describe pathologic conditions of the digestive system and the associated indications and contraindications for massage.

After completing this section, the student will be able to perform the following:

- Define *digestion*.
- Explain emotional eating.
- Locate and describe the organs of the digestive system.
- Describe the effects of autonomic nervous system on digestion.
- Describe the sequence of the digestive process.
- Define *nutrition*.
- List and explain the role of the main food groups.
- Define the *citric acid cycle*.
- Define *metabolic rate*.
- Describe the results of increased or decreased metabolic rate.
- Determine indications and contraindications of massage to digestive system pathology.

Digestion is a physiologic process that involves the intake and assimilation of nutrients and the **elimination** of waste (Figures 12-5 and 12-6). The intake of food is much more than a means of obtaining nutrients for the growth, repair, and maintenance of the body. Eating is a pleasurable activity and a social event that involves many neurochemical interactions. Food choices can have effects on health risks. Biologic drives for food, especially foods high in fat and simple carbohydrates or sugars, played an important part in early human survival. These foods, which are rare in nature, supply quick and sustaining energy sources. An overabundance of fat and sugar, which are no longer rare in our society, feeds the biologic cravings we still have even though the energy required to acquire these food sources has decreased. The result is an epidemic of obesity.

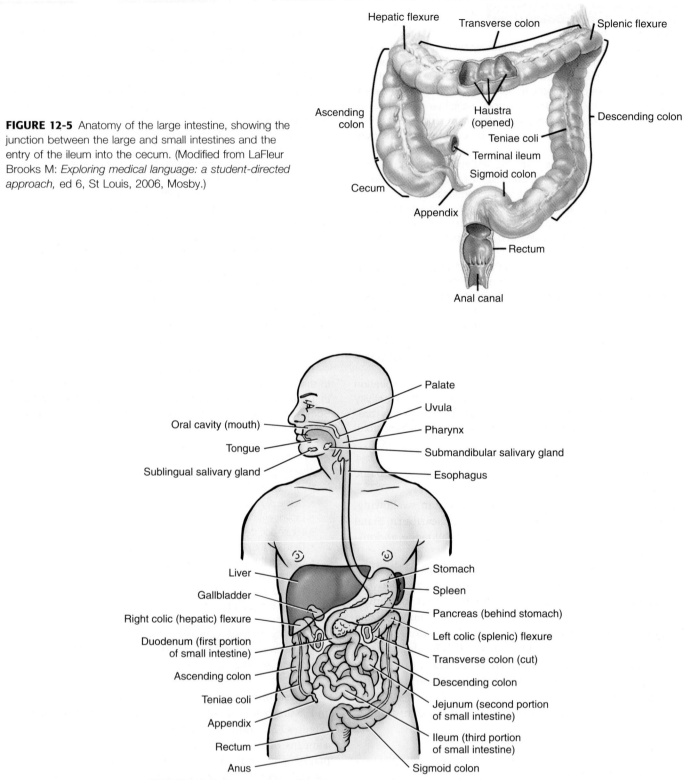

FIGURE 12-5 Anatomy of the large intestine, showing the junction between the large and small intestines and the entry of the ileum into the cecum. (Modified from LaFleur Brooks M: *Exploring medical language: a student-directed approach,* ed 6, St Louis, 2006, Mosby.)

FIGURE 12-6 Organs of the digestive system and some associated structures.

Emotional eating is one type of substitution for touch and loving relationships with others because it stimulates similar chemicals. Foods such as chocolate and other fat-carbohydrate combinations, along with some forms of protein, generate serotonin and other feel-good neurochemicals as effectively as a hug does. Food behaviors can become as addictive as any

other pleasurable activity. Exercise also produces these neurochemicals, so moderate exercise programs are good for mood as well as weight management. Because biologic tendencies favor energy conservation, and our biologic patterns are designed for survival in a more primitive environment, the internal drive toward movement and activity was originally used to provide shelter, food, and protection. In modern times we find ourselves needing to move for the sake of movement, not because it is directly critical to our survival. This is a physiologically confusing process and may be part of the reason that many people are not motivated to exercise.

Eating special foods or fasting as a cleansing and purification process is at the heart of many social and religious rituals. What would a holiday be without all the food? Healing practices usually involve the **ingestion** of a healing herb or brew. Mating behaviors often involve food and feeding behaviors, such as drinking one milkshake with two straws or sharing a romantic dinner. A popular tradition in Western wedding ceremonies calls for the bride and groom to feed each other wedding cake. One of the first acts of parental bonding is feeding the infant. Our lips and tongues remain forever sensitive to sensory stimulation connected with soothing and pleasurable behaviors. The act of eating stimulates these areas and provides comfort and sensory stimulation, as do childhood thumb sucking and adult kissing.

Even the processes of elimination and the social constraints and rules about the passage of intestinal gas become important. Is a belch rude behavior that is best kept private, or a compliment after a good meal? One cause of chronic constipation in Western society is the social stigma involved with the act of having a bowel movement.

Food itself is interesting. Whether the food source is plant or animal, the life force is transferred from one being to another. Eating is the giving of one life for the continuation of another. "What greater gift is there than laying down your life for another?" Human beings are at the top of the food chain, so regardless of what we eat, many lives—plant and animal—have been sacrificed so that we may live. Ancient peoples and those who still attempt to live in the old ways remember this. The act of asking for a blessing of food is a ritual of respect and a way to honor the life force given so that we may live. As we explore the parts and process of the digestive system ever so briefly in this text, the student would do well to remember the bigger picture involved in the intake of food and water and the process of receiving energy from one so that another may live.

Organs and Structures of the Digestive System

The digestive system is one long tube with accessory organs. It starts at the mouth, extends through the body, and ends at the anus. This tube is known as the *gastrointestinal tract* and also referred to as the *alimentary canal*. The gastrointestinal tract is about 30 feet long and contains several special structures in its length. The entire lining is a mucous membrane made up of three layers of tissues: epithelium, connective tissue, and smooth muscle.

The digestive tract consists of the mouth, pharynx, esophagus, stomach, small intestine, large intestine, rectum, and anus. Accessory structures include the salivary glands, pancreas, liver, and gallbladder. The abdomen, or abdominal cavity, contains the major organs of digestion. The cavity is lined with a serous membrane called the *peritoneum*. The

portion of the peritoneum lying against the body wall is the parietal peritoneum; the portion surrounding each organ is the visceral peritoneum. The peritoneal cavity is the fluid-filled space between the parietal and visceral peritoneum. It decreases friction as the viscera move.

In the embryo the peritoneum is a large sac that lines the abdominal cavity. The beginnings of viscera are outside the sac. As they develop, they push into the peritoneum in varying degrees. Some organs are covered with peritoneum on only the anterior surface; they are referred to as *retroperitoneal*. Other organs are covered completely with peritoneum except for the small area where the peritoneum attaches; they are referred to as *intraperitoneal*.

The peritoneum covering most of the small intestine is called *mesentery*. The mesocolon is peritoneum that binds the transverse colon and sigmoid colon of the large intestine to the posterior abdominal wall. A double-layered sheet or fold of peritoneum is called the *omenta*. The lesser omentum connects the stomach and duodenum to the liver. The greater omentum extends from the stomach to the transverse colon. Fat stored in the greater omentum accounts for much of the girth in obesity. Peritoneal ligaments consist of double layers of peritoneum. They connect organs with other organs or the abdominal wall and may contain blood vessels or remnants of blood vessels. The greater omentum is divided into three peritoneal ligaments: the gastrocolic ligament, the apron-like part attached to the transverse colon; the gastrosplenic ligament, the left part that connects the spleen to the greater curvature of the stomach; and the gastrophrenic ligament, the superior part that attaches to the diaphragm.

Mouth

The mouth is the oral cavity and makes up the first portion of the gastrointestinal tract. It includes the lips, cheeks, tongue, hard and soft palates, teeth, and salivary glands.

The tongue is a large, strong muscle that mixes the food particles with saliva and helps us swallow. It is the location of the taste buds (see Chapter 5).

The palate forms the roof of the mouth. The anterior hard part is the partition between the oral and nasal cavities and consists of the palatine and maxillae bones. The posterior soft portion is the partition between the oropharynx and nasopharynx.

Teeth are accessory structures used to bite off and mechanically break up large pieces of food into smaller ones that can be swallowed. These bonelike structures are actually calcified connective tissue covered with enamel.

Salivary glands are located inside the mouth. They provide secretions that keep the mucous membrane of the mouth moist and that lubricate food so that it is easier to swallow. Saliva is mainly water mixed with small amounts of salts and organic substances. One of these is the enzyme amylase, which breaks down carbohydrates. Another enzyme is lingual lipase, which begins lipid digestion. Smell, sight, taste, and the thought of food stimulate parasympathetic nerve fibers to increase the secretion of saliva. Food that has been mechanically chewed and mixed with saliva is referred to as a *bolus.*

Pharynx

The pharynx is a cavity located at the back of the mouth; it receives the bolus from the mouth.

Esophagus

The esophagus is a 10-inch muscular, collapsible tube directly behind the trachea. It extends from the pharynx to the stomach. The opening into the stomach is the esophageal hiatus, and at the point of attachment is a thickened region called the *cardiac sphincter*, which keeps the entrance to the stomach closed and prevents gastric regurgitation.

Stomach

The stomach is a J-shaped saclike organ that is actually an enlargement of the gastrointestinal tract. Its widest part is located beneath the diaphragm. The narrow distal end lies under the liver and empties into the duodenum. The stomach receives the bolus from the esophagus and continues the digestion process. With the addition of more liquids, the bolus breaks down and becomes a semiliquid known as *chyme*. The stomach contains folds called *rugae* that enable it to expand as food is ingested. The walls of the stomach contain gastric glands that secrete the hormone gastrin and gastric juices, including hydrochloric acid, protein-digesting enzymes, mucus, and water. The digestion of proteins begins in the stomach.

The pylorus is the part of the stomach that narrows to connect with the duodenum. The stomach ends at the pyloric sphincter, a muscle that regulates the flow of chyme into the small intestine. Some gastric cells have histamine receptors. Irritation of the stomach appears to liberate histamine, a potent stimulator of gastric acid secretion. Cimetidine (Tagamet) competes with histamine for receptor sites, thus blocking the secretion of acid and making it an effective medication for treating ulcers.

Small Intestine

The small intestine is a coiled muscular tube that is approximately 24 to 30 feet long. The small intestine consists of three parts:

1. The duodenum (du-o-DE-num) is the shortest portion, making up the first 10 inches of the small intestine. The duodenum forms a C-shaped curve, circling the head of the pancreas, at which point it becomes the jejunum. Ducts from the liver, gallbladder, and pancreas enter this structure.
2. The jejunum (je-JU-num) continues from the duodenum for the next 7 to 8 feet.
3. The ileum (IL-e-um) makes up the final 12 feet of the small intestine. The ileum connects the small intestine to the large intestine at the ileocecal valve or sphincter.

Numerous glands located in the walls of the small intestine provide secretions for the digestive process, the primary function of the jejunum. The small intestine receives the chyme from the stomach and continues the digestive process using intestinal juices containing enzymes secreted by the small intestine as well as secretions from the pancreas, liver, and gallbladder. The complete chemical digestion of carbohydrates, lipids, and proteins is finished in the small intestine.

Ninety percent of the **absorption** of food takes place in the small intestine; the other 10% occurs in the stomach and large intestine. Absorption is the movement of food molecules from the digestive tract to the cardiovascular and lymphatic systems so they can be transported to the cells of the body.

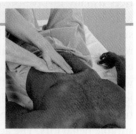

Practical Application

A general and nonspecific massage application that targets digestive support involves a firm but nonpainful broad-based kneading and rolling of the abdomen. The goal is to support normal sliding of the internal organs and peristalsis. Deep prodding and poking of the abdomen should be avoided.

Pancreas

The pancreas is about 5 inches long and 1 inch wide. It lies behind the stomach and is connected to the duodenum by two pancreatic ducts. Most of the pancreas functions as an exocrine gland, producing pancreatic juices containing digestive enzymes. About 1% of the cells of the pancreas, the islets of Langerhans, are scattered throughout the pancreas and secrete the hormones insulin, glucagon, and somatostatin.

Liver

The largest gland of the body, weighing about 3 pounds, the liver lies under the diaphragm in the upper right quadrant. The liver has many functions, including the following:

1. It is active in protein metabolism.
2. It breaks down fatty acids and stores the fat we need for fuel.
3. It removes glucose from the blood and stores it as glycogen when blood sugar levels are high, converting it back to glucose when blood sugar levels are low.
4. It secretes bile, which is important in the digestion of lipids.
5. It stores vitamins A, B_{12}, D, E, K, iron, and copper.
6. It detoxifies the blood by removing drugs and hormones.
7. It converts amino acids into glucose or fatty acids, depending on the needs of the body.
8. It destroys old red blood cells.

Gallbladder

The gallbladder is a small 3- to 4-inch sac that lies on the undersurface of the liver; its function is to store and concentrate bile. The gallbladder releases bile into the small intestine by way of the cystic duct.

Large Intestine

The large intestine is a muscular tube, about 4 to 5 feet long and $2\frac{1}{2}$ inches in diameter. The large intestine has few digestive functions but does reabsorb water and electrolytes, manufacture vitamins, and form and store the feces until defecation occurs. The large intestine, also called the *colon*, consists of eight parts:

1. The cecum begins as a blind pouch about 3 inches long; it receives the digested matter from the ileum of the small intestine.
2. The appendix is a narrow, twisted, close-ended tube attached to the cecum. The appendix contains lymphatic tissue, but its function has not been defined clearly.
3. The ascending colon goes up on the right side of the abdomen to the underside of the liver, where it curves toward the left. This curve is known as the *hepatic flexure.*
4. The transverse colon goes across the abdomen from the hepatic flexure to the spleen, where it turns downward at the splenic flexure.
5. The descending colon extends down the left side of the abdomen from the splenic flexure to about the top of the iliac crest.
6. The sigmoid colon forms an S-shaped curve beginning at the left iliac crest and continuing to the middle of the abdomen, where it connects the descending colon to the rectum.
7. The rectum is a straight, 5- to 6-inch continuation of the sigmoid colon, beginning at about the level of S3.
8. The anal canal is the last inch of the rectum, and it ends at the anus, a sphincter muscle of smooth and skeletal muscle that controls the involuntary and voluntary elimination of feces.

The colon contains large numbers of bacteria. They break down bile pigments, which results in the brown color of feces, and they produce some B vitamins and vitamin K.

Medicines often are given as rectal suppositories because the colon has great absorptive capacity. Feces is undigested matter that is eliminated from the body.

A colostomy is an artificial opening between the colon and skin of the abdomen for the evacuation of feces. Usually done to relieve tumor obstruction, physicians can perform a colostomy as a temporary measure when inflammation or trauma is present.

Nerves

Parasympathetic stimulation by the vagus and pelvic nerves (from the sacral part of the spinal cord) increases peristalsis and the secretion of mucus, which protects the intestinal wall. Sympathetic stimulation has the opposite effects.

Digestion

The function of the digestive system is to break down foods so that they can be assimilated by the body. Digestion begins in the mouth and ends in the small intestine (Figure 12-7) and is accompanied by digestive enzymes that split large food particles into substances small enough to pass through the wall of the digestive tract into the blood and lymph capillaries. The gastrointestinal tract contains glands that secrete mucus and digestive enzymes (Table 12-1).

The rhythmic contraction of smooth muscle, called **peristalsis**, propels products of digestion along the tract from the

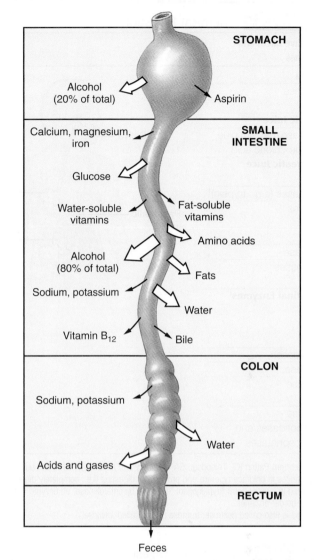

FIGURE 12-7 Absorption sites in the digestive tract. The size of the *arrow* at each site indicates the amount of absorption of a particular substance at that site. Most absorption occurs in the intestines, particularly the small intestine. (From Patton KT, Thibodeau GA: *Anatomy and physiology,* ed 6, St Louis, 2007, Mosby.)

esophagus to the anus (Figure 12-8). This is a form of mechanical digestion.

Box 12-2 shows the four essential steps in the process of digestion. *Digestion secretion* generally refers to the release of various substances from the exocrine glands that serve the digestive system (Table 12-2). Digestive secretion includes the release of saliva, gastric juice, pancreatic juice, bile, and intestinal enzymes.

Citric Acid Cycle

The citric acid cycle (Krebs cycle) is the main pathway by which food energy is released by cells to manufacture their own energy-rich adenosine triphosphate (ATP). The citric acid cycle is a complex transformation process. The end result of many chemical reactions is energy for cellular function (Figure 12-9).

Table 12-1 Chemical Digestion

Digestive Juices and Enzymes	Substance Digested (or Hydrolyzed)	Resulting Product*
Saliva		
Amylase	Starch (polysaccharide)	Maltose (a double sugar, or disaccharide)
Gastric Juice		
Protease (pepsin) plus hydrochloric acid	Proteins	Partially digested proteins
Pancreatic Juice		
Proteases (e.g., trypsin)[†]	Proteins (intact or partially digested)	Peptides and **amino acids**
Lipases	Fats emulsified by bile	**Fatty acids, monoglycerides,** and **glycerol**
Amylase	Starch	Maltose
Nucleases	Nucleic acids (DNA, RNA)	Nucleotides
Intestinal Enzymes[‡]	Peptides	Amino acids
	Sucrose (cane sugar)	**Glucose** and **fructose**[§] (simple sugars, or monosaccharides)
Peptidases		
Sucrase		
Lactase	Lactose (milk sugar)	**Glucose** and **galactose** (simple sugars)
Maltase	Maltose (malt sugar)	**Glucose**
Nucleotidases and phosphatases	Nucleotides	Nucleosides

Modified from Patton KT, Thibodeau GA: *Anatomy and physiology,* ed 7, St Louis, 2010, Mosby.
*Substances in boldface type are end products of digestion (i.e., completely digested nutrients ready for absorption).
[†]Secreted in inactive form (trypsinogen); activated by enterokinase, an enzyme in the intestinal brush border.
[‡]Brush-border enzymes.
[§]Glucose is also called dextrose; fructose is also called *levulose.*

Box 12-2 Steps in the Digestion Process

First Step
Ingestion: Food enters the mouth (i.e., eating).

Second Step
Digestion: The mechanical and chemical breakdown of food from its complex form into simple molecules.

Third Step
Absorption: The movement of the simple molecules from the digestive tract into the cardiovascular or lymphatic systems; vitamins and minerals are absorbed in the small intestine; amino acids, simple sugars, and small fatty acids pass through the intestinal villi into the bloodstream; larger fatty acids are reconstituted to fats in the intestinal wall and pass into the specialized lymphatic capillaries; capillaries of the intestinal villi become venules and then veins, and finally the large portal vein carries absorbed foodstuffs to the liver; the liver converts these substances into compounds required for body functions.

Fourth Step
Elimination (egestion): Removal and release by defecation of solid waste products (feces) from food that cannot be digested or absorbed.

Nutrition

Nutrition is the use of food for growth and maintenance of the body. Poor nutrition has an effect on general health, stress responses, and sleeping. For most people, nutritional problems result from not following dietary recommendations. In the elderly, decreased ability to digest and assimilate food may result in poor nutrition. Others may have diseases that can cause nutritional deficiencies. Food affects mood. Mood influences feelings. Behavior supports feelings, and the whole issue of food is often an emotional topic.

The basics of good nutrition include eating a diet high in vegetables, grains, legumes, and fruits that are fresh, clean, and grown in nutrient-rich soil. Human protein requirements are moderate and may be met by food from animal or nonanimal sources. Fat and sugar requirements in the diet are small, but human beings have a strong urge for fats and sweets. An ideal diet is low to moderate in unsaturated fats (avoid hydrogenated fats), sugars, and protein, with the bulk of the calories coming from complex carbohydrates. These recommendations vary with differing genetic predispositions, ages, and

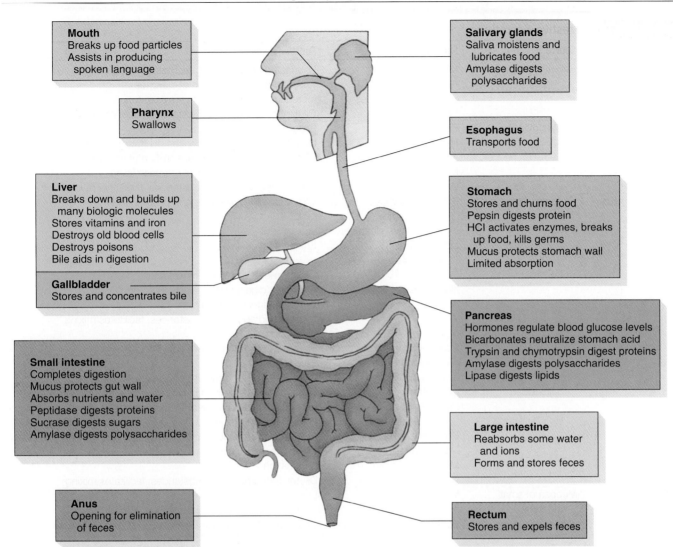

Mouth
Breaks up food particles
Assists in producing
spoken language

Salivary glands
Saliva moistens and
lubricates food
Amylase digests
polysaccharides

Pharynx
Swallows

Esophagus
Transports food

Liver
Breaks down and builds up
many biologic molecules
Stores vitamins and iron
Destroys old blood cells
Destroys poisons
Bile aids in digestion

Gallbladder
Stores and concentrates bile

Stomach
Stores and churns food
Pepsin digests protein
HCl activates enzymes, breaks
up food, kills germs
Mucus protects stomach wall
Limited absorption

Pancreas
Hormones regulate blood glucose levels
Bicarbonates neutralize stomach acid
Trypsin and chymotrypsin digest proteins
Amylase digests polysaccharides
Lipase digests lipids

Small intestine
Completes digestion
Mucus protects gut wall
Absorbs nutrients and water
Peptidase digests proteins
Sucrase digests sugars
Amylase digests polysaccharides

Large intestine
Reabsorbs some water
and ions
Forms and stores feces

Anus
Opening for elimination
of feces

Rectum
Stores and expels feces

FIGURE 12-8 Summary of digestive function. (From Patton KT, Thibodeau GA: *Anatomy and physiology,* ed 6, St Louis, 2007, Mosby.)

states of health, which influence the ratio among fats, proteins, and carbohydrates that best suits an individual.

The food we eat is only as good as the soil in which it is grown or the food the animals were fed. Many suggest that much of the soil used in agriculture is worn out, depleted, and toxic because of the continuous use of artificial fertilizers and pesticides and that the land has been overused and denied rest time to replenish itself. If this is the condition of the soil, what is the nutritional value of the food grown in it? Food is most nutritious when freshly harvested and ripe. Food eaten a day after harvest has already lost a substantial number of nutrients. Food, mostly fruit, picked green is not as nutritious as fruit allowed to ripen on the vine. All food-preservation methods result in loss of the nutritional value of the food. Under ideal conditions, we would harvest all of our food an hour before we eat it, but this is not possible for most of us. We have to make a trade-off between convenience and nutrition.

Many persons take nutritional supplements, and many opinions exist on this topic. It must be remembered that these are supplements to our diet and should not be expected to replace proper food intake. The closer a supplement is to a real food, the better the body is able to use it. Supplements usually are best taken with food to maximize absorption and use.

For the intestinal tract to function effectively, it is necessary to eat dietary fiber. Fiber is especially important for colon health. When combined with water, fiber expands or bulks in the colon, making the stool easier to pass.

Drinking a sufficient quantity of pure water is important for optimal body function. Recommendations are for at least 64 ounces of water per day for efficient body function.

Main Food Groups

Proteins

Proteins are large, high-molecular-weight substances containing carbon, hydrogen, oxygen, and nitrogen and small amounts of other elements. Proteins break down into amino acids, which the body then absorbs. The body's metabolic requirements include 24 amino acids. Most can be manufactured in the liver from other amino acids, but eight cannot. These eight are referred to as *essential amino acids:* phenylalanine, valine, threonine, leucine, isoleucine, methionine, tryptophan,

Table 12-2   Digestive Secretions

	Source	Substance	Functional Role
Saliva	Salivary glands	Mucus	Lubricates bolus of food; facilitates mixing of food
		Amylase	Enzyme; begins digestion of starches
		Sodium bicarbonate	Increases pH (for optimum amylase function)
		Water	Dilutes food and other substances; facilitates mixing
Gastric juice	Gastric glands	Pepsin	Enzyme; digests proteins
		Hydrochloric acid	Denatures proteins; decreases pH (for optimum pepsin function)
		Intrinsic factor	Protects and allows later absorption of vitamin B_{12}
		Mucus	Lubricates chyme; protects stomach lining
		Water	Dilutes food and other substances; facilitates mixing
Pancreatic juice	Pancreas (exocrine portion)	Proteases (trypsin, chymotrypsin, collagenase, elastase)	Enzymes; digest proteins and polypeptides
		Lipases (lipase, phospholipase)	Enzymes; digest lipids
		Colipase	Coenzyme; helps lipase digest fats
		Nucleases	Enzymes; digest nucleic acids (RNA and DNA)
		Amylase	Enzyme; digests starches
		Water	Dilutes food and other substances; facilitates mixing
		Mucus	Lubricates
		Sodium bicarbonate	Increases pH (for optimum enzyme function)
Bile	Liver (stored and concentrated in gallbladder)	Lecithin and bile salts	Emulsify lipids
		Sodium bicarbonate	Increases pH (for optimum enzyme function)
		Cholesterol	Excess cholesterol from body cells, to be excreted with feces
		Products of detoxification	From detoxification of harmful substances by hepatic cells, to be excreted with feces
		Bile pigments (mainly bilirubin)	Products of breakdown of heme groups during hemolysis, to be excreted with feces
		Mucus	Lubrication
		Water	Dilutes food and other substances; facilitates mixing
Intestinal juice	Mucosa of small and large intestine	Mucus	Lubrication
		Sodium bicarbonate	Increases pH (for optimum enzyme factor)
		Water	Small amount to carry mucus and sodium bicarbonate

From Thibodeau GA, Patton KT: *Anatomy and physiology,* ed 7, St Louis, 2010, Mosby.

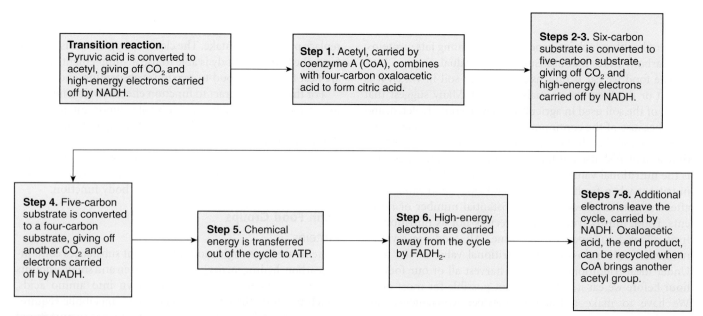

FIGURE 12-9 Citric acid cycle. The transition reaction prepares each pyruvic acid molecule to enter the citric acid cycle, yielding a pair of high-energy electrons and a CO_2 molecule. Coenzyme A (CoA) picks up the acetyl group thus formed and takes it into the citric acid cycle proper, which is described here as a recurring series of eight steps. *NADH,* The reduced form of nicotinamide adenine dinucleotide (NAD^+). (Adapted from Patton KT, Thibodeau GA: *Anatomy and physiology,* ed 7, St Louis, 2010, Mosby.)

and lysine. In addition, histidine and arginine are required for growth and development. Dietary proteins include animal products and bean and grain combinations.

Proteins are the chief structural components of the body. Enzymes, some hormones, muscle tissue, and a substantial portion of chromosomes are proteins. Proteins are essential components of the cell membrane. Important compounds such as epinephrine and acetylcholine are derived from amino acids.

Carbohydrates

Carbohydrates have as basic components carbon, hydrogen, and oxygen in precise proportions. Complex carbohydrates are long chains of sugar molecules found in rice, vegetables, and so on. These long chains are called *polysaccharides.* Simple carbohydrates are sugars and consist of single sugar molecules called *monosaccharides,* or double sugar molecules, called *disaccharides.* Animal starch, or glycogen, is the form glucose takes for storage in liver and muscle. All carbohydrates are digested into one of several types of monosaccharides. All types of monosaccharides are converted into glucose by the liver because glucose is the main fuel for the manufacture of ATP in the cells.

Lipids

Lipids, or triglycerides, are broken down into fatty acids and glycerol by the digestive system. A fatty acid is a molecule consisting of a chain of carbons with no double bonds (saturated) or several double bonds (unsaturated). The unsaturated fats most closely resemble body fat and are more easily assimilated and used. Saturation (addition of hydrogen molecules) makes fat more solid and less desirable in the diet. Linoleic acid is an example of a fatty acid essential to human nutrition. In addition to serving as a reservoir of stored energy, fats are essential components of many hormones, the cell membrane, and the myelin sheath of the nerve fiber. Dietary fats are found in nuts, seeds, oils, and animal products.

Vitamins

Vitamins are growth factors needed in small amounts for daily body metabolism. They are classified as fat soluble or water soluble. Many vitamins act as enzyme activators and are called *coenzymes.* The fat-soluble vitamins are more toxic because excess amounts are stored in the fat tissue and are not excreted readily. Water-soluble vitamins, however, are absorbed and excreted more easily (Table 12-3).

Table 12-3 Functions and Sources of Vitamins

Vitamin	Function	Food Source	Adult RDA
Fat Soluble			
Vitamin A	Healthy mucous membranes, skin, hair; essential for bone development and growth; component for the pigments in retina needed for night vision	Milk and cheese; yellow, orange, green vegetables	800-1000 µg
Vitamin D	Formation and development of bones and teeth; assists in absorption of calcium	Fortified milk, fish oils; made in skin when exposed to sunlight	5-10 µg
Vitamin E	Conserves certain fatty acids; aids in protection against cell membrane damage	Whole grains, wheat germ, vegetable oils, nuts, green leafy vegetables	8-10 µg
Vitamin K	Needed for synthesis of factors essential in blood clotting	Green leafy vegetables, cabbage; synthesized by bacteria in intestine	65-80 µg
Water Soluble			
Thiamine (B_1)	Release of energy from carbohydrates and amino acids; growth; proper functioning of nervous system	Whole grains, legumes, nuts	1.5 mg
Riboflavin (B_2)	Helps transform nutrients into energy; involved in citric acid cycle	Whole grains, milk, green vegetables, nuts	1.7 mg
Niacin (B_3)	Helps transform nutrients into energy; involved in glycolysis and citric acid cycle	Whole grains, nuts, legumes, fish, liver	20 mg
Pyridoxine (B_6)	Involved in amino acid metabolism	Legumes, poultry, nuts, dried fruit, green vegetables	2 mg
Cyanocobalamin (B_{12})	Aids in formation of red blood cells; helps in nervous system function	Dairy products, eggs, fish, poultry	2 µg
Pantothenic acid	Part of coenzyme A; functions in steroid synthesis; helps in nutrient metabolism	Legumes, nuts, green vegetables, milk, poultry	7 mg
Folic acid	Aids in formation of hemoglobin and nucleic acids	Green vegetables, legumes, nuts, fruit juices, whole grains	200 µg
Biotin	Fatty acid synthesis; movement of pyruvic acid into citric acid cycle	Eggs; made by intestinal bacteria	0.3 mg
Ascorbic acid (C)	Important in collagen synthesis; helps maintain capillaries; aids in absorption of iron	Citrus fruits, tomatoes, green vegetables, berries	60 mg

µg, Microgram; *mg,* milligram.
From Applegate E: *The anatomy and physiology learning system,* ed 4, Philadelphia, 2011, Saunders.

Table 12-4	Functions and Sources of Selected Minerals		
Mineral	Function	Food Source	Adult RDA
Calcium	Component of bones and teeth; muscle contraction; blood clotting	Dairy products, green vegetables, legumes, nuts	800-1000 µg
Chloride	Acid-base balance of the blood; component of hydrochloric acid in the stomach	Table salt, milk, eggs, meat	750 mg
Phosphorus	Component of bones and teeth; component of adenosine triphosphate and nucleic acids; component of cell membranes	Legumes, dairy products, nuts, poultry, lean meats	800 mg
Sodium	Regulates body fluid volume; nerve impulse conduction	Table salt is biggest source of sodium in diet	500 mg
Potassium	Body fluid balance; muscle contraction; nerve impulse conduction	Fruits, legumes, nuts, vegetables; widely distributed	2000 mg
Magnesium	Component of some active enzymes; releases energy from nutrients	Whole grains, legumes, green vegetables, nuts	280-350 mg
Iron	Component of hemoglobin and myoglobin; releases energy from nutrients	Whole grains, nuts, legumes, poultry, fish, lean meats	10-15 mg
Iodine	Component of thyroid hormones	Iodized table salt, dairy products, fish	150 µg
Zinc	Component of several enzymes; formation of proteins; wound healing	Legumes, poultry, nuts, whole grains, fish, lean meats	12-15 mg
Fluoride	Healthy bones and teeth	Fluoridated water is best source	1.5-4.0 mg

µg, Microgram; *mg,* milligram.
From Applegate E: *The anatomy and physiology learning system,* ed 4, Philadelphia, 2011, Saunders.

Minerals

Minerals are important for the formation of the bones and teeth and the function of muscle, blood, and nerve cells. They are vital to overall mental and physical well-being. Minerals act as catalysts for many biological reactions within the body, including muscle response, the transmission of messages through the nervous system, and the utilization of nutrients in food.

Vitamins cannot be assimilated without the aid of minerals. Although the body can manufacture a few vitamins, it cannot manufacture a single mineral. All tissue and internal fluids contain varying quantities of minerals (Table 12-4 and Box 12-3).

Metabolic Rate

The metabolic rate is the catabolic rate, or rate of energy release. The **basal metabolic rate** (BMR) is not the minimum metabolic rate and does not indicate the smallest amount of energy that must be expended to sustain life. BMR does indicate, however, the smallest amount of energy expenditure that can sustain life and also maintain the waking state and a normal body temperature in a comfortably warm environment. The BMR is the rate of energy expenditure under basal conditions; that is, when an individual:

- Is awake but lying down and not moving.
- Has not eaten for 18 to 23 hours.
- Is in a comfortably warm environment.

The BMR is not identical for all individuals because of the influence of the following factors.

Size

BMR is calculated on the basis of the individual's height and weight. A large individual has more surface area and a greater BMR than a small individual.

Sex

Men oxidize their food approximately 5% to 7% faster than women, so a male has a BMR greater than a female of the same size. This gender difference in BMR results from the difference in the proportion of body fat, which is determined by sex hormones. Women tend to have a higher percentage of body fat (and thus a lower total lean mass) than men. Fat tissue is less metabolically active than lean tissues such as muscle. Also, testosterone, found in much higher levels in men, increases metabolic rate. Women who are pregnant or lactating, however, have a greatly increased BMR.

Age

The younger the individual, the higher the BMR for a given size and sex.

Thyroid Hormones

Thyroid hormones (T_3 and T_4) stimulate basal metabolism. Homeostasis depends on having thyroid hormones within normal ranges.

Body Temperature

An increase in body temperature increases BMR. A decrease in body temperature (hypothermia) has the opposite effect.

Drugs

Stimulants increase the BMR, and depressants decrease the BMR.

Energy Balance and Body Weight

The total metabolic rate is the amount of energy used or expended by the body in a given time. The BMR usually constitutes about 55% to 60% of the total metabolic rate. The energy used to do all kinds of skeletal muscle work contributes

Nutritional Databases

The National Institutes of Health sponsors two databases, one through the Office of Dietary Supplements (http://ods.od.nih.gov), the other through the National Center for Complementary and Alternative Medicine (http://nccam.nih.gov). Both provide safety and effectiveness information about supplements that is free of commercial influence. The Consumer Reports database allows consumers to check herbal medicines that might be effective for specific health problems.

The basics of balanced nutrition are explained in the Department of Agriculture's guide to good eating. These newer recommendations have reconfigured the previous six-section MyPyramid guide into MyPlate (www.ChooseMyPlate.gov). MyPlate illustrates the five food groups that are the building blocks for a healthy diet by using a place setting for a meal. The idea is to think about what goes on your plate or in your cup or bowl before you eat. The segmented place setting provides the proper proportions for how much of each food group you should be eating at each meal. A list of suggestions for each food group are also provided as well as how much is needed, what constitutes a serving size, the health benefits and nutrients, and tips to help you eat from that food group. Daily food plans based on demographic (e.g., moms, preschoolers), sample menus and recipes, and a SuperTracker to help you plan, analyze, and track your diet and physical activity, are all also included.

The USDA, in conjunction with the Department of Health and Human Services, also publishes The Dietary Guidelines for Americans, which describes a healthy diet as one that:

- Emphasizes fruits, vegetables, whole grains, and fat-free or low-fat milk and milk products
- Includes lean meats, poultry, fish, beans, eggs, and nuts
- Is low in saturated fats, trans fats, cholesterol, salt (sodium), and added sugars.

The recommendations in the Dietary Guidelines and in MyPlate are for the general public over 2 years of age. MyPlate helps individuals use the Dietary Guidelines to:

- Make smart choices from every food group.
- Find balance between food and physical activity.
- Get the most nutrition out of calories.
- Stay within daily caloric needs.

The Dietary Guidelines were updated in 2010 and are available at www.DietaryGuidelines.gov.

to the total metabolic rate. The metabolic rate increases for several hours after a meal, apparently because of the energy needed to metabolize foods.

The body attempts to maintain a state of energy balance; its energy input should equal its energy output. Energy input per day equals the total calories (kilocalories) in the food ingested per day. Energy output equals the total metabolic rate expressed in kilocalories. Energy intake versus output determines body weight.

Body weight remains constant (except for possible variations in water content) when the body maintains energy balance. Weight increases when energy input exceeds energy output, and the body synthesizes and stores fat. It decreases when energy input is less than energy output.

Pathologic Conditions of the Digestive System

Digestive diseases can affect all organs and function of the digestive system. These disorders have many causes, including acute and chronic infections, cancer, adverse effects of drugs and toxins, genetic predisposition, birth defects, and lifestyle choices. In many cases the cause of the disease is unknown.

Constipation

Constipation is difficulty in passing stools or an incomplete or infrequent passage of hard stool. Among the causes are dehydration, insufficient dietary fiber intake, intestinal obstruction, diverticulitis, and tumors. Functional impairment of the colon may occur in elderly or bedridden clients who fail to respond to the urge to defecate. Backache and headache may be present. Constipation and diarrhea are common side effects of many medications. Increasing fluid, dietary fiber, and exercise may be helpful. Stool softeners may be prescribed for the constipation. Education about regular bowel habits may be necessary.

Hemorrhoids

Hemorrhoids are dilated varicose veins of the anus. They can be due to constipation; straining to defecate causes the anal veins to become varicosed. Hemorrhoids also often appear during pregnancy and delivery. External hemorrhoids lie distal to the anorectal margin; internal hemorrhoids lie proximal. Occasionally, a thrombus or clot forms, resulting in a painful, bluish mass. Hemorrhoids may cause pain, but the usual symptom is bleeding and itching caused by the drying up of the protective mucus. The primary treatment is sitz baths, steroid creams or suppositories, and stool softeners. The clot may be removed surgically under local anesthesia. Hemorrhoids also are treatable by laser to seal the blood vessels, cryosurgery, or surgical removal.

Gastroenteritis

Gastroenteritis is a general term for irritation, inflammation, or infection of the gastrointestinal tract. If the stomach is involved, the condition is called *gastritis*. Hemorrhagic gastritis is characterized by bleeding erosions and also is called *acute erosive gastritis* or *multiple gastric erosions*. It can occur without any apparent reason. It is associated, however, with aspirin ingestion, burns, traumatic injury, surgery, shock, liver disease, respiratory problems, and septicemia and can cause vomiting and diarrhea and lead to dehydration.

If the intestine is affected, the condition is called *enteritis*. Usually the stomach and intestine are involved, so the term *gastroenteritis* applies. The most common cause is a virus, which can be passed from person to person. This stomach flu usually lasts 24 to 36 hours. If the cause is a bacterial toxin, the condition is food poisoning. Occasionally, bacterial infection or, rarely, protozoal infection, such as that involved in dysentery, causes enteritis. Food poisoning, caused by toxic foods, poisonous mushrooms, and so on, is implicated in many cases. Gastroenteritis can become dangerous if infectious organisms or toxic substances enter the bloodstream.

The inflammation also may result from illness or dietary changes, especially when food and water are ingested in foreign countries, or may result from extended use of antibiotics.

Diarrhea and generalized cramping abdominal pain are symptoms of the condition. Primary treatment is rehydration and relaxing the hyperactive bowel. Ingesting only fluids for 24 hours relaxes the intestine because food stimulates gastrointestinal hormone release and peristalsis. Several compounds slow the bowel: bismuth subsalicylate (Pepto-Bismol), diphenoxylate with atropine (Lomotil), and anticholinergic antispasmodics such as dicyclomine (Bentyl). If a stool culture shows a bacterial or protozoal infection, an antibiotic or antiprotozoal is given.

Reflux Esophagitis (Gastroesophageal Reflux)

Reflux esophagitis is the regurgitation of gastric acid up through an open esophageal sphincter, causing heartburn. This is usually caused by problems with control of the esophageal sphincter that may be due to a hiatal hernia or another, less common pathologic condition. However, reflux esophagitis also may be caused by physical corrosion resulting from components in the diet, such as tobacco, alcohol, and acidic food. Lying flat or bending over often aggravates the discomfort, and sitting upright relieves it. Reflux esophagitis commonly occurs in obese persons. Inflammation or ulceration of the esophagus is present. Primary treatment is weight loss if the person is overweight, which decreases the pressure on the abdominal structures and relieves the hiatal hernia, and the use of an antacid.

Peptic Ulcer Disease

A peptic ulcer is a gastric or duodenal ulcer that affects the lining of the esophagus, stomach, or duodenum. The sore can perforate the wall of the digestive tract. The term *peptic* means that pepsin is involved. Risk factors include being male, smoking, genetic predisposition, alcohol use, and stress. There is also a correlation with a bacterial infection caused by the organism *Helicobacter pylori*. Increased secretion of hydrochloric acid and pepsin and decreased tissue resistance contribute to the process. The normal protective mechanisms of the duodenal and gastric mucosa against hydrochloric acid and pepsin are blocked, and excessive vagal stimulation is present. The ulcer causes pain and may erode a vessel and cause bleeding. The ulcer may perforate the intestinal or stomach wall, causing peritonitis and shock. Recent studies indicate that a bacterial infection may cause many ulcers, and treatment involves the use of antibiotics.

Common signs and symptoms of peptic ulcer disease include the following:
- Heartburn or burning pain $\frac{1}{2}$ hour to 2 hours after a meal, relieved by antacids
- Vomiting of brownish-black material (the color of coffee grounds) or the passage of dark stools, indicating the presence of blood after perforation
- Tenderness on palpation of the epigastric region of the abdomen
- Nausea, weight loss, and decreased appetite, which are also signs that may indicate gastric cancer

Antacids such as magnesium-aluminum hydroxide mixtures (Maalox, Mylanta) are useful. Cimetidine (Tagamet) or ranitidine (Zantac) inhibit gastric acid secretion. Stopping smoking, decreasing or stopping alcohol consumption, and using stress-management techniques also are indicated.

Appendicitis

Appendicitis is an inflammation of the appendix, usually caused by bacterial infection. Signs and symptoms often begin with discomfort in the umbilical region that becomes painful and localized in the lower right quadrant, with fever, nausea, and vomiting. The appendix may be inflamed or abscessed and may burst. If the appendix bursts, the pain initially decreases because of the pressure release, but the bacteria spread to the abdominal cavity, resulting in peritonitis, which is infection of the peritoneal membrane and potentially fatal.

Hernia

A hernia is the protrusion of soft tissues through a tear or weak spot in the abdominal muscle wall. Herniae can occur anywhere but are most common in the abdomen. In a hiatal hernia the intestines bulge through an opening in the diaphragm. A more common type is inguinal hernia, which produces a bulging of the abdominal organs down the inguinal canal, often into the scrotum of males or labia of women. Males experience this most often, and herniation can occur at any age. Women may experience a femoral hernia below the groin, often caused by changes that occur during pregnancy. A reducible hernia is one in which the protruding organ can be manipulated back into the abdominal cavity naturally by lying down or by manual reduction through a surgical opening in the abdomen. A strangulated hernia is one in which the hernia is not reducible, and blood flow to the affected organ (e.g., the intestine) is blocked, which may result in obstruction and gangrene. The individual usually experiences pain and vomiting, and immediate surgical repair is required.

Malabsorption and Intolerance Syndromes

Malabsorption syndromes involve poor absorption of nutrients and can be caused by deficiency of digestive enzymes, inadequate transport of nutrients, abnormalities in the structure of the intestine because of disease or surgery, or a hypersensitivity reaction to a particular food. Wheat, corn, and dairy products are the most common foods to cause malabsorption syndrome, and elimination diets may be beneficial. Malabsorption can result from cystic fibrosis, diabetes mellitus, dietary intolerance such as celiac disease, reaction to dietary gluten, or lactose intolerance as a result of lactase deficiency.

Irritable Bowel Syndrome

Irritable bowel syndrome is also known as *spastic*, or *irritable*, *colon*. Symptoms include abdominal pain, alternating constipation and diarrhea, nausea, and gas. Poor diet, tension, and emotional problems can induce irritable bowel syndrome. Peristaltic action is not well coordinated and results in changes in the pattern of bowel movements. Primary treatment includes a diet high in fiber, restriction of alcohol and tobacco, a psyllium laxative such as Metamucil, and perhaps an anticholinergic medications such as dicyclomine. A comprehensive stress management program is beneficial.

Inflammatory Bowel Disease

Two inflammatory diseases of the gastrointestinal tract affect mainly young men and women between the ages of 20 and 40, causing ulcerative lesions and thickening of the intestinal wall. The cause of both is unknown, but autoimmunity may be a factor. Ulcerative colitis affects primarily the sigmoid colon, with symptoms of lower abdominal pain and bloody diarrhea. Ulcers actually develop inside the large intestine. Regional enteritis is a chronic inflammation of the intestine, most commonly the ileum, and is known as *Crohn's disease.* It presents symptoms of cramping, right lower quadrant pain, and intermittent diarrhea. One or two attacks may occur, or they may occur regularly. The body does not absorb nutrients and loses weight. The primary treatment for both is an adequate diet, antibiotic therapy, and steroids. Occasionally, surgical removal of the ileum is necessary.

Diverticular Disease

Diverticula are small, saclike outpouchings of the intestinal wall found in weak areas of the colon near the locations of vessels. Most occur in the sigmoid colon. When multiple diverticula are present, the condition is called *diverticulosis.* If they become inflamed and infected, the condition is called *diverticulitis.* Perforation of a diverticular sac may cause peritonitis. Symptoms are similar to those of irritable bowel syndrome, except that patients with peritonitis may have a fever and acute onset of symptoms. Primary treatment consists of a high-fiber diet, increased intake of fluids, a bulk-forming laxative such as psyllium (Metamucil), and an antibiotic. Severe cases may require hospitalization.

Cirrhosis

Cirrhosis is the infiltration of connective tissue into the functioning cells of the liver that causes slow deterioration of the liver (Figure 12-10). End-stage signs and symptoms include jaundice, portal hypertension, and fluid accumulation in the peritoneal cavity. The most common cause is alcoholism, although cirrhosis also occurs in hepatitis. Cirrhosis interrupts many systemic functions. If the disease is not too far advanced and causal factors can be eliminated, liver regeneration capacity is good.

Gallbladder Disease

Gallbladder disease (cholelithiasis) is almost always the result of a gallstone composed of bile salts and cholesterol lodged in the cystic duct. A fatty meal often precedes an attack because the presence of fat stimulates contraction of the gallbladder. Signs and symptoms are as follows:

- Pain in the right upper quadrant of the abdomen, often radiating to the right scapula or upper back
- Nausea and vomiting
- Fever

Gallbladder colic is pain caused by a stone that temporarily obstructs the cystic duct or common bile duct. Cholecystitis

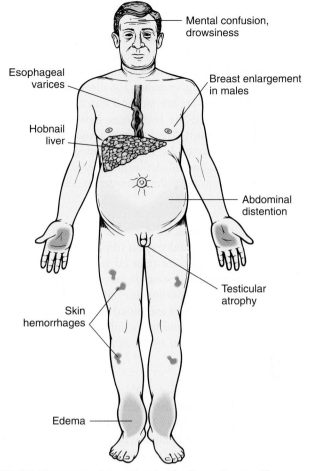

FIGURE 12-10 Symptoms of cirrhosis. (From Frazier MS, Drzymkowski J: *Essentials of human disease and conditions,* ed 4, St Louis, 2008, Saunders.)

is inflammation of the gallbladder caused by obstruction of the cystic duct or common bile duct (choledocholithiasis or common bile duct stone). Cholangitis is infection.

Treatment of mild cases of gallbladder disease involves using an analgesic and eliminating fatty foods from the diet. If infection is present, antibiotics are used. Surgical removal of the gallbladder may be necessary.

Obstructions

An obstruction is a partial or complete closure of the small or large intestine. As a result, chyme backs up, the intestinal walls expand, local arteries may be compressed, and ischemic bowel disease can result. Obstructions may be caused by any of the following:

- Adhesion: Bands of fibrous tissue resulting from previous inflammation or surgical scars that grow between and around the loops of intestine can cause strangulation.
- Hernia: The intestine protrudes through a weakness in the abdominal wall; if the loop of intestine becomes trapped or strangulated, a medical emergency exists.
- Tumors: Growths, such as those seen in colon cancer, can obstruct the intestine.
- Volvulus: A knotting or twisting can cause strangulation in the intestine.

Cystic Fibrosis

Cystic fibrosis is a genetic disease involving exocrine gland dysfunction. Secretions from the pancreas, mucous glands of the respiratory tract, and sweat glands are affected. Without production of pancreatic enzymes, the digestive tract cannot break down food and absorb fats and nutrients. Rarely does a child survive beyond the teen years; most die as a result of pulmonary infections. Treatment is a high-protein, high-calorie diet accompanied by the replacement of pancreatic enzymes. Antibiotics and inhalation and physical therapies are useful. Continuous home pulmonary care is often necessary.

Pancreatitis

Most cases of acute pancreatitis involve alcoholism and gallstones. Lipase, amylase, and trypsin (digestive enzymes) back up in the pancreas and are released into the surrounding tissue. This causes autodigestion of the pancreas and necrosis of tissues, including the peritoneum. Massive destruction of tissue accompanied by fluid and blood loss may lead to shock and death. Signs and symptoms include the following:

- Intense pain in the center of the upper abdomen radiating to the back
- Nausea and vomiting
- Distended, tender abdomen, with the seated position more comfortable than the supine position
- Elevated amylase and lipase levels in the bloodstream

Acute pancreatitis is a medical emergency. If the condition is suspected, immediate referral is necessary.

Chronic pancreatitis may occur after acute pancreatitis, gallstones, or alcohol abuse. Pancreatic function decreases and ultimately stops, and insulin and other pancreatic enzymes and hormones are no longer produced. Pain may be intense, although some patients with chronic pancreatitis do not experience any pain. A drastic treatment is removal of a portion of the pancreas.

Colon Cancer

Colon cancer is the most common cancer and usually affects the lowest part of the rectum. Males and females are equally susceptible. Tumors in the ascending colon usually cause rectal bleeding; those in the descending colon cause constipation and obstructive symptoms. Polyps and ulcerative colitis are important risk factors. Screening for blood in the stool and sigmoidoscopy detect most lesions; 70% are located in the sigmoid colon and rectum. Treatment usually involves surgical removal of the bowel or removal of a section of the bowel, with the ends reattached to maintain a passageway.

Stomach Cancer

Stomach cancer is one of the more common causes of cancer death. Causal factors include chronic gastritis and exposure to environmental chemicals. Onset is slow and insidious, with little advanced warning or detection mechanisms. Indigestion appears; other signs and symptoms are unexplained weight loss, epigastric pain, palpable upper abdominal mass, and iron-deficiency anemia resulting from gastric bleeding.

INDICATIONS/CONTRAINDICATIONS for Therapeutic Massage

A client with shoulder pain (referred), abdominal pain, or referred back pain may have one of several gastrointestinal disorders. In such cases, referral is necessary for proper diagnosis. Many gastrointestinal diseases are bacterial or viral and are contagious. The practitioner should take appropriate precautions to maintain sanitary practice. Most chronic gastrointestinal diseases have a strong correlation with stress. The intestinal tract is highly responsive to changes in autonomic function and endocrine patterns. The influence of the vagus nerve is extensive, and research indicates that therapeutic massage influences vagal function. Sympathetic arousal changes peristaltic action and can send the intestinal tract into all kinds of dysfunction. Comprehensive stress management programs, including therapeutic massage methods, are often effective in managing these conditions.

A specific type of massage to the large intestine can assist in managing constipation. The practitioner can teach this method to the client for self-care. Such massage is contraindicated in inflammatory bowel disease, and the practitioner should obtain permission from the physician treating any other conditions. The massage consists of short, scooping strokes firmly against the abdomen beginning on the left, always directed toward the rectum. Progress continues along the length of the large intestine to the cecum in a fashion of two steps forward and one step back because the direction of the force is down and back toward the rectum. Beginning at the cecum on the right may push fecal material into a large mass, especially at the flexure (Figure 12-11).

URINARY SYSTEM AND FLUID ELECTROLYTE BALANCES

SECTION OBJECTIVES

Chapter objectives covered in this section:
11. List the functions of the urinary system.
12. List and describe the components of the urinary system.
13. Describe urinary function and the processes of fluid electrolyte balances.
14. Describe pathologic conditions of the urinary system and the associated indications and contraindications for massage.

After completing this section, the student will be able to perform the following:
- List and locate the organs of the urinary system.
- Describe the roles of water in the body.
- Define *hydrostatic force.*
- Explain the role of the hypothalamus in fluid regulation.
- Explain the function of osmoreceptors and baroreceptors.
- Describe electrolyte balance.
- Define *pH,* and explain the relationship of pH to homeostasis.
- Identify indications and contraindications of massage for urinary pathology.

The urinary system consists of two kidneys, two ureters, one bladder, and one urethra (Figure 12-12). The kidneys maintain homeostasis by filtering waste products from the blood and keeping the proper amount of water and electrolytes in the blood. Urine passes out of the kidneys and down through the ureters to the bladder for storage. When the

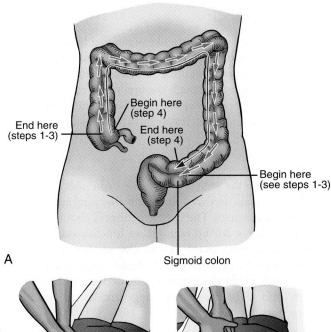

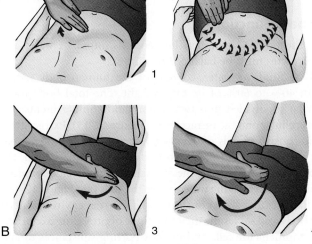

FIGURE 12-11 A, Colon with flow pattern arrows. All massage manipulations are directed in a clockwise fashion. The manipulations begin in the lower left-hand quadrant (on the left side of the illustration) at the sigmoid colon. The methods progressively contact all of the large intestine because they eventually end up encompassing the entire colon area. **B,** Abdominal sequence. The direction of flow for emptying of the large intestine and colon is as follows: *1,* Massage down the left side of the descending colon using short strokes directed to the sigmoid colon. *2,* Massage across the transverse colon to the left side using short strokes directed to the sigmoid colon. *3,* Massage up the ascending colon on the right side of the body using short strokes directed to the sigmoid colon. End at the right side ileocecal valve located in the lower right-hand quadrant of the abdomen. *4,* Massage the entire flow pattern using long, light to moderate strokes from ileocecal valve to sigmoid colon. Repeat sequence.

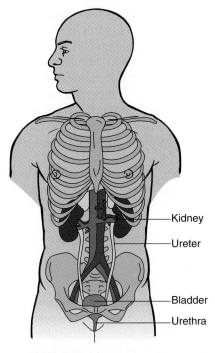

FIGURE 12-12 Urinary system.

bladder reaches a certain volume, it triggers the urge to void. The bladder expels urine through the urethra.

Functions of the Urinary System

The urinary system has the following important functions:
- Conservation of water
- Maintenance of the normal concentration of electrolytes
- Regulation of the acid-base balance
- Regulation of blood pressure
- Activation of vitamin D

The kidneys filter and eliminate most waste. In the average person the kidneys filter about 100 liters of blood per day, reabsorbing 99 liters of filtrate and leaving about 1 liter of urine. Substances secreted from the capillaries into the tubular filtrate include hydrogen, potassium, and ammonia.

Micturition (voiding, urination) is a parasympathetic action modified by voluntary control. It is initiated when afferent impulses from stretch receptors in the bladder stimulate the sacral portion of the spinal cord. The detrusor muscle contracts, and the sphincter relaxes.

Organs of the Urinary System
Kidneys

The kidneys are two reddish-brown, bean-shaped organs located on the posterior wall of the abdomen against the back of the body wall musculature, just above the waist. They are embedded in fat and located at about the spinal level of T11 to L3 on each side of the vertebral column. The right kidney is lower than the left because of its displacement by the liver. On top of each kidney is an adrenal gland.

The inside of a kidney is divided into a cortex, medulla, and pelvis. The cortex and medulla contain approximately 1 million nephrons, specialized tube-shaped filters that reabsorb or excrete substances to form urine. A nephron consists of a Bowman's capsule; a glomerulus, which is composed of a group of capillaries; and a renal tubule. Water and small solids in the blood pass across the membrane of the capillaries and enter the tubule. From there they travel through smaller loops and tubules to the collecting cups. Necessary substances such as water and electrolytes are returned to the blood, whereas the urine drains through ducts and eventually reaches the ureters.

The renal artery, renal vein, and ureters enter or exit the kidneys at the renal hilus. Although sympathetic and parasympathetic nerve fibers are present in the kidneys, the important component is sympathetic, causing vasoconstriction and the release of renin, a substance important in blood pressure control.

Kidneys and Homeostasis

Although we think of the kidneys as organs of excretion, they are more than that. The kidneys do remove wastes, but they also remove normal components of the blood that are present in greater-than-normal concentrations. When excessive water, sodium ions, calcium ions, and so on are present, the excess quickly passes out in the urine. Moreover, the kidneys step up their reclamation of these same substances when they are present in the blood in less-than-normal amounts. Thus the kidneys continuously regulate the chemical composition of the blood within narrow limits. The kidneys are one of the major homeostatic devices of the body.

The kidneys produce erythropoietin, a hormone released in response to lowered levels of oxygen in the blood, and calcitriol (vitamin D₃), the active form of vitamin D that is involved in calcium assimilation. The kidneys also contribute to the acid-base balance.

Practical Application

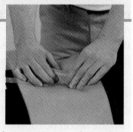

Massage therapy does not interact as directly with the urinary system as specifically as it does with the respiratory and digestive systems. Indirectly, massage influences the autonomic nervous system, which in turn regulates aspects of blood pressure regulation. The influence of massage on the autonomic nervous system also influences the endocrine system, which in turn influences urinary function.

Ureters

The ureters are two narrow tubes extending from the kidney and connecting to the bladder. The two ureters lie on top of the psoas muscles. Each is a tube about 12 inches long, $\frac{1}{8}$ to $\frac{1}{4}$ inch in diameter, and abundantly supplied with nerves. Peristalsis moves urine down into the bladder. Ureter walls contain muscle cells that help move the urine into the bladder. As the bladder fills, it presses against the ureters, compressing them and thus preventing a reverse flow of urine.

Urinary Bladder

The bladder is a muscular, baglike organ that lies in the pelvis and is a reservoir of urine. Urine flows continuously into the bladder from the ureters until a sufficient quantity of urine is collected for disposal through the urethra. When the bladder is distended by about 1 cup of urine, the signal to empty the bladder occurs, and the detrusor muscle causes the bladder to contract.

Urethra

The urethra is the tube that carries urine away from the bladder. The male urethra is about 8 inches long and serves to pass urine and semen. The female urethra is about $1\frac{1}{2}$ inches long, lies anterior to the vagina, and functions only to pass urine. The opening at the end of the urethra is called the *meatus*. The close proximity of the female urethra to the anus allows anal bacteria to migrate up the urethra to the bladder, ureters, and kidneys, predisposing females to ascending urinary tract infections.

Urinary Function

For the body to maintain homeostasis, input of water and electrolytes must be balanced by output.

The fluid, or water, content of the human body ranges from 40% to 60% of its total weight. The total body water can be subdivided into two major fluid compartments: the extracellular and the intracellular (Figure 12-13). Extracellular fluid consists mainly of the plasma found in the blood vessels, the interstitial fluid that surrounds the cells, the lymph, the cerebrospinal fluid, and the specialized joint fluids. *Intracellular fluid* refers to the water inside the cells (see Figure 12-13).

Extracellular fluid constitutes the internal environment of the body and serves the dual functions of providing a constant environment for cells and of transporting substances to and

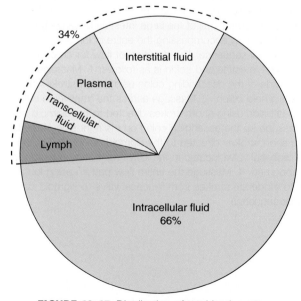

FIGURE 12-13 Distribution of total body water.

34%
Interstitial fluid
Plasma
Transcellular fluid
Lymph
Intracellular fluid 66%

Functions of Water in Human Physiology

- Water provides a medium for chemical reactions.
- Water is crucial for the regulation of chemical and bioelectric distributions within cells.
- Water transports substances such as hormones and nutrients.
- Water aids in oxygen transport from lungs to body cells.
- Water aids in carbon dioxide transport from body cells to lungs.
- Water dilutes toxic substances and waste products and transports them to the kidneys and the liver.
- Water distributes heat around the body.

Table 12-5   Percentage of Water in the Body Tissues

Tissue	Percentage of Water
Blood	83.0
Kidneys	82.7
Heart	79.2
Lungs	79.0
Spleen	75.8
Muscle	75.6
Brain	74.8
Intestine	74.5
Skin	72.0
Liver	68.3
Skeleton	22.0
Adipose tissue	10.0

Table 12-6   Where Water Is Lost from the Body (Healthy Adult)

Organ	Mode of Water Loss	Percentage of Loss
Kidneys	Urine	62
Skin	Diffusion and sweat	19
Lungs	Water vapor	13
Gastrointestinal tract	Feces	6

from them. Intracellular fluid facilitates intracellular chemical reactions that maintain life. With the exception of plasma, fluid volumes are proportionately larger in infants and children than in adults. The function of the urinary system is to maintain the fluid environment of the body.

Fluid regulation is essential to homeostasis. If water or electrolyte levels rise or fall beyond normal limits, many bodily functions are impaired. Dehydration is the most common imbalance. Maintaining normal pH levels is also important for normal body functioning because small changes in pH can produce major disruptions in metabolism.

Water Balance

Water is a component of all living things and often is referred to as "the universal biologic solvent." Only liquid ammonia is able to dissolve more substances than water.

Water acts to minimize temperature changes throughout the body because of its high specific heat. A considerable amount of energy is needed to break the hydrogen bonds between water molecules to make the water molecules move faster (i.e., increase the temperature of water). Therefore water can absorb a great deal of heat without rapidly changing its own temperature.

Box 12-4 lists the many important functions of water in the body.

The water content of the body tissues varies. Adipose tissue (fat) has the lowest percentage of water; the skeleton has the second lowest water content. Skeletal muscle, skin, and the blood are among the tissues that have the highest content of water in the body (Table 12-5).

The total water content of the body decreases most dramatically during the first 10 years of life and continues to decline through old age, at which time water content may be only 45% of the total body weight. Men tend to have higher percentages of water (about 65%) than women (about 55%), mainly because of their increased muscle mass and smaller amount of subcutaneous fat.

The water in the body is in a constant state of motion, shifting between the two major fluid compartments and being continuously lost from and taken into the body. In a normal, healthy human being, water input equals water output. Maintaining this ratio is of prime importance in maintaining health. Approximately 90% of the water is taken in by the gastrointestinal tract in the form of food and liquids. The remaining 10% is called *metabolic water* and is produced as the result of various chemical reactions in the cells of the tissues. Table 12-6 shows the routes by which the healthy adult loses water.

The amount of water lost by way of the kidneys is under hormonal control. The average amount of water lost and consumed per day is approximately 2.5 liters in a healthy adult.

The walls of the blood vessels form barriers to the free passage of fluid between interstitial fluid and blood plasma. At the capillaries these walls are only one cell thick. These capillary walls are generally permeable to water and small solutes but impermeable to large organic molecules such as proteins. Thus the blood plasma tends to have a higher concentration of such molecules than the interstitial fluid. Much of this interstitial fluid becomes lymph, which eventually finds its way back into the bloodstream (see Chapter 11). Because water and small solutes such as sodium, potassium, and calcium can be exchanged freely between the blood plasma and the interstitial fluid, the action of the kidneys on the blood regulates these electrolytes. This exchange depends mainly on the hydrostatic and osmotic forces of these fluid compartments.

Hydrostatic Forces

Liquid exerts force by pushing against a surface, such as a dam in a river or the wall of a blood vessel. The pressure of blood in the capillaries is a major hydrostatic force in the human body, and it functions as a filter because the pressure of the fluid is higher at the arterial end of the capillary than at the venous end. The pressure of the interstitial fluid is negative (−5 mm Hg) because the lymphatic system is continuously taking up the excess fluid forced out of the capillaries.

Osmotic Pressure

Osmotic pressure is the attraction of water to large molecules such as proteins. Because proteins are more abundant within the blood vessels than outside of them, the concentration of proteins in the blood tends to attract water from the interstitial space.

Overall, near equilibrium exists between the fluids forced out of the capillaries and the fluids reabsorbed, because the lymphatic system collects the excess fluid forced out at the artery end and eventually drains it back into the veins at the base of the neck.

A similar situation exists between the interstitial fluid and the intracellular fluid, although ion pumps and carriers complicate the process. Generally, water movement is substantial in both directions, but ion movement is restricted and depends on active transport by way of the pumps. Nutrients and oxygen, because they are dissolved in water, move passively into cells; waste products and carbon dioxide move out of cells.

The mechanisms that regulate body fluids are centered in the hypothalamus, which also receives input from the digestive tract that helps to control thirst. Antidiuretic hormone (ADH) regulates body fluid volume, extracellular osmosis, and many other areas. Primary among them is increasing the permeability of the collecting tubules in the kidneys, thus allowing more water to be reabsorbed by the kidneys. If the body is short of fluid intake (as during sleep), the urine is concentrated, so it is darker and low in volume. When an individual is overhydrated, the urine is diluted, so it is pale or colorless and high in volume, and ADH is absent.

The production of ADH is triggered primarily by osmoreceptors and baroreceptors (pressure receptors); secondary triggers include stress, pain, hypoxia, and extreme exercise.

Osmoreceptors

Osmoreceptors are stimulated by dehydration. This may occur because of fluid loss or lack of fluid intake, or it may be relative dehydration in which the body loses no overall water content but gains sodium ions. The precise location of the osmoreceptors is as yet unclear, but they appear to be in the hypothalamus or the third ventricle of the brain.

The thirst response is connected to the activity of the osmoreceptors, but the actual mechanism is not understood completely. The moistening of the mucosal linings of the mouth and pharynx seems to initiate some sort of neurologic response that sends a message to the thirst center of the hypothalamus. Perhaps more important, stretch receptors in the gastrointestinal tract appear to transmit nerve messages to the thirst center of the hypothalamus that inhibit the thirst response.

Baroreceptors

Changes in the circulating volume of body fluid also stimulate ADH secretion. The result is an increase or decrease in internal pressure, which is monitored by baroreceptors. If the normal volume of water in the body is reduced by 8% to 10% because of hemorrhage or excessive perspiration, ADH is secreted. Pressure receptors located in the atria of the heart and in the pulmonary artery and vein relay their messages to the hypothalamus by way of the vagus nerve.

Electrolyte Balance

An electrolyte is any chemical that dissociates into ions when dissolved in a solution. Ions can be positively charged (cations) or negatively charged (anions). The major electrolytes found in the human body are as follows:

Sodium (Na^+)
Potassium (K^+)
Calcium (Ca^{2+})
Magnesium (Mg^{2+})
Chloride (Cl^-)
Phosphate (HPO_4^{2-})
Sulfate (SO_4^-)
Bicarbonate (HCO_3^-)

Sodium and chloride are the major electrolytes in the interstitial fluid and blood plasma. Potassium and phosphate are the major electrolytes in the intracellular fluid.

Sodium Balance

Sodium balance plays an important role in the excitability of muscles and neurons and is also crucially important in regulating fluid balance in the body. The kidneys closely regulate sodium levels.

Potassium Balance

Potassium is the major electrolyte in intracellular fluid, where its level of concentration is 28 times that in extracellular fluid. Like sodium, potassium is important to the correct functioning of excitable cells, such as muscles, neurons, and sensory receptors. Potassium is also involved in the regulation of fluid levels within the cell and in maintaining the correct pH balance of the body. The pH balance of the body also affects potassium levels. In acidosis, potassium excretion decreases, whereas the opposite occurs in alkalosis.

Calcium and Phosphorus Balance

Calcium is found mainly in the extracellular fluids, whereas phosphorus is found mainly in the intracellular fluids. Both are important in the maintenance of healthy bones and teeth.

Calcium is important in the transmission of nerve impulses across synapses, the clotting of blood, and the contraction of muscles. If calcium levels fall below normal, muscles and nerves become more excitable.

Recall from Chapter 6 that decreased levels of calcium in the body stimulate the parathyroid gland to secrete parathyroid hormone, which increases the calcium and phosphate levels in the interstitial fluids by releasing these minerals from reservoirs lodged in the bones and the teeth. Parathyroid hormone also decreases calcium excretion by the kidneys. If the levels of calcium in the body become too high, the thyroid gland releases calcitonin that inhibits the release of calcium and potassium from the bones. Calcitonin also inhibits the absorption of calcium from the gastrointestinal tract and increases calcium excretion by the kidneys.

Phosphorus is required for the synthesis of nucleic acids and high-energy compounds such as ATP. Phosphorus is also important in the maintenance of pH balance.

Magnesium Balance

Most magnesium is found in the intracellular fluid and in bone. Within cells, magnesium functions in the sodium-potassium pump and as an aid to enzyme action. It plays a role in muscle contraction, action potential conduction, and bone and teeth production. Aldosterone controls magnesium concentrations in the extracellular fluid. Low magnesium levels result in the secretion of more aldosterone, which increases magnesium reabsorption by the kidneys.

Chloride Balance

Chloride is the most plentiful extracellular electrolyte. Its extracellular concentration is 26 times that of its intracellular concentration. Chloride ions are able to diffuse easily across plasma membranes, and their transport is linked closely to sodium movement, which also explains the indirect role of aldosterone in chloride regulation. When sodium is reabsorbed, chloride follows passively. Chloride helps to regulate osmotic pressure differences between fluid compartments and is essential in pH balance. The chloride shift within the blood helps to move bicarbonate ions out of the red blood cells and into the plasma for transport. In the gastric system, chlorine and hydrogen combine to form hydrochloric acid.

pH Balance

Recall from Chapter 1 that pH level is a measurement of the hydrogen concentration of a solution. Lower pH values indicate higher hydrogen concentration, or higher acidity. Higher pH values indicate lower hydrogen concentration, or higher alkalinity. The relative number of hydrogen ions is referred to as *pH balance,* or *acid-base balance.* Hydrogen ion regulation in the fluid compartments of the body is critically important to health. Even a slight change in hydrogen ion concentration can result in a significant alteration in the rates of chemical reactions and can affect the distribution of sodium, potassium, and calcium ions and the structure and function of proteins.

The normal pH of the arterial blood is 7.4, whereas that of the venous blood is 7.35. The venous blood has a lower pH because it has a higher concentration of carbon dioxide, which dissolves in water to make a weak acid called *carbonic acid.* When the pH in the arterial blood changes, one of two conditions may result: acidosis or alkalosis. Acidosis occurs when the hydrogen ion concentration in the arterial blood increases and the pH therefore decreases. Alkalosis occurs when the hydrogen ion concentration in the arterial blood decreases and the pH therefore increases.

Sources of hydrogen ions in the body include the carbonic acid previously mentioned; sulfuric acid (a by-product in the breakdown of proteins); phosphoric acid (a by-product of protein and phospholipid metabolism); ketone bodies produced by the metabolism of fat; and lactic acid (a product formed in skeletal muscle during exercise).

Of all the acids formed by or introduced into the body, about half of them are neutralized by the ingestion of alkaline foods. The remaining acid is neutralized by three major systems: chemical buffers, the respiratory system, and the kidneys. Chemical buffers have an instantaneous effect on pH changes. They are effective in minimizing pH changes but do not entirely eliminate them. Within cells, chemical buffers generally take about 2 to 4 hours to minimize changes in pH. The respiratory system also helps to minimize pH changes; there, the effects occur within minutes. Renal regulation is able to return the pH to absolute normal but requires hours or several days.

Pathologic Conditions of the Urinary System

Disease of the urinary system primarily affects the kidneys and bladder. Because the kidneys maintain homeostasis by filtering waste products from the blood and keeping the proper amount of water and electrolytes in the blood, any pathology of the kidneys has bodywide effects. Bladder infections are common. One function of the urinary system is to allow urine to leave the body. If the structures that carry the urine become blocked, bladder and kidney damage can occur.

Clinical Problems with Fluid Balance

The fluid balance in the body can be upset in many ways, all of which can cause severe problems and even death.

Dehydration

Obviously, dehydration occurs when water is unavailable (Figure 12-14). However, conditions such as diarrhea, severe vomiting, excessive sweating, bleeding, and surgical removal of body fluids also can result in dehydration. There are three types. Hypertonic dehydration occurs when the fluid loss results in an increase in electrolyte levels, causing the blood pressure to fall and the blood to become thicker, which can result in heart failure. Isotonic dehydration results in no perceptible difference from the normal electrolyte balance and may lead to hypotonic dehydration, in which the fluid and electrolyte losses keep pace with each other. Any intake of pure water alters the fluid electrolyte balance because this results in too much water and not enough electrolytes. Thus replacing the body fluid with a balanced preparation of electrolytes and water is important in cases of severe diarrhea.

Problems in the production of urine also can lead to dehydration. Impaired ability to concentrate urine can be caused by the following:

Damage to the medulla of the kidneys: Inadequate water reabsorption occurs, and the urine is too dilute, resulting in fluid loss.

Inadequate ADH production: Inadequate ADH production occurs in diabetes insipidus. Individuals suffering from this disorder may eliminate as much as 5 to 20 liters ($8\frac{1}{2}$ to 34 pints) of urine per day. In the psychologic disorder known as *polydipsia,* the sufferer is obsessed with drinking (usually water), which results in dilution of the plasma,

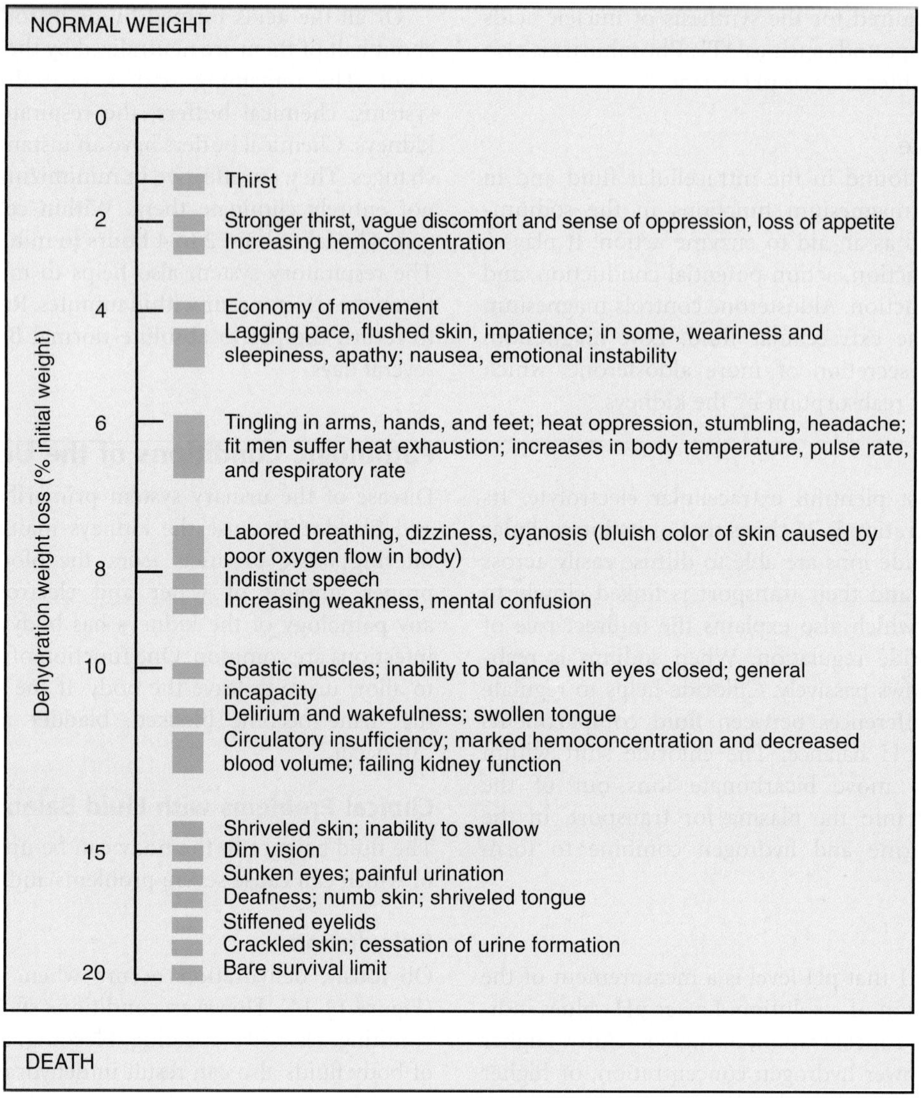

NORMAL WEIGHT

Dehydration weight loss (% initial weight)

0

Thirst

2 — Stronger thirst, vague discomfort and sense of oppression, loss of appetite
Increasing hemoconcentration

4 — Economy of movement
Lagging pace, flushed skin, impatience; in some, weariness and
sleepiness, apathy; nausea, emotional instability

6 — Tingling in arms, hands, and feet; heat oppression, stumbling, headache;
fit men suffer heat exhaustion; increases in body temperature, pulse rate,
and respiratory rate

Labored breathing, dizziness, cyanosis (bluish color of skin caused by
poor oxygen flow in body)
8 — Indistinct speech
Increasing weakness, mental confusion

10 — Spastic muscles; inability to balance with eyes closed; general
incapacity
Delirium and wakefulness; swollen tongue
Circulatory insufficiency; marked hemoconcentration and decreased
blood volume; failing kidney function

Shriveled skin; inability to swallow
15 — Dim vision
Sunken eyes; painful urination
Deafness; numb skin; shriveled tongue
Stiffened eyelids
Crackled skin; cessation of urine formation
20 — Bare survival limit

DEATH

FIGURE 12-14 The effects of dehydration. (From Thibodeau GA, Patton KT: *Anatomy and physiology,* ed 6, St Louis, 2007, Mosby.)

causing artificial lowering of the osmolarity and decreasing ADH secretion.

Solute diuresis in individuals suffering from diabetes mellitus: Elevated blood sugar levels can make the kidneys unable to reabsorb water, which results in excess fluid loss.

In any of the aforementioned conditions, fluid balance must be maintained; otherwise, dehydration or even hypovolemic shock, caused by insufficient volume of body fluid, may occur.

Edema

Edema is a condition in which an excess of fluid exists in the interstitial compartment. The condition often results in tissue swelling and is common whenever lymphatic blockage occurs. It is also caused by impaired ability of the body to dilute the urine and by renal failure, especially the early stages of acute renal failure and the later stages of chronic renal failure.

Liver failure can result in inefficient metabolism of aldosterone, a hormone that controls sodium levels. Heart failure means that the production of aldosterone is enhanced because

of the lowering of the blood pressure. The result is the same as in liver failure. Excessive ADH secretion is a rare condition that may occur because of tumors in the lung, brain, or pancreas, resulting in increased reabsorption of water.

To test for edema, apply steady pressure with the thumb on the lower leg for 10 to 20 seconds. If a depression remains after removal of the pressure, fluid retention is indicated (Figure 12-15).

Urinary Tract Infections

The following symptoms are warning signs of urinary tract infection:

- Increased urge and frequency of urination (usually small amounts of urine)
- Pain or burning sensation with urination
- Pain in the lower abdomen or back
- Blood visible in the urine
- Fever and chills
- Rapid heart rate
- Nausea and vomiting

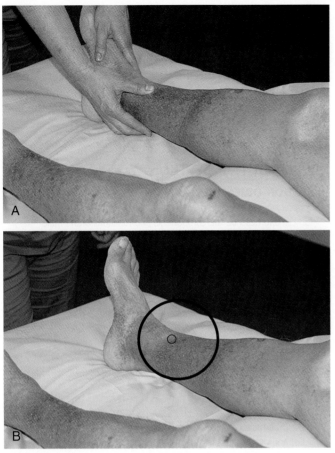

FIGURE 12-15 A, Test for edema. **B,** Identification of pitting edema.

The following suggestions decrease the risk of urinary tract infections:

- Drink plenty of fluids.
- Lie on the left side to increase kidney efficiency and output.
- Wear cotton underwear.
- Avoid tight-fitting clothes.
- Keep the vaginal area clean: Always wipe from front to back after urinating or having a bowel movement.
- Avoid perfumed soaps and panty liners.

Bladder Infections (Cystitis)

Bladder infections (cystitis) are common, particularly in girls and women, in whom the infection usually is caused by bacteria that have spread from the perineal region into the bladder. Symptoms include pain in the lower abdomen, stinging or burning during urination, frequent urination of only small amounts (frequency). Another symptom is a continuous, sometimes uncontrollable urge to urinate (urgency). Antibiotics such as nitrofurantoin (Macrodantin), sulfa-containing agents such as trimethoprim/sulfamethoxazole (Bactrim, Septra), and synthetic penicillins (ampicillin or amoxicillin) are effective. Cranberry juice also seems to be beneficial in managing bladder infection because it prevents the *Escherichia coli* organism from adhering to bladder walls.

Pyelonephritis

Pyelonephritis is an infection of the kidney that affects the nephrons, or filtering units. Bacteria may reach the kidney from the bladder or by spreading through the bloodstream from another infected site, such as the tonsils, middle ear, sinuses, or prostate. Common symptoms are flank and back pain, usually on one side; abdominal pain that moves into the groin; and fever, sometimes with chills and nausea. Treatment includes the use of an appropriate antibiotic. If not treated, pyelonephritis may become chronic and lead to kidney failure.

Incontinence

Urinary incontinence is the inability to control urination. Commonly caused by weak pelvic floor muscles or nerve damage, factors include age, infection, obesity, brain or spinal cord lesion, damage to the nerves to the bladder, or injury to the sphincter (which usually occurs during childbirth). Stress incontinence is urine leakage during coughing, straining, sneezing, and so on, when stress is placed on the muscles. This condition is improved by strengthening the pelvic floor muscles. Urge incontinence is feeling the need to void frequently; it may be caused by irritation or infection or may result from the decrease in the amount of estrogen in a woman's body during and after menopause, which can weaken pelvic floor muscles and reduce the size of the mucous membranes, resulting in both stress and urge incontinence.

Kidney Stones

Kidney stones are small crystalline substances that develop in the kidney. Most kidney stones, also called *calculi,* consist of calcium, but some contain amino acids, uric acids, and other excretory products. The most common cause of stone formation is dehydration; most kidney stones occur during the summer. Other factors are urinary tract infection, impaired tubular reabsorption of calcium, gout, family history, medications such as diuretics, dietary imbalances, and immobilization. Excessive intake of calcium does not lead to kidney stones. Kidney stones are usually undiscovered until one passes into a ureter, causing sudden, excruciating flank pain. Nausea and vomiting may occur. Treatment includes increasing fluid intake to help pass the stone if it is small enough to pass through the ureter. If the stone is too large, surgical removal may be necessary, or the stone may be crushed by an ultrasonic beam or shock wave.

Obstruction

Obstruction of the urethra, causing retention of urine, is most common in older men who have prostate problems. (The reproductive section of this chapter discusses the topic in further detail.)

Glomerulonephritis

Glomerulonephritis is a group of diseases involving antigen-antibody reactions affecting the glomeruli. The antigen may be an external one, such as beta-hemolytic streptococci, or may involve an autoimmune reaction. The most common type occurs after a streptococcal infection, such as pharyngitis, tonsillitis, or impetigo, when antibodies react with streptococci. Immune complexes are deposited in the glomeruli. For mild cases without bacterial infections, treatment is bed rest and salt restriction. Streptococcal infections require antibiotic treatment, whereas autoimmune reactions require treatment with immunosuppressant medications or steroids.

Kidney Failure

Kidney failure, also known as *renal failure,* is the inability to excrete waste products and retain electrolytes. In acute kidney failure the kidneys suddenly stop working, commonly because of acute glomerulonephritis, allergic reactions to medications, shock, or obstruction. Waste products back up in the blood. Kidney failure may cause hypertension, edema, dehydration, and itching of the skin because of the accumulation of waste products in the blood vessels of the skin. The buildup of excessive amounts of nitrogen wastes in the blood is known as *uremia.* Chronic kidney failure is caused by a gradual decrease in kidney function, often as a result of inflammation, glomerulonephritis, or diabetes mellitus. As in the acute stage, the kidneys are unable to excrete waste products or water, and these substances back up in the blood and tissues. In the chronic stage, scar tissue builds up in the kidneys, and they are unable to function. Scarring leads to end-stage kidney failure in which the kidneys are unable to function at all—a life-threatening situation.

Signs and symptoms include the following:

- Weakness and fatigue resulting from sodium, potassium, and calcium abnormalities, such as anemia and acidosis
- Hypertension
- Itching caused by the accumulation of waste products in skin vessels
- Dehydration caused by water loss
- Generalized edema

Treatment includes cautious administration of amino acids, adequate calories, sodium, and calcium, as well as antihypertensive medication. Severe anemia caused by kidney failure may require blood transfusions. The body can survive with only one functioning kidney. If both kidneys fail, however, hemodialysis, the filtering of wastes from blood using a machine, is required. A kidney transplant may be necessary. Of organ transplant procedures, kidney transplants are among the most successful. Careful matching of blood and genetic types, as well as up-to-date immunosuppressive drug therapy, may result in long-term survival rates.

REPRODUCTIVE SYSTEM

SECTION OBJECTIVES

Chapter objectives covered in this section:

15. List and describe the components and functions of the male reproductive system.
16. List and describe the components and functions of the female reproductive system.
17. Explain the three stages of pregnancy and the process of lactation.
18. Describe pathologic conditions of the reproductive system and the associated indications and contraindications for massage.

After completing this chapter, the student will be able to perform the following:

- List the organs of the male reproductive system.
- Trace the movement of sperm from the seminiferous tubules to ejaculation.
- Describe the endocrine and nervous system control over the male reproductive system.
- Describe male contraceptive methods.
- List and describe the organs of the female reproductive system.
- Describe the process of menstruation.
- Describe endocrine and nervous system control over the female reproductive system.
- Explain female contraceptive methods.
- Describe the stages of pregnancy.
- Explain the birth process.
- Define *lactation.*
- Determine indications and contraindications of massage for reproductive system pathology.

The continuation of the species is the biologic function of the reproductive system, yet sexuality is more than reproduction and more than genitals. This last section, the reproductive system, connects the study of the body to the beginning, the cell. The essence of reproduction is the duality of yin/yang and male/female; at the moment of conception, two cells create one whole.

The most obvious differences between males and females are in the construction and functions of the reproductive systems, but even in the differentiation, a continuity exists. The same hormones from the hypothalamus stimulate ovaries and testes. Musculature is similar, as is nervous system distribution. The main difference lies in development of the sex cells (ovum and sperm), the anatomy required to deliver the sperm to the ovum, and the organs to house the developing infant. The difference is not so prevalent in young children before puberty or in those in their mature years (i.e., after 60 or so), but during the reproductive years the differences, and in some ways the gender behaviors, are more evident.

INDICATIONS/CONTRAINDICATIONS for Therapeutic Massage

Urinary System

Therapeutic massage may slightly increase blood volume flow in general through the kidneys by way of mechanical and reflexive processes. In healthy individuals, massage therapy supports the filtration process of blood by potentially increasing blood flow in general. However, in those with kidney disease, the increased volume can strain the kidneys' functioning. Therefore general contraindications exist for anyone with kidney disease. Therapeutic massage modalities may be useful for pain and stress management, but only with the careful supervision of the treating physician.

Acute infectious processes contraindicate massage until the infection has run its course. Massage therapy may be used in chronic infection as part of a supervised treatment plan. Stress contributes to incontinence, so any form of stress management helps somewhat with both stress and urge incontinence. Remember that incontinent clients require easy access to the restroom.

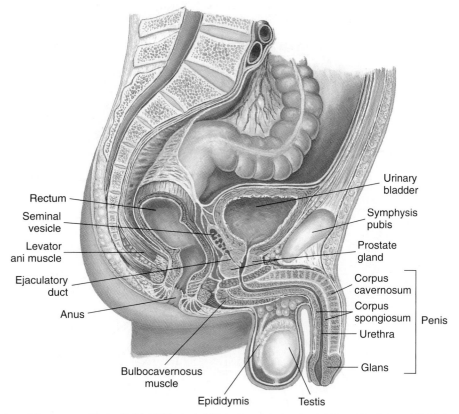

FIGURE 12-16 Male pelvic organs. (From Seidel HM et al: *Mosby's guide to physical examination,* ed 7, St Louis, 2011, Mosby.)

Male Reproductive System

The male reproductive system consists of the testicles, epididymis, vas deferens, ejaculatory duct, urethra, penis, and scrotum (Figure 12-16). The two testicles are enclosed in an external sac called the *scrotum.*

Tiny seminiferous tubules in the testicles produce sperm. The production of sperm is called *spermatogenesis.* Sperm cells travel from the testicles into the epididymis, where they mature. Sperm then moves into the vas deferens, which extends upward into the body cavity, over the symphysis pubis and around the urinary bladder to connect with the two seminal vesicles.

The seminal vesicles produce and secrete a viscous fluid that makes up most of the semen and joins with the sperm to pass from the vas deferens into the ejaculatory duct. The ejaculatory duct passes through the prostate gland and joins with the urethra. The prostate gland is actually a group of small glands that surround the urethra as it exits the bladder; it produces a milky alkaline fluid that becomes a component of semen.

The duct of the bulbourethral, or Cowper's, glands connects to the urethra below the prostate. These two small glands secrete a thick lubricating fluid, which is also a component of semen. On ejaculation, semen flows through the urethra to the outside of the body.

The penis is composed of a meshwork of erectile tissue, meaning it is able to become firm by engorgement with blood. It consists of a shaft, the end of which is covered with a loose flap of skin called the *prepuce,* or *foreskin.* This foreskin often is removed in a surgical process called *circumcision.* The end

of the penis is called the *glans penis.* The penis functions to deposit sperm cells into the vagina.

Hormonal and Nervous System Control

Follicle-stimulating hormone (FSH) and luteinizing hormone (LH) from the pituitary gland control testicular function. FSH stimulates sperm production, whereas LH stimulates the secretion of testosterone from interstitial cells. Gonadotropin-releasing hormone from the hypothalamus stimulates the production of FSH and LH.

Before puberty males produce little testosterone because no releasing hormone is secreted. During adolescence the hypothalamus matures, and gonadotropin-releasing hormone stimulates the production of FSH and LH. The number of interstitial cells is increased by LH, and acceleration occurs in the production of testosterone, which increases the synthesis of protein in cells, creating an anabolic effect. Male secondary sex characteristics appear. Body growth accelerates; muscle and bone mass increase; the penis and scrotum enlarge; the larynx develops and the voice deepens; and hair appears on the face, chest, axillae, abdomen, and pubis.

Hormones stimulate the sebaceous glands of the skin, increasing the likelihood of acne. Testosterone stimulates the male sexual drive, or libido, and boys may begin to exhibit more aggressive social behavior. The production of sperm accelerates. Testosterone and sperm are produced throughout life, but levels gradually diminish after age 40. Spermatogenesis takes place at a temperature lower than body temperature, so the testes are located in the scrotal sac, where

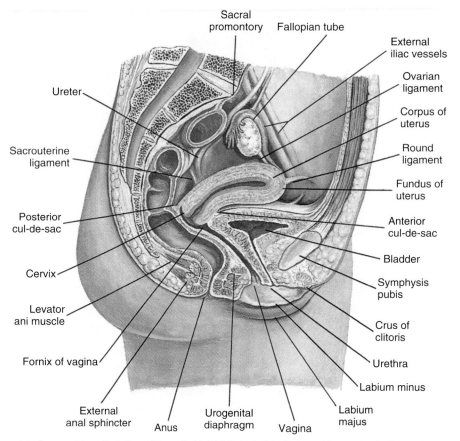

FIGURE 12-17 Female pelvic floor, midsagittal view. (From Seidel HM et al: *Mosby's guide to physical examination,* ed 7, St Louis, 2011, Mosby.)

the temperature is cooler, although during cold weather the cremaster muscle contracts and elevates the testes closer to the body.

Erection is a parasympathetic response in which arteries of the penis dilate and veins constrict, allowing blood flow into the erectile tissue but blocking venous outflow. A variety of stimuli cause erection. Emission involves the contraction of the epididymis, the vas deferens, the prostate, and the seminal vesicles. Semen moves into the urethra. Ejaculation consists of contraction of the muscles at the base of the penis (bulbocavernosus, ischiocavernosus), which propels approximately 3 mL of semen through the penile urethra at high pressure.

Male Contraceptive Methods

Several contraceptive methods are available for men: abstinence, the condom, the condom with spermicidal jelly or foam, withdrawal, and vasectomy. The condom alone and the withdrawal method are not reliable. The condom with a spermicide is a fairly reliable method. In addition, the condom protects against some, but not all, sexually transmitted infections. Vasectomy is performed in a physician's office with the area under local anesthesia; the procedure involves removing a 2-cm piece of the vas deferens and tying the remaining ends. A vasectomy is considered a permanent method of sterilization, even though the cut ends can be rejoined; reattainment of fertility occurs in fewer than 50% of cases after rejoining.

Female Reproductive System

The female reproductive system is designed for childbearing. The system consists of two ovaries, two fallopian tubes, a uterus, and a vagina. Also included in the system are the external genitalia and the mammary glands (Figure 12-17).

Internal Organs

The two ovaries are held in position, one on each side of the uterus, by several ligaments. The largest of these ligaments is called the *broad ligament;* it holds the ovaries in close proximity to the fallopian tubes.

The ovaries are solid glands that produce the hormones estrogen and progesterone. The cortex of the ovaries contains numerous small masses of cells called ovarian (graafian) follicles. Each follicle contains an ovum.

Each funnel-shaped fallopian tube is about 4 inches long and serves as a duct to transport the ovum to the uterus, or womb, a hollow, muscular organ in the shape of an inverted pear. It lies between the urinary bladder and the rectum. The upper part of the uterus is the fundus; the middle part is the corpus; the lower, narrow portion is the cervix, which opens into the vagina. The uterus receives the ovum and allows the embryo to grow and develop into a fetus. The inner lining is a soft, spongy layer, the endometrium, the surface of which is shed each month during menstruation. Uterine contractions at the end of the **gestation** period push the fetus into the vagina.

The vagina is a flexible, fibromuscular tube about $3\frac{1}{2}$ inches long that receives the sperm from the male and serves as the birth canal. The region between the vagina and anus is the clinical perineum and may tear during the birth process because of overstretching.

The vagina has a dual function: sexual intercourse and the delivery of a baby. Mucus in the vagina during nonsexual times comes from uterine glands. During sexual arousal Bartholin's glands secrete mucus into the vagina. During orgasm the muscular layer of the vagina contracts, moving semen into the cervix. Changes in the vaginal mucosa reflect cyclic endocrine changes that may be used to determine times of increased fertility.

External Organs

The external organs of the female reproductive system include the labia majora, labia minora, clitoris, mons pubis, vestibule, vaginal orifice, and Bartholin's (vestibular) glands. The aforementioned external genitalia are known collectively as the *vulva*. The mons pubis, located over the symphysis pubis, becomes covered with hair during puberty.

Each Bartholin's gland opens into the mucosal surface near the superior portion of the labia minora. The gland discharges a clear secretion during sexual arousal. Cysts and abscesses are common in these glands.

The mammary glands (breasts) are accessory organs that produce and secrete milk after pregnancy. They are included in the integument and are discussed in Chapter 11.

Beginning with puberty and for the next 35 to 40 years, the ovaries undergo cyclic changes in which a certain number of ovarian follicles develop. When one ovum completes the developmental process, it is released into one of the fallopian tubes. If fertilization does not occur, the developed ovum disintegrates and a new cycle begins.

A series of hormonal events takes place approximately every 28 days. Known as the menstrual cycle, day number 1 begins with the first day of uterine bleeding, called *menses* or *menstruation*. Cyclic hormonal changes occur in the pituitary, uterus, ovaries, and vagina. As in the male, FSH and LH from the pituitary gland affect the gonads. FSH stimulates the growth of the follicle containing the egg and the secretion of female hormones called *estrogens* and *progesterone*. The main estrogen is estradiol, responsible for female secondary sex characteristics, growth of the maturing follicle, growth of the uterine lining (endometrium), and negative feedback control of FSH. LH has two main functions: ovulation and formation of the corpus luteum (from the old follicle). The corpus luteum secretes estrogen and another group of hormones, the progestins. The main progestin, progesterone, is responsible for the secretory phase of the uterine cycle, glandular growth in the breast, and negative feedback control of LH.

In the female, as in the male, almost no gonadal hormones are formed before age 9 or 10. As the hypothalamus matures, gonadotropin-releasing hormone stimulates production of FSH and LH. In response, the ovaries produce estradiol and then progesterone. Breast buds and pubic hair appear at about age 11. The breasts grow, and axillary hair appears; the adrenal cortex is responsible for initial axillary and pubic hair growth in both sexes. The uterus and vagina enlarge. Uterine bleeding (the menarche) begins about 2 years after breast bud development and is often sporadic for several months. Ovulation takes place after the menarche.

As puberty progresses, the hips broaden, the forearms diverge more at the elbows, and scant body hair but much head hair are evident. The voice retains a high-pitched quality. Estradiol is not as anabolic as testosterone, so muscular development, bone size, and general body growth are not as great as in the male. Estrogens cause the skin to have a smooth texture. Prepubertal characteristics such as voice pitch, head hairline, sparse body hair (compared with that of the male), and distribution of body fat are retained and accentuated. Estradiol and testosterones are responsible for the female libido. In mammals, estrogens induce mating behavior, receptiveness of the female for the male, and nesting and maternal characteristics. As in the male, libido is influenced by cerebral control. Libido increases at ovulation and sometimes during menstruation.

At about the age of 40 or 50, a decrease in the responsiveness of the ovaries to FSH and LH occurs and is accompanied by irregular menstrual cycles. This is menopause. Although levels of estradiol and progesterone decrease, it is common for there to be little change in libido.

The autonomic nervous system exerts influence over the female reproductive system; as in the male, sexual arousal is a parasympathetic function, and orgasm is a sympathetic activation. Sympathetic deviances can interfere with ovulation and menstruation and thus are implicated in menstrual disorders and infertility.

Female Contraceptive Methods

In contrast to men, women have available a multitude of contraceptive methods. Tying or cauterizing the fallopian tubes, known as *tubal ligation*, is a permanent procedure. As with the vasectomy, even though the ends of the cut and tied fallopian tubes may be rejoined later, fertility decreases. Tubal ligation by cauterization is almost impossible to reverse. Currently used methods of birth control are the birth control pill, injections of hormones, implanted hormone-releasing devices, the intrauterine device, the diaphragm, spermicidal agents, abstinence, and the rhythm method. The most reliable methods are the pill, injections and implants, the condom plus a spermicidal agent, the intrauterine device, and the diaphragm with a spermicidal agent, in decreasing order of effectiveness. In some women, especially smokers older than 35, the pill contributes to venous thromboembolism. In others the pill may cause weight gain. The condom with a spermicidal agent has the added benefit of protection from some, but not all, sexually transmitted infections.

Pregnancy

Fertilization is the penetration of the egg by a sperm, restoring the diploid number (46) of chromosomes. Fertilization usually occurs as the egg moves down the fallopian tube. The ovum contains one X chromosome. A sperm contains an X or a Y chromosome, so the male determines the sex of the baby. If a male sperm (Y) reaches the egg, a male baby results; if a female sperm (X) reaches the egg, a female baby is produced. After the head of the sperm enters the egg, the tail detaches, and the ovum prohibits the entrance of other sperm. The chromosomes of egg and sperm nuclei arrange themselves at the two poles of the fertilized egg, and it begins to divide.

Gestation takes approximately 10 lunar months (9 calendar months) and is divided into trimesters.

First Trimester

Various physiologic changes occur during the first trimester, along with radical hormonal changes. The changes influence mood, digestion, sleep, and energy levels.

Early pregnancy is a different experience for each woman. Actual menstruation stops, but slight bleeding may occur throughout the first trimester, which is why some women often do not realize they are pregnant until about 3 months into the pregnancy. About 7 days after conception, implantation bleeding may occur. This bleeding is rare but normal; vaginal spotting is caused by the formation of new blood vessels. The urge to urinate occurs more frequently because the uterus begins to enlarge and press down on the bladder. Hormonal changes such as megabursts of progesterone result in the retention and release of more water.

Most women feel changes in their breasts. The breasts may swell, tingle, throb, or hurt because of the developing milk glands and the increased blood supply to the breasts. The veins become more pronounced and visible. The nipples enlarge and become more erect, and the areolae darken and become broader. Some women notice early on that their nipples feel sensitive and sore.

Fatigue is another major symptom at this stage. It begins after the first missed period and persists until the fourteenth to twentieth week of pregnancy. The need for sleep increases. About 10 hours of sleep per night is suggested during the first trimester.

Increased levels of progesterone also may cause the pregnant woman to feel faint and be constipated. The progesterone dilates the smooth muscle of the blood vessels and causes blood to pool in the legs, and more blood begins to flow to the uterus, which can cause low blood pressure and may result in fainting. Standing or sitting for long periods of time tends to trigger faintness. Lying flat and doing exercises that get the blood circulating prevent this.

Progesterone also relaxes the smooth muscles of the small and large intestines, slowing down the digestive process and leading to constipation. Lower back pain also occurs because the expanding uterus might put pressure on the sciatic nerve.

Between 60% and 80% of all women suffer nausea and vomiting in the first trimester. Discomfort that begins in the morning, often called *morning sickness,* can persist 24 hours a day for the first few weeks of pregnancy. Sometimes the nausea is not bad enough to cause vomiting but is an ever-present condition that can be controlled by eating dry crackers or juice.

Numerous other symptoms accompany morning sickness, including an aversion to certain tastes or smells. Changes in hormone levels somehow affect the stomach lining and stomach acids, causing the nausea. An empty stomach aggravates the nausea. Also, a strong connection exists between nausea and low blood sugar levels. Eating well is important during pregnancy. Some women require a vitamin supplement; some women must discontinue taking vitamin supplements to relieve or prevent other symptoms.

Fitness and exercise are important, but in moderation.

Second Trimester

In the second trimester the woman settles into the pregnant state, develops maternal feelings, and often has a general sense of well-being. Appetite increases, blood volume increases, and the body places additional workload on all physiologic functions.

Increased blood in the vaginal area causes more vaginal secretions and discharge. Progesterone depresses the central nervous system and may cause moodiness or depression. The hormones that slow down the intestinal tract also relax the sphincter between the stomach and esophagus, allowing stomach juices to flow up into the esophagus. Reflux of stomach juices into the esophagus causes a burning sensation in the middle of the chest that is called *heartburn.* As the uterus grows, it crowds the intestines, and heartburn may get much worse.

By week 15 the baby weighs almost 2 oz. The bones are growing, and the muscle movement is increasing. The pregnant woman probably does not feel the baby moving yet, and the first movements feel like flutters. A soft, fine hair called *lanugo* covers the baby. The neck of the baby becomes longer, and the head can move. The arms move freely in front of the body, and the hands can grasp each other. Ultrasound has picked up babies actually sucking their thumbs by this time.

Table 12-7 provides an approximation of weight distribution during pregnancy. This distribution varies with each mother and increases with twins, triplets, and quadruplets. With multiple babies, the weight of each baby is lower.

The amount of blood circulating throughout the body, especially in the areas of the vagina and rectum, continues to increase. New vessels form, but they are not strong and often bulge or swell in the vaginal area, rectum, and legs, and varicose veins may form around the labia, vagina, and legs.

Table 12-7 Weight Gain during Pregnancy	
Area of Gain	**Amount of Gain**
Mother (at Term)	
Uterus	2-3 lb
Breasts	1-3 lb
Blood volume	3-5 lb
Body fluid	1-3 lb
Fat, protein, etc.	5-8 lb
Baby (at 9 Months)	
Baby	7-8 lb
Amniotic fluid	2-2½ lb
Placenta	1-1½ lb
Total	**22-32 lb**

When the vessels in the rectum swell, hemorrhoids develop and may protrude out of the rectum with strenuous bowel movements.

By 21 weeks the baby weighs almost 1 lb and is nearly 10 to 11 inches long. Every system is progressing in development. The primitive structures of the brain have been developed for some time. Now the fine details of the nerve pathways in the brain are forming. Nerve cells that allow the baby's brain to receive and transmit messages are forming layers in the brain. This process continues at a much slower rate for another 3 months.

The baby is able to hear sounds from outside of the body and is aware of the constant rhythm created by the mother's beating heart as well as the swishing and gurgling of fluids inside her body. The baby's eyes remain fused shut. By the end of week 21, the layers of the retina have developed and the skin is forming a white coating called *vernix caseosa,* a fatty film that protects the baby's skin from breakdown in the amniotic fluid. Vernix also prevents the loss of water and electrolytes from the baby into the amniotic fluid. The permanent ridges that form the fingers, hands, and feet are now developed, and the fingernails and toenails are getting harder.

The baby is swallowing more than 2 tsp of amniotic fluid per day, and by the end of the pregnancy may be swallowing nearly 2 cups of amniotic fluid per day. The digestive system has developed, and the digestive processes are beginning. Stool called *meconium* forms in the bowel. The air sacs in the lungs, called *alveoli,* are beginning to emerge.

In the pregnant woman the progesterone that has slowed the digestive system affects the gallbladder in much the same way. The gallbladder takes a longer time to empty, allowing bile salts to accumulate in the system and absorb through the skin. This causes significant itching that is particularly noticeable around the navel, entire belly, chest, neck, face, and sometimes hands.

The growing uterus and baby put a lot of pressure on the two main blood vessels that lead into and out of the heart, the vena cava and the aorta. Pressure occurs when lying flat on the back. The side-lying position is best.

As the pregnancy progresses, the capillaries become more permeable and have a tendency to leak water. When the capillaries leak water, the result is an increase in water retention, or edema. Some edema is normal in pregnancy, but edema that increases all over the body, particularly in the legs, arms, lower back, and face, could indicate a serious problem requiring immediate referral to a physician.

Following are suggestions and cautions to ease the discomforts of swelling:

- Drink plenty of fluids to stimulate the kidneys.
- Avoid tight-fitting clothing, especially socks, hose, pant legs, and waistbands.
- Avoid standing or sitting in one place for long periods of time.
- Rest with the legs elevated on a chair or pillow.
- Lie down on the left side to increase kidney function.
- Increase protein intake to pull the fluid back into the vessels.

- Exercise such as walking and swimming increases circulation and lymphatic movement of water back into the vessels.
- Do not take diuretics for water retention in pregnancy.

The renal system changes in pregnant women. The kidneys produce more urine, and the bladder has decreased tone. The same progesterone that alters other systems influences the urinary system and makes it less efficient. As a result, many pregnant women have a tendency to develop urinary tract infections, which can become serious and cause not only pain and discomfort but also preterm labor. If untreated, a mild urinary tract infection can lead to a serious bladder or kidney infection that could require hospitalization and treatment with intravenous antibiotics.

At the end of the second trimester, the baby is at a milestone in development. The eyes are no longer fused shut; the fine details of optic nerve development, peripheral vision, and focus are present. Hearing has completely developed. The brain is functioning at a higher level, as are all of the baby's senses: sight, hearing, taste, touch, and smell. The baby has developed a schedule of sorts, moving while awake and being still while asleep. An early sucking reflex is present, although the ability to suck and swallow will not be present until about 34 weeks. The baby is also practicing the motions needed for breathing.

Third Trimester

The last trimester finds the mother-to-be heavy with the baby, and postural changes are evident. Internal organs are crowded. Physiologic systems are strained by the need to sustain mother and baby. The mother's connective tissue structure softens to permit the expansion needed for the birth. This is a time of rest and waiting (Figure 12-18).

The third trimester begins after about 26 weeks of pregnancy. During these last 3 months, the baby continues to grow and develop. Although a baby might survive if born during the early to middle part of the last trimester, these months are critical to the development of organs such as the lungs and the brain.

The baby is now about 15 inches long and weighs around 3 pounds. The baby may suck the thumb, hiccup, and respond to stimuli such as light, pain, and sounds.

The mother's lower abdomen may hurt from time to time, and she may have an occasional brief contraction in which the uterus hardens and then returns to normal. Vaginal discharge may become heavier, and the mother may feel breathless for no apparent reason and have difficulty sleeping. Colostrum, the early form of milk, may leak from the breasts, and the mother may feel apprehensive or excited about the coming labor and delivery.

By the eighth month the baby has grown to about 18 inches and weighs approximately 5 lb. He or she can see and hear. The lungs are still immature, but many other organs are well developed. Brain growth is especially rapid during this time. At some point during the eighth month, the baby shifts into a position he or she will maintain until birth.

By 36 weeks the baby is about 20 inches long, weighs 6 to 7 lb, and will gain about ½ lb a week until delivery. The baby's

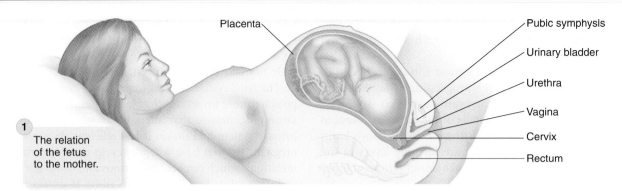

Placenta
Pubic symphysis
Urinary bladder
Urethra
Vagina
Cervix
Rectum

1 The relation of the fetus to the mother.

FIGURE 12-18 Fetus in utero. (From Thibodeau GA, Patton KT: *Structure and function of the body*, ed 14, St Louis, 2012, Mosby.)

lungs are mature. Movement often slows down because of the cramped space and head-down position in the pelvis.

The pregnant woman's backache and heaviness increase, the abdomen may itch, and the pelvis may be uncomfortable. After the baby drops, breathing and eating become easier, but urinary urge increases. Uterine contractions may increase and feel more intense.

Birth

The exact stimulus for birth is unknown, but increased fetal activity seems to play a role. Oxytocin stimulates contraction of the uterus, causes delivery of the placenta after expulsion of the fetus, and promotes parental bonding with the baby.

Prelabor

Prelabor can begin any time during the last few weeks or last days of pregnancy. The mother also may get diarrhea and possibly a severe backache, both precursors to early labor. The diarrhea empties the intestinal tract before actual labor begins, and painless Braxton Hicks contractions may begin to be more frequent.

At this stage the cervix softens and may start to thin out a little, which allows it to dilate slightly. The woman experiences some mucous, bloody discharge called *bloody show,* which means that the mucus plug sealing the cervical opening is now pink, or blood-streaked, and is leaking discharge.

As the baby's head presses down against the amniotic membranes containing fluid, the membranes may break in what is known as "breaking the water," the classic prelabor symptom. Women expect this event to be like a flood of water suddenly rushing out of their vaginas, and it commonly happens that way, but the fluid also may just trickle out. The fluid normally is clear and odorless. Some women think that they have wet their pants when this happens. If the water has not broken at this point, it probably will during more active labor.

Early Labor

Prelabor slowly unfolds into early labor. This phase lasts about 7 or 8 hours. Early labor and active labor also are known as the first stage of labor. Early labor is characterized by contractions that cause the cervix to dilate 3 to 4 cm. These contractions can feel wavelike. They build up and then recede. They are mildly intense and begin in the lower back.

They also can feel like heavy menstrual cramps. The contractions occur between 5 and 20 minutes apart, become more intense each time they occur, last anywhere from 30 to 45 seconds, get longer each time they occur, and occur more closely together.

Active Labor

Active labor is similar to early labor but is far more pronounced. This phase lasts from 3 to 5 hours. Now the contractions occur every 2 to 4 minutes and last as long as 60 seconds. They may be moderately or extremely painful, depending on the woman. The physician could administer an epidural, a painkiller that numbs from the breasts down, at this point. In natural childbirth this type of procedure is not used. Whether or not she receives an epidural, the mother will have a very strong urge to push, much like the urge to push during a bowel movement. The mother also may start to feel warm or get chills.

Transition Phase

The transition phase proceeds to delivery and lasts anywhere from 30 to 90 minutes. Active labor has been in progress for approximately 3 hours. The mother is likely tired and frustrated; may have no idea what time it is; may be shaking, hiccupping, vomiting, or having chills; may have cold feet and dry mouth and lips; and may be hyperventilating, moaning, crying, or screaming. She has a tremendous urge to push and experiences rectal pressure. Contractions are intense, occurring every 30 seconds and lasting 90 seconds. The cervix is almost fully dilated. Some women may want to use the bathroom, which will help them to relax and encourage pushing.

Delivery: Bearing Down

Instead of holding back the urge to push, the woman actually gets to push. At this phase the hardest part is pushing out the head. As the head emerges, the woman may feel intense burning and stinging sensations. The vagina is like a huge elastic band that stretches for this event.

Episiotomy

An episiotomy is a minor surgical procedure in which the physician makes an incision in the perineum, the area between the rectum and vagina. The episiotomy enlarges the opening for vaginal births, making it easier for the baby's head to come out.

A routine episiotomy cuts through skin, vaginal mucosa, and three layers of muscle in an otherwise sensitive area. The side effects include pain, bleeding, a breakdown of stitches, and delayed healing. Many doctors believe that a little natural tearing, which often takes place without the episiotomy, not only heals much more quickly than a surgical procedure but is less painful.

Any medical emergency during delivery can be a reason for an episiotomy. For example, an episiotomy might be deemed necessary when the baby's heartbeat becomes abnormal during pushing, when delivery must be facilitated because the baby is premature or breech, and whenever forceps are necessary (e.g., if the head is in an awkward position). The procedure is also necessary when the delivery of the baby's head is progressing at a rate or manner that will badly tear the perineum or when the vagina is not stretching. But for the majority of normal, vaginal deliveries, episiotomy is not necessary.

Cesarean Birth

A cesarean section, or C-section, is a surgical procedure that is essentially an abdominal delivery. Cesarean section is considered major pelvic surgery that usually involves a spinal or epidural anesthetic (only in some cases is a general anesthetic necessary). The surgeon makes a vertical or horizontal incision just above the pubic hair and then (usually) cuts horizontally through the uterine muscle and eases the baby out. Sometimes this second cut is vertical, known as the "classic incision." The second cut, into the uterine muscle, affects the viability of a vaginal birth after a prior cesarean delivery. With a horizontal cut, women have gone on to have normal second vaginal births.

In some instances, the pregnant woman knows in advance that she will have a cesarean section. The pelvis may be too small; or the cervix may have irreparable scarring, because of previous pelvic surgery, that prevents dilation; or an emergency situation may be detected in utero (in the womb) that requires immediate removal of the fetus. In these cases, the problem usually does not appear until labor.

Placenta

The placenta is known as the *afterbirth, birth of placenta,* or just the *third stage of labor.* In a vaginal delivery, whether or not an episiotomy has been performed, the uterus contracts enough to loosen the placenta from the uterine wall after the birth of the baby. These contractions may be painful, but they are mild compared with the previous contractions. The placenta then slips out with one or two pushes. The uterus then continues to contract against exposed blood vessels where the placenta used to be as a natural way to control bleeding.

Hormones secreted by the placenta, including chorionic gonadotropin and other substances having estrogenic, progestational, or adrenocorticoid activity, play important roles during pregnancy. Parental bonding with the infant immediately after birth is important. The touch, sound, and smell of parents and infant in the first hours of birth establish biologic and emotional bonds. The hormone oxytocin seems to play a role in this bonding process for both mothers and fathers.

Lactation

The main physiologic function of the mammary glands is to provide proper nutrition for the baby, as well as to protect the infant from infections during the first few months of life by transferring antibodies from mother to baby. The breasts enlarge substantially after the second month of pregnancy because of increased amounts of estrogens and progesterone. Prolactin causes the production and secretion of milk. The actual ejection (letdown) of milk from the nipple requires suckling and the release of oxytocin from the posterior pituitary gland. The cry of the infant, and in some cases emotional responses, may cause oxytocin release and lactation. Because milk production is based on demand, lactation persists for months, even years, if suckling continues. The breasts secrete a yellow fluid, colostrum, during the last part of pregnancy and for the first day or two after delivery. Colostrum has a high protein content and contains antibodies. The breasts start to secrete milk 1 to 3 days after delivery (Figure 12-19).

Practical Application

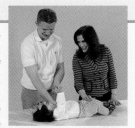

Massage therapy can be supportive during pregnancy, labor, delivery, lactation, and the eventual return of the body to a nonpregnant state. Massage can even support conception by creating relaxation in the body. During the pregnancy the main goal is stress management, sleep support, and management of some of the muscular and skeletal discomforts of pregnancy.

Pathologic Conditions of the Reproductive System
Abnormal Pregnancy
Bleeding

Not all bleeding means that a miscarriage is imminent. Nevertheless, although some bleeding during early pregnancy is fairly common, it is still not normal. A woman with bleeding that requires heavy-duty pads that need to be changed frequently should report the condition immediately. Other signs and symptoms, including cramps, pain in the abdomen, fever, weakness, and possibly vomiting, are serious. The blood may have clumps of tissue in it and have an unusual odor. Another kind of bleeding is brown, intermittent or continuous vaginal spotting or light bleeding accompanied by severe abdominal or shoulder pain. Finally, light bleeding that continues for more than 3 days may also indicate an intrauterine problem requiring evaluation.

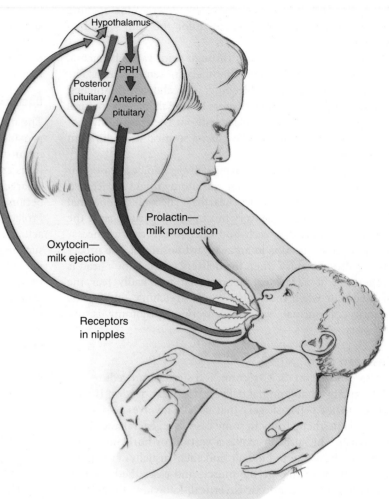

Hypothalamus

PRH

Posterior
pituitary   Anterior
pituitary

Prolactin—
milk production

Oxytocin—
milk ejection

Receptors
in nipples

FIGURE 12-19 Stimulus for lactation. (From Applegate E: *The anatomy and physiology learning system,* ed 4, Philadelphia, 2011, Saunders.)

PRH = Prolactin releasing hormone

Miscarriage

Heavy bleeding and cramping at any time between the end of the second month to the end of the third month are classic signs of miscarriage. Cramps without any bleeding are also a danger sign of miscarriage. The bleeding may be heavy enough to soak several pads in an hour, or it may be manageable and more like a heavy period. Cramping may occur with passing clots, which are dark red clumps that look like small pieces of raw beef liver. Sometimes grayish or pinkish tissue is passed. A miscarriage also can take place with persistent, light bleeding and milder cramping at this stage.

Several kinds of spontaneous abortions can occur:

Threatened abortion: The cervix still is closed, but the woman has cramps, bleeding, or staining. The doctor performs a physical examination, checks the fetal heartbeat, and may prescribe bed rest. In some cases the bleeding stops, and the pregnancy continues normally.

Inevitable abortion: In this case, nature has taken its course already and the process of miscarriage has started. Bleeding is heavy, cramps increase, and the cervix begins to dilate, expelling everything still intact: the fetus, amniotic sac, and placenta, accompanied by a great deal of blood.

Incomplete abortion: In this condition the uterus has spontaneously expelled some, but not all, pregnancy tissue. Usually what remains are fragments of the placenta. The condition is correctable with a dilation and curettage procedure to clean out the uterus and help it heal.

Complete abortion: Complete abortion occurs when all pregnancy tissue passes spontaneously. Although dilation and curettage may be indicated, the procedure usually is not necessary.

Missed abortion: The fetus dies in the uterus but is not expelled. Symptoms that something is wrong may not be apparent. Instead, all of the pregnancy symptoms gradually disappear. It is common for the physician to diagnose missed abortion during a routine examination when the fetal heartbeat is no longer audible. Treatment depends on the duration of the pregnancy.

The reason for miscarriage usually has to do with a fetus self-terminating because of improper development or genetic problems.

Ectopic Pregnancy

An ectopic pregnancy occurs when the fetus fails to implant itself in the uterus and starts to develop in the fallopian tube. Ectopic pregnancies are dangerous. Rupture of the tube could be a life-threatening situation. The classic symptoms of ectopic pregnancy are sharp abdominal cramps or pains on one side. The pains may start out as dull aches that get more severe. Neck pains and shoulder pains are also common. The woman also may experience a menstrual type of bleeding along with the pain, but the pain is the most obvious sign. The problem with an ectopic pregnancy is that a woman may not realize she is pregnant.

Women in groups at high risk for ectopic pregnancy generally have the following characteristics:
- They are users of intrauterine devices.
- They have histories of pelvic inflammatory disease.
- They have histories of pelvic surgery resulting in scarring that may block the tube and prevent the fertilized egg from traveling to the uterus.
- They have histories of ectopic pregnancies.
- Their pregnancies result from assisted contraception techniques in which gametes or embryos have been injected into the fallopian tubes.

Preeclampsia, Toxemia, and Pregnancy-Induced Hypertension

Preeclampsia is a disease that occurs only during pregnancy. The terms *preeclampsia, pregnancy-induced hypertension,* and *toxemia* are essentially interchangeable. The complications of preeclampsia are swelling, high blood pressure, poor kidney function, poor liver function, pulmonary edema, the presence of protein in the urine, and possible seizure. A poor blood supply to the baby decreases the baby's nutrients, interfering with development. Preeclampsia occurs in 5% to 10% of all pregnancies and can appear without warning at any time during pregnancy or labor or in the early postpartum period. This disease also can be chronic, gradually becoming worse over time. Preeclampsia may be mild or severe, but the only cure is delivery of the baby.

Hyperemesis Gravidarum

Hyperemesis gravidarum is severe nausea and vomiting during pregnancy that results in dehydration and the loss of at least 10 lb. Women in this state may be unable to eat or drink anything for days. They may require intravenous hydration and may have abnormalities in blood chemical levels. Hyperemesis gravidarum is exhausting and emotionally distressing but usually has no effect on the developing fetus.

Bartholin's Cyst

Bartholin's glands are located on each side of the vaginal opening. Obstruction of a duct sometimes occurs because of a bacterial infection that makes the area painful and swollen. Treatment may require drainage.

Breast Lumps

Most breast lumps are not cancerous, although the incidence of cancer increases with age (see Chapter 11). However, clients should be referred to their physician for evaluation of any new lumps or masses, either in the axillae or breasts.

Cervical Cancer

Cervical cancer is the third most common malignancy in women, after breast and colon cancer. Cervical dysplasia is a change in the cells of the cervix. Some of these abnormal cells can develop into cancerous cells. Early detection and treatment by removing or destroying the cells may prevent cancer. Factors contributing to the development of cervical cancer are as follows: becoming sexually active at an early age; having multiple sexual partners; having genital herpes; and, possibly, previous infection with human papillomavirus (HPV). Cervical cancer that is not treated in the early stages can spread into other tissues, especially lymph nodes and the uterus. Vaccines are now available that may prevent infection with various strains of HPV and prevent some forms of cervical cancer.

Cervicitis

Cervicitis is inflammation of the cervix. Acute cervicitis usually is caused by the same organisms that cause vaginitis (fungus, bacteria, or protozoa). Symptoms vary and may include redness, bleeding, pelvic pain, and discharge.

Chronic cervicitis is a recurrent inflammation of the cervix, commonly causing pelvic pain, often with a heavy discharge. Treatment of cervicitis is medication if it is caused by organisms or cauterization if the condition becomes chronic.

Endometriosis

Endometriosis is a disease in which endometrial tissue is present in nonuterine locations, such as on the intestines or ovaries or even in the fallopian tubes. Endometriosis occurs most often in women between the ages of 25 and 50, especially if they have borne no children. Although symptoms may be mild, common symptoms are heavy menstrual periods, intense back or pelvic pain, painful menstruation (dysmenorrhea), and painful intercourse (dyspareunia). Pregnancy often eliminates the problem. Birth control pills may help because they cause a change in the endometrial tissue. Sometimes surgical intervention is necessary.

Infertility

Infertility is a decrease in the ability to conceive, whereas sterility is a total loss of the ability to conceive. Infertility may be temporary and can result from structural or functional problems in the man, the woman, or both. Common causes in men are impotence (the inability to have an erection), a decrease in sperm number, or abnormalities in sperm anatomy and motility. In women common causes include lack of ovulation; disorders of the fallopian tubes (often the result of a previous infection); and abnormal mucus secretion by the cervix, which creates an environment hostile to sperm. A low sperm count may be caused by excessive use of alcohol, tobacco, and caffeine; poor nutrition; and fatigue. Men should not wear tight underwear because it pulls the testes close to the body, increasing the temperature and decreasing the sperm count. Clomiphene citrate is sometimes effective in inducing ovulation in

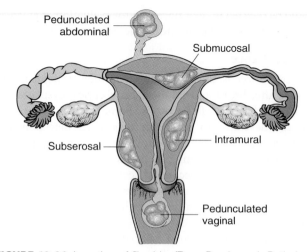

FIGURE 12-20 Location of fibroids. (From Damjanov I: *Pathology for health professions,* ed 3, St Louis, 2006, Saunders.)

women. Surgery may help to correct tubal scarring. The administration of estrogen may restore normal cervical mucus. Generalized stress can be a cause of infertility.

Uterine Disorders

A myoma, or fibroid, is a benign tumor in the uterus that grows inside the uterine muscle wall or attaches to the wall (Figure 12-20). This tumor may be small, grow slowly, and cause no symptoms. Tumors that grow large or rapidly cause heavy bleeding. If blood loss is extensive, anemia may occur. Fibroids are the most common disorder of the uterus. Occurring in late reproductive years, these tumors are estrogen-dependent. Prolonged or abnormal menstrual bleeding is usually the first sign. Treatment may be dietary for the anemia. In the rare cases in which the tumor grows large enough to cause severe bleeding, a hysterectomy is required.

Polyps are small growths of the endometrium extending into the body of the uterus. They are common in all age groups, especially in women with no children. The main symptom is increased menstrual bleeding between periods or postmenopausal bleeding. Removal of the polyps by a uterine curet (curettage) is indicated if symptoms are problematic. Cervical polyps occur when the lining of the cervix develops growths that hang outside the cervix.

Dysfunctional uterine bleeding is abnormal bleeding throughout much of the 28-day cycle. The main form of diagnosis and treatment is dilation and curettage.

Vaginitis

Vaginitis is inflammation of the vagina. Signs and symptoms are vaginal discharge, itching (pruritus), and irritation. A foul odor or itching or a yellow or green discharge may indicate a vaginal infection. A curdlike white discharge with itching probably indicates a yeast infection, which is treatable. A foul-smelling discharge or one that is yellow or green could indicate a more serious infection.

Yeast vaginitis (candidiasis, moniliasis) is a common infection caused by the fungus *Candida albicans.* The infection

responds to an antifungal ointment such as miconazole (Monistat) or nystatin or tablets of fluconazole (Diflucan).

Trichomonas vaginitis (trichomoniasis) is caused by a protozoal parasite that may infect the urinary tract of both sexes and is a sexually transmitted organism. Metronidazole (Flagyl) is effective. The sexual partner also may require treatment.

Vaginitis caused by species of the *Gardnerella* genus (formerly called *Haemophilus*) is a bacterial infection of the vagina. It responds to metronidazole or clindamycin.

Prostate Disorders

Prostatitis is an infection of the prostate, usually resulting from a urinary tract infection. Perineal pain, fever, chills, painful urination, and a tender prostate on rectal examination are common signs. If bacteria are causing the prostatitis, treatment with an antibiotic is indicated. Chronic prostatitis commonly occurs in older men with enlarged prostate glands.

Benign prostatic hypertrophy is the enlargement of the prostate, a disorder that occurs in males 45 years and older; it may be caused by a decrease in the ratio of testosterone to estrogen. As testosterone declines, estrogen produced by the adrenal cortex seems to stimulate the central portion of the prostate, causing an overgrowth of prostate tissue. The amount of the enlargement is not as important as its ability to compress the urethra, which causes problems with urination, such as straining, dribbling, and sometimes urinary retention. Medical treatment, including catheterization and surgery, is indicated in the most severe cases. The herb saw palmetto has been shown to be beneficial in decreasing hypertrophy.

Prostatic cancer is the most common malignancy in men after skin cancer. It grows slowly, is commonly asymptomatic, and is usually found during a physical checkup. Early-stage cancer is usually slow growing, whereas in later stages metastasis to bone commonly occurs, particularly in the thoracic and lumbar vertebrae and the sacrum. Symptoms include urinary retention if obstruction has taken place and lower back pain if metastasis has occurred. Primary treatment depends on the age of the person and stage of the cancer; it may focus on relieving symptoms or removing the cancer by prostatectomy, radiation therapy, or removal of the testes because testosterone stimulates cancer cells.

Sexually Transmitted Infections

Sexually transmitted infections include vaginal infections, hepatitis B infection, nongonococcal urethritis or chlamydia, genital warts, herpes genitalis, acquired immunodeficiency syndrome, gonorrhea, syphilis, and body lice. Most of these diseases have been discussed elsewhere in the text.

Gonorrhea is an infectious disease caused by a bacterium. It is becoming more resistant to antibiotics because mutant strains have developed. Gonorrhea infects the urethra of both sexes, producing urethritis several days after exposure. The person may show no signs or mild symptoms, which the person ignores while the bacteria spread.

In men, gonorrhea affects primarily the urethra, where it can cause scarring. If untreated, the bacteria can infect and inflame the prostate or the epididymis. Symptoms include difficult urination and a cloudy discharge.

In women, gonorrhea usually infects the cervix, causing cervicitis. Untreated gonorrhea may infect the uterus or fallopian tubes, causing scarring that may result in infertility. Involvement of the tubes and surrounding pelvic area is called *pelvic inflammatory disease.* If gonorrhea travels to the abdominal cavity, it can cause peritonitis. Signs and symptoms of gonorrhea in women include fever, abnormal bleeding, cloudy vaginal discharge, bilateral pelvic pain (usually during the menses), and tenderness on movement of the cervix (stretching the broad ligament).

Untreated gonorrhea in both sexes can infect the bloodstream, causing blood poisoning, and can spread to the skin, bones, joints, and tendons.

Syphilis is a bacterial infection transmitted sexually or from mother to fetus. The frequency of infections declined with the discovery of penicillin but, as with gonorrhea, resistant strains are appearing. Syphilis appears in three stages:

Stage 1: Painless sores appear on the skin and are treated primarily with antibiotics.

Stage 2: A skin rash, which may be helped by antibiotics (stages 1 and 2 are highly contagious), appears.

Stage 3: Referred to as *late syphilis,* stage 3 is not as contagious, except when blood is exchanged between two persons. If the person does not recognize the symptoms of stages 1 or 2, the third stage can flare at any time and affect the brain, nervous system, aorta, and other organs of the body. Syphilis cannot be reversed in the third stage.

Herpes simplex is a virus that causes painful blisters and small ulcers in and around the mouth and the genital area. Type 1 usually infects the upper body, and type 2 affects the genital area. Type 2 is a common sexually transmitted disease. The primary infection lasts about 1 to 4 weeks.

Recurrent lesions are less painful and debilitating, often emerging every month or two and lasting 7 to 10 days. The blisters form and then break open, remaining open for 2 to 3 weeks. The open blisters are painful. Herpes is transmitted when it is active—that is, when the lesions are present and up to 7 days afterwards. Lesions recur in some affected persons. In others, recurrence takes place once or twice and never again.

Fever, emotional stress, the menses, sunlight, infections, and trauma may activate herpes lesions. Genital lesions in women consist of painful vesicles and erosions on the labia, vagina, or cervix. In men the lesions are commonly located on the penis. The antiviral drug acyclovir (Zovirax) is effective.

SUMMARY

On completion of the last set of justification exercises, you, the student, should be familiar with a logical model of reasoning that honors intuition as well as the emotions and perceptions of the persons involved. As with all knowledge, you must question the process, make it your own, and improve it. This model is only a framework; however, the model helps you become more objective and addresses questions and issues that you may not think of on your own. It is good to consider various perspectives and then make your own best decisions.

The respiratory, digestive, urinary, and reproductive systems contribute to the complete function of the body as a whole. These systems concern the movement of energy, water, and air and the creation of new life inside and outside of the body. They reveal the interconnectedness involved in being alive and, with these systems, the need for interaction outside of yourself as you breathe in air, take in food and water, and connect with another to produce life.

INDICATIONS / CONTRAINDICATIONS for Therapeutic Massage

Reproductive System

As with all acute infections, massage is contraindicated until any infectious diseases of the reproductive system have run their course. Massage in clients with malignancies is contraindicated unless the appropriate health care professional provides approval and supervision. Therapeutic massage during a normal pregnancy is part of a wellness program, with accommodation for the changes in the pregnant woman. The practitioner should obtain permission from the supervising health care professional. Certainly, anyone working with pregnant women regularly should learn more about pregnancy and fetal development than is provided in this text. Most reproductive-system conditions present regional contraindications. As with most chronic illness and pain, therapeutic massage offers generalized support for homeostasis and can offer palliative or comfort care for the maintenance of these conditions (Activity 12-1).

@volve

http://evolve.elsevier.com/Fritz/essential
Activity 12-1 Read a case study about an asthmatic client and answer a few follow-up questions.
Activity 12-2 Drag-and-drop labeling exercises on the Evolve site help you review the structures of the systems of the body discussed in this chapter.
Activity 12-3 Reinforce your knowledge of the system structures by playing a Tetris game on Evolve.
Additional Resources:
Scientific animations and Electronic Coloring Book Weblinks
Remember to study for your certification and licensure exams! Review questions for this chapter are located on Evolve.

Evolve Activity 12-2

Evolve Activity 12-3

✏ ACTIVITY 12-1

We must be able to explain and justify the therapeutic value of the work we do. The following activity will assist you in developing the skills to explain the effectiveness of therapeutic massage to clients and other health care professionals. Use the clinical reasoning model that follows to accomplish this task. The focus should be the primary modality or modalities applied to the reproductive system.

Methods/Applications

1. What are the facts?
   a. Which system is involved, and which structures of that system can be reached directly or indirectly?
   b. Which of these structures are most affected by this massage?
   c. Which physiologic functions are affected by this approach?
   d. When the treatment is applied, what changes in function will occur in:
      (1) this system?
      (2) the whole body?
   e. What is considered normal or balanced function?
   f. How are the functions of this system related to the homeostasis of the body?
   g. What has worked or has not worked?
   h. Where could you find information that would support the use of this modality as a therapeutic intervention?
   i. What research is available to support the use of the therapeutic intervention?
   j. How does the intervention support a healthy state?
   k. Under which pathologic or dysfunctional conditions is the therapeutic massage most likely to be beneficial?
2. What are the possibilities?
   a. What do the data suggest?
   b. What are the reasons for using the proposed method?
   c. What are the possible interventions?
   d. List at least three applications of massage that would affect the structure and function of the system involved.

   e. What are other ways to look at the situation?
   f. What other methods could provide similar benefits?
3. What is the logical outcome of therapeutic intervention?
   a. What would be the logical progression of the symptom pattern, contributing factors, and current behaviors?
   b. What are the benefits and drawbacks of each intervention suggested?
      Benefits:
      Drawbacks:
   c. What are the costs in terms of time, resources, and finances?
   d. What is likely to happen if the modality is not used?
   e. What is likely to happen if the modality is used?
4. For the intervention proposed, what would be the effect on the persons involved, specifically the client, practitioner, and other professionals working with the client?
   a. How does each person involved (including, besides the aforementioned, the client's family and support system) feel about the possible interventions?
   b. Does the practitioner feel qualified to work with the situation and apply the identified modality to the particular person?
   c. Does a feeling of cooperation and agreement exist among all those involved, and how would the practitioner recognize this feeling?

Justification

Using the information developed in the clinical reasoning model, present a clear, concise statement of how the ways in which the particular soft-tissue or movement modality would be beneficial in supporting the particular body system in a healthy condition or as part of a treatment plan for a pathologic or dysfunctional condition. On the basis of the preceding information, give a brief summary of the effectiveness of the modality for this system.

Workbook Section

Short Answer

1. What are the parts of the upper and lower respiratory tract?
   _____
   _____
   _____
   _____
   _____

2. How does the nose affect the breathing pattern when we sleep?
   _____
   _____
   _____
   _____
   _____
   _____
   _____

3. What happens in our bodies to prevent food from going into our lungs while we are swallowing?
   _____
   _____
   _____
   _____
   _____
   _____
   _____
   _____

4. How does the diaphragm work to help us breathe?
   _____
   _____
   _____
   _____
   _____
   _____
   _____
   _____

5. Describe the mechanics of relaxed breathing.
   _____
   _____
   _____
   _____
   _____
   _____
   _____

6. What is a normal respiratory rate, and how can it be affected?
   _____
   _____
   _____
   _____
   _____
   _____

7. Where does digestion begin and end?
   _____
   _____
   _____
   _____

8. List the organs of digestion.
   _____
   _____
   _____

9. What are the steps in digestion, and what does each involve?
   _____
   _____
   _____
   _____
   _____
   _____
   _____
   _____
   _____

10. What are the main food groups, and why is each important? Give two examples of each.
    _____
    _____
    _____
    _____
    _____
    _____
    _____
    _____

11. What are the organs of the urinary system, and where are they located?
    _____
    _____
    _____
    _____
    _____
    _____
    _____

12. How much urine does the average person produce per day?

_____

_____

_____

13. What are the parts of the male reproductive system?

_____

_____

_____

14. What are the parts of the female reproductive system?

_____

_____

_____

_____

_____

_____

15. What are the divisions of the gestational period in the human being, and what are the primary features of each period?

_____

_____

_____

_____

_____

_____

Fill in the Blank

(1) _____ is the movement of air in and out of the lungs, the exchange of oxygen and carbon dioxide between the lungs and blood, and the exchange between blood and body tissues.

(2) _____ is the exchange of oxygen and carbon dioxide between the lungs and the bloodstream.

The lower two thirds of the (3) _____ is composed mostly of cartilage. The upper third, or bridge of the nose, is formed of two small hard nasal bones. The tip of the nose is the apex, and the nostrils are the (4) _____.

The (5) _____ is the actual space inside the external and internal nose structures. It is separated into left and right sides by the septum, a partition composed of cartilage and bone. At the upper portion of the nasal cavity, three thin, curled bones, the (6) _____, or conchae, project inward from the two outer walls.

Venous areas called (7) _____ are located on the turbinates.

The (8) _____ are four groups of air-filled spaces that open into the frontal, ethmoid, sphenoid, and maxillary bones of the skull. The (9) _____ is the continuation of the nasal cavity into the throat, or pharynx. The (10) _____, or voice box, connects the

pharynx to the trachea. Its structure consists of cartilage, ligaments, connective tissue, muscles, and the vocal cords. The vocal cords and the spaces between the cords are located inside the _____ (11).

The (12) _____, or windpipe, is the main airway to the lungs. It is a 4- to 5-inch tube that begins at the glottis and ends at the junction of the two main bronchi near the level of the sternal angle.

The two (13) _____ are the primary organs of respiration. These soft, spongy, highly vascular structures are separated into the left and right lungs by the mediastinum. The (14) _____ is a dome-shaped sheet of muscle attached to the thoracic wall that separates the lungs and thoracic cavity from the abdominal cavity.

The (15) _____, or chest cavity, is the upper region of the torso enclosed by the sternum, ribs, and thoracic vertebrae. It contains the lungs, heart, and great vessels.

The (16) _____, or (17) _____, contains the major organs of digestion. The cavity is lined with a mucous membrane, the (18) _____, the function of which is to prevent friction.

Products of digestion are propelled along the tract from the esophagus to the anus by the rhythmic contraction of smooth muscle called (19) _____. The term *digestive secretion* generally refers to the release of various substances from the (20) _____ that serve the digestive system. Digestive secretion includes the release of saliva, gastric juice, pancreatic juice, bile, and intestinal juice.

The citric acid cycle is the main pathway by which food energy is released by cells to manufacture their own energy-rich (21) _____

(22) _____ is a constituent of all living things. The water content of the tissues of the body varies. Adipose tissue (fat) has the lowest percentage of water; the (23) _____ has the second lowest water content.

The testicles contain tiny seminiferous tubules that produce (24) _____. The (25) _____ gland surrounds the urethra and produces a milky alkaline fluid.

The (26) _____ are solid glands that produce the hormones estrogen and progesterone. The external female genitalia are known collectively as the (27) _____.

Gestation takes approximately 10 lunar months (9 calendar months) and is divided into (28) _____. The hormone (29) _____ stimulates contraction of the uterus. Prelabor can begin any time in the last few weeks or last days of pregnancy. The (30) _____ at this stage softens and may start to thin out a little, which allows it to dilate (open up) slightly. As the baby's head presses down against the amniotic membranes containing fluid, the membranes may break, producing what is known as (31) _____. This is the classic prelabor symptom.

Exercise

In the illustration of the digestive system below, write the name of each part of the system next to its corresponding letter. Then color the illustration.

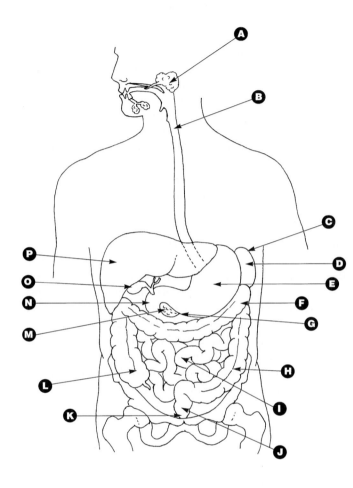

Anus
Cecum
Descending colon
Diaphragm
Duodenojejunal flexure
Duodenum
Esophagus
Gallbladder
Ileum
Liver
Pancreas
Parotid gland
Rectum
Spleen
Stomach
Transverse colon

A. _____
B. _____
C. _____
D. _____
E. _____
F. _____
G. _____
H. _____
I. _____
J. _____
K. _____
L. _____
M. _____
N. _____
O. _____
P. _____

Assess Your Competencies

Review the following objectives for this chapter:
1. List and describe the components and function of the respiratory system.
2. Explain the mechanics of breathing.
3. Describe pathologic conditions of the respiratory system and the associated indications and contraindications for massage.
   - Define respiration.
   - Explain external and internal respiration.
   - Locate and describe the organs of the respiratory system.
   - List the nerves and vessels of the respiratory system.
   - Locate the muscles involved in respiration.
   - Explain the mechanisms of breathing.
   - Define lung volume.
   - Explain the transport of oxygen and carbon dioxide.
   - Describe the central nervous system control of breathing.
   - List the reflexes of the respiratory system.
   - Determine indications and contraindications of massage to respiratory system pathology.
4. Describe how the decisions about what and when to eat influence health.
5. List and describe the components of the digestive system.
6. Describe the process of digestion.
7. Explain the importance of nutrition.
8. List and describe the main food groups.
9. Explain metabolic rate, energy balance, and body weight.
10. Describe pathologic conditions of the digestive system and the associated indications and contraindications for massage.
    - Define *digestion*.
    - Explain emotional eating.
    - Locate and describe the organs of the digestive system.
    - Describe the effects of autonomic nervous system on digestion.
    - Describe the sequence of the digestive process.
    - Define nutrition.
    - List and explain the role of the main food groups.

- Define the *citric acid cycle.*
- Define *metabolic rate.*
- Describe the results of increased or decreased metabolic rate.
- Determine indications and contraindications of massage to digestive system pathology.

11. List the functions of the urinary system.
12. List and describe the components of the urinary system.
13. Describe urinary function and the processes of fluid electrolyte balances.
14. Describe pathologic conditions of the urinary system and the associated indications and contraindications for massage.
    - List and locate the organs of the urinary system.
    - Describe the roles of water in the body.
    - Define *hydrostatic force.*
    - Explain the role of the hypothalamus in fluid regulation.
    - Explain the function of osmoreceptors and baroreceptors.
    - Describe electrolyte balance.
    - Define *pH,* and explain the relationship of pH to homeostasis.
    - Identify indications and contraindications of massage for urinary pathology.

15. List and describe the components and functions of the male reproductive system.
16. List and describe the components and functions of the female reproductive system.
17. Explain the three stages of pregnancy and the process of lactation.
18. Describe pathologic conditions of the reproductive system and the associated indications and contraindications for massage.
    - List the organs of the male reproductive system.
    - Trace the movement of sperm from the seminiferous tubules to ejaculation.
    - Describe the endocrine and nervous system control over the male reproductive system.
    - Describe male contraceptive methods.
    - List and describe the organs of the female reproductive system.
    - Describe the process of menstruation.
    - Describe endocrine and nervous system control over the female reproductive system.
    - Explain female contraceptive methods.
    - Describe the stages of pregnancy.
    - Explain the birth process.
    - Define *lactation.*
    - Determine indications and contraindications of massage for reproductive system pathology.

Next, on a separate piece of paper or using an audio or video recorder, prepare a short narrative that reflects how you would explain this content to a client and how the information relates to how you would provide massage. See the example in Chapter 1 on p. 22. When read or listened to, the narrative should not take more than 5 to 10 minutes to complete. Simpler is better. Use examples, tell stories, and use metaphors. It is important to understand that there is no precisely correct way to complete this exercise. The intent is to help you identify how effectively you understand the content and how relevant your application is to massage therapy. An excellent learning activity is to work together with other students and share your narratives. Also share these narratives with a friend or family member who is not familiar with the content. If the person can understand what has been written or recorded by you, that indicates that you understand it. There are many different ways to complete this learning activity. Yes, it may be confusing to do this, but that's all right. Out of confusion comes clarity. By the time you've done this 12 times, once for each chapter in this book, you will be much more competent.

Professional Application

What education and information does a massage practitioner need in order to work with pregnant women?

Muscle Quick Reference Guide

ⓔ http://evolve.elsevier.com/Fritz/essential

This chart is an abbreviated, simplified description of the main muscles and referred pain patterns encountered during massage application. Detailed information is provided in Chapters 9 and 10.

Muscle Name	Function/Action	Trigger Point Referred Pain Pattern*
Muscles of the Face and Head		
Muscles of Facial Expression	Move scalp forward and backward; assist in raising the eyebrows and wrinkling the forehead; draw the eyebrows downward and medially; and create transverse wrinkles over the bridge of the nose.	Galea aponeurotica, muscles over the eyebrows, eyes, ears, nose, and scalp above the ears
Auricular (ear) muscles	Move the ear.	None identified
Eye muscles	Open and close the eyelids; provide intrinsic movement of the eyeball.	Superior orbital area above the eyelid
Muscles that move the mouth	Move lips; aid in mastication; force air out between the lips; and compress the cheek against the teeth.	
Muscles of mastication (chewing)	Move the mouth; close the jaw; provide side-to-side movement and biting; and elevate the mandible.	Near and in the zygomatic arch; anterior, medial, and posterior along the inferior aspect of the muscles near the tendinous junction at the coronoid process of the mandible; temporal region, eyebrow, upper teeth, cheek, and temporomandibular joint; back of the throat, into the ear; upper and lower jaw, the ear, and the eyebrow
Muscles of the Neck		
Posterior Triangle of the Neck		
Longus colli and longus capitus	Bend the neck forward (flexion); oblique portion bends neck laterally; inferior portion rotates neck to the opposite side; control acceleration of cervical extension, lateral extension, and contralateral rotation; and provide dynamic stabilization of the cervical spine.	These muscles are difficult to palpate, and thus no specific trigger point locations have been identified. However, the pain from the trigger points in the muscles presents as a sore throat, difficulty swallowing, and tightness in the posterior neck muscles.
Scalene Group		
Anterior scalene	Bends the cervical portion of the vertebral column forward (flexion) and laterally; also rotates to the opposite side and assists in elevation of the first rib, thus functioning as an accessory muscle of respiration; checks (decelerates) cervical lateral flexion and rotation; and stabilizes the cervical spine.	Pectoral region, rhomboid region, and the entire length of the arm into the hand
Middle scalene	Acting from above, helps to raise the first rib, thus functioning as an accessory muscle of respiration; acting from below, bends the cervical part of the vertebral column to the same side; assists flexion of the neck; checks (decelerates) cervical lateral flexion and rotation; and stabilizes the cervical spine.	Pectoral region, rhomboid region, and the entire length of the arm into the hand

*The most common location of trigger points is in the belly of the muscles or at the attachments.

Continued

Muscle Name	Function/Action	Trigger Point Referred Pain Pattern*
Posterior scalene	When the second rib is fixed, bends the lower end of the cervical portion of the vertebral column to the same side (lateral flexion); when the upper attachment is fixed, helps to elevate the second rib, thus functioning as an accessory muscle of respiration; checks (decelerates) cervical lateral flexion and rotation; and stabilizes the cervical spine.	Pectoral region, rhomboid region, and the entire length of the arm into the hand
Sternocleidomastoid	Assists in flexing the cervical portion of the vertebral column forward, elevating the thorax, and extending the head at the atlantooccipital joint; stabilizes the head; and resists forceful backward movement of the head, tilts the head, rotates the head, and simultaneously acts to control rotation.	Several trigger points are located in the entire length of both divisions of the muscle: head and face, particularly the occipital region, ear, and forehead. Autonomic nervous system phenomena and proprioceptive disturbances are common.
Deep Posterior Cervical Muscles		
Splenius capitis and splenius cervicis	Extend head and neck, draw head dorsally and laterally and rotate head to the same side; check and control cervical flexion and contralateral rotation; and stabilize the cervical spine.	Belly of the muscles closer to the head; to the top of the skull (the pain often feels as though it is inside the head), to the eye, and into the shoulder
Erector Spinae Group		
Spinalis thoracis, cervicis, and capitis Longissimus thoracis, cervicis, and capitis Iliocostalis lumborum, thoracis, and cervicis	Extend, rotate, and laterally flex the vertebral column and head; assist with anterior tilt elevation and rotation of the pelvis and spinal stabilization; control and decelerate vertebral flexor rotation and lateral flexion; and stabilize the lumbar spine primarily.	Scapular, lumbar, abdominal, and gluteal areas; bandlike headache into the eyes; stiff neck
Oblique Muscles, Transversospinalis Group		
Semispinalis thoracis, cervicis, and capitis Multifidus Rotatores Intertransversarii lumborum, thoracis, and cervicis Interspinales	This group of muscles extends the motion segments of the back; rotates the thoracic, cervical, and lumbar vertebral joints; and stabilizes the vertebral column.	Scapular, lumbar, abdominal, and gluteal areas; bandlike headache into the eyes; stiff neck
Suboccipital Muscles		
Suboccipital muscles Rectus capitis posterior major and minor Obliquus capitis superior and inferior	As a group these muscles extend and rotate the head in small, precise movements. More often these muscles isometrically function as stabilizers of the head and provide proprioceptive input about head position. These muscles are also important postural muscles and are neural reporting stations on balance and proprioceptive monitors of cervical spine and neck position.	Belly of the muscle, located with deep palpation at the base of the skull, around the ear on the same side; sensation of compressed junction of skull and neck; bandlike headache
Muscles of the Torso		
Muscles of the Thorax and Posterior Abdominal Wall		
Diaphragm	Participates in respiration; during inspiration (breathing in), diaphragmatic contractions increase the capacity of the thoracic cavity; controls expiration as the diaphragm relaxes; and during breath holding, assists in stabilizing the lumbar and pelvic floor.	None identified
Serratus posterior superior	Assists in lifting the ribs during inspiration.	Under the scapula near the insertion of the muscle on the ribs and under the upper portion of the scapula
Serratus posterior inferior	Depresses last four ribs (9-12). Some studies disagree that this is the function, finding no electromyographic activity of this muscle during respiration. Seems to act as a stabilizer during forced expirations such as coughing.	Nagging ache in the area of the muscle

*The most common location of trigger points is in the belly of the muscles or at the attachments.

Muscle Name	Function/Action	Trigger Point Referred Pain Pattern*
External intercostal muscles	Elevate ribs and draw adjacent ribs together; lift ribs, increasing the volume of the thoracic cavity—ipsilateral torso rotation; and stabilize the thorax.	The intercostal muscles can develop trigger points, which are located by palpating the muscles between the ribs. Pain spans the intercostal segment, especially noticed with deep breathing or rotational movement.
Internal intercostal muscles	Depress ribs and draw adjacent ribs together, decreasing volume of thoracic cavity—ipsilateral torso rotation; stabilize the thorax.	The intercostal muscles can develop trigger points, which are located by palpating the muscles between the ribs. Pain spans the intercostal segment, especially noticed with deep breathing or rotational movement.
Innermost intercostal muscles	The muscles of this small group attach to the internal aspects of two adjoining ribs. They are believed to act with the internal intercostal muscles.	The intercostal muscles can develop trigger points, which are located by palpating the muscles between the ribs. Pain spans the intercostal segment, especially noticed with deep breathing or rotational movement.
Transversus thoracis	Draws anterior portion of the ribs caudally (reduces thoracic cavity); stabilizes the rib cage.	None identified
Quadratus lumborum	Draws last rib downward; flexes lumbar vertebral column laterally to the same side; acts to elevate and anteriorly tilt the pelvis; acting bilaterally, extends the lumbar spine and assists forced exhalation, as when coughing; restrains and checks lateral flexion; and assists normal inhalation by stabilizing the diaphragm and the twelfth rib and stabilizing the lumbar area.	Gluteal and groin area, sacroiliac joint and greater trochanter: These points are implicated in most low back pain. The dual function of lumbar stabilization (isometric function) and respiration (concentric function) can cause severe pain in the low back with a cough or sneeze if these trigger points are active. Low back pain often is related more to maintenance of posture than trigger point activity; therefore a common finding is corresponding pain patterns in the muscles that laterally flex the head and neck, such as the scalenes.
Psoas major and psoas minor	With origin fixed, flex the hip joint by flexing the femur on the pelvis; may assist in lateral rotation of the hip joint; acting bilaterally, flex the hip joint by flexing the trunk on the pelvis; can assist extension of the lumbar spine, increasing lumbar lordosis; acting unilaterally, may assist in lateral flexion of the trunk toward the same side; restrain and check trunk and hip extension and contralateral flexion of the trunk; control tendency of lordosis; and stabilize the lumbar spine and help to maintain upright posture.	Entire lumbar area into the superior gluteal region; front of the thigh; menstrual aching; can mimic appendicitis. Shortening is a major cause of low back pain. If tension or trigger point activity is located at insertion, pain can mimic a groin pull. Because of postural reflexes, muscles that flex the head and neck are facilitated with psoas activation. A common correlation exists between neck pain and stiffness and psoas pain and low back stiffness. Massage often must address both areas in sequence to be effective.
Iliacus	Flexes the hip joint; may assist in lateral rotation and abduction of the hip joint; with insertion fixed and acting bilaterally flexes the hip joint by flexing the trunk on the femur; tilts pelvis forward (anterior) when legs are fixed; decelerates hip extension; and stabilizes the pelvis.	Inner border of the ilium behind the anterior superior iliac spine.

Muscles of the Anterior Abdominal Wall

Muscle Name	Function/Action	Trigger Point Referred Pain Pattern*
Transversus abdominis	Constricts and compresses the abdomen, increasing intraabdominal pressure, and supports the abdominal viscera; assists in forced expiration.	Pain located throughout the area but concentrated more in the external circle of the abdominal wall rather than toward the middle near the umbilicus
Internal abdominal oblique	Compresses the abdominal cavity (some isometric abdominis activity); assists with posterior tilt of the pelvis; flexes the vertebral column, bringing the costal cartilage toward the pubis; laterally bends and ipsilaterally rotates the vertebral column (brings the shoulder of the opposite side forward); and restrains trunk extension.	Pain located throughout the area but concentrated more in the external circle of the abdominal wall rather than toward the middle near the umbilicus

Continued

Muscle Name	Function/Action	Trigger Point Referred Pain Pattern*
External abdominal oblique	Compresses the abdominal cavity (some isometric activity); assists in forced expiration; with both sides acting, flexes the vertebral column, bringing the pubis toward the xiphoid process of sternum; laterally bends and brings the shoulder of the same side forward; and restrains trunk extension.	Pain located throughout the area but concentrated more in the external circle of the abdominal wall rather than toward the middle near the umbilicus
Rectus abdominis	Flexes the vertebral column, bringing the sternum toward the pelvis; compresses the abdominal cavity; assists with posterior tilt of the pelvis (some isometric activity); assists in forced expiration; and restrains trunk extension.	Trigger points often found in the rectus abdominis just below the umbilicus on either side of the linea alba and near the attachment on the ribs. Pain is referred in local area or to groin.
Muscles of Scapular Stabilization		
Trapezius	Upper trapezius elevates and rotates scapula and the shoulder and, with the shoulder fixed, can assist in drawing the head backward and laterally to tilt the chin; the middle portion adducts (retracts) the scapula, draws back the acromion process; lower fibers depress the scapula; the entire muscle, acting bilaterally, assists extension of the cervical and thoracic spine; upper trapezius restrains and controls flexion, lateral flexion, and rotation of the neck and head. Middle trapezius controls and restrains scapular abduction (protraction). Lower trapezius restrains scapular elevation and rotates the scapula. Trapezius stabilizes the scapula and cervical spine.	Neck behind the ear and to the temple; subscapular area; acromial pain
Rhomboid major and rhomboid minor	Adduct (retract) and elevate the scapula and also rotate it downward so that the glenoid cavity faces down toward the feet; restrain protraction and upward rotation of the scapula; stabilize the scapula.	At the attachment point near the scapular border; scapular region
Levator scapulae	Raises the scapula and draws it medially; with the scapula fixed, performs lateral flexion and rotates the neck to the same side; bilaterally extends the neck; restrains and controls head and neck flexion, scapular depression, and lateral flexion of the cervical spine; and stabilizes cervical/scapular function.	Belly of the muscle just as it begins the rotation and at the attachment near the scapula; angle of the neck and along the vertebral border of the scapula; stiff neck in rotation
Pectoralis minor	Assists in drawing the scapula forward (protraction) around the chest wall; rotates the scapula to depress the point of the shoulder; assists in forced inspiration; restrains scapular retraction; and stabilizes the scapula during movement.	Near the attachment at the coracoid process and at the belly of the muscle; may mimic angina with pain in front of the chest from the shoulder and down the ulnar side of the arm into the fingers
Serratus anterior	Abducts (protracts) the scapula; rotates the scapula so that the glenoid cavity faces cranially (toward the head); raises the ribs with the scapula fixed and therefore is an accessory muscle of respiration; controls scapular retraction; and holds the medial border of the scapula firmly against the thorax and prevents winging of the scapula.	Along the midaxillary line near the ribs; side and back of the chest and down the ulnar aspect of the arm into the hand; may result in shortness of breath and pain during inhalation
Muscles of the Musculotendinous (Rotator) Cuff		
Supraspinatus	Abducts the arm; restrains adduction of the arm; and acts to stabilize the humeral head in the glenoid cavity during movements of the shoulder joint.	Shoulder, deltoid, and down the arm to the elbow, often experienced as a dull ache

*The most common location of trigger points is in the belly of the muscles or at the attachments.

Muscle Name	Function/Action	Trigger Point Referred Pain Pattern*
Infraspinatus	Provides lateral or external rotation of the arm at the shoulder; restrains and controls internal (medial) rotation of the arm at the shoulder; and acts to stabilize the humeral head in the glenoid cavity during movements of the shoulder joint.	Deep into the shoulder and deltoid area, down the arm, suboccipital area, medial border of the scapula, with limits reaching behind back
Teres minor	Provides adduction and lateral (external) rotation of the arm; restrains internal (medial) rotation of the arm; and acts to stabilize the humeral head in the glenoid cavity during movements of the shoulder joint.	Posterior deltoid region. Client often experiences limited range of motion when reaching behind the back, such as putting hands in back pocket of pants.
Subscapularis	Rotates humerus medially (internal rotation) and draws it forward and down when the arm is raised; restrains lateral (external) rotation of the arm; and stabilizes the humeral head in the glenoid cavity during movement of the shoulder.	Access is through the axilla near the attachment at the humerus and in the belly of the muscle. Pain in posterior deltoid, scapular region, triceps area, and into the wrist often is mistaken for bursitis because pain often refers to insertion at shoulder.
Muscles of the Shoulder Joint		
Deltoid	Provides flexion and extension and medial and lateral rotation of the arm and abduction of the arm. Anterior deltoid restrains and controls extension and external rotation of the arm. Middle deltoid restrains arm adduction. Posterior deltoid restrains flexion and internal rotators and horizontal adduction of the arm. Deltoid stabilizes glenohumeral joint during arm movement.	Deltoid region and down the lateral side of the arm
Pectoralis major	With proximal attachment (origin) fixed, adducts and draws the humerus forward (flexion) and horizontally and medially (internally) rotates it; with insertion fixed and arm abducted, assists in elevating the thorax (as in forced inspiration); controls arm extension, horizontal abduction, and external rotation; and stabilizes the shoulder during overhead activity.	Chest and breast and down the ulnar aspect of the arm to the fourth and fifth fingers
Subclavius	Draws the clavicle forward and down; stabilizes the clavicle.	Chest and breast and down the radial aspect of the arm to the fourth and fifth fingers
Latissimus dorsi	With proximal attachment (origin) fixed, medially or internally rotates, adducts, and extends the humerus; depresses the shoulder girdle and assists in lateral flexion of the trunk; with insertion fixed, assists in tilting the pelvis anteriorly and laterally; acting bilaterally, assists in hyperextending the spine and tilting the pelvis anteriorly; controls abduction, flexion, and external (lateral) rotation of the humerus; and stabilizes the lumbar and pelvic area by maintaining tension on the thoracolumbar fascia.	Posterior axillary area just as the muscle begins to twist around the teres major; belly of the muscle near the rib attachments; just below the scapula and into the ulnar side of the arm; anterior deltoid region and abdominal oblique area
Teres major	Medial or internal rotation, adduction, and extension of the arm; upward rotation of the scapula; controls and restrains flexion, abduction, and external rotation of the arm; and stabilizes the glenohumeral joint.	Near the musculotendinous junction at both attachments; posterior deltoid region and down the dorsal portion of the arm
Coracobrachialis	Flexion and adduction of the humerus; controls extension and abduction of the scapula; stabilizes the shoulder.	Front of shoulder, posterior aspect of the arm down the triceps and dorsal forearm in the hand

Continued

Muscle Name	Function/Action	Trigger Point Referred Pain Pattern*
Muscles of the Elbow and Radioulnar Joints		
Biceps brachii	Provides flexion of the humerus. The long head may assist with abduction if the humerus is laterally rotated. The short head assists arm adduction. With proximal attachment (origin) fixed, flexes the forearm toward the humerus and supinates the forearm; with insertion fixed, flexes the elbow joint, moving the humerus toward the forearm, as in a pull-up or chin-up; restrains and controls elbow extension and extension of the humerus; stabilizes the humerus at the shoulder and the elbow joint during full extension; and stabilizes the elbow when flexed and holding a weight.	Front of the shoulder at the anterior deltoid region and into the scapular region; also into the antecubital space or the front of the elbow
Brachialis	Flexes the elbow joint; restrains and controls elbow extension; stabilizes the elbow in full extension and fixed flexion.	Primarily to the thumb, with some pain in the anterior deltoid area and at the elbow
Brachioradialis	Flexes the elbow joint after brachialis and biceps initiate movement; assists in pronation and supination of the forearm to midposition; restrains and controls elbow extension; and stabilizes the elbow in full extension and fixed flexion.	Wrist and base of the thumb in the web space between the thumb and index finger and to the lateral epicondyle at the elbow
Pronator teres	Pronates the forearm; assists in flexing the elbow joint; controls supination of the forearm; and stabilizes the elbow joint and radioulnar joint.	Radial side of the forearm into the wrist and thumb. Pain may mimic carpal tunnel syndrome.
Supinator	Supinates the forearm; assists with flexion of the forearm at the elbow when the hand is held halfway between supination and pronation; restrains and controls pronation of the forearm; and stabilizes the elbow and radioulnar joint.	Lateral epicondyle and dorsal aspect of the arm (pain mimics tennis elbow); near the radius in the antecubital space; thumb area
Pronator quadratus	Provides pronation of the forearm; restrains and controls supination of the forearm.	Belly of muscle; active supination
Triceps brachii	Extension of the forearm; in addition, the long head adducts and assists in extension of the humerus; restrains elbow flexion and arm abduction and flexion; stabilizes the elbow in extension and fixed flexion to allow carrying weight in the hands; and assists in stabilizing the glenohumeral joint.	Length of posterior arm
Anconeus (elbow)	Assists the triceps in extension of the elbow joint; balances elbow flexion; and stabilizes the joint capsule of the elbow.	Elbow at lateral epicondyle
Muscles of the Wrist and Hand Joints		
Anterior Flexor Group: Superficial Layer		
Flexor carpi radialis	Flexes and abducts the wrist (radial deviation); may assist in pronation of the forearm and flexion of the elbow; restrains and controls extension and adduction of the wrist; and stabilizes the wrist.	Into the wrist and fingers; occasionally into the elbow
Palmaris longus	Flexes the wrist; may assist in flexion of the elbow and pronation of the forearm; restrains wrist extension; and tenses the palmar fascia.	Into the wrist and fingers; occasionally into the elbow
Flexor carpi ulnaris	Flexes and adducts (ulnar deviation) the wrist; may assist in elbow flexion; controls and restrains wrist extension and abduction; and stabilizes the wrist.	Into the wrist and fingers; occasionally into the elbow

*The most common location of trigger points is in the belly of the muscles or at the attachments.

Muscle Name	Function/Action	Trigger Point Referred Pain Pattern*
Flexor digitorum superficialis	Flexes the proximal interphalangeal joints of the second through fifth digits; assists in flexion of the wrist; restrains and controls finger extension; stabilizes wrist and hand joints; flexes the metacarpophalangeal joints; flexes the forearm at the elbow.	Into the wrist and fingers; occasionally into the elbow
Flexor digitorum profundus	Flexes the distal interphalangeal joints of the second through fifth digits; assists in flexion of the proximal interphalangeal and metacarpophalangeal joints; assists in adduction of the index, ring, and little fingers and in flexion of the wrist; restrains and controls extension of the fingers; and stabilizes the fingers.	Into the wrist and fingers; occasionally into the elbow
Flexor pollicis longus	Flexes interphalangeal joint of the thumb; assists in flexion of the metacarpophalangeal and carpometacarpal joints; restrains thumb; and stabilizes the thumb.	Thumb
Posterior Extensor Group: Superficial Layer		
Extensor carpi radialis longus	Extends and adducts (ulnar deviation) the wrist; may assist in flexion of the elbow and pronation and supination of the forearm; restrains and controls wrist flexion and abduction; and stabilizes the wrist	From the lateral epicondyle at the elbow down the dorsum of the forearm to various parts of the hand, especially to the web of the thumb and elbow joint
Extensor carpi radialis brevis	Extends the wrist and assists in abduction (radial deviation) of the wrist and weak flexion of the forearm; restrains and controls wrist flexion and adduction; and stabilizes the wrist.	From the lateral epicondyle at the elbow down the dorsum of the forearm to various parts of the hand, especially to the web of the thumb
Extensor digitorum	Extends the metacarpophalangeal joints; extends the interphalangeal joint of the second through fifth digits (with the lumbricales and interossei); assists in extension of the wrist; restrains and controls wrist and finger flexion; and stabilizes the wrist.	From the lateral epicondyle at the elbow down the dorsum of the forearm to various parts of the hand, especially to the web of the thumb
Extensor digiti minimi	Extends the metacarpophalangeal and (with the interosseous and lumbrical muscles) the interphalangeal joints of the little finger; assists in abduction of the little finger; controls and restrains flexion and adduction of the little finger; and stabilizes the joints of the little finger.	From the lateral epicondyle at the elbow down the dorsum of the forearm to various parts of the hand, especially to the web of the thumb
Extensor carpi ulnaris	Extends and adducts (ulnar deviation) the wrist; controls wrist flexion and abduction; and stabilizes the wrist.	From the lateral epicondyle at the elbow down the dorsum of the forearm to various parts of the hand, especially to the web of the thumb
Extensor pollicis brevis	Extends and abducts the carpometacarpal joint of the thumb; extends the metacarpophalangeal joint; assists in abduction (radial deviation) of the wrist; restrains flexion of the thumb and adduction of the wrist; and stabilizes the thumb.	From the lateral epicondyle at the elbow down the dorsum of the forearm to various parts of the hand, especially to the web of the thumb
Posterior Extensor Group: Deep Layer		
Abductor pollicis longus	Abducts and extends the carpometacarpal joint of the thumb; abducts (radial deviation) and assists in wrist flexion and supination of the forearm; controls thumb adduction; and stabilizes the thumb and wrist.	To the web of the thumb
Extensor pollicis longus	Extends the interphalangeal joint and assists in extension of the metacarpophalangeal and carpometacarpal joints of the thumb; assists in abduction (radial deviation) and extension of the wrist; restrains thumb and wrist flexion; and stabilizes the thumb and wrist.	To the web of the thumb

Continued

Muscle Name	Function/Action	Trigger Point Referred Pain Pattern*
Extensor indicis	Extends the metacarpophalangeal joint and (with the lumbrical and interosseous muscles) extends the interphalangeal joints of the index finger; may assist in adduction of the index finger and supination of the forearm; restrains, stabilizes, and controls flexion of the index finger; and extends the hand at the wrist.	Dorsum of the forearm to various parts of the hand
Intrinsic Muscles of the Hand		
Thenar Eminence Muscles		
Opponens pollicis	Abducts at the carpometacarpal joint of the thumb; flexes at the carpometacarpal joint; aids in opposition of the thumb to each of the other digits; controls and restrains adduction of the thumb; and stabilizes the thumb.	Into the thumb and the wrist
Abductor pollicis brevis	Abducts and aids in opposition of the thumb; controls and restrains adduction of the thumb; and stabilizes the thumb.	Into the thumb and the wrist
Flexor pollicis brevis	Flexes the proximal phalanx of the thumb; assists in opposition of the thumb; restrains and controls extension of the thumb; and stabilizes the thumb.	Into the thumb and the wrist
Hypothenar Muscles		
Opponens digiti minimi	Provides flexion and slight rotation of the carpometacarpal joint of the little finger; helps to cup the palm of the hand; and stabilizes the little finger.	Little finger and wrist
Abductor digiti minimi manus	Abducts the metacarpophalangeal joint of the little finger; controls and restrains adduction and flexion of the little finger; and stabilizes the little finger.	Little finger and wrist
Flexor digiti minimi (brevis manus)	Flexes the metacarpophalangeal joint of the little finger; assists in opposition of the little finger to the thumb; controls extension of the little finger; and stabilizes the little finger.	Little finger and wrist
Deep Muscles of the Hand		
Adductor pollicis	Adducts the thumb and aids in opposition; restrains thumb abduction; and stabilizes the thumb.	Thumb
Palmar interossei	Adducts the index, ring, and little fingers toward the middle digit; assists in restraining abduction of the fingers; and stabilizes the hand.	Into the associated finger
Dorsal interossei manus	Abducts the index, middle, and ring fingers from the midline of the hand.	Into the associated finger
Lumbricals manus	Extends the interphalangeal joints and simultaneously flexes the metacarpophalangeal joint of the second through fifth digits.	Into the associated finger
Muscles of the Gluteal Region		
Gluteus maximus	Extends and laterally rotates the hip joint; upper fibers assist abduction of the hip; lower fibers assist in adduction of the hip joint; with femur fixed, assists in extension of the trunk and posterior tilt of the pelvis; the gluteus maximus is active primarily during strenuous activity, such as running, jumping, and climbing stairs; restrains and controls hip and trunk flexion and medial rotation and abduction/adduction of the hip. These muscles are important postural muscles that help maintain the upright posture, stabilize the pelvis, and provide tension to the iliotibial tract to keep the fascial band taut.	Regionally into the gluteal area, especially to the ischial tuberosity, the tip of the greater trochanter, and the sacrum

*The most common location of trigger points is in the belly of the muscles or at the attachments.

Muscle Name	Function/Action	Trigger Point Referred Pain Pattern*
Gluteus medius	Abducts the hip joint; anterior fibers medially rotate and assist in flexion of the hip joint and anterior tilt of the pelvis; posterior fibers laterally rotate and assist in extension of the hip joint and posterior tilt of the pelvis; restrains adduction, medial/lateral rotation and flexion/extension of the hip; and stabilizes the pelvis when a person is standing on one foot.	Along the musculotendinous junction at the iliac crest; low back, posterior crest of the ilium to the sacrum, and to the posterior and lateral areas of the buttock into the upper thigh
Gluteus minimus	Abducts the hip joint; anterior fibers medially rotate and assist in flexion of the hip joint and anterior tilt of the pelvis; posterior fibers laterally rotate and assist in extension of the hip joint and posterior tilt of the pelvis; restrains adduction, medial/lateral rotation and flexion/extension of the hip; and stabilizes the pelvis when a person is standing on one foot.	Lower lateral buttock and down the lateral to posterior aspect of the thigh, knee, and leg to the ankle
Tensor fasciae latae	Flexes, medially rotates, and abducts the hip joint; assists in anterior pelvic tilt; extends the knee; restrains hip extension and lateral rotation; tenses the iliotibial tract, counterbalancing the backward pull of the gluteus maximus on the iliotibial tract; and stabilizes the pelvis and knee.	Localized in the hip and down the lateral side of the leg to the knee
Deep Lateral Rotators		
Piriformis Obturator internus and obturator externus Gemellus superior and gemellus inferior	Provide lateral rotation and abduction of the hip joint when the thigh is flexed; restrain medial rotation and adduction of the hip; and stabilize the hip joint.	The belly of each muscle can house trigger points. Sacroiliac region, entire buttock, and down the posterior thigh to just above the knee
Quadratus femoris	Laterally rotates the hip joint and adducts the thigh; restrains internal rotation and abduction of the hip joint; and stabilizes the hip joint.	The main trigger points are near the attachments and the insertion. Tension in this muscle may cause deep hip and groin pain.
Muscles of the Posterior Thigh		
Semimembranosus	Flexes the knee and medially rotates the knee joint when the knee is semiflexed; moves the medial meniscus posteriorly during knee flexion; extends and assists in medial rotation and adduction of the hip joint; posteriorly tilts the pelvis; restrains and controls knee extension and lateral rotation; assists in controlling flexion and lateral rotation of the hip; and stabilizes the knee and hip complex.	Several areas in the belly of each muscle and at the musculotendinous junction closer to the knee; ischial tuberosity, back of the knee, and the entire posterior leg to midcalf
Semitendinosus	Flexes the knee and medially rotates the knee joint when the knee is semiflexed; extends and assists in medial rotation and adduction of the hip joint; restrains and controls knee extension and lateral rotation; assists in controlling flexion and lateral rotation of the hip; and stabilizes the knee and hip complex.	Several areas in the belly of each muscle and at the musculotendinous junction closer to the knee; ischial tuberosity, back of the knee, and the entire posterior leg to midcalf
Biceps femoris	Flexes and laterally rotates the knee joint when the knee is semiflexed; long head also extends and assists in lateral rotation of the hip joint and posteriorly tilts the pelvis; restrains and controls knee extension and medial rotation; also restrains hip flexion and medial rotation; and stabilizes the hip and knee complex.	Several areas in the belly of each muscle and at the musculotendinous junction closer to the knee; ischial tuberosity, back of the knee, and the entire posterior leg to midcalf
Muscles of the Medial Thigh		
Pectineus	Adducts, flexes, and assists in medial rotation of the hip joint and anterior tilt of the pelvis; restrains abduction, extension, and lateral rotation of hip; and stabilizes the hip.	Deep in the groin into the medial thigh and downward to the knee and shin. Pain may mimic hamstring tension.

Continued

Muscle Name	Function/Action	Trigger Point Referred Pain Pattern*
Adductor brevis	Adducts and assists in flexing the hip joint anteriorly and tilts the pelvis; restrains and controls abduction and extension of the hip; and stabilizes the hip and trunk in the standing position.	Deep in the groin into the medial thigh and downward to the knee and shin. Pain may mimic hamstring tension.
Adductor longus	Adducts and assists in flexing the hip joint and anteriorly tilts the pelvis; restrains and controls abduction and extension of the hip; and stabilizes the hip and trunk in the standing position.	Deep in the groin into the medial thigh and downward to the knee and shin. Pain may mimic hamstring tension.
Adductor magnus	Adducts the hip joint and posteriorly tilts the pelvis; upper portion medially rotates and flexes, whereas the lower portion extends the hip joint; restrains and controls hip abduction; and stabilizes the trunk, pelvis, and hip.	Deep in the groin into the medial thigh and downward to the knee and shin. Pain may mimic hamstring tension.
Gracilis	Adducts and flexes the hip joint; assists with anterior tilt of the pelvis; flexes the knee and medially rotates the knee joint when the knee is semiflexed; controls and restrains hip abduction and extension and knee extension and lateral rotation; and assists in controlling and stabilizing the valgus angulation of the knee and stabilizing the pelvic and knee complex.	Deep in the groin into the medial thigh and downward to the knee and shin. Pain may mimic hamstring tension.
Muscles of the Anterior Thigh		
Sartorius	Flexes, laterally rotates, and abducts the hip joint; also weakly flexes the torso toward the pelvis when the leg is fixed and anteriorly and laterally tilts the pelvis; flexes and assists in medial rotation of the knee joint; controls and restrains extension, medial rotation, and adduction of the hip and assists in restraining trunk extension; at the knee, restrains and controls extension and lateral rotation of the knee; and stabilizes the knee and hip complex.	Into the hip and medial knee
Quadriceps Femoris Group		
Rectus femoris	Extends the knee joint; flexes the hip joint; anteriorly tilts the pelvis; restrains and controls knee flexion and hip extension; and stabilizes the knee and hip complex.	Into the hip and knee
Vastus lateralis	Extends the knee joint and exerts a lateral pull on the patella; controls and restrains knee flexion and medial pull of patella; and stabilizes iliotibial tract and knee.	Into the hip and lateral knee
Vastus medialis	Extends the leg and draws the patella medially, particularly the lower oblique aspect of the muscle (vastus medialis oblique) with attachment into the adductor magnus; controls and restrains knee flexion and lateral movement of patella; and stabilizes the knee and patella.	Entire anterior thigh, with concentration at the knee
Vastus intermedius	Extends the knee joint; restrains and controls knee flexion; and stabilizes the knee and patella.	Into the knee
Muscles of the Anterior and Lateral Leg		
Anterior Muscles		
Tibialis anterior	Provides dorsiflexion of the ankle joint; assists in inversion and adduction of the foot. Note: Combined action of inversion and adduction results in supination. Restrains and controls plantar flexion and eversion of the foot. Stabilizes the ankle.	Down the leg to the ankle and into the toes

*The most common location of trigger points is in the belly of the muscles or at the attachments.

Muscle Name	Function/Action	Trigger Point Referred Pain Pattern*
Extensor digitorum longus	Extends the phalanges of the second through fifth digits; assists in dorsiflexion of the ankle joint and eversion and abduction of the foot; restrains and controls flexion of the toes, plantar flexion, and inversion of the ankle and foot; and stabilizes the ankle and foot.	Down the leg to the ankle and into the toes
Extensor hallucis longus	Extends the metatarsophalangeal joint of the great toe; also assists in inverting and adducting (supination) the foot and dorsiflexing the ankle joint; restrains and controls flexion of the great toes, eversion of the foot, and plantar flexion of the ankle; and stabilizes the great toe and assists in stabilizing the ankle.	Down the leg to the ankle and into the toes
Fibularis (peroneus) tertius	Dorsiflexes the ankle joint; everts and abducts (pronates) the foot; assists in controlling and restraining plantar flexion of the ankle and inversion of the foot; and assists in stabilizing the ankle.	Down the leg to the ankle
Lateral Muscles		
Fibularis (peroneus) longus and fibularis (peroneus) brevis	Everts and abducts (pronates) the foot; assists in plantar flexion of the ankle joint; restrains and controls dorsiflexion of the ankle and inversion of the foot; and stabilizes the ankle.	To the lateral malleolus and the heel
Posterior Leg Muscles		
Popliteus	Assists in restraining knee extension; stabilizes the knee.	To the back of the knee
Tibialis posterior	Inverts the foot; assists in plantar flexion of the ankle joint; restrains and controls eversion of the foot and dorsiflexion of the ankle; and stabilizes the ankle.	Down the posterior leg to the heel and the sole of the foot into the plantar surface of the toes; can be a factor in knee pain and restricted mobility of the knee and ankle
Flexor digitorum longus	Flexes the joints of the second through fifth digits; assists in plantar flexion of the ankle joint and inversion and adduction (supination) of the foot; restrains and controls extension of the toes; assists in controlling dorsiflexion of the ankle and eversion of the foot; and stabilizes the ankle and toes.	Down the posterior leg to the heel and the sole of the foot into the plantar surface of the toes; can be a factor in knee pain and restricted mobility of the knee and ankle
Flexor hallucis longus	Flexes the joints of the great toe; provides plantar flexion of the ankle joint and inverts the foot; restrains extension of the great toe and assists in controlling dorsiflexion of the ankle and eversion of the foot; and stabilizes the great toe, ankle, and foot.	Down the posterior leg to the heel and the sole of the foot into the plantar surface of the great toe
Plantaris	Provides plantar flexion of the ankle joint; assists in flexion of the knee joint; restrains dorsiflexion of the ankle and assists in controlling extension of the knee; and assists in stabilizing the ankle/knee complex.	Can be a factor in knee pain and restricted mobility of the knee and ankle.
Soleus	Provides plantar flexion of the ankle joint and assists inversion of the foot at the ankle; restrains and controls dorsiflexion and eversion of the ankle; and stabilizes the leg over the foot and ankle.	Down the posterior leg to the heel and the sole of the foot into the plantar surface of the toes; can restrict mobility of the ankle
Gastrocnemius	Provides plantar flexion of the ankle joint; assists in flexion of the knee joint and inversion of the foot; restrains and controls dorsiflexion of the ankle and extension of the knee; stabilizes the knee and ankle complex and is involved in maintaining balance in static standing.	Down the posterior leg to the heel and the sole of the foot into the plantar surface of the toes; can be a factor in knee pain and restricted mobility of the knee and ankle

Continued

Muscle Name	Function/Action	Trigger Point Referred Pain Pattern*
Muscles of the Foot		
Dorsal Aspect		
Extensor digitorum brevis	Extends the interphalangeal and metatarsophalangeal joints of the second through fourth toes.	The entire foot with areas concentrated at the toes, the ball of the foot, and the heel
Plantar Aspect: Superficial Layer		
Abductor hallucis	Abducts and assists in flexion of the metatarsophalangeal joint of the great toe.	The entire foot with areas concentrated at the large toe, the ball of the foot, and the heel
Flexor digitorum brevis	Flexes the proximal interphalangeal joints and assists in flexion of the metatarsophalangeal joints of the second through fifth toes.	The entire foot with areas concentrated at the toes, the ball of the foot, and the heel
Abductor digiti minimi pedis	Abducts and assists in flexing the metatarsophalangeal joint of the fifth toe.	The entire foot with areas concentrated at the small toe
Plantar Aspect: Second Layer		
Quadratus plantae	Modifies the line of pull of the flexor digitorum longus and assists in flexion of the second through the fifth digits.	The entire foot
Lumbricales pedis	These muscles flex the metatarsophalangeal joints and extend the interphalangeal joints of the second through the fifth digits.	Several areas concentrated in the belly of each muscle; the entire foot with areas concentrated at the large toe, the ball of the foot, and the heel
Plantar Aspect: Third Layer		
Flexor hallucis brevis	Flexes metatarsophalangeal joint of the great toe.	The entire foot with areas concentrated at the large toe
Adductor hallucis	Adducts and assists in flexion of the metatarsophalangeal joint of the great toe.	The entire foot with areas concentrated at the large toe
Flexor digiti minimi pedis	Flexes the metatarsophalangeal joint of the fifth toe.	The entire foot with areas concentrated at the little toe
Plantar Aspect: Fourth Layer		
Plantar interossei	These muscles adduct the third, fourth, and fifth toes toward an axis through the second toe; assist in flexion of the metatarsophalangeal joints of the third through fifth toes.	Trigger points seem to follow the bellies of the muscles
Dorsal interossei pedis	These muscles abduct the second, third, and fourth toes from a longitudinal axis through the second toe; also assist in flexion of the metatarsophalangeal joints of the second through the fourth digits and extension of interphalangeal joints of the second through fourth digits.	Trigger points seem to follow the bellies of the muscles

*The most common location of trigger points is in the belly of the muscles or at the attachments.

Diseases/Conditions and Indications/Contraindications for Massage Therapy

Disease/Condition	Indications/Contraindications for Massage Therapy	Chapter Reference
Aneurysm An aneurysm is a weakening and bulging of the wall of a blood vessel, usually an artery. Aneurysms occur most often in the abdominal aorta and the brain.	Treatment is contraindicated. Refer client immediately to a physician.	4

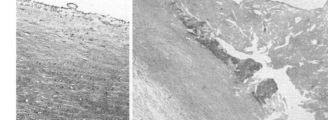

FIGURE B-1 Micrographs of aneurysms. (From Tsang VT et al: Interruption of the aorta with multilobulated arch aneurysms, *J Thorac Cardio Surg* 133(4): 1092-1093, 2007.)

Asthma Acute asthma is spasmodic constriction of the smooth muscle in the bronchial tubes. This is sometimes called an *asthmatic attack*. Chronic asthmas involve inflammation in the bronchial tubes along with excessive mucus production.	Massage is indicated for clients with asthmas as long as they are not having an asthmatic attack. Between episodes, massage can be beneficial for general stress management and relief of tension in muscles.	12

Continued

Disease/Condition	Indications/Contraindications for Massage Therapy	Chapter Reference

Atherosclerosis

This is a condition in which arteries become inelastic because of the development of plaques. Because of the inelasticity, atherosclerosis is also called *hardening of the arteries.* Plaque buildup in the walls of the arteries that supply the heart is referred to as *coronary artery disease (CAD).* If enough plaque builds up, blood flow can become obstructed, leading to a heart attack or stroke. Because the plaque has a rough surface, thrombosis (formation of a clot in an unbroken blood vessel) can occur. The clot can obstruct blood flow in the area in which it develops, or it can break off and become an embolus.

Mild atherosclerosis is an indication for massage. Advanced atherosclerosis may be a contraindication for massage, but the gentle resting of hands on the body used in some forms of touch systems might be indicated with supervision.

11

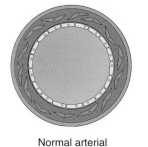
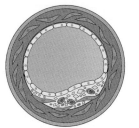
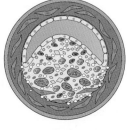

Normal arterial lumen   Atherosclerotic plaque deposit   Advanced arterial atherosclerotic disease

FIGURE B-2 Atherosclerosis. (From Frazier MS, Drzymkowski JW: *Essentials of human diseases and conditions*, ed 4, St. Louis, 2008, Saunders.)

Bell's palsy

This palsy causes partial or total paralysis of the facial muscles on one side as the result of inflammation or injury to the seventh cranial nerve.

Massage approaches can reduce stress. The practitioner must gauge the intensity and duration of any massage application so as not to overtax an already stressed client, aggravating the condition. Shorter, more frequent treatments may be indicated.

5

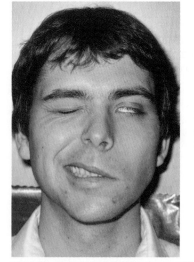

FIGURE B-3 Bell's palsy. (From Neville BW et al: *Oraland maxillofacial pathology*, ed 3, St. Louis, 2009, Saunders. Courtesy Dr. Bruce Brehm.)

Breathing pattern disorder

This disorder is complex and involves altered breathing patterns. It is associated with stress and anxiety.

Therapeutic massage approaches and moderate application of movement therapies such as tai chi, yoga, and aerobic exercise assist with normalizing breathing patterns and altering mood, feelings, and behavior.

12

Disease/Condition	Indications/Contraindications for Massage Therapy	Chapter Reference
Bursitis This is inflammation of the bursae, especially those located between the bony prominences and a muscle or tendon such as in the shoulder, elbow, hip, and knee. It usually results from trauma and repetitive use.	Therapeutic massage can help manage pain and support an increase in range of motion. However, massage directly over the bursae is contraindicated.	8
Cancer *Dysplasia* is the term for a change in normal body cells. Some of these abnormal cells can develop into cancerous cells. Some types of abnormal cells grow slowly and can be treated easily; other types are aggressive and invasive malignancies that can spread to other parts of the body. Common types of cancer include lung cancer, breast cancer, colorectal cancer, leukemia, bone cancer, melanoma (malignant skin cancer), prostate cancer, and stomach cancer.	If the cancer is detected and successfully treated before metastasis, the client can receive any type of massage therapy. However, massage for clients with malignancies is contraindicated unless the client's health care professional gives approval and supervision. If approval and supervision for massage is given, the practitioner must adjust treatments for any radiation therapy, chemotherapy, or surgical procedures the client is undergoing. As with most chronic illness and pain, therapeutic massage offers the client palliative or comfort care and may be helpful in reducing stress stemming from the cancer and cancer treatments the client is receiving. Sometimes clients with colorectal cancer have colostomies. If so, the practitioner needs to adjust treatments to accommodate the colostomy bag.	Multiple
Carpal tunnel syndrome This syndrome results from irritation of the meridian nerve as it passes under the transverse carpal ligament into the wrist. Symptoms include pain, numbness, tingling, and weakness in the part of the hand innervated by the median nerve, namely the thumb, the first and second finger, half the third finger, and the palm of the hand proximal to these digits.	Various forms of massage application can reduce muscle spasms, lengthen shortened muscles, and soften and stretch connective tissue, restoring a more normal space around the nerve and possibly alleviating impingement. When massage is combined with other appropriate methods, surgery may not necessary. If surgery is performed, the practitioner must manage adhesions appropriately and keep soft tissues surrounding the healing surgical area supple to prevent reentrapment of the nerve. Before doing any work near the site of a recent incision, the practitioner must obtain approval from the client's physician. In general, work close to the surgical area can begin after the stitches have been removed and all inflammation is gone. As healing progresses, soft-tissue methods can be used to address the forming scar more directly. Direct work on a new scar usually is safe 8 to 12 weeks into the healing period.	5

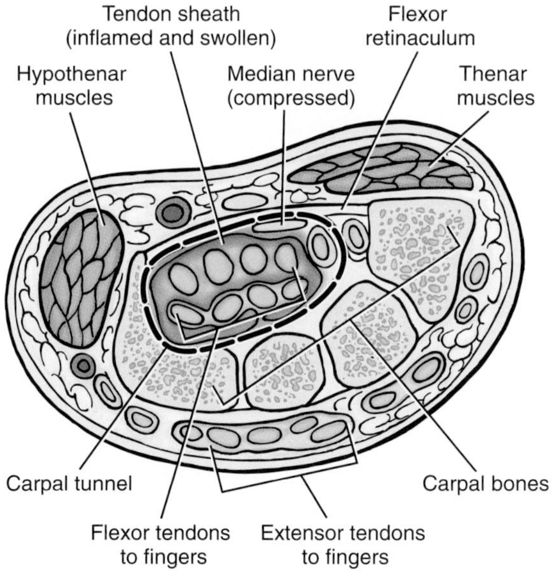

Tendon sheath (inflamed and swollen)   Flexor retinaculum

Hypothenar muscles   Median nerve (compressed)   Thenar muscles

Carpal tunnel   Carpal bones

Flexor tendons to fingers   Extensor tendons to fingers

FIGURE B-4 Cross-section of wrist affected by carpal tunnel syndrome.

Continued

Disease/Condition	Indications/Contraindications for Massage Therapy	Chapter Reference

Contusion

A muscle bruise results from trauma to the muscles and involves local internal bleeding and inflammation.

Direct work over the area of injury is contraindicated regionally until all signs of inflammation have dissipated.

9

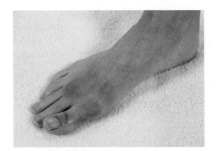

FIGURE B-5 Contusion. (From Fritz S: *Mosby's fundamentals of therapeutic massage*, ed 5, St. Louis, 2013, Mosby.)

Coronary artery disease

See Atherosclerosis.

Decubitus ulcer

Also called *bed sores* or *pressure ulcers,* decubitus ulcers are caused by impaired blood circulation to the skin. The impairment is due to pressure of the body against a surface such as a bed, cast, or wheelchair. The impaired blood flow leads to necrosis (tissue death) and a subsequent high risk of infection.

Massage can be beneficial in preventing the development of decubitus ulcers. Once the tissue has been damaged, however, the risk of infection is high, so massage is regionally contraindicated. However, massaging around the edges of the affected area may stimulate blood flow to assist in healing.

11

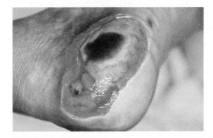

FIGURE B-6 Pressure ulcer, showing tissue necrosis. (From Potter PA, Perry AG: *Fundamentals of nursing*, ed 7, St. Louis, 2009, Mosby.)

Disease/Condition	Indications/Contraindications for Massage Therapy	Chapter Reference
Diabetes mellitus This disease results from the pancreas not producing any insulin (type I) or not producing enough insulin (type II). **FIGURE B-7** Complications of diabetes mellitus. (From Damjanov I: *Pathology for the health professions,* ed 4, St Louis, 2012, Saunders.)	Massage for clients who have diabetes should be a supportive part of an overall treatment program. It should be performed under medical supervision. Impaired blood circulation, especially in the extremities, and neuropathy often accompany diabetes mellitus. The massage therapist should refer the client for immediate medical care if any tissue changes are noted. In pain management of diabetic neuropathy, gentle massage techniques can prove beneficial for short-term reduction of pain symptoms.	6

Continued

Disease/Condition	Indications/Contraindications for Massage Therapy	Chapter Reference
Dislocation Dislocation is displacement of the bones of a joint; a subluxation is a partial dislocation.	Massage and bodywork are contraindicated locally over a trauma area until healing is complete. Massage methods are beneficial in supporting the rest of the body during the healing process, especially in managing compensation patterns caused by immobilizing the area. Massage and other forms of bodywork can also help manage secondary muscle tension.	8
Diverticular disease Diverticula are small, saclike outpouchings of the intestinal wall in weak areas of the colon. Diverticulosis is the development of these pouches. Diverticulitis is inflammation caused by infection of these pouches. Abdominal pain or referred back pain may indicate gastrointestinal disorders, including diverticular disease.	clients should be referred to their physicians for proper diagnosis. If the client has been diagnosed with diverticulosis, deep abdominal massage is contraindicated. If the client has been diagnosed with diverticulitis, massage is contraindicated.	12

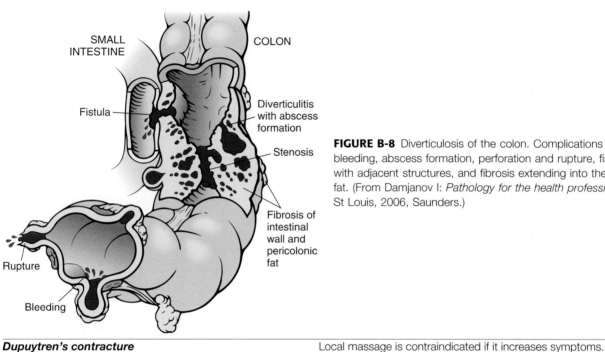

SMALL INTESTINE

COLON

Fistula

Diverticulitis with abscess formation

Stenosis

Fibrosis of intestinal wall and pericolonic fat

Rupture

Bleeding

FIGURE B-8 Diverticulosis of the colon. Complications include bleeding, abscess formation, perforation and rupture, fistula formation with adjacent structures, and fibrosis extending into the pericolonic fat. (From Damjanov I: *Pathology for the health professions,* ed 3, St Louis, 2006, Saunders.)

Disease/Condition	Indications/Contraindications for Massage Therapy	Chapter Reference
Dupuytren's contracture This disorder results from the shrinking and thickening of the palmar fascia. The contracture pulls on the tendons of the ring finger and occasionally the little finger, causing them to be permanently flexed.	Local massage is contraindicated if it increases symptoms.	9
Edema In this condition excessive fluid accumulates within the interstitial spaces. Edema can be caused by electrolyte or protein imbalances or obstruction in the cardiovascular or lymphatic systems. With pitting edema tissues do not immediately spring back after being touched.	Massage is contraindicated for most types of edema. However, edema resulting from subacute soft-tissue injury, standing for long periods of time, or short-term immobility can be alleviated by massage as long as there is no other factor contraindicating treatment application.	12

Disease/Condition	Indications/Contraindications for Massage Therapy	Chapter Reference
Fibromyalgia This syndrome causes symptoms of widespread pain or aching, persistent fatigue; generalized morning stiffness; nonrestorative sleep; and multiple tender points.	General massage approaches seem to work best to help reduce pain and restore sleep patterns. The client should avoid any form of therapy that causes therapeutic inflammation, including intense exercise and stretching programs, until healing mechanisms in the body are functioning. If tender points have been injected with antiinflammatory medications, anesthetics, or other substances, the practitioner should not massage over these areas.	9

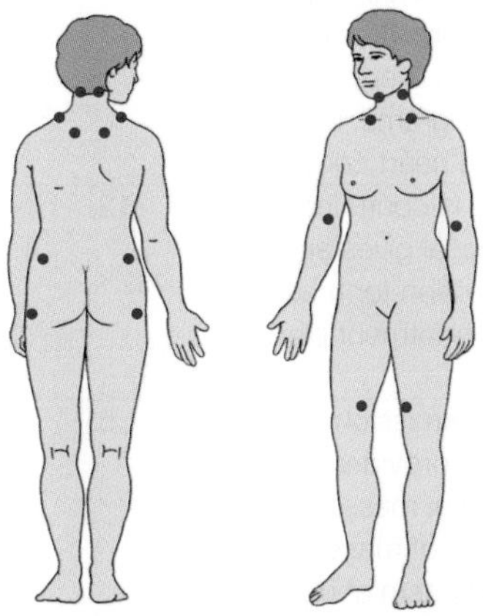

FIGURE B-9 Fibromyalgia tender points. (From Shiland BJ: *Mastering healthcare terminology,* ed 2, St Louis, 2006, Mosby.)

Disease/Condition	Indications/Contraindications for Massage Therapy	Chapter Reference
Gallbladder disease (cholelithiasis) The disease almost always results from a gallstone composed of bile salts or cholesterol lodged in the cystic duct. Abdominal pain or referred back pain may indicate one of several gastrointestinal disorders.	In such cases, referral is necessary for proper diagnosis.	12

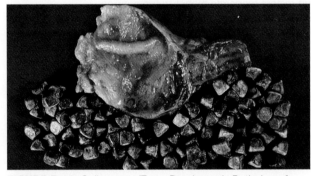

FIGURE B-10 Gallstones. (From Damjanov I: *Pathology for the health professions,* ed 4, St Louis, 2012, Saunders.)

Disease/Condition	Indications/Contraindications for Massage Therapy	Chapter Reference
Headache Pain occurs in the forehead, eyes, jaw, temples, scalp, skull, occiput, or neck.	Massage therapy is effective in treating muscle tension headache but much less so with migraine or cluster headaches. However, massage can relieve secondary muscle tension headache caused by the pain of the primary headache. Because headache is often stress induced, stress management in all forms usually is indicated for chronic headaches.	4

Continued

Disease/Condition	Indications/Contraindications for Massage Therapy	Chapter Reference
Heart attack A heart attack, also known as a *myocardial infarction,* is permanent damage to the myocardium caused by obstructed blood flow through the coronary arteries to the tissues.	Massage is contraindicated for clients recovering from recent heart attacks, but the gentle resting of hands on the body used in some forms of touch systems might be indicated with supervision. Once clients have completely recovered, if approval for massage is given by the client's health care provider, the practitioner may develop treatment plans according to the client's vitality. Comprehensive stress management programs, including therapeutic massage, can help manage heart conditions.	11
Hepatitis Hepatitis is an inflammation of the liver. It is usually, but not always, caused by viral infection. Acute hepatitis is contraindicated for massage.	Massage for clients with chronic hepatitis is contraindicated unless the client's health care professional gives approval and supervision. If approval and supervision for massage is given, the practitioner must develop treatment plans according to the client's vitality.	12
Herniated disk Herniated disk occurs when the fibrocartilage surrounding the intervertebral disk ruptures, releasing the nucleus pulposus.	Massage should not be performed until permission is given by the client's primary health care provider. Once permission has been given, regional massage is contraindicated. However, various forms of massage are important in managing the muscle spasm and pain surrounding the area of the herniated disk. The muscle spasms serve the stabilizing and protective function of guarding. Without some protective spasm, the nerve could be damaged further; however, too much muscle spasm increases the discomfort. The therapeutic treatment goals should be to reduce pain and excessive tension and restore moderate mobility while allowing the resourceful compensation produced by the muscle tension pattern.	5

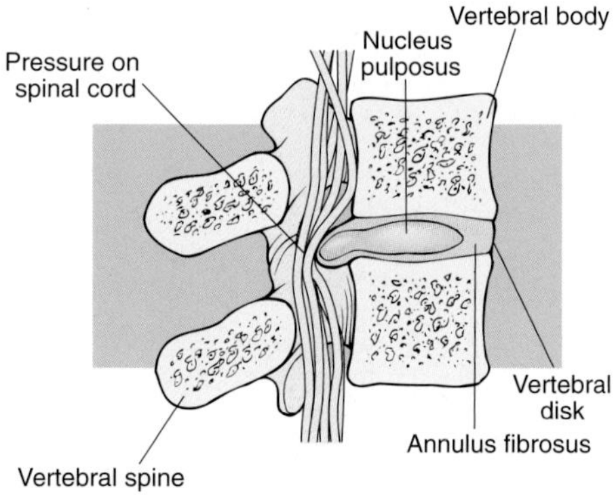

FIGURE B-11 Lateral view of a herniated disk, showing pressure on the spinal cord. (From Frazier MS, Drzymkowski JW: *Essentials of human diseases and conditions,* ed 4, St. Louis, 2008, Saunders.)

Disease/Condition	Indications/Contraindications for Massage Therapy	Chapter Reference
Hypertension This is the medical term for high blood pressure.	For borderline or mild hypertension, massage may be beneficial for managing stress and well being. However, if the hypertension is due to more serious conditions in the body, massage may be contraindicated. Hypertension that results from other cardiovascular diseases may be contraindicated for massage, but the gentle resting of hands on the body used in some forms of touch systems might be indicated with supervision.	11
Irritable bowel syndrome (IBS) IBS is also called *spastic,* or *irritable, colon.*	Most chronic gastrointestinal diseases, including IBS, have a strong correlation to stress. Comprehensive stress management programs, including therapeutic massage, can help manage these conditions.	12

Disease/Condition	Indications/Contraindications for Massage Therapy	Chapter Reference
Joint injuries Pain and swelling of joint injury can be overcome with the judicious and short-term use of pain medication, antiinflammatory medications, and appropriate rehabilitation exercise.	Massage, myofascial release, and trigger point work are often effective after the acute phase (2 to 3 days post injury). The application of ice along with rehabilitation exercise is beneficial. However, ice is contraindicated for some conditions and therefore should be used with caution. Management and rehabilitation of joint problems is a long-term process that often requires a multidisciplinary approach. Although direct work over an area that is actively healing is contraindicated unless supervised by the client's health care team, massage and other forms of soft-tissue work, coupled with movement therapies, can manage compensatory patterns that develop because of casting and other forms of immobilization.	8

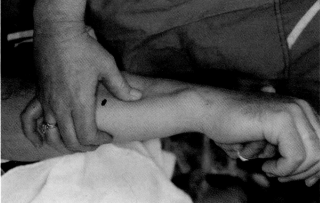

FIGURE B-12 Joint injury. (From Marcotte AL, Osterman AL: Longitudinal radioulnar dissociation: identification and treatment of acute and chronic injuries, *Hand Clinics* 23(2): 195-208, 2007.)

Disease/Condition	Indications/Contraindications for Massage Therapy	Chapter Reference
Kidney failure See Renal failure.		
Meningitis Meningitis is a bacterial or viral infection in the meninges, mainly in the subarachnoid fluid.	Because unusual or unexplained stiff neck is a symptom of encephalitis, clients with this condition should be immediately referred to their physicians for diagnosis. Infectious processes are contraindicated for massage.	4
Multiple sclerosis This involves the destruction of myelin sheaths around sensory and motor neurons in the central nervous system.	Supervised massage can be an effective part of a comprehensive long-term care program. Stress management also is an important component of an overall care program for any chronic disease. Massage and other forms of bodywork can help manage secondary muscle tension caused by the alteration of posture and the use of equipment such as wheelchairs, braces, and crutches. Treatments should be developed according to the client's vitality.	5

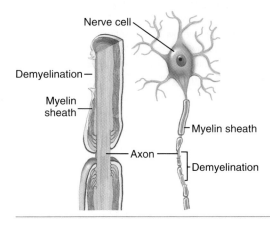

FIGURE B-13 Nerve sheath demyelination seen in multiple sclerosis. (From Shiland BJ: *Mastering healthcare terminology,* ed 3, St Louis, 2010, Mosby.)

Continued

Disease/Condition	Indications/Contraindications for Massage Therapy	Chapter Reference
Muscle spasms (entrapment) and shortening Muscle spasms are involuntary contractions of skeletal muscle. They are considered to be low-intensity, long-lasting contractions. However, their contractions may compress nerves traveling through them. This is referred to as *entrapment*. Examples of entrapments include thoracic outlet syndrome and piriformis syndrome.	Various forms of massage are important in managing muscle spasms and pain. The muscle spasms may serve the stabilizing and protective function of guarding. Without some protective spasm, the nerve could be damaged further; however, too much muscle spasm increases the discomfort. The therapeutic treatment goals should be to reduce pain and excessive tension and restore moderate mobility while allowing the resourceful compensation produced by the muscle tension pattern. Because of the joint structures involved, therapeutic massage should be incorporated into a total treatment program with supervision by the appropriate health care professional.	5
Muscle strain Strain is an injury to skeletal muscles from overexertion or trauma and can range from mild to severe.	Direct work over the area of injury is contraindicated regionally until all signs of inflammation have dissipated. The use of ice and gentle range of motion can support healing. The therapeutic treatment goals should be to reduce pain and excessive tension caused by compensating postural distortions.	9

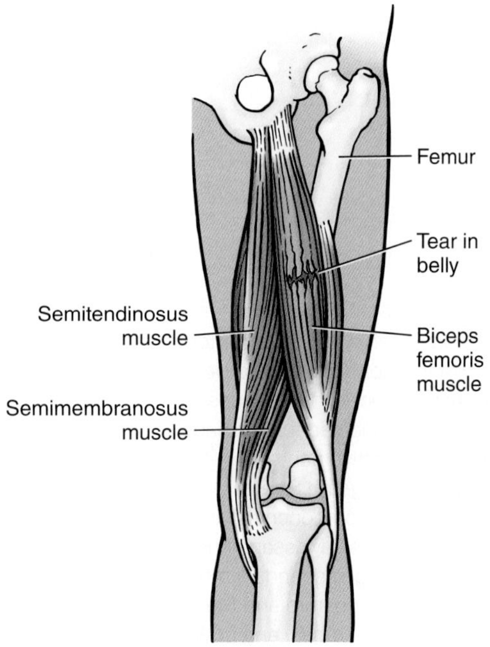

Femur

Tear in belly

Semitendinosus muscle

Biceps femoris muscle

Semimembranosus muscle

FIGURE B-14 Muscle strain. (From Fritz S: *Mosby's fundamentals of therapeutic massage*, ed 5, St. Louis, 2013, Mosby.)

Disease/Condition	Indications/Contraindications for Massage Therapy	Chapter Reference
Neuropathy Neuropathy is the inflammation or degeneration of the peripheral nerves. Nerve pain is difficult to manage and does not respond well to analgesics.	Massage may provide short-term pain relief by causing changes in neurotransmitter levels and stimulation of alternate nerve pathways, resulting in hyperstimulation analgesia and counterirritation. Any therapy that increases mood-elevating and pain-modulating mechanisms makes coping with nerve pain easier for short periods.	5

Disease/Condition	Indications/Contraindications for Massage Therapy	Chapter Reference
Osgood-Schlatter disease This disease occurs when the tibial tubercle becomes inflamed or separates from the tibia because of irritation caused by the patellar tendon pulling on the tubercle during periods of rapid growth or overuse of the quadriceps.	Regional massage may be contraindicated if inflammation or necrosis is present. Methods that relax and lengthen the muscle and soften the connective tissue are appropriate.	7

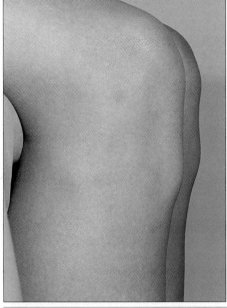

FIGURE B-15 Osgood-Schlatter disease. (From Hochberg MC et al: _Rheumatology_, ed 4, Edinburgh, 2008, Mosby.)

Disease/Condition	Indications/Contraindications for Massage Therapy	Chapter Reference
Osteoarthritis A degenerative joint disease, osteoarthritis is the breakdown of joints caused by normal wear and tear.	Because the progression and flare-ups of the disease are often stress related, the generalized gentle stress reduction methods provided by massage therapy may be beneficial in long-term management of the condition, if supervised as part of a total care program. The practitioner should avoid frictioning techniques or any other forms of bodywork that cause inflammation.	8
Osteogenesis imperfecta This group of hereditary disorders appears in newborns and young children. The bones are deformed and fragile as a result of demineralization and defective formation of connective tissue. If skeletal problems create or are part of a permanent condition, supportive care is required.	Massage methods are helpful in managing compensatory muscle spasms and connective tissue changes. Any type of compressive force or joint movement methods are contraindicated for a fragile skeletal structure, regardless of the cause, unless carefully supervised by the appropriate medical professionals. Light, superficial methods, such as resting the hands on the body, used in some forms of touch systems, might be indicated, again with supervision.	7

Continued

Disease/Condition	Indications/Contraindications for Massage Therapy	Chapter Reference
Osteomyelitis Osteomyelitis is infection in the bone that most commonly affects children and adults older than age 50.	Because this is an infectious disease, massage is contraindicated until permission is given by the client's primary health care provider.	7

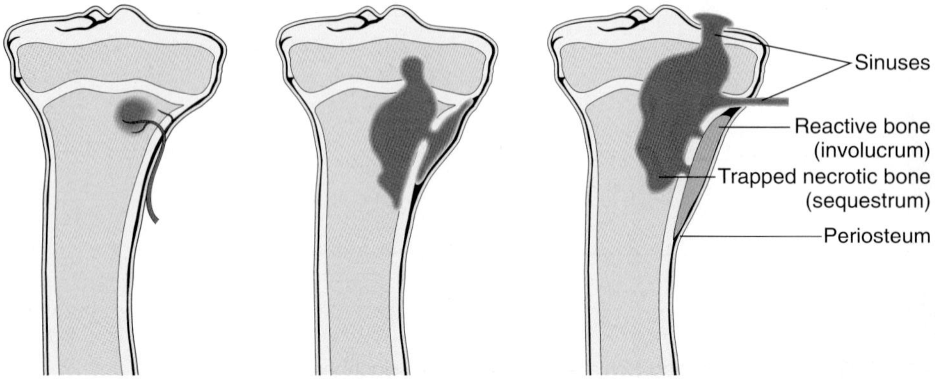

FIGURE B-16 Osteomyelitis. The bacteria reach the metaphysic through the nutrient artery. Bacterial growth results in bone destruction and formation of an abscess. From the abscess cavity, the pus spreads. The pus destroys the bone and sequesters parts of it in the abscess cavity. Reactive new bone is formed around the focus of inflammation. (From Damjanov I: *Pathology for the health professions,* ed 4, St Louis, 2012, Saunders.)

Disease/Condition	Indications/Contraindications for Massage Therapy	Chapter Reference
Osteonecrosis (ischemic necrosis) Osteonecrosis is the death of a segment of bone, usually caused by insufficient blood flow to the area.	Necrosis usually is a localized condition that requires regional avoidance of the involved bone area. Because massage provides the generalized effect of enhanced local circulation, massaging around the edges of the affected area may be beneficial. However, massage is contraindicated unless supervised by the client's primary health care provider.	7
Osteoporosis This disorder is caused by loss of bone mass and density as a result of endocrine imbalances and poor calcium metabolism. The bones become depleted of calcium, other minerals, and protein.	A fragile skeletal structure, regardless of the cause, is a contraindication for any type of compressive force or joint movement methods. Light, superficial methods, such as gentle resting of the hands used in some forms of touch systems, might be indicated.	7
Paget's disease (osteitis deformans) This is a chronic disorder in which healthy bone is quickly reabsorbed and replaced with fibrous connective tissue that never completely calcifies.	A fragile skeletal structure, regardless of the cause, is a contraindication for any type of compressive force or joint movement methods. Light, superficial methods, such as gentle resting of the hands used in some forms of touch systems might be indicated.	7

Disease/Condition	Indications/Contraindications for Massage Therapy	Chapter Reference

Parkinson's disease

In this disease neurons that release the neurotransmitter dopamine in the brain degenerate, thus slowing or stopping its release.

Because massage has been shown to increase dopamine activity, its use is indicated for managing Parkinson's disease and tremor. In addition, massage therapy and other forms of soft-tissue manipulation may help manage secondary muscle tension.

4

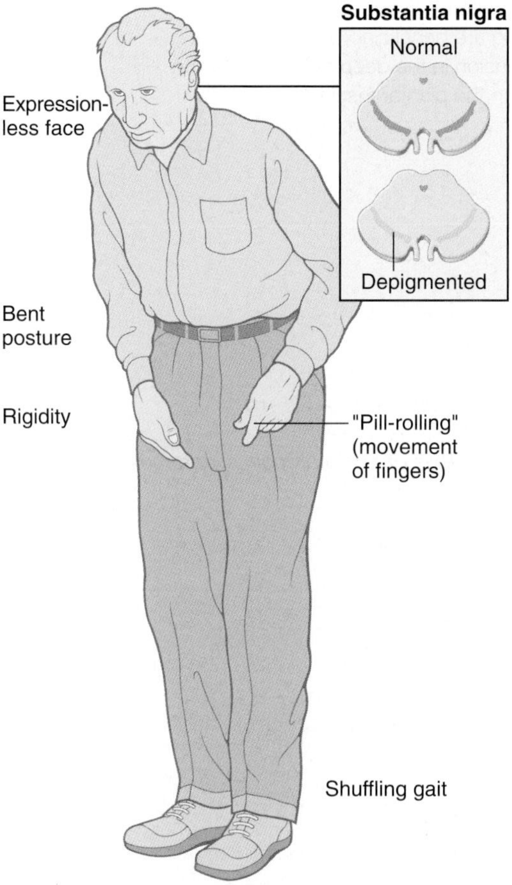

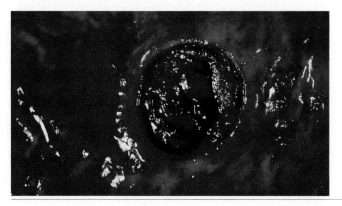

Expression-less face

Bent posture

Rigidity

Substantia nigra

Normal

Depigmented

"Pill-rolling" (movement of fingers)

Shuffling gait

FIGURE B-17 Signs and symptoms of Parkinson's disease. (From Damjanov I: *Pathology for the health professions,* ed 4, St Louis, 2012, Saunders.)

Peptic ulcer

A gastric or duodenal ulcer affects the lining of the esophagus, stomach, or duodenum. Ulcers result from tissue damage that never heals because of constant irritation or because healing mechanisms are impeded.

Deep abdominal massage is contraindicated for clients with peptic ulcers. Most chronic gastrointestinal diseases have a strong correlation to stress. Comprehensive stress management programs, including therapeutic massage methods, are often effective in managing stress.

12

FIGURE B-18 Peptic ulcer. (From Damjanov I: *Pathology for the health professions,* ed 4, St Louis, 2012, Saunders.)

Continued

Disease/Condition	Indications/Contraindications for Massage Therapy	Chapter Reference
Piriformis syndrome In this syndrome a hypertonic piriformis muscle compresses the sciatic nerve passing through it, resulting in sciatica-like symptoms.	Massage methods help relieve muscle entrapment of the nerve by relaxing and lengthening the muscles.	9
Plantar fasciitis The condition results from repeated microscopic injury to the plantar fascia and surrounding myofascial structures. Acute-phase plantar fasciitis responds to rest and ice.	After the inflammation has diminished, soft-tissue methods that address the connective tissue of the plantar fascia and gentle stretching are beneficial. Techniques that release muscular tension in the deep calf muscles can help reduce strain on the plantar fascia.	9

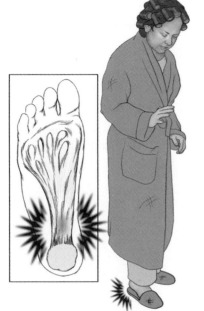

FIGURE B-19 Plantar fasciitis. (From Waldman S: *Atlas of common pain syndromes,* Philadelphia, 2002, Saunders.)

Disease/Condition	Indications/Contraindications for Massage Therapy	Chapter Reference
Preeclampsia Also termed *pregnancy-induced hypertension* or *toxemia,* the condition is a complication of pregnancy characterized by increasing hypertension, protein in the urine, and edema.	Massage is contraindicated.	12
Renal failure Also known as *kidney failure,* this disorder involves the inability of the kidneys to function normally. It may be acute or chronic, and it can be life threatening.	Massage therapy is contraindicated for both acute and chronic renal failure.	12

Disease/Condition	Indications/Contraindications for Massage Therapy	Chapter Reference
Rheumatoid arthritis This crippling condition is characterized by swelling of the joints in the hands, feet, and other parts of the body as a result of inflammation and overgrowth of the synovial membranes and other joint tissues.	Because the progression and flare-ups of the disease are often stress related, generalized gentle stress reduction massage may be beneficial in long-term management of the condition, if supervised as part of a total care program. The practitioner should avoid frictioning techniques or any other forms of bodywork that cause inflammation.	8

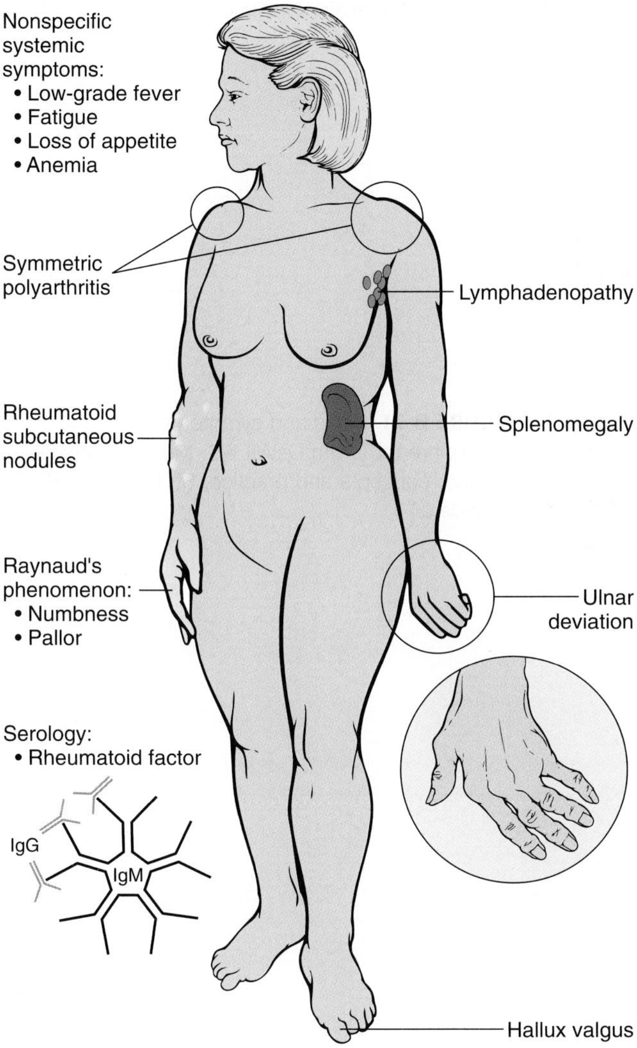

Nonspecific systemic symptoms:
- Low-grade fever
- Fatigue
- Loss of appetite
- Anemia

Symmetric polyarthritis

Lymphadenopathy

Rheumatoid subcutaneous nodules

Splenomegaly

Raynaud's phenomenon:
- Numbness
- Pallor

Ulnar deviation

Serology:
- Rheumatoid factor

IgG

IgM

Hallux valgus

FIGURE B-20 Signs and symptoms of rheumatoid arthritis. *IgG,* Immunoglobulin G; *IgM,* immunoglobulin M. (From Damjanov I: *Pathology for the health professions,* ed 4, St Louis, 2012, Saunders.)

Continued

Disease/Condition	Indications/Contraindications for Massage Therapy	Chapter Reference
Rotator cuff tear Tears often are caused by repeated impingement, overuse, or other conditions that weaken the rotator cuff and eventually cause partial or complete tears.	Massage techniques applied to acute myofascial tears are contraindicated. However, massage therapy may be indicated in the rehabilitative process and as part of a supervised treatment protocol. Massage may be able to help manage and improve compensatory patterns.	9
Schizophrenia Schizophrenia is the most common mental disorder and includes a large group of psychotic disorders characterized by gross distortion of reality; disturbances of language and communication; withdrawal from social interaction; and disorganization and fragmentation of thought, perception, and emotional reaction.	Therapeutic massage may be supportive in a multidisciplinary approach to treatment because such methods influence neurotransmitters. However, supervision by the client's health provider is necessary.	4

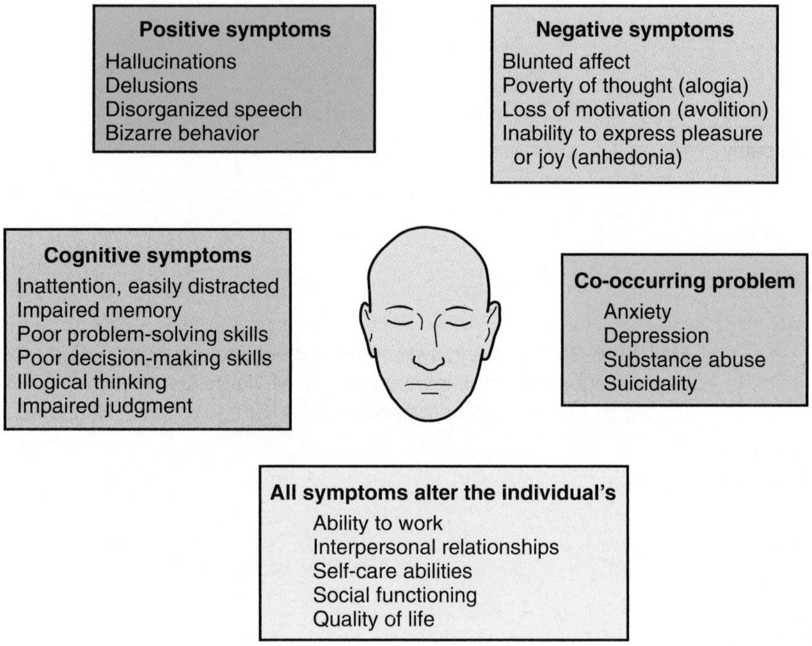

Positive symptoms
Hallucinations
Delusions
Disorganized speech
Bizarre behavior

Negative symptoms
Blunted affect
Poverty of thought (alogia)
Loss of motivation (avolition)
Inability to express pleasure or joy (anhedonia)

Cognitive symptoms
Inattention, easily distracted
Impaired memory
Poor problem-solving skills
Poor decision-making skills
Illogical thinking
Impaired judgment

Co-occurring problem
Anxiety
Depression
Substance abuse
Suicidality

FIGURE B-21 Signs and symptoms of schizophrenia. (From DeWit SC: Medical-surgical nursing: concepts and practice, St. Louis, 2009, Saunders.)

All symptoms alter the individual's
Ability to work
Interpersonal relationships
Self-care abilities
Social functioning
Quality of life

Disease/Condition	Indications/Contraindications for Massage Therapy	Chapter Reference

Sciatica

This is inflammation of the sciatic nerve. It originates in the low back or hip and radiates down the leg.

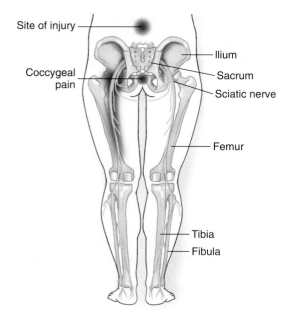

Site of injury
Coccygeal pain
Ilium
Sacrum
Sciatic nerve
Femur
Tibia
Fibula

FIGURE B-22 Sciatica. (From Shiland BJ: *Mastering healthcare terminology,* ed 3, St Louis, 2010, Mosby.)

Massage treatments should be developed on the basis of the cause of sciatica. If it is caused by a herniated disk, massage should not be performed until permission is given by the client's primary health care provider. Once permission has been given, regional massage is contraindicated. However, various forms of massage are important in managing the muscle spasm and pain surrounding the area of the herniated disk. The muscle spasms serve the stabilizing and protective function of guarding. Without some protective spasm, the nerve could be damaged further; however, too much muscle spasm increases the discomfort. If the cause is piriformis syndrome, then regional massage is indicated. Whether the cause of sciatica is a herniated disk or piriformis syndrome, the therapeutic treatment goals should be to reduce pain and excessive tension and restore moderate mobility while allowing the resourceful compensation produced by the muscle tension pattern.

5

Shingles

This is a painful outbreak of the herpes zoster virus along sensory neurons. Herpes zoster is the same virus that causes chickenpox. After an episode of chickenpox, the virus retreats to the dorsal root ganglia, where the immune system usually keeps it in check. Sometimes, however, the virus is able to overcome the immune system, and shingles result. Blisters form along the peripheral nerves associated with the dorsal root ganglia that house the virus.

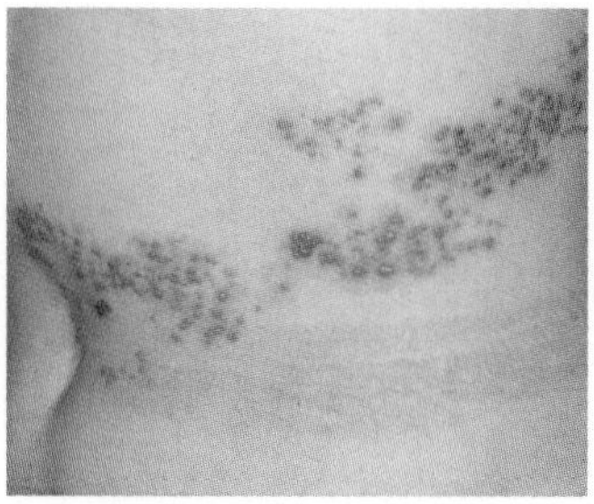

Because it is so painful, massage is contraindicated in the acute stages. After the blisters have healed and the pain has gone away, massage is indicated.

5

FIGURE B-23 Shingles. (From Habif T: *Clinical dermatology,* ed 4, St. Louis, 2004, Mosby.)

Continued

Disease/Condition	Indications/Contraindications for Massage Therapy	Chapter Reference
Spinal cord injury Spinal cord injury involves damage to the spinal cord. The damage usually results from trauma but can also result from tumors or bony growths in the spinal canal. Loss of motor function in the lower extremities is paraplegia; loss of motor function in both the upper and lower extremities is quadriplegia.	Massage is an effective part of a comprehensive, supervised rehabilitation and long-term care program. Massage and other forms of bodywork can help manage secondary muscle tension resulting from the alteration of posture and the use of equipment such as wheelchairs, braces, and crutches. Specifically focused massage can help manage difficulties with bowel paralysis. Because massage increases local blood flow, it can help prevent or manage decubitus ulcers.	4

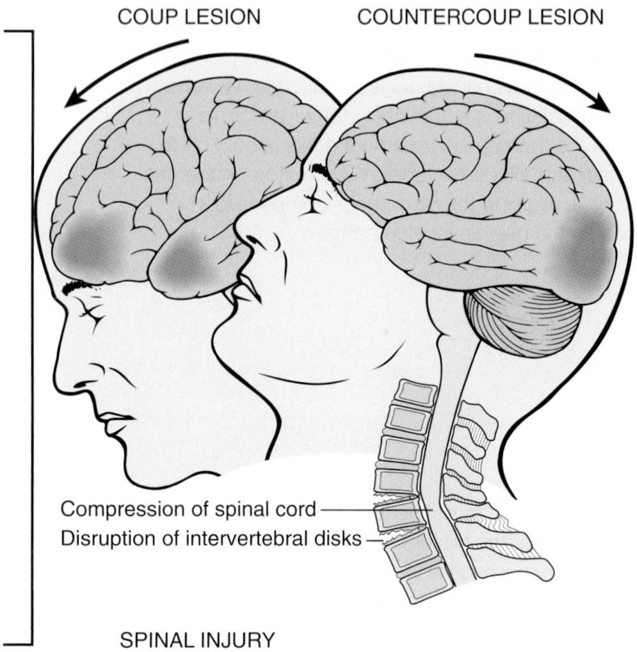

COUP LESION   COUNTERCOUP LESION

Compression of spinal cord
Disruption of intervertebral disks

SPINAL INJURY

FIGURE B-24 Spinal cord trauma. A coup lesion of the brain occurs at the site of impact, whereas a countercoup lesion is diametrically opposite to the coup lesion. The spinal cord lesion depicted here is caused by hyperextension. (From Damjanov I: *Pathology for the health professions,* ed 4, St Louis, 2012, Saunders.)

Disease/Condition	Indications/Contraindications for Massage Therapy	Chapter Reference
Spondylolisthesis In this condition a vertebra becomes displaced anteriorly. It can occur almost anywhere on the space, but it happens most often in the lower spine.	Various forms of massage are important in managing the muscle spasm and pain in the accompanying backache. The muscle spasms serve the stabilizing and protective function of guarding. Without some protective spasm, the nerve could be damaged further; however, too much muscle spasm increases the discomfort. The therapeutic treatment goals should be to reduce pain and excessive tension and restore moderate mobility while allowing the resourceful compensation produced by the muscle tension pattern. Because of the joint structures involved, therapeutic massage should be incorporated into a total treatment program with supervision by the appropriate health care professional.	8

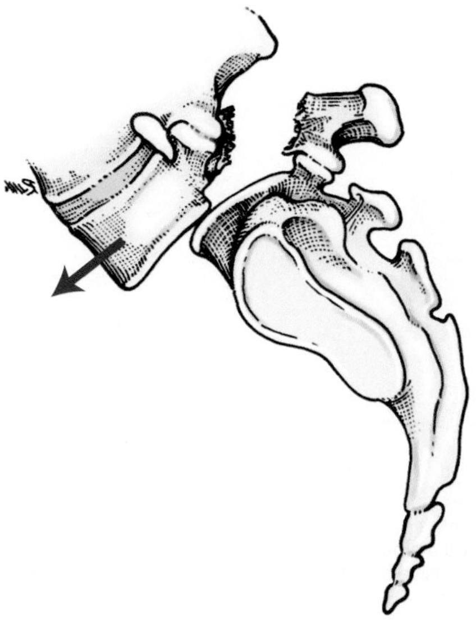

FIGURE B-25 Spondylolisthesis. (In Neumann DA: *Kinesiology of the musculoskeletal system: foundations for physical rehabilitation*, ed 2, St Louis, 2010.)

Continued

Disease/Condition	Indications/Contraindications for Massage Therapy	Chapter Reference
Stroke Stroke is sudden loss of neurologic function caused by a vascular injury to the brain. The interrupted blood supply causes brain tissue to die. Stroke is a medical emergency requiring immediate referral.	Once the client is recovering, massage and bodywork can be an effective part of a supervised comprehensive care program. Massage and other forms of bodywork can help manage secondary muscle tension resulting from the alteration of posture and the use of equipment such as wheelchairs, braces, and crutches.	4

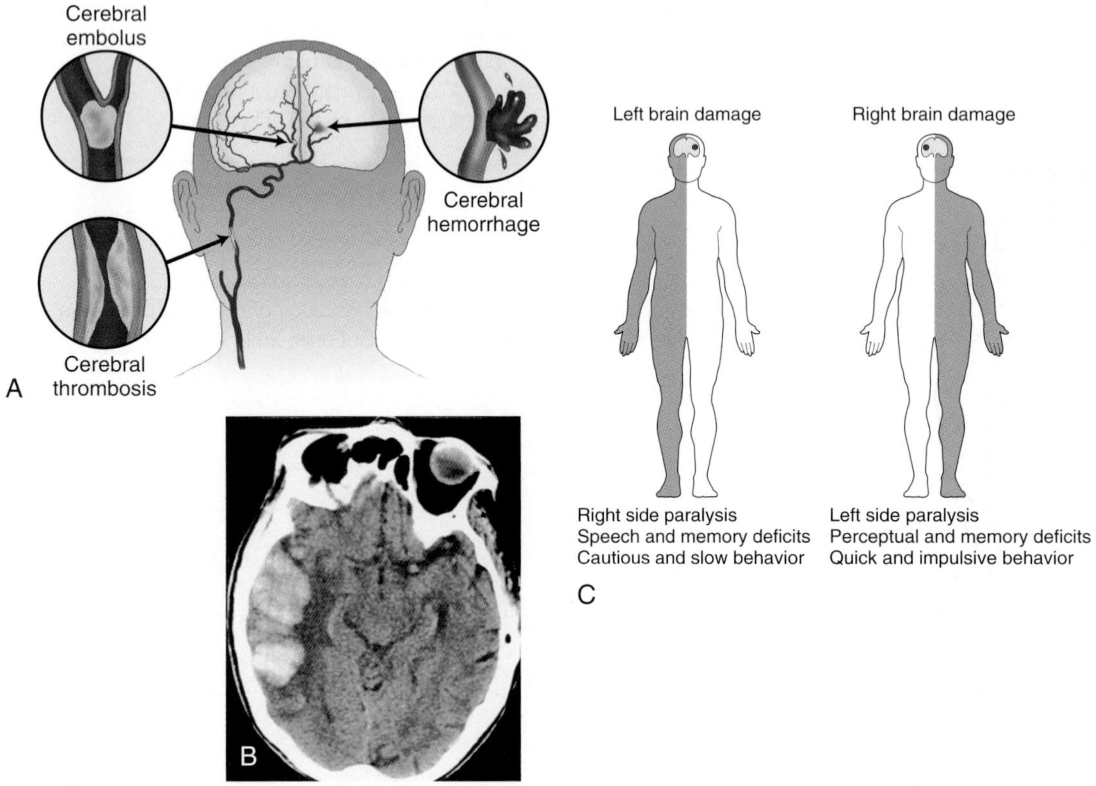

FIGURE B-26   Cerebrovascular accident (CVA). **A,** Events causing stroke. **B,** Magnetic resonance imaging showing hemorrhagic stroke in right cerebrum. **C,** Areas of the body affected by CVA. (**A,C** from Shiland BJ: *Mastering healthcare terminology,* ed 3, St Louis, 2010, Mosby; **B** from Black J: *Medical-surgical nursing,* ed 8, St. Louis, 2009, Saunders.)

Disease/Condition	Indications/Contraindications for Massage Therapy	Chapter Reference
Tendinitis/tenosynovitis Tendinitis is inflammation of a tendon; tenosynovitis is inflammation of a tendon sheath.	Any massage methods that increase the inflammatory response are contraindicated. In the acute phase the use of ice and gentle movement are indicated. Chronic conditions may benefit from methods that elongate the connective tissue structures, relieving the irritation that caused the inflammation in the area.	9

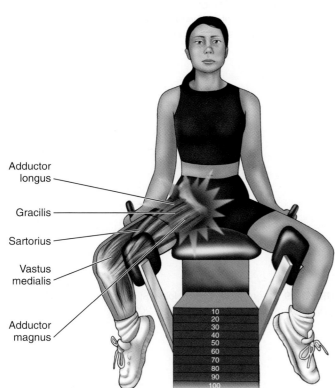

Adductor longus
Gracilis
Sartorius
Vastus medialis
Adductor magnus

FIGURE B-27 Tendinitis/tenosynovitis. (From Waldman S: *Atlas of uncommon pain syndromes*, ed 2, Philadelphia, 2008, Saunders.)

| ***Thoracic outlet syndrome***
This syndrome occurs when the brachial plexus and blood supply of the arm become entrapped, resulting in shooting pains, weakness, and numbness. | Massage methods help relieve muscle entrapment of nerves by relaxing and lengthening the muscles. | 9 |

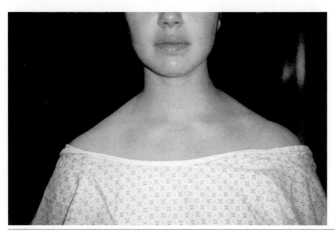

FIGURE B-28 Thoracic outlet syndrome. (From Lederman RJ: Peripheral neuropathies in instrumental musicians, *Phys Med Rehab North Am* 17(4): 761-779, 2006.)

Continued

Disease/Condition	Indications/Contraindications for Massage Therapy	Chapter Reference
Thrombosis A thrombus is a blood clot. The process of forming a clot in an unbroken blood vessel is called *thrombosis*. A blood clot, bubble of air, fat from broken bones, or a piece of debris transported by the bloodstream is called an *embolus*. When an embolus becomes lodged in a blood vessel smaller in diameter than it is, this situation is called an *embolism*. For example, an embolus that becomes lodged in the lungs is called a *pulmonary embolism*. The major danger of thrombosis and embolisms is that they block vital blood flow to tissues. A common place for thrombosis is in the lower extremities because gravity impedes venous return. This is called a *deep venous thrombosis* (DVT), and it may cause inflammation in the tissues.	Massage therapy is contraindicated regionally and possibly generally because of the pain associated with thrombosis and because massage can further damage debilitated tissues. Clients who are prone to thrombosis take anti-coagulant medications such as heparin or warfarin. These medications made the client more susceptible to bruising so lighter pressure is indicated during massage, and, of course, avoiding the area in which the thrombus is located.	11

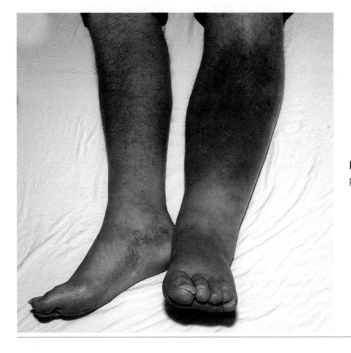

FIGURE B-29 Thrombosis. (From Noble S: Other problems in palliative care, *Medicine* 36(2): 100-104, 2008.)

Disease/Condition	Indications/Contraindications for Massage Therapy	Chapter Reference
Torticollis Also called *wry neck,* this condition involves a spasm or shortening of one of the sternocleidomastoid muscles.	Management of torticollis with massage therapy involves relaxing the neck, releasing trigger points, stretching the contracted muscles, and improving range of motion. Pressure on the blood vessels and nerves deep to the sternocleidomastoid should be avoided.	9

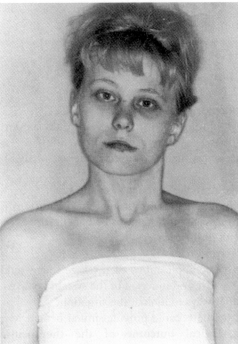

FIGURE B-30 Torticollis in 18-year-old girl. (From Tachdjian MO: *Pediatric orthopedics*, p. 68, Philadelphia, 1972, Saunders.)

Disease/Condition	Indications/Contraindications for Massage Therapy	Chapter Reference
Vertigo Vertigo is the sensation that the body or environment is spinning or swaying.	Movement therapies can help or aggravate vertigo; therefore the practitioner must take care to design an individual therapeutic program on the basis of the client's history. Massage methods can deal effectively with muscle tension and diminish anxiety and nausea, but the benefit is temporary because the symptoms return with a recurrence of vertigo.	5
Whiplash Whiplash is an injury to the soft tissues of the neck caused by sudden hyperextension or flexion (or both) of the neck.	Massage treatment during the acute phase is contraindicated unless closely supervised by a physician or other qualified health care professional. Massage methods are valuable as part of rehabilitation in the subacute phase and can help restore function if the condition is chronic. Extension injury is more severe and requires more carefully applied massage techniques.	9

At the end of Chapters 11 and 12, the student was asked to consider massage as a therapeutic intervention and to use the clinical reasoning model to justify the effectiveness of the massage method in supporting balanced functioning of each system involved. One can use this same approach to justify the use of therapeutic massage when dealing with disease or dysfunction. Students must be able to explain and justify the ways in which therapeutic massage is beneficial in supporting optimal function and how massage can manage an existing condition or support a return to health if a pathologic condition exists.

In completing the clinical reasoning activities, the student will need to refer to other sections of this text. Section Two, Systems of Control, is particularly useful. The student also will need knowledge of the therapeutic massage approach being justified. (See *Mosby's Fundamentals of Therapeutic Massage*, edition 5, 2013.)

These exercises, when well thought out, should help the student understand the connection between what is done (the therapeutic massage method) and what is affected (the change in physiology). Because what is done (the massage method) depends on where it is done (the anatomy), putting all the pieces together in an explanation of the benefits of massage will help the student not only to understand the process but also to educate others. This is particularly important when developing goal-oriented and outcome-based treatment plans for massage application.

Therapeutic Massage: Clinical Reasoning Model for Problem Solving and Justification

1. **What are the facts?**
   a. Which system is involved, and which structures of that system can be reached directly and indirectly?
   b. Which of these structures are most affected by this massage?
   c. Which physiologic functions are affected by massage?
   d. When the treatment is applied, what changes in function will result in
      (1) this system
      (2) the whole body
   e. What is considered normal or balanced function?
   f. How are the functions of this system related to the homeostasis of the body?

g. What has worked or has not worked?
   h. Where could you find information that would support the use of massage as a therapeutic intervention?
   i. What research is available to support the use of therapeutic massage?
   j. How does the massage support a healthy state?
   k. Under which pathologic or dysfunctional conditions is therapeutic massage most likely to be beneficial?

2. **What are the possibilities?**
   a. What do the data suggest?
   b. List at least three applications of massage that would affect the structure and function of the system involved.
   c. What are other ways to look at the situation?
   d. What other methods could provide similar benefits?

3. **What is the logical outcome of the therapeutic intervention?**
   a. What would be the logical progression of the symptom pattern, contributing factors, and current behavior?
   b. What are the benefits and drawbacks of using therapeutic massage as suggested?
   c. What are the costs in terms of time, resources, and finances?
   d. What is likely to happen if massage is not used?
   e. What is likely to happen if massage is used?

4. **What would be the effect on the persons involved if massage intervention was used, specifically the client, the practitioner, and other professionals working with the client?**
   a. How does each person involved (including, besides the foregoing, the client's family and support system) feel about therapeutic massage?
   b. Does the practitioner feel qualified to work with the situation and apply massage to the particular person?
   c. Does a feeling of cooperation and agreement exist among all those involved? How would the practitioner recognize this feeling?

Justification

Using the information developed in the clinical reasoning model, present a clear, concise, valid statement of how massage would be beneficial in supporting the particular body system in a healthy condition or as part of a treatment plan for a pathologic or dysfunctional condition.

Example of the Clinical Reasoning Process Used to Create a Justification Statement

The following example applies this process to the muscular system.

1. **What are the facts?**

   a. Which system is involved, and which structures of that system can be reached directly and indirectly?
   The muscles and associated connective tissue are involved, along with various nerves and sensory receptors. The circulation to the muscles is affected as well.

   b. Which of these structures are most affected by this massage?

   c. Which physiologic functions are affected by massage?

   d. When the treatment is applied, what changes in function will result in
   (1) this system
   (2) the whole body
   Muscle tension patterns and reflexes may be restored to balanced function if imbalances exist. Connective tissue may normalize, usually by becoming more pliable, although specific methods can be used to firm lax connective tissue. Circulation will be normalized.

   e. What is considered normal or balanced function?
   The muscles maintain posture, produce movement, stabilize joints, and generate heat efficiently without wasting energy. The muscles should be able to respond to activation of the sympathetic portion of the autonomic nervous system and then return to a relaxed state.

   f. How are the functions of this system related to the homeostasis of the body?
   The pumping action of muscle contraction supports blood and lymph circulation. Maintenance of a constant internal heat is an important part of muscle action. Support of posture and joint stability provides space for internal organs and efficient operation without restriction. Movement is used to obtain air and food and to ensure survival.

   g. What has worked or has not worked?
   Many different forms of massage produce beneficial results for the muscles. The basic approaches include compression, lifting, kneading, tapping, and horizontal gliding, along with various forms of active and passive movement and muscle contraction methods. The intensity, duration, and rhythm of massage applications depend on the desired results. Therapeutic massage could relax the muscles, reduce pain, increase blood and lymph circulation, increase nutrition to the muscles, and encourage repair of muscles. However, the benefits of extremely painful massage application may be diminished by activation of the defensive mechanisms of the body.

   h. Where could you find information that would support the use of massage as a therapeutic intervention?
   Textbooks; research institutes; various medical, nursing, physical therapy, chiropractic, and bodywork journals; professional organizations; clinical application by other professionals; and the Internet.

   i. What research is available to support the use of therapeutic massage?
   - American Massage Therapy Association (AMTA) Data Base: www.amtamassage.org
   - Field T: *Touch therapy,* Edinburgh, 2000, Churchill Livingstone
   - Greenman P: *Principles of manual medicine,* ed 2, Baltimore, 1996, Williams & Wilkins
   - MedLine: *http://www.medline.com*
   - Yates J: *Physiological effects of therapeutic massage and their application to treatment,* ed 2, Vancouver, 1999, British Columbia Massage Therapist Association
   - Leon Chaitow: Although not a researcher, this author effectively translates research into useful application.

   j. How does the massage support a healthy state?
   The various types of sensory stimulation provided by massage result in alteration of the nervous system control mechanisms toward more balanced function. The more mechanical normalization of associated connective tissue supports pliability and stability of the muscles. Massage supports circulation.

   k. Under which pathologic or dysfunctional conditions is the therapeutic massage most likely to be beneficial?
   Increased or decreased muscle tension from daily mechanical and emotional stress. Management of pain resulting from such alterations. Compression on nerves or vessels from increased muscle tension and the resulting pain and dysfunction.

2. **What are the possibilities?**

   a. What do the data suggest?
   The data suggest (1) normal muscle function needs support to maintain health, (2) the development of muscle problems that could be reversed readily, restoring the system to health, or (3) a serious pathologic condition that requires several interventions.

   b. List at least three applications of massage that would affect the structure and function of the system involved.
   Compression spreads muscle fibers, affects proprioception, and increases circulation. The "tense, relax, and lengthen" techniques affect reflex mechanisms. Tapping at the muscle tendon strengthens muscles through its effect on the tendon organ. Kneading mechanically increases connective tissue ground substance pliability.

   c. What are other ways to look at the situation?
   The muscle symptoms could be a reflection of a pathologic neurologic condition; medications may be influencing the muscle system; or emotional armoring in the muscles may provide effective coping patterns. A pathologic condition of the connective tissue may be present. Muscle tension patterns may be appropriate compensation patterns for joint instability or bone fragility.

   d. What other methods could provide similar benefits?
   Various forms of aerobic exercise; stretching programs (e.g., yoga); physical therapy; and medications.

3. **What is the logical outcome of the therapeutic intervention?**

   a. What would be the logical progression of the symptom pattern, contributing factors, and current behavior?

Increased muscle tension is a waste of energy, a common source of pain, and often interferes with sleep patterns. Any long-term sleep interference affects the restorative processes of the body. More serious pathologic conditions could result from the increased levels of stress.

b. What are the benefits and drawbacks of using therapeutic massage as suggested?

Benefits:

Massage is pleasurable, often easily accepted by the client, and effective in short-term symptom control of muscle dysfunction.

Massage can replace or reduce the use of palliative types of medication such as muscle relaxants and analgesics.

Drawback:

Massage is not curative and requires continual maintenance intervention to support benefits.

c. What are the costs in terms of time, resources, and finances?

Compared with other interventions, massage is cost-effective even for long-term intervention. Weekly or biweekly 1-hour sessions can produce sustainable results. A maintenance schedule, once goals have been achieved, can be less intensive and therefore less costly. Massage professionals are found easily in most areas. Home and office care often are available.

d. What is likely to happen if massage is not used?

Muscle tension could increase and the symptoms worsen. More serious pathologic conditions could develop.

e. What is likely to happen if massage is used?

Daily stress management and support for healthy function of the muscle system could be achieved, and use of over-the-counter or prescription medications could be reduced.

4. **What would be the effect on the persons involved if massage intervention was used, specifically the client, the practitioner, and other professionals working with the client?**

a. How does each person involved (including, besides the foregoing, the client's family and support system) feel about therapeutic massage?

Touch intervention can be nurturing to many clients; however, those who have experienced many of the various forms of touch trauma may not have predictable responses to the intense duration of touch in the form of massage. Health care professionals still are confused about the benefits and applications of massage. The practitioner may have issues of countertransference with the client that would need to be addressed.

b. Does the practitioner feel qualified to work with the situation and apply massage to the particular person?

Depending on the practitioner's training and the client's therapeutic goals, as well as the support of other health care or training professionals, most situations can be addressed effectively with some sort of massage intervention. The more complex the situation, the more support and training are required.

c. Does a feeling of cooperation and agreement exist among all those involved? How would the practitioner recognize this feeling?

Support and cooperation depend on shared knowledge and the ability to educate in the benefits of massage. Free exchange of information with the client's permission and the client's willingness to participate would indicate cooperation.

Note: The previous questions stimulate thought processes and support more effective information gathering. The information then is evaluated, organized, and condensed to form a short, concise, and valid justification statement.

Justification

Therapeutic massage provides a pleasurable, easily accessible, cost-effective approach to support normal function of the muscular system. Massage increases circulation and waste removal from the muscles, maintains normal connective tissue structures, encourages appropriate neuromuscular interaction, and enhances general restorative functions.

The practitioner can manage muscle tension and pain syndromes effectively using massage as a treatment method. The general benefits listed are important in the treatment of these conditions. Massage can provide some of the same short-term benefits as medication for muscle tension and pain without the side effects.

Glossary

Abduction Lateral movement away from the midline of the trunk.

Absorption The movement of food molecules from the digestive tract to the cardiovascular and lymphatic systems so they can be transported to the cells of the body.

Acceleration The rate of change in speed.

Acetylcholine A neurotransmitter that stimulates the parasympathetic nervous system and the skeletal muscles and is involved in memory.

Acne A chronic inflammation of the sebaceous glands and hair follicles caused by interactions among bacteria, sebum, and sex hormones.

Active transport The transport of substances into or out of a cell using energy.

Activities of daily living Normal daily living activity, such as eating, bathing, dressing, grooming, going to work, performing housekeeping duties, and engaging in leisure activities.

Acupuncture The practice of inserting needles at specific points on meridians, or channels, to stimulate or sedate energy flow to regulate or alter body function. A branch of Chinese medicine, acupuncture is the art and science of manipulating the flow of Qi, the basic life force, and of xue, the blood, body fluids, and nourishing essences. Western medicine uses acupuncture primarily to reduce pain. Acupressure, which uses digital pressure, follows the same Asian principles.

Acute diseases Disease that has a specific beginning and signs and symptoms that develop quickly, last a short time, and then disappear.

Acute pain Pain that is usually temporary, of sudden onset, and easily localized. Acute pain can be a symptom of a disease process or a temporary aspect of medical treatment. Acting as a warning signal, acute pain activates the sympathetic nervous system.

Adduction A medial movement toward the midline of the body.

Adenosine triphosphate (ATP) A compound that stores energy in the muscles. When ATP is broken down during catabolic reactions, it releases energy.

Adrenergic Stimulation of the sympathetic nervous system causing a release of epinephrine and similar neurotransmitters and hormones.

Afferent Toward a center or point of reference.

Afferent nerves Sensory nerves that link sensory receptors with the central nervous system and transmit sensory information.

Agonist A muscle that causes or controls joint motion through a specified plane of motion; also known as a *mover*.

Alimentary canal The tube-shaped portion of the digestive system known as the *gastrointestinal tract*, the alimentary canal is about 30 feet long and contains several special structures throughout its length.

All-or-none response The property of a muscle fiber (cell) which, when stimulated to contract, contracts to its full ability or does not contract at all.

Alopecia Hair loss or baldness on parts or all of the body.

Amphiarthrosis A slightly movable joint that connects bone to bone with fibrocartilage or hyaline growth cartilage. The two types in the human body are symphyses and synchondroses.

Amyotrophic lateral sclerosis Also called *Lou Gehrig's disease.* A progressive disease that begins in the central nervous system and involves the degeneration of motor neurons and the subsequent atrophy of voluntary muscle.

Anabolism Chemical processes in the body that join simple compounds to form more complex compounds of carbohydrates, lipids, proteins, and nucleic acids. The processes require energy supplied from adenosine triphosphate.

Anaplasia Meaning "without shape," the term describes abnormal or undifferentiated cells that fail to mature into specialized cell types. Anaplasia is a characteristic of malignant cells.

Anatomic position A standard position in which the person stands upright with the feet slightly apart, arms hanging at the sides, and palms facing forward with thumbs outward.

Anatomic range of motion The amount of motion available to a joint based on the structure of the joint and determined by the shape of the joint surfaces, joint capsule, ligaments, muscle bulk, and surrounding musculotendinous and bony structures. The anatomic range of motion is the limit of passive range of motion.

Anatomy The study of the structures of the body and the relationship of its parts.

Androgens Male sex hormones.

Anemia A decrease in the normal number of red blood cells or in the amount of hemoglobin or iron in the blood.

Aneurysm A permanent dilation of part of a blood vessel caused by weakness or damage to its structure. The most common sites of aneurysms are the aorta and the arteries of the brain.

Antagonist A muscle usually located on the opposite side of a joint from the mover (agonist) and having the opposite action. The antagonist must lengthen when the mover contracts and shortens.

Anterior pelvic rotation Anterior movement of the upper pelvis; the iliac crest tilts forward in a sagittal plane.

Antibodies Serum proteins of the immunoglobulin class that are secreted by plasma cells.

Antigen Any substance that causes the body to produce antibodies.

Aorta The large artery that carries oxygen and nutrients out of the heart.

Apical surface The surface of epithelial cells that is exposed to the external environment.

Apocrine A type of sweat gland that discharges a thicker and more odoriferous form of sweat.

Aponeurosis A broad, flat sheet of fibrous connective tissue.

Appendicular skeleton The part of the skeleton composed of the limbs and their attachments.

Arterioles The smallest arteries.

Arteriosclerosis A term meaning "hardening of the arteries;" refers to arteries that have lost their elasticity.

Artery A blood vessel that transports oxygenated blood from the heart to the body or deoxygenated blood from the heart to the lungs.

Arthritis The most common type of joint disorder, *arthritis* literally means "inflammation of the joint."

Arthrokinematics Movement of bone surface in the joint capsule including roll, spin, and slide.

Articulation A place where two or more bones meet to connect parts and allow for movement in the body. Also called A joint.

Ascending tracts Tracts in the spinal cord that carry sensory information to the brain.

Atherosclerosis A condition in which fatty plaque is deposited in medium-sized and large arteries.

Atom The smallest particle of an element that retains and exhibits the properties of that element. Atoms are made up of protons, neutrons, and electrons.

Atrium One of the two small, thin-walled upper chambers of the heart.

Atrophy A decrease in the size of a body part or organ caused by a decrease in the size of the cells.

Attachments Connections of skeletal muscles to bones; often referred to as the *origin* and *insertion.*

Autonomic nervous system A division of the peripheral nervous system composed of nerves that connect the central nervous system to the glands, heart, and smooth muscles to maintain the internal body environment.

Avulsion Injury to a ligament or tendon involving tearing off of its attachment.

Axial skeleton The axis of the body; the axial skeleton consists of the head, vertebral column, ribs, and sternum.

Axis Series of glands that signal each other in a sequence

Axon A single elongated projection from the nerve cell body that transmits impulses away from the cell body.

Balance The ability to control equilibrium. Two types of balance are static, or still, balance and dynamic, or moving, balance.

Ball-and-socket joint Joint that allows movement in many directions around a central point. Ball-and-socket joints are ball-shaped convex surfaces fitted into concave sockets. This type of joint gives the greatest freedom of movement but also is the most easily dislocated.

Basal metabolic rate The rate of energy expenditure of the body in a quiet, resting, fasting state.

Basal surface The tissue surface that faces the inside of the body.

Basement membrane A permeable membrane that attaches epithelial tissues to the underlying connective tissues.

Benign (be-NINE) Usually describing a noncancerous tumor that is contained and does not spread. More broadly, it can also be defined by a term such as *nonthreatening* to cover instances when the tumor is not associated with cancer.

Biologic rhythm The internal, periodic timing component of an organism, also known as a *biorhythm.*

Biomechanics The principles and methods of mechanics applied to the structure and function of the human body.

Blood A thick red fluid that provides oxygen, nourishment, and protection to the cells and carries away waste products.

Blood pressure The measurement of pressure exerted by the blood on the walls of the blood vessels. The highest pressure exerted is called *systolic pressure,* which results when the ventricles contract. Diastolic pressure, the lowest pressure, results when the ventricles relax.

Brain The largest and most complex unit of the nervous system, the brain is responsible for perception, sensation, emotion, intellect, and action.

Brainstem The inferior, primitive portion of the brain that contains centers for vital functions and reflex actions, such as vomiting, coughing, sneezing, posture, and basic movement patterns.

Breathing pattern disorder A complex set of behaviors that leads to overbreathing without the presence of a pathologic condition.

Buffers Compounds that prevent the hydrogen ion concentration from fluctuating too much and too rapidly to alter the pH.

Bursa A flat sac of synovial membrane in which the inner sides of the sac are separated by a fluid film. Bursae are located where moving structures rub over each other and are considered high-friction areas.

Bursitis Inflammation of a bursa.

Callus An area of thickened, hardened skin that develops in an area of friction or region of recurrent pressure.

Cancer Malignant, nonencapsulated cells that invade surrounding tissue. They often break away, or metastasize, from the primary tumor and form secondary cancer masses.

Capillary The smallest blood vessel; found between arteries and veins. Capillaries allow the exchange of gases, nutrients, and waste products.

Carbohydrates Sugars, starches, and cellulose composed of carbon, hydrogen, and oxygen.

Cardiac cycle A synchronized sequence of events that takes place during one full heartbeat.

Cardiac muscle fibers Smaller, striated, involuntary muscle fibers (cells) in the heart that contract to pump blood.

Cardiac output The amount of blood pumped by the left ventricle in 1 minute.

Carotene A yellow pigment found in the dermis that provides a natural yellow tint to the skin of some individuals.

Cartilage A form of flexible connective tissue. Types of cartilage include hyaline, fibrocartilage, and elastic cartilage.

Catabolism Chemical processes in the body that release energy as complex compounds are broken down into simpler ones.

Catecholamines A group of neurotransmitters involved in sleep, mood, pleasure, and motor function.

Cell The basic structural unit of a living organism. A cell contains a nucleus and cytoplasm and is surrounded by a membrane.

Center of gravity An imaginary midpoint or center of the weight of a body or object, where the body or object could balance on a point.

Central nervous system The brain and spinal cord and their coverings.

Cerebellum The second largest part of the brain, the cerebellum is involved with balance, posture, coordination, and movement.

Cerebrospinal fluid A clear, colorless fluid that flows throughout the brain and around the spinal cord, cushioning and protecting these structures and maintaining proper pH balance.

Cerebrum The largest of the brain divisions, the cerebrum consists of two hemispheres that occupy the uppermost region of the cranium. The cerebrum receives, interprets, and associates incoming information with past memories and then transmits the appropriate motor response.

Cerumen A sticky substance released by glands in the ear. Also known as *earwax,* cerumen protects the ear from the entry of foreign material and repels insects.

Ceruminous glands Modified apocrine glands found in the external ear canal that secrete cerumen.

Chakra A wheel-like energy center believed to receive, assimilate, and express life force energy.

Charting The process of keeping a written record of a client or patient. The most effective charting methods follow clinical reasoning, which emphasizes a problem-solving approach. Many systems of charting are used, but they all have similar components based on the POMR (problem-oriented medical record) and SOAP (subjective, objective, analysis/assessment, and plan).

Chemical properties Properties that demonstrate how a substance reacts with other substances or responds to a change in the environment.

Chronic diseases Conditions with a vague onset, develop slowly, and last for a long time, sometimes for life. Some chronic disorders are initiated by an acute injury/disease.

Chronic pain Pain that continues or recurs over a prolonged time, usually for more than 6 months. The onset may be obscure, and the character and quality of the pain may change over time. Chronic pain usually is poorly localized and not as intense as acute pain, although for some the pain is exhausting and depressing.

Circadian rhythms Biologic rhythms that work in a 24-hour period to coordinate internal functions such as sleep.

Circumduction Circular movement of a limb, combining the movements of flexion, extension, abduction, and adduction, to create a cone shape.

Closed kinematic chain The positioning of joints in such a way that motion at one of the joints is accompanied by motion at an adjacent joint.

Close-packed position The position of a synovial joint in which the surfaces fit precisely together and maximal contact between the opposing surfaces occurs. The compression of joint surfaces permits no movement, and the joint possesses its greatest stability.

Collagen A protein substance composed of small fibrils that combine to create the connective tissue of fasciae, tendons, and ligaments. Collagen constitutes approximately one fourth of the protein in the body.

Collagenous fibers Strong fibers with little capacity for stretch. They have a high degree of tensile strength, which allows them to withstand longitudinal stress.

Collaterals Branches from an axon that allow communication among neurons.

Combining vowel A vowel added between two roots or a root and a suffix to make pronunciation of the word easier.

Communicable diseases Infectious diseases that spread through contact with infected individuals; also called a contagious disease.

Compact (dense) bone The hard portion of bone that protects spongy bone and provides the firm framework of the bone and the body.

Compounds Substances made up of different kinds of atoms

Concentric action A contraction in which the muscle shortens with tone because its contractile force is greater than the opposing force at the attachments of the muscle. Concentric contractions are contractions of a mover (agonist) wherein it creates the movement of a body part.

Concentric contraction The action of a prime mover or agonist by which a muscle develops tension as it shortens to provide enough force to overcome resistance, described as *positive contraction.*

Concentric function A contraction in which the muscle shortens with tone because its contractile force is greater than the opposing force at the attachments of the muscle. Concentric contractions are contractions of a mover (i.e., an agonist) wherein it creates the movement of a body part.

Condyle A rounded projection at the end of a bone.

Condyloid (condylar) joint Joint that allows movement in two planes, but one motion predominates. The joint resembles a condyle, which is a rounded protuberance at the end of a bone forming an articulation.

Congenital diseases Condition present at birth, not acquired during life.

Connective tissue The most abundant type of tissue in the body. It supports and holds together the body and its parts, protects the body from foreign matter, and is organized to transport substances throughout the body.

Contractility The ability of a muscle to shorten forcibly with adequate stimulation. This property sets muscle apart from all other types of tissue.

Contracture The chronic shortening of a muscle, especially the connective tissue component.

Contusion A bruise.

Corn A painful, conical thickening of skin over bony prominences of the feet caused by continued pressure and friction on normally thin skin. Soft corns are those located in moist areas, such as between the toes.

Coronary arteries The arteries that supply oxygenated blood to the heart muscle itself; they are located in grooves between the atria and ventricles and between the two ventricles.

Coronary veins Veins that return the deoxygenated blood from the heart to the right atrium.

Cortisol A glucocorticoid also known as *hydrocortisone.* Levels of stress often are measured by cortisol levels.

Cramps Painful muscle spasms or involuntary twitches that involve the whole muscle.

Cranial nerves Twelve pairs of nerves that originate from the olfactory bulbs, thalamus, visual cortex, and brainstem. They transmit information to and from the sensory organs of the face and the muscles of the face, neck, and upper shoulders as well as organs of the thorax and abdomen.

Creep The slow movement of viscoelastic materials back to their original state and tissue structure after release of a deforming force.

Cytoplasm Material enclosed by the cell membrane.

Cytoskeleton A framework of proteins inside the cell providing flexibility and strength.

Cytosol The fluid that surrounds the nucleus or organelles inside the cell membrane.

Deep fascia A coarse sheet of fibrous connective tissue that binds muscles into functional groups and forms partitions, called *intermuscular septa,* between muscle groups.

Degenerative joint disease Osteoarthritis.

Dendrites Branching projections from the nerve cell body that carry signals to the cell body.

Deoxyribonucleic acid (DNA) Genetic material of the cell that carries the chemical "blueprint" of the body.

Depression Downward or inferior movement.

Dermatitis A general term for acute or chronic skin inflammation characterized by redness, eruptions, edema, scaling, and itching.

Dermatome A cutaneous (skin) section supplied by a single spinal nerve.

Dermis The deep layer of skin that contains collagen and elastin fibers, which provide much of the structure and strength of the skin.

Descending tracts Tracts in the spinal cord that carry motor information from the brain to the spinal cord.

Developmental anatomy How anatomy changes over the life cycle.

Diagnosis When a licensed medical professional categorizes a disease by identifying its signs and symptoms.

Diagonal abduction Movement of a limb through a diagonal plane directly across and away from the midline of the body.

Diagonal adduction Movement of a limb through a diagonal plane toward and across the midline of the body.

Diaphragm A dome-shaped sheet of muscle attached to the thoracic wall that separates the lungs and thoracic cavity from the abdominal cavity. As the chest cavity enlarges, the diaphragm moves downward and flattens to create a vacuum that allows air to flow into the lungs. As the chest contracts and the diaphragm relaxes, the diaphragm arches upward, helping air to flow out of the lungs.

Diarthrosis A freely movable synovial joint.

Diffusion Movement of ions and molecules from an area of higher concentration to that of a lower concentration.

Digestion The mechanical and chemical breakdown of food from its complex form into simple molecules.

Disease An abnormality in functions of the body, especially when the abnormality threatens well-being.

Disharmony Distortions in health that result when the functions or systems are neither balanced nor working optimally. In Chinese medicine, disharmony can be created by the imbalance of the Six Pernicious Influences or the Seven Emotions.

Disk herniation A pathologic condition that occurs when the fibrocartilage that surrounds the intervertebral disk ruptures, releasing the nucleus pulposus that cushions the vertebrae above and below. The resultant pressure on spinal nerve roots may cause pain and damage the surrounding nerves.

Dopamine A catecholamine found in the brain and autonomic system. Generally a stimulant, dopamine is involved in emotions and moods and in regulating motor control and the executive functioning of the brain.

Dorsal root Also called the *posterior root.* Posterior attachment of a spinal nerve to the spinal cord. Transmits sensory information into the spinal cord.

Dorsiflexion (dorsal flexion) Movement of the ankle that results in the top of the foot moving toward the anterior tibia.

Dosha Physiologic function; described in Ayurveda.

Dynamic force Force applied to an object that produces movement in or of the object.

Eccentric action A contraction in which the muscle lengthens with tone because its contractile force is less than the opposing force at the attachments of the muscle. Eccentric contractions are contractions of an antagonist that usually restrain or control the action of the prime mover. Eccentric contractions sometimes are described as *negative contractions.*

Eccentric contraction The action of an antagonist by which a muscle lengthens while under tension and changes in tension to control the descent of the resistance. Eccentric contractions may be thought of as controlling movement against gravity or resistance and are described as *negative contractions.*

Eccrine A type of sweat gland that releases a watery fluid known as *sweat,* which cools the body and provides minor elimination of metabolic waste.

Edema The accumulation of abnormal amounts of fluid in tissue spaces.

Efferent Away from a center or point of reference.

Efferent nerves Motor nerves that transmit motor impulses; they link the central nervous system to the effectors outside it.

Effort The force applied to overcome resistance.

Elastic fibers Connective tissue fibers that are extensible and elastic. They are made of a protein called *elastin,* which returns to its original length after being stretched.

Elasticity The ability of a muscle to recoil and resume its original resting length after being stretched.

Elastin A connective tissue fiber type that has elastic properties and allows flexibility of connective tissue structures.

Element Substance containing only a single kind of atom.

Elevation Upward or superior movement.

Elimination (egestion) The removal and release of undigested and unabsorbed food as solid waste products.

Endocrine glands Ductless glands that secrete hormones directly into the bloodstream.

Endocytosis The cellular process of engulfing particles located outside the cell membrane into a cell by forming vesicles.

Endoplasmic reticulum A network of intracellular membranes in the form of tubes that is connected to the nuclear membrane.

Endorphins Peptide hormones that mainly work like morphine to suppress pain. They influence mood, producing a mild euphoric feeling such as is seen in runner's high.

Endoskeleton The bony support structure found inside the human body that accommodates growth.

Endosteum A thin membrane of connective tissue that lines the marrow cavity of a bone.

Energy The capacity to work; work is the movement of or a change in the physical structure of matter.

Enteric nervous system The enteric nervous system (ENS) is a subdivision of the peripheral nervous system (PNS) that controls the digestive system.

Entrainment A coordination or synchronization to an internal or external rhythm, especially when a person responds to certain patterns by moving in a manner that is coordinated with those patterns.

Enzyme Protein that speeds up chemical reactions but is not consumed or altered in the process

Epicondyle A bony projection above a condyle.

Epidemiology The field of science that studies the frequency, transmission, occurrence, and distribution of disease in human beings.

Epidermis The superficial layer of skin; composed of epithelial tissue in sublayers called *strata.*

Epilepticus A continuous seizure.

Epinephrine A catecholamine released by the nervous system and involved in fight-or-flight responses such as dilation of blood vessels to the skeletal muscles. Epinephrine is classified as a hormone when secreted by the adrenal gland.

Epithelial tissues A specialized group of tissues that cover and protect the surface of the body and its parts, line body cavities, and form glands. Epithelial tissue usually is found in areas that move substances into and out of the body during secretion, absorption, and excretion.

Erythrocytes Red blood cells that contain hemoglobin and function to transport oxygen to the cells and carbon dioxide away from the cells.

Essential tremor A chronic tremor that does not result from any other pathologic condition.

Etiology The study of the factors involved in the development of disease, including the nature of the disease and the susceptibility of the person.

Eversion Movement of the sole of the foot outward away from the midline.

Excitability The ability of a muscle to receive and respond to a stimulus.

Exocrine glands Glands that secrete hormones through ducts directly into specific areas. Exocrine glands are part of the endocrine system.

Exocytosis The movement of substances out of a cell.

Extensibility The ability of a muscle to be stretched or extended.

Extension A movement that increases the angle between two bones, usually moving the body part back toward the anatomic position.

External respiration The exchange of oxygen and carbon dioxide between the lungs and the bloodstream.

External rotation Rotary movement around the longitudinal axis of a bone away from the midline of the body. Also known as *rotation laterally, outward rotation,* and *lateral rotation.*

Facet A smooth, flat surface on a bone.

Facilitated diffusion The transport of substances by carriers to which the substance binds to move the substance into a cell along the concentration gradient without energy.

Fascia A fibrous or loose type of connective tissue; a fibrous membrane covering, supporting, and separating muscles; the subcutaneous tissue that connects the skin to the muscles.

Feedback loop A self-regulating control system in the body that receives information, integrates that information, and provides a response to maintain homeostasis. Negative feedback reverses the original stimulus, whereas positive feedback enhances and maintains the stimulus.

Fibrocartilage A connective tissue that permits little motion in joints and structures. It is found in places such as the intervertebral disks and the menisci of the knees.

Fibromyalgia A syndrome with symptoms of widespread pain or aching, persistent fatigue, generalized morning stiffness, non-restorative sleep, and multiple tender points. A disrupted sleep pattern, coupled with the dysfunction of myofascial repair mechanisms, seems to be a factor.

Fibrous joint An articulation in which fibrous tissue connects bone directly to bone.

Fistula A tract that is open at both ends, through which abnormal connections occur between two surfaces.

Fixator A stabilizing muscle located at a joint or body part that contracts to fix, or stabilize, the area, enabling another limb or body segment to exert force and move. The fixator also may be described as a muscle (or other force) that stops one attachment of a muscle from moving so that the other attachment of the muscle must move.

Flaccid A term used to describe a muscle with decreased or absent tone.

Flexion A movement that decreases the angle between two bones as the body part moves out of the anatomic position.

Fontanels Areas of the skull of an infant in which the bone formation is incomplete. The fontanels allow for compression of the skull as the infant travels through the birth canal and expansion as the brain grows.

Foramen An opening in a bone, such as the foramen magnum of the skull.

Force Push or pull on an object in an attempt to affect motion or shape.

Fossa A depression in the surface or at the end of a bone.

Free nerve endings Sensory receptors that detect itch and tickle sensations.

Frontal (coronal) plane A vertical plane that divides the body into anterior and posterior (front and back) parts.

Gait The rhythmic and alternating motions of the legs, trunk, and arms resulting in the propulsion of the body.

Gait cycle Subdivided into the stance phase and swing phase, this cycle begins when the heel of one foot strikes the floor and continues until the same heel strikes the floor again.

Gallbladder A small 3- to 4-inch sac that stores and concentrates bile.

Ganglion Cystic, round, usually nontender swellings located along tendon sheaths or joint capsules.

General adaptation syndrome The method the body uses to mobilize different defense mechanisms when threatened by actual or perceived harmful stimuli.

Gestation The period of fetal growth from conception until birth.

Gibbus An angular deformity of a collapsed vertebra, the causes of which include metastatic cancer and tuberculosis of the spine.

Gliding joints Known also as *synovial planes,* gliding joints allow only a gliding motion in various planes.

Gray matter Unmyelinated nervous tissue in the central nervous system.

Gross anatomy The study of body structures visible to the naked eye.

Ground substance The medium in which the cells and protein fibers are suspended. Ground substance is usually clear and colorless and has the consistency of thick syrup.

Half-life The amount of time required for half of a drug or hormone to be eliminated from the bloodstream.

Health A condition of homeostasis resulting in a state of physical, emotional, social, and spiritual well-being; the opposite of disease.

Heart A hollow, cone-shaped, muscular organ responsible for pumping blood. It is about the size of a fist and is located in the mediastinum of the thoracic cavity.

Heart rate The number of cardiac cycles in 1 minute. In the average, healthy person the rate works out to be 60 to 70 cycles or beats per minute.

Heart sounds The two main sounds resulting from the closure of the valves. Murmurs are extra sounds, such as those resulting from faulty valves.

Heart valves Four sets of valves that keep the blood flowing in the correct direction through the heart.

Hemoglobin The oxygen-carrying, red-colored molecule in the blood.

Hemorrhage The passage of blood outside of the cardiovascular system.

Hernia Weakness in a muscle or structure that allows for protrusion of a muscle, organ, or structure through the resulting opening.

Herpes simplex A DNA virus that causes painful blisters and small ulcers in and around the mouth and on the genital area.

High-energy bonds Covalent bonds created in specific organic substrates in the presence of enzymes.

Hinge joint Joint that allows flexion and extension in one plane, changing the angle of the bones at the joint, like a door hinge.

Histamine A neurotransmitter that is considered a stimulant. Histamine is released by the mast cells as part of the inflammatory process and can cause itching.

Homeostasis The relatively constant state of the internal environment of the body that is maintained by adaptive responses. Specific control and feedback mechanisms are responsible for adjusting body systems to maintain this state.

Horizontal abduction Movement of the humerus in the horizontal plane away from the midline of the body. Also known as *horizontal extension* or *transverse abduction.*

Horizontal adduction Movement of the humerus in the horizontal plane toward the midline of the body. Also known as *horizontal flexion* or *transverse adduction.*

Hyaline cartilage The thin covering of articular connective tissue on the ends of the bones in freely movable joints in the adult skeleton. Hyaline cartilage forms a smooth, resilient, low-friction surface for the articulation of one bone with another, distributes forces, and helps absorb some of the pressure imposed on the joint surfaces.

Hyperalgesia An increased sensitivity to pain.

Hyperextension A movement that takes the body part further in the direction of the extension, further out of anatomic position.

Hypermobility A range of motion of a joint greater than would be permitted normally by the structure. Hypermobility may result, leading to instability. Some hypermobility may be present without instability if sufficient dynamic stabilization is present

Hyperplasia An uncontrolled increase in the number of cells of a body part.

Hypersecretion The excessive release of a hormone.

Hypertension An increase in systolic and diastolic pressures.

Hypertrophy An increase in the size of a cell, which results in an increase in the size of a body part or organ.

Hyperventilation Abnormally deep or rapid breathing in excess of physical demands.

Hypomobility A range of motion of a joint less than what would be permitted normally by the structure. Hypomobility results in restricted range of motion.

Hyposecretion The insufficient release of a hormone.

Hypotension A decrease in systolic and diastolic pressures. Hypotension is an important manifestation of shock, which causes inadequate blood supply to vital organs.

Hypothalamic-pituitary-adrenal (HPA) axis Complex set of direct influences and feedback interactions among the hypothalamus, the pituitary gland and the adrenal glands

Idiopathic Refers to diseases with undetermined causes.

Immunity Resistance to disease; the immune system is a functional system rather than an organ system in the anatomic sense.

Impermeable The quality of not permitting entry of a substance.

Incontinence The inability to control urination or defecation, most often because of weak pelvic floor muscles or nerve damage.

Inertia The property of matter in which it remains at rest or in uniform motion in the same straight line unless acted on by some external force.

Inflammation A protective response of the tissues to irritation or injury that may be chronic or acute. The four primary signs are redness, heat, swelling, and pain.

Inflammatory response A sequence of events that involves chemical and cellular activation that destroys pathogens and aids in repairing tissues.

Ingestion Taking food into the mouth.

Inherited diseases Conditions due to genetics.

Inorganic compounds Chemical structures that do not have carbon and hydrogen atoms as the primary structure.

Insertion The attachment of a muscle that moves (or usually moves) when the muscle contracts. The insertion of a muscle is usually the distal attachment of the muscle. For muscles located on the axial body, the insertion is usually the superior attachment of the muscle or the part of the muscle that attaches farthest from the midline, or center, of the body.

Integument The skin and its appendages: hair, sebaceous and sweat glands, nails, and breasts.

Internal respiration The exchange of gases between the tissues and blood.

Internal rotation Medial rotary movement of a bone. Also known as *rotation medially, inward rotation,* and *medial rotation.*

Interphase The period during which a cell grows and carries on its internal activities but is not yet dividing.

Intractable pain The continuation of chronic pain without active disease present or when chronic pain persists even with treatment.

Inversion Movement of the sole of the foot inward toward the midline.

Ion pumps Carriers that transport charged particles into or out of a cell using energy.

Ischemia A temporary deficiency or decreased supply of blood to a tissue.

Isometric action A contraction in which the muscle stays the same length with tone because its contractile force equals that of the opposing force at the attachments of the muscle. The muscle tenses but does not produce movement. Isometric contractions are usually contractions of a fixator/stabilizer muscle (or neutralizer muscle) that acts to stabilize or fix a body part in position while another joint action is occurring.

Isometric contraction The action of the prime mover that occurs when tension develops within the muscle but no appreciable change occurs in the joint angle or the length of the muscle. Movement does not occur.

Isometric function A contraction in which the muscle stays the same length with tone because its contractile force equals that of the opposing force at the attachments of the muscle. The muscle tenses but does not produce movement. Isometric contractions are usually contractions of a fixator/stabilizer muscle (or neutralizer muscle) that acts to hold (i.e., stabilize or fix) a body part in position while another joint action is occurring.

Isotonic action The action of the muscle that occurs when tension develops in the muscle while it shortens or lengthens.

Isotonic contraction The action of the prime mover that occurs when tension develops in the muscle while it shortens or lengthens.

Joint capsule A connective tissue structure that connects the bony components of a joint.

Joint play The involuntary movement that occurs between articular surfaces that is separate from the axial range of motion of a joint produced by muscles. Joint play is an essential component of joint motion and must occur for normal functioning of the joint.

Kapha dosha Physiologic function that blends the water and earth elements.

Keratin The fibrous protein produced in the epidermis that protects our skin and makes it waterproof.

Kinematics A branch of mechanics that involves the aspects of time, space, and mass in a moving system.

Kinesiology The study of movement that combines the fields of anatomy, physiology, physics, and geometry and relates them to human movement.

Kinesthesia The sense of movement of body parts

Kinetic chain An integrated functional unit. The kinetic chain is made up of the myofascial system (muscle, ligament, tendon, and fascia), articular (joint) system, and nervous system. Each of these systems works interdependently to allow structural and functional efficiency in all three planes of motion: sagittal, frontal, and transverse.

Kinetics Those forces causing movement in a system.

Kyphosis A condition of exaggeration of the thoracic curve.

Lateral flexion (side bending) Movement of the head or trunk laterally away from the midline. Abduction of the spine.

Lateral recumbency (side-lying) Lying horizontally on the right or left side.

Least-packed position Joint capsule is at its most lax. Joints assume least-packed position when they are inflamed.

Leukocytes White blood cells that protect the body from pathogens and remove dead cells and substances.

Lever A solid mass such as a crowbar or a person's arm that rotates around a fixed point called the *fulcrum.* The rotation is produced by a force applied to a lever at some distance from the fulcrum.

Ligaments Dense bundles of parallel connective tissue fibers, primarily collagen, that connect bones and strengthen and stabilize the joint.

Lipids Organic compounds that have carbon, hydrogen, and oxygen atoms but in a different proportion than that of carbohydrates.

List A lateral tilt of the spine.

Locomotion Moving from one place to another; walking.

Loose-packed position The position of a synovial joint in which the joint capsule is most lax and the joint is least stable. Joints tend to assume this position to accommodate the increased volume of synovial fluid when inflammation occurs.

Lordosis A condition of exaggeration of the normal lumbar curve.

Lower respiratory tract The larynx, trachea, bronchi, and alveoli.

Lungs The primary organs of respiration. The lungs are soft, spongy, highly vascular structures separated into the left and right lungs by the mediastinum. Each lung is separated into lobes. The right lung has three lobes: upper, middle, and lower; the left lung has two lobes: upper and lower.

Lymph Fluid derived from interstitial fluid; contains lymphocytes, returns plasma proteins that have leaked out through capillary walls, and transports fats from the gastrointestinal system to the bloodstream.

Lymph nodes Small, round structures distributed along the network of lymph vessels; they filter wastes and pathogens out of lymph.

Lysosome Cell organelle that is part of the intracellular digestive system.

Matrix The basic substance between the cells of a tissue. Matrix is composed of amorphous ground substance consisting of molecules that expand when water molecules and electrolytes bind to them. As much as 90% of connective tissue is ground substance. Fibers make up the other component of matrix.

Maximal stimulus The point at which all motor units of a muscle have been recruited and the muscle is unable to increase in strength.

Mechanical receptors Sensory receptors that detect changes in pressure, movement, temperature, or other mechanical forces.

Mechanics The branch of physics dealing with the study of forces and the motion produced by their actions.

Medical terminology Terms used to accurately describe the human body, medical treatments and conditions, and processes of health care in a science-based manner

Meiosis A type of cell division in which each daughter cell receives half the normal number of chromosomes from the parent cell, forming two reproductive cells.

Melanin The pigment that colors our skin and works as a natural sunscreen to protect us from ultraviolet rays by darkening our skin.

Membrane A thin, sheetlike layer of tissue that covers a cell, an organ, or some other structure; that lines a tube or a cavity; or that divides or separates one part from another.

Metabolism Chemical processes in the body that convert food and air into energy to support growth, distribution of nutrients, and elimination of waste.

Metabolites Molecules synthesized or broken down inside the body by chemical reactions.

Microorganisms Small life forms that may be damaging to the body or interfere with its function.

Microvilli Small projections of the cell membrane that increase the surface area of the cell.

Micturition The clinical term for urination or voiding.

Mitochondria Rod- or oval-shaped cell organelles that provide energy for cellular activity.

Mitosis Cell division in which the cell duplicates its DNA and divides into two identical daughter cells.

Mixed nerves Nerves that contain sensory and motor axons.

Mole Also known as a *nevus,* a mole is a benign pigmented skin growth formed of melanocytes.

Molecule A combination of two or more atoms. A molecule is the smallest portion of a substance that can exist separately without losing the physical and chemical properties of that substance.

Monoplegia Paralysis of a single limb or a single group of muscles.

Motion A change in position with respect to some reference frame or starting point

Motor point The location where the motor neuron enters the muscle and where a visible contraction can be elicited with a minimal amount of stimulation. Motor points most often are located in the belly of the muscle.

Motor unit A motor neuron and all of the muscle fibers it controls.

Muscle tissue A specialized form of tissue that contracts and shortens to provide movement, maintain posture, and produce heat.

Myasthenia gravis A disease that usually affects muscles in the face, lips, tongue, neck, and throat but can affect any muscle group.

Myelin A white, fatty insulating substance formed by the Schwann cells that surrounds some axons. Also produced in the central nervous system by oligodendrocytes.

Myogloblin A red pigment similar to hemoglobin that stores oxygen within the muscle cells.

Myotome A skeletal muscle or group of skeletal muscles that receives motor axons from a particular spinal nerve.

Negative feedback system A control mechanism that provides a stimulus to decrease a function, such as a fire alarm, which causes a series of reactions that work to reduce the fire.

Neoplasm The abnormal growth of new tissue. Also called a *tumor,* a neoplasm may be benign or malignant.

Nerve A bundle of axons or dendrites or both.

Nervous tissue A specialized tissue that coordinates and regulates body activity. It can develop more excitability and conductivity than other types of tissue.

Neuroendocrine system Interactions between the nervous system and the endocrine system

Neurolemma Also called *Schwann's membrane, sheath of Schwann,* and *endoneural membrane.* The outer cell membrane of a Schwann cell that encloses the myelin sheath found on certain peripheral nerves. It is essential in the regeneration of injured axons.

Neuroglia Specialized connective tissue cells that support, protect, and hold neurons together.

Neurons Nerve cells that conduct impulses.

Neurotransmitters Chemical compounds that generate action potentials when released in the synapses from presynaptic cells.

Neurovascular bundle A spinal nerve, artery, deep vein, and deep lymphatic vessel bound together by connective tissue, traveling the same pathway in the body.

Nociceptors Sensory receptors that detect painful or intense stimuli.

Norepinephrine A catecholamine primarily involved in emotional responses. Norepinephrine is found in the central nervous system and the sympathetic division of the autonomic nervous system and causes constriction of blood vessels in the skeletal muscles.

Nucleic acids The two types of nucleic acid are deoxyribonucleic acid (DNA) and ribonucleic acid (RNA).

Nutrients Essential elements and molecules obtained from the diet and that are required by the body for normal body function.

Nutrition The use of food for growth and maintenance of the body.

Open kinematic chain A position in which the ends of the limbs or parts of the body are free to move without causing motion at another joint.

Opportunistic pathogens Organisms that cause disease only when the immunity is low in a host.

Opposition Movement of the thumb across the palmar aspect to make contact with the fingers.

Organelles The basic components of a cell that perform specific functions within the cell.

Organic compounds Substances that have carbon and hydrogen as part of their basic structure.

Origin The attachment of a muscle that does not move (or usually does not move) when the muscle contracts. The origin of a muscle is usually the proximal attachment of the muscle. For muscles located on the axial body, the origin is usually the inferior attachment of the muscle or the part of the muscle that attaches closest to the midline, or center, of the body.

Osmosis Diffusion of water from a region of lower concentration of solution to a region of higher concentration of solution across the semipermeable membrane of a cell.

Osteokinematics The movement of bones as opposed to the movement of articular surfaces; also known as *range of motion.*

Osteoporosis A disorder of the bones in which a lack of calcium and other minerals and a decrease in bone protein leaves the bones soft, fragile, and more likely to break.

Oxygen debt The extra amount of oxygen that must be taken in to remove the buildup of lactic acid from anaerobic respiration of glucose (to convert lactic acid to glucose or glycogen).

Pain An unpleasant sensation. Pain is a complex, personal, subjective experience with physiologic, psychological, and social aspects. Because pain is subjective, it is often difficult to explain or describe.

Paraplegia Paralysis of the lower portion of the body and of both legs.

Parasympathetic nervous system The energy conservation and restorative system associated with what commonly is called the *relaxation response.*

Passive transport Transportation of a substance across the cell membrane without the use of energy.

Pathogenesis The development of a disease.

Pathogenicity The ability of the infectious agent to cause disease.

Pathogens Disease-causing organisms; are a type of infectious agent.

Pathologic range of motion The amount of motion at a joint that fails to reach the normal physiologic range or exceeds normal anatomic limits of motion of that joint.

Pathology The study of disease as observed in the structure and function of the body.

Pericardium A double-membrane, serous sac that surrounds and protects the heart.

Periosteum The thin membrane of connective tissue that covers bones except at articulations.

Peripheral nervous system The system of somatic and autonomic neurons outside the central nervous system. The peripheral nervous system comprises the afferent (sensory) division and the efferent (motor) division.

Peristalsis Rhythmic contraction of smooth muscles that propel products of digestion along the tract from the esophagus to the anus.

Peritoneum The mucous membrane that lines the abdominal cavity to prevent friction from the organs.

Phagocytosis The process of endocytosis followed by digestion of the vesicle contents by enzymes present in the cytoplasm.

Phantom pain A form of pain or other sensation experienced in the missing extremity after a limb amputation.

Pharmacology The study of medications and their uses in treating or preventing a disease.

Pharynx The throat.

Phospholipid bilayer Cell membrane made up of lipids, carbohydrates, and proteins.

Physiologic range of motion The amount of motion available to a joint determined by the nervous system from information provided by joint sensory receptors. This information usually prevents a joint from being positioned such that injury could occur.

Physiology The study of the processes and functions of the body involved in supporting life.

Piezoelectric Ability to produce electrical current when deformed or compressed, especially in a crystalline substance such as bone matrix. Also means that when electric currents pass through them, these substances deform slightly and vibrate.

Pitta dosha Physiologic function that combines fire and water.

Pivot joint A bony projection from one bone fits into a ring formed by another bone and ligament structure to allow rotation around its own axis in one plane.

Plantar flexion An extension movement of the ankle that results in the foot and toes moving away from the body.

Plasma A thick, straw-colored fluid that makes up about 55% of the blood.

Plastic range The range of movement of connective tissue that is taken beyond the elastic limits. In this range the tissue permanently deforms and cannot return to its original state.

Plexus A network of intertwining nerves that innervates a particular region of the body.

Polio A viral infection first of the intestines and then (for about 1% of exposed persons) the anterior horn cells of the spinal cord.

Posterior pelvic rotation Posterior movement of the upper pelvis; the iliac crest tilts backward in a sagittal plane.

Prefix A word element added to the beginning of a root to change the meaning of the word.

Pressure The amount of force on a specific area.

Process Any prominent bony growth that projects out from the bone.

Prognosis The expected outcome in a client who has a disease.

Pronation Internal rotary movement of the radius on the ulna that results in the hand moving from the palm-up to the palm-down position.

Prone Lying horizontal with the face down.

Proprioceptors Sensory receptors that provide the body with information about position, movement, muscle tension, joint activity, and equilibrium.

Proteins Substances formed from amino acids.

Protraction Forward movement remaining in a horizontal plane.

Psoriasis A common, chronic skin disease characterized by reddened skin covered by dry, silvery scales. Psoriasis most often is found on the scalp, elbows, knees, back, or buttocks.

Pulmonary trunk The large artery that carries blood to the lungs to release carbon dioxide and take in oxygen.

Pulmonary veins The four veins from the lungs that bring oxygen-rich blood to the left atrium.

Qi Also spelled *Chi, Qi* refers to the life force.

Quadriplegia Paralysis or loss of movement of all four limbs.

Quality of life An individual's perceptions of his or her position in life in the context of the culture and value systems in which the person lives and in relation to his or her goals, expectations, standards, and concerns.

Reciprocal inhibition Stimulation of an antagonist muscle to inhibit action in the prime mover.

Reciprocal innervation The circuitry of neurons that allows reciprocal inhibition to take place. The massage therapist can use reciprocal innervation therapeutically to assist in muscle relaxation.

Reduction Return of the spinal column to the anatomic position from lateral flexion. Adduction of the spine.

Referred pain Pain felt in a surface area far from the stimulated organ.

Reflex An automatic, involuntary reaction to a stimulus.

Reflex arc The pathway that a nerve impulse follows in a reflex action.

Regional anatomy The study of the structures of a particular area of the body.

Remission The reversal of signs and symptoms that may occur in clients who have chronic diseases. Remission can be temporary or permanent.

Resistance Resistance opposes force.

Respiration The movement of air in and out of the lungs, the exchange of oxygen and carbon dioxide between the lungs and blood, and the exchange between blood and body tissues.

Respiratory rate The number of breaths in 1 minute.

Resting tone The state of tension in resting muscles.

Reticular fibers Delicate connective tissue fibers that occur in networks and support small structures, such as capillaries, nerve fibers, and the basement membrane. Reticular fibers are made of a specialized type of collagen called *reticulin*.

Retraction Backward movement in a horizontal plane.

Reverse action When a muscle contracts and the attachment that normally stays fixed (the origin) moves, and the attachment that usually moves (the insertion) stays fixed.

Ribonucleic acid Ribonucleic acid (RNA) is a type of nucleic acid. It is transcribed (copied) from DNA by enzymes. RNA carries information from DNA to ribosomes, where it is read and translated so cells can make the proteins necessary for body functions.

Root A word element that contains the basic meaning of the word.

Rotation Partial turning or pivoting in an arc around a central axis.

Rupture The tearing or disruption of connective tissue fibers that takes place when they exceed the limits of the plastic range.

Saddle joint Joint that is convex in one plane and concave in the other with the surfaces fitting together like a rider on a saddle.

Schwann cell A specialized cell that forms myelin.

Scoliosis A lateral curvature of the spine.

Sebaceous glands The oil glands found in the skin.

Sebum The oily substance secreted by sebaceous glands that prevents dehydration, softens skin and hair, and slows the growth of bacteria.

Serotonin A neurotransmitter that works primarily as an inhibitor in the central nervous system, is synthesized into melatonin, and affects our sleep and moods.

Sesamoid bones Round bones that often are embedded in tendons and joint capsules. The largest of these is the patella.

Seven Emotions The Asian concept that joy, anger, fear, fright, sadness, worry, and grief are emotional responses that may trigger disharmony in the body, mind, or spirit under certain conditions.

Shock An inadequate blood supply to vital organs, causing reduced function in these organs.

Signs Objective changes that can be seen or measured by someone other than the client.

Sinus A tract leading from a cavity to the surface.

Sinuses Four groups of air-filled spaces that open into the internal nose. They are located in the frontal, ethmoid, sphenoid, and maxillary bones of the skull. They lighten the weight of the skull and play a role in sound production.

Six Pernicious Influences The Asian concept that heat, cold, wind, dampness, dryness, and summer heat, which are natural climate changes, may induce disease under certain conditions.

Skeletal muscle fibers Large, cross-striated cells that make up muscles connected to the skeleton; under voluntary control of the nervous system.

Sliding filament mechanism The process describing skeletal muscle contraction in which the thick and thin filaments slide past one another.

Smooth muscle fibers Muscle fibers that are neither striated nor voluntary. These muscle cells help regulate blood flow through the cardiovascular system, propel food through the digestive tract, and squeeze secretions from glands.

SOAP notes The acronym refers to subjective, objective, analysis or assessment, and plan, the four parts of the written account of record keeping.

Somatic nervous system A system of nerves that keeps the body in balance with its external environment by transmitting impulses among the central nervous system, skeletal muscles, and skin.

Somatic pain Pain that arises from the body wall. Superficial somatic pain comes from the stimulation of receptors in the skin, whereas deep somatic pain arises from stimulation of receptors in skeletal muscles, joints, tendons, and fasciae.

Spastic Term used to describe a muscle with excessive tone.

Spinal cord The portion of the central nervous system that exits the skull and extends into the vertebral column. The two major functions of the spinal cord are to conduct nerve impulses and to be a center for spinal reflexes.

Spinal nerves Thirty-one pairs of mixed nerves, originating in the spinal cord and emerging from the vertebral column; they are part of the peripheral nervous system

Spongy (cancellous) bone The lighter-weight portion of bone, which is made up of trabeculae.

Stabilizer A force or an object that helps maintain a position. Stabilization is essential to assess movement patterns accurately.

Standard Precautions Safety measures established by the Centers for Disease Control and Prevention. The precautions were instituted to prevent the spread of bacterial and viral infections by setting up specific methods of dealing with human fluids and waste products.

Static force Force applied to an object in such a way that it does not produce movement.

Status epilepticus A medical emergency characterized by a continuous seizure lasting longer than 30 minutes.

Stress Any external or internal stimulus that requires a change or response so as to prevent an imbalance in the internal environment of the body, mind, or emotions. Stress may be any activity that makes demands on mental and emotional resources. Some responses to stress may stimulate neurons of the hypothalamus to release corticotropin-releasing hormone.

Subacute Diseases that have characteristics that fall between those described as acute or chronic.

Suffix A word element added to the end of a root to change the meaning of the word.

Superficial fascia The subcutaneous tissue that comprises the third layer of skin; consists of loose connective tissue and contains fat or adipose tissue.

Supination External rotary movement of the radius on the ulna that results in the hand moving from the palm-down to the palm-up position.

Supine Lying horizontal with the face up.

Surface anatomy The study of internal organs and structures as they can be recognized and related to external features.

Suture A synarthrotic joint in which two bony components are united by a thin layer of dense fibrous tissue.

Sweat glands The sudoriferous glands in the skin; they are classified as apocrine or eccrine depending on their location and structure.

Sympathetic nervous system The part of the autonomic nervous system that provides for most of the active function of the body; when the body is under stress, the sympathetic nervous system predominates with fight-or-flight responses.

Symphysis A cartilaginous joint in which the two bony components are joined directly by fibrocartilage in the form of a disk or plate.

Symptoms The subjective changes noticed or felt only by the client or patient.

Synapse A space between neurons or between a neuron and an effector organ.

Synarthrosis A limited-movement, nonsynovial joint.

Synchondrosis A joint in which the material used for connecting the two components is hyaline cartilage.

Syndesmosis A fibrous joint in which two bony components are joined directly by a ligament, cord, or aponeurotic membrane.

Syndrome A group of different signs and symptoms that identify a pathologic condition, especially when they have a common cause.

Synergist Movers of a joint other than the prime mover(s); that is, assistant, secondary, or emergency movers. *Synergists* may be more broadly defined as any muscle that helps the action occur (i.e., also may be fixator, neutralizer, or support muscles, as well as other movers).

Synovial fluid A thick, colorless lubricating fluid secreted by the joint cavity membrane.

Synovial joints Freely moving joints allowing motion in one or more planes of action.

Systemic anatomy The study of the structure of a particular body system.

Tao An ancient philosophic concept that represents the whole and its parts as one and the same.

Tendinitis Inflammation of a tendon.

Tenosynovitis Inflammation of a tendon sheath.

Terminology A vocabulary used by people involved in a specialized activity or field of work. Also, the study of the meaning of words used in a language.

Thermal receptors Sensory receptors that detect changes in temperature.

Thorax Also known as the *chest cavity.* The thorax is the upper region of the torso. It is enclosed by the sternum, ribs, and thoracic vertebrae and contains the lungs, heart, and great blood vessels.

Threshold stimulus The stimulus at which the first observable muscle contraction occurs.

Tissue A group of similar cells combined to perform a common function.

Tone The state of tension in resting muscles.

Trabeculae An irregular meshing of small, bony plates that makes up spongy bone; its spaces are filled with red marrow.

Tracts Collections of nerve fibers in the brain and spinal cord that have a common function.

Trigger points A hyperirritable locus within a taut band of skeletal muscle, located in the muscular tissue or its associated fascia. The spot is painful on compression and can evoke characteristic referred pain and autonomic phenomena.

Trochanter One of two large bony processes found only on the femur.

Tropic (or trophic) hormones Hormones produced by the endocrine glands that affect other endocrine glands.

Tubercle A small rounded process on a bone.

Tuberosity A large rounded protuberance on a bone.

Tumor Also referred to as a *neoplasm,* a tumor is a growth of new tissues that may be benign or malignant.

Ulcer A round, open sore of the skin or mucous membrane.

Ultradian rhythms Biologic rhythms that repeat themselves at a rate that ranges from 90 minutes to every few hours.

Upper respiratory tract The nasal cavity and all its structures and the pharynx.

Upward rotation Scapular motion that turns the glenoid fossa upward and moves the inferior angle superiorly and laterally away from the spinal column.

Vata dosha Physiologic function formed from ether and air.

Vector The direction of the force.

Veins Blood vessels that collect blood from the capillaries and transport it back to the heart.

Vena cava One of two large arteries that returns poorly oxygenated blood to the right atrium of the heart.

Ventral root Also called the *anterior root.* Anterior attachment of a spinal nerve to the spinal cord. Transmits motor information away from the spinal cord.

Ventricles The two large lower chambers of the heart; they are thick-walled and are separated by a thick interventricular septum.

Venules Small blood vessels that connect capillaries to veins.

Virulent A quality of organisms that readily cause disease.

Visceral pain Pain that results from the stimulation of receptors or an abnormal condition in the viscera (internal organs).

Viscoelasticity The combination of resistance offered by a fluid to a change of form and the ability of material to return to its original state after deformation.

Whiplash An injury to the soft tissues of the neck caused by sudden hyperextension or flexion of the neck (or both).

White matter Myelinated nerve tissue in the central nervous system

Word elements The parts of a word; the prefix, root, and suffix.

Yellow elastic cartilage Cartilage that is more opaque, flexible, and elastic than hyaline cartilage and is distinguished further by its yellow color. The ground substance is penetrated in all directions by frequently branching fibers.

Yin/yang Yin and yang are terms used to describe polar relationships. Yin/yang refers to the dynamic balance between opposing forces and the continual process of creation and destruction. Yin/yang reflects the natural order and duality of the whole universe and everything in it, including the individual.

Works Consulted

Alfaro-LeFevre R: *Critical thinking and clinical judgment: a practical approach to outcome-focused thinking*, ed 4, St. Louis, 2009, Elsevier.

Anderson SK: *The practice of shiatsu*, St. Louis, 2008, Mosby.

An outline of Chinese acupuncture: the Academy of Traditional Chinese Medicine, Peking, 1975, Foreign Languages Press.

Applegate E, Thomas P: *The anatomy and physiology learning system*, ed 4, Philadelphia, 2011, Saunders Elsevier.

Arnheim DD, Prentice WE: *Principles of athletic training*, ed 12, New York, 2006, McGraw-Hill.

Basmajian JV, DeLuca CJ: *Muscles alive: their functions revealed by electromyography*, ed 5, Baltimore, 1985, Williams & Wilkins.

Basmajian JV, Nyberg R: *Rational manual therapies*, Baltimore, 1993, Williams & Wilkins.

Bates B: *Bates' guide to physical examination and history taking*, ed 9, Philadelphia, 2005, Lippincott, Williams & Wilkins.

Berryman N, Lovelace-Chandler V, Soderberg GL, Zabel RJ: *Muscle and sensory testing*, ed 2, St. Louis, 2005 Elsevier.

Birch SJ, Felt RL: *Understanding acupuncture*, New York, 1999, Churchill Livingstone.

Brennan R: *The Alexander technique workbook: your personal system for health, poise and fitness*, London, 2003, Vega Books.

Bullock BL, Rosendahl PP: *Pathophysiology: adaptations and alterations in function*, ed 4, Philadelphia, 1996, JB Lippincott.

Butler DS: *Mobilization of the nervous system*, Melbourne, 1991, Churchill Livingstone.

Cailliet R: *Neck and arm pain*, ed 3, Philadelphia, 1991, FA Davis.

Cailliet R: *Shoulder pain*, ed 3, Philadelphia, 1991, FA Davis.

Cailliet R: *Knee pain and disability*, ed 3, Philadelphia, 1992, FA Davis.

Cailliet R: *Hand pain and impairment*, ed 4, Philadelphia, 1994, FA Davis.

Cailliet R: *Low back pain syndrome*, ed 5, Philadelphia, 1995, FA Davis.

Cailliet R: *Soft tissue pain and disability*, Philadelphia, 1996, FA Davis.

Cailliet R: *Foot and ankle pain*, ed 3, Philadelphia, 1997, FA Davis.

Cassar M-P: *Handbook of massage therapy: a complete guide for the student and professional massage therapist*, Boston, 1999, Butterworth-Heinemann.

Cavallaro Goodman C, Fuller KS: *Pathology: implications for the physical therapist*, ed 3, St. Louis, 2005, Elsevier.

Chaitow L: *The acupuncture treatment of pain*, Rochester, Vt., 1990, Healing Arts Press.

Chaitow L: *The book of natural pain relief*, New York, 1995, Harper Paperbacks.

Chaitow L: *Modern neuromuscular techniques*, ed 2, New York, 2003, Churchill Livingstone.

Chaitow L: *Muscle energy techniques*, ed 3, New York, 2007, Churchill Livingstone.

Chaitow L, Delany J: *Clinical application of neuromuscular techniques*, ed 2, vol 1, *The upper body*, London, 2008, Churchill Livingstone.

Chaitow L, Delany J: *Clinical application of neuromuscular techniques*, vol 2, *The lower body*, London, 2002, Churchill Livingstone.

Clayton BD, Stock YN: *Basic pharmacology for nurses*, ed 14, St. Louis, 2007, Mosby.

Damjanov I: *Pathology for the health-related professions*, ed 3, Philadelphia, 2006, Saunders.

Di Lima SN, Painter SJ, Johns LT, editors: *Orthopaedic patient education resource manual*, Gaithersburg, Md., 2001, Aspen (three-ring binder with CD ROM).

Dossey L: *Space, time and medicine*, Boston, 1982, Random House.

Drake R et al: *Gray's anatomy for students*, ed 2, Philadelphia, 2010, Churchill Livingstone.

Freeman LW, Lawlis GF: *Mosby's complementary and alternative medicine: a research-based approach*, ed 2, St. Louis, 2004, Mosby.

Furlan AD et al: Massage for low back pain, *Clin J Pain* 18(3):154-163, 2002.

Gould BE: *Pathophysiology for the health professions*, ed 3, St. Louis, 2009, Elsevier.

Greene DP, Roberts SL: *Kinesiology: movement in the context of activity*, St. Louis, 1999, Elsevier.

Greenman PE: *Principles of manual medicine*, ed 3, Baltimore, 2003, Williams & Wilkins.

Gunn C: *Bones and joints*, ed 5, New York, 2007, Churchill Livingstone.

Gurevich D: *Russian medical massage*, Flint, Mich., 1992 (self published).

Heinerman J: *Healing powers of herbs*, ed 2, Boca Raton, Fla., 2004, Globe Communications.

Hislop HJ, Montgomery J: *Daniel and Worthingham's muscle testing: techniques of manual examination*, ed 8, Philadelphia, 2007, Saunders.

Hooper J, Teresi D: *The three-pound universe*, New York, 1986, Dell.

Huan Z, Rose K: *Who can ride the dragon?* Brookline, Mass., 1999, Paradigm Publications.

Jacobs PH, Anhalt TS: *Handbook of skin clues of systemic diseases*, ed 2, Philadelphia, 1992, Lea & Febiger.

Kasper DL et al: *Harrison's principles of internal medicine*, ed 16, New York, 2004, McGraw-Hill.

Keirsey D, Bates M: *Please understand me: character and temperament types*, ed 2, Del Mar, Calif., 1984, Prometheus Nemesis.

Keirsey D, Bates M: *Please understand me: temperament in leading*, Del Mar, Calif., 1996, Prometheus Nemesis.

Kendall F: *Florence Kendall's muscle testing video library*, vols 1-5, Baltimore, (no date), Williams & Wilkins.

Kisner C, Colby LA: *Therapeutic exercise: foundations and techniques*, ed 5, Philadelphia, 2007, FA Davis.

Leadbeater CW: *The chakras*, Wheaton, Ill., 1927, Theosophical Publishing House.

Le Blanc-Louvry I et al: Does mechanical massage of the abdominal wall after colectomy reduce postoperative pain and shorten the duration of ileus? Results of a randomized study, *J Adv Nurs* 38(1):68-73, 2002.

Maciocia G: *The foundations of Chinese medicine*, ed 2, New York, 2005, Churchill Livingstone.

Mahan LK, Escott-Stump S: *Krause's food & nutrition therapy*, ed 12, St. Louis, 2010, Elsevier.

Marieb EN: *Human anatomy and physiology*, ed 7, Redwood City, Calif., 2006, Benjamin/Cummings.

Masunaga S, Ohashi W: *Zen shiatsu: how to harmonize yin and yang for better health*, Tokyo, 1977, Japan Publications.

McCance KL, Huether SE, Brashers VL: *Pathophysiology, the biologic basis for disease in adults and children*, ed 6, St. Louis, 2010, Elsevier.

McCraty R, Tiller WA, Atkinson M: Head-heart entrainment: a preliminary survey. Paper presented at the Key West Brain-Mind, Applied Neurophysiology, EEG Biofeedback 4th Annual Advanced Colloquium, Key West, Fla, Feb 1996 (website): www.heartmath.org/research/research-papers/HeadHeart/index.html. Accessed August 29, 2007.

Mennell JM: *The musculoskeletal system: differential diagnosis from symptoms and physical signs*, Gaithersburg, Md., 1992, Aspen.

Millenson JR: *Mind matters: psychological medicine in holistic practice*, Seattle, 1995, Eastland Press.

Muscolino JE: *The muscular system manual, the skeletal muscles of the human body*, ed 3, St. Louis, 2010, Mosby.

Myers TW: *Anatomy trains: myofascial meridians for manual and movement therapists*, ed 2, New York, 2009, Churchill Livingstone.

Netter FH: *The Ciba collection of medical illustrations*, Summit, N.J., 1991, Ciba-Geigy Corporation.

Netter FH: *The Ciba collection of medical illustrations*, ed 2, Summit, N.J., 1992, Ciba-Geigy Corporation.

Neumann DA: *Foundations for rehabilitation*, ed 2, St. Louis, 2010.

Neumann DA: *Kinesiology of the musculoskeletal system, foundations for rehabilitation*, ed 2, St. Louis, 2009, Elsevier.

Nikola RJ: *Creatures of water: hydrotherapy textbook*, Salt Lake City, 1995, Europa Therapeutic.

Nix S: *Williams' basic nutrition & diet therapy*, ed 13, St. Louis, 2009, Elsevier.

Norkin CC, Levangie PK: *Joint structure and function*, ed 2, Philadelphia, 1992, FA Davis.

Northrup C: *Women's bodies, women's wisdom*, New York, 1994, Bantam Books.

Oschman JL: What is healing energy? III. Silent pulses, *J Bodywork Movement Ther* 1(3):179, 1997.

Patton KT, Thibodeau GA: *Anatomy and physiology*, ed 7, St. Louis, 2010, Elsevier.

Peckenpaugh NJ: *Nutrition essentials and diet therapy*, ed 10, St. Louis, 2008, Elsevier.

Premkumar K: *Pathology A to Z: a handbook for massage therapists*, Calgary, Alberta, 1996, VanPub Books.

Premkumar K: *The massage connection: anatomy, physiology & pathology*, Calgary, Alberta, 1997, VanPub Books.

Price SA, Wilson LM: *Pathophysiology, clinical concepts of disease processes*, ed 6, St. Louis, 2003, Mosby.

Quinn L, Gordon J: *Functional outcomes documentation for rehabilitation*, ed 2, St. Louis, 2003, Elsevier.

Rattray F, Ludwig L: *Clinical massage therapy: understanding, assessing, and treating over 70 conditions*, Toronto, 2000, Talus.

Seeley RR, Stephens TD, Tate P: *Essentials of anatomy and physiology*, ed 6, St. Louis, 2006, McGraw-Hill.

Selye H: *The stress of life*, New York, 1978, McGraw-Hill.

Sieg K, Adams S: *Illustrated essentials of musculoskeletal anatomy*, ed 4, Gainesville, Fla., 2002, Megabooks.

Simons D: Understanding effective treatments of myofascial trigger points, *J Bodywork Movement Ther* 6(2):2002.

Smith LK, Weiss E, Lehmkuhl L: *Brunnstrom's clinical kinesiology*, ed 5, Philadelphia, 1996, FA Davis.

Sorrentino SA: *Mosby's textbook for nursing assistants*, ed 7, St. Louis, 2008, Mosby.

Standring S: *Gray's anatomy: the anatomical basis of medicine and surgery*, ed 39, Edinburgh, 2005, Churchill Livingstone.

Stanway A: *The new natural family doctor*, Berkeley, Calif., 1987, North Atlantic Books.

Stevens A, Lowe JS, Young B: *Wheater's basic histopathology*, ed 4, New York, 2003, Churchill Livingstone.

Sun C: *Chinese bodywork: a complete manual of Chinese therapeutic massage*, Berkeley, Calif., 1993, Pacific View Press.

Thibodeau GA, Patton KT: *Structure and function of the body*, ed 14, 2012, Mosby.

Thibodeau GA, Patton KT: *Anatomy and physiology*, ed 7, St. Louis, 2010, Mosby.

Thibodeau GA, Patton KT: *The human body in health and disease*, ed 4, St. Louis, 2005, Mosby.

Thomas CL: *Taber's cyclopedic medical dictionary*, ed 16, Philadelphia, 1985, FA Davis.

Thompson GW, Floyd RT: *Manual of structural kinesiology with dynamic movement*, ed 14, St. Louis, 2000, Mosby.

Timmons BH, Ley R: *Behavioral and psychological approaches to breathing disorders*, New York, 1994, Plenum Press.

Tortora GJ, Grabowski SR: *Principles of anatomy and physiology*, ed 11, New York, 2005, Wiley.

Trew M, Everett T: *Human movement: an introductory text*, ed 5, New York, 2006, Churchill Livingstone.

Whitney EN, Rolfes SR: *Understanding nutrition*, ed 11, Minneapolis, 2007, West.

Whittle MW, Cline WM: *Gait Analysis, an introduction*, ed 4, St. Louis, 2007, Elsevier.

Wiseman N, Feng Y: *A practical dictionary of Chinese medicine*, ed 2, Brookline, Mass., 1998, Paradigm.

Yates J: *A physician's guide to therapeutic massage: its physiological effects and their application to treatment*, Vancouver, 1990, Massage Therapist Association of British Columbia.

Young B et al: *Wheater's functional histology*, ed 5, New York, 2006, Churchill Livingstone.

Zahourek J: *Myologik: an atlas of human musculature in clay*, vols 1-5, Zoologik Systems Kinesthetic Anatomy Maniken, Loveland, Colo., 1996, Zahourek Systems.

Zi N: *The art of breathing*, Glendale, Calif., 1997, Vivi.

Zukav G: *The dancing wu li masters*, New York, 1980, Bantam Books.

RECOMMENDED READINGS

Anderson SK: *The practice of shiatsu*, St. Louis, 2008, Mosby.

Chaitow L: *Palpation and assessment skills: assessment and diagnosis through touch*, ed 2, New York, 2003, Churchill Livingstone.

Chaitow L, Fritz S: *A massage therapist's guide to understanding, locating and treating myofascial trigger points*, Edinburgh, 2007, Churchill Livingstone.

Chaitow L, Fritz S: *A massage therapist's guide to lower back and pelvic pain*, London, 2008, Churchill Livingstone.

Chaitow L, Fritz S: *A massage therapist's guide to treating headaches and neck pain including DVD*, Edinburgh, 2009, Churchill Livingstone.

Chaitow L: *Cranial manipulation, theory and practice with CD-ROM*, ed 2, Edinburgh, 2005, Churchill Livingstone.

Chaitow L: *Muscle energy techniques with DVD-ROM*, ed 3, Edinburgh, 2007, Churchill Livingstone.

Chaitow L: *Positional release techniques with DVD-ROM*, ed 3, Edinburgh, 2008, Churchill Livingstone.

Chaitow L: *Fibromyalgia syndrome, a practitioner's guide to treatment*, ed 3, London, 2010, Churchill Livingstone.

Chaitow L, Lovegrove Jones R: *Chronic pelvic pain and dysfunction, practical physical medicine*, London, 2011, Churchill Livingstone.

Chaitow L: *Palpation and assessment skills, assessment through touch*, ed 3, London, 2010, Churchill Livingstone.

Chaitow L: *Modern neuromuscular techniques with DVD*, ed 3, London, 2011, Churchill Livingstone.

Chaitow L, Delany J: *Clinical application of neuromuscular techniques, practical case study exercises*, Edinburgh, 2006, Churchill Livingstone.

Chaitow L, Delany J: *Clinical application of neuromuscular techniques*, vol 1, *the upper body*, ed 2, Edinburgh, 2008, Churchill Livingstone.

Chaitow L, DeLany J: *Clinical application of neuromuscular techniques*, vol 2, *the lower body*, ed 2, Edinburgh, 2012, Churchill Livingstone.

Fritz S: *Mosby's fundamentals of therapeutic massage*, ed 5, St. Louis, 2013, Mosby.

Fritz S: *Sports and exercise massage, comprehensive care in athletics, fitness, and rehabilitation*, St. Louis, 2006, Elsevier.

Fritz S: *Mosby's fundamentals of therapeutic massage*, ed 4, St. Louis, 2010, Elsevier.

Fritz S, Grosenbach J: *Mosby's essential sciences for therapeutic massage, anatomy, physiology, biomechanics and pathology*, ed 3, St. Louis, 2008, Elsevier.

Fritz S: *Mosby's PDQ for massage therapists*, ed 2, St. Louis, 2009, Elsevier.

Fritz S: *Business and professional skills for massage therapy*, St. Louis, 2010, Elsevier.

Fritz S: *Mosby's massage therapy review*, ed 3, St. Louis, 2010, Elsevier.

Fritz S, Chaitow L, Hymel G: *Clinical massage in the healthcare setting*, St. Louis, 2008, Elsevier.

Fritz S, Chaitow L: *The massage therapist's guide to pain management with CD-ROM*, St. Louis, 2011, Elsevier.

Hymel G: *Research methods for massage and holistic therapies*, St. Louis, 2006, Mosby.

Lowe WW: *Orthopedic massage*, ed 2, Edinburgh, 2009, Churchill Livingstone.

Lowe WW: *Functional assessment in massage therapy*, ed 3, Sisters, Ore., 1997, OMERI.

Maciocia G: *The foundations of Chinese medicine*, ed 2, New York, 2005, Churchill Livingstone.

Mosby's dictionary of medicine, nursing, and health professions, ed 7, St. Louis, 2006, Mosby.

Muscolino JE: *Flashcards for bones, joints and actions of the human body*, ed 2, St. Louis, 2011, Mosby.

Muscolino JE: *Musculoskeletal anatomy flashcards*, ed 2, St. Louis, 2010, Mosby.

Muscolino J: *Know the body: muscle, bone, and palpation*, St. Louis, 2011, Mosby.

Muscolino J: *Kinesiology*, ed 2, St. Louis, 2011, Mosby.

Muscolino J: *The muscular system manual, the skeletal muscles of the human body*, ed 3, St. Louis, 2010, Mosby.

Muscolino J: *Mosby's trigger point flip chart with referral patterns and stretching*, St. Louis, 2009, Mosby.

Muscolino J: *The muscle and bone palpation manual with trigger points, referral patterns and stretching*, St. Louis, 2009, Mosby.

Myers TW: *Anatomy trains: myofascial meridians for manual and movement therapists*, ed 2, New York, 2009, Churchill Livingstone.

Salvo SG: *Mosby's pathology for massage therapists*, ed 2, St. Louis, 2009, Mosby.

Thompson DL: *Hands heal: Communication, documentation, and insurance billing for manual therapists*, ed 4, 2011, Lippincott, Williams, and Wilkins.

Index

Note: Page numbers followed by f, t, and b refer to figures, tables, and boxes.

Abbreviations, 62-63, 62t
Abdominal arteries, 568f, 574
Abdominal breathing, 503
Abdominal cavity, 63, 66, 66f
Abdominal quadrants, 66, 67f
Abdominal regions, 66, 67f
  biomechanics of, 502
Abdominal thrusts, 611b
Abdominal wall muscles, 350, 351f-352f, 502
  anterior/anterolateral, 361-364, 362f-364f
  biomechanics of, 502
  posterior, 350, 351f-352f, 354-360
Abdominopelvic cavity, 63, 66f
Abducens nerve, 136f, 136t-137t
Abduction, 69, 70f-74f, 74, 247-249, 248f
  diagonal, 249
  of fingers, 524
  of glenohumeral joint, 509-510
  of hip, 528, 528t, 531
    muscle firing patterns in, 496
  horizontal, 249
    of shoulder, 509-510
  of scapula, 509, 512-513
  of wrist, 518
Abductor digiti minimi, 526
Abductor digiti minimis manus, 454, 454f
Abductor digiti minimis pedis, 410, 410f
Abductor digiti quinti pedis, 537
Abductor hallucis, 409, 409f
Abductor pollicis brevis, 452, 452f, 518
Abductor pollicis longus, 449, 449f, 518, 525-526
Abortion, spontaneous, 642
Absorption, 6
Acceleration, force and, 470
Accessory movements, 245, 245f
Accessory muscles of breathing, 503
Accessory nerve, 136f, 136t-137t
Acetabulum, 214, 218f, 262
Acetylcholine, 108, 148b
Achilles tendon reflex, 144
Aching pain, 40
Acid-base balance, 631
Acidity, 10, 10f, 631
Acne, 556
Acquired immunodeficiency syndrome (AIDS), 595-596
Acromegaly, 182
Acromioclavicular joint, 508
  close-packed position of, 248t
  least-packed position of, 247t
  movements of, 508
  palpation of, 257
  structure of, 255, 256f
Acromioclavicular ligament, 255, 255f-256f
Acromion, 210b, 211f
ACTH, 175, 176f, 177
Actin, 283, 289-291, 290f
Action potential, 103-105
  conduction of, 105, 105f-106f
Active joint movement, 272
  assisted, 272
  resistive, 272
Active transport, 11
Activities of daily living (ADLs), 75
Acupressure, 43, 152b
Acupuncture, 36b, 80-81
  autonomic nervous system and, 150-152
  connective tissue effects of, 15b, 81-85
  effects of, 15b, 81-85
  fascia and, 152
  indications for, 81b
  mechanism of action of, 81, 152b

Acupuncture (Continued)
  needle grasp in, 15b
  for pain, 43, 81b
Acupuncture points, 80-81, 85, 150-152, 292b
  meridians and, 85, 85f, 86b, 87
Acute disease, 30
Acute erosive gastritis, 623
Acute pain, 39, 39b
Acute pancreatitis, 626
Adam's apple, 606
Adaptation, 25
Adaptive capacity, 25
Addiction, 118b, 124
Addison's disease, 182, 187, 597t
Adduction, 69, 70f-74f, 74, 247-249, 248f
  diagonal, 249
  of fingers, 524
  of glenohumeral joint, 509-510
  of hip, 528, 528t, 532
  horizontal, 249
    of shoulder, 509-510, 516
  of scapula, 509
  of shoulder, 509-510, 516
  of thumb, 525
  of wrist, 518
Adductor brevis, 385, 385f, 529
Adductor hallucis, 413, 413f, 537
Adductor longus, 386, 386f, 529
Adductor magnus, 386, 386f, 529
Adductor pollicis, 456, 456f
Adductor tubercle, 219f
Adenoids, 586
Adenosine triphosphate (ATP), 9-10
  muscle action in, 287-288, 290-293
Adhesions, 15
  intestinal, 625
Adhesive capsulitis, 276-277
Adipose cells, in connective tissue, 15
Adipose tissue, 16, 17f, 170b
Adrenal cortex, 177
Adrenal glands, 169f, 177-178
  disorders of, 186-187
  in stress response, 47b, 48f, 177-178
Adrenal medulla, 177
Adrenaline, 177
Adrenocorticotropic hormone (ACTH), 175, 176f, 177
Afferent, 27
Age/aging
  cancer and, 33
  longevity and, 50-51
  physiology of, 50
  as risk factor, 30
Agonist muscles, 304
AIDS, 595-596
Air sinuses, 202, 203f, 606
Airway obstruction, 611
  Heimlich maneuver for, 611b
Alar ligament, 267f
Aldosterone, 177-178, 178b
Alimentary canal, 615
Alkalinity, 10, 10f, 631
Alkalosis, respiratory, 610
Allergic reactions, 32, 595, 595b
  to foods, 624
All-or-none response, in muscle contraction, 289
Alopecia, 561
Alpha-adrenergic blockers, 158
Alveoli, 605f
Alzheimer's disease, 126
Amino acids, 10
  essential, 619-621

Amphiarthroses, 242-243, 242f
Amputation, phantom pain and, 42-43
Amylase, 615, 618t
Amylin, 176
Amyotrophic lateral sclerosis (ALS), 126
Anabolism, 9
Anaerobic respiration, in muscle contraction, 293
Anal sphincter, external, 367, 367f
Analgesics, 43-44, 44b
Anaphylactic shock, 595b, 596
Anaplasia, 33
Anastomoses (arteriovenous shunts), 567
Anatomic planes, 69, 69f
Anatomic position, 63, 63f, 66, 69
Anatomic range of motion, 246
Anatomic terminology, 63-75, 285. See also
    Terminology.
  for muscles and muscle attachments, 284-285, 285b, 304-307
  for posterior regions of trunk, 65-66
  for regional and surface anatomy, 63
  for structural plan, 63-65
Anatomy, 4-5. See also Structural organization of body.
  definition of, 4
  developmental, 4
  gross, 4
  physiology and, 4-5
  regional, 4, 63, 65f
  surface, 4, 63, 65f
  systemic, 4
  tube-within-tube structure and, 63, 66f
Anatomy Trains: Myofascial Meridians for Manual and Movement Therapists (Myers), 294b, 301-303
Ancient healing practices. See Traditional medicine.
Anconeus, 439, 439f
Androgens, 178-179
Anemia, 575, 580
  bone marrow suppression, 581
  hemolytic, 597t
  nutritional, 580-581
  pallor in, 555
  pernicious, 597t
  sickle cell, 583
Aneurysms, 125, 580
Angina pectoris, 576-577
Angiomas, 560
Ankle, 213
  biomechanics of, 535-537
  bones of, 213, 220f, 221, 221b
  close-packed position of, 248t
  dorsiflexion of, 70f-74f, 75, 248-249, 264b, 536, 537f
  eversion of, 70f-74f, 75, 249, 536, 537f, 541
  inversion of, 70f-74f, 75, 249, 536, 537f, 540
  joints of, 264-265, 264b, 265f, 535-537
  least-packed position of, 247t
  ligaments of, 264, 265f
  movements of, 70f-74f, 241, 264, 264b, 535-537
  muscles of, 537
  palpation of, 265-266
  range of motion of, 271b
  sprains of, 275-277, 276f
  structure of, 535-537
Ankle-jerk reflex, 144
Ankylosing spondylitis, 277
Annular ligament of radius, 257, 257f
Antagonist muscles, 289, 295, 304, 418
Anterior, definition of, 67, 68f
Anterior clinoid process, 202f-203f
Anterior compartment syndrome, 461
Anterior corticospinal tracts, 123b

Anterior cruciate ligament, 262, 263f
Anterior deltoid, 510
Anterior inferior iliac spine, 218f
Anterior longitudinal ligament, 206, 206f, 266, 267f-268f
Anterior oblique ligament, 258
Anterior pelvic tilt, 249, 260, 475
Anterior pituitary hormones, 174-175, 174b, 176f
Anterior rotation, of hip, 474f, 527, 528t
Anterior sacroiliac ligament, 259, 261f
Anterior scalene, 333-334, 333f
Anterior sternoclavicular ligament, 255
Anterior superior iliac spine, 214, 218f
Antibiotics, for muscle disorders, 459-460
Antibodies, 590, 593-594
Antidepressants, 161
    for muscle disorders, 459-460
Antidiuretic hormone (ADH), 175, 175b, 176f
    deficiency of, 631-632
Antigens, 590
Antigravity muscles, 475
Antineoplastics, 33-34
Anus, 617, 619f
Anxiety, 127-128, 161
Aorta, 562f, 563
Aortic bodies, 609
Aortic valve, 563, 563f
Apical ligament of dens, 267f
Apical surface, 14
Apnea, 609
    infant, 612
    sleep, 611
Apocrine glands, 555
Aponeurosis, 298
    deltoid, 508-509
Appendicitis, 624
Appendicular, definition of, 64
Appendicular skeleton, 199, 200f-201f
    bones of, 209-213
Appendix, 617
Apple shape, health risks for, 32f
Arachnoid mater, 120, 120f
Arches, of foot, 213, 220f, 265-266, 536, 543f
Arcuate pubic ligament, 259
Ardnt-Schultz law, 300b
Areolar (loose) tissue, 16, 17f
Arm. See also Upper extremity.
    definition of, 209
Aromatherapy, 157b
    for pain, 44
Arrhythmias, 576
Arterial blood flow, stimulation of, 566b, 567f
Arterial inflammation, 580
    temporal, 580
Arteries, 563, 565
    of abdomen, 568f, 574
    definition of, 565
    of head and neck, 568f, 573
    of lower extremity, 568f, 574
    middle cerebral, 121, 121f
    principal, 568f
    structure of, 565, 566f
    therapeutic compression of, 566b, 567f
    of trunk, 568f, 574
    types of, 565
    of upper extremity, 568f, 573
    vertebral, 205
Arteriole(s), 562-563, 565, 566f
    blood pressure and, 571
Arteriole tone, 571
Arteriosclerosis, 572, 579
Arteriovenous shunts (anastomoses), 567
Arteritis, 580
    temporal, 580
Arthritis
    crystal-induced, 275
    infectious, 276
    osteoarthritis, 244b, 274, 274f
    rheumatoid, 246
Arthrokinematics, 245, 245f, 272
Articular (hyaline) cartilage, 16, 17f, 195-197, 238, 238f.
    See also Cartilage.
Articulations. See Joint(s).
Ascending tracts, 122-123, 122f
Ascorbic acid, 621t
Asian five-element theory, 25, 26f

Assessment
    biomechanical. See Biomechanical assessment.
    physical, 91
Asterion, 202f-203f
Asthma, 610
Asymptomatic infections, 591
Atherosclerosis, 579, 579f
Athlete's foot, 559
Atlantoaxial joint, 266, 267f
Atlantooccipital joint, 266, 267f
Atlas, 207f, 208
Atoms, 7, 7t, 9f
Atopic dermatitis, 561
ATP (adenosine triphosphate), 9-10
    muscle action in, 287-288, 290-293
Atrial natriuretic factor, 180
Atrioventricular valves, 563, 563f
Atrium, 562f, 563, 564f
Atrophy, 13, 50
Auditory bones, 154, 154f, 202, 202f-203f
Auricle, 153-154, 154f
Auricularis, 312, 312f
Auricularis posterior, 312, 312f
Auricularis superior, 312, 312f
Autoimmune diseases, 32, 181, 596-597, 597t
Autonomic nervous system, 100, 134, 147-152
    divisions of, 100, 147-150
        enteric, 100, 134, 147, 147t
        parasympathetic, 100, 134, 147-150, 149f, 151t, 177b
        sympathetic, 100, 134, 147-150, 149f, 151t, 177b
    drugs affecting, 158
    fight-or-flight response and, 46, 148
    functions of, 147
    meridians and, 150-152
    neurotransmitters of, 147t, 148b
    receptors of, 148b
    in stress response, 46, 48f
    yin/yang and, 150-152
Avulsion, 239
Avulsion fractures, 214, 224f
Axial, definition of, 64
Axial skeleton, 199, 200f-201f, 202-209
Axillary sheath, 299f
Axis, 207f, 208
Axis of rotation, 470
Axons, 101, 102f
Ayurveda, 25-27, 26b, 26f, 81. See also Chakras;
    Traditional medicine.

B cells, 593-594
Back muscles, 335-349, 335f-336f
    deep, 335-349, 335f-336f
    intermediate, 335f-336f
    oblique (transversospinales group), 342-346, 342f-346f
    suboccipital, 347-349, 348f-349f
    superficial, 335f-336f
    vertical (erector spinae group), 338-340, 338f-340f
Back pain, 223b, 277, 527
Back-shu points, 150-152
Bacterial infections, of skin, 556, 557f-558f
Balance, 152b, 155, 473, 474f
    duality of, 4
Baldness, 561
Ball-and-socket joints, 250, 253f
Baroreceptors, 630
    blood pressure and, 573, 573b
Bartholin's cysts, 643
Bartholin's glands, 637
Basal cell carcinoma, 557f-558f, 560
Basal ganglia, 111
Basal metabolic rate (BMR), 622
Basal surface, 14
Base pairs, 8b, 8f
Basement membrane, 14
Basophils, 576
Bed bugs, 559
Behavior
    body chemistry of, 106-109, 109b
    pain, 109-110
Bell's palsy, 160
Bending, biomechanics of, 240-242, 244f, 478
Benign prostatic hypertrophy, 644
Benign tumors, 33, 33f
Beta-adrenergic drugs, 158

Biaxial joints, 250, 253f
Biceps brachii, 435-439, 435f, 510, 518
Biceps femoris, 380, 380f, 529, 535
Biceps reflex, 144
Bifurcate ligament, 265f
Bilateral arm adductor test, 492
Bilateral leg adductor test, 492-493
Bile, 620t
Bile duct, in hepatic triad, 575
Biofeedback, for pain, 44
Biologic rhythms, 28-29, 29f
    circadian, 28
    melatonin and, 179-180, 187
    ultradian, 28
Biology, 58b
Biomechanical assessment, 494-537
    clinical reasoning in, 498
    of joints, 494-498
    range of motion in, 498
    resistance in, 498
    stabilization in, 498
Biomechanical dysfunctions, 537-546
    degrees of, 545-546
    joint-related, 544-545
    myofascial-related, 543
    neuromuscular-related, 543
    nonoptimal motor function, 543, 545
    postural deviations, 542-543, 545f
    regional postural muscular imbalance, 543, 545
    stages of, 546
Biomechanics, 69, 468-549. See also Joint
        movement(s).
    of abdomen, 502
    of ankle, 535-537
    balance and, 473, 474f
    of bending, 240-242, 244f, 478
    of clavicle, 508
    connective tissue and, 300-301, 300b-301b
    definitions of, 193, 193b
    of elbow, 517-518, 519f-525b
    equilibrium and, 473
    of fingers, 518-526
    of foot, 535-537
    force and, 469-470
    of hand, 518-526
    of head and neck, 500-501
    of hip, 526-529
    kinetic chains and, 294, 476-494
    of knee, 533-534
    laws of, 300b
    mechanical advantage and disadvantage and,
        471-472, 472f
    muscle firing patterns and, 297-298, 494
    of pelvic girdle, 526-529
    posture and, 473-476, 475f
    of shoulder region, 508-510
    of sitting, 478
    skeletal system and, 192-233
    of spine, 501-502, 501f
    stability and, 473
    of standing, 478, 479f
    of thorax, 501-503
    of trunk, 501-503
    vs. kinesiology, 469
    of walking, 478-480, 480f-482f
    of wrist, 518-526
Biotin, 621t
Bipennate muscles, 295, 296f
Bipolar neurons, 102, 103b
Birth control pills, 637
Birth process, 628
Bladder, 627f, 628
    infections of, 633
Bleeding, 582-583
    dysfunctional uterine, 644
    during pregnancy, 641
Blind spot, 156
Blood, 16, 17f, 575-576
    components of, 575-576
    disorders of, 580-583
    production of, 575
    viscosity of, 572-573
Blood cells
    platelets, 576
    red, 575, 609
    white, 575-576

Blood flow
   arterial, stimulation of, 566b, 567f
   cardiac, 563-564, 564f
   hydrostatic pressure and, 572
   venous return and, 568-570, 570f
   viscosity and, 572-573
Blood gases, 609
Blood pressure, 570-573, 572b
   baroreceptors and, 573, 573b
   elevated, 579
      in pregnancy, 643
Blood supply
   of heart, 563, 564f, 568-570
   of liver, 574-575
   of lung, 607
   of skin, 554
Blood types, 575
Blood vessels. *See also* Vascular system.
   of brain, 121, 121f
   types of, 563. *See also* Arteries; Arteriole(s);
      Capillaries; Veins; Venules.
Bloom's Taxonomy, 284b
Body, tensegrity of, 301-303, 302f
Body cavities, 63, 65-66, 66f
Body map, 63-68, 63f. *See also* Structural organization
      of body.
Body movements. *See* Joint movement(s).
Body planes, 69-75, 69f
   cardinal, 247-248, 248f
Body positions. *See* Position(s).
Body rhythms. *See* Biologic rhythms.
Body types, health risks for, 32f
Body water. *See also* Fluid.
   distribution of, 628, 628f, 629t
   functions of, 629t
   loss of, 632f
   metabolic, 629
Body weight, 622-623
   in pregnancy, 638t
Boils, 556, 557f-558f
Bonds. *See* Chemical bonds.
Bone(s), 16, 17f, 194-197. *See also* Skeletal system.
   age-related changes in, 197
   of ankle, 213, 220f, 221b
   of appendicular skeleton, 209-213
   auditory, 154, 154f, 202, 202f-203f
   avulsion of, 239
   of axial skeleton, 199, 200f-201f, 202-209
   characteristics of, 193-194
   classification, 197
   compact (dense), 195, 196f
   as connective tissue, 238
   cranial, 202, 202f-203f, 204b, 267f
   cube-shaped, 197
   demineralization of, 224
   depressions and openings in, 198
   development of, 195
   of elbow, 211-212, 212b, 213f-214f
   facial, 202, 202f-203f, 204b
   of fingers, 211-212
   flat, 197
   of foot, 213, 220f-221f, 221, 221b, 535
   of forearm, 212, 214f
   functions of, 193-194
   growth and repair of, 197
   of hand, 211-212, 216f
   of hip, 211, 214b, 218f, 221f
   infections of, 225
   irregular, 197
   of knee, 213, 215, 219f, 221f, 262b
   lacrimal, 204b
   long, 197
   of lower extremity, 211-213, 214b-215b, 218f-221f,
      221b
   of neck, 203-206, 207f
   necrosis of, 224-225
   of pectoral girdle, 209, 210b, 211f
   piezoelectric qualities of, 194, 194b, 198b
   radiation effects on, 224
   repair of. *See* Bone healing.
   sesamoid, 194, 197
   short, 197
   of shoulder, 209, 211f, 217f, 256f
   of spine. *See* Vertebrae.
   spongy (cancellous), 195, 196f
   structure of, 194-195

Bone(s) *(Continued)*
   tensegrity of, 301-303, 302f
   thoracic, 209, 209b, 210f
   tuberculosis of, 225
   tumors of, 225
   of upper extremity, 209-211, 211f, 212b, 213f-214f,
      216f-217f
   of wrist, 211-212, 216f
Bone healing, 39f
   piezoelectric effect and, 194, 194b, 198b
Bone marrow, 195
Bone marrow suppression anemia, 581
Bone spurs, 274
Bone stimulators, 198b
Bone tissue, 194-195, 196f
Bony end feel, 246
Bony landmarks, 197-199
Bony processes
   joint-forming, 198-199
   of scapula, 210b, 213f
   of skull, 199, 202f-203f
   spinous, 204, 205f-206f
   of sternum, 209, 209b, 210f
   for tendon/ligament attachment, 199
   of ulna, 212, 214f
Boundaries, maintenance of, 5
Bow legs, 533-534
Brachial plexus, 137, 139f
   injuries of, 159
Brachialis, 436, 436f, 518
Brachioradialis, 436, 436f, 518
Bradycardia, 576
Bradypnea, 609
Brain. *See also under* Cerebral.
   blood vessels of, 121, 121f
   integrative/associative functions of, 113-118, 116f
   meninges of, 119-120, 120f
   motor areas of, 101f
   sensory areas of, 101f
   structure of, 111-121, 112f-114f, 114t-115t. *See also*
      specific structures.
   ventricles of, 120, 120f
Brain aneurysms, 125
Brain dominance, 111, 112f
Brain tumors, 126
Brainstem, 112f-113f, 119
Breast
   cancer of, 560-561
   development of, 637
   disorders of, 560-561
   fibrocystic disease of, 560
   lumps in, 643
   mammary glands of, 555
Breastfeeding, 641
Breathing. *See also* Respiration.
   control of, 609
   diaphragmatic (abdominal), 503
   exhalation in, 607, 608f
   inhalation in, 607, 608f
   mechanics of, 607-610, 608f
   muscles of, 350-369, 351f-352f, 502-503, 607-610,
      607f-608f
   reflexes in, 609-610
   during sleep, 605
   thoracic, 503
Breathing pattern disorder, 161, 609, 612-613
Bright pain, 40
Broad ligament, 636
Broca's area, 111-113, 114f
Bronchi, 605f, 606
Bronchioles, 606
Bronchoconstriction, 607
Bronchodilation, 607
Bruise, muscle, 461
Buccinator, 318, 318f
Buffers, 10
Bulbospongiosus, 368-369, 368f
Bulbourethral glands, 635, 635f
Burning pain, 40
Burns, 561
Bursae, 238, 244b. *See also* Connective tissue.
   of knee, 264
Bursitis, 273
Café coronary, 611
Calcaneofibular ligament, 265f
   of ankle, 264

Calcaneus, 220f, 221
Calcification, 195
Calcitonin, 176
Calcium balance, 630-631
Calculi, urinary, 633
Callus, 220, 222, 559-560
Canals, in bone, 198
Cancellous bone, 195, 196f
Cancer
   bone, 225
   breast, 560-561
   causative factors in, 33b
   cell growth in, 33
   cervical, 643
   colon, 626
   Hodgkin's disease, 588
   leukemia, 588
   lung, 611
   lymphoma, 588
   metastasis in, 33
   pathogenesis of, 32-34
   prostate, 644
   skin, 557f-558f, 560
   stomach, 626
   treatment of, 33-34
   warning signs of, 33, 33b
Candidiasis, 559
   vaginal, 644
Capillaries, 563, 565-567, 566f
   definition of, 565
   lymph, 584, 584f-585f
   permeability of, 629
   structure of, 566f
Capital extension, 503
Capital extensors, 500
Capital flexion, 504
Capital flexors, 500
Capital movement, 501
Capitulum, 212, 217f
Capsular end feel, 246
Capsular ligaments, 237
Carbohydrates, 10, 621
Carbon dioxide, 609
Carbon monoxide poisoning, 612
Carbuncles, 550
Carcinogens, 33
Cardiac arrhythmias, 576
Cardiac conduction system, 564-565
Cardiac cycle, 564
Cardiac input, 568-569
Cardiac muscle, 286-287, 287f
   innervation of, 291
Cardiac muscle fibers, 16
Cardiac output, 565
Cardiac sphincter, 616
Cardiac valves, 563f, 564-565
   dysfunction of, 576
Cardinal planes of body, 247-248, 248f
Cardiomyopathy, 597t
Cardiovascular system, 562-583. *See also* Heart;
      Vascular system.
   disorders of, 576-583, 583b
   massage contraindications for, 583b
Carotene, 555
Carotid bodies, 609
Carotid canal, 202f-203f
Carpal tunnel syndrome, 159
Carpals, 211, 212b, 216f
Carpometacarpal joint, 258
   close-packed position of, 248t
   least-packed position of, 247t
Carrier-mediated transport, 11
Cartilage, 16, 238. *See also* Connective tissue.
   articular (hyaline), 16, 17f, 195-197, 238, 238f
   elastic, 16, 17f, 238
   fibrocartilage, 16, 17f, 238
   piezoelectric effect on, 17b
   tumors of, 225
Cartilaginous joints, 242-243
Casts, 276
Catabolism, 9
Catecholamines, 108, 124, 177b
Cauda equina, 121f, 122
Causalgia syndrome, 161
CD4 T cells, 594
   in HIV infection, 595-596

Cecum, 617
Cell(s), 13
    cancer, 33
    functions of, 13
    muscle, 13, 16
    nerve, 18
    size of, 13
    structure of, 11-12, 12f
Cell cycle, 13
Cell differentiation, 13
Cell division, 13
Cell matrix, 13-14
Cell membrane, 11, 12f. *See also under* Membrane.
Cellulitis, 556
Center of gravity, 473
Central nervous system. *See also* Brain; Nervous system;
        Spinal cord.
    components of, 100
    drugs affecting, 123-124
    pathologic conditions of, 124-128
Central sulcus, 113
Cerebellum, 112f, 119, 120b
    rocking and, 120b
Cerebral aneurysms, 125
Cerebral cortex, 111, 114f, 114t-115t
Cerebral palsy, 125
Cerebrospinal fluid, 102, 120
Cerebrovascular accident, 124-125
Cerebrovascular disease, 125
Cerebrum, 111-113, 112f-114f
    frontal lobe of, 111-113, 114f, 114t-115t
    gyri, sulci, and fissures of, 113
    insula of, 113, 114f
    limbic system of, 113
    occipital lobe of, 113, 114f, 114t-115t
    parietal lobe of, 113, 114f, 114t-115t
    temporal lobe of, 113, 114f, 114t-115t
Cerumen, 555
Ceruminous glands, 555
Cervical cancer, 643
Cervical extension, 501, 504
Cervical flexion, 505
Cervical movements, 501
Cervical plexus, 135, 138f, 159
    injuries of, 159
Cervical polyps, 644
Cervical region, 66
Cervical rotation, 505-506
Cervical vertebrae, 203-206, 207f, 208, 208b. *See also*
        Spine; Vertebrae.
    movements of, 266
Cervicitis, 643
Cervix, 636
Cesarean birth, 641
Chakras, 26, 26f, 51
    endocrine glands and, 170-171, 172f, 179
    life cycle and, 51
    location of, 172f
Channels. *See* Meridians.
Charting, 91
    databases for, 91
    problem-oriented medical record in, 91
    SOAP notes in, 90-91
    terminology for, 76b
Cheek bones, 202f-203f, 204b
Chemical agents, disease-causing, 32
Chemical bonds, 7-8
    covalent, 7, 9f
    high-energy, 9-10
    hydrogen, 7-8
    ionic, 7, 9f
    polar covalent, 7-8
Chemical messengers, 107b. *See also* Neurotransmitters.
Chemical properties, 6-7
Chemical reactions, 8, 9f
    anabolic, 9
    catabolic, 9
Chemistry, 58b
Chest. *See under* Thoracic; Thorax.
Chewing, muscles for, 320-322, 320f-322f
Chicken pox, 556-558
Childbirth, 628
Chinese medicine. *See* Traditional Chinese medicine.
Chloride balance, 631
Choking, 611
    Heimlich maneuver for, 611b

Cholecystokinin, 108, 180
Chondroblasts, 195
Chondrosarcomas, 225
Chondrosternal joints, 268
Chordae tendineae, 563
Chorea, 127
Choroid, 155f, 156
Chronic bronchitis, 610-611
Chronic disease, 30
Chronic inflammation, 37
Chronic obstructive pulmonary disease (COPD),
        610-611
Chronic pain, 39, 39b
Chronic pancreatitis, 626
Chyme, 616
Ciliary body, 155f, 156
Circadian rhythms, 28, 29f
    melatonin and, 179-180, 187
Circle of Willis, 121, 121f
Circular muscles, 295, 296f
Circulation
    blood, 6. *See also* Blood flow.
    lymphatic, 6, 586, 587b, 587f
Circumcision, 635
Circumduction, 75, 249
Cirrhosis, 625, 625f
Cisterna chyli, 586
Citric acid cycle, 617, 620f
Clavicle, 210b, 211f, 217f
    biomechanics of, 508
Cleavage lines, of skin, 553, 554f
Cleft palate, 223
Clinical reasoning, 3b, 90-92, 90b
    in biomechanical assessment, 498
    in charting, 91
    in data analysis, 91, 92b
    in data collection, 91
    in treatment planning, 91-92
Closed fractures, 214, 224f
Close-packed position, 246-247, 247f, 248t
Clubfoot, 223
Cluster headaches, 127
Coccygeal plexus, 353f
Coccygeus, 366, 366f
Coccyx, 66, 205, 207f, 208b
Cochlea, 153
Coenzymes, 621
Cold application, for pain, 44
Cold sores, 558
Colds, 610
Collagen, 14, 237, 237f
Collagenous fibers, 14
Collar bone (clavicle), 210b, 211f, 217f
    biomechanics of, 508
Colloids, 300b
    thixotropy of, 17b, 301, 301b
Colon, 614f, 616, 619f
    cancer of, 626
    structure of, 614f
Colostomy, 617
Combining vowels, 59
Comminuted fractures, 215, 224f
Common cold, 610
Communicable diseases, 30
Communication, ethical issues in, 59
Compact bone, 195, 196f
Complementary and alternative medicine, 170b.
        See also Traditional medicine.
Complete fractures, 215, 224f
Complex regional pain syndrome, 161
Compound(s), 7
    inorganic, 10
    organic, 10
Compound fractures, 214, 220, 224f
Compression, 240, 242f
    arterial, 566b, 567f
Compression fractures, 215, 224f
Compression neuropathies, 158-162
Compression syndromes, 158-162
Concentric action, 288-289, 288f, 304
    muscle dysfunction in, 459
Concussions, 125
Conditioned reflex, 140-142. *See also* Reflex(es).
Condoms, 636
Conductivity, 6
Condyles, 198

Condyloid joints, 250, 253f
Cones, 156
Congenital diseases, 30
Congestive heart failure, 577-578
Connective tissue, 14-16, 17f, 235-240. *See also specific*
        types.
    acupuncture effects on, 15b, 81-85
    adipose, 16, 17f
    biomechanical forces on, 300-301, 300b-301b
    bone, 238
    bursae, 238
    cartilage, 238
    cell types in, 15, 15t
    characteristics of, 298-300
    collagen in, 14, 237, 237f
    creep in, 238, 301, 301b
    dense irregular, 16, 17f
    dense regular, 16, 17f
    distribution of, 15, 15t
    elastin in, 237, 237f
    fascia. *See* Fascia.
    fiber types in, 14-15
    functions of, 298-300
    ground substance of, 17b
    laxity of, 239
    lengthening of, 239
    ligaments, 197, 237-238
    loading/unloading of, 301-302, 301b
    loose (areolar), 16, 17f
    manipulation of, 15, 15b, 17b
    muscles and, 298-303
    of nerves, 134, 135f
    pathologic changes in, 303
    plastic range of, 239-240
    practical applications for, 17b
    repair of, 303
    shortening of, 239-240
    structure of, 14-15, 236, 298
    tendons, 238
    tensegrity of, 301-303, 302f
    types of, 15-16
    water content of, 303
Connective tissue growth factor, 555-556
Connective tissue matrix, 298
Connective tissue membranes, 16
Connective tissue sheaths, 289f, 298, 299f
Conn's syndrome, 186-187
Conoid ligament, 255f
Consciousness, 113, 117b
    altered states of, 117, 117b
Constipation, 623
    massage for, 626b, 627f
Contact dermatitis, 557f-558f, 561
Contraception
    female, 637
    male, 636
Contractility, of muscle, 287. *See also* Muscle
        contraction.
Contracture(s), 460
    Dupuytren's, 460
    Volkmann's ischemic, 460
Contralateral, definition of, 68
Contralateral reflexes, 145
Contusion, muscle, 461
Convergent muscles, 295, 296f
Convulsions, 126-127
COPD (chronic obstructive pulmonary disease),
        610-611
Coracobrachialis, 431, 431f, 510
Coracoclavicular ligament, 255f-256f
Coracohumeral ligament, 255
Coracoid fossa, 211f
Coracoid process, 210, 211f, 217f
Cornea, 155, 155f
Corns, 560
Coronal (frontal) plane, 69, 69f, 247, 248f
Coronal suture, 202, 202f-204f, 254, 254f
Coronary arteries, 562f, 563-564
Coronary artery disease, 579, 579f
Coronoid fossa, 211-212, 213f
Coronoid process, 212, 214f, 217f
Corpus luteum, 637
Corrugator supercilii, 310, 310f
Corticosteroids, synthetic, 182
    for muscle disorders, 459-460
Corticotropin-releasing hormone, 170t

Cortisol, 47b, 177-178, 178b
Costal angle, 209
Costochondral joints, 268
Costoclavicular ligament, 255, 256f
Costospinal joints, 268, 270f
Costotransverse facet, 268f
Costotransverse joints, 268, 270f
Costotransverse ligaments, 268
Costovertebral facet, 268f
Costovertebral joints, 268, 270f
Cough reflex, 609
Counterirritation, for pain, 40, 41f
Counternutation, 249, 260b
Covalent bonds, 7, 9f
Cowper's glands, 635, 635f
Cramps, 460
Cranial bones, 202, 202f-203f, 204b, 267f
Cranial cavity, 65, 66f
Cranial nerves, 134-135, 136f, 136t-137t. *See also* Nerve(s).
Cranial sutures, 202, 202f-204f, 242-243, 243b, 254, 254f
    palpation of, 254
Cranial-sacral rhythm, 120b, 527
Craniosacral system, pelvic girdle and, 527
Creep, 238, 301, 301b
Cremaster, 364, 364f
Crests, 199
Cretinism, 183
Critical thinking, 3b, 90, 90b
    in charting/documentation, 91
Crohn's disease, 625
Crossed extensor reflex, 145, 297
Cross-fiber friction, 242
Croup, 610
Crystal-induced arthritis, 275
Cube-shaped bones, 197
Cuboid bone, of ankle, 199, 220f
Cun, 87
Cuneiform bones, of ankle, 220f, 221b
Cupping, 87
Cushing's disease, 186
    secondary, 182
Cushing's syndrome, 186
Cutaneous membranes, 14
Cyanocobalamin, 621t
Cyanosis, 555
Cyst(s)
    Bartholin's, 643
    sebaceous, 560
Cystic fibrosis, 611, 626
Cystitis, 633
Cytokines, 594
Cytoplasm, 11, 12f
Cytoskeleton, 11
Cytosol, 11
Cytotoxic T cells, 594

Data analysis, 91, 92b
Data collection, 91
Databases, for charting, 91
Decubitus ulcers, 559
Deep, definition of, 68
Deep fascia, 298
Deep pain, 40
Deep tendon reflexes, 122, 144, 297
Deep transverse perineals, 367, 367f
Deep vein thrombosis, 581
Degenerative disorders, 32, 126, 244b
Degenerative joint disease, 244b, 274f, 277
Dehydration, 631-632, 633f
    effects of, 632f
    routes of fluid loss in, 629t
Delivery, obstetric, 640
Deltoid aponeurosis, 508-509
Deltoid ligament, 264, 265f
Deltoid muscle, 428-431, 428f
    anterior, 510
    middle, 510
    posterior, 510
Dementia, 126
    Alzheimer's, 126
Dendrites, 101, 102f
Dense bone, 195, 196f
Dense irregular tissue, 16, 17f
Dense regular tissue, 16, 17f

Deoxyribonucleic acid (DNA), 8b, 8f, 11
Depolarization, 103-104
Depressant drugs, 124
Depressed fractures, 215, 224f
Depression (motor), 70f-74f, 75, 249
    of scapula, 509, 514
Depression (psychological), 127, 161
Depressor anguli oris, 314, 314f
Depressor labii inferioris, 317, 317f
Dermatitis, 557f-558f, 561
Dermatomes, 42, 42f, 138-139, 141f
Dermatophytosis, 557f-558f, 559
Dermis, 553, 553f
Descending tracts, 122-123, 122f, 123b
Developmental anatomy, 4
Deviated septum, 606
Dextral (dextro), 68
Diabetes insipidus, 183, 631-632
Diabetes mellitus
    complications of, 185-186, 186f
    dehydration in, 632
    type I (insulin-dependent), 185, 597t
    type II (non–insulin-dependent), 185
Diabetic ketoacidosis, 161, 185
Diabetic neuropathy, 161
Diagnosis, 30
Diagonal abduction, 249
Diagonal adduction, 249
Diaphragm, 350, 354, 354f, 502-503, 606-610, 607f
Diaphragmatic breathing, 503
Diarrhea, 624
Diarthroses. *See* Synovial joints.
Diastole, 564
Diastolic pressure, 571
Dictionaries, medical, 59-62
Diencephalon, 112f, 114f, 118
Diet. *See also* Nutrition.
    food groups in, 619-622
Diffusion, 11
Digastric, 326, 326f
Digestion, 6, 613, 617
    absorption sites in, 617f
    citric acid cycle in, 617, 620f
    nutrition and, 618-623
    organs of, 619f
    peristalsis in, 617
    steps in, 618b
Digestive enzymes and juices, 615-616, 618t
Digestive system, 613-626
    disorders of, 623-626, 626b
    hormones of, 180
    organs of, 614f, 615-617
    psychosocial aspects of, 614-615
Directional sense, 152b
Directional terms, 67-68, 68f
Disaccharides, 621
Disease. *See also specific diseases.*
    acute, 30
    autoimmune, 32, 181, 596-597, 597t
    causes of, 30-36, 30b
    chronic, 30
    communicable, 30
    congenital, 30
    definition of, 30
    diagnosis of, 30
    epidemiology of, 30
    etiology of, 30
    idiopathic, 30
    immunodeficiency, 32
    inflammatory, 37b
    inherited, 30
    mechanisms of, 29-36
    pathogenesis of, 30
    pathology of, 30
    prognosis of, 30
    remission in, 30
    risk factors for, 30, 30b
    signs of, 30
    stress-induced, 30, 49b
    subacute, 30
    symptoms of, 30
Disharmony, 87
Disk
    intervertebral. *See* Intervertebral disks.
    optic, 156
Dislocations, 235

Displaced fractures, 224f
Distal, definition of, 67, 68f
Distal interphalangeal joints
    of foot, 264f, 265, 536, 536f
    of hand, 243f, 259
        close-packed position of, 248t
        least-packed position of, 247t
Distal tibiofibular joint, 264-265
Distraction, for pain, 43
Diverticular disease, 625
DNA (deoxyribonucleic acid), 8b, 8f, 11
Documentation. *See* Charting.
Dominance, brain, 111, 112f
Dopamine, 108, 109b, 148b
Dorsal, definition of, 67, 68f
Dorsal cavities, 63, 65
Dorsal interosseous, 526
Dorsal root ganglion, 135
Dorsal roots, 122
Dorsal sacroiliac ligament, 259, 261f
Dorsiflexion, 70f-74f, 75, 248-249, 264b, 536, 537f, 540
Doshas, 26
Double helix, 8b, 8f
Double stance, 480
Dowager's hump (hyperkyphosis), 209, 223, 223f, 277
Downward rotation, 249
Drowning, 612
Drug(s)
    affecting central nervous system, 123-124
    for cancer, 33-34
    for infections, 32b
    mood-altering, 109
    psychotropic, 109
Drug addiction, 118b, 124
Drug tolerance, 124
Dual innervation, 147
Duality
    of balance, 4
    definition of, 4
    of wholeness, 4
    yin/yang and. *See* Yin/yang.
Duchenne's muscular dystrophy, 462-463
Duodenal ulcers, 624
Duodenum, 614f, 616
Dupuytren's contracture, 460
Dura mater, 120, 120f
Dwarfism, 182-183
Dynamic force, 286
Dynorphins, 108

Ear
    immune defenses of, 591
    muscles of, 312, 312f
    ossicles of, 154, 154f, 202, 202f-203f
    structure of, 153-154, 154f
    vestibular apparatus of, 119b, 155
Eardrum, 154, 154f
Earth science, 58b
Earwax, 555
Eating, 613. *See also* Diet; Food; Nutrition.
    psychosocial aspects of, 614-615
Eccentric action, 288f, 289, 304
    muscle dysfunction in, 459
Eccrine glands, 554-555
Ecthyma, 556
Ectomorphs, 32f
Ectopic pregnancy, 643
Eczema, 557f-558f, 561
Edema, 586-587, 632, 633f
    pulmonary, 611
Efferent, 27
Effort, 99b-100b
    force and, 470
Ejaculation, 636
Ejaculatory duct, 635, 635f
Elastic cartilage, 16, 17f, 238
Elastic fibers, 15, 237, 237f
Elasticity, 238
    of fascia, 301, 301b
    of muscle, 287
Elastin, 15, 237, 237f
Elbow
    biomechanics of, 517-518
    bones of, 211-212, 212b, 213f-214f
    close-packed position of, 248t
    extension of, 520

Elbow *(Continued)*
  flexion of, 519
  golfer's, 273
  joints of, 257-258, 257f-258f, 517-518
  least-packed position of, 247t
  ligaments of, 257-258, 257f
  movements of, 70f-74f, 257-258, 258f, 517-518, 519b-525b
  muscles of, 433-439, 433f-434f, 518
  palpation of, 258
  pitcher's, 273
  range of motion of, 271b
  structure of, 257, 257f-258f
  tennis, 273
Electrical stimulation
  bone effects of, 194, 194b, 198b
  cartilage effects of, 17b
Electrocardiogram, 564-565
Electrolyte balance, 630-631
Electron, 7, 9f
Electron shells, 7, 9f
Elements, chemical, 7, 7t
Elephantiasis, 587
Elevation, 70f-74f, 75, 249
  of pelvis, 507
  of scapula, 509, 513
Elimination, 613
  psychosocial aspects of, 615
Ellipsoid joints, 250, 253f
Embolus, 581-582
Emissary foramen, 202f-203f
Emotional eating, 614-615
Emotions, 116
Emphysema, 610-611
Encephalitis, 128
End feel, 246
Endarteritis obliterans, 580
Endocarditis, 578
Endocardium, 562-563, 566f
Endocrine axis, 170
Endocrine disorders, 181-182
  adrenal, 186-187
  of hypersecretion, 173, 181
  of hyposecretion, 173, 181-182
  nonglandular, 182
  pancreatic, 185-186
  parathyroid, 184-185
  pineal, 187
  pituitary, 182-183
  primary vs. secondary, 173
  thyroid, 183-184, 183f, 184t
Endocrine system, 167-191
  chakras and, 170-171, 172f, 179
  functions of, 168
  glands of, 168-169, 169f. *See also specific glands.*
  hormones of. *See* Hormones.
  negative feedback in, 168, 169f, 173
  nervous system and, 99, 168, 170, 177b
  overview of, 167-168
Endocytosis, 11
Endometrial polyps, 644
Endometriosis, 643
Endometrium, 636
Endomorphs, health risks for, 32f
Endomysium, 289f, 298
Endoneurium, 134, 135f
Endoplasmic reticulum, 11-12, 12f
Endorphins, 44b, 108, 110, 180-181
Endoskeleton, 193
Endosteum, 195, 196f
Energy
  definition of, 8
  kinetic, 8
  muscles and, 286
  potential, 8
Energy balance, 622-623
Energy levels, atomic, 9f
Energy patterns, 18. *See also* Yin/yang.
Engrams, 116
Enkephalins, 44b, 108, 110
Enteric nervous system, 100, 134, 147, 147t
Enteritis, 623-624
Entrainment, 565
Entrapment neuropathies, 159
Environmental risk factors, 30
  for cancer, 33

Enzymes, 10
  digestive, 615-616, 618t
Eosinophils, 576
Epicardium, 562-563, 566f
Epicondyles, 199
  of femur, 215, 219f
  of humerus, 209, 213f, 217f
Epidemiology, 30
Epidermis, 553, 553f
Epidural hematoma, 125
Epidural space, 120, 120f
Epiglottis, 609
Epilepsy, 126-127
Epimysium, 289f, 298
Epinephrine, 108, 177
Epineurium, 134, 135f
Episiotomy, 640-641
Epithelial tissue, 14, 14f, 17f
Equilibrium, 155, 473
Erect position, 66
Erection, 636
Erector pili, 554
Erector spinae group, 338-340, 338f-340f
Erysipelas, 556
Erythrocytes, 575
  oxygen transport by, 609
Erythropoietin, 180
Esophagitis, reflux, 624
Esophagus, 614f, 616, 619f
Essential amino acids, 619-621
Essential substances, 87
Essential tremor, 127
Estradiol, 637
Estrogen, 178-179, 637
Ethical issues, in communication, 59
Ethmoid bone, 204b
Ethmoid sinus, 202, 203f
Etiology, 30
Eustachian tube, 154, 154f
Eversion, 70f-74f, 75, 249, 536, 537f, 541
Excitability, muscle, 287
Excretion, 6
Exocrine glands, 168
Exocytosis, 11
Exophthalmos, 183
Expiratory reserve volume, 609
Extensibility, of muscle, 287
Extension, 69, 70f-74f, 247-249, 248f, 418
  capital, 500, 503
  cervical, 501, 504
  of elbow, 520
  of fingers, 523
  of glenohumeral joint, 509-510
  of hip, 528, 528t, 531
  hyperextension and, 70f-74f, 74
  of knee, 534, 539
    muscle firing patterns in, 497
  of shoulder, 509-510, 515
  of spine, 501
  of toe, 536, 541
  of trunk, 506
  of wrist, 518, 522
Extensor carpi radialis brevis, 446, 446f, 518
Extensor carpi radialis longus, 445, 445f, 518
Extensor carpi ulnaris, 447, 447f, 525
Extensor digiti minimi, 447, 447f, 525-526
Extensor digitorum, 446, 446f, 525-526
Extensor digitorum brevis, 408, 408f
Extensor digitorum longus, 396, 396f, 537
Extensor hallucis longus, 397, 397f
Extensor indicis, 525-526
Extensor pollicis brevis, 448-450, 448f, 525-526
Extensor pollicis longus, 449, 449f, 525-526
External, definition of, 68
External anal sphincter, 367, 367f
External auditory meatus, 202f-203f
External intercostals, 356, 356f, 502-503
External oblique, 363, 363f, 502
External occipital protuberance, 202f-203f
External pterygoid, 321, 321f
External respiration, 604
External rotation. *See also* Rotation.
  of hip, 532
  of knee, 534
  of shoulder, 517
Exteroceptors, 141, 142f

Extracellular fluid, 13, 628-629, 628f
Exudates, inflammatory, 34, 34b
Eye
  immune defenses of, 591
  muscles of, 156, 313, 313f
  structure of, 155-156, 155f

Facet(s)
  bony, 199
  vertebral, 205, 205f, 266, 268f
Facet capsular ligament, 268f
Facial bones, 202, 202f-203f, 204b
Facial muscles, 307-322, 308f
  expression, 309-310
Facial nerve, 136f, 136t-137t
  Bell's palsy of, 160
Factors, in blood typing, 575
Fallopian tubes, 636
Fascia, 298-303
  biomechanical forces on, 300-301, 300b-301b, 303
  characteristics of, 298-300
  as colloid, 300b
  deep, 298
  elasticity of, 301, 301b
  functions of, 298-300
  innervation of, 146-147, 149-150
  of leg, 393
  loading/unloading of, 301-302, 301b
  meridians and, 152
  pathologic changes in, 303
  of pectoral region, 350
  pliability of, 301
  prevertebral, 299f
  repair of, 303
  superficial, 298, 553-554
  tensegrity of, 301-303, 302f
  of thigh, 299f
  water content of, 303
Fascia lata, 299f
Fascicles, 298
Fasciitis, plantar, 213, 222
Fascioscapulohumeral dystrophy, 462
Fast-twitch fibers, 291-293
Fats, dietary, 621
Fatty acids, 621
Feedback, positive, 27-28
Feedback loops, 27-28, 27f. *See also* Negative feedback.
  biological rhythms and, 28, 29f
  in endocrine system, 168, 169f, 173
  negative feedback and, 27, 27f
Feet. *See* Foot.
Female reproductive system, 636-641, 640f
  external organs of, 637
  internal organs of, 636-637
Femur, 213, 215, 219f, 221f
Fertilization, 637-638
Fibers
  collagenous (white), 14
  elastic (yellow), 15, 237, 237f
  muscle. *See* Muscle fibers.
  reticular, 14
Fibrocartilage, 16, 17f, 238
Fibrocystic disease of breast, 560
Fibroid tumors, 644
Fibromyalgia, 460
Fibrous exudates, 34b
Fibrous joints, 240f, 242-243
Fibula, 213, 215, 219f, 221f
Fibular (lateral) collateral ligament, 262, 263f
Fibularis (peroneus) brevis, 399, 399f, 537
Fibularis (peroneus) longus, 399, 399f, 537
Fibularis (peroneus) tertius, 397, 397f
Fight-or-flight response, 46, 148
Filariasis, lymphatic, 587
Filtration, 11
Finger(s)
  abduction of, 524
  adduction of, 524
  biomechanics of, 518-526
  bones of, 211-212
  extension of, 523
  flexion of, 523
  joints of, 258-259, 259f, 518
  movements of, 70f-74f, 258-259, 518
  palpation of, 259
Fingernails, 554, 554f

First aid, for choking, 611b
Fissure(s)
  in bone, 198
  in brain, 113
  superior orbital, 202f-203f
Fissure of Rolando, 113
Fissure of Sylvius, 113
Fistulas, 37
Five-element theory, 25, 26f, 88, 89f, 89t
Fixator (stabilizer) muscles, 295, 297-298, 304, 494
Flaccid paralysis, 123, 124b
Flaccidity, muscle, 140, 461
Flat bones, 197
Flexibility, vs. stability, 236, 236b, 239
Flexion, 69, 70f-74f, 247-249, 248f, 418
  capital, 500, 504
  cervical, 505
  dorsal, 70f-74f, 75, 248-249, 264b, 536, 537f, 540
  of elbow, 519
  of fingers, 523
  of glenohumeral joint, 509
  of hip, 528, 528t, 530
  of knee, 534, 538
    muscle firing patterns in, 496
  lateral, 74, 249
  lumbar, 501
  plantar, 75, 248-249, 264b, 536, 537f
  of scapula, 515
  of shoulder, 515
  of spine, 501
  of thumb, 525
  of toe, 536, 541
  of trunk, 495, 507
  of wrist, 518, 522
Flexor carpi radialis, 441, 441f, 518
Flexor carpi ulnaris, 442, 442f, 518, 525
Flexor digiti minimi brevis, 526
Flexor digiti minimi manus, 455, 455f
Flexor digiti minimi pedis, 413, 413f
Flexor digiti quinti brevis pedis, 537
Flexor digitorum brevis, 409, 409f, 537
Flexor digitorum longus, 403, 403f, 537
Flexor digitorum profundus, 444, 444f, 525-526
Flexor digitorum superficialis, 443, 443f, 525-526
Flexor hallucis brevis, 412-413, 412f, 537
Flexor hallucis longus, 403, 403f, 537
Flexor pollicis brevis, 453, 453f
Flexor pollicis longus, 444, 444f, 525-526
Flexor reflexes, 144-145, 297, 297b
Fluid. See also Water.
  extracellular, 628-629, 628f
  interstitial, 629
  intracellular, 628, 628f
Fluid homeostasis, 628-631, 632f
  baroreceptors in, 630
  disorders of, 631-632
  hydrostatic forces in, 629-630
  kidneys in, 628
  osmoreceptors in, 630
  osmotic pressure in, 630
Fluid loss, 631-632, 633f
  effects of, 632f
  routes of, 629t
Fluid viscosity, 238, 572-573
Folic acid, 621t
Follicle-stimulating hormone (FSH), 175, 176f, 635, 637
Fontanelles, 203, 204f
Food. See also Diet; Eating; Nutrition.
  absorption of, 616
Food groups, 619-622
Food intolerances, 624
Food poisoning, 623-624
Foot, 213
  arches of, 213, 220f, 265, 536, 543f
  athlete's, 559
  biomechanics of, 535-537
  bones of, 213, 220f-221f, 221, 221b, 535
  clubbed, 223
  dorsiflexion of, 70f-74f, 75, 248-249, 264b, 536, 537f, 540
  eversion of, 70f-74f, 75, 249, 536, 537f, 541
  intrinsic muscles of, 406-415, 407f
  inversion of, 70f-74f, 75, 249, 536, 537f, 540
  joints of, 264f-265f, 265, 535-537
  movements of, 249, 264b, 535-537
  muscles of, 406-415, 407f, 537

Foot (Continued)
  palpation of, 265-266
  range of motion of, 271b
  structure of, 535-537, 536f
Foramen, 198
  emissary, 202f-203f
  infraorbital, 202f-203f
  intervertebral, 204, 205f
  mental, 202f-203f
Foramen lacerum, 202f-203f
Foramen magnum, 121, 202f-203f
Foramen ovale, 202f-203f
Foramen rotundum, 202f-203f
Foramen spinosum, 202f-203f
Force, 469-470. See also Biomechanics.
  acceleration and, 470
  dynamic, 286
  effort and, 470
  inertia and, 470
  levers and, 470-472, 472f-473f
  mechanical advantage/disadvantage and, 471-472, 472f
  muscles and, 286
  pressure and, 470
  resistance and, 470
  speed and, 470
  static, 286
  vectors and, 470
Forces, mechanical. See Mechanical forces.
Forearm
  bones of, 212, 214f. See also Radius; Ulna.
  movements of, 70f-74f, 249, 258, 258f
  muscles of, 433-439, 433f-434f
  pronation of, 70f-74f, 75, 248-249, 258, 258f, 521
  supination of, 75, 248-249, 258, 258f, 521
Forebrain (cerebrum), 111-113, 112f-114f
Foreskin, 635, 635f
Fossa, 198
  coracoid, 211f
  coronoid, 211-212, 213f
  glenoid, 211f
  iliac, 218f
  infraspinous, 210, 211f
  intercondylar, 215, 219f
  olecranon, 211-212, 213f
  pituitary, 202f-203f
  radial, 211-212, 213f
  subscapular, 210
  supraspinous, 210, 211f
  temporal, 202f-203f
Fossa ovalis, 299f
Fovea capitis, 215, 219f
Fracture(s), 214-222, 224f
  avulsion, 214, 224f
  comminuted, 215, 224f
  complete, 215, 224f
  compound (open), 214, 220, 224f
  compression, 215, 224f
  depressed, 215, 224f
  displaced, 224f
  greenstick, 215, 224f
  healing of, 39f, 194, 194b, 220, 222-224
  impacted, 215, 224f
  incomplete, 215
  longitudinal, 224f
  oblique, 224f
  simple (closed), 214, 224f
  stress, 215
  transverse, 224f
  treatment of, 220
  of wrist, 211
Free nerve endings, 143
Frictioning techniques, 36b, 239, 242
  cross-fiber friction in, 242
Frontal bone, 202f-203f, 204b
Frontal lobe, 111-113, 114f, 114t-115t
Frontal (coronal) plane, 69, 69f, 247, 248f
Frontal sinus, 202, 203f
Frozen shoulder, 276-277
Fulcrum, 470
Fuller, R. Buckminster, 301
Functional block, 544-545
Functional muscle groups, 294-295, 295b, 477-478.
  See also Kinetic chain(s).
Functional position, 66, 69

Fungal infections, of skin, 557f-558f, 559
Furuncles (boils), 556, 557f-558f

GABA (gamma-aminobutyric acid), 108, 110b, 147t
Gait. See also Walking.
  definition of, 480
  kinetic chain protocol for, 483b-493b
  muscle firing patterns and, 494
  Trendelenburg, 529
Gait cycle, 480
  stance phase of, 480, 481f
  swing phase of, 480, 482f
Gallbladder, 614f, 616, 619f
  disorders of, 625
Gamma motor neurons, 146-147
Gamma-aminobutyric acid (GABA), 108, 110b, 147t
Ganglia, 277
  basal, 111
  dorsal root, 135
Gases, 7
  blood, 609
Gastric cancer, 626
Gastric juice, 616, 618t, 620t
Gastric ulcers, 624
Gastrin, 180
Gastritis, acute erosive, 623
Gastrocnemius, 405, 405f, 534-535, 537
Gastrocolic ligament, 615
Gastroenteritis, 623-624
Gastroesophageal reflux, 624
Gastrointestinal disorders, 623-626
  massage contraindications for, 626b
Gastrointestinal hormones, 180
Gastrointestinal tract, 614f, 615-617. See also Digestive
  system.
Gastrophrenic ligament, 615
Gastrosplenic ligament, 615
Gate-control theory of pain, 41f, 80-81
Gemellus inferior, 377, 377f, 529
Gemellus superior, 376, 376f, 529
General adaptation syndrome, 46, 47b, 48f, 170, 171b
Genetic factors
  in cancer, 33
  in disease, 30, 32
  in stress response, 49
Geniohyoid, 327, 327f
Genitourinary tract. See also Reproductive system.
  immune defenses of, 592
Geoscience, 58b
German measles, 558
Gestation period, 636. See also Pregnancy.
Gibbus, 277
Gigantism, 182
Glands. See Endocrine system and specific types.
Glans penis, 635, 635f
Glasgow Coma Scale, 113
Glenohumeral joint, 255, 255f, 508-509
  biomechanics of, 508-509
  close-packed position of, 248t
  least-packed position of, 247t
  movements of, 508-509
  muscles of, 510
  palpation of, 257
  structure of, 255, 255f, 508-509
Glenohumeral ligament, 255, 255f
Glenoid fossa, 211f
Glenoid labrum, 508
Gliding joints, 250, 253f
Glomerulonephritis, 597t, 633-634
Glossopharyngeal nerve, 136f, 136t-137t
Glottis, 609
Glucagon, 177
Glucocorticoids, 177
  in stress response, 47b, 48f
Glucose
  deficiency of, 185
  in diabetes mellitus, 185-186
  glucagon and, 177
  insulin and, 167, 176
  in muscle contraction, 291-293
Glutamate, 108
Gluteal muscles, 369-392, 370f, 529
Gluteal tuberosity, 219f
Gluteus maximus, 299f, 371-373, 371f, 529
Gluteus medius, 372, 372f, 529
Gluteus minimus, 372, 372f

Glycoproteins, 303
Glycosaminoglycans, 303
Goiter, 183
Golfer's elbow, 273
Golgi apparatus (complex), 12, 12f
Golgi tendon organs, 143
Gomphoses, 243
Gonadocorticoids, 177-178
Gonadotropin-releasing hormone, 170t
Gonorrhea, 644-645
Gout, 275
Gracilis, 387, 387f, 529, 534-535
Graves' disease, 183, 597t
Gray matter
  of brain, 111
  of spinal cord, 122
Great vessels, 562f, 563
Greater omentum, 615
Greater sciatic notch, 218f
Greater trochanter, 215, 219f, 221f
Greater tubercle, 217f
Greenstick fractures, 215, 224f
Grooves, in bone, 198
Gross anatomy, 4
Ground substance, 17b, 237, 298
Growing pains, 224
Growth, 6
Growth hormone, 174, 174b, 176f
Growth hormone–releasing hormone, 170t
Growth plates, 197
Guillain-Barré syndrome, 160
Gyri, cortical, 113

Habits, 118
Hair, 554
  loss of, 561
Hair cells, 155
Hair root plexuses, 142
Half-life, of hormones, 171-172
Hallucinogens, 124
Hamstring group, 378-380, 379f-380f, 529, 534-535
Han re, 87
Hand
  bones of, 211-212, 216f
  joints of, 258-259, 259f, 518
  ligaments of, 258
  movements of, 258-259, 518
  muscles of, 439-450, 440f, 518-526
    intrinsic, 451-458, 451f
  palpation of, 259
Hard palate, 615
Hashimoto's disease, 183
Head. See also under Cranial; Facial.
  arteries of, 568f, 573
  biomechanics of, 500-501
  bony framework of, 202, 202f-203f, 204b
  muscles of, 307-322, 308f, 500-501
  veins of, 569f, 574
Head (of bone), 199
Head trauma, 125
Headaches, 127, 162
  muscle tension, 162, 460
Healing
  fracture, 39f
  muscle, 294, 294b
  stages of, 36b
  tissue repair in, 36b-37b
  wound, 38f, 555-556
Hearing, 153-155
  mechanics of, 154
Heart. See also under Cardiac; Cardiovascular.
  apex of, 563f
  blood flow through, 564-565, 564f
  blood supply to, 563, 564f, 568-570
  conduction system of, 564-565
  disorders of, 576-578
  entrainment and, 565
  structure of, 562-565, 562f
  venous return to, 568-570, 570f
Heart attack, 577, 577f
Heart disease, 576-578
  massage contraindications in, 583b
Heart failure, 577-578
Heart murmurs, 565
Heart rate, 564, 576
Heart sounds, 565

Heart valves, 563f, 564-565
  dysfunction of, 576
Heat
  in inflammation, 34, 35f
  from muscle contraction, 293
Heat application, for pain, 44
Heberden's nodes, 274
Heimlich maneuver, 611b
Helper T cells, 594
Hematemesis, 583
Hematoma
  epidural, 125
  fracture, 220
  subdural, 125
Hematopoiesis, 575
Hematuria, 583
Hemiparesis, 124
Hemoglobin, 575
  skin color and, 555
Hemolytic anemia, 597t
Hemophilia, 583
Hemoptysis, 583
Hemorrhage, 582-583. See also Bleeding.
Hemorrhagic exudates, 34b
Hemorrhoids, 623
Hemothorax, 606
Hepatic artery, 574-575
Hepatic flexure, 617
Hepatic portal system, 574-575
Hepatic triad, 575
Hepatitis, 596
Hernias, 624-625
Herniated disk, 159, 245, 269f
Herpes simplex, 160, 558, 645
Herpes zoster (shingles), 160, 557f-558f, 558
Hiccups, 607b, 610
High-energy bonds, 9-10
Hilton's law, 244, 300b
Hinge joints, 250, 253f
Hip
  abduction of, 528, 528t, 531
    muscle firing patterns in, 496
  adduction of, 528, 528t, 532
  biomechanics of, 526-529
  bones of, 211, 214b, 218f, 221f
  close-packed position of, 248t
  extension of, 531
    muscle firing patterns in, 495
  flexion of, 530
  joints of, 259-260, 261f, 526-529
  least-packed position of, 247t
  movements of, 70f-74f, 527-528, 528t
  muscles of, 527-529, 527f
  palpation of, 260-262
  range of motion of, 271b, 527
  rotation of, 532-533
  structure of, 526-529
Histamine, 108
Histiocytes, 300
History taking, 91
HIV/AIDS, 595-596
Hives, 561
Hodgkin disease, 588
Holter monitor, 564-565
Homeopathy, 594b
Homeostasis, 4, 24-27
  adaptive capacity and, 25
  Ayurveda and, 25-27
  feedback loops in, 27-28, 27f
  fluid. See Fluid homeostasis.
  practical applications for, 26b, 28b-29b
  sources of disturbances in, 30-36
  traditional Chinese medicine and, 25
Hooke's law, 300b
Horizontal abduction, 249
  of glenohumeral joint, 509-510
  of shoulder, 509-510
Horizontal adduction, 249
  of glenohumeral joint, 509-510
  of shoulder, 516
Horizontal plane, 234, 248, 248f
Hormones, 171-173. See also Endocrine system and
    specific hormones.
  adrenal, 47b, 48f, 177-178
  anterior pituitary, 174-175, 174b, 176f
  functions of, 171

Hormones (Continued)
  gastrointestinal, 180
  half-life of, 171-172
  hypersecretion of, 168, 173, 181
  hyposecretion of, 168, 173, 181-182
  hypothalamic, 170t
  neurotransmitters and, 99, 106, 108b, 168
  overview of, 167-168
  pancreatic, 176-177
  parathyroid, 176
  pineal, 179-180
  posterior pituitary, 169-170, 176f
  secretion of, 172
  sex, 178-179, 635-637
  stress, 47b, 48f
  target cells for, 172-173, 173f
  thymic, 180
  thyroid, 176
  tissue, 34b, 169-170, 181
  tropic, 169
  types of, 171, 171t
Human immunodeficiency virus (HIV) infection,
    595-596
Human papillomavirus infection, 643
Humeroradial joint, 517-518
Humeroulnar joint, 517-518
Humerus, 209-212, 213f, 217f
Hunchback (hyperkyphosis), 209, 223, 223f, 277
Huntington's chorea, 127
Hyaline cartilage, 16, 17f, 195-197, 238, 238f
Hydration, 301
Hydrogen bonds, 7-8
Hydrostatic forces, 629-630
Hydrostatic pressure, 572
Hyoid bone, 202
Hyperalgesia, 38
Hyperemesis gravidarum, 643
Hyperextension, 70f-74f, 74
Hyperkyphosis, 209, 223, 223f, 277
Hyperlordosis, 209, 223, 223f, 277, 475
Hypermobility, 246
Hyperparathyroidism, 184-185
  osteitis fibrosa cystica and, 224
Hyperplasia, 32-34
Hyperpnea, 609
Hypersensitivity, 32, 595, 595b
  to foods, 624
Hypertension, 579
  pregnancy-induced, 643
Hyperthyroidism, 183-184, 183f, 184t, 597t
Hypertonicity, muscle, 140
Hypertrophy, 13
Hyperventilation, 161, 609, 612-613
Hypnosis, for pain, 44
Hypochondriasis, 117b
Hypoglossal canal, 202f-203f
Hypoglossal nerve, 136f, 136t-137t
Hypomobility, 246
Hypoparathyroidism, 184-185
Hypothalamic hormones, 170t
  in stress response, 47b, 48f
Hypothalamic-pituitary-adrenal (HPA) axis, 170
Hypothalamus, 112f, 118, 168-169, 169f, 170t
  in stress response, 47b, 48f
Hypothenar muscles, 454-455, 454f
Hypothyroidism, 183-184, 183f, 184t
Hypotonicity, muscle, 140
Hysteresis, 301, 301b

Idiopathic disease, 30
Ileum, 614f, 616
Iliac crest, 214, 218f
Iliac fossa, 218f
Iliacus, 360, 360f
Iliocostalis cervicis, 338, 338f
Iliocostalis lumborum, 338, 338f
Iliocostalis thoracis, 338, 338f
Iliofemoral ligament, 259-260, 261f
Iliolumbar ligament, 261f
Iliopectineal line, 218f
Iliopsoas, 529
Iliosacral motion, 249, 260b
Iliotibial band, 299f, 393
Ilium, 214, 218f
Imagery, for pain, 43
Immobilization, 276-277

Immune response, 27, 589-597
  hypersensitive, 32, 595, 595b, 624
  inflammation in, 34, 592-593, 593f. See also
    Inflammation.
  nonspecific (innate), 589-593
  specific, 589-590, 593-594, 593f, 593t
  stress and, 49
  suppressed/deficient, 32, 595
    in HIV/AIDS, 595-596
Immune system, 589-597
  components of, 589-590, 589f
  disorders of, 595-597
  massage contraindications for, 596b
  mind-body connection in, 594-595
  nonspecific defenses in, 591-593
  specific defenses in, 589-590, 593-594, 593f, 593t
Immunization, 594b
Immunodeficiency diseases, 32, 595
  HIV/AIDS, 595-596
Impacted fractures, 215, 224f
Impermeable membranes, 11
Impetigo, 556, 557f-558f
Impingement neuropathies, 158
Incomplete fractures, 215
Incontinence, 633
Incubation period, 590-591
Incus, 154, 154f, 202f-203f
Inertia, force and, 470
Infant apnea, 612
Infant skull, 203, 204f
Infections. See also specific sites and types.
  asymptomatic, 591
  latent, 591
  microorganisms causing, 27, 32, 32b, 590
  opportunistic, 32, 590, 595
  prodrome in, 590-591
  stages of, 590-591
  subclinical, 591
Infectious arthritis, 276
Infectious mononucleosis, 588
Infectious polyneuritis, 160
Inferior, definition of, 68-69, 68f
Inferior articular facet, 268f
Inferior pubic ligament, 259
Inferior pubic ramus, 218f
Inferior vena cava, 563
Infertility, 597t, 643-644
Inflammation, 34, 34b, 35f, 592-593, 593f
  chronic, 37
  controlled therapeutic, 36b, 239. See also Frictioning
    techniques.
  in healing process, 36b
  in immune response, 592-593, 593f
  mediators of, 34b, 35f
  practical applications for, 36b
  signs of, 34, 35f
Inflammatory bowel disease, 597t, 625
Inflammatory disease, 37b
Inflammatory exudates, 34, 34b
Inflammatory joint disease, 273-275
Inflare, 260
Influenza, 610
Infrahyoid muscles, 328-332, 328f-330f
Infraorbital foramen, 202f-203f
Infraspinatus, 424, 424f, 510
Infraspinous fossa, 210, 211f
Inguinal ligament, 261f, 299f
Inguinal ring, 299f
Inherited diseases, 30
Inhibin, 179
Inion, 202f-203f
Inorganic compounds, 10
Insertions, 285. See also Muscle attachments.
Inspiratory reserve volume, 609
Instep, 213
Insula, 113, 114f
Insulin, in diabetes mellitus, 185-186
Insulin reaction, 185
Insulin-like growth factor, 180
Integumentary system. See also Breast; Hair; Nails;
    Sebaceous glands; Skin; Sweat glands.
  functions of, 553
  pathologic conditions of, 556-562
  structure of, 552-556, 553f-554f
Interclavicular ligament, 255
Intercondylar eminence, 215, 219f

Intercondylar fossa, 215, 219f
Intercostal muscles, 502-503, 607-610, 607f-608f
  external, 356, 356f
  innermost, 357
  internal, 356, 356f
Intermediate muscle fibers, 293
Intermuscular septa, 298
Internal, definition of, 68
Internal auditory meatus, 202f-203f
Internal intercostal muscles, 356, 356f
Internal oblique, 362, 362f, 502
Internal pterygoid, 322, 322f
Internal respiration, 604
Internal rotation. See also Rotation.
  of hip, 533
  of knee, 534
  of shoulder, 517
Internal sense, 152b
International standards, for terminology, 285
Interneurons, 101-102, 103b
Interoception, 152b
Interossei dorsalis manus, 457, 457f, 526
Interossei dorsalis pedis, 415, 415f, 537
Interossei palmares, 456, 456f
Interossei plantares, 414-415, 414f, 537
Interphalangeal joints
  close-packed position of, 248t
  of foot, 264f, 265, 536, 536f. See also Toe(s).
  of hand, 243f, 259. See also Finger(s).
  least-packed position of, 247t
Interphase, 13
Interspinalis cervicis, 346, 346f
Interspinalis lumborum, 346, 346f
Interspinalis thoracis, 346, 346f
Interspinous ligaments, 206, 206f, 266, 267f-268f
Interstitial fluid, 13, 629
Intertarsal joints, 265
Intertransversarii cervicis, 345, 345f
Intertransversarii lumborum, 345, 345f
Intertransversarii thoracis, 345, 345f
Intertransverse ligaments, 206, 206f, 266, 267f-268f
Intertrochanteric crest, 219f
Intertrochanteric line, 219f
Intervertebral disks, 205, 205f-206f, 501
  herniated, 159, 245, 269f
  joints of, 266, 267f
  spinal nerve root compression and, 159
Intervertebral foramen, 204, 205f
Intestinal adhesions, 625
Intestinal enzymes, 616, 618t, 620t
Intestinal obstruction, 625
Intestines. See also Large intestine; Small intestine.
  immune defenses of, 592
Intracellular fluid, 11, 13, 628, 628f
Intractable pain, 39
Intraperitoneal organs, 615
Intrinsic muscles
  of foot, 406-415, 407f, 537
  of hand, 526
Intuition, 80
Inverse stretch reflexes, 144
Inversion, 70f-74f, 75, 249, 536, 537f, 540
Ion pumps, 11
Ionic bonds, 7, 9f
Ions, 103
Ipsilateral, definition of, 68
Ipsilateral reflex arc, 144
Iris, 155f, 156
Irregular bones, 197
Irritable bowel syndrome, 624-625
Ischemic compression, 292b
Ischemic necrosis, of bone, 224-225
Ischial ramus, 218f
Ischial tuberosity, 218f
Ischiocavernosus, 368, 368f
Ischiofemoral ligament, 259-260, 261f
Ischium, 214, 218f
Islets of Langerhans, 169f, 176, 616
Isometric contraction, 288, 288f, 304
  muscle dysfunction in, 459
Isotonic contraction, 288-289, 288f

Jejunum, 614f, 616
Jin ye, 87
Jing, 87

Jing luo, 87
Jock itch, 559
Joint(s), 234-282. See also Skeletal system and specific
    joints.
  of ankle, 264-265, 264b, 265f, 535-537
  ball-and-socket, 250, 253f
  biaxial, 250, 253f
  biomechanics of, 468-549. See also Biomechanical
    assessment; Biomechanical dysfunctions;
    Biomechanics.
  bony processes and, 198-199
  cartilaginous, 242-243
  characteristics of, 236
  condyloid (ellipsoid), 250, 253f
  connective tissue and, 235-240
  of elbow, 257-258, 257f-258f, 517-518
  fibrous, 240f, 242-243
  of finger, 258-259, 259f, 518
  of foot, 264f-265f, 265, 535-537
  gliding, 250, 253f
  of hand, 258-259, 259f, 518
  hinge, 250, 253f
  of hip, 259-260, 261f, 526-529
  immune-related disorders of, 275
  infectious disorders of, 275
  inflammatory disorders of, 273-275
  injuries of, 275-277
  of knee, 262-264, 262b, 263f
  movement-related disorders of, 273
  overview of, 235-244
  pathologic conditions of, 273
  of pelvis, 259, 260b, 261f, 526-529
  pivot, 250, 253f
  saddle, 250, 253f
  of shoulder, 255-257, 255f, 508-509
  of skull, 245, 254f
  of spine, 266-268, 267f-269f, 501-502, 501f
  stability vs. mobility of, 236, 236b, 239
  structure of, 198-199
  synovial, 242-244, 242f, 244b, 248-250
  thoracic, 268-269, 270f, 501-503
  of thumb, 258-259, 259f, 518
  of toe, 536
  triaxial, 250, 253f
  types of, 242-243, 248-250, 253f
  uniaxial, 250, 253f
  of wrist, 518
Joint cancer, 244
Joint capsule, 237, 238f
  of knee, 262
Joint cavity, 244
Joint immobility, from connective tissue shortening,
    240
Joint injuries, mechanical forces causing, 240-242
Joint kinesthetic receptors, 143
Joint movement(s), 69-75, 244-253
  accessory, 245, 245f
  active, 272
  of ankle, 70f-74f, 241, 264, 264b, 535-537
  arthrokinematic, 245, 245f, 272
  assessment of, 494-498
  biomechanics of, 498-537. See also Biomechanics and
    specific joints.
  cardinal planes of body and, 247-248, 248f
  of clavicle, 508
  definition of, 5
  descriptive terms for, 248, 249b
  of elbow, 70f-74f, 257-258, 258f, 517-518, 519b-525b
  of fingers, 70f-74f, 258-259, 518
  of foot, 249, 264b, 535-537
  of hand, 258-259, 518
  of hip, 70f-74f, 527-528, 528t
  integration into massage, 270-273
  joint play and, 245, 272
  of knee, 70f-74f, 262, 534
  measurement of, 248, 251f-252f
  osteokinematic, 245-246, 246b, 272
  overview of, 270-271, 272b
  passive, 272
  of pelvis, 249, 259-260, 260b, 526-528, 528f-529f,
    528t
  range of motion and. See Range of motion (ROM).
  of shoulder, 70f-74f, 249, 255, 508-510
  of spine, 501-502, 501f
  of temporomandibular joint, 254
  terminology for, 69-75

Joint movement(s) (Continued)
  of thumb, 70f-74f, 248-249
  of wrist, 70f-74f, 249, 258, 518
Joint movement methods
  application of, 273
  hand placement in, 273
  types of, 272-273, 272b
Joint play, 245, 272
Joint positions, 246-247
  close-packed, 246-247, 247f, 248t
  loose-packed, 246-247, 247f
Joint space narrowing, 244b
Joint stability, close-packed position and, 246-247, 247f,
    248t
Jugular foramen, 202f-203f

Kapha dosha, 26
Kaposi's sarcoma, 557f-558f
Keratin, 553
Keratitis, seborrheic, 560
Ketoacidosis, diabetic, 161, 185
Kidney
  in fluid homeostasis, 628
  functions of, 628
  structure of, 627-628, 627f
Kidney disease, massage contraindications for, 634b
Kidney failure, 634
Kidney stones, 633
Killer T cells, 594
Kinematic chains, 250-253, 253b
  closed, 250-252
  open, 252-253
Kinematics, 69
Kinesiology, 69-75
  biomechanics of, 469
  definitions of, 69, 193, 193b
  joints and, 234-282
  skeletal system and, 192-233
Kinesthesia, 143, 152b, 153
Kinetic chain(s), 294, 476-494, 477f
  inner unit of, 477-478
  outer unit of, 478
  in postural stabilization, 478
  sitting, standing, and bending and, 478
Kinetic chain protocol
  for gait, 483b-493b
  for postural stabilization, 474b
Kinetic energy, 8
Kinetics, 69
Knee
  bones of, 213, 215, 219f, 221f, 262b
  close-packed position of, 248t
  extension of, 534, 539
    muscle firing patterns in, 497
  flexion of, 534, 538
    muscle firing patterns in, 496
  joint capsule of, 262, 534
  joints of, 262-264, 262b, 263f
  least-packed position of, 247t
  ligaments of, 262, 262b, 263f, 533-534
  menisci of, 215, 262, 263f, 533
  movements of, 70f-74f, 262, 534
  muscles of, 534-535
  palpation of, 262-264
  range of motion of, 271b, 478
  rotation of, 534, 536f
  screw-home mechanism of, 534, 536f
  structure of, 262b, 533-534
Kneecap. See Patella.
Knee-jerk reflex, 144
Knock-knees, 533-534, 536f
Kyphosis, 206, 208f. See also Spinal curves.

Labia majora, 637
Labia minora, 637
Labor, 640
Labrum
  glenoid, 508
  of hip, 260
Labyrinth
  bony, 154, 154f
  membranous, 154, 154f
Lacrimal bones, 204b
Lacrimal glands, 155f, 156
Lactase, 618t
Lactation, 641

Lambdoid suture, 202, 202f-204f, 254, 254f
Language, 113-116
  brain areas for, 111-116, 114f
Large intestine, 614f, 616, 619f
  cancer of, 626
  structure of, 614f
Laryngitis, 606
Larynx, 605f, 606
Latent infections, 591
Lateral, definition of, 68, 68f
Lateral collateral ligament, 262, 263f, 533-534
Lateral condyle
  of femur, 215, 219f, 221f, 262
  of tibia, 215, 219f, 221f, 262
Lateral corticospinal tracts, 123b
Lateral epicondyle
  of femur, 215, 219f
  of humerus, 209, 213f, 217f
Lateral epicondylitis, 273
Lateral fissure, 113
Lateral flexion, 74, 249, 501
Lateral longitudinal arch, 213, 220f, 536
Lateral malleolus, 197-199, 221f
Lateral (external) pterygoid, 321, 321f
Lateral pterygoid plate, 202f-203f
Lateral recumbent position, 67, 67f
Lateral reticulospinal tracts, 123b
Lateral rotation, 69, 75, 248-249
  of glenohumeral joint, 510
  of hip, 527-528, 528t, 532
  of shoulder, 517
Lateral supracondylar line, 219f
Lateral supracondylar ridge, 219f
Lateral temporomandibular ligament, 254, 254f
Lateral tilt, 507
Latissimus dorsi, 430, 430f, 510
Learning, 116-118
  memory and, 116-117, 116b
Left arm extensor test
  for contralateral extensors, 485
  for unilateral extensors, 490
Left arm flexor test
  for contralateral flexors, 483
  for unilateral flexors, 488
Left lateral flexion, 74
Left leg extensor test
  for contralateral extensors, 486
  for unilateral extensors, 491
Left leg flexor test
  for contralateral flexors, 484
  for unilateral flexors, 489
Left rotation, 75
Leg. See also Lower extremity.
  anterior, muscles of, 393, 394f, 395-397
  bones of, 213, 215, 219f, 221f
  definition of, 209
  fascia of, 393
  lateral, muscles of, 393, 399, 399f
  posterior, muscles of, 400-405, 401f
Legg-Calvé-Perthes disease, 225
Lengthening, muscle, 239
Length-tension relationships, 290-291, 290f, 477
Leptin, 170b
Lesser sciatic notch, 218f
Lesser trochanter, 215, 219f, 221f
Lesser tubercle, 217f
Leukemia, 588
Levator anguli oris, 318, 318f
Levator ani, 366, 366f
Levator labii superioris, 316, 316f
Levator labii superioris alaeque nasi, 317, 317f
Levator scapulae, 420, 420f, 509
Levers, 470-472
  first-class, 471, 472f
  second-class, 471-472, 473f
  third-class, 472, 473f
Levo, 68
Lice, 559
Life, characteristics of, 5-6
Life cycle, 49-51. See also Age/aging.
  biologic, 51
  chakra system and, 51
  longevity and, 50-51
  psychological, 51
Life force, eating and, 615
Lifestyle factors, in disease, 30

Ligaments, 197, 237-238. See also Connective tissue and
    specific ligaments.
  of ankle, 264, 265f
  bony attachments for, 199
  capsular, 237
  of elbow, 257-258, 257f
  of hand, 258
  of knee, 262, 262b, 263f, 533-534
  laxity of, 239
  of pelvis, 259, 261f
  peritoneal, 615
  proprioceptors for, 295
  rupture of, 239
  of shoulder, 255, 255f-256f, 257
  of spine, 206, 206f, 266, 267f-269f
  structure of, 237-238
  tears of, 275-277, 276f
  of temporomandibular joint, 254, 254f
  of thorax, 268-269
  of thumb, 258
  vertebral, 206, 206f
  of wrist, 258
Ligamentum flavum, 206, 206f, 266, 267f-268f
Ligamentum nuchae, 266, 267f
Limbic system, 113, 114f, 114t-115t, 116, 119
Linea aspera, 215, 219f, 221f
Lines, 199
Lipases, 618t
Lipids, 10, 621
Lipomas, 560
Liquids, 7
List, spinal, 277
Liu fu, 87
Liu qi, 87-88
Liver, 614f, 616, 619f. See also under Hepatic.
  portal system of, 574-575
Loading/unloading, 301, 301b
Lock-and-key model, 172-173, 173f
Locked position, 246-247, 247f, 248t
Locomotion. See Walking.
Long bones, 197
Long plantar ligament, 265f
Longevity, 50-51
Longissimus capitis, 339, 339f
Longissimus cervicis, 339, 339f
Longissimus thoracis, 339, 339f
Longitudinal fractures, 224f
Longus capitis, 332, 332f
Longus colli, 331, 331f
Loose (areolar) tissue, 16, 17f
Loose-packed position, 246-247, 247t
Lordosis, 206, 208f, 475. See also Spinal curves.
Lou Gehrig's disease, 126
Low back pain, 223b, 277, 527
Lower crossed syndrome, 543, 544f
Lower extremity. See also Leg.
  arteries of, 568f, 574
  bones of, 211-213, 214b-215b, 218f-221f, 221b
  definition of, 209
  veins of, 569f, 574
Lower motor neuron injuries, 123, 124b, 138
Lower respiratory tract, 605f, 613
LSD, 124
Lumbar flexion, 501
Lumbar plexus, 137, 140f
  injuries of, 159
Lumbar region, 66
  biomechanics of, 502, 528t
Lumbar vertebrae, 205, 207f, 208, 208b
  biomechanics of, 502
Lumbosacral angle, 502
Lumbricales manus, 458, 458f, 526
Lumbricales pedis, 411, 411f, 537
Lung
  blood supply of, 607
  cancer of, 611
  immune defenses of, 592, 605
  nerve supply of, 607
  structure of, 605f, 606
Lung volumes, 609
Lunula, 554, 554f
Luteinizing hormone (LH), 175, 176f, 635, 637
Lymph, 629
Lymph nodes, 584-585, 584f
Lymph nodules, 586
Lymph vessels, 584, 584f-585f

Lymphangion, 586
Lymphatic drainage, 586
   stimulation of, 586, 587b, 587f
Lymphatic filariasis, 587
Lymphatic malformations, 588, 588b
Lymphatic pumps, 586
Lymphatic system, 583-588
   components of, 584, 584f
   disorders of, 586-588
   massage contraindications for, 588b
Lymphedema, 587-588
Lymphocytes, 27, 575, 593-594
Lymphomas, 588
Lysosomes, 12

Macrophages, in connective tissue, 15
Macules, 556f
Magnesium balance, 631
Magnetoreception, 152b
Malabsorption, 624
Male contraception, 636
Male reproductive system, 635-636, 635f
Malignant melanoma, 560
Malignant tumors, 33, 33f. *See also* Cancer.
Malleus, 154, 154f, 202f-203f
Malnutrition, 32
   bone abnormalities in, 225-226
   myopathy in, 463
Maltase, 618t
Mammary glands, 555, 637
Mandible, 202f-203f, 204b
Marmas, 81
Massage therapy
   components of, 58
   definition of, 58, 170b
   frictioning techniques in, 36b, 239, 242
Masseter, 320, 320f
Mast cells, in connective tissue, 15
Mastectomy, 560-561
Mastication, muscles of, 320-322, 320f-322f
Mastoid process, 202f-203f
Matrix, 13-14
Matter, 7
Maxilla, 202f-203f, 204b
Maxillary sinus, 202, 203f
Maximal stimulus, for muscle contraction, 291
Measles, 558-559
Meatus, 198
   external auditory, 202f-203f
   internal auditory, 202f-203f
   nasal, 604-605
Mechanical advantage/disadvantage, 471-472, 472f
Mechanical forces, 240-242. *See also* Biomechanics;
      Force.
   bending, 240-242, 244f
   compression, 240, 242f
   shear, 240f, 242
   tension, 240, 243f
   torsion, 240f, 242
Mechanical receptors, 142-143
Mechanics, 69. *See also* Biomechanics.
Mechanoreceptors, 142, 153
Mechanotransduction, 15b
Medial, definition of, 68, 68f
Medial collateral ligament
   of ankle, 264
   of elbow, 257, 257f
   of knee, 262, 263f, 533-534
Medial condyle
   of femur, 215, 219f, 221f, 262
   of tibia, 215, 219f, 221f, 262
Medial epicondyle
   of femur, 215, 219f
   of humerus, 209, 213f, 217f
Medial epicondylitis, 273
Medial longitudinal arch, 213, 220f, 265
Medial malleolus, 197-199, 215, 219f, 221f
Medial (internal) pterygoid, 322, 322f
Medial reticulospinal tracts, 123b
Medial rotation, 69, 75, 249. *See also* Rotation.
   of glenohumeral joint, 510
   of hip, 248, 533
   of shoulder, 517
   of thumb, 525
Medial supracondylar line, 219f
Medial supracondylar ridge, 219f

Medical dictionaries, 59-62
Medical records. *See* Charting.
Medical terminology, 59-63, 107b. *See also*
      Terminology.
   abbreviations in, 62-63, 62t
   anatomic, 63-68
   directional, 67-68, 68f
   reference resources for, 59-62
   word elements in, 59, 60t-61t
Medications. *See* Drug(s).
Meditation, 115b, 117
Medulla oblongata, 112f, 119
   vascular system and, 573
Meiosis, 13
Meissner's corpuscles, 142, 153
Melanin, 553, 555
Melanocyte-stimulating hormone, 175, 176f
Melanoma, 560
Melatonin, 118, 179-180
   biologic rhythms and, 179-180, 187
   in seasonal affective disorder, 187
   sleep and, 179-180, 187
Melena, 583
Membrane(s)
   basement, 14
   cell (plasma), 11
   cutaneous, 14
   mucous, 14
   serous, 14
   synovial, 16
Membrane depolarization, 103-104
Membrane permeability, 11
Membrane potentials, 103-104
Membrane transport
   active, 11
   carrier-mediated, 11
   passive, 11
   vesicular, 11
Memory, 116
   learning and, 116-117, 116b
   state-dependent, 117b
Meninges, 119-120, 120f
Meningitis, 128
Menisci, 215, 262, 263f, 533
Menopause, 637
Menorrhagia, 583
Menstrual cycle, 637
Mental foramen, 202f-203f
Mentalis, 319, 319f
Meridians, 85, 85f, 86b, 87, 294b
   autonomic nervous system and, 150-152
   fascia and, 152
Merkel's disks, 143, 153
Mesencephalon (midbrain), 119
Mesentery, 615
Mesomorphs, 32f
Metabolic myopathies, acquired, 463
Metabolic rate
   basal, 622
   total, 622-623
Metabolic water, 629
Metabolism, 6, 8-10
   muscle, 287-288, 291-293
Metabolites, 9
Metacarpals, 211, 212b, 216f
Metacarpophalangeal joint, 243f, 258, 518
Metastasis, 33
Metatarsals, 220f, 221
Metatarsophalangeal joint, 264f, 265, 536
   close-packed position of, 248t
   least-packed position of, 247t
Metrorrhagia, 583
Microcirculation, 567
Microorganisms
   disease-causing, 27, 32, 32b, 590
   nonharmful, 590
Microvasculature, 563, 565-567
Microvilli, 12
Midbrain, 112f, 119
Middle cerebral arteries, 121, 121f
Middle deltoid, 510
Middle scalene, 333, 333f
Midtarsal joint
   close-packed position of, 248t
   least-packed position of, 247t
Migraine, 127

Minerals
   dietary, 622, 622t
   piezoelectric, 17b, 194, 194b, 198b
Miscarriage, 642
Mitochondria, 12, 12f
Mitochondrial DNA (mtDNA), 8b
Mitosis, 13
Mitral valve, 563, 563f
   dysfunction of, 576
Mnemonics, 192b
Mobility, vs. stability, 236, 236b, 239
Models, 92b
Molecules, 7
   polar, 7-8, 9f
Moles, 559
Molluscum contagiosum, 559
Moment, 470-471
Monocytes, 575-576
Mononucleosis, 588
Monoplegia, 126
Monosaccharides, 621
Monosynaptic reflex arc, 144
Mood-altering drugs, 109
Motion. *See also* Joint movement(s).
   definition of, 69
Motor areas of brain, 101f
Motor descending tracts, 122-123, 122f, 123b
Motor end plate, 291
Motor function, nonoptimal, 543, 545
Motor neurons, 101-102, 103b
   gamma, 146-147
   injuries of, 123, 124b, 138
Motor points, 84f, 291, 292b
Motor unit, 291, 291f
Mouth, 614f, 615
   functions of, 619f
   immune defenses of, 591-592
   muscles of, 314-319, 314f-319f
   structure of, 614f, 615
Movements. *See* Joint movement(s).
Mover muscles, 295, 297-298, 304
   in muscle firing patterns, 494
Moxibustion, 36b, 88
Mucosa-associated lymph tissue, 586
Mucous membranes, 14
Multifidus, 343, 343f
Multipennate muscles, 295, 296f
Multiple gastric erosions, 623
Multiple sclerosis, 160, 597t
Multipolar neurons, 102, 103b
Multiunit muscle, 287
Murmurs, 565
Muscarinic receptors, 148b
Muscle(s), 283-467
   abdominal wall. *See* Abdominal wall muscles.
   agonist, 304
   of ankle, 537
   antagonist, 289, 295, 304, 418
   of anterior leg, 393, 394f, 395-397
   antigravity, 475
   of back. *See* Back muscles.
   biomechanical forces on, 300-301, 300b-301b
   blood supply of, 293
   of breathing, 350-369, 351f-352f, 502-503, 607-610,
      607f-608f
   cardiac, 286-287, 287f, 291
   circular, 295, 296f
   connective tissue and, 298-303, 299f. *See also* Fascia.
   contractility of, 287. *See also* Muscle contraction.
   contusions of, 461
   convergent, 295, 296f
   of ear, 312, 312f
   elasticity of, 287, 301
   of elbow, 433-439, 433f-434f, 518
   energy and, 286
   excitability of, 287
   extensibility of, 287
   of eye, 156, 313, 313f
   facial, 307-322, 308f
   fixator (stabilizer), 295, 297-298, 304, 494
   flaccid, 140, 461
   of foot, 406-415, 407f, 537
   force and, 286
   of forearm, 433-439, 433f-434f
   functional characteristics of, 287-288
   functions of, 286, 474b

Muscle(s) (Continued)
 gluteal, 369-392, 370f, 529
 of hand, 439-450, 440f, 518-526
 of head, 307-322, 308f
 of hip, 527, 527f
 hypertonic, 146
 hypotonic, 146
 information sources for, 304, 418
 innervation of, 291
 in kinetic chain, 477-478. See also Kinetic chain(s).
 of knee, 534-535
 of lateral leg, 393, 399, 399f
 layers of, 304, 305f-306f
 lengthening of, 239, 292b
 length-tension relationship in, 290-291, 290f, 477
 loading/unloading of, 301, 301b
 of mastication, 320-322, 320f-322f
 metabolism in, 287-288, 291-293
 of mouth, 314-319, 314f-319f
 mover, 295, 297-298, 304
   in muscle firing patterns, 494
 multiunit, 287
 names of, 284-285, 304-307
 of neck. See Neck, muscles of.
 neutralizer, 295, 304
 palpation of, 307
 parallel, 295, 296f
 pathologic conditions of. See Muscle disorders.
 pelvic, 353f, 365-369
 pennate, 295, 296f
 perineal, 353f, 365-369, 367f
 of posterior leg, 393, 400-405, 401f
 prime movers, 304, 494
 proprioceptors for, 295-297
 repair of, 294, 294b
 shapes of, 295
 shortening of, 295
   contractures and, 460
 of shoulder. See Shoulder, muscles of.
 smooth, 286-287, 287f, 291. See also Smooth muscle.
 striated involuntary, 286
 structure of, 286-298, 289f
 support, 295
 synergist, 295, 418
 tensegrity of, 301-303, 302f
 terminology for, 284-285, 304-307
 of thigh. See Thigh, muscles of.
 tight, 288
 of torso, 350-369, 351f-353f
 trigger points in, 81, 82f-83f
 types of, 284, 286-287
 of wrist, 439-450, 440f, 518-526
Muscle action, 288-289, 304. See also Muscle
     contraction.
 ATP in, 287-288, 290-293
 concentric, 288-289, 288f, 304
 eccentric, 288f, 289, 304
 isometric, 288, 288f, 304
 isotonic, 288-289, 288f
 reverse, 285, 381, 433
Muscle activation sequences. See Muscle firing patterns.
Muscle attachments, 298-303
 insertions, 285
 origins, 285
 terminology for, 285, 285b
Muscle belly, 298, 300f
Muscle cells, 13, 16
Muscle contraction. See also Muscle action.
 all-or-none response in, 289
 concentric, 459
 descriptions of, 418
 eccentric, 459
 energy sources for, 291-293
 isometric, 459
 maximal stimulus for, 291
 physiology of, 283, 289-290, 290f
 sliding filament mechanism in, 289-290, 290f
 threshold stimulus for, 291
 treppe and, 291
Muscle cramps, 460
Muscle disorders, 458-463
 infectious, 462
 massage for, 459
 medications for, 459-460
 myopathies, 462-463
 pathogenesis of, 458-459

Muscle fatigue, 293
Muscle fibers, 16-18, 291-293
 intermediate, 293
 red (slow-twitch), 291-293
 smooth, 16-18
 structure of, 289-294, 289f-290f
 white (fast-twitch), 291-293
Muscle firing patterns, 297-298, 494
 assessment of, 494, 495b-497b
 dysfunctional, 494
 interventions for, 494, 495b-497b
Muscle groups, functional, 294-295, 295b, 477-478.
     See also Kinetic chain(s).
Muscle pain, 40. See also Pain.
Muscle reflex, 144
Muscle relaxants, 459-460
Muscle spasms, 140, 460-461
 pain-spasm-pain cycle and, 27-28, 40, 40f
Muscle spindles, 143, 295
Muscle strain, 461-462
Muscle tension, 288
 stress-induced, 460
Muscle tension headaches, 162, 460
Muscle tissue, 16-18, 17f, 286-289
Muscle tone, resting, 291
Muscolino, Joseph, 304
Muscular dystrophy, 462-463
Muscular pump, 569, 570b, 570f
The Muscular System Manual: The Skeletal Muscles of
     the Human Body (Muscolino), 304
Musculoskeletal system, 193. See also Bone(s); Joint(s);
     Muscle(s).
Musculotendinous cuff. See Rotator cuff.
Musculotendinous junction, 298
Music therapy, for pain, 44
Myasthenia gravis, 160-161, 597t
Myelin, 102, 105
Myelitis, 128
Mylohyoid, 327, 327f
Myers, Tom, 294b, 301-303
Myocardial infarction, 577, 577f
Myocarditis, 578
Myocardium, 562-563, 566f
Myofascial complex, 300b
Myofascial continuity, 301, 302f
Myofascial integration, 301-303, 302f
Myofibrils, 289, 290f
Myoglobin, 289, 291-293
Myomas, 644
Myoneural junction, 291
Myopathies, 462-463
Myosin, 283, 289-291, 290f
Myositis, 462
Myotactic units, 294-295, 295b
Myotomes, 139
Myxedema, 183, 597t

Nails, 554, 554f
Naming systems, anatomical, 285. See also
     Terminology.
Narcotic analgesics, 44
Nasal bones, 202f-203f, 204b, 604-605
Nasal cavity, 604-606, 605f
Nasal conchae, 204b
Nasal septum, 605-606
Nasalis, 310, 310f
Nasion, 202f-203f
Natural killer cells, 593
Navicular bone, 220f, 221
Near-drowning, 612
Neck. See also under Cervical.
 arteries of, 568f, 573
 biomechanics of, 500-501
 bones of, 203-206, 207f. See also Vertebrae.
 movements of, 266
 muscles of, 323-334, 323f-324f
   of anterior triangle, 325-327, 326f-327f
   deep posterior, 337, 337f
   infrahyoid, 328-332, 328f-330f
   of posterior triangle, 331f-332f
   scalene, 333-334, 333f-334f
 veins of, 569f, 574
 whiplash injury of, 461
 wry, 461
Necrosis, bone, 224-225
Needle grasp, in acupuncture, 15b

Negative feedback, 27, 27f
 biological rhythms and, 28, 29f
 in endocrine system, 168, 169f, 173
Neoplasms, 32-34. See also Cancer; Tumors.
Nerve(s)
 connective tissue of, 134, 135f
 cranial. See Cranial nerves.
 peripheral
   injuries of, 158-162
   structure of, 135f, 150
 repair/regeneration of, 102-103, 104f
 spinal. See Spinal nerve(s); Spinal nerve roots.
Nerve compression syndromes, 158-162
Nerve entrapment, 159
Nerve impingement, 158
Nerve impulse, 103-105
 conduction of, 105, 105f-106f
Nerve map, 42, 42f
Nerve plexuses, 135-137
 brachial, 137, 139f, 159
 cervical, 135, 138f, 159
 hair root, 142
 injuries of, 158-159
 lumbar, 137, 140f
   injuries of, 159
 sacral, 137, 140f, 353f
   injuries of, 159
Nerve root compression, 159
Nervous system, 98-132
 divisions of, 100, 101f. See also Autonomic
     nervous system; Central nervous system;
     Parasympathetic nervous system; Peripheral
     nervous system; Sympathetic nervous system.
 endocrine system and. See Neuroendocrine
     system.
 functions of, 100
 overview of, 100
 structure of, 100
Nervous tissue, 18, 18f
Neuralgia, 161
 trigeminal, 161-162
Neurochemicals, 105-106, 107b-108b
 behavior and, 106-109
Neuroendocrine system, 99, 168, 170, 177b
 organs of, 168
Neuroglia, 18, 102-103, 104f
Neuroimmunomodulation, 594-595
Neurolemma, 102
Neuromas, 138
Neuromodulators, 106, 107b-108b
 behavior and, 106-109
Neuromuscular junction, 291
Neuromuscular spindles, 143, 295
Neurons, 18, 100-102, 102f, 103b
 motor. See Motor neurons.
 spinal cord, 123
Neuropathy, 158-162
 compression, 158-162
 entrapment, 159
 impingement, 158
Neuropeptides, 107b
Neurotransmitters, 99, 105-106, 107b-108b
 addiction and, 118b
 of autonomic nervous system, 147t, 148b
 behavior and, 106-109
 of enteric nervous system, 147t
 feel-good, 118b
 hormones and, 99, 106, 108b, 168
 practical applications for, 110b
Neurotrophic ulcers, 559
Neurovascular bundle, 135
Neutralizer muscles, 295
Neutrons, 7
Neutrophils, 575
Newtonian vs. quantum view, 171b
Newton's third law, 300b
Niacin, 621t
Nicotinic receptors, 148b
Nitric oxide, 108, 147t
Nociception, 152b
Nociceptors, 37-40, 143
Nodes of Ranvier, 105, 106f
Nodules, 556f
Non-Hodgkin's lymphoma, 588
Noradrenaline, 177
Norepinephrine, 108, 177

Nose, 604-606, 605f. *See also under* Nasal.
  air sinuses of, 202, 203f, 606
  immune defenses of, 592
  structure of, 157f
Notch, 198
  supraorbital, 202f-203f
Nuchal ligament, 206, 206f
Nuclear DNA, 8b
Nucleic acids, 8b, 8f, 11
Nucleotides, 8b
Nucleus
  atomic, 7, 9f
  cell, 12, 12f
Nutation, 249, 260b
Nutrients, 10
Nutrition, 618-623
  energy balance and, 622-623
  food groups and, 619-622
  guidelines for, 623b
  inadequate, 32, 225-226, 463
  weight and, 622-623
Nutritional anemias, 580-581
Nutritional databases, 623b
Nutritional disorders, 32
  bone abnormalities in, 225-226
  myopathy in, 463
Nutritional supplements, 619

Oblique capitis inferior, 349, 349f
Oblique capitis superior, 349, 349f
Oblique fractures, 224f
Oblique popliteal ligament, 262, 263f
Obstructive sleep apnea, 612
Obturator externus, 375, 375f, 529
Obturator foramen, 218f
Obturator internus, 375, 375f, 529
Occipital bone, 202f-203f, 204b
Occipital condyle, 202f-203f
Occipital lobe, 113, 114f, 114t-115t
Occipitofrontalis, 309, 309f
Oculomotor nerve, 136f, 136t-137t
Oculopelvic reflex, 297
Olecranon fossa, 211-212, 213f
Olecranon process, 212, 214f, 217f
Olfaction, 157
Olfactory nerve, 136f, 136t-137t, 605
Omentum, 615
Omohyoid, 329, 329f
Open fractures, 214, 220, 224f
Opiates
  natural, 44b, 108, 110
  pharmaceutical, 44
  receptors for, 110, 110b
Opponens digiti minimi, 454-455, 454f, 526
Opportunistic infections, 32, 590
  in AIDS, 595
Opposition, of thumb, 249, 258, 518, 525
Optic canal, 202f-203f
Optic disk, 156
Optic nerve, 136f, 136t-137t
Oral cavity. *See* Mouth.
Oral contraceptives, 637
Orbicularis oculi, 313, 313f
Orbicularis oris, 314, 314f
Orbit, 156
Organ of Corti, 153-154
Organ systems, 18
Organelles, 11-12, 12f
Organic compounds, 10
Organizational physiology, 4
Origins, 285. *See also* Muscle attachments.
Osgood-Schlatter disease, 224
Osmoreceptors, 630
Osmosis, 11
Osmotic pressure, 630
Osseous tissue, 194-195, 196f
Ossicles, 154, 154f, 202, 202f-203f
Ossification, 195
Osteitis deformans, 224
Osteitis fibrosa cystica, 224
Osteoarthritis, 244b, 274, 274f
  of spine, 277
Osteoblasts, 195
Osteochondritis dissecans, 225
Osteochondroma, 225
Osteogenesis, 195

Osteogenesis imperfecta, 223
Osteokinematics, 245-246, 246b, 272
Osteonecrosis, 224-225
Osteophytes, 274
Osteoporosis, 224
Osteosarcoma, 225
Otoliths, 155
Outflare, 260
Oval window, 154, 154f
Ovaries, 169f, 178-179, 636
Overuse injuries, 273
  of foot, 213, 222
Ovulation, 636
Oxygen debt, 293
Oxygen transport, 609
Oxytocin, 108, 175, 176f

Pacemakers, 564-565
Pacinian corpuscles, 142, 153
Paget disease, 224
Pain, 37-44
  aching, 40
  acute, 39, 39b
  assessment of, 43
  back, 223b, 277, 527
  bright, 40
  burning, 40
  chronic, 39, 39b
  counterirritation for, 40, 41f
  deep, 40
  gate-control theory of, 41f, 80-81
  from growth spurts, 224
  headache, 127, 162, 460
  increased sensitivity to, 38
  in inflammation, 34, 35f
  intractable, 39
  meaning of, 39, 39b
  muscle, 40
  perception of, 37-40, 43, 44b, 152b
  phantom, 42-43
  pricking, 40
  referred, 40-42, 41f-42f
  sacroiliac, 527
  severity of, 43
  somatic, 23, 40
  trigger points and, 81, 82f-83f
  types of, 40
  visceral, 40-42, 41f
Pain behavior, 109-110
Pain management, 43-44, 44b
Pain medications, 44
Pain receptors, 37-44, 143
Pain sensations, 37-40
Pain sense, 152b
Pain threshold, 43
Pain tolerance, 43
Pain-spasm-pain cycle, 27-28, 40, 40f
Palatal process, 202f-203f
Palate, 615
  cleft, 223
Palatine bone, 202f-203f, 204b
Pallor, 555
Palmar, definition of, 68
Palmar interosseous, 526
Palmaris longus, 441, 441f, 518
Palpation
  of ankle, 265-266
  of cranial sutures, 254
  of elbow, 258
  of foot, 265-266
  of hip, 260-262
  of knee, 262-264
  of muscles, 307
  of pelvis, 260-262
  of ribs, 269
  of shoulder, 256-257
  of temporomandibular joint, 254, 254f
  of thoracic joints, 269
Pancreas, 169f, 176-177, 614f, 616, 619f
  disorders of, 185-186, 626
Pancreatic juice, 616, 618t, 620t
Pancreatitis, 626
Panic disorder, 161
Pantothenic acid, 621t
Papules, 556f
Parallel muscles, 295, 296f

Paralysis, 276
  facial, 160
  flaccid, 123, 124b
  in paraplegia, 126
  in quadriplegia, 124
  spastic, 123, 124b
  in spinal cord injury, 125-126
  in stroke, 124
Paranasal sinuses, 202, 203f, 606
Paraplegia, 126
Parasitic infections, of skin, 557f-558f, 559
Parasympathetic blockers, 158
Parasympathetic nervous system, 100, 134, 147-150, 177b
  structure and function of, 148-149, 149f, 151t
Parathormone, 176
  imbalance of, 184-185
Parathyroid glands, 169f, 176
  disorders of, 184-185
Parietal bone, 202f-203f, 204b
Parietal lobe, 113, 114f, 114t-115t
Parietal membranes, 66
Parietooccipital fissure, 113
Parkinson's disease, 127
Passive joint movement, 272
Passive transport, 11
Patella, 213, 215, 219f, 221f, 262, 533
  bones of, 221f
  tracking of, 535
Patellar groove, 215, 219f
Patellar ligament, 262, 263f
Patellar reflex, 144
Patellar tendon, 533
Patellofemoral joint, 262-264, 262b, 263f
Pathogen(s), 27, 32, 32b, 590
  opportunistic, 32, 590
Pathogenesis, 30
Pathogenicity, 32
Pathology, 30
  definition of, 4
Pathophysiology, 4
Pavlov, Ivan, 141
PCP (phencyclidine), 124
Pear shape, health risks for, 32f
Pectineus, 385, 385f, 529
Pectoral girdle
  bones of, 209, 210b, 211f
  muscles of, 350, 351f-352f
Pectoralis major, 429, 429f, 510
Pectoralis minor, 421, 421f, 509, 511, 607-610, 607f-608f
Pediculosis, 559
Pelvic cavity, 63, 66, 66f
Pelvic floor, 353f, 365
Pelvic girdle/pelvis, 211, 214b, 218f
  biomechanics of, 526-529
  craniosacral system and, 476
  elevation of, 507
  functions of, 260b
  joints of, 259, 260b, 261f, 526-529
  ligaments of, 259, 261f
  movements of, 249, 259-260, 260b, 526-528, 528f-529f, 528t
  muscles of, 353f, 365-369
  palpation of, 260-262
  rotation of, 526-528, 528t-529f, 528t, 534f-535f
Pelvic inflammatory disease, 645
Pelvic tilt
  anterior, 249, 260, 475
  lateral, 507, 527-528
  posterior, 249, 260, 475
  posture and, 475
Penis, 635, 635f
Pennate muscles, 295, 296f
Peptic ulcer disease, 624
Peptidases, 618t
Peptides, 10
Pericarditis, 578
Pericardium, 562, 566f
Perimysium, 289f, 298
Perineal muscles, 353f, 365-369, 367f
Perineurium, 134, 135f
Periosteum, 195, 196f
Peripheral nerves. *See also* Nerve(s).
  connective tissue of, 134, 135f
  injuries of, 158-162. *See also* Neuropathy.

Peripheral nerves *(Continued)*
    repair/regeneration of, 102-103, 104f
    structure of, 135f, 150
Peripheral nervous system, 133-166. *See also* Nervous
        system.
    components of, 100, 134
    divisions of, 100. *See also* Autonomic nervous system;
        Somatic nervous system.
    subdivisions of, 134
Peripheral neuropathy. *See* Neuropathy.
Peripheral resistance, 572
Peripheral vascular system, 566f
Peristalsis, 617
Peritoneal cavity, 615
Peritoneal ligaments, 615
Peritoneum, 615
Pernicious anemia, 597t
Peroneus brevis, 399, 399f, 537
Peroneus longus, 399, 399f, 537
Peroneus tertius, 397, 397f
Peroxisomes, 12
Perthes disease, 225
Pes anserinus, 535
Peyer's patches, 586
pH, 10, 10f
pH balance, 631
Phagocytosis, 15
Phalanges
    of foot, 196f, 221. *See also* Toe(s).
    of hand, 70f-74f, 211, 212b, 216f, 258-259, 259f.
        See also Finger(s); Thumb.
Phantom pain, 42-43
Pharmacology, 30. *See also* Drug(s).
Pharyngitis, 610
Pharynx, 605f, 606, 614f, 616, 619f
Phencyclidine (PCP), 124
Phenylethylamine (PEA), 108
Phlebitis, 581
Phonation, 606
Phospholipid bilayer, 11, 11f
Phosphorus balance, 630-631
Phrenic nerve, 607
Physical agents, disease-causing, 32
Physical assessment, 91
Physical properties, 7
Physics, 58b
Physiology, 4-5
    anatomy and, 4-5
    definition of, 4
    organizational, 4
    systemic, 4
Pia mater, 120, 120f
Piezoelectric effect
    on bone, 194, 194b, 198b
    on cartilage, 17b
Pineal gland, 112f, 118, 169f, 179-180
    disorders of, 187
Pinna, 153-154, 154f
Piriformis, 374-377, 374f, 527, 529
Pitcher's elbow, 273
Pitta dosha, 26
Pituitary fossa, 202f-203f
Pituitary gland, 169f, 173-180, 176f
    disorders of, 182-183
    in stress response, 47b, 48f
Pituitary hormones
    anterior pituitary, 174-175, 174b, 176f
    posterior pituitary, 169-170, 176f
Pivot joints, 250, 253f
Placebo response, 43
Placenta, 641
Planes, body, 69-75, 69f
    cardinal, 247-248, 248f
Plantar, definition of, 68
Plantar aponeurosis, 213
Plantar calcaneofibular ligament, 265f
Plantar fasciitis, 213, 222
Plantar flexion, 75, 248-249, 264b, 536, 537f
Plantar ligaments, 265f
Plantar warts, 559
Plantaris, 404, 404f, 535
Plaque, cutaneous, 556f
Plasma, 576
Plasma membrane, 11, 12f
Plastic range, 239-240
Plasticity, 301, 301b

Platelets, 576
Platysma, 290-291, 319f
Pleural cavity, 606
Pleurisy, 611
Plexuses. *See* Nerve plexuses.
Pneumonia, 610
Pneumothorax, 606
Points
    acupressure, 152b
    acupuncture, 80-81, 85
    common characteristics of, 81
    marmas, 81
    motor, 84f
    in traditional Chinese medicine, 84f, 85, 86b, 87
    trigger, 81, 82f-83f, 89b, 292b
Polar covalent bonds, 7-8
Polar molecules, 7-8, 9f
Poliomyelitis, 160, 462
Pollack, Gerald, 303
Polycythemia, 575, 583
Polydipsia, 631-632
Polyps, endometrial, 644
Polysaccharides, 621
Pons, 112f, 119
Popliteus, 402-405, 402f, 534-535
Portal system, 574-575
Portal vein, 574-575
Position(s)
    anatomic, 63, 63f, 66, 69
    erect, 66
    functional, 66, 69
    lateral recumbent, 67, 67f
    prone, 66, 67f
    supine, 66, 67f
Positive feedback, 27-28
Postcentral gyrus, 113, 114f, 114t-115t
Posterior, definition of, 67, 68f
Posterior clinoid process, 202f-203f
Posterior cruciate ligament, 262, 263f
Posterior deltoid, 510
Posterior inferior iliac spine, 218f
Posterior longitudinal ligament, 206, 206f, 266,
        267f-268f
Posterior meniscofemoral ligament, 262, 263f
Posterior oblique ligament, 258
Posterior pelvic tilt, 249, 260, 475
Posterior pituitary hormones, 169-170, 176f
Posterior rotation, of hip, 474f, 527, 528t
Posterior scalene, 334, 334f
Posterior sternoclavicular ligament, 255
Posterior superior iliac spine, 214, 218f
Postisometric relaxation, 145b
Postpolio syndrome, 462
Postural deviations, 542-543, 545f
Postural reflexes, 297
Postural stabilization, kinetic chains and, 474b, 478
Posture, 473-476, 475f. *See also* Spinal curves.
    in anterior view, 476
    in lateral view, 476
    in posterior view, 476
Potassium balance, 630
Potassium ions, 103
Potential energy, 8
Pott's disease, 225
Prana, 17b, 286
Precapillary sphincters, 567
Precentral gyrus, 111-113, 114f, 114t-115t
Preeclampsia, 643
Preexisting conditions, 30
Prefixes, 59, 60t
Pregnancy, 637-640
    bleeding in, 641
    disorders of, 641-643
    ectopic, 643
    fertilization and, 637-638
    first trimester of, 638
    hypertension in, 643
    massage therapy in, 645b
    miscarriage in, 642
    preeclampsia in, 643
    second trimester of, 638-639
    third trimester of, 639-640
    toxemia in, 643
    vomiting in, 643
    weight gain in, 638t
Prelabor, 640

Premotor cortex, 114t-115t
Prepuce, 635, 635f
Pressure, force and, 470
Prevertebral fascia, 299f
PRICE mnemonic, 43, 43b
Pricking pain, 40
Primary hyperparathyroidism, 185
Prime movers, 304
    in muscle firing patterns, 494
Problem-oriented medical record, 91
Procallus, 220
Procerus, 309, 309f
Processes. *See* Bony processes.
Prodrome, 590-591
Progesterone, 178-179, 637
Prognosis, 30
Prolactin, 175, 176f
Prolactin-inhibiting factor, 170t
Prolactin-releasing hormone, 170t
Pronation, 70f-74f, 75, 248-249, 258, 258f, 521
Pronator quadratus, 438, 438f, 518
Pronator teres, 437, 437f, 518
Prone position, 66, 67f
Proprioception, 143
    definition of, 150
    gamma motor neurons in, 146-147
    vs. kinesthesia, 153
Proprioceptors, 141, 142f, 143, 295-297
    types of, 143
Proprio-neuro-facilitation stretching, 297b
Prostaglandins, 34b, 169-170, 181
Prostate, 635f
    cancer of, 644
    disorders of, 644
Prostatitis, 644
Protease, 618t
Proteins, 10
    dietary, 619-621
Proteoglycans, 303
Protons, 7
Protraction, 75, 249
Proximal, definition of, 67, 68f
Proximal interphalangeal joints, 243f, 259
    close-packed position of, 248t
    of foot, 264f, 265, 536, 536f
    least-packed position of, 247t
Pseudofolliculitis barbae, 561
Psoas major, 359, 359f, 527
Psoas minor, 360, 360f
Psoriasis, 557f-558f, 561
Psychological disorders, 161
Psychoneuroimmunology, 49
Psychophysiology, 49
Psychotropic drugs, 109
Pterygoid hamulus, 202f-203f
Pterygoideus lateralis, 321, 321f
Puberty
    female, 637
    male, 635-636
Pubic symphysis. *See* Symphysis pubis.
Pubis, 214, 218f
Pubofemoral ligament, 259-260, 261f
Pulmonary arteries, 562f, 563
Pulmonary edema, 611
Pulmonary embolism, 581-582
Pulmonary infarction, 582
Pulmonary valve, 563, 563f
Pulmonary veins, 563
Pulse, 570-573, 572b
Purulent exudates, 34b
Pus, 34b
Pustules, 556f
Pyelonephritis, 633
Pyloric sphincter, 616
Pylorus, 616
Pyramidalis, 364, 364f
Pyridoxine, 621t

Q angle, 533, 534f-535f
Qi, 17b, 87-88, 286
Qi heng zhi fu, 88
Qi qing, 88
Qigong, 88
Quadratus femoris, 376, 376f, 529
Quadratus lumborum, 358, 358f
Quadratus plantae, 411, 411f, 537

Quadriceps (Q) angle, 533, 534f-535f
Quadriceps femoris group, 380-392, 388f-392f, 533, 535, 535f
Quadriplegia, 124
Quality of life
    definition of, 76
    terminology for, 76, 79b
    WHO domains for, 76, 77b-79b
Quantun vs. Newtonian view, 171b
Quartz, 194, 194b

Radial collateral ligament, 257-258, 257f
Radial deviation, 248-249
Radial fossa, 211-212, 213f
Radial tuberosity, 217f
Radiation therapy, bone effects of, 224
Radiocarpal joint, 258
Radiohumeral joint, 257, 257f
    close-packed position of, 248t
    least-packed position of, 247t
Radioulnar joints, 258
    close-packed position of, 248t
    least-packed position of, 247t
    movements of, 518, 519b-525b
    muscles of, 433-439, 433f-434f, 518
    structure of, 517-518
Radius, 209-212, 214f, 217f
Range of motion (ROM), 245-246. See also specific joints.
    active joint movements and, 272
    anatomic barriers and, 271
    anatomic motion and, 246
    assessment of, 248, 251f-252f, 271, 498
    definition of, 245
    end feel and, 246
    factors affecting, 270-272
    limits of, 246
    normal, 271b
    passive joint movements and, 272
    pathologic, 246, 246b
    pathologic barriers to, 271
    physiologic (active), 246
    physiologic barriers to, 271
    restoration of, 234
Raphe, 298
Rash, in measles, 558-559
Raynaud's disease/phenomenon, 580
Razor bumps, 561
Receptors
    opiate, 110, 110b
    pain, 37-44, 143
    sensory, 141-143
    touch, 153
Reciprocal inhibition, 144
Reciprocal innervation, 144
Rectum, 617, 619f
Rectus abdominis, 363, 363f, 502, 607-610, 607f
Rectus capitis posterior major, 348, 348f
Rectus capitis posterior minor, 348, 348f
Rectus femoris, 389, 389f, 529
Red blood cells, 575
    oxygen transport by, 609
Red fibers, 291-293
Redness, in inflammation, 34, 35f
Reduction, 501
Referred pain, 40-42, 41f-42f
Reflex(es), 139-140
    Achilles tendon, 144
    biceps, 144
    in breathing, 609-610
    complex (conditioned), 140-142
    contralateral, 145
    cough, 609
    crossed extensor, 145, 297
    deep tendon, 122, 144, 297
    definition of, 139-140
    flexor, 144-145, 297
    inverse stretch, 144
    ispsilateral, 144
    massage effects and, 146b
    monosynaptic, 144
    muscle, 144
    oculopelvic, 297
    patellar, 144
    postural, 297
    simple (unconditioned), 140

Reflex(es) (Continued)
    sneeze, 609
    somatic, 143-144, 296, 297f
    somatosomatic, 141
    somatovisceral, 141
    stretch, 144, 145b, 296-297
    tendon, 144, 145b, 297
    triceps, 144
    types of, 140-141
    viscerosomatic, 141
    viscerovisceral, 141
    withdrawal, 297, 297b
Reflex arcs, 143-145
    deep tendon, 122
    monosynaptic, 144
    somatic, 296, 297f
    tendon, 122
Reflux esophagitis, 624
Refractory period, 104-105, 105b
Regional anatomy, 4, 63, 65f
Relaxin, 179
REM sleep, 118b
Remission, 30
Renal calculi, 633
Renal disease, massage contraindications for, 634b
Renal failure, 634
Repetitive stress injuries, 273
    of foot, 213, 222
Reproduction, 6. See also Pregnancy.
Reproductive system, 634-645
    female, 636-641, 636f, 640f
    immune defenses of, 592
    male, 635-636, 635f
Resistance
    force and, 470
    in joint assessment, 498
Respiration, 6, 604. See also Breathing.
    aerobic, 291-293
    anaerobic, 293
    external, 604
    internal, 604
    rib cage in, 269, 270f
Respiratory alkalosis, 610
Respiratory center, 609
Respiratory muscles, 350-369, 351f-352f, 502-503, 607-610, 607f-608f
Respiratory pump, 569, 570b, 570f
Respiratory rate, 609
Respiratory system, 604-613
    carbon dioxide in, 609
    immune defenses of, 592, 605
    lower respiratory tract, 605f, 613
    massage contraindications for, 613b
    organs of, 604-607, 605f
    oxygen transport in, 609
    upper respiratory tract, 605f, 613
Responsiveness, 5
Resting muscle tone, 291
Reticular activating system, 118-119
Reticular fibers, 14
Retina, 155f, 156
Retraction, 75, 249
Retroperitoneal organs, 615
Retroviruses, 595
Reverse action, 285, 381, 433
Rheumatic fever, 578, 597t
Rheumatic heart disease, 578, 597t
Rheumatoid arthritis, 246, 597t
Rheumatoid inflammatory disorder, 277
Rhomboid major, 419, 419f, 509-510
Rhomboid minor, 420, 420f, 509-510
Riboflavin, 621t
Ribonucleic acid (RNA), 8b, 8f, 11
Ribosomes, 8b, 12, 12f
Ribs, 209, 209b, 210f
    movements of, 269, 270f
    palpation of, 269
Rickets, 225-226
Right arm extensor test
    for contralateral extensors, 485
    for unilateral extensors, 490
Right arm flexor test
    for contralateral flexors, 483
    for unilateral flexors, 488
Right lateral flexion, 74

Right leg extensor test
    for contralateral extensors, 487
    for unilateral extensors, 491
Right leg flexor test
    for contralateral flexors, 484
    for unilateral flexors, 489
Right lymphatic duct, 584, 584f
Right rotation, 74-75
Righting reflex, 297
Ringworm, 557f-558f, 559
Risk factors, 30, 30b
Risorius, 315, 315f
RNA (ribonucleic acid), 8b, 8f, 11
Rocking, 120b
Rods, 156
Roll, 245, 245f
Root(s)
    spinal nerve, 122
    word, 59, 60t-61t
Root chakra, 179
Root hair plexuses, 142
Rosacea, 561
Rotation, 70f-74f, 74-75, 248-249
    axis of, 470
    cervical, 505-506
    downward, 249
    of glenohumeral joint, 509-510
    of hip, 528, 528t, 532-533
    of knee, 534, 536f
    lateral, 69, 248-249
    left, 75
    medial, 69, 248-249
    of pelvis, 526-528
    right, 74-75
    of scapula, 509, 513
    of shoulder, 517
    spinal, 501
    of thumb, 525
    transverse, 248
    of trunk, 507
    upward, 249
Rotator cuff
    muscles of, 422-425, 423f
    palpation of, 257
    tears of, 462
Rotatores, 344, 344f
Rough endoplasmic reticulum, 11-12, 12f
Round window, 154, 154f
Rubella, 558
Rubrospinal tracts, 123b
Ruffini's end-organs, 142-143, 153
Rugae, 616
Ruptures, 239

Saccules, 119b
Sacral plexus, 137, 140f, 353f
    injuries of, 159
Sacral region, 66
Sacroiliac joint, 214, 218f
    movements of, 249, 260b, 262, 526
    structure of, 259, 261f, 526, 526f
Sacroiliac ligament, 259, 261f
Sacroiliac motion, 260b, 500
Sacroiliac pain, 527
Sacrospinalis muscles, 338-340, 338f-340f
Sacrospinous ligament, 259, 261f
Sacrotuberous ligament, 259, 261f
Sacrum, 205, 207f, 208
Saddle joints, 250, 253f
Sagittal plane, 69, 69f, 247-248, 248f
Sagittal suture, 202, 202f-204f, 254, 254f
Saliva, 620t
Salivary glands, 614f, 615, 619f
Saltatory conduction, 105, 106f
Sarcomeres, 289, 290f
Sartorius, 388, 388f, 529, 534-535
Scabies, 557f-558f, 559
Scalene muscles, 333-334, 333f-334f, 502-503, 607-610, 607f
Scapula, 210b, 211f
    abduction of, 512-513
    assessment of, 511b-517b
    depression of, 514
    elevation of, 513
    flexion of, 515
    movements of, 508-509, 511b-517b

Scapula *(Continued)*
  stabilizing muscles of, 415-421, 416f-417f
  upward rotation with abduction of, 513
Scapular winging, 511b-517b
Scapulothoracic junction, 509
Scheuermann disease, 225
Schizophrenia, 128
Schwann cells, 102, 102f
Science
  branches of, 58b
  definition of, 58
Scientific terminology, 59-63. *See also* Terminology.
Sclera, 155, 155f
Scleroderma, 561
Scoliosis, 209, 223f, 277, 475
  functional, 277
Screw-home mechanism, 534, 536f
Scurvy, 226
Seasonal affective disorder, 187
Sebaceous cysts, 560
Sebaceous glands, 554
Seborrheic dermatitis, 561
Seborrheic keratitis, 560
Secondary hyperparathyroidism, 185
Secretin, 180
Secretion, 6
Seizures, 126-127
Sella turcica, 202f-203f, 204
Selye, Hans, 46, 47b, 80, 170, 171b
Semicircular canals, 155
Semilunar valves, 563, 563f
Semimembranosus, 379, 379f, 529, 535
Seminal vesicles, 635, 635f
Semispinalis capitis, 342, 342f
Semispinalis cervicis, 342, 342f
Semispinalis thoracis, 342, 342f
Semitendinosus, 379, 379f, 529, 535
Sensory areas of brain, 101f
Sensory ascending tracts, 122-123, 122f
Sensory neurons, 101-102, 103b
Sensory receptors, 122-123, 141-143
  adaptation of, 142-143
  exteroceptors, 141, 142f
  joint kinesthetic, 143
  mechanical, 142-143
  proprioceptors, 141, 142f, 143, 154
  somatic, 141, 142f
  thermal, 143
Serotonin, 108, 110, 147t
Serous exudates, 34b
Serous membranes, 14
Serratus anterior, 421, 421f, 509-510, 510f, 607-610, 607f
Serratus posterior inferior, 355, 355f, 607-610, 607f
Serratus posterior superior, 355, 355f, 607-610, 607f
Sesamoid bones, 194, 197
Sex determination, 637-638
Sex hormones, 178-179
  female, 637
  male, 635-636
Sexual development
  in female, 637
  in male, 635-636
Sexually transmitted diseases, 644-645
Shear and friction, 242
Shear forces, 240f, 242
Sheathed tendons, 238
Shells, electron, 7, 9f
Shen, 88
Shin splints, 222
Shingles, 160, 557f-558f, 558
Shock, 580
  anaphylactic, 595b, 596
Short bones, 197
Short plantar ligament, 265f
Shortening, of connective tissue, 239-240
Shoulder
  biomechanics of, 508-510
  bones of, 209, 211f, 217f, 256f
  extension of, 515
  flexion of, 497, 515
  frozen, 276-277
  horizontal abduction of, 510
  horizontal adduction of, 509-510, 516
  joints of, 255-257, 255f, 508-509
  ligaments of, 255, 255f-256f, 257

Shoulder *(Continued)*
  movements of, 70f-74f, 249, 255, 508-510, 509t, 511b-517b
  muscles of, 509-510
    rotator cuff, 422-425, 423f
    for scapular stabilization, 415-421, 416f-417f
    of shoulder joint, 426-431, 427f
  palpation of, 256-257
  range of motion of, 271b
  rotation of, 517
  stability of, 508
Shoulder blade. *See* Scapula.
Shoulder girdle
  biomechanics of, 508-509
  movements of, 509t
  muscles of, 509-510
Shunts, arteriovenous, 567
Si shi, 88
Sickle cell disease, 583
Side bending, 74, 249, 501
SIDS (sudden infant death syndrome), 612
Sight. *See* Vision.
Signs, of disease, 30
Simple fractures, 214, 224f
Singultus (hiccups), 607b, 610
Sinistral (sinistro), 68
Sinus(es), 198
  in chronic inflammation, 37
  nasal air, 202, 203f, 606
Sinusitis, 610
Sitting, biomechanics of, 478
Skeletal muscle, 286-287. *See also* Muscle(s).
  functions of, 286
Skeletal muscle pump, 569, 570b, 570f
Skeletal system, 192-233
  age-related changes in, 197
  components of. *See* Bone(s); Cartilage; Joint(s); Ligaments; Skeleton.
  demineralization disorders of, 224
  developmental disorders of, 222-224
  functions of, 193-194
  infectious diseases of, 225
  necrotic disorders of, 224-225
  nutritional disorders of, 225-226
  traumatic disorders of, 214-222, 224f
  tumors of, 225
Skeleton. *See also* Bone(s).
  appendicular, 199, 200f-201f, 209-213
  axial, 199, 200f-201f, 202-209
Skin
  bacterial infections of, 556, 557f-558f
  benign tumors and growths of, 559-560
  blood supply of, 554
  burns of, 561
  cancer of, 557f-558f, 560
  color of, 555
  fungal infections of, 557f-558f, 559
  immune defenses of, 591
  lesions of, 556f-558f
  parasitic infections of, 557f-558f, 559
  structure of, 553-555, 553f
  ulcers of, 559, 572f
  viral infections of, 556-559, 557f-558f
Skin cleavage lines, 553, 554f
Skin disorders, 556-562, 557f-558f
  massage contraindications for, 562b
Skin tags, 560
Skin wounds, healing of, 38f, 555-556
Skull, 202, 202f-203f, 204b. *See also under* Cranial.
  bones of, 202, 202f-203f, 204b, 267f
  of infant, 203, 204f
  joints of, 245, 254f
Sleep, 118b-119b
  head-body moving cycle in, 605
  melatonin and, 179-180, 187
Sleep apnea, 611
Slide, 245, 245f
Sliding filament mechanism, 289-290, 290f
Slow-twitch fibers, 291-293
Small intestine, 614f, 616, 619f
Smell, 157
Smooth endoplasmic reticulum, 11-12, 12f
Smooth muscle, 286-287, 287f
  innervation of, 291
  multiunit, 287
  visceral, 287

Smooth muscle fibers, 16-18
Sneezing, 609
SOAP notes, 90-91
Sodium balance, 630
Sodium ions, 103
Sodium-potassium pump, 11
Soft end feel, 246
Soft palate, 615
Soleus, 404, 404f, 537
Solids, 7
Soma/somato, 64
Somatic nervous system, 100, 134
  sensory receptors of, 141-143
Somatic pain, 40
  superficial, 23
Somatic reflex arc, 143-144, 296, 297f
Somatosomatic reflexes, 141
Somatostatin, 108, 170t, 176
Somatotropin, 174, 176f
Somatovisceral reflexes, 141
Sore throat, 610
Spasms, 140, 460-461
  pain-spasm-pain cycle and, 27-28, 40, 40f
Spastic colon, 624-625
Spastic paralysis, 123, 124b
Speed, force and, 470
Spermatogenesis, 635-636, 635f
Sphenoid bone, 202f-203f, 204b
Sphenoid sinus, 202, 203f
Sphenomandibular ligament, 254
Sphincter(s), 295, 296f
  cardiac, 616
  external anal, 367, 367f
  precapillary, 567
  pyloric, 616
Sphincter ani externus, 367, 367f
Spin, 245, 245f
Spina bifida, 222
Spinal cord, 121-123
  functions of, 121
  segments of, 121
  structure of, 111f, 121-123, 121f-122f
Spinal cord injury, 125-126
  respiratory failure in, 607
Spinal curves, 206-209, 208f, 475
  abnormal, 209, 223, 223f, 277, 475
  primary, 475
Spinal nerve(s), 121-122, 134-139, 137f, 137t. *See also* Nerve(s).
  injuries of, 137-138
Spinal nerve roots, 122
  compression of, 159
Spinal rotation, 501
Spinal tracts
  ascending, 122-123, 122f
  descending, 122-123, 122f, 123b
Spinalis capitis, 340, 340f
Spinalis cervicis, 340, 340f
Spinalis thoracis, 340, 340f
Spine. *See also under* Vertebrae; Vertebral; Vertebral column.
  age-related changes in, 197
  close-packed position of, 248t
  disorders of, 277
  extension of, 501
  flexion of, 501
  joints of, 266-268, 267f-269f, 501-502, 501f
  least-packed position of, 247t
  ligaments of, 206, 206f, 266, 267f-269f
  movements of, 249, 266, 501-502, 501f, 528t
  muscles of, 500-501
  palpation of, 266-268
  tuberculosis of, 225
Spinous processes, 199, 204, 205f-206f
Spleen, 585
Splenius capitis, 304-458, 337f
Splenius cervicis, 304-458, 337f
Splints, 276
Spondylitis, 277
Spondylolisthesis, 277
Spondylosis, 277
Spongy bone, 195, 196f
Sprains, 275-277, 276f
Spring ligament, 265f
Springy block, 246
Squamous cell carcinoma, of skin, 557f-558f, 560

Squamous suture, 202, 204f, 254, 254f
Stability, 473
   vs. mobility, 236, 236b, 239
Stabilization, in joint assessment, 498
Stabilizer muscles, 295, 297-298, 304, 494
Stance phase, of gait cycle, 480, 481f
Standard Precautions, 552-556
Standing, biomechanics of, 478, 479f
Stapes, 154, 154f, 202f-203f
State-dependent memory, 117b
Static force, 286
Status epilepticus, 127
Stem cells, 555-556, 575
Sternoclavicular joint
   close-packed position of, 248t
   least-packed position of, 247t
   movements of, 508
   palpation of, 256
   structure of, 255, 256f
Sternoclavicular ligaments, 255, 256f
Sternocleidomastoid, 325, 325f, 607, 607f-608f
   shortening/spasm of, 461
Sternocostal joints, 268-269, 270f
Sternocostal pectoralis, 510
Sternohyoid, 328, 328f
Sternothyroid, 329, 329f
Sternum, 209, 209b, 210f
Steroids, 171, 171t
   synthetic, 182
      for muscle disorders, 459-460
Stimulant drugs, 124
Stomach, 614f, 616, 619f, 626
   cancer of, 626
   immune defenses of, 592
   ulcers of, 624
Strain (mechanical), 301b
Strain (muscle), 461-462
Stratum fibrosum, 244
Stratum synovium, 244
Strep throat, 610
Stress, 45-49
   adaptation to, 25, 48-49
   adrenal hormones in, 47b, 48f, 177-178, 178b
   biomechanical, 301b
   definition of, 25, 30
   general adaptation syndrome and, 46, 47b, 48f, 148,
      170, 171b
   muscle tension due to, 460
   perception of, 46-49
Stress fractures, 215
Stress load, 45-46, 47f
Stress management, 48-49
   massage therapy in, 49b, 174b-175b
   medical assistance in, 49
   multidisciplinary approach in, 49
Stress response, 46, 47b, 48f
   catecholamines in, 177b
Stress-induced diseases, 30, 49b
Stretch reflexes, 144, 145b
   inverse, 144
Stretching, proprio-neuro-facilitation, 297b
Striated involuntary muscle, 286
Stroke, 124-125
Structural organization of body, 6-19, 7f, 63-75. See also
      Anatomy.
   body map and, 63-68, 63f
   body regions and surface anatomy and, 63, 65f
   at chemical level, 6-11
   at organ level, 18
   at organelle level, 11-12
   at organism level, 18-19
   at system level, 18
   at tissue level, 13-18, 17f
Study tips, 3b
Stylohyoid muscle, 326, 326f
Styloid process, 202f-203f, 211-212, 214f
Stylomandibular ligament, 254, 254f
Subacute disease, 30
Subarachnoid space, 120, 120f
Subclavius, 429, 429f
Subclinical infections, 591
Subcutaneous layer, 553-554
Subdural hematoma, 125
Subdural space, 120, 120f
Sublingual salivary glands, 614f, 615, 619f
Submandibular salivary glands, 614f, 615, 619f

Suboccipital muscles, 347-349, 348f-349f
Subscapular fossa, 210
Subscapularis, 425, 425f, 510
Subtalar joint, 264-265
   close-packed position of, 248t
   least-packed position of, 247t
Sucrase, 618t
Sudden infant death syndrome (SIDS), 612
Sudoriferous glands, 554-555
Suffixes, 59, 61t
Sugars, 10
Sulci, cortical, 113
Superficial, definition of, 68
Superficial fascia, 315f, 553-554
Superficial inguinal ring, 299f
Superficial somatic pain, 23
Superior, definition of, 68-69, 68f
Superior articular facet, 268f
Superior orbital fissure, 202f-203f
Superior pubic ligament, 259
Superior pubic ramus, 218f
Superior tibiofemoral joint, 533
Superior vena cava, 563
Supination, 75, 248-249, 258, 258f, 521
Supinator, 437, 437f, 518
Supine position, 66, 67f
Support muscles, 295
Suprahyoid muscles, 325-327, 326f-327f
Supraorbital notch, 202f-203f
Supraspinatus, 424-425, 424f, 510
Supraspinous fossa, 210, 211f
Supraspinous ligament, 206, 206f, 266, 267f-268f
Surface anatomy, 4
Sutures, cranial, 202, 202f-204f, 242-243, 243b, 254,
      254f
   palpation of, 254
Swayback (hyperlordosis), 209, 223, 223f, 277, 475
Sweat glands, 554-555
Swell bodies, 605
Swelling, in inflammation, 34, 35f
Swing phase, of gait cycle, 480, 482f
Sympathetic nervous system, 100, 134, 147-150,
      177b
   structure and function of, 147-148, 149f, 151t
Symphysis pubis, 214, 218f, 243
   movements of, 259, 260b, 526
Symptoms, 30
Synapses, 99, 105, 107f
Synaptic cleft, 105, 107f
Synarthroses, 242-243
Synchondrosis, 243
Syndesmoses, 243
Syndromes, 30
Synergist muscles, 295, 418
Synergistic dominance, 494
Synovial cavity, 244
   of knee, 264, 534
Synovial fluid, 195-197, 238, 244, 244b, 534
Synovial joints, 242-244, 242f, 244b
   types of, 248-250
Synovial membranes, 16
Synovial plane joint, 250, 253f
Syphilis, 645
Systemic anatomy, 4
Systemic lupus erythematosus, 597t
Systemic physiology, 4
Systemic sclerosis, 561
Systems of control, 18
Systole, 564
Systolic pressure, 571

T cells, 593-594
   in HIV infection, 595-596
Tachycardia, 576
Tachypnea, 609
Tactile receptors, 153
Tailbone (coccyx), 66, 205, 207f, 208b
Talipes, 223
Talocalcaneal joint, 264-265
Talocrural joint, 264
Talofibular ligaments, 264, 265f
Talonavicular ligament, 265f
Talus, 215, 220f, 221
Target cells, 172-173, 173f
Tarsal bones, 220f, 221

Tarsometatarsal joint, 265
   close-packed position of, 248t
   least-packed position of, 247t
Taste, 156, 156f
Taste buds, 156, 156f
Teeth, 615
   gomphosis joints and, 243
Temperature sense, 152b
Temporal arteritis, 580
Temporal bone, 202f-203f, 204b
Temporal fossa, 202f-203f
Temporal lobe, 113, 114f, 114t-115t
Temporalis, 321, 321f
Temporomandibular joint, 254, 254f
   close-packed position of, 248t
   least-packed position of, 247t
Tendon(s), 238. See also Connective tissue.
   bony attachments for, 199
   musculotendinous junction and, 298
   origin of, 298
   proprioceptors for, 295
   rupture of, 239
   sheathed, 238
   structure of, 238
Tendon reflexes, 144, 145b, 297
Tennis elbow, 273
TENS (transcutaneous electrical nerve stimulation), 43
Tensegrity, 301-303, 302f
Tensile stress injuries, 240
Tension forces, 240, 243f
Tension headaches, 162, 460
Tensor fascia lata, 299f, 373, 373f, 529, 535
Teres major, 431, 431f, 510
Teres minor, 425, 425f
Terminologia Anatomica, 285
Terminology, 57-97, 285
   anatomic. See Anatomic terminology.
   definitions of, 58, 58b
   in documentation, 76b
   international standards for, 285
   for kinesiology, 69-75
   medical, 59-63. See also Medical terminology.
   for movement, 69-75
   practical applications for, 59b, 68b, 76b, 79b, 107b
   quality-of-life, 76, 77b-79b
   tips for learning, 58b
   for traditional medicine, 80, 87b-88b
Testes, 169f, 178-179, 635, 635f
Testosterone, 635-636
Thalamus, 112f, 118
Thenar eminence muscles, 452-453, 452f
Thermal receptors, 143
Thermo sense, 152b
Thiamine, 621t
Thigh
   bones of, 213, 219f
   fascia of, 299f
   muscles of
      adductor group, 380, 385f-387f
      of anterior and medial compartments, 369,
         382f-384f
      deep lateral rotators at hip, 374-377, 374f
      hamstring group, 378-380, 379f-380f
      of posterior compartment, 369, 378f
      quadriceps femoris group, 380-392, 388f-392f
Thixotropy, 17b, 301b
Thoracic bones, 209, 209b, 210f
Thoracic breathing, 503
Thoracic cage, palpation of, 269
Thoracic cavity, 66, 66f
Thoracic duct, 584, 584f
Thoracic joints, 268-269, 270f, 501-503
Thoracic ligaments, 268-269
Thoracic muscles, 350
Thoracic region, 66
Thoracic vertebrae, 205, 207f, 208, 208b
   biomechanics of, 501-502
Thoracotomy, 606
Thorax, 607
   biomechanics of, 501-503
Threshold stimulus, for muscle contraction, 291
Throat, 605f, 606, 614f, 616
   sore, 610
   strep, 610
Thrombocytopenia, 583
Thrombophlebitis, 581

Thrombosis, 581, 581f
  deep vein, 581
Thrush, 559
Thumb
  adduction of, 525
  close-packed position of, 248t
  flexion of, 525
  joints of, 258-259, 259f, 518
  least-packed position of, 247t
  ligaments of, 258
  medial rotation of, 525
  movements of, 70f-74f, 248-249
  opposition of, 249, 258, 518, 525
  palpation of, 259
Thymus, 169f, 180, 585
Thyrohyoid, 330, 330f
Thyroid cartilage, 606
Thyroid gland, 169f, 176, 176f
  disorders of, 183-184, 183f, 184f
Thyroid-stimulating hormone (TSH), 174-175, 176f
Thyrotoxicosis, 183, 183f, 184t
Thyrotropin-releasing hormone, 170t
Thyroxine, 176
  functions of, 184t
  hypersecretion of, 183, 183f, 184t
  hyposecretion of, 168, 183f, 184t
Tibia, 213, 215, 219f, 221f
Tibial (medial) collateral ligament, 262, 263f, 533-534
Tibial tuberosity, 215, 219f, 221f
Tibialis anterior, 395-397, 395f, 537
Tibialis posterior, 402, 402f, 537
Tibiofemoral joint, 262-264, 262b, 263f
  superior, 533
Tibiofibular ligament, 265f
Tic douloureux, 161-162
Tidal volume, 609
Tinea corporis, 557f-558f, 559
Tinea cruris, 559
Tinea pedis, 559
Tissue, 13-18
  connective, 14-16, 17f. See also Connective tissue.
  epithelial, 14, 14f, 17f
  muscle, 16-18, 17f
  nervous, 18, 18f
Tissue hormones (prostaglandins), 34b, 169-170, 181
Toe(s)
  bones of, 196f, 221
  extension of, 542
  flexion of, 541
  joints of, 536
  movements of, 70f-74f, 536-537, 541-542
Toenails, 554, 554f
Tolerance, drug, 124
Tongue, 615
Tonic neck reflex, 297
Tonsillitis, 610
Tonsils, 568, 586
Tooth. See Teeth.
Torque, 470-471
Torsion forces, 240f, 242
Torso, 65
  muscles of, 350-369, 351f-353f
Torticollis, 461
Total body water, 629-631
Total metabolic rate, 622-623
Touch, 153
  importance of, 174b
  physiology of, 552
Touch receptors, 153
Toxemia of pregnancy, 643
Toxic myopathies, 463
Trachea, 606
  immune defenses of, 592
Tracts. See Spinal tracts.
Traditional Chinese medicine, 4, 26b
  acupuncture in. See Acupuncture.
  five-element theory and, 25, 26f, 80, 89f, 89t
  homeostasis and, 25
  jing luo in, 87
  points and meridians in, 84f, 85, 86b, 87
  terminology for, 80, 87b-88b
  yin/yang and, 4-5, 5f, 5t, 18, 25, 80, 87. See also Yin/yang.
Traditional medicine
  altered states of consciousness and, 117
  Ayurveda, 25-27, 26b, 26f, 81

Traditional medicine (Continued)
  Chinese. See Traditional Chinese medicine.
  definition of, 80
  organ relationships in, 88-89
  piezoelectric substances and, 194, 194b, 198b
  practical applications for, 80b, 89b
  terminology for, 80, 87b-88b
Transcutaneous electrical nerve stimulation (TENS), 43
Transient ischemic attack, 125
Transition phase, of childbirth, 640
Transmembrane potential, 11
Transverse arch, 213, 265-266, 536
Transverse fractures, 224f
Transverse friction massage, 36b
Transverse humeral ligament, 255f
Transverse ligament
  of atlas, 267f
  of knee, 262, 263f
  of shoulder, 255f
Transverse plane, 69, 69f, 248, 248f
Transverse rotation, 248
  of hip, 474f, 528, 528t
Transverse scapular ligament, 255f
Transversospinales group, 342-346, 342f-346f
Transversus abdominis, 362, 362f, 502
Transversus perinei, 367, 367f
Transversus thoracis, 357, 357f, 607-610, 607f
Trapezius, 418-421, 418f, 509, 510f
Trapezoid ligament, 255f
Traumatic brain injury, 125
Treatment planning, 91-92
Tremors, 127
Trendelenburg gait, 529
Treppe, 291
Triaxial joints, 250, 253f
Triceps brachii, 438, 438f, 518
Triceps reflex, 144
Trichinosis, 462
Tricuspid valve, 563, 563f
Trigeminal nerve, 136f, 136t-137t
Trigeminal neuralgia, 161-162
Trigger points, 81, 82f-83f, 89b, 292b
Triglycerides, 621
Triiodothyronine, 176
  functions of, 184t
  hypersecretion of, 183, 183f, 184t
  hyposecretion of, 183-184, 183f, 184t
Trochanters, 199
Trochlea, 199, 212, 217f
Trochlear groove, 215, 219f
Trochlear nerve, 136f, 136t-137t
Trochlear notch, 212, 214f
Tropic hormones, 169
Trunk, 65
  arteries of, 568f, 574
  biomechanics of, 501-503
  extension of, 506
  flexion of, 507
    muscle firing patterns in, 495
  movements of, 70f-74f
  posterior region of, 65-66
  rotation of, 507
  veins of, 569f, 574
Tubal ligation, 637
Tubercles, 199
Tuberculosis, 611
  of bone, 225
Tuberosities, 199
Tumors, 32-34
  benign, 33, 33f
  bone, 225
  brain, 126
  cartilage, 225
  fibroid, 644
  malignant, 33, 33f. See also Cancer.
  skin, 559-560
Tuning forks, 198b
Tympanic membrane, 154, 154f

Ulcer(s), 37
  decubitus, 559
  neurotrophic, 559
  peptic, 624
  skin, 556f, 559

Ulcerative colitis, 597t, 625
Ulna, 209-212, 214f, 217f
Ulnar collateral ligament, 257-258, 257f
Ulnar deviation, 248-249
Ultradian rhythms, 28, 29f
Uniaxial joints, 250, 253f
Unipennate muscles, 295, 296f
Unipolar neurons, 102, 103b
Unlocked position, 246-247, 247t
Unohumeral joint, 257, 257f
Upper crossed syndrome, 543, 544f
Upper extremity
  arteries of, 568f, 573
  bones of, 209-211, 211f, 212b, 213f-214f, 216f-217f
    definition of, 209
    veins of, 569f, 574
Upper motor neuron injuries, 123, 124b, 138
Upper respiratory tract, 605f, 613
  immune defenses of, 592
Upward rotation, 249
Ureter, 627f, 628
Urethra, 627f, 628
Urinary calculi, 633
Urinary incontinence, 633
Urinary obstruction, 633
Urinary system, 626-634
  disorders of, 631-634
  functions of, 627
  organs of, 627-628, 627f
  structure of, 626-627, 627f
Urinary tract infections, 632-633
Urticaria, 561
Uterus, 636
  disorders of, 644
Utricles, 119b

Vaccination, 594b
Vagina, 637
Vaginitis, 644
Vagus nerve, 98, 135b, 136f, 136t-137t
Valgus, definition of, 68
Valgus deformity, 533-534, 536f
Valves, heart, 563f, 564-565
Varicella, 556-558
Varicose veins, 579-580, 580f
Varus, definition of, 68
Varus deformity, 533-534
Vas deferens, 635, 635f
Vascular resistance, 572
Vascular system, 565-575. See also Arteries; Arteriole(s); Capillaries; Veins; Venules.
  disorders of, 578-580
  massage contraindications for, 583b
  medulla oblongata and, 573
  peripheral, 566f
Vasectomy, 636
Vasoactive intestinal peptide, 108, 147t
Vasoconstriction, in inflammation, 34b, 35f
Vasodilation, in inflammation, 34b, 35f
Vasopressin, 175, 175b, 176f
Vastus intermedius, 535
Vastus lateralis, 390, 390f, 535
Vastus medialis, 391, 391f, 535
Vata dosha, 26
Vectors, 470
Veins, 562-563, 567-568
  definition of, 565
  of head and neck, 569f, 574
  of lower extremities, 569f, 574
  principal, 569f
  structure of, 566f, 567
  of trunk, 569f, 574
  of upper extremities, 569f, 574
  varicose, 579-580, 580f
Venous pumping mechanisms, 568-570, 570f
Venous return, 568-570, 570f
  stimulation of, 570b, 571f
Ventral, 67, 68f
Ventral cavities, 63, 66
Ventral corticospinal tracts, 123b
Ventral roots, 122
Ventricles
  cardiac, 562f, 563, 564f
  cerebral, 120, 120f
Venules, 562-563

Vertebrae. *See also under* Spinal; Spine.
  cervical, 203-206, 207f, 208b, 266
  ligaments of, 206, 206f
  lumbar, 205, 207f, 208b, 502
  movements of, 266, 501-502
  sacral, 205, 207f, 208b
  structure of, 203-205, 206f-207f
  thoracic, 205, 207f, 208b, 501-502
Vertebral arteries, 205
Vertebral cavity, 65, 66f
Vertebral column. *See also under* Spinal; Spine.
  age-related changes in, 197
  movements of, 249, 266
Vertebral ligaments, 206, 206f
Vertigo, 162
Vesicles, 556f
Vesicular transport, 11
Vessels. *See* Blood vessels; Lymph vessels.
Vestibular sense, 152b, 155
Vestibular system, 119b, 155
Vestibulocochlear nerve, 136f, 136t-137t
Viral infections
  of nerves, 160
  of skin, 556-559, 557f-558f
Virulence, 32
Viscera, 66
Visceral membranes, 66
Visceral muscle, 287
Visceral nervous system. *See* Autonomic nervous
    system.
Visceral pain, 40
  referred, 40-42, 41f
Viscerosomatic reflexes, 141
Visceroviscoral reflexes, 141
Viscoelasticity, 301b
  of connective tissue, 238-240
Viscoplasticity, 301, 301b
Viscosity, 238, 572-573
Vision, 155-156
Visual orientation, 156b
Vital capacity, 609
Vitamin(s), 621
  as coenzymes, 621
  fat-soluble, 621t
  functions of, 621t

Vitamin(s) (*Continued*)
  sources of, 621t
  water-soluble, 621t
Vitamin A, 621t
Vitamin C, deficiency of, bone abnormalities in, 226
Vitamin D, 621t
  deficiency of, rickets and, 225-226
Vitiligo, 557f-558f, 561-562
Vocabulary. *See* Terminology.
Voice box, 605f, 606
Volar, definition of, 68
Volkmann's ischemic contracture, 460
Volvulus, 625
Vomer, 204b
Vomiting, in pregnancy, 643
Vowels, combining, 59
Vulva, 637

Walking. *See also* Gait.
  biomechanics of, 478-480, 480f-482f
Walking cycle, 479-480
Warts, 557f-558f, 559
Water. *See also* Fluid.
  in body tissues, 628, 628f, 629t
  metabolic, 629
Weight, 622-623
  in pregnancy, 638t
Wernicke's area, 113, 114f, 114t-115t
Western science, 26b
Whiplash, 461
White blood cells, 575-576
White cartilage (fibrocartilage), 16, 17f, 238
White fibers
  collagenous, 14
  muscle, 291-293
White matter
  of brain, 111
  of spinal cord, 122
Winging, scapular, 511b-517b
Withdrawal reflex, 297, 297b
Wolff's law, 300b
Work, 8
World Health Organization (WHO), quality-of-life
    domains of, 76, 77b-79b
Wound healing, 38f, 555-556

Wrist
  abduction of, 518
  adduction of, 518
  biomechanics of, 518-526
  bones of, 211-212, 216f
  close-packed position of, 248t
  extension of, 518, 522
  flexion of, 518, 522
  fractures of, 211
  joint of, 258
  least-packed position of, 247t
  ligaments of, 258
  movements of, 70f-74f, 249, 258, 518
  muscles of, 439-450, 440f, 518-526
  palpation of, 259
  range of motion of, 271b
  structure of, 258-259
Wry neck, 461
Wu xing, 88
Wu zang, 88

Xiphoid process, 209, 209b, 210f
Xu shi, 88
Xue, 88
Xun, 87

Yang organs, 18
Yeast infections, 559
  vaginal, 644
Yellow (elastic) cartilage, 16, 17f, 238
Yellow (elastic) fibers, 15, 237, 237f
Ying, 88
Yin/yang, 4-5, 5f, 5t, 18, 25b, 80, 87. *See also* Traditional
    Chinese medicine.
  autonomic nervous system and, 150-152
  homeostasis and, 25
  life cycle and, 50
  meridians and, 85f, 87
Yin/yang organs, 18

Zheng xie, 88
Zygomatic bones, 202f-203f, 204b
Zygomaticus major, 315, 315f
Zygomaticus minor, 316, 316f
Zygopophyseal (facet) joints, 266, 267f